Complications
in Surgery

Complications in Surgery

EDITORS

■ MICHAEL W. MULHOLLAND, MD, PHD

Frederick A. Coller Distinguished Professor of Surgery and Chairman; Surgeon-in-Chief, Department of Surgery, University of Michigan, Ann Arbor, Michigan

■ GERARD M. DOHERTY, MD

N. W. Thompson Professor of Surgery; Chief of Endocrine Surgery; Section Head of General Surgery, University of Michigan, Ann Arbor, Michigan

Dec 2005
Ann Arbor
All the best
M Mulholland

Dec 2005
To Amir
With best regards –
Ger Doherty

LIPPINCOTT WILLIAMS & WILKINS
A **Wolters Kluwer** Company

Philadelphia • Baltimore • New York • London
Buenos Aires • Hong Kong • Sydney • Tokyo

Acquisitions Editor: Brian Brown
Developmental Editor: Julia Seto
Project Manager: Fran Gunning
Manufacturing Manager: Ben Rivera
Marketing Manager: Adam Glazer
Creative Director: Doug Smock
Production Services: Laser Words Pvt. Limited
Printer: Edwards Brothers

Library of Congress Cataloging-in-Publication Data

Complications in surgery / editors, Michael W. Mulholland, Gerard M. Doherty.
     p. ; cm.
Includes bibliographical references and index.
ISBN 0-7817-5316-3
1. Surgery—Complications. I. Mulholland, Michael W. II. Doherty, Gerard M.
[DNLM: 1. Intraoperative Complications. 2. Postoperative Complications. 3. Surgical
Procedures, Operative—adverse effects. WO 181 C7367 2005]
RD98.C63 2005
617'.01—dc22

2005012468

Care has been taken to confirm the accuracy of the information presented and to describe generally accepted practices. However, the authors, editors, and publisher are not responsible for errors or omissions or for any consequences from application of the information in this book and make no warranty, expressed or implied, with respect to the currency, completeness, or accuracy of the contents of the publication. Application of this information in a particular situation remains the professional responsibility of the practitioner.

The authors, editors, and publisher have exerted every effort to ensure that drug selection and dosage set forth in this text are in accordance with current recommendations and practice at the time of publication. However, in view of ongoing research, changes in government regulations, and the constant flow of information relating to drug therapy and drug reactions, the reader is urged to check the package insert for each drug for any change in indications and dosage and for added warnings and precautions. This is particularly important when the recommended agent is a new or infrequently employed drug.

Some drugs and medical devices presented in this publication have Food and Drug Administration (FDA) clearance for limited use in restricted research settings. It is the responsibility of health care providers to ascertain the FDA status of each drug or device planned for use in their clinical practice.

The publishers have made every effort to trace copyright holders for borrowed material. If they have inadvertently overlooked any, they will be pleased to make the necessary arrangements at the first opportunity.

To purchase additional copies of this book, call our customer service department at (800) 639-3030 or fax orders to (301) 824-7390. International customers should call (301) 714-2324. Lippincott Williams & Wilkins customer service representatives are available from 8:30 AM to 6:00 PM, EST.

Visit Lippincott Williams & Wilkins on the Internet at LWW.com.

10 9 8 7 6 5 4 3 2

To our wives, Patricia and Faith

Contents

Preface ix
Acknowledgments xi
Contributors xiii

SECTION 1: INSTITUTIONAL ISSUES 1

1 Surgical Complications 3
Michael W. Mulholland, Gerard M. Doherty

2 Contemporary Surgical Training 5
Seth W. Wolk, Leslie W. Ottinger

3 Future Surgical Training 9
Paul G. Gauger

4 Continuing Education for Practicing Surgeons 18
Richard E. Burney, R. Van Harrison

5 Surgical Credentials 25
Mary E. Klingensmith

6 Assessing Surgical Quality with Structure and
Process of Care Measures 30
John D. Birkmeyer

7 Assessing Surgical Quality with Clinical Outcomes
Measures 45
Darrell A. Campbell, Jr., William G. Henderson,
Shukri F. Khuri

SECTION 2: MANAGEMENT OF SURGICAL COMPLICATIONS 57

8 Assessment of Perioperative Risk 59
Debabrata Mukherjee, Kim A. Eagle

9 Anesthesia Complications 69
Paul E. Kazanjian

10 Complications of Wound Healing 102
Michael G. Franz

11 Surgical Site Infections 114
Gerard M. Doherty

12 Septic Shock 126
Stewart C. Wang

13 Hypovolemic Shock 136
Saman Arbabi

14 Fluid and Electrolyte Abnormalities 144
Bradley D. Freeman

15 Acute Renal Failure 150
Kareem D. Husain, Craig M. Coopersmith

16 Pulmonary Complications 157
Mark R. Hemmila

17 Cardiac Complications 174
Wendy L. Wahl

18 Abnormalities in Coagulation 185
Alvin H. Schmaier

19 Complications of Nutritional Support 195
Daniel H. Teitelbaum, Imad F. Btaiche, Saleem Islam

20 Complications of Immunosuppression 212
Niraj M. Desai, Matthew J. Koch

SECTION 3: COMPLICATIONS OF THORACIC SURGERY 225

21 Complications of Intubation, Tracheotomy, and
Tracheal Surgery 227
Kevin Fung, Norman D. Hogikyan

22 Complications of Esophageal Surgery 245
Andrew C. Chang, Mark D. Iannettoni

23 Complications of Pulmonary and Chest Wall
Surgery 264
Harvey I. Pass, Shane Yamane

24 Complications of Extracorporeal Circulation 277
Jennifer S. Lawton

25 Complications of Surgical Coronary
Revascularization 286
Traves D. Crabtree, Marc R. Moon

26 Complications of Valvular Cardiac Surgery 298
    Steven F. Bolling

27 Complications of Thoracoscopy 306
    Michael A. Smith, Richard J. Battafarano

SECTION 4: COMPLICATIONS OF VASCULAR SURGERY 315

28 Complications of Arterial Surgery 317
    Gilbert R. Upchurch, Jr., Jonathan L. Eliason, James C. Stanley

29 Complications of Venous Disease and Therapy 337
    Thomas W. Wakefield, Peter K. Henke

30 Complications of Endovascular Therapy 357
    Matthew J. Eagleton, Sunita D. Srivastava

SECTION 5: COMPLICATIONS OF GASTROINTESTINAL SURGERY 383

31 Complications of Gastric Surgery 385
    Michael W. Mulholland

32 Complications of Hepatic Surgery 407
    James A. Knol

33 Complications of Biliary Surgery 423
    Lisa M. Colletti

34 Complications of Pancreatic Surgery 463
    Diane M. Simeone

35 Complications of Intestinal Surgery: Small Bowel 477
    Arden M. Morris

36 Complications of Appendectomy and Colon and Rectal Surgery 498
    Emina H. Huang

37 Complications of Abdominal Wall and Hernia Operations 523
    Michael G. Franz

38 Complications of Laparoscopic Surgery 546
    Kathleen M. Diehl

SECTION 6: COMPLICATIONS OF ENDOCRINE AND ONCOLOGIC SURGERY 557

39 Complications of Adrenal Surgery 557
    Paul G. Gauger

40 Complications of Thyroid and Parathyroid Surgery 575
    Gerard M. Doherty

41 Complications in Endocrine Pancreatic Surgery 594
    Terry C. Lairmore

42 Complications of Breast Surgery 603
    Lisa A. Newman

43 Complications of Soft-tissue Tumor Surgery 619
    Adam I. Riker, Vernon K. Sondak

44 Complications of Lymphadenectomy 628
    Alliric I. Willis, Jeffrey F. Moley

SECTION 7: COMPLICATIONS OF TRANSPLANTATION 637

45 Complications of Renal Transplantation 639
    Robert M. Merion

46 Complications of Liver Transplantation 655
    Juan D. Arenas, Jeffrey D. Punch

47 Complications of Pancreatic Transplantation 665
    Dixon B. Kaufman

48 Complications of Pulmonary Transplantation 683
    Christine L. Lau, Bryan F. Meyers

49 Complications of Heart Transplantation 700
    Francis D. Pagani

SECTION 8: COMPLICATIONS OF PEDIATRIC SURGERY 723

50 Surgical Complications in Newborns 725
    Ronald B. Hirschl

51 Surgical Complications in Children 764
    James D. Geiger

Index 787

Preface

Surgical therapy is inherently risky. All surgeons seek to balance an operation's potential benefit and risk with the disease being treated. The best surgeons display a combination of knowledge, technical skill, and clinical judgment. Knowledge begins with a thoughtful appraisal of the medical literature. Operative technical ability develops from an understanding of the process of surgery with comprehension of both the operation's objectives and the steps needed to meet them. Clinical judgment may be developed individually from experience, but it is also acquired from the distilled experience of others. Surgical judgment and understanding crucially depend on a detailed reading of the surgical literature and the expertise of others.

In recent years it has become clear that surgical results depend not only on individual technical facility and judgment but also on the system in which a surgeon treats patients. Institutional parameters, the organization of clinical care, and teamwork play key roles in assuring that patients receive care that is both safe and efficacious. In many instances the setting of care is as important in clinical outcomes as the individual surgeon.

Complications in Surgery is organized to cover both the broad concepts of surgical care and the complications relevant to operations on specific organs. Surgical epidemiology, operative technique, and disease pathophysiology are each essential in contemporary surgical practice; each is emphasized in this new textbook. In selecting contributors to *Complications in Surgery*, the editors sought surgeons who had significant clinical experience with the diseases and the operations described. In addition, the authors chosen are active contributors to new clinical knowledge and to the contemporary practice of surgery. The editors believe that *Complications in Surgery* is a truly new book—new in concept and new in scope. We hope that our readers will find that the book combines unique elements of modern surgical practice and that it will be genuinely educational.

Michael W. Mulholland, MD, PhD
Frederick A. Coller
Distinguished Professor of Surgery
  and Chairman
Surgeon-in-Chief
Department of Surgery
University of Michigan

Gerard M. Doherty, MD
N. W. Thompson Professor of Surgery
Chief of Endocrine Surgery
Section Head of General Surgery
University of Michigan

Acknowledgments

We are very grateful to the outstanding group of contributors who we believe are unchallenged in their understanding and experience in these areas of surgery. We appreciate their precious time and effort on this project. We are privileged to have worked with Holly Fischer, M.F.A., who did the original drawings. Her carefully detailed drawings clarify and add detail to the contributors' text. Finally, we have enjoyed wonderful support from Brian Brown and Lisa McAllister at Lippincott Williams & Wilkins who gently guided this process. It has been a pleasure for us to work with such a dedicated group of individuals.

MWM
GMD

Contributors

SAMAN ARBABI, MD, MPH Assistant Professor, Department of Surgery, University of Michigan, Ann Arbor, Michigan

JUAN D. ARENAS, MD Surgical Director, Liver Transplantation, Department of General Surgery, Henry Ford Health System, Detroit, Michigan

RICHARD J. BATTAFARANO, MD, PHD Assistant Professor of Surgery, Division of Cardiothoracic Surgery, Washington University School of Medicine; Attending Surgeon, Division of Cardiothoracic Surgery, Barnes-Jewish Hospital, St. Louis, Missouri

JOHN D. BIRKMEYER, MD George D. Zuidema Professor of Surgery, Department of Surgery, University of Michigan, Ann Arbor, Michigan

STEVEN F. BOLLING, MD Professor of Surgery, Section of Cardiac Surgery, University of Michigan, Ann Arbor, Michigan

IMAD F. BTAICHE, PHARMD, BCNSP Clinical Assistant Professor of Pharmacy, Department of Clinical Sciences, University of Michigan College of Pharmacy; Clinical Pharmacist–Nutrition Support, Department of Pharmacy Services, University of Michigan, Ann Arbor, Michigan

RICHARD E. BURNEY, MD Professor of Surgery, Department of Surgery, University of Michigan, Ann Arbor, Michigan

DARRELL A. CAMPBELL, JR., MD Henry King Ransom Professor of Surgery; Chief of Clinical Affairs, Department of Surgery, University of Michigan, Ann Arbor, Michigan

ANDREW C. CHANG, MD Assistant Professor, Department of Surgery, University of Michigan, Ann Arbor, Michigan

LISA M. COLLETTI, MD C. Gardner Child Professor, Department of Surgery; Chief, Division of Gastrointestinal Surgery, University of Michigan, Ann Arbor, Michigan

CRAIG M. COOPERSMITH, MD Associate Professor, Departments of Surgery and Anesthesiology, Washington University School of Medicine; Attending Physician, Barnes-Jewish Hospital, St. Louis, Missouri

TRAVES D. CRABTREE, MD Assistant Professor, Department of Cardiothoracic Surgery, Washington University School of Medicine, St. Louis, Missouri

NIRAJ M. DESAI, MD Assistant Professor, Department of Surgery, Washington University School of Medicine, St. Louis, Missouri

KATHLEEN M. DIEHL, MD Assistant Professor of Surgery, Department of Surgery, University of Michigan, Ann Arbor, Michigan

GERARD M. DOHERTY, MD N. W. Thompson Professor of Surgery; Chief of Endocrine Surgery; Section Head of General Surgery, University of Michigan, Ann Arbor, Michigan

KIM A. EAGLE, MD Albion Walter Hewlett Professor of Internal Medicine; Clinical Director, Cardiovascular Center, Division of Cardiovascular Medicine, Department of Internal Medicine, University of Michigan, Ann Arbor, Michigan

MATTHEW J. EAGLETON, MD Assistant Professor of Surgery, Section of Vascular Surgery, University of Michigan, Ann Arbor, Michigan

JONATHAN L. ELIASON, MD Clinical Assistant Professor, Department of Surgery, University of Texas Health Science Center, San Antonio, Texas; Staff Vascular Surgeon, Department of Surgery, Wilford Hall Medical Center, Lackland AFB, Texas

MICHAEL G. FRANZ, MD Assistant Professor, Department of Surgery, University of Michigan, Ann Arbor, Michigan

BRADLEY D. FREEMAN, MD Associate Professor, Department of Surgery, Washington University School of Medicine, St. Louis, Missouri

KEVIN FUNG, BA, MD, FRCS(C) Assistant Professor, Department of Otolaryngology, Division of Head and Neck Oncology & Reconstructive Surgery, University of Western Ontario, London Health Sciences Center, Westminster Campus, London, Ontario, Canada

PAUL G. GAUGER, MD Associate Professor, Departments of Surgery and Medical Education, University of Michigan, Ann Arbor, Michigan

JAMES D. GEIGER, MD Associate Professor, Department of Surgery, University of Michigan, Ann Arbor, Michigan

R. VAN HARRISON, PHD Professor, Department of Medical Education, University of Michigan, Ann Arbor, Michigan

MARK R. HEMMILA, MD Assistant Professor, Department of Surgery, University of Michigan, Ann Arbor, Michigan

WILLIAM G. HENDERSON, MPH, PHD Professor, Department of Preventive Medicine & Biometrics, Colorado Health Outcomes Program, University of Colorado, Aurora, Colorado

PETER K. HENKE, MD Assistant Professor, Section of Vascular Surgery, University of Michigan, Ann Arbor, Michigan

RONALD B. HIRSCHL, MD Professor, Department of Surgery, University of Michigan, Ann Arbor, Michigan

NORMAN D. HOGIKYAN, MD, FACS Associate Professor, Department of Otolaryngology, Division of Head and Neck Surgery; Director, Vocal Health Center, University of Michigan, Ann Arbor, Michigan

EMINA H. HUANG, MD Assistant Professor, Department of Surgery; Chief, Division of Colorectal Surgery, University of Michigan, Ann Arbor, Michigan

KAREEM D. HUSAIN, MD Resident, Department of Surgery, Barnes-Jewish Hospital, St. Louis, Missouri

MARK D. IANNETTONI, MD, MBA Ehrenhaft Professor of Cardiothoracic Surgery; Chairman, Division of Cardiothoracic Surgery, University of Iowa Carver College of Medicine, Iowa City, Iowa

SALEEM ISLAM, MD Assistant Professor, Division of Pediatric Surgery, University of Mississippi Medical School; Attending Surgeon, Pediatric Surgery, Blair E. Batson Hospital for Children, Jackson, Mississippi

DIXON B. KAUFMAN, MD, PHD Professor, Department of Surgery, Northwestern University, Feinberg School of Medicine; Director, Pancreas Transplantation, Northwestern Memorial Hospital, Chicago, Illinois

PAUL E. KAZANJIAN, MD Clinical Assistant Professor, Department of Anesthesiology, University of Michigan, Ann Arbor, Michigan

SHUKRI F. KHURI, MD Professor of Surgery, Department of Surgery, Harvard Medical School, Boston, Massachusetts; Chief, Cardiothoracic Surgery, VA Healthcare System, West Roxbury, Massachusetts

MARY E. KLINGENSMITH, MD Assistant Professor, Department of Surgery, Washington University School of Medicine; Staff Surgeon, Department of Surgery, Barnes-Jewish Hospital, St. Louis, Missouri

JAMES A. KNOL, MD Associate Professor, Department of Surgery, University of Michigan, Ann Arbor, Michigan

MATTHEW J. KOCH, MD Assistant Professor, Department of Medicine, Washington University School of Medicine; Medical Staff, Barnes-Jewish Hospital, St. Louis, Missouri

TERRY C. LAIRMORE, MD Professor of Surgery, Texas A & M System Health Sciences Center, College of Medicine; Director, Division of Surgical Oncology, Scott and White Hospital, Temple, Texas

CHRISTINE L. LAU, MD Assistant Professor, Section of Thoracic Surgery, University of Michigan, Ann Arbor, Michigan.

JENNIFER S. LAWTON, MD Assistant Professor of Surgery, Department of Cardiothoracic Surgery, Washington University School of Medicine and Barnes-Jewish Hospital St. Louis, Missouri

ROBERT M. MERION, MD Professor, Department of Surgery, University of Michigan, Ann Arbor, Michigan

BRYAN F. MEYERS, MD Associate Professor, Department of Surgery, Washington University School of Medicine, St Louis, Missouri

JEFFREY F. MOLEY, MD Professor, Department of Surgery, Washington University School of Medicine; Associate Director, Siteman Cancer Center, St. Louis, Missouri

MARC R. MOON, MD Associate Professor, Division of Cardiothoracic Surgery, Washington University School of Medicine, St. Louis, Missouri

ARDEN M. MORRIS, MD, MPH Assistant Professor, Department of Surgery, University of Michigan, Ann Arbor, Michigan

DEBABRATA MUKHERJEE, MD, MS Tyler Gill Professor of Interventional Cardiology; Director, Peripheral Vascular Interventions, Division of Cardiovascular Medicine, University of Kentucky, Lexington, Kentucky

MICHAEL W. MULHOLLAND, MD, PHD Frederick A. Coller Distinguished Professor of Surgery and Chairman; Surgeon-in-Chief, Department of Surgery, University of Michigan, Ann Arbor, Michigan

LISA A. NEWMAN, MD, MPH, FACS Associate Professor, Department of Surgery, University of Michigan; Director, Breast Cancer Center, University of Michigan Comprehensive Cancer Center, Ann Arbor, Michigan

LESLIE W. OTTINGER Formerly Associate Professor, Department of Surgery, Harvard Medical School; Formerly Visiting Surgeon and Director, Program in General Surgery, Massachusetts General Hospital, Boston, Massachusetts

FRANCIS D. PAGANI, MD, PHD Associate Professor of Surgery, Section of Cardiac Surgery, University of Michigan, Ann Arbor, Michigan

HARVEY I. PASS, MD   Professor of Surgery and Oncology, Department of Surgery and Oncology, Wayne State University; Chief of Thoracic Oncology, Department of Oncology, Karmanos Cancer Institute and Harper Hospital, Detroit, Michigan

JEFFREY D. PUNCH, MD   Associate Professor; Chief, Division of Transplantation, Department of Surgery, University of Michigan, Ann Arbor, Michigan

ADAM I. RIKER, MD, FACS   Assistant Professor, Department of Surgery, University of South Florida College of Medicine; Assistant Professor of Surgery, Department of Cutaneous Oncology, H. Lee Moffitt Cancer Center & Research Institute, Tampa, Florida

ALVIN H. SCHMAIER, MD   Professor, Department of Internal Medicine and Pathology; Director, Coagulation Laboratory, Department of Pathology, University of Michigan, Ann Arbor, Michigan

DIANE M. SIMEONE, MD   Associate Professor, Departments of Surgery and Molecular and Integrative Physiology, University of Michigan, Ann Arbor, Michigan

MICHAEL A. SMITH, MD   Assistant Professor, Cardiothoracic Surgery, Keck School of Medicine, University of Southern California, Los Angeles, California

VERNON K. SONDAK, MD   Professor, Departments of Surgery and Interdisciplinary Oncology, University of South Florida; Program Leader, Cutaneous Oncology, H. Lee Moffitt Cancer Center & Research Institute, Tampa, Florida

SUNITA D. SRIVASTAVA, MD   Assistant Professor, Department of Surgery, University of Michigan, Ann Arbor, Michigan

JAMES C. STANLEY, MD   Professor of Surgery, Section of Vascular Surgery, Co-director, Cardiovascular Center, University of Michigan, Ann Arbor, Michigan

DANIEL H. TEITELBAUM, MD   Professor, Department of Surgery, University of Michigan, Ann Arbor, Michigan

GILBERT R. UPCHURCH, JR., MD   Associate Professor, Department of Surgery, University of Michigan, Ann Arbor, Michigan

WENDY L. WAHL, MD   Clinical Associate Professor, Department of Surgery, University of Michigan, Ann Arbor, Michigan

THOMAS W. WAKEFIELD, MD, RVT   S. Martin Lindenauer Professor of Vascular Surgery; Section Head of Vascular Surgery, Department of Surgery, University of Michigan, Ann Arbor, Michigan

STEWART C. WANG, MD, PHD   Associate Professor, Department of Surgery, University of Michigan, Ann Arbor, Michigan

ALLIRIC I. WILLIS, MD   Surgical Oncology Fellow; Active Staff, Department of Surgical Oncology, Fox Chase Cancer Center, Philadelphia, Pennsylvania

SETH W. WOLK, MD   Clinical Associate Professor, Department of Surgery, University of Michigan; Staff Surgeon, Department of Surgery, St. Joseph Mercy Hospital, Ann Arbor, Michigan

SHANE YAMANE, MD   Cardiothoracic Fellow, Department of Cardiothoracic Surgery, Wayne State University and Harper Hospital, Detroit, Michigan

Institutional Issues

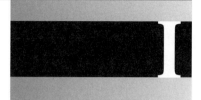

Surgical Complications

Michael W. Mulholland   Gerard M. Doherty

Surgical care has always focused on balancing risk and benefit. In traditional surgical teaching, operative complications represent risk, and cure rates or palliation of symptoms represent benefit. For the past several decades, surgical attention has been directed to avoiding complications by development of meticulous operative techniques and to early detection of postoperative problems, with rapid efforts to minimize undesirable events. Although surgical complications are often obvious and clearly tied to the act of surgical intervention, issues of risk have traditionally been a private matter between an individual surgeon and an individual patient.

The traditional view of surgical risk and benefit is no longer adequate. Risk still properly begins with an assessment of intraoperative problems and postoperative events. Surgical risk in contemporary practice also includes consideration of balancing complementary, sometimes competing, techniques and achieving results that optimize physical, occupational, and societal goals. Modern surgeons must appreciate the appropriate sequence and combination of operative and nonoperative therapy. Judicious utilization of resources is now a consideration. Not just physical healing, but also patient satisfaction is required.

The relationship of an individual surgeon to an individual patient, still central to surgical care, has become overlaid with increased scrutiny and with additional societal expectations. Standards of expected outcomes for groups of patients require evidence-based practice and have made both seniority and experience less important. Surgical care must be provided within financial constraints. Societal

interest in surgical outcomes is expressed in a recent Institute of Medicine report detailing "unnecessary" deaths resulting from surgical complications (1).

American society's investment in health care is enormous and growing. In 1997, health services made up approximately 14% of gross domestic product (GDP), or $1.1 trillion. By 2007, this figure is estimated to grow to $2 trillion, or 16% of GDP (2). The Agency for Healthcare Research and Quality has identified top-priority conditions for the next decade, including cancer, diabetes mellitus, emphysema, HIV infection, hypertension, ischemic heart disease, stroke, and gallstones. Many of these conditions are highly relevant to contemporary surgical practice. In treating patients with these conditions, the 21st-century health care system must adapt and focus increasingly on provision of care that is

safe
effective
patient-centered
timely
efficient
equitable (3).

New knowledge related to the practice of surgery has increased exponentially during the past decade. Surgical studies are also more sophisticated, requiring the reader to know about patient selection, statistical analysis, and molecular biology. The number of drugs, surgical devices, and technological support systems has expanded as well. In this context it is impossible for any one clinician to synthesize all of the information necessary for effective, evidence-based practice. No surgeon can read, organize,

Michael W. Mulholland, Gerard M. Doherty: University of Michigan, Ann Arbor, MI 48109

and recall the current volumes of clinically important information (3).

The revolution in information technology (IT) has a potential to accelerate greatly changes in surgical care and make that care both more effective and safer. Reduction in surgical complications will require effective use of the available scientific database. Evidence from laboratory experiments, clinical trials, epidemiology, and health services research must be instantly available to clinicians. The Institute of Medicine has identified five major areas in which IT can contribute to safer health care delivery: (i) access to the medical knowledge base; (ii) computer-aided decision support systems; (iii) collection and sharing of clinical information; (iv) reduction in errors; and (v) enhanced patient and clinician communication (3).

The Internet has created a tide in medical consumerism. In 2000 an estimated 70 million Americans sought online health care information, and the number is growing (4). Medical IT users demand both sound information and convenience in all areas of health commerce. Medical information systems hold great promise for reducing surgical complications. An informed patient is a safer patient.

Knowledge, technical skill, and judgment are foundations of safe surgical care, but they do not always prevent complications. Patients are frequently injured because of flaws in the design of medical systems. Recognition of the importance of the system in which care is received has caused a reexamination of surgical culture. A system of surgical accountability that blames individuals has a poor prospect of significant improvement. Contemporary surgical morbidity and mortality conferences must reflect this realization. Prevention, reporting, analysis, and minimization of surgical harm can occur only in environments of learning, not of blame and reprisal.

These considerations imply that a focus on surgical complications will remain a major endeavor for surgical practitioners. These changes also mean that new texts on this subject must include new perspectives to remain relevant to contemporary practice.

REFERENCES

1. Institute of Medicine. In: Kohn LT, Corrigan JM, Donaldson MS, eds. *To err is human: building a safer health system*. Washington, DC: National Academy Press; 2000.
2. Smith S, Freeland M, Heffler S, et al. The next ten years of health spending: What does the future hold? *Health Affairs* 1998; 17:129–140.
3. Institute of Medicine. In: Richardson WC, ed. *Crossing the quality chasm*. Washington, DC: National Academy Press; 2003.
4. Cain MM, Mittman R, Sarasohn-Kahn J, et al. *Health e-people: the online consumer experience*. Oakland, CA: Institute for the Future, California Health Care Foundation; 2000.

Contemporary Surgical Training

Seth W. Wolk   Leslie W. Ottinger

A central goal of resident education is improvement of patient care. To this end, training programs must produce well-trained and competent physicians. This chapter examines the process by which surgical training programs have arrived at their present state, the pressures that they have experienced over the last two decades, and projections for the future.

Programs for training residents in the United States, accredited by the Accreditation Council for Graduate Medical Education (ACGME) and its subcommittee, the Residency Review Committee (RRC) in Surgery, have a high degree of uniformity. These similarities reflect the effective efforts of the RRC and the American Board of Surgery (ABS) during the last four decades. The length, content, structure, and aims of the programs and their relationship to residents in training have all been the subject of increasing scrutiny and regulation by these organizations.

During the 19th and early 20th centuries, the usual education of a young surgeon was at the hands of a preceptor, with whom the trainee exchanged services for instruction and experience. Today's programs still have an important component of direct personal relationship between teachers of surgery and their students. All surgeons can list a few such key figures in their surgical educations. These intense personal bonds constitute a central and critical part of every residency training program. Modern trainees have access to a wide range of preceptors with central interests in clinical surgery, investigation, and health-care management. In the minds of many applicants, the presence of

gifted preceptors remains a characteristic that differentiates superior programs from lesser ones.

The establishment of the Johns Hopkins Hospital surgery training program, under the guidance of William Stewart Halstead in the last decades of the 19th century, is often cited as an important turning point in the education of surgeons. Patterned on training in Germany, this program brought well-qualified applicants to an institution highly supportive of them under the mantle of a great educator. Training clinical surgeons was only one component of the program. Halstead also sought to train surgeons for surgical investigation and for leadership positions, an effort in which he was remarkably successful. The program was uniquely centered, with full-time staff and residents supported by the hospital. The program was "pyramidal" in structure, with selection pressure continuing during training so as to produce a few truly outstanding academic surgeons.

By the last half of the 19th century, the best surgical education was found within the structure of medical schools, even if still in the hands of preceptors. A seminal change occurred with the formalization of training in hospitals, often with university affiliations, with the institution progressively assuming responsibility. This university-based system represented the second step in the evolution of the current training system.

By the mid-20th century, clearly defined residency programs had emerged in surgery. These were eventually lengthened to 5 years, the length of training needed to impart the necessary knowledge, technical skill, and clinical maturity for the independent practice of surgery. During the mid-20th century, many strong programs emerged. These programs were invariably developed by a superior clinical surgeon with a central interest in surgical

Seth W. Wolk: St. Joseph Mercy Hospital, Ann Arbor, MI 48106
Leslie W. Ottinger: Harvard Medical School, Boston, MA 02115

education. The excellence of any individual program was apt to reflect the ideas and innovation of the department chairperson and his or her willingness to commit departmental resources to educational effort. Despite increasing uniformity of residency programs, the chairperson and his or her relationship to the surgical training program and residents are factors well understood by applicants, and they remain primary considerations when comparing residency programs.

The most recent stage in the evolution of surgery programs reflects the work of the ABS and the RRC in Surgery. Both have had major and increasing impact during the last three decades. Changing requirements for Board certification, uniformity in length, and structured operative experience of residents have improved marginal and faltering programs and brought them to a higher standard. The RRC has used requirements for accreditation, formulated for the same purpose, to introduce innovations and to shift emphasis in the training experience of residents. New disciplines have been given a carefully defined importance.

Shifts such as increasing time spent by residents in outpatient settings and limitation of working hours have greatly modified many programs. Because of the possible failure of trainees to meet the requirements for examination for certification and the far-reaching consequences of loss of accreditation, the ABS and RRC have enormous power to bring about change. One worrisome consequence is that opportunities for innovation and for emphasis on a hospital's particular strengths in training residents have been stripped away and all programs are being brought increasingly to a single, standard level. In this way the ABS and RRC have assumed an overwhelming responsibility, and this often leaves department chairpersons and program directors struggling just to meet requirements with little opportunity to meet their own standards of excellence.

Although training programs have always felt the effects of societal influences, these pressures began to exert considerable force in the early 1980s. Dramatic changes in reimbursement for in-hospital patient care that began with the Medicare programs of the 1960s accelerated dramatically with the introduction of Diagnostic Related Groups and culminated in the Balanced Budget Act in 1997. These changes resulted in major decreases in reimbursement and substantially increased pressure on teaching hospitals for fiscal efficacy, resulting in a strain to maintain the educational mission of these institutions. Faculty members have also experienced considerable pressure to increase clinical productivity, which has often resulted in a decreased ability to provide teaching to residents in all settings, including the outpatient clinic, the in-hospital services, and the operating room. The result is in an increasingly difficult environment in which faculty are unable to provide high-quality resident education. Attending staff face their own increasing pressures to become more cost-effective and clinically

productive. Teaching walk rounds have virtually disappeared from most institutions. There is also less time and patience in the operating room to allow residents to perform operative procedures or parts of them.

Resident salaries and benefits have generally kept pace with inflation. However, over the last two decades, the debt levels of general surgery residents following to their undergraduate and medical school education have risen dramatically. Increasing financial indebtedness has multiple insidious effects, influencing both a trainee's ability to take time from clinical training years to perform research in a laboratory setting and ultimate career decisions based on length of training years in additional post-general surgery fellowships. Various solutions have been proposed, including scholarship programs from professional surgical organizations and consideration by the ABS to modify the length of general surgery training programs. The latter includes continuing the basic 5-year program for trainees destined to become general surgeons, as well as proposals for "3 + 3 or 4 + 2" integrated programs for trainees who will become pediatric, vascular, or cardiothoracic surgeons. Although promising, these proposals all have significant drawbacks. These include the need for early and accurate designation of trainees into different paths balanced with the ability to maintain flexibility. The impact on a particular general surgical training program of "losing" a senior-level resident into a fellowship training program might also be substantial. There is also the difficult problem that a method must be found to provide these trainees with senior experience in the middle years of a 5-year general surgery program.

In the last two decades, there has also been a significant increase in the influence the ACGME has had in the day-to-day running of surgical training programs. In July 2001, the ACGME initiated a 10-year timeline for full implementation of a curriculum, including evaluation strategies for six competencies for residency training programs throughout the United States. These competencies are patient care, medical knowledge, practice-based learning and improvement, interpersonal skills and communication, professionalism, and systems-based practice. The new ACGME competencies will serve to shift the focus of graduate medical education from the educational process to evidence of residents' learning and patient outcomes (1). The RRC's choices of what is important and what is not and the necessity of emphasizing these in the design of programs might further limit innovation and flexibility.

The federal government has also indirectly influenced general surgery training programs by pursuing an agenda to increase the number of primary care physicians being trained. Financial pressures and incentives have been placed on US medical schools to actively push students toward primary care specialties and away from surgical careers. At many schools this effort has permeated down to the admissions committee level, with fewer applicants who express an interest in specialized fields being accepted.

Many medical schools over the last decade have decreased the time students spend during their third and fourth years on surgery rotations. Surgery is often given a small part in the curriculum and exposure to clinical surgery and surgeons is increasingly limited. So far, US medical schools have given little support to incorporating the ACS recommendation of a curricular path designated for students interested in surgical fields. Attracting well-qualified individuals to general surgery programs will likely become more challenging. The total number of categorical general surgery positions in the United States has remained relatively stable for the last two decades. However, the number of US medical school graduates applying to these positions has declined substantially in the last decade. International medical graduates will likely fill many of these positions. Surgery educators must continue to attract not only the type of individuals who can excel in longer duty hours and the more stressful environment of surgical practice but, just as important, also those who have a passion for creativity and investigation. This latter group is responsible for many of the innovations that keep the profession healthy and thriving.

The hallmark of surgical training has been the commitment on the part of both faculty and resident to patient care without regard to time, day of the week, hours worked, or on-call schedule. The patient's welfare comes first (2). The relationship between quality of care and continuity of care has been well documented and, indeed, serves as the basis for one of the most fundamental ethical principles of our profession: commitment to the total care of our patients (3). The implementation of the ACGME duty hour restrictions will affect these aspects of surgical training. As Frank R. Lewis has summarized, "there are few issues on which the profession and the public are so far apart as work hours limitations, as a result of a dangerous degree of misunderstanding on both sides. The simple fact that resident work hours has become a federal issue potentially requiring regulation by Congress is an index of how anomalous the issue has become" (4). Surgical educators acknowledge that resident hours have to be reduced and the lay public needs to be educated so they do not believe the superficial and incorrect logic that resident work hours are related to medical errors in the hospital. Legislators need to understand that when medical responsibility by a single individual is sacrificed, less vigilant patient care is sure to result. There is simply no way that the complexity and subtlety of observations made by an experienced clinician of a sick patient can be translated into a "sign-out sheet" or verbally transmitted. There is a real, but subtle, difference in the ethical and professional responsibility felt by conscientious surgeons toward a patient on whom they have operated versus that felt by physicians who have never seen the patient before and have no prior knowledge of the patient (4).

Faculty must increase the efficiency of resident education, given the reduction in the total amount of time available.

Efforts to minimize the tasks that serve no educational or clinical value but that occupy residents' workdays need to continue while still giving residents sufficient exposure to the details of surgical care.

Surgical faculty members need to acknowledge that duty hour restrictions might bring beneficial effects. Board pass rates, case numbers, and patient outcomes need to be measured before definitive conclusions can be made (5). Resident attitudes toward work hours will also need to be understood. Initial studies have shown that a reduction in work hours has had subjective and objective benefits on quality of life and resident education (6).

Residents might feel pressured to violate the duty hour restrictions imposed by faculty supervisors or made to feel guilty for a duty hours infraction because they are conscientiously motivated to follow and care for their patients (4). Given that the main purpose of these statutes stems from a desire to improve patient care, further outcomes-based studies to assess the effects on patients in surgical resident training are urgently needed (7).

The Complication Conference has played an important role in surgical education. Although the conduct and atmosphere of this conference might vary greatly from institution to institution, the dual goal of open peer review and education is standard (8). The conference is a required component of resident training under program requirements stated by the RRC. Typically, the Complication Conference is held weekly and attended by faculty and residents, with the latter presenting patients who have experienced adverse events. Subsequent discussion commonly focuses on alternative strategies that might have minimized the likelihood of an adverse event. Historically, the Complication Conference was used to monitor surgical practice. Recently, it has been used as an educational tool for house staff and as a platform for improving surgical practice. Current evidence suggests that complication conferences might not be fulfilling either role well (9). Investigators reported that residents had a lower opinion of the educational value of complication conferences than did faculty (10). They also stated that the improvement in the Complication Conference that residents most wished to see was a decrease in defensiveness and blame. Certainly, the moderator of this conference must promote an educational atmosphere, as well as a willingness of physicians to accept appropriate responsibility and to discuss such events with peers (11).

Defining and measuring quality are complex tasks. The most widespread strategy for quality assessment in surgery uses the departmental Complication Conference, which traditionally involves case-finding methods. This approach to quality assessment uses peer review of cases. Although the historic and educational roles of the Complication Conference are indisputable, case-finding strategies for quality assessment have several limitations, including emphasis on outliers and fault-finding, focus on individual performance rather than organizational processes, emphasis on individual events rather than patterns of outcomes, and focus on early complications rather than long-term results (12).

The key feature of peer review is the involvement of physicians formulating a judgment about the quality of care on a case-by-case basis. One criticism of this approach is its focus on physician performance, minimizing the contributions of nonphysicians and organizational processes more generally (13). An emphasis on changing physician behavior through inspection focuses on blame and fault-finding rather than on the recognition of patterns of errors, which might reflect problems related to other components of the health care system (12). Although the likelihood that a complication would be reported at the conference increased with the severity of the complication, the majority of less medically severe but more common, negative outcomes were not reviewed (12).

There have been attempts to use prospective outcomes data to improve Morbidity and Mortality (M & M) Conferences (9). These authors demonstrated the feasibility of this format, resulting in an opportunity to examine local practice trends and to identify departmental practice improvement opportunities. Limitations stated were the initial startup costs for development of an outcomes registry ($20,000 to $30,000), as well as the need for local expertise of a surgeon with extensive prior experience in working with clinical and administrative databases. Medical–legal concerns about the documentation of patient safety issues and worry over public disclosure of data often hinder the accurate portrayal of the postoperative course and subsequent tabulation of data (14). Despite these concerns, the M & M Conference, if fulfilling its role, is one of the most powerful educational tools in surgical residency training programs.

Research is needed to understand the short-range and long-range impact of the expected changes and to tell leaders how to improve the quality of surgical residency education and appropriately adjust to demands so that professional excellence as well as an appropriate balance between service, education, and quality of life is achieved. Redesigning residents' roles to meet the new work hour requirements will require teaching hospitals to reengineer systems of patient care. Stakeholders, whether they are faculty, residents, other health professionals, patients, or hospital administrators, must understand the pressures that have been placed on surgical training programs in recent years. Efforts need to be made to preserve those components of a residency program considered critical to maintain the quality of education, whereas inefficiencies in both the educational and service aspects of the residency programs must be reviewed and addressed. Changes in resident education will require increased financial support as well as a reevaluation of currently existing resources (15).

General surgery training programs have changed considerably over the last 100 years and will likely do so at a considerably faster pace, given the professional and societal pressures thrust upon them. However, the heart of surgical training programs will remain in placing residents in the position to take responsibility for making and implementing decisions about the care of individual surgical patients. It will remain the obligation of the program to ensure that the resident has the opportunity and knowledge to do this with benefit for the patient. This requirement requires the next senior person in the system to have specific knowledge of each resident and the ability to provide ready and effective assistance when needed. It is the exercise of this kind of responsibility in a structured educational environment that leads to development of wise and capable surgeons.

REFERENCES

1. Dunnington GL, Reed GW. Addressing the new competencies for resident's surgical training. *Acad Med* 2003;78:14–21.
2. Greenfield LJ. Limiting resident duty hours. *Am J Surg* 2003; 185:10–12.
3. Zinner MJ. Surgical residencies: Are we still attracting the best and the brightest? *Bull Am Coll Surg* 2002;87:20–25.
4. Lewis FR. Should we limit resident work hours? *Ann Surg* 2003;237:458–459.
5. Chao L, Wallack MK. Limits on resident work hours. *Ann Surg* 2003;237(4):256–257.
6. Whang EE, Mello MM, Ashley SW, et al. Implementing resident work hour limitations. Lessons from the New York State experience. *Ann Surg* 2003;4:449–455.
7. Barden BB, Specht MC, McCarter MD. Effects of limited work hours on surgical training. *J Am Coll Surg* 2002;195:531–538.
8. Thompson JS, Prior MA. Quality assurance and morbidity and mortality conference. *J Surg Res* 1992;52:97–100.
9. Hamby LS, Birkmeyer JD, Birkmeyer C, et al. Using prospective outcomes data to improve morbidity and mortality conference. *Curr Surg* 2000;57:384–388.
10. Harbison SP, Regehr G. Faculty and resident opinions regarding the role of morbidity and mortality conference. *Am J Surg* 1999;177:136–139.
11. Wu AW, Folkman S, McPhee SJ. Do house officers learn from their mistakes? *J Am Med Assoc* 1991;265:2089–2094.
12. Feldman L, Barkun J. Measuring postoperative complications in the general surgery patients using an outcomes-based strategy: comparison with complications presented at morbidity and mortality rounds. *Surgery* 1997;122:711–720.
13. Laffel G, Blumenthal D. The case for using industrial quality management science in health care organizations. *J Am Med Assoc* 1989;262:2869–2873.
14. Martin RC, Brennan MF, Jacques DP. Quality of complication reporting in the surgical literature. *Ann Surg* 2002;235:803–813.
15. DaRosa DA, Bell RH, Dunnington GL. Residency program models, implications and evaluation: results of a think tank consortium on resident work hours. *Surgery* 2003;133:13–23.

Future Surgical Training

3

Paul G. Gauger

"You can never plan the future by the past."
Edmund Burke

■ **INTRODUCTION 9**

■ **WHY SURGICAL TRAINING IS CHANGING 9**
Increase in Number and Complexity
of Procedures 9
The Emergence of General Surgery Subspecialty
Practice 10
An Evolution in the Way We Learn and Teach 11
External Regulation of the Profession and the
Educational Process 11
A Health Care System in Crisis 12
The Social Contract of Medicine and Changes in the
Doctor–Patient Relationship 12
Personal Economic Factors 12
Generational Values and Lifestyle Considerations 12
Threats to Patient Safety and the Quality and
Continuity of Care 12
Decreased Operative Experience of Graduating Surgical
Residents 13
Threats to Professional Values 13

■ **HOW WILL SURGICAL TRAINING CHANGE? 13**
Early Specialization Programs 13
Length of Training Issues 14
Novel Residency Structures and Physician Extenders 14
New Methods of Feedback and Assessment 15
Educational Integration 15
Simulation Training 15

■ **CONCLUSION 17**

■ **REFERENCES 17**

Paul G. Gauger: University of Michigan, Ann Arbor, MI 48109

INTRODUCTION

Three prominent themes characterize American medicine today. There has been an explosive increase in basic knowledge underlying clinical practice. There is a crisis in the manner in which we deliver health care. And recent technologic advances are so fundamentally complex as to require major reassessment and change in accepted educational paradigms (1). All these factors have affected the long-standing model of American surgical training to create a unique crisis in surgical education. Table 3-1 contains an incomplete assessment of the factors that cause this crisis.

Although every generation laments changes, it is not an overstatement to say that surgical training is undergoing more changes and challenges than ever before. As a field steeped in tradition and inherited wisdom, surgery has been slow to embrace change, but, viewed from the proper perspective, much of the change is welcome and necessary. Change must be managed to assure that the values of the profession are preserved. To do so, it is critically important to understand the internal and external forces that have led to this point. Selected influences are examined below within the context of surgical training, and the manner in which educational programs will have to adapt are delineated.

WHY SURGICAL TRAINING IS CHANGING

Increase in Number and Complexity of Procedures

There have been remarkable advances in the last decades in the understanding of diseases and in options for treatment.

TABLE 3-1
MEDICAL EDUCATION ISSUES, INFLUENCES, AND RESPONSIBILITIES

General Educational Issues

- Explosive increase in medical knowledge
- Competitive imbalance between work load and educational opportunity
- Need for new training paradigms
- ACGME outcome project (competencies)
- Changing expectations of patients and society
- Changes in educational techniques and technology (Internet, simulation, etc.)
- Sources of innovation outside academic medicine (industry R & D)
- Focus on documentation instead of delivery of care

Policy, Administrative, and Financial Issues

- Decreased number of applicants for training
- Changes in applicant quality
- Changing demographics of applicant pool
- Increased medical school dependence on clinical revenue
- Decreased reimbursement for graduate medical education
- Decreased faculty professional reimbursement
- Length of training programs
- Increased indebtedness of trainees
- Increased fraction of foreign medical graduates in training programs

Specific Surgical Training Issues

- Ensuring broad exposure to surgical subspecialties
- Increased technologic sophistication and dependency on procedures
- Assessing surgical competency
- RRC mandates/standards for case volume during training
- Continuity of care/work load
- Disenchantment with specialty among practitioners

Personal Issues for Trainees

- Increased indebtedness of graduates
- Low pay
- Lack of overtime compensation
- Lack of retirement benefits
- Length and intensity of training
- Balance between work load and personal time
- Decreased income as practitioner to repay loan burden

ACGME, Accreditation Council for Graduate Medical Education; R & D, research and development; RRC, Residency Review Committee.
From Zelenock GB: Presidential address: Medical education: Thoughts on the training of physicians and surgeons. *J Vasc Surg* 2003;37:921–929, with permission.

For some diseases surgical intervention is becoming less common (e.g., peptic ulcer disease), but for many others factors such as earlier detection are making some operations more common (e.g., colon cancer). For nearly all examples, the breadth of therapeutic options has increased significantly. The emergence of laparoscopic and endoscopic technologies has greatly amplified this trend. The present-day graduating surgical resident is responsible for demonstrating exposure to an ever-increasing list of procedures. Demonstrated competency in these areas is another issue.

The Emergence of General Surgery Subspecialty Practice

General surgery has gradually changed from a broad and flexible specialty responsible for "the skin and its contents"

to a more limited definition. Many of the operations formerly performed by the general surgeon are now being performed by a general surgeon with additional fellowship training or declared interest. The rise in vascular surgery, endocrine surgery, and colorectal surgery are examples of this increase in subspecialization. These changes have a bearing on the curriculum redesign required to facilitate specialization and fellowship training.

As surgical training represents a microcosm of medical practice, it was to be expected that the sweeping changes of the last 30 to 40 years have had downstream effects. Medical practice has been transformed into medical industry. Declining professional reimbursement, an increased pace of clinical practice, and dehumanization of the physician–patient relationship have taken their toll on practicing physicians. The medical profession is occasionally demoralized, confused, and cynical. Perhaps amplified by the perception that surgeons are working harder and being paid less than those in other specialties, dissatisfaction and frustration might be vocally and visibly expressed during the daily routine. As a result, young, enthusiastic, impressionable medical students and trainees find themselves analyzing their interactions with established surgeons and asking, "Why would I want to do what they do when they don't even want to do what they do?"

The business of medicine can be so all-consuming that surgeons might find themselves more concerned with the business of coding, billing, and reimbursement than with taking care of patients. Patients sense this, and accordingly, trust is eroded (2). Media exploitation, public perception and dissatisfaction, and the medical liability crisis further test this relationship. This strain is often visible to medical students.

Although trends suggesting declining interest in surgical careers over the last few years appeared to portend significant problems, recent match statistics suggest that the trend might be reversing (Table 3-2). It is likely that limitations on duty hours are attracting students who previously would have been too concerned about lifestyle issues to pursue surgical training. Additionally, in many segments of the profession, this trend was noted, analyzed, and specifically addressed with interventions intended to demonstrate the pleasure, reward, and satisfaction associated with a surgical career (3).

An Evolution in the Way We Learn and Teach

Advances in medical practice, especially those that depend on advanced technologies, require skills neither selected for nor taught in medical schools and residencies. In contrast to the prodigious increase in medical knowledge that occurs every year, our ability to comprehend and then assimilate this knowledge into medical practice is constrained. Even the evolution of clinical practice has been driven by technology. Consider the incorporation of endoscopic, laparoscopic, and robotic technology into current surgical practice. It has been a challenge for practicing surgeons to learn and master the requisite new skills and more difficult to decide how best to teach these skills to surgeons in training. Academic medicine no longer has a monopoly on innovation and research. Many technological advances are driven by industry, which changes the dynamics of education and requires an ongoing interaction with commercial entities.

Because declining reimbursement exacerbates the economic crisis in surgical practice, a nearly constant attention to one's practice is required. Taking dedicated time for education and self-improvement is increasingly difficult. Additionally, surgical departments are the clinical engines that drive the hospital's financial mission—especially in academic health centers. As such, the pace of surgical practice is often breakneck and the time for learning, teaching, reflection, and innovation is critically diminished. This pace hurts both faculty and residents. As the educational environment has changed, so has educational technology. As computer-based and Internet-enabled educational programs continue to improve, it is clear that they will soon be the means to provide educational content at an individualized pace, document content exposure, and evaluate content mastery. The ability to simulate both patients and procedures has exponentially increased educational opportunities for the present and the future.

External Regulation of the Profession and the Educational Process

When external forces regulate a profession, it nearly always means that the profession has not adequately managed to do so itself. Surgeons have done an inadequate job of articulating why the practice of surgery and the implicit training are different and must remain different from other specialties. Therefore, surgical training is now subject to the same group of regulations as all other specialties. In the wake of frequent and often poorly coordinated regulation from agencies such as the Accreditation Council for Graduate Medical Education (ACGME), the Residency Review Committee (RRC), and the American Board of Surgery (ABS), many program directors find themselves mired in regulations and pressing changes.

Work hour regulations have become highly politicized. Although the original impetus might have been the Libby Zion case in New York State, the issue has grown in the public eye to center around concerns of sleep deprivation and inadequate supervision. The 2000 Institute of Medicine report, *To Err Is Human: Building a Safer Health System*, claimed that medical errors resulted in >1 million

TABLE 3-2
PERCENTAGE OF OPEN SURGICAL RESIDENCY SLOTS FILLED[a,b]

	2000 Positions		2001 Positions		2002 Positions		2003 Positions		2004 Positions	
	% U.S.	% Total	% U.S.	% Total	% U.S.	% Total	% U.S.	% Total	% U.S.	% Total
Categorical	85.4	98.5	78.8	93.5	75.3	94.4	82.7	99	84.8	99.8
Preliminary	37.4	55.2	37.9	55.5	38.6	58.1	42.1	64.4	42.6	65.1

[a]The % U.S. columns indicate the % of positions filled by US medical graduates.
[b]The % total columns indicate the % of positions filled by US and foreign medical graduates.

patient injuries and nearly 100,000 patient deaths each year (4). Although many possible contributors to medical errors were considered, this report implied a relationship to physician workload, fatigue, lack of alertness, and sleep deprivation. Education has become a casualty of this public and political discourse. The time that residents are engaging in sanctioned educational activities are counted against the work hours limit, exacerbating the educational dilemma.

A Health Care System in Crisis

It is an accepted observation that the crisis environment is especially severe in the academic health centers (5). For this reason, the crises more directly impact undergraduate, graduate, and continuing medical education. The Balanced Budget Act of 1997 exacerbated these problems—especially for graduate medical education (GME)—and has severely curtailed educational resources (6). Still, direct and indirect federal funds flow to hospitals—in part to support and subsidize graduate medical education.

The Social Contract of Medicine and Changes in the Doctor–Patient Relationship

The pressures that have led to a perturbed relationship between physicians and patients are complicated. A few decades ago, patients covered under Medicare and Medicaid understood that their care might be provided by physicians in training under the supervision of senior physicians. This relationship was an accepted part of the social contract of medicine. Patients knew that they were participants in the educational process of the profession (7). Increasing affluence and consumerism, dissatisfaction with the insurance industry and the "medical machine," and a general increase in a sense of entitlement and empowerment in the American patient population have altered these expectations. Many patients are no longer interested or willing to serve an educational role. Many expect their care to be delivered by the most highly skilled practitioner available. Some might misunderstand the process of supervision and question or refuse the participation of trainees in the provision of care.

Personal Economic Factors

The definition of residents' jobs is ambiguously mired in a no-man's land between student and employee. This confusion is used as justification for low salaries, lack of retirement benefits, and inadequate work facilities and support systems. For decades the residency years served as a rite of passage and these conditions were tolerated. It was understood that the prestige and affluence afforded to physicians in practice would act as eventual compensation. An increasing number of current medical school graduates do not seek additional training and instead leverage their M.D. degree for success in related fields. As college friends find early success and

happiness in fields that require only a fraction of the education and dedication that medicine does, it becomes even more difficult to run the gauntlet of surgical training.

An especially difficult factor in this economic equation is medical school graduate indebtedness. Many students continue to carry loan debt from undergraduate education. The average debt level of graduating American medical students is nearly $100,000. Because most residents do not accrue retirement savings, each additional year of training threatens lifetime earning potential. Surgical residents, by virtue of extensive training and decreasing remuneration, are disproportionately disadvantaged.

Generational Values and Lifestyle Considerations

It is the archetype of the surgeon to be dedicated to patients at any expense. Most of the great surgeons of the last century had an unflagging dedication to their patients and their careers. However, such dedication, while benefiting patients, often penalized marriage and family life. The current generation of men and women pursuing a career in surgery has begun to reject some of these values. It is the pervasive sentiment of this generation that personal happiness is a right to be claimed. Where happiness cannot be guaranteed from one's career alone, it might be found in leisurely pursuit of other interests and in a fulfilling family life. These characteristics are influencing the growth of "lifestyle" specialties such as dermatology and anesthesiology.

Threats to Patient Safety and the Quality and Continuity of Care

Society, through its regulatory agencies, has determined that surgical training must change to protect patients from overly tired physicians and medical errors. The consequences of these externally managed changes might not be fully apparent for years (8). The limitation of duty hours and the resulting increase in information transfer (patient handoffs) and an emerging "shift work" mentality might create a decrease in patient satisfaction from further dilution of the physician–patient relationship and in patient safety, as defined by an increase in "near-misses" or medical errors. The field of error analysis has clearly shown that errors occur in systems that are designed in a way that unintentionally enables the error. Although residents previously were largely responsible for the longitudinal care of patients, this care now occurs in spurts and intervals. This care model necessitates frequent transfer of encapsulated medical information and simultaneously discourages individual reassessment of the patient when called upon for intervention or judgment of some sort. Patient rounds are occasions in which latent errors are enabled.

A recent survey of surgeons in training indicated that the majority felt that they should be allowed to work >80 hours per week (9). Perhaps this response indicates some discomfort with interrupted continuity of care and challenges to professional values. Threshold limitations of work hours, no matter whether they are well reasoned or completely arbitrary, undercut the importance of continuity of care, a principle highly valued by surgeons and one that is absolutely critical to inculcate in future practitioners. Temporal restraints have no place in the definition of a profession or professional behaviors. It is paradoxical that duty-hour regulations are being assimilated into the structure of surgical residency at the same time that professionalism is one of the ACGME Educational Outcomes (Competencies) to be separately taught and measured (10). This juxtaposition of values will require major attention and vigilance in the structure and the practice of surgical training.

Many developed nations have restrictions on duty hours of physicians in training. It is impossible to completely extrapolate these experiences to American surgery because of differences in patient and societal expectations, as well as differences in traditions and values. In general, maintaining excellent quality surgical training appears to be possible, largely because of an increase in the number of educational resources and technologies, which can facilitate more efficient content assimilation and skill mastery (11). In Sweden, the duty-hour limit has been 40 hours per week for 30 years, and patient outcomes appear not to have suffered as a result. Because of the limited hours and thus, ultimately, limited exposure, the training period has become structured around time-targeted competency goals (12). Curricula have been tightly tailored for specific training programs.

Decreased Operative Experience of Graduating Surgical Residents

With the increased breadth of operative procedures to master during graduate medical training, decreasing the work hours in which to be exposed to these procedures is inopportune. Novel solutions will be required. A very practical question is whether the hours off duty are hours lost from mastering operations and preoperative and postoperative care. Several studies that characterize the time and work flow of surgical residents have discovered a large amount of time spent in noneducational activities (13). There is a large opportunity to streamline and redesign surgical residency. "Hours worked" is a poor surrogate for determining "work done," and a large fraction of the traditional duties of residents needs to be transferred to nonphysician clinicians and ancillary staff. If it is not accurate to say that residents have been the *engine* of the academic health center, they traditionally have been the *drivetrain*. As residents learn to work *smarter* rather than *harder*, hospitals must also readjust.

Although limitation of duty hours for surgical training in Sweden has not damaged patient outcomes, it has changed the level of experience and the end product of surgical training. A period of junior specialist practice follows

residency training to enhance skills, and subspecialization is very common. Perhaps this factor has preserved excellent patient outcomes, but emergency general surgery operations have suffered because few broadly trained surgeons remain (12). It seems likely that our own system might eventually come to mimic these changes and adjustments. Without an accompanying overhaul of the national (GME) administrative and reimbursement structure and limitations, patient outcomes might ultimately suffer.

Another question centers on how to determine competency. The assumption inherent in the current model of American surgical training is that repeated exposure to patient care and specific operations assures competency. Competency is a relative concept. How many cholecystectomies are enough? Should the goal be to do as many operations as possible? Can one perform too many operations before ideal learning no longer occurs? Should these definitions be individualized for different residents? The overarching question is whether the graduating resident meeting RRC requirements is really prepared for active surgical practice and whether the answer is different for community practice.

Threats to Professional Values

For many years the nature of surgical training was a paradox. The fact that surgical training was so hard, both mentally and physically punishing, so relentless and lengthy, was the thing that made it so unique, so valuable, and so worthy. Surgeons were imbued with professional values such as altruism and lifetime learning and continuous self-improvement. Most illustrative of this value system was the continuity of care, which permeated surgical practice. Surgeons knew it, patients knew it, and other physicians knew it. As the current model of training involves limitation of work hours and a shift in clinical practice toward outpatient and short-stay procedures, surgical residents are increasingly operating on patients whom they have not previously met or evaluated. Similarly, other residents and faculty address complications when they occur. Aside from losing the opportunity to learn about the continua of disease and healing, the overall doctor–patient relationship becomes compartmentalized, and as such, is diminished. As care is more frequently provided in shifts, it becomes more difficult to inculcate professional qualities.

HOW WILL SURGICAL TRAINING CHANGE?

Early Specialization Programs

In 2003, the ABS approved a pilot training scheme called the Early Specialization Program (ESP). This program is meant to enable residency directors in general surgery, pediatric surgery, and vascular surgery (but not thoracic surgery) to create specific curricular tracks, which lead to dual certification in 6 instead of 7 years. In concept, the fourth clinical year serves as a general surgery chief year and the last 2 years have a concentrated experience in the subspecialty. Both portions of the program need to take place at a single institution, and the pilot requires both a carefully defined curriculum and specific metrics to determine whether the ESP is a success or failure. To date, pediatric surgery training programs have not embraced this model and vascular surgery training programs are tentatively considering ESP's. The American Board of Thoracic Surgery (ABTS) approved a similar pilot program in 2001. This latter resolution determined that certification by the ABS is optional and that other pathways to ABTS certification could be developed. Specifically, the Thoracic Surgery Directors Association would develop categorical integrated 6-year programs. Another pathway will potentially be a 3-year thoracic surgery residency to follow a defined 3-year general surgery curriculum. Again, thoracic surgery training programs have ultimately been very hesitant to embrace some of these potential changes.

These changes are meant to redefine the training of vascular surgeons, pediatric surgeons, and thoracic surgeons. The standard curriculum of the general surgery residency will also need to be rearranged to provide a consistent core exposure for those residents tracked into specialties, while redefining the fourth- and fifth-year curricula for residents remaining in general surgery. Although many are concerned about the further disintegration of general surgery that this change might cause, it is conceivable that it could reaffirm general surgery as a destination instead of an in-transit experience. If the final years are to be preserved as advanced experiences in general surgery (complex hepatobiliary cases, oncology cases, endocrine procedures, etc.), careful attention will need to be paid to the redesign of the curriculum required to facilitate the ESPs in order to preserve experiences for those pursuing a career in general surgery.

Length of Training Issues

The trend to support earlier specialization and consolidation of surgical training could not have come at a more awkward time. The impact of the 80-hour workweek on resident education is not yet completely defined. On the basis of the experience in New York State over the last decade, it seems possible to provide solid surgical training in the setting of limited work hours. If the ESP is to succeed in the context of limited work hours, the program director position will become even more challenging. All rotation experiences will need to be planned and provided with the education–service balance clearly tipped toward the former.

It has been suggested that if surgical experience is meant to stay the same, then limitation of the weekly work schedule would require additional years of training. This calculus is oversimplified. Training extension will almost certainly not occur because of the limits of the current GME funding structure that dictates the maximum term of reimbursable training to be 5 years. Such an expansion of training, especially without reconsideration of the personal economic disadvantages incurred, would certainly make the field of surgery less attractive to medical students.

Novel Residency Structures and Physician Extenders

If residencies could be redesigned to form the ideal training system with unlimited financial and political support, they would likely look vastly different. However, the immediately necessary changes must be made within the matrix of current resources and restrictions. A number of reengineering solutions have been suggested that manage immediate regulatory issues while variably balancing educational needs (14). An *Apprenticeship Model* is built around sequential close working relationships with mentor faculty who are chosen for both their skills as teachers and the educational value of their practice. This model theoretically minimizes in-house time on call and results in early intensive technical skills training. The *Mastery (Case-Based) Model* proposes that residents develop knowledge and skills associated with predefined diseases and operations. A logistical challenge, this type of program would assign cases to residents on the basis of individual educational needs. This type of residency would potentially be most flexible in terms of advancement, "job-sharing," and overall training time. Another proposed model is based on the *Night Float System*. This is a more traditional team-based system in which some residents provide patient care only during the night shift (on a rotating basis). This schedule obviously is meant to facilitate most of the other residents going home, but, admittedly, it sublimates the educational value of the rotation to the service component. Because it is a temporary and equally distributed experience, it might be a legitimate trade-off.

As the pace of clinical practice increases with the aging of the population and the impending shortage in physicians and as the overall length of training is very unlikely to change, it is clear that many new members of the patient care team will be required. Nurse practitioners and physician assistants have already added substantially to both inpatient and outpatient settings. Often the cost of these practitioners is borne by the hospitals that have long benefited from a seemingly inexhaustible and inexpensive workforce in the resident pool. It will take careful attention by program directors and chairmen to deploy these additional professionals in duties that decrease the "service" expectations of physicians in training while increasing the "education" opportunities. In short, we have a responsibility to assure that physician *extenders* do not become physician *replacements*. However, the model in which physician assistants are charged only with dictations and paperwork while surgical residents spend all day operating carries an inherent danger that we will be breeding a generation of "incomplete" surgeons, which will eventually decrease our respect and stature as a profession. Incorporation of these nonphysician clinicians will eventually lead to reforms in the inadequate pay and benefit structure of residents as the differences in their training and their level of commitment will become more evident.

New Methods of Feedback and Assessment

One of the basic premises of surgical training is that facts must be learned. Those residents most successful in surgical training are often not those with the largest selection of facts at the ready but those who are facile at finding accurate information when knowledge deficiencies are encountered. In response to the growing body of medical knowledge and practical limits to the capacity to learn and memorize, technology has fostered robust and available decision support. Surgical decision making increasingly utilizes handheld computing and electronic resources for access to the best evidence for clinical practice. Residency programs will become less focused on teaching residents what to know and think and more on how to find the answers they need from trusted sources when a gap in their knowledge and experience is encountered. This approach is a much more appropriate androgogic model for lifelong learning and for the continual quest for improvement that defines the surgical profession.

The ways that residents and practicing physicians are evaluated will change substantially. Surgical training has long used a model of evaluation that assessed skills globally and assumed transfer of competency from one skill set to another. The ACGME outcome project has already changed this issue by requiring a much more specific and granular way of rating competency in defined domains. The final format of the related evaluation instruments and methods is still unsettled. The level of feedback will be increased to close the loop between education and assessment. One can imagine that the steep slope of the learning curve during surgical residency can be increased even further by individualized, supportive, and specific feedback provided in defined areas. Computers will provide some of this feedback during exercises in decision analysis and in procedural simulations.

No longer will subjective assessment of skills, knowledge, and attitude be sufficient for evaluation during residency training. Competency will be defined by measurable criteria, and these data will be used for decisions regarding graded responsibility and for promotions and advancement through the training schemes. If these strategies are adequately operationalized, residencies might eventually be competency-driven (and relatively time-independent) instead of time-driven (and relatively competency-independent). For this change to occur, the rigid limitations of GME funding need to be redesigned significantly. Implementation

will ultimately require accurately defining the key elements of surgical training, establishing quantifiable metrics, stringently measuring performance against criteria, and reporting outcomes throughout the career of a surgeon (15).

Educational Integration

A shift in where and by whom residents are trained will likely occur. There is very likely to be a shortage of qualified physicians in the years to come (16). It is probable that the total number of slots for training will increase and these will most likely be incremental additions at larger, better-coordinated programs. As the complexity of the surgical field and the prevalence of subspecialty practice increase, many residents will pursue additional fellowship training. It is inevitable that the operative experience of fellows will compete with that of residents. Successful management of this competition will require an increase in the coordination that occurs within and between training programs, especially in light of the curricular implications of the ESPs if they are ultimately accepted and implemented. For example, programs with an active vascular surgery fellowship might choose to have general surgery residents rotate at active programs without a fellowship.

Another aspect of educational coordination will involve taking full advantage of scientific and clinical expertise, where and when it exists. Distance learning via the Internet and live telesurgery transmissions make this a very tangible possibility. As the body of surgical knowledge increases, and as the multidisciplinary aspect of clinical care becomes more prominent, better coordination between undergraduate, graduate, and continuing medical curricula will need to be defined. Because the advanced technology aspects of surgical practice impact the spectrum of caregivers, the educational process will often involve teams. Because of patient-safety issues, the costs of this education will likely be shifted to hospitals.

Simulation Training

To fully develop the skills of surgeons, live patients are absolutely necessary. Of course, there is an obligation to provide optimal treatment and ensure patient safety and best outcomes. Balancing these two needs represents a fundamental ethical tension in surgical education (17). Other professions that are typified by long stretches of routine shattered infrequently by high-hazard, high-acuity crises, such as the aviation industry, the military, and the nuclear power industry, have long ago institutionalized simulation-based training. Medical education has been slow to embrace simulation for reasons of cost, complacency, and lack of rigorous determination of reliability and construct validity. Focused by the patient safety movement, the face validity of simulation education is overwhelming. Many recent articles in the ethics literature have condemned the use of sedated or dying patients for training in examinations or basic procedures, again highlighting the role for simulation-based training (18).

The first attempted surgical simulations utilizing virtual reality took place a decade ago. Since then, computer power has rapidly improved, as has the quality of procedural simulation both in terms of visual fidelity and enhancements such as haptic feedback. The digital aspect of these computer-based simulations allows robust data capture to provide immediate performance assessment and feedback. Although the literature establishing the construct validity and the reliability of these education and assessment tools is relatively limited, it is growing exponentially. Professional organizations have begun to seriously consider the potential of these tools to revolutionize the surgical training and certification processes (19,20).

Although the advent and diffusion of laparoscopic surgery was soon followed by curricula and guidelines for training, the specific metrics of evaluation were lacking. Owing to efforts in such diverse locations as Scotland, Canada, and the United States, sophisticated analyses of psychomotor skills have led to objective structured assessments for technical skills. Currently, there is no standardized threshold level that residents are expected to attain, and there is no consensus on metrics of performance, methods of evaluation, or the significance of these measurements when applied to clinical outcomes (15,20). This experience in teaching standard surgical skills has not been fully realized in surgical simulation technology. For a curriculum based on accepted criteria in the training

and evaluation of technical skills on a simulator, Satava has recommended the following steps: (i) development of standardized definitions/taxonomy of technical skills (e.g., metrics); (ii) definitions/taxonomy of errors; (iii) establishment of core outcomes/results reporting; and (iv) development of a comprehensive curriculum. The curriculum should include (i) didactic information (lecture, multimedia, etc.) of the relevant anatomy and correct performance of the skills being taught; (ii) definition and description of the errors the simulator will detect; (iii) pretest documentation that the student understands the information; (iv) performance of the simulation with immediate feedback after errors; (v) a final report on performance; and (vi) a longitudinal record of the performances over time as well as comparison to peer levels (15).

Currently, simulation-based training and assessment is available for such diverse procedures as general laparoscopy, laparoscopic cholecystectomy, hysteroscopy, bronchoscopy, esophagoduodenoscopy, endoscopic retrograde cholangiopancreatography, endoscopic ultrasound, arthroscopy, endoscopic sinus surgery, endovascular surgery, and others (Fig. 3-1). For most of these applications, the procedure being simulated requires interaction with an image. The image serves as the basis for the simulation. For that reason, simulation of open operations, where the interaction with tissue uses many senses, is years away—or perhaps unattainable. As impressive as some of the currently available simulators are, it is fascinating to consider that the field is generally at the same stage of

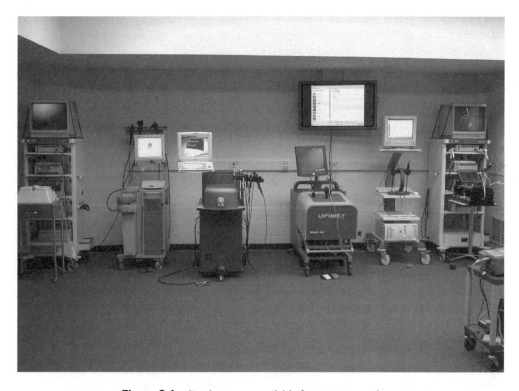

Figure 3-1 Simulators are available for many procedures.

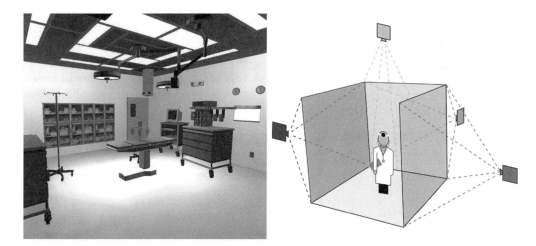

Figure 3-2   Simulated environments may be important to increase the fidelity (sense of realism) when interacting with simulated patients or procedures. Interactive virtual reality environments such as the operating room (*left panel*) can be projected into the CAVE environment (*right panel*) to create an immersive virtual environment.

development as the first flight simulator (20). It took nearly 20 years for the field of flight simulation to develop into a standard part of flight training and certification, so we will likely continue to see significant advances in surgical simulation. In addition, the ability to simulate interactive environments with technologies such as the CAVE (Cave Automatic Virtual Environment) (Fig. 3-2) and the geowall stereoscopic projection system will have the potential to increase fidelity and to enhance evaluation of performance under stress.

CONCLUSION

Change is upon us and the opportunities are numerous to further improve the system of surgical training in the United States. We must now be proactive in order to improve the field and enhance the aspects of surgery that we cherish. As characterized by an improvement in the ratio of resident education to resident service and the incorporation of physician extenders into the clinical enterprise, and as enhanced by computer-based learning and simulation, the future of surgical training is quite bright.

REFERENCES

1. Zelenock GB. Presidential address: medical education: thoughts on the training of physicians and surgeons. *J Vasc Surg* 2003; 37:921–929.
2. Russell TR. What is the future of surgery? *Arch Surg* 2003; 138:825–831.
3. Mulholland MW. Program increases medical student interest in surgical careers. *Bull Am Coll Surg* 2003;88:25–27.
4. Kohn L, Corrigan J, Donaldson ME. *To err is human: building a safer health system.* Washington, DC: National Academic Press; 2000.
5. Kassirer JP. Academic medical centers under siege. *N Engl J Med* 1994;331:1370–1371.
6. Inglehart JK. Medicare's declining payments to physicians. *N Engl J Med* 2001;346:1924–1930.
7. Ludmerer KM. *A time to heal.* New York: Oxford University Press; 1999.
8. Russell RCG. Limitations of work hours: the U.K. experience. *Surgery* 2003;134:19–22.
9. Underwood W, Boyd AJ, Fletcher KE, The Executive Committee of the American College of Surgeons-Candidate Associate Group, Lypson ML. Viewpoints from generation X. A survey of candidate and associate viewpoints on resident duty-hour regulations. *J Am Coll Surg* 2004;198:989–993.
10. Fischer JE. Continuity of care: a casualty of the 80-hour work week. *Acad Med* 2004;79:381–383.
11. Romanchuk K. The effect of limiting residents' work hours on their surgical training: a Canadian perspective. *Acad Med* 2004;79:384–385.
12. Ihse I, Haglund U. The Swedish 40-hour workweek: How does it affect surgical care? *Surgery* 2003;134:17–18.
13. Brasel KJ, Pierre AL, Weigelt JA. Resident work hours. What they are really doing. *Arch Surg* 2004;139:490–494.
14. DaRosa DA, Bell RH, Dunnington GL. Residency program models, implications, and evaluation: results of a think tank consortium on resident work hours. *Surgery* 2003;133:13–23.
15. Satava RM. Disruptive visions. Surgical education. *Surg Endosc* 2004;18:779–781.
16. Cooper RA, Getzen TE, McKee JH, et al. Economic and demographic trends signal an impending physician shortage. *Health Affairs* 2002;21:140–154.
17. Ziv A, Wolpe PR, Small SD, et al. Simulation-based medical education: an ethical imperative. *Acad Med* 2003;78:783–788.
18. Rosenson J, Tabas JA, Patterson P. Teaching invasive procedures to medical students. *J Am Med Assoc* 2004;291:119–120.
19. Seymour NE, Gallagher AG, Roma SA, et al. Virtual reality training improves operating room performance. *Ann Surg* 2002;236:458–464.
20. Satava RM. Accomplishments and challenges of surgical simulation. Dawning of the next-generation surgical education. *Surg Endosc* 2001;15:232–241.

Continuing Education for Practicing Surgeons

4

Richard E. Burney   R. Van Harrison

■■■ **BRIEF HISTORY OF CME 19**

■■■ **SOURCES AND CHARACTERISTICS OF HIGH-QUALITY, EFFECTIVE CME 19**

■■■ **PRINCIPLES OF ADULT EDUCATION AND LEARNING 19**

■■■ **PREPARING FOR RECERTIFICATION AND RECREDENTIALING REQUIREMENTS 22**

■■■ **INDUSTRY, ETHICS, AND CME 22**

■■■ **CONCLUSION AND RECOMMENDATIONS: A BALANCED PORTFOLIO OF CME 23**

■■■ **REFERENCES 23**

CME consists of educational activities that serve to maintain, develop, or increase the knowledge, skills, and professional performance and relationships a physician uses to provide services for patients, the public, or the profession. The content of CME is that body of knowledge and skills generally recognized and accepted by the profession as within the basic medical sciences, the discipline of clinical medicine, and the provision of health care to the public (1).

In the broadest sense, continuing medical education (CME) for surgeons is the acquisition of new knowledge

Richard E. Burney, R. Van Harrison: University of Michigan, Ann Arbor, MI 48109

and skills after completing residency or fellowship training. Once beyond the structured environment of postgraduate training, all surgeons face the ongoing challenge of maintaining their general medical knowledge base, keeping up with changes in basic pathophysiology of disease, learning about new pharmacotherapeutic agents, becoming acquainted with new or improved surgical techniques, improving day-to-day medical and surgical care practices, acquiring new technical skills, and learning how to use new devices and apply new technology in their daily lives. All these things are part of CME and professional development (also referred to as "life-long learning"). Continued learning is a requisite to good practice and to the prevention of complications that can occur when education is deficient. Surgeons have a professional obligation to continue their education and to maintain competence throughout their surgical careers (2).

A narrower view of CME is the enterprise managed by the Accreditation Council for Continuing Medical Education (ACCME). ACCME's mission is to identify, develop, and promote standards for quality of CME. ACCME accredits eligible institutions that sponsor CME programs. It thereby oversees the quality of CME offerings for which physicians receive American Medical Association Physician Recognition Award (AMA-PRA) category 1 credits, which in turn are mandated by various state and local administrative entities as part of their regulatory and licensing requirements. CME may be mandated as well as a requirement for credentialing within a hospital or health care organization. Of course, the primary purpose for seeking continuing education is to improve patient care, not to satisfy licensing and other mandates. For those motivated to learn, the accumulation of

CME credits presents less of a problem than does the proper documentation of that CME for administrative purposes.

BRIEF HISTORY OF CME

At the turn of the 20th century, on July 3, 1900, Sir William Osler gave an address in London entitled "The Importance of Post-Graduate Study," in which he emphasized the importance of lifelong learning for professional competence. This event is generally accepted as the birth of CME (3). Since then the importance of advancing the profession by providing opportunities for individual practitioners to acquire new information and improve skills has never been questioned. The American College of Surgeons was founded in 1913 to develop, among other things, a broad and continuing program for surgical education. One of the chief purposes of medical societies, surgical associations, and specialty societies has been to sponsor journals in which to publish and disseminate new information. University-based postgraduate courses were developed in the 1930s. In the past 50 years, academic medical centers and medical and surgical specialty organizations have increasingly played larger roles in providing continuing education programs that offer learning opportunities for practicing physicians.

In the early 1970s, several trends made CME a focus of additional attention. First, the expansion of scientific information made medical practice more complex while offering hope for cure of previously untreatable medical problems. Second, patients and their advocates began to call attention to failures in medical practice and the costs associated with medical malpractice began to rise and be recognized as a major societal problem. Third, educational psychologists began to define and analyze adult educational processes more scientifically and identify those that were most effective. Finally, the American Medical Association, in response to these pressures and on the basis of the assumption that lack of information was a remediable cause of physician failure, proposed that physicians voluntarily obtain 50 hours of CME per year in order to maintain proficiency. Physicians who did so were eligible for a physician recognition award (PRA).

Another response related to these pressures was the introduction of new regulations by state governments. By 1978, 13 states, beginning with New Mexico and Michigan, had passed laws that made 50 hours per year of CME mandatory for relicensure and other states were poised to do so. This mandatory CME requirement led to an expansion of entrepreneurial CME offerings. An increasing amount of time and money was swiftly invested in providing education opportunities for physicians, sometimes in vacation settings and often of questionable educational value. At the same time, mandatory CME had the salutary effect of encouraging hospitals to devote funds and attention to providing CME for medical staff members.

SOURCES AND CHARACTERISTICS OF HIGH-QUALITY, EFFECTIVE CME

Diffusion and acquisition of new knowledge occurs through a variety of mechanisms and stimuli, both formal and informal. A list of the most common, readily available sources of continuing education is shown in Table 4-1. Only a small number of these are formal CME offerings. The most common and frequently unmentioned source of new information is informal discussion with colleagues. Most surgeons obtain new information by asking questions of their colleagues. In the right circumstances, this is one of the chief sources of reliable, practical information.

Regular general information gathering through reading of relevant journals and reports is a simple yet basic way to expand one's knowledge base. Every surgeon must set aside time to read a selection of journals and other sources of written information. Computer and Internet-based educational materials are proliferating and readily available from a variety of sources.

Attendance at a selection of local, regional, or national professional meetings, at which a broad range of information is offered and at which one can share information and questions with colleagues, is similarly important. Awareness of new knowledge induces questions that lead to more directed or focused learning and application of selected new knowledge into practice. High-quality skill acquisition courses offered through universities, professional societies, and industry facilitate the skill acquisition needed to apply new knowledge.

PRINCIPLES OF ADULT EDUCATION AND LEARNING

To deal with the rapid pace of change in professional practice in our quickly changing world, one must learn about learning. An understanding of how adults learn will help one select a balance of learning activities that will be most efficient and effective. A number of models have been developed for the complex processes involved in learning (4). Most education models suggest at least four prerequisites for effective continuing education and learning to occur.

- **Motivation:** The first and most important is the intrinsic motivation to question oneself, to learn, and to improve. The student should have a question to be answered, be aware of a deficiency or an inadequacy to be corrected, or have a similar, strong motivation to learn or change behavior. Dilemmas and questions encountered in daily practice are prime sources of motivation, but not the only ones. Competitive pressures and strategic planning also motivate.
- **Objective:** The student must have a clear goal or objective in mind for applying that new knowledge or

TABLE 4-1

READILY AVAILABLE SOURCES OF CONTINUING MEDICAL EDUCATION

Informal discussion or consultation with colleagues
Textbooks and journals
       Reading only
       Reading + CME quiz
Hospital/Intramural conferences and committees
       Teaching conferences
       Morbidity and mortality
       Multidisciplinary committee (e.g., Tumor Board)
       Journal club
       Quality assurance/quality improvement committee
Computer (CD/DVD) and Internet-based educational programs
       Hospital/Medical school sponsored
Specialty society-provided (e.g., Society of Colon and Rectal Surgeons)
Industry-sponsored and commercial sites
Professional meetings
       American College of Surgeons
Clinical Congress
Postgraduate courses
Regional meetings
Special skills courses (e.g., Advanced Trauma Life Support)
Specialty society meetings
       Special skills courses, and so on
Surgical association meetings
University-sponsored postgraduate courses
Skills/Technology acquisition courses (with or without commercial funding)
       University-based (e.g., sentinel node biopsy)
       Professional society-based (e.g., ultrasound)
       Industry-sponsored (e.g., advanced laparoscopy)

skill—i.e., know how the new information will be put to use.

- **Practice:**   The student must have the opportunity not only to read and hear about what is to be learned but also to apply or practice the new behavior in an appropriate simulation context or environment, both to gain familiarity with it and to gain insight into it.
- **Application and feedback:**   Finally, the student must apply the new behavior or practice promptly on a regular basis and there must be timely evaluation or feedback through data collection and analysis of outcomes on the success or failure of the new behavior.

For an individual, the phases of learning that bring about behavior change may be summarized as awareness, agreement, adoption, and adherence (5).

- **Awareness:**   Individuals become aware of new ideas through reading, searching Internet sites, attending meetings, discussing matters with colleagues, and confronting clinical dilemmas on a daily basis.
- **Agreement:**   Individuals must intellectually agree that new information is appropriate and worthwhile. Sometimes new and important information is not

accepted rapidly, particularly when it calls for a change in behavior. New pain-management approaches and techniques have been available for over a decade, but surgeons are only now slowly accepting them.

- **Adoption:**   Having agreed that new information is valid, individuals must decide to adopt that information into their practices. Adopting a new idea might require making changes in day-to-day practices and in the related practices of those around them.
- **Adherence:**   The cycle of learning is complete when individuals regularly apply the changes in practice, examine the outcomes over time, and make modifications to improve practice.

Table 4-2 displays four types of continuing education activity in the form of a continuum, the level of personal engagement required for each, how each relates to the general prerequisites for adult learning and to the individual phases of learning outlined above, and some of the advantages and disadvantages of each. The types of CME activity may be summarized as follows:

- **General information:**   A surgeon's intrinsic motivation to increase knowledge leads to scanning journals

TABLE 4-2
TYPES OF CME ACTIVITIES AND THEIR CHARACTERISTICS

Type of Activity	Level of Engagement	General Prerequisites for Learning	Phases of Individual Learning	Advantages and Limitations

General Awareness
General reading
Informal discussion
Listening at conference
Viewing a video
	Passive learning
	Unfocused
		Motivation	Awareness	Broad content covered
				Introduces
				  unknown issues
				Limited expense
				Limited likelihood
				  of producing
				  change by itself

Answering Questions
Consultation with colleague
Literature search
Problem-based learning
  activities
Interaction with others
	Active learning
	More focused
		Motivation
		Objective
			Awareness
			Agreement
				Focus on practical
				  issues
				Must be aware
				  of issue
				Limited expense
				Somewhat likely
				  to produce change

Skill Training
Preparation and interaction
Role playing or simulation
Skill practice/demonstration
Testing/evaluation
	Interactive learning
	Skill acquisition
	  course
		Motivation
		Objective
		Practice
			Awareness
			Agreement
			Adoption
				Focus on priority
				  skills
				Often meaningful
				  direct or
				  indirect expense
				Likely to produce
				  specific change

Performance Review
Regular data collection,
  analysis, and evaluation
Regular feedback regarding
  performance or outcome
Prompt application of change
  or skill into daily practice
  with feedback
	Participation in
	  research or
	  clinical trial
	Organized change
	  initiative
		Motivation
		Objective
		Practice
		Application and
		  feedback
			Awareness
			Agreement
			Adoption
			Adherence
				Focus on specific
				  activities
				Often requires
				  supporting
				  infrastructure and
				  related expense
				Very likely to
				  produce specific
				  change

and attending weekly lectures, annual update programs, and general review courses. These passive activities are important in providing an awareness of new knowledge but are the least likely to bring insight into current problems or by themselves induce change in behavior.

- **Answering questions:** Settings that demand active participation, presentation, discussion, or argument help the surgeon determine the usefulness of new information and to decide whether to accept it. Active participation includes directed reading or a literature search designed to answer specific questions.

- **Skill training:** Having a specific goal and participating in a course that offers a setting for learning and practice under expert monitoring and assistance provide excellent in-depth learning, including practice and adoption of new skills. Highly successful postgraduate courses, such as the American College of Surgeons Advanced Trauma Life Support course, embody these characteristics of active learning and participation by motivated participants. Courses that teach new surgical techniques, such as laparoscopic and robotic surgery, are also common.

- **Performance review:** Reviews of practice through morbidity and mortality conferences, examination of complication rates, personal databases, or case logs that record outcomes, and other methods of feedback help assure ongoing improvement in practice.

An organized plan for continuing education and professional development must have a balance across the various types of CME activities. Time, location, and practicality demand that much CME time will be devoted to broad, information-gathering activities, such as scanning for new information in discussions, reading, conferences, and regular meetings. In so doing, one continuously gathers information that is potentially applicable to all aspects of one's surgical practice. This will help motivate in-depth study of a few areas each year. Skill acquisition courses, although highly effective, are expensive, time consuming, and resource intensive. They should be carefully selected to fill in known gaps or to improve clinical practice in which a scan of the environment suggests it is deficient. Only a limited amount of time and resources can be devoted to these, and they should therefore fit carefully into one's overall plan for professional development. Ordinarily, one can only learn, adopt, implement, and evaluate new skills one at a time. Ideally, at the end of each year one should be able to record the things that have been learned that have improved clinical practices and patient care.

PREPARING FOR RECERTIFICATION AND RECREDENTIALING REQUIREMENTS

All surgeons certified by the American Board of Surgery (ABS) after 1976 must recertify every 10 years to maintain their certification. At present, recertification requires passing a written multiple-choice test of factual knowledge. The content for this examination can be found primarily in standard textbooks and recent surgical literature. The American College of Surgeons offers a similar, voluntary knowledge test, called Surgical Education and Self-Assessment Program (SESAP), to help surgeons maintain this knowledge base. The SESAP is offered as an educational program to help surgeons maintain current knowledge in clinical surgery and is promoted as a study guide for the ABS certification and recertification exams (6). Prerequisites for eligibility to take a recertifying examination are 100 hours of CME (at least 60 hours category 1 credit) in the two years prior to the examination. Completion of SESAP provides 60 hours category 1 credit.

The recertification process has not yet required demonstration of clinical competence or skill beyond this written examination. No secure, reliable means currently exists for gathering national data about actual practices or outcomes for uniform assessment of competence or skill acquisition, or both (7). However, in the future, recertification is expected to include some aspect of demonstration of clinical competence. The public demand for more evidence of competence in practice is inspiring appreciable professional effort toward the exploration and development of methods to demonstrate competence.

The American Board of Medical Specialties (ABMS) in 1999 adopted a new description of the "competent physician." The general competencies defined by the ABMS are

- medical knowledge
- patient care
- interpersonal and communication skills
- professionalism
- practice-based learning and improvement
- systems-based practice.

As a functional complement to this new definition, the ABMS adopted in September 2002 a new program for "maintenance of certification" (8). The four components of this program are

- evidence of professional standing
- evidence of commitment to life-long learning and involvement in periodic self-assessment
- evidence of cognitive expertise
- evidence of evaluation of performance in practice.

In addition to the current requirements for evidence of CME and of successful completion of a test of practice-related knowledge, the ABMS will require that the applicant hold an unrestricted license to practice and demonstrate evidence of having participated in performance evaluation and self-assessment. Physicians will be asked to demonstrate "that they can assess the quality of care they provide compared to peers and national benchmarks and then apply the best evidence or consensus recommendations to improve that care using follow-up assessments" (9). The ABMS anticipates a several-year transition as individual certifying boards and specialty societies develop resources that will enable physicians to demonstrate these competencies.

The American College of Surgeons recently announced plans to develop an Internet-based "practice-based learning and improvement" website (10). The site will help surgeons develop a personal learning portfolio that links personal practice data to that of others. Comparing personal data with others' data is expected to provide helpful feedback to surgeons regarding their performance. The Society of American Gastrointestinal Endoscopic Surgeons (SAGES) has developed a similar program for surgical activity and outcomes reporting (11).

INDUSTRY, ETHICS, AND CME

The availability of industry-sponsored CME opportunities and the inducements to participate in such activities might make it difficult for physicians to avoid crossing the threshold of ethical behavior. The offering of gifts and inducements to modify behavior is an ancient and powerful tool for influencing others. Surgeons should seek the information and training that will best serve their patients. Subsidies and inducements can cause a surgeon to choose a convenient CME activity instead of one with more important content. If a surgeon accepts a free trip to learn to use a piece of equipment or learn a new technique, that surgeon will feel a sense of obligation to a person or company.

In the pursuit of new skills, surgeons must be cognizant of potential ethical issues and conflicts of interest. Advances in surgical technique require acquisition of new equipment and learning new technical skills. Cooperation with sales representatives and manufacturers *after* purchasing decisions have been made is essential for learning how to use new tools and equipment safely. Purchase agreements might include the cost of such training. It is inappropriate, however, to accept direct personal benefits, such as money, food, or lodging, provided by salespersons or device manufacturers as part of CME programs that are primarily designed to encourage surgeons to purchase or use their equipment. Such participation is unethical because the inducements of personal benefits to the surgeon conflict with the surgeon's impartiality in selecting learning activities and equipment that best meet the needs of patients.

A professional relationship between medical professionals and commercial representatives that avoids accepting gifts, inducements, product endorsements, or other forms of commercial co-option can and must be maintained at all times. This does not inhibit manufacturers from advertising or sponsoring educational activities. They may ethically sponsor CME programs that are voluntary and open to all, do not bias program content, and contain no individual inducements. In 2003, commercial sources provided 65% of the financial revenue for the 697 national providers of CME accredited by ACCME (12). To help surgeons avoid unethical behavior in pursuit of new skills and techniques, the American College of Surgeons has promulgated standards for advanced courses in new technologies and also guidelines for collaboration of industry and surgical organizations in support of research and continuing education (13,14).

CONCLUSION AND RECOMMENDATIONS: A BALANCED PORTFOLIO OF CME

To keep abreast of new knowledge, to acquire new skills, and to avoid becoming obsolete, every surgeon should have a plan for life-long learning and professional development using principles of effective adult education and behavior change. This will require an investment of time and effort and involve a mixture of active and passive learning experiences. As with any investment, an organized plan and a balanced portfolio of CME and professional development activities will pay more dividends than a random one.

An organized plan should include a balance across types of learning activities that include

- general information awareness
- answering questions
- skill training
- performance review.

Scanning for new information includes reading a selection of medical and surgical journals regularly. In a teaching environment, a "journal club" stimulates regular reading. It is important to have a group of professional surgical colleagues with whom to interact on a regular basis to exchange ideas and information. Local and regional surgical societies and specialty societies serve this purpose. One should take advantage of CME offerings sponsored by professional societies and academic centers, which are more likely than industry-sponsored events to be free of bias, and regularly choose some topics identified by this kind of scanning activity for in-depth study on the basis of self-evaluation and on goals that are both personal and institutional. One should choose focused courses that fill a gap in knowledge, give needed information, engage participants in active learning experiences, and impart information and skills that have immediate practical application.

Whenever possible, one should try to introduce new technologic applications in conjunction with colleagues and have a plan to evaluate the outcomes of the changes that have been made. This is always the most difficult yet most critically important component of the improvement cycle. Errors and complications persist in clinical practice when surgeons are unwilling to record and confront their actual outcomes and hold them up against relevant benchmarks. In the future recredentialing and recertification requirements might make this kind of examination of personal performance mandatory. Professional societies are developing new learning tools and Internet-based programs by which they hope to facilitate this process. Maintaining a learning program that combines both previously available and emerging types of educational activities will help surgeons continue to provide high-quality care as cognitive requirements, skills, and standards of care evolve throughout their careers.

REFERENCES

1. *ACCME glossary of terms and abbreviations.* Chicago, IL: Accreditation Council on Continuing Medical Education; 2000. Available at www.accme.org/sec_docs_f.asp.
2. The American College of Surgeons. Code of professional conduct. *J. Am. Coll. Surg* 2003;197(4):603–604.
3. Rosof AB, Felch WC, eds. *Continuing medical education: a primer,* 2nd ed. Westport, CT: Praeger; 1992.
4. Mann DV, Gelula MH. How to facilitate self-directed learning. In: Davis D, Barnes BE, Fox R, eds. *The continuing professional development of physicians: from research to practice.* Chicago, IL: American Medical Association Press; 2003.
5. Pathman DE, Konrad TR, Freed GL, et al. The awareness-to-adherence model of the steps to clinical guideline compliance: the case of pediatric vaccine recommendations. *Med Care* 1996; 34(9):873–889.
6. *Surgical education and self-assessment program.* Chicago, IL: American College of Surgeons; 2003. Available at www.facs.org/fellows_info/sesap/sesap.html.
7. Landon BE, Normand ST, Blumenthal DM, et al. Physician clinical performance assessment: prospects and barriers. *JAMA* 2003;290(9):1183–1189.

8. *Principles for transitioning from recertification to maintenance of certification.* Chicago, IL: American Board of Medical Specialties; 2002. Available at www.abms.org/MOC.asp.

9. *Evaluating practice performance for MOC.* Chicago, IL: American Board of Medical Specialties; 2002. Available at www.abms.org/MOC.asp.

10. Sachdeva AK. Acquisition and maintenance of surgical competence. *Semin Vasc Surg* 2002;15(3):182–190.

11. *SAGES online outcome initiative.* Los Angeles, CA: Society of American Gastrointestinal Endoscopic Surgeons; 1999. Available at www.sages.org/outcomes.html.

12. *ACCME annual report data.* Chicago, IL: Accreditation Council for Continuing Medical Education; 2004. Available at www.accme.org.

13. American College of Surgeons. Standards for advanced courses in new technologies. *Bull Am Coll Surg* 1998;83:36.

14. Committee on Ethics, American College of Surgeons. Guidelines for collaboration of industry and surgical organizations in support of research and continuing education. *Bull Am Coll Surg* 2001;86:30–31.

Surgical Credentials

5

Mary E. Klingensmith

■ INTRODUCTION 25

■ BOARD CERTIFICATION 25

■ STEPS LEADING TO BOARD CERTIFICATION 26
Prerequisites 26
The Examination Process 26

■ RECERTIFICATION 26

■ FAILURE TO PASS BOARD EXAMINATIONS 26
Qualifying Examination 26
Certifying Examination 27

■ CANADIAN AND INTERNATIONAL TRAINEES 27

■ SUBSPECIALTY CERTIFICATION 27

■ HOSPITAL PRIVILEGING 27

■ HOSPITAL CREDENTIALS COMMITTEES 28

■ APPLYING FOR PRIVILEGES 28

■ RECREDENTIALING 28

■ DENIAL OF PRIVILEGES 28

■ MAINTENANCE OF CERTIFICATION 29
MOC Time Line 29

■ REFERENCES 29

Mary E. Klingensmith: Washington University School of Medicine, Saint Louis, MO 63110

INTRODUCTION

The processes leading to Board certification and hospital credentialing are often confusing to surgical trainees or those new to the American health care system. This chapter will seek to outline these two areas, pointing out where they overlap and how they relate to the requirements for residency training in surgery. Evolving issues in credentialing and the certification process will also be discussed with regard to the maintenance of certification initiative.

BOARD CERTIFICATION

The American Board of Surgery (ABS) is a member of the American Board of Medical Specialties (ABMS). The ABMS is the umbrella organization for 24 medical specialty boards. In early 2003, more than 85% of all licensed physicians in the United States were certified by at least one ABMS member board (1). Thus, board certification status is clearly recognized as a critical component of the professional dossier of all physicians in the United States, surgeons included.

The ABS was founded in 1937 as a private, voluntary, nonprofit organization with three primary purposes:

1. To conduct examinations of acceptable candidates who seek certification or recertification by the Board;
2. To issue certificates to all candidates meeting the Board's requirements and satisfactorily completing its prescribed examinations;
3. To improve and broaden the opportunities for graduate education and training of surgeons (2).

According to ABS definitions, the term "general surgery" is comprehensively yet specifically defined as "a discipline having a central core of knowledge embracing anatomy, physiology, metabolism, immunology, nutrition, pathology, wound healing, shock and resuscitation, intensive care and neoplasia, which are common to all surgical specialties…(as defined this way), a General Surgeon…has, during their training, acquired knowledge and experience related to the diagnosis, preoperative, operative, and postoperative management, including the management of complications…(in the following) essential content areas…"(2):

1. Alimentary Tract
2. Abdomen and Its Contents
3. Breast, Skin, and Soft Tissue
4. Endocrine System
5. Head and Neck Surgery
6. Pediatric Surgery
7. Surgical Critical Care
8. Surgical Oncology
9. Trauma/Burns
10. Vascular Surgery.

To be admitted to the Board certification process, the program director must endorse a candidate's application, adding a statement that attests to an applicant's appropriate educational experience in the above areas and that signifies the applicant has the judgment, knowledge, and skills to be considered for Board certified status.

STEPS LEADING TO BOARD CERTIFICATION

Prerequisites

Candidates for Board certification must have completed training in an accredited general surgery residency program. Accredited programs must meet standards set forth by the Accreditation Council for Graduate Medical Education (ACGME). Within the ACGME, each specialty has its own Residency Review Committee (RRC). Individual RRCs collaborate with the specialty board (i.e., ABS) to determine the components that shall be deemed essential for a program to be accredited. Accredited programs produce graduates that are potentially Board eligible.

As part of a process overseen by both the ABS and RRC, a minimum number of cases in each of the essential content areas listed above is determined for Board examination admissibility. Residents must keep track of the operations they perform during training, as they count toward these minimum numbers. Upon completion of training, these case logs must be submitted to the ABS as part of the initial application for Board examination. This application also includes areas in which the trainee must list the rotation schedules for the 5 years of general surgery training to demonstrate that the trainee has acquired adequate experience in each of the essential content areas.

Other requirements for certification in surgery include "satisfactory moral and ethical standing," active practice in surgery with admitting privileges in an accredited health care organization (or currently in pursuit of additional graduate education in surgery or a surgical subspecialty), and permanent licensure to practice medicine in a state or jurisdiction of the United States or Canada. All of these prerequisite components are represented on the initial application for Board certification.

The Examination Process

After the ABS has accepted the initial application, the applicant is eligible for the examination process. This has two parts. A written examination (called the *Qualifying Examination*) is given in October of the year following completion of training. If the candidate passes this exam, an oral exam (the *Certifying Examination*) follows. This exam is given in several cities around the United States, with examinees directed to the nearest test site; exam dates vary from January to October of the year following the written exam. If the examinee passes the oral exam, a certificate signifying Board Certification in Surgery and designating the examinee as a diplomat of the ABS is issued.

[A more thorough review of this information is available on the ABS website (www.absurgery.org), which is updated annually. Readers are encouraged to access this information frequently during surgical training to stay abreast of any changes in Board examination admissibility requirements that might occur.]

RECERTIFICATION

The certificate issued by the Board is valid for up to 10 years. In order to maintain certification, a recertification exam is required. This exam can be taken as early as 7 years following certificate issuance but no later than 10. According to the ABS, "The purpose of Recertification is to demonstrate to the profession and the public, through periodic evaluations, that the surgical specialist has maintained continuing qualifications on a currently acceptable level in the Diplomat's chosen area of practice. The ABS believes that such periodic evaluation of its Diplomats is in their own interest as well as in the public interest"(3). The recertification process is being expanded in scope, to "maintenance of certification"; see the final section of this chapter for more information.

FAILURE TO PASS BOARD EXAMINATIONS

Qualifying Examination

Applicants have five opportunities to take the qualifying examination within a 5-year period following approval of the initial application. Applicants who are unable to pass the exam after these five attempts or who fail to apply to take the examination within 3 years of completing residency training are allowed eligibility only if they complete a defined "readmissibility pathway."

The ABS recently expanded the readmissibility process to include two options. In the first, candidates must complete a "Structured Year" in an ACGME-approved residency program, which is essentially an additional year of training designed by the residency program and approved in advance by the ABS. The second, alternate pathway recently created by the ABS involves a three-step educational process. First, candidates must complete the most recent version of the American College of Surgeons Surgical Education and Self-Assessment Program (SESAP). Second, candidates must take a 100-question examination derived from the clinical management section of the In-Training/Surgical Basic Science Examination and achieve a minimum score predetermined by the ABS. Finally, a 200-question examination derived from the latest two versions of SESAP must be taken, and examinees must also score above a predetermined minimum. Once either of these two pathways is completed, the applicant must apply for readmission and supply operative logs, letters of reference from hospitals in which the applicant currently practices, and documentation of 100 hours of continuing medical education (CME) activity.

Certifying Examination

Candidates have five opportunities to take the certifying examination in the 5 years following successful completion of the qualifying examination (this was recently increased from three attempts in 5 years). If the applicant is unsuccessful in passing the certifying examination, an additional year of training (the "Structured Year," as described above) is required to gain readmission.

[This information is covered in greater depth on the ABS website (www.absurgery.org), *which is updated annually. Readers are encouraged to access this information frequently to stay abreast of changes that might occur in the readmission criteria.]*

CANADIAN AND INTERNATIONAL TRAINEES

Applicants who have trained in Canada in university residency programs in surgery, which are accredited by the Royal College of Physicians and Surgeons, are deemed eligible for Board exam admissibility. The other Board requirements (noted above in the "Prerequisites" section) must also be met.

Applicants from abroad are not granted credit for their training or practice experiences directly, no matter how accomplished. On a case-by-case basis, the ABS will consider granting partial credit for training abroad only upon the request of a program director of an accredited residency program in the United States. This program director must have observed the applicant as a junior resident for 9 to 12 months and desire to advance the applicant to a higher level in that program. This credit is not transferable to another program and is not granted until the applicant successfully completes the accredited residency-training program. Applicants from Canadian programs must have completed all of their training in Canada and will not be admitted to the Board certification process if some of that training was in countries outside of the United States or Canada. Thus, all international applicants must spend at least some portion of their professional training in a US residency program in order to be Board eligible.

SUBSPECIALTY CERTIFICATION

The ABS also sponsors specialty certifications in the areas of vascular surgery, pediatric surgery, surgery of the hand, and surgical critical care. For subspecialty certification in these areas, applicants must also hold certification in general surgery. The American Board of Colon and Rectal Surgery (www.abcrs.org) and the American Board of Thoracic Surgery (www.abts.org) sponsor subspecialty certification in their respective areas. The certifying examinations in these subspecialties are taken after fellowship training. Currently, there is no separate certification board for transplant surgery, gastrointestinal surgery, oncologic surgery, or minimally invasive surgery, although fellowship programs in these areas offer certificates at the completion of such additional training. These certificates signify that the bearer has completed training in the subspecialty area. Oversight of these programs is done by individual societies whose membership determines the program requirements; the degree of oversight can vary widely among the specialties.

HOSPITAL PRIVILEGING

The provision of the rights to individual surgeons to admit and treat patients is determined on a local level by individual hospitals or health-care organizations. To be eligible for the credentialing process, applicants must show either Board certification (or eligibility)—which is required by the vast majority of hospitals—or evidence of residency training or practice experience in the area for which the applicant desires privileges. It is unusual for academic medical centers to grant clinical privileges to surgeons who are not Board certified. Conversely, some hospitals in areas of the United States with large populations of underserved patients do occasionally grant privileges without the requirement for Board certification if all other requirements are met.

Before the credentialing process can begin, applicants must possess an unrestricted state medical license, federal and state Drug Enforcement Administration (DEA) numbers, and various identifying numbers needed for charge reimbursement: Medicare/Medicaid provider numbers, UPINs (unique provider identification numbers), and federal and state tax identification numbers. The hospital credentialing committee can usually supply the list of requirements and provide applications to secure these various items. Most hospitals also require applicants to simultaneously complete paperwork for the various insurance companies and HMOs (health maintenance organizations) in their area to insure reimbursement for services once practice begins.

HOSPITAL CREDENTIALS COMMITTEES

Hospitals determine the criteria for credentialing in the various practice areas. Typically, several surgeons from different disciplines serve on a surgical credentialing committee, which is chaired by the hospital's chief of surgery. This individual is ultimately responsible for determining that an applicant has met the criteria set by the committee and possesses the knowledge, judgment, and skills necessary to perform the requested clinical activities.

The Joint Council on Accreditation of Healthcare Organizations (JCAHO) outlines the process for credentialing and delineation of clinical privileges this way: "the credentialing process includes a series of activities designed to collect relevant data that will serve as the basis for decisions regarding…delineation of clinical privileges for individual members of the medical staff…the required information should include data on qualifications such as licensure and training experience [and] data on actual performance that [are] collected and assessed initially and in an ongoing process" (4).

Uniform standards exist for privileges in various areas. These are often sponsored by specialty societies. For instance, in the field of minimally invasive surgery, the Society of American Gastrointestinal Endoscopic Surgeons (SAGES) has a credentials committee that updates and expands the suggested criteria for privileges in various areas of minimally invasive surgery as a resource for hospital credentialing committees (www.sages.org).

APPLYING FOR PRIVILEGES

Individuals applying for privileges must submit information requested by the hospital committee. Typically, this includes documentation of training and experience in the relevant areas, including case lists and a summary letter from the residency program director attesting to the accuracy of the list and to the applicant's ability. Other information, such as education, licensure information, and proof of Board certification, are also required.

The applicant must also make specific requests for privileges in a given area. For instance, permission to perform

vascular procedures or minimally invasive abdominal procedures must be specifically requested and granted before the applicant may perform such operations. Obviously, the applicant should be able to demonstrate adequate training in the areas of practice requested. Often, such requests are facilitated by an application checklist format, in which procedures of various types are grouped together to facilitate a surgeon's request for privileges, say, in vascular surgery, that would encompass a typical practice in that area.

If an applicant does not have experience in an area for which privileges are requested, options are available to provide preliminary or provisionary privileges. Such a situation might arise for procedures developed after an individual completed formal residency training (as occurred with a large number of practicing surgeons with the advent of laparoscopic cholecystectomy in the late 1980s and early 1990s). In the absence of formal residency training in the procedure, documentation of attendance of a didactic course dedicated to the procedure that includes hands-on instruction (in animal or cadaver lab or live operating room) plus planned proctor/mentor experience might be sufficient for preliminary privileging. Some credentialing bodies accept practical experience as a first assistant in such procedures, with documentation from a mentor or preceptor required. It is important to be aware of the requirements of individual credentialing committees to ensure the best chance that privileges will be granted.

Although it's not always a requirement of an individual hospital, the surgeon requesting privileges in a given area should consider carefully institutional support for programmatic procedures. This support has proven to be especially important in the area of bariatric surgery, in which multidisciplinary care of the patient has been associated with improved patient outcome (5).

RECREDENTIALING

Some hospitals will grant preliminary privileges to surgeons during the first year, with a request for reapplication after 1 year. Increasingly, at the time of reapplication, surgeons are being asked to provide information regarding the outcome of their work as evidence to support the granting of full privileges.

The recredentialing process is thereafter an annual or a biannual event. Most hospitals also require CME credits in the area of practice and expertise to demonstrate continued efforts at practice improvement.

DENIAL OF PRIVILEGES

Individuals applying for privileges in a given area should be certain they possess the qualifications for work in that area. If privileges are denied, the appeals process outlined by the hospital credentials committee should be followed. However, applicants should be aware that if a formal denial of privileges is returned, such information is reported to the National Practitioner Databank and kept as part of that practitioner's permanent file.

MAINTENANCE OF CERTIFICATION

The ABMS is leading an effort termed the Maintenance of Certification © (MOC) program, an initiative that has been several years in the making. The process has evolved as the member boards of the ABMS have collectively agreed that the "snapshot" evaluation of physicians that is available through the current system of certification and recertification does not capture a physician's true competency and efforts at practice assessment and improvement. When fully integrated, the MOC process will encompass recertification.

MOC has four primary components (6):

1. Evidence of professional standing
2. Evidence of a commitment to life-long learning and involvement in periodic self-assessment processes
3. Evidence of cognitive expertise
4. Evidence of evaluation of performance in practice.

The evaluation process of physician practice performance (item 4) is based on the six competency areas recently defined by the ACGME for residency training (medical knowledge, patient care, interpersonal and communication skills, professionalism, practice-based learning and improvement, and systems-based practice). Eventually, evaluation based on the six competency areas will be a seamless process that begins in residency training and continues throughout a surgeon's career.

The portion of MOC involving critical self-assessment and improvement is central to the effort. According to the ABMS, this approach is preferable to regulatory inspections and will also provide more meaningful data than traditional health outcomes studies, which are limited in their power to discriminate true physician performance because of the limited case numbers an individual might have and the wide variability in patient populations (6).

MOC Time Line

The ABMS assembly adopted the basic premise for MOC in March 2000. Since then assessment implementation guidelines for the four component areas were formulated (March 2002). MOC will be initiated with consideration of the first three content areas: professional standing, lifelong learning and self-assessment, and cognitive expertise. Each of the 24 member boards of the ABMS was required to submit final plans for incorporation of these three areas by July 1, 2003. Evaluation of physician practice performance was scheduled for inclusion by December 31, 2004, with rollout of the fully described MOC slated to begin shortly thereafter (6).

Although this process is a paradigm shift for many of the ABMS member boards, the end product, when realized, will be of great benefit: "...It will help to reduce medical errors and enhance the quality of care provided by physicians, and lead to better patient healthcare outcomes" (6).

REFERENCES

1. ABMS website. Available at: www.abms.org. Accessed on November 7, 2003.
2. The American Board of Surgery. Booklet of Information, July 2003–June 2004. Available at: www.absurgery.org. Accessed on November 10, 2003, 10.
3. The American Board of Surgery. Booklet of Information, July 2003–June 2004. Available at: www.absurgery.org. Accessed on November 10, 2003, 25.
4. Joint Commission on Accreditation of Health Care Organizations (JCAHO). The credentialing process. *CAMH: Comprehensive accreditation manual for hospitals.* Oakbrook Terrace, IL: JCAHO; 2000:MS5-7.
5. American College of Surgeons. Recommendations for facilities performing bariatric surgery. *Bull Am Coll Surg* 2000; 85(9):20–23.
6. ABMS website. Available at: www.abms.org. Accessed on November 17, 2003.

Assessing Surgical Quality with Structure and Process of Care Measures

John D. Birkmeyer

■■■■ INTRODUCTION 30

■■■■ EVIDENCE LINKING STRUCTURE OF CARE TO
SURGICAL OUTCOMES 31
Hospital-level Variables 31
Surgeon-level Variables 33
The Relative Importance of Hospital and Surgeon
Factors 35

■■■■ EVIDENCE LINKING PROCESS OF CARE TO
SURGICAL OUTCOMES 35

■■■■ STRUCTURE AND PROCESS MEASURES AS
QUALITY INDICATORS: POLICY
CONSIDERATIONS 39

■■■■ IMPROVING THE QUALITY OF QUALITY
MEASUREMENT 42

■■■■ REFERENCES 43

INTRODUCTION

At least 20,000 patients die every year in the United States while undergoing elective surgery (1). A much larger number of patients experiences other complications. Efforts to reduce surgical morbidity and mortality can take two basic tacks. First, surgical patients can be directed toward hospitals or surgeons likely to have the best results—so-called evidence-based referral. For example, the Leapfrog Group, a large coalition of public and private purchasers, is using a variety of incentives to concentrate certain surgical procedures in selected hospitals (2). Second, efforts can be made to improve the quality of surgical care at all hospitals. With this goal in mind, for example, the National Surgical Quality Improvement Program (NSQIP) has been tracking surgical morbidity and mortality rates for all hospitals of the Department of Veterans Affairs (3). Although evidence-based referral and quality improvement strategies differ in many important respects, the success of both strategies depends on reliable, provider-specific measures of surgical quality.

The most direct measures of surgical quality are risk-adjusted morbidity and mortality rates. Numerous regional and national quality improvement programs have demonstrated the feasibility of tracking such measures for

John D. Birkmeyer: University of Michigan, Ann Arbor, MI 48109

hospitals performing coronary artery bypass grafting (CABG) (4,5). For other procedures, however, the value of measuring procedure-specific morbidity and mortality rates for individual hospitals is less clear, primarily due to sample-size limitations. Unless a procedure is both common and associated with a relatively high complication rate, it is impossible to determine whether observed differences in performance among hospitals reflect random variation or real differences in quality. With the notable exception of CABG, few procedures meet both criteria. Of course, sample size and thus precision can be improved if morbidity and mortality rates are assessed after aggregating all major surgical procedures performed in a given hospital—the approach taken by NSQIP. However, performance measures that are not procedure-specific are considerably less useful for either evidence-based referral or targeting quality improvement efforts.

For this reason, it is important to consider surgical quality in two other domains: structure and process (6). Structural measures, the most prominent of which is procedure volume, include a very broad group of variables that reflect the setting in which care is delivered. Process measures, which reflect the particulars of care that patients actually receive (e.g., use of perioperative β-blockers), have long served as quality indicators in other specialties and might be equally useful in surgery (7). In this chapter the evidence linking structure and process measures to surgical outcomes is reviewed. Policy implications of using structure and process measures to reflect surgical quality are then considered.

EVIDENCE LINKING STRUCTURE OF CARE TO SURGICAL OUTCOMES

Structural measures include a broad list of variables reflecting the setting or system in which care is delivered. Many of these variables are best considered at the hospital level, reflecting, directly or indirectly, its physical plant and resources or staff coordination and organization. Other structural variables describe attributes associated with the relative expertise of individual physicians.

Hospital-level Variables

Volume

Procedure volume—the frequency with which a given procedure is performed by the surgeon or hospital—is by far the most recognizable structural variable. A considerable body of evidence has accrued linking volume to surgical outcomes, particularly operative mortality. In one of the earliest studies, Lee et al. reviewed mortality rates with appendectomy, peptic ulcer surgery, and prostatectomy in England and Wales between 1951 and 1954 (8). Mortality rates in patients undergoing these procedures at small

hospitals were approximately double those observed at larger, teaching hospitals. In a seminal study done more than 20 years later, Luft et al. documented the importance of hospital procedural volume and became among the first to advocate regionalization of high-risk procedures (9). Subsequent population-based studies by Flood et al. confirmed that procedural volume was a more important determinant of surgical mortality rates than teaching status or other correlated hospital characteristics (10,11).

Over the past 20 years, hundreds of articles have examined the relative importance of hospital volume with different procedures. Recently, two structured literature reviews have synthesized this large body of work (12,13), each supporting the premise that high-volume hospitals have substantially lower mortality rates with many surgical procedures. Dudley et al. performed a systematic literature search to identify all studies published between 1988 and 1998 examining correlations between hospital volume and mortality for numerous surgical and medical conditions (13). After applying several additional methodologic criteria, the authors identified 72 articles addressing 40 different procedures and diagnoses. Because some articles examined more than one procedure/diagnosis, a total of 127 unique volume–outcome analyses were represented in these studies. The large majority of studies suggested better outcomes at high-volume hospitals (Table 6-1). Of the 127 analyses, 123 (96%) noted lower mortality at high-volume hospitals (80% statistically significant). Only four (3%) found higher mortality rates at high-volume hospitals, but none of these findings were statistically significant. For each procedure/diagnosis, Dudley et al. identified the single highest quality study on the basis of explicit criteria. Factors considered included quality of case mix adjustment, sample size and number of hospitals included, data currency, and other variables. On the basis of findings from the single best studies, mortality was found to be significantly lower at high-volume hospitals for elective abdominal aortic aneurysm (AAA) repair, lower extremity bypass, CABG, coronary angioplasty, heart transplantation, pediatric cardiac surgery, pancreatic cancer surgery, esophageal cancer surgery, and cerebral aneurysm surgery.

A second structured literature review was performed by Halm et al., in a report commissioned by the Institute of Medicine (12). The authors identified all volume–outcome studies for five procedure groups: CABG, pediatric cardiac surgery, carotid endarterectomy, AAA repair, and cancer surgery. Of the 88 studies identified, 77% found statistically significant associations between higher volume and better outcomes. The remaining 23% did not, but no study demonstrated statistically significant associations in the opposite direction. The authors described wide variation in the methodologic quality of volume–outcome studies and noted the predominance of studies based on administrative data (with attendant concerns about the adequacy of risk adjustment). However, the 16 studies with the highest quality scores in the Halm review—each using clinical data

TABLE 6-1

SUMMARY OF FINDINGS OF VOLUME–OUTCOME STUDIES IN STRUCTURED LITERATURE REVIEW

		Number of Studies			
Procedure	Total	High Volume SS Better	NS Trend Toward High Volume Better	NS Trend Toward High Volume Worse	High Volume SS Worse
CABG	11	9	2	0	0
Coronary angioplasty	6	6	0	0	0
Elective AAA repair	9	9	0	0	0
Carotid endarterectomy	9	6	3	0	0
Pancreatic resection	8	8	0	0	0
Esophagectomy	2	2	0	0	0
All others	82	62	16	4	0
Overall	**127**	**102**	**21**	**4**	**0**

SS, statistically significant; NS, nonsignificant; CABG, coronary artery bypass grafting; AAA, abdominal aortic aneurysm.
From Dudley RA, Johansen KL, Brand R, et al. Selective referral to high volume hospitals: Estimating potentially avoidable deaths. *JAMA* 2000;283:1159–1166, with permission.

for risk adjustment—all demonstrated statistically significant lower mortality rates at high-volume hospitals.

Although the conclusions of these two reviews are consistent and compelling, many of the volume–outcome studies on which they are based are either outdated or restricted to specific states or regions that might not be broadly representative. To provide a national view of the relative importance of hospital volume with different procedures, Birkmeyer et al. examined operative mortality in 2.5 million Medicare patients undergoing one of 14 different cancer or cardiovascular procedures (14). To categorize volume with each procedure, hospitals were ranked in order of increasing total hospital volume (average procedures per year), and then five volume groups were defined by selecting whole number annual volume cutpoints that most closely sorted patients into five evenly sized groups: Very Low, Low, Medium, High, and Very High. Regression techniques were then used to describe relationships between hospital volume and mortality (in-hospital or within 30 days), adjusting for patient characteristics.

Hospital volume was related to both observed and adjusted operative mortality rates for all 14 procedures ($p < 0.001$). The importance of hospital volume varied markedly by procedure (Fig. 6-1). For example, with pancreatic resection, adjusted mortality rates at very-low-volume hospitals were 12.5% higher (in absolute terms) than at very-high-volume hospitals (16.3% vs. 3.8%, respectively). Relatively large risk differences were also observed for esophagectomy (11.9%) and pneumonectomy (5.4%). Absolute differences in adjusted mortality rates between very-low- and very-high-volume hospitals were between 2% and 5% for gastrectomy, cystectomy, (nonruptured) abdominal aneurysm repair, and aortic and mitral valve replacement and <2% for CABG, lower extremity bypass, colectomy, lobectomy, nephrectomy, and carotid endarterectomy.

In that study, the nature of the volume–outcome "curve" also varied widely by procedure. For several procedures (including CABG, valve replacement, and pancreatic resection), mortality declined monotonically with each stratum of increasing hospital volume. For others (including elective AAA repair, gastrectomy, and pneumonectomy), mortality differences were most apparent at volume extremes, whereas hospitals in intermediate volume strata had similar mortality rates.

Although most volume–outcome studies have focused primarily on operative mortality, volume has also been linked to other outcomes, including risks of nonfatal complications. For example, studies have reported that higher-volume hospitals (or surgeons) have lower rates of late urinary stricture after radical prostatectomy, nonfatal complications after total hip replacement, and stroke after carotid endarterectomy (15–17). Hospital volume also seems to be related to improved long-term survival after cancer surgery. Recent studies, most relying on the Medicare-SEER linked databases, have demonstrated that patients receiving care at high-volume hospitals have better late survival after cancer surgery than patients at lower-volume centers (18–23). Finlayson et al. used decision analysis to estimate the cumulative effect of volume-related difference in operative and long-term mortality rates on patient life expectancy (24). Overall, patients gained 0.6, 1.2, and 1.7 years of life expectancy by selecting a high-volume hospital over a lower-volume center for surgery for colon, lung, and pancreatic cancer, respectively.

Intensive Care Unit Staffing

A large proportion of surgical patients, particularly those experiencing serious complications, receive care in the intensive care unit (ICU). Because these patients have high

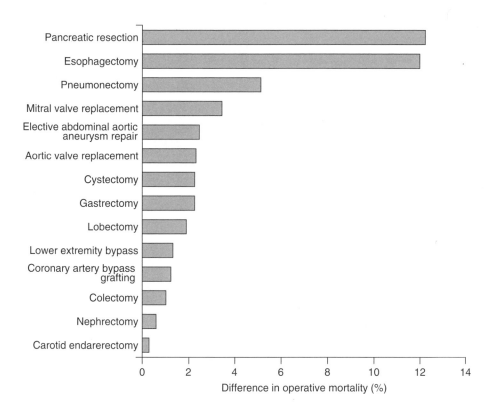

Figure 6-1 Absolute differences in adjusted operative mortality rates between very-low- and very-high-volume hospitals. Based on US Medicare population, 1994–99. (From Birkmeyer JD, Siewers AE, Finlayson EV, et al. Hospital volume and surgical mortality in the United States. *N Engl J Med* 2002;346:1128–1137, with permission.)

mortality rates, it should not be surprising that structural variables reflecting the quality of ICU care might affect surgical outcomes.

The most prevalent studies in this area have focused on ICU staffing and, in particular, the importance of board-certified intensivists. In one systematic review of the literature, Pronovost et al. assessed mortality at hospitals with so-called low-intensity ICU physician staffing (no intensivist or elective intensivist consultation only) and with high-intensity staffing (mandatory intensivist consultation or "closed" ICU with all care directed by intensivist) (25). High-intensity staffing was associated with lower hospital mortality in 16 of 17 studies (94%) (Fig. 6-2). Overall, the relative risk for hospital mortality with high-intensity staffing was 0.71 (95% CI, 0.62 to 0.82). Similar reductions in ICU mortality rates were also noted. Studies included in this review were very heterogeneous and all observational in nature. Many were based on comparisons of mortality rates before and after establishment of staffing changes at individual hospitals; others relied on "cross-sectional" designs, comparing mortality rates at hospitals with different staffing patterns during a single period of time. Despite their heterogeneity, these studies are remarkable in the consistency of their findings.

Other Variables

Evidence is growing that high nurse-staffing levels are associated with better surgical outcomes (26–28). Aiken et al. studied relationships between nurse staffing and operative

mortality in a broad population of over 230,000 general, vascular, and orthopedic surgery patients (29). After controlling for both patient and other hospital characteristics, patients treated in hospitals with eight patients or more per nurse were 31% more likely to die perioperatively in relative terms (0.5% higher in absolute terms) than patients in hospitals with four patients per nurse. Nurse-staffing levels were more strongly related to mortality among patients experiencing complications. In a follow-up study by the same authors, hospitals in which a high proportion of nurses held a bachelor's degree or higher also had lower operative mortality rates (30).

Resource availability might predict outcomes with some procedures. In one study from the Department of Veterans Affairs' NSQIP (31), site visits were conducted at 10 VA hospitals with lower than expected mortality rates and 10 with worse than expected mortality. Site visit teams, which included surgeons, nurses, and study epidemiologists, were blinded to the performance status of each hospital. Hospitals with lower than expected mortality rates were more likely to have up-to-date technology and equipment in their ICUs and tended to rely more heavily on interdisciplinary teams in patient management.

Surgeon-level Variables

Surgeon Volume

Although most research has focused on hospital volume, a large number of studies has explored associations between surgeon volume and mortality with various procedures.

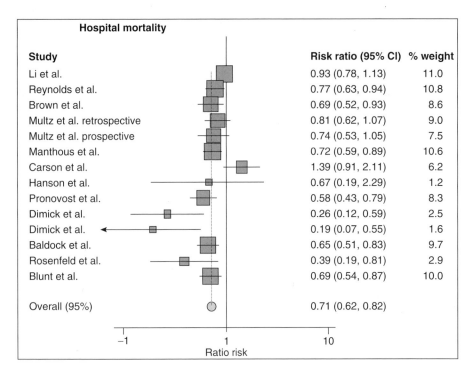

Figure 6-2 In-hospital mortality associated with high-intensity vs. low-intensity ICU physician staffing. (From Pronovost PJ, Angus DC, Dorman T, et al. Physician staffing patterns and clinical outcomes in critically ill patients: a systematic review. *JAMA* 2002;288: 2151–2162, with permission.)

Most have documented significant (inverse) relationships between the two (15,32–35). For example, in New York State, patients undergoing carotid endarterectomy by low-volume surgeons were twice as likely to die perioperatively (2.0%) than patients treated by high-volume surgeons (0.9%) (35).

In the largest study to date, Birkmeyer et al. used national Medicare data to examine the relationship between surgeon volume and operative mortality with eight different cardiovascular procedures and cancer resections in the national Medicare population (36). Surgeon volume was inversely related to operative mortality with all eight procedures. As with hospital volume, the magnitude of surgeon volume–outcome relationships varied markedly by procedure in terms of both absolute mortality rates and adjusted odds ratios of mortality. Comparing low-volume with high-volume surgeons, adjusted odds ratios of mortality ranged from only 1.24 (lung resection) to 3.61 (pancreatic resection).

Subspecialty Training

There is also a growing body of research examining the importance of surgeon training, particularly subspecialty fellowship training or board certification, or both (37,38). For example, patients with rectal cancer managed by board-certified colorectal surgeons had lower recurrence rates and improved long-term survival compared to patients managed by other general surgeons (37). Many studies in this area have failed to account adequately for potentially confounding variables. Fellowship-trained

subspecialists are more likely to have more specialized practices and thus higher volume with specific procedures. They are also more likely to practice in higher-volume tertiary care centers, which might also have better patient outcomes.

However, several studies suggest that subspecialty training might be an independent predictor of favorable outcomes. For example, Goodney et al. studied operative mortality in US Medicare patients undergoing resection for lung cancer (38). Board-certified cardiothoracic surgeons had lower overall mortality rates (5.9%) than general surgeons (7.6%). These specialty-related differences were partly attenuated by surgeon volume, hospital volume, and other characteristics, but did not disappear after controlling for these other variables. In another study of carotid endarterectomy in New York State, vascular surgeons had lower rates of 30-day stroke or death than did neurosurgeons or general surgeons, differences that persisted after controlling for their higher procedure volumes (39).

Although subspecialty training might be important for many procedures, training at a prestigious program does not necessarily imply better outcomes for patients. Hartz et al. examined CABG mortality rates among surgeons who completed their general surgery and/or cardiothoracic surgery training at prestigious hospitals, as determined by *US News & World Report* rankings (40). Mortality rates did not differ between such surgeons and those trained elsewhere, including abroad. Interestingly, the more important surgeon attribute was years out of training. Cardiac surgeons between 5 and 10 years out of training had slightly lower mortality rates than more junior surgeons and substantially lower mortality than surgeons 20 or more years out of training.

The Relative Importance of Hospital and Surgeon Factors

Whether surgical outcomes depend more on the surgeon performing the operation or the hospital in which it is performed is difficult to establish. To date, only a small proportion of structural variables potentially related to surgical outcomes have been examined, and rarely in a head-to-head fashion. Most studies tend to focus on hospital-level or surgeon-level variables that are easily measured, such as procedure volume, board certification, or nurse staffing levels. Although such variables are sometimes powerful predictors of morbidity and mortality, they no doubt serve primarily as proxies for the finer elements of structure or process of care that lead directly to better outcomes at the patient level.

Nonetheless, studies assessing the relative importance of hospital and surgeon volume might provide useful insights. Many have assumed the former to be the more important factor. Because they tend to be much larger facilities, high-volume hospitals have a broader range of specialist and technology-based services, better-staffed ICUs, and other resources not available at smaller centers. By virtue of these resources, high-volume hospitals might be better equipped to deliver the complex perioperative care required by patients undergoing high-risk surgery.

A recent study by Birkmeyer et al., however, did not confirm the preeminent role of hospital volume (36). On the basis of data from the 1998–99 national Medicare population, low-volume surgeons had higher mortality rates than high-volume surgeons across a wide spectrum of eight cardiovascular procedures and cancer resections, even after accounting for hospital volume (Fig. 6-3). Adjusting for hospital volume attenuated the strength of surgeon volume–outcome relationships to some degree, but the effect of surgeon volume remained statistically significant for seven of the eight procedures.

In contrast, for many procedures surgeon volume largely mediated the hospital volume. Without accounting for surgeon volume, hospital volume was inversely related to operative mortality with seven of the eight procedures ($p = 0.20$ for carotid endarterectomy, $p < 0.001$ for others). After adjusting for surgeon volume, however, higher hospital volume remained a significant predictor of decreased mortality for only four procedures. In fact, high hospital volume predicted increased mortality for carotid endarterectomy after accounting for surgeon volume. For many procedures, surgeon volume accounted for a large proportion of apparent differences in operative mortality between high-volume and low-volume hospitals. With elective AAA repair, for example, adjusted odds ratios of mortality by hospital volume fell from 1.40 to 1.17 after adjusting for surgeon volume. Thus, surgeon volume accounted for 57%

of the apparent difference in mortality between low-volume and high-volume hospitals. The proportion of the apparent hospital volume effect attributable to surgeon volume varied by procedure, from 100% with carotid endarterectomy and aortic valve replacement to only 24% with lung resection.

From a clinical perspective, it is not surprising that the relative importance of surgeon and hospital volume varies by procedure. With carotid endarterectomy, for example, technical skill and use of specific intraoperative processes (e.g., intra-arterial shunts, patch angioplasty)—factors primarily associated with the operating surgeon—are important determinants of operative mortality. In contrast, the importance of other hospital-based services is relatively low. Most carotid endarterectomy patients do not require intensive postoperative management, and length of stay is typically just overnight. For these reasons the preeminent role of surgeon volume with this procedure has strong face validity. With lung resection, in contrast, patients rarely die because of direct technical complications of the procedure itself (e.g., bleeding, bronchial stump leak); they die from cardiac events, pneumonia, and respiratory failure. Hospital-based services (e.g., intensive care, pain management, respiratory, and nursing care) are very important and lengths of stay are relatively long. Thus, it is not surprising that hospital volume was more important than surgeon volume with this procedure. Of course, these two procedures represent the extremes. For many high-risk procedures, factors related to both surgeon volume and hospital volume seem to be important.

Apart from their varying associations with mortality rates for different procedures, hospital and surgeon volume might also have different effects on different types of complications. Katz et al. studied outcomes in >70,000 Medicare patients undergoing total hip replacement between 1995 and 1996 (17). Hospital volume, but not surgeon volume, was an independent predictor of operative mortality. Higher surgeon volume, but not hospital volume, was independently associated with decreased risks of hip dislocation and deep wound infection. Again, these findings make sense clinically. The most common cause of death after this procedure is myocardial infarction. Thus, variation in mortality rates might primarily reflect the quality of anesthesia or cardiology services, which might be more closely associated with the hospital than the operating orthopedist. Conversely, it is not surprising that surgeon volume will be more important than hospital volume in explaining variable rates of surgical site complications

EVIDENCE LINKING PROCESS OF CARE TO SURGICAL OUTCOMES

Process of care variables reflect different components of the care that patients actually receive before, during, or after a surgical intervention. Relative to structure variables,

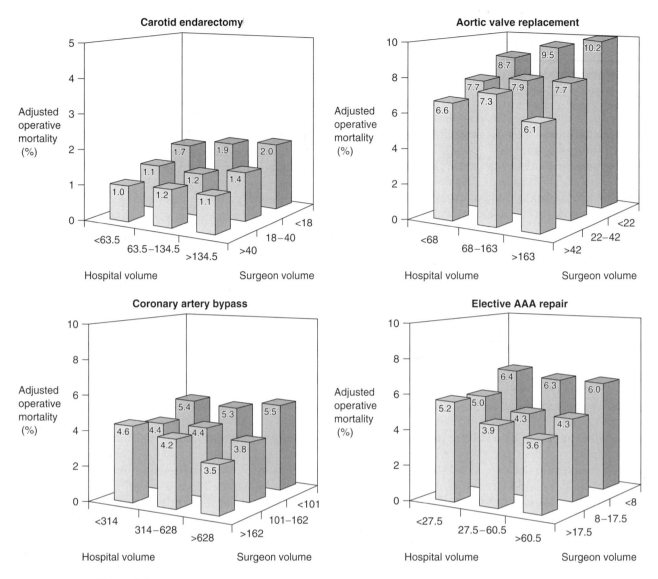

Figure 6-3 Adjusted in-hospital/30-day mortality in Medicare patients (1998–99), by tercile of total hospital and surgeon volume (Medicare and non-Medicare) for four cardiovascular procedures (A) and four cancer resections (B). Owing to small sample sizes (*n* <20), mortality rates for high-volume surgeons in low hospital volumes are not shown for esophagectomy and pancreatic resection. AAA, abdominal aortic aneurysm. (From Birkmeyer J, Stukel T, Siewers A, et al. Surgeon volume and operative mortality in the United States. *N Engl J Med* 2003; 349:2117–2127, with permission.)

processes of care have a more direct effect on patient outcomes. They might also constitute the causal pathway underlying apparent associations between structural variables and outcomes. For example, Hannan et al. performed a prospective clinical study of patients undergoing carotid endarterectomy at six hospitals in New York State (39). In that study vascular surgeons had substantially lower 30-day rates of operative stroke or death than did general surgeons or neurovascular surgeons. However, the investigators also found that use of intraarterial shunting, eversion endarterectomy techniques, patching of the arteriotomy, and protamine were associated with lower complication rates. Greater adoption of these four processes of care by vascular surgeons explained in large part their better outcomes.

A full accounting of processes of care related to surgical outcomes is beyond the scope of this chapter. Many procedure-specific processes are considered elsewhere in this book. Among processes that cut across procedures, a large number have high levels of evidence supporting their effectiveness. For example, the Agency for Healthcare Research and Quality (AHRQ) recently commissioned a critical review of hospital-based practices related to patient safety (41). Many practices identified by this review pertain to perioperative care, which are summarized in Table 6-2, according to strength of evidence supporting their effectiveness and the magnitude of their potential benefits. These include the use of sterile barriers and ultrasound guidance in preventing complications

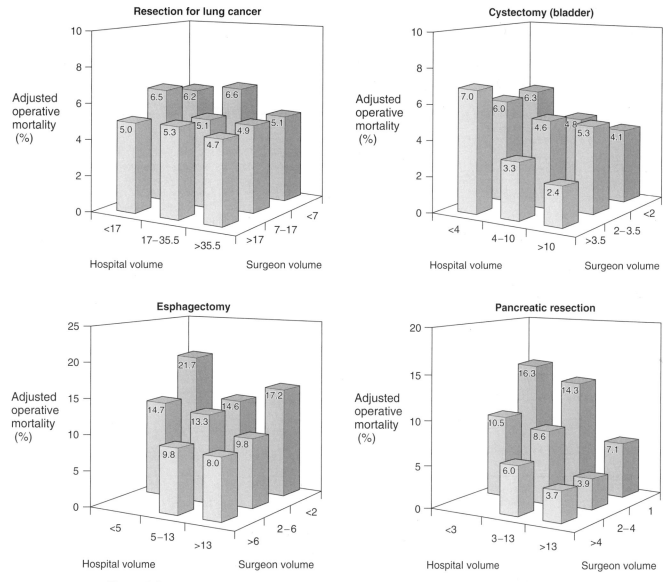

Figure 6-3 (continued).

Venous Thromboembolism Prophylaxis

with central venous lines, early enteral nutrition and gut decontamination in critically ill patients, stress ulcer prophylaxis, and practices aimed at reducing wrong-site procedures.

A few specific processes of care warrant additional comment because of their wide applicability or their high potential to reduce rates of serious complications, or both. Not surprisingly, some of these processes are also used widely as quality indicators in both public reporting and quality improvement initiatives.

Venous Thromboembolism Prophylaxis

The risks of postoperative venous thromboembolism (DVT) and pulmonary embolism (PE) vary widely according to both procedure and patient risk factors. In high-risk general-surgery patients, however, rates of proximal DVT and PE might exceed 20% and 10%, respectively (42). Numerous studies show that both low dose unfractionated heparin (LDUH) and low molecular weight heparin (LMWH) reduce the risk of clinically important venous thromboembolism (43). Pooled results from 46 randomized trials show that prophylaxis of general surgical patients with LDUH compared with placebo reduced the risk of DVT (as determined by imaging) by 68%, from 25% to 8% (42). LMWH had comparable efficacy to LDUH overall but was possibly more effective for preventing proximal DVT and PE. In the same meta-analysis, both intermittent pneumatic compression and elastic stockings significantly reduced the overall incidence of

TABLE 6-2

EXAMPLES OF PROCESS MEASURES ASSOCIATED WITH SURGICAL OUTCOMES, ACCORDING TO STRENGTH OF SCIENTIFIC EVIDENCE SUPPORTING THEM AND THE COST AND COMPLEXITY OF IMPLEMENTING THEM

Implementation Cost/Complexity	Strength of the Evidence/Magnitude of Potential Benefit				
	Greatest	**High**	**Medium**	**Lower**	**Lowest**
Low	Appropriate venous thromboembolism prophylaxis	Use of supplemental perioperative oxygen	H₂ antagonists for stress ulcer prophylaxis	Early analgesics in patients with acute abdomen (without compromising diagnostic accuracy)	Use of preanesthesia checklists
	Use of perioperative β-blockers in patients at risk for cardiac events	Selective decontamination of digestive tract	Protocols/ nomograms for intravenous heparin titration	Intraoperative monitoring of vital signs/oxygenation	Counting sharps, instruments, and sponges
	Appropriate use of antibiotic wound prophylaxis	Use of silver alloy-coated urinary catheters	Maintenance of perioperative normothermia		Sucralfate for stress ulcer prophylaxis
	Antibiotic-impregnated central venous catheters				
Medium or high	Early nutritional support in critically ill patients		Barrier precautions (via gowns and gloves, dedicated equipment, dedicated personnel)	Tunneling short-term central venous catheters	"Sign your site" protocols
	Use of real-time ultrasound guidance during central line insertion		Perioperative glucose control		Catheter changes as prophylaxis against central line infections

Adapted from Making health care safer: A critical analysis of patient safety practices. Rockville, MD: Agency for Healthcare Quality and Research; 2001.

DVT, but not proximal DVT or PE, in general surgical patients.

Prophylactic Antibiotics

A large body of Level 1A evidence supports the premise that the administration of appropriate prophylactic antibiotics can prevent surgical site infections. As summarized in the AHRQ report on patient safety (44), seven meta-analyses and two structured literature reviews have synthesized >100 randomized controlled clinical trials assessing the effectiveness of prophylactic antibiotics. Although these studies focused on different antibiotic regimens and surgical populations, all concluded that perioperative antibiotics prevent surgical site infection. When compared with single dose prophylaxis, multiple-dose prophylaxis generally did not result in significant additional benefit. Two national organizations, the Centers for Disease Control and Prevention (CDC) and the American Society for Health System Pharmacists, have compiled detailed guidelines regarding the administration of prophylactic antibiotics across a broad range of procedures (45,46).

Prophylactic β-blockers

Cardiac events, including myocardial infarction, are among the most common causes of mortality in patients undergoing major surgery, particularly peripheral vascular surgery. As summarized in one recent review (47), five randomized clinical trials have assessed the effectiveness of perioperative β-blockers, generally consisting of therapeutic dosing prior to induction of anesthesia and continuation of targeted, postoperative therapy (generally to heart rates <70 beats per minute). Although the trials varied markedly in terms of study populations and intervention protocols, four of the five showed substantial reductions in rates of perioperative cardiac ischemia. Two of the three focusing on mortality as a primary endpoint also found substantial risk reductions. For example, in one study of male veterans undergoing major noncardiac surgery, patients receiving perioperative β-blockers had a nearly 55% relative reduction in all-cause mortality at 2 years (48). The sole trial not to report significant benefits with perioperative β-blockers was relatively small and enrolled lower-risk patients than the other trials (49).

Intensive Insulin Therapy for Critically Ill Patients

Postoperative hyperglycemia is common in surgical patients, particularly those who are critically ill. However, the clinical importance of hyperglycemia had not been well established until a recent randomized controlled trial of intensive insulin therapy in critically ill patients was published. In that study 1,548 patients in the ICU were randomized to traditional therapy (subcutaneous insulin dosed on a "sliding scale") or intensive insulin therapy (continuous, intravenous insulin dosed to main blood glucose between 80 and 110 mg per dL) (50). Intensive insulin therapy reduced mortality almost 50%, from 8.0% with conventional treatment to 4.6%. Benefits of a similar magnitude have been reported in a nonrandomized study of cardiac surgery patients (51). Although randomized clinical trials focusing on other patient groups are clearly needed, the potential benefit of tight perioperative glucose control could be substantial.

STRUCTURE AND PROCESS MEASURES AS QUALITY INDICATORS: POLICY CONSIDERATIONS

Ongoing Initiatives

There is growing interest in using both structure and process measures as quality indicators. Structural measures, particularly procedure volume, are most commonly used in the context of evidence-based hospital referral, the most visible of these being led by the Leapfrog Group, a large coalition of public and private health care purchasers currently representing >40 million patients. Since it was launched in 2000, the Leapfrog Group has been using a variety of incentives to encourage patients to seek care at hospitals with computerized order-entry systems for inpatients, intensivist-staffed ICUs, and high volumes with selected surgical procedures or neonatal intensive care (52). In the 2003 update of the surgical standards, minimum hospital volume criteria remain in place for CABG, percutaneous coronary interventions (PCI), elective AAA repair, esophagectomy, and pancreatic resection. For three procedures, however, the Leapfrog Group now requires direct outcomes assessment (risk-adjusted mortality for CABG and PCI) or acceptable compliance with selected process measures (perioperative β-blockers with elective AAA repair), or both (Table 6-3).

Although also used as criteria for evidence-based referral, process measures are more often associated with quality improvement initiatives. For example, the AHRQ, in cooperation with various experts and other organizations, has developed a list of quality indicators for surgical care (Table 6-4). Although they also include mortality and volume measures for selected procedures, some quality indicators are process measures—for example, use of laparoscopy in patients requiring cholecystectomy and avoidance of incidental appendectomy in the elderly. Individual states (e.g., Texas) or large health plans collect information on these measures as part of their quality reporting systems. Similarly, the Joint Commission on Accreditation of Healthcare Organizations (JCAHO) might soon begin asking hospitals to provide information on the use of prophylactic antibiotics with surgical procedures. In this context, provider-specific performance data are collected and reported primarily to incentivize corrective action by hospitals, not to encourage patients to select alternate hospitals.

Although each type of measure has its advantages, structure and process measures also have drawbacks as quality indicators (53). For contrast, Table 6-5 lists the strengths and weaknesses of the two measures, relative to direct outcomes assessment.

Strengths and Weaknesses of Structural Measures

From a measurement perspective, structural measures have several attractive features as indicators of surgical quality. As already described, many of these variables are strongly related to surgical outcomes. Some structural measures have strong face validity for patients, essential for the success of public reporting and evidence-based referral initiatives. Procedure volume, in particular, is considered very important by many patients, who rarely ask their surgeons about their complication rates but often ask, "Do you do this procedure often?"

The primary advantage of structural variables, however, is expediency. Compared to direct outcomes assessment, structural variables, including procedure volume, can be assessed easily and inexpensively, often with administrative data. Such information is already widely available on the World Wide Web (e.g., www.healthgrades.com).

Among the downsides, the scientific evidence assessing the importance of structural measures is flawed. Unlike process measures, which can often be evaluated in randomized clinical trials, most structural measures can only be assessed in observational studies. Thus, it is often difficult to rule out differences in patient case mix across hospitals as an explanation for observed associations between structure and outcomes. Second, in contrast to process measures, many structural measures are not readily actionable, which limit their ultimate effectiveness as a means toward quality improvement. For example, a small hospital can increase how many of its high-risk patients receive perioperative β-blockers but cannot readily make itself a high-volume center for a given procedure or convert to an intensivist-model ICU.

Finally, and most importantly, structural variables are imperfect proxies for quality—they reflect average results for large groups of providers, not for individuals. For example,

TABLE 6-3

LEAPFROG GROUP CRITERIA FOR EVIDENCE-BASED HOSPITAL REFERRAL, 2003

Procedure	Volume Standard	Process Measures	Outcomes Measures
Pancreatic resection	11/yr	None	None
Esophageal resection	13/yr	None	None
AAA repair	50/yr	Perioperative β-blockers in >80% eligible patients	None
Coronary artery bypass grafting			
NY, NJ, PA, CA[a]	None	(β-blockers, use of IMA, aspirin, and lipid lowering therapy)[b]	Must be in the lowest quartile of mortality rates
Other states	450/yr	(β-blockers, use of IMA, aspirin, and lipid lowering therapy)[b]	Must participate in STS database *AND* have mortality rate below the national average
Percutaneous coronary intervention			
NY, NJ, PA, CA[a]	None	(Aspirin on discharge, intervention within 90 minutes for AMI)[b]	Must be in the lowest quartile of mortality rates
Other states	400/yr	(Aspirin on discharge, intervention within 90 minutes for AMI)[b]	Must participate in ACC database *AND* have mortality rate below the national average

[a]NY, NJ, PA, CA have prospective outcomes registries for coronary artery bypass grafting and percutaneous coronary interventions.
[b]Used in partial credit algorithms for hospitals not meeting the criteria for full adherence to the Leapfrog EHR standards.
AAA, abdominal aortic aneurysm; IMA, internal mammary artery; AMI, acute myocardial infarction; STS, Society of Thoracic Surgery; ACC, American College of Cardiology.

TABLE 6-4

QUALITY INDICATORS FOR VARIOUS SURGICAL PROCEDURES PROMOTED BY THE AGENCY FOR HEALTHCARE RESEARCH AND QUALITY

Procedure	Type of Measure		
	Structure	Process	Outcome
Abdominal aortic aneurysm repair	Volume		Mortality
Appendectomy, incidental		Avoidance of procedure in elderly	
Carotid endarterectomy	Volume		
Coronary artery bypass grafting	Volume		Mortality
Cholecystectomy		Proportion performed laparoscopically	
Craniotomy			Mortality
Esophageal resection	Volume		Mortality
Hip replacement			Mortality
Pancreatic resection	Volume		Mortality
Pediatric heart surgery	Volume		Mortality

Adapted from the Agency for Healthcare Research and Quality (AHRQ) Guide to Inpatient Quality Indicators, available at http://www.qualityindicators.ahrq.gov.

TABLE 6-5

TRADE-OFFS OF USING STRUCTURE, PROCESS, OR OUTCOME MEASURES AS QUALITY INDICATORS

	Structure	Process	Outcomes
Examples	Procedure volume	Perioperative β-blockers in high-risk surgical patients	Morbidity and mortality rates
	Fellowship-trained surgeons	Perioperative antibiotics as wound infection prophylaxis	Functional health status
	Intensivist-staffed ICUs		Patient satisfaction
Primary advantage(s)	Expedient, inexpensive proxies of surgical outcomes	Reflect care that patients actually receive—might seem "fairer" to providers	Acceptance from surgeons—the "bottom line" of what they do
	Some measures (i.e., volume) resonate with patients	Actionable from provider perspective, clear link to quality improvement activities	Outcomes measurement alone might improve quality
Disadvantages	Most variables not actionable from provider perspective	Little information about which processes are important for specific procedures	Inadequate caseloads at most hospitals for measuring procedure-specific outcomes with adequate precision
	Imperfect proxies for outcomes—reflect average results for large groups of providers, not individuals		Outcome measures that are not procedure-specific less useful for evidence-based referral or quality improvement

ICUs, intensive care units.

many low-volume hospitals have excellent performance, whereas many high-volume centers are poor performers. Thus, even if all high-risk procedures were concentrated in high-volume hospitals, there would remain substantial variation in quality across hospitals and thus opportunity for improvement.

Strengths and Weaknesses of Process Measures

As potential quality indicators, process of care measures have several attractive features. Their effectiveness is often supported by high-level evidence (e.g., randomized clinical trials) and, as described earlier, can be large in magnitude. Because they often apply to broad groups of surgical patients and are often underutilized (e.g., perioperative β-blockers), efforts focusing on process measures could have very large benefits from a population perspective. Second, process variables reflect the care that patients actually receive and thus might be perceived by providers as "fairer" measures of quality than structural measures, important for hospital and surgeon acceptance.

Finally, and most importantly, process of care measures are generally actionable and link directly to outcomes measurement activities. For example, investigators and clinicians at six hospitals in northern New England have maintained a prospective clinical registry for CABG and

other cardiac procedures since 1987 (5). They identified numerous process of care measures linked to lower operative mortality, including use of an internal mammary graft, continuing aspirin through surgery, and maintaining a hematocrit of 24% or higher while "on pump." As a result of systematic efforts to increase the use of these practices and timely feedback of performance data to clinicians, operative mortality rates across the region fell by almost half during the 1990s, a decline significantly greater than observed in regions of the United States without similar quality improvement initiatives in place (54).

Among the downsides, process measures require the ability to accurately identify eligible patient populations—that is, the right denominator. Many processes known to be effective in general might not be appropriate for all patients undergoing a given procedure (e.g., β-blockers in patients with bradyarrhythmias or severe left ventricular dysfunction). Because it implies the need for clinical data, process measurement can be labor intensive and expensive.

A second major limitation of process measures is the relative lack of evidence about which processes are important for specific procedures. Much of the existing literature on processes of care focuses on general perioperative care. However, many of the most serious adverse events occurring after surgery are specific to the surgical site—anastamotic leaks, bleeding, infection, and so on.

Although high-leverage technical processes have been elucidated for some procedures (notably CABG and carotid endarterectomy), few procedures have been as carefully studied and thus major knowledge gaps remain.

IMPROVING THE QUALITY OF QUALITY MEASUREMENT

No single measure of surgical quality is optimal for every situation. As reviewed earlier, the value of structure and process measures depends to a large extent on whether the primary goal is redirecting patients to the best hospitals (evidence-based referral) or improving care everywhere (quality improvement). It is also important to consider the attributes of the surgical procedure being assessed. Two factors are particularly important: (i) the baseline risks of the procedure and (ii) how commonly it is performed at individual hospitals (Fig. 6-4). Measuring quality for procedures that are both low risk and uncommonly performed (Quadrant III) should receive low priority. Many high-risk procedures, like esophagectomy and pancreatic resection (Quadrant IV), are performed too infrequently at the vast majority of hospitals to support direct outcomes assessment. Thus, procedure volume, a structural measure highly correlated with mortality for many of these procedures, is likely the only practical quality indicator. Quality for procedures that are both common and relatively high risk (e.g.,

CABG, Quadrant II) is best assessed directly using risk-adjusted measures of morbidity and mortality. Quality improvement consortiums designed to accomplish this task are also ideal platforms for measuring process variables and linking them to outcomes. Measuring quality is perhaps most problematic for common but relatively low-risk procedures (e.g., laparoscopic cholecystectomy, Quadrant I). For these procedures, volume and other structural measures are not known to be major determinants of outcomes. Low baseline rates of mortality or other serious complications preclude measuring outcomes with sufficient precision. Thus, quality for these procedures is best judged by process measures, where available, or by patient-centered outcome measures (e.g., functional health status).

Improving the quality of quality measurement will require better information about high-leverage processes of care with different procedures. As described earlier, most high-level evidence linking process to surgical outcomes pertains to the medical aspects of perioperative care, not the technical aspects of specific procedures that determine their success. A better understanding of such processes is essential if successes achieved with CABG are to be replicated in other areas.

Finally, we must be careful that surgical quality is not considered too narrowly. Quality in health care can be described as "doing the right things right." This chapter (and debates about surgical quality in general) focuses on only the latter component of this aphorism—how well the procedure was

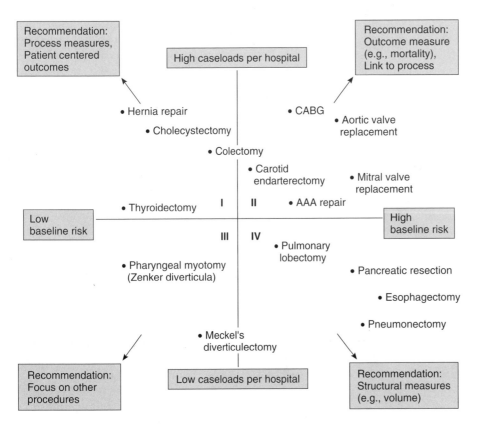

Figure 6-4 Recommendations for when to focus on structure, process, or outcomes. CABG, coronary artery bypass grafting; AAA, abdominal aortic aneurysm. [From Birkmeyer JD, Birkmeyer NJ, Dimick JB. Measuring the quality of surgical care: Structure, process, or outcomes? *J Am Coll Surg* 2004 (*in press*), with permission.]

performed (i.e., doing things right). However, as suggested by wide geographic variation in the use of different procedures in the United States (55), the quality of the decision to operate in the first place (i.e., doing the right thing) might be an equally important issue in surgical care. Thus, a full accounting of surgical quality will require measures of appropriateness and how well patient preferences are incorporated in clinical decisions, not just how well they do after surgery.

REFERENCES

1. Goodney PP, Siewers AE, Stukel TS, et al. Is cancer surgery getting safer? National trends in operative mortality, 1994–1999. *J Am Coll Surg* 2002;195:219–227.
2. Birkmeyer JD, Finlayson EV, Birkmeyer CM. Volume standards for high-risk surgical procedures: potential benefits of the Leapfrog initiative. *Surgery* 2001;130:415–422.
3. Khuri SF, Daley J, Henderson W. The Department of Veterans Affairs' NSQIP: the first national, validated, outcome-based, risk-adjusted, and peer-controlled program for the measurement and enhancement of the quality of surgical care. National VA Surgical Quality Improvement Program. *Ann Surg* 1998;228:491–507.
4. Hannan EL, Kilburn H Jr, Racz M, et al. Improving the outcomes of coronary artery bypass surgery in New York State. *JAMA* 1994;271:761–766.
5. O'Connor GT, Plume SK, Morton JR. Results of a regional prospective study to improve the in-hospital mortality associated with coronary artery bypass grafting. *JAMA* 1996;275:841–846.
6. Donabedian A. Evaluating the quality of medical care. *Milbank Memorial Fund Q* 1966;44:166–206.
7. Ferguson TB Jr, Peterson ED, Coombs LP, et al. Use of continuous quality improvement to increase use of process measures in patients undergoing coronary artery bypass graft surgery: a randomized controlled trial. *JAMA* 2003;290:49–56.
8. Lee JAH, Morrison SL, Morris JN. Fatality from three common surgical conditions in teaching and non-teaching hospitals. *Lancet* 1957;ii:785–790.
9. Luft HS, Bunker JP, Enthoven AC. Should operations be regionalized? The empirical relation between surgical volume and mortality. *N Engl J Med* 1979;301:1364–1369.
10. Flood AB, Scott WR, Ewy W. Does practice make perfect? Part I: The relation between hospital volume and outcomes for selected diagnostic categories. *Med Care* 1984;22(2):98–114.
11. Flood AB, Scott WR, Ewy W. Does practice make perfect? Part II: The relation between volume and outcomes and other hospital characteristics. *Med Care* 1984;22(2):115–125.
12. Halm EA, Lee C, Chassin MR. Is volume related to outcome in health care? A systematic review and methodologic critique of the literature. *Ann Intern Med* 2002;137:511–520.
13. Dudley RA, Johansen KL, Brand R, et al. Selective referral to high volume hospitals: Estimating potentially avoidable deaths. *JAMA* 2000;283:1159–1166.
14. Birkmeyer JD, Siewers AE, Finlayson EVA, et al. Hospital volume and surgical mortality in the United States. *N Engl J Med* 2002;346:1128–1137.
15. Begg CB, Reidel ER, Bach PB. Variations in morbidity after radical prostatectomy. *N Engl J Med* 2002;346:1138–1144.
16. Cebul RD, Snow RJ, Pine R, et al. Indications, outcomes, and provider volumes for carotid endarterectomy. *JAMA* 1998;279:1282–1287.
17. Katz JN, Losina E, Barrett J. Association between hospital and surgeon procedure volume and outcomes of total hip replacement in the United States Medicare population. *J Bone Joint Surg* 2001;83:1622–1629.
18. Bach PB, Cramer LD, Schrag D, et al. The influence of hospital volume on survival after resection for lung cancer. *N Engl J Med* 2001;345:181–188.
19. Birkmeyer JD, Warshaw AL, Finlayson SR, et al. Relationship between hospital volume and late survival after pancreaticoduodenectomy. *Surgery* 1999;126:178–183.

20. Gillis CR, Hole DJ. Survival outcome of care by specialist surgeons in breast cancer: a study of 3,786 patients in the west of Scotland. *Br Med J* 1996;312:145–153.
21. Hodgson DC, Fuchs CS, Ayanian JZ. Impact of patient and provider characteristics on the treatment and outcomes of colorectal cancer. *J Natl Cancer Inst* 2001;93(7):501–515.
22. Sainsbury R, Haward B, Rider L, et al. Influence of clinician workload and patterns of treatment on survival from breast cancer. *Lancet* 1995;345:1265–1270.
23. Schrag D, Cramer LD, Bach PB, et al. Influence of hospital procedure volume on outcomes following surgery for colon cancer. *JAMA* 2000;284(23):3028–3035.
24. Finlayson EV, Birkmeyer JD. Effects of hospital volume on life expectancy after selected cancer operations in older adults: a decision analysis. *J Am Coll Surg* 2003;196:410–417.
25. Pronovost PJ, Angus DC, Dorman T, et al. Physician staffing patterns and clinical outcomes in critically ill patients: a systematic review. *JAMA* 2002;288:2151–2162.
26. Dang D, Johantgen ME, Pronovost PJ, et al. Postoperative complications: does intensive care unit staff nursing make a difference? *Heart Lung: J Acute Crit Care* 2002;31(3):219–228.
27. Dimick JB, Swoboda SM, Pronovost PJ, et al. Effect of nurse-to-patient ratio in the intensive care unit on pulmonary complications and resource use after hepatectomy. *Am J Crit Care* 2001; 10(6):376–382.
28. Pronovost PJ, Dang D, Dorman T, et al. Intensive care unit nurse staffing and the risk for complications after abdominal aortic surgery. *Effect Clin Pract* 2001;4:199–206.
29. Aiken LH, Clarke SP, Sloane DM, et al. Hospital nurse staffing and patient mortality, nurse burnout, and job dissatisfaction [comment]. *JAMA* 2002;288(16):1987–1993.
30. Aiken LH, Clarke SP, Cheung RB, et al. Educational levels of hospital nurses and surgical patient mortality. *JAMA* 2003; 290(12):1617–1623.
31. Daley JM, Forbes G, Young M, et al. Validating risk-adjusted surgical outcomes: Site visit assessment of process and structure. *J Am Coll Surg* 1997;185:341–351.
32. Schrag D, Panageas KS, Riedel E, et al. Hospital and surgeon procedure volume as predictors of outcome following rectal cancer resection. *Ann Surg* 2002 (*submitted*).
33. Harmon JW, Tang DG, Gordon TA, et al. Hospital volume can serve as a surrogate for surgeon volume for achieving excellent outcomes in colorectal resection. *Ann Surg* 1999;230:404–411.
34. Hannan EL, Siu AL, Kumar D, et al. The decline in coronary artery bypass graft surgery mortality in New York State: the role of surgeon volume. *JAMA* 1995;273:209–213.
35. Hannan EL, Popp AJ, Tranmer B, et al. Relationship between provider volume and mortality for carotid endarterectomies in New York state. *Stroke* 1998;29:2292–2297.
36. Birkmeyer J, Stukel T, Siewers A, et al. Surgeon volume and operative mortality in the United States. *N Engl J Med* 2003; 349:2117–2127.
37. Porter GA, Soskolne CL, Yakimets WW, et al. Surgeon-related factors and outcome in rectal cancer. *Ann Surg* 1998;227: 157–167.
38. Goodney P, Lucas FL, Stukel T, et al. Surgeon specialty and operative mortality with lung resection. *Ann Surg* 2004 (*in press*).
39. Hannan EL, Popp AJ, Feustel P. Association of surgical specialty and processes of care with patient outcomes for carotid endarterectomy. *Stroke* 2001;32:2890–2897.
40. Hartz AJ, Kuhn EM, Pulido J. Prestige of training program and experience of bypass surgeons as factors in adjusted patient mortality rates. *Med Care* 1999;37:93–103.
41. Agency for Healthcare Research and Quality. *Making health care safer: a critical analysis of patient safety practices.* Rockville, MD: Agency for Healthcare Research and Quality; 2001.
42. Geerts WH, Heit JA, Clagett GP, et al. Prevention of venous thromboembolism. *Chest* 2001;119:132S–175S.
43. Kleinbart J, Williams MV, Rask K. Prevention of venous thromboembolism. *Making health care safer: a critical analysis of patient safety practices.* Rockville, MD: Agency for Healthcare Research and Quality; 2001:333–348.
44. Auerbach AD. Prevention of surgical site infections. *Making health care safer: a critical analysis of patient safety practices.* Rockville, MD: Agency for Healthcare Research and Quality; 2001:231–243.

45. American Society of Health-System Pharmacists. ASHP therapeutic guidelines on antimicrobial prophylaxis in surgery. *Am J Health Syst Pharm* 1999;56:1839–1888.

46. Mangram AJ, Horan TC, Pearson ML, et al. Guideline for prevention of surgical site infection, 1999. Centers for Disease Control and Prevention (CDC) Hospital Infection Control Practices Advisory Committee. *Am J Infect Control* 1999;27:97–132.

47. Auerbach AD, Goldman L. Beta-blockers and reduction of cardiac events in noncardiac surgery: scientific review. *JAMA* 2002;287(11):1435–1444.

48. Mangano DT, Layug EL, Wallace A, et al. Effect of atenolol on mortality and cardiovascular morbidity after noncardiac surgery. Multicenter study of perioperative ischemia research group. *N Engl J Med* 1996;335:1713–1720.

49. Urban MK, Markowitz SM, Gordon MA, et al. Postoperative prophylactic administration of beta-adrenergic blockers in patients at risk for myocardial ischemia. *Anesth Analg* 2000;90:1257–1261.

50. van den Berghe G, Wouters P, Weekers F, et al. Intensive insulin therapy in the critically ill patients. *N Engl J Med* 2001;345:1359–1367.

51. Furnary AP, Zerr KJ, Grunkemeier GL, et al. Continuous intravenous insulin infusion reduces the incidence of deep sternal wound infection in diabetic patients after cardiac surgical procedures. *Ann Thorac Surg* 1999;67:352–360.

52. Birkmeyer JD, Wennberg DE, Young M. et al. *Leapfrog safety standards: potential benefits of universal adoption.* Washington, DC: The Business Roundtable; 2000.

53. Birkmeyer JD, Birkmeyer NJ, Dimick JB. Measuring the quality of surgical care: Structure, process, or outcomes? *J Am Coll Surg* 2004 (*in press*).

54. Peterson ED, DeLong ER, Jollis JG, et al. The effects of New York's bypass surgery provider profiling on access to care and patient outcomes in the elderly [comment]. *J Am Coll Cardiol* 1998;32:993–999.

55. Wennberg JE. *Dartmouth atlas of health care.* Chicago: American Hospital Publishing, Inc; 1996.

Assessing Surgical Quality with Clinical Outcomes Measures

7

Darrell A. Campbell, Jr.   *William G. Henderson*
Shukri F. Khuri

■■■ CRITICAL ELEMENTS IN THE COMPARATIVE EVALUATION OF SURGICAL QUALITY: NSQIP AS A MODEL USING CLINICAL OUTCOMES 46

■■■ HOW RISK ADJUSTMENT INFLUENCES THE EVALUATION OF SURGICAL CARE QUALITY 49

■■■ RESULTS REPORTING USING THE O/E RATIO AT THE INSTITUTIONAL LEVEL 51

■■■ LINKING STRUCTURE AND PROCESS TO CLINICAL OUTCOME 52

■■■ LINKING COORDINATION OF CARE TO CLINICAL OUTCOME: THE NSQIP EXPERIENCE 52

■■■ MEASUREMENT AND QUALITY IMPROVEMENT 53

■■■ THE APPLICATION OF NSQIP TO THE PRIVATE SECTOR 54

■■■ MAKING A BUSINESS CASE FOR QUALITY USING NSQIP 54

■■■ NEXT STEPS IN THE EVOLUTION OF THE NSQIP 55

■■■ REFERENCES 56

Early in the 20th century there was considerable resistance to the idea that surgical results should be measured. Surgeons succeeded on the basis of social position, appearance, or important friends. When E. A. Codman, a surgeon at Massachusetts General Hospital, proposed a heretical notion that surgical quality should be carefully and systematically measured, the profession roundly criticized and ostracized him (1). Codman advocated an "end results system," in which each patient at discharge was issued an "end results card" that was meant to monitor the complications and efficiency of the surgical procedure. In Codman's words, "the end results system is merely the common sense notion that every hospital should follow every patient it treats, long enough to determine whether or not the treatment has been successful and then to inquire 'if not, why not?' with a view to preventing a similar failure in the future." Thus, what is now referred to as "outcomes research" originated in the mind of a trouble-making surgeon.

Darrell A. Campbell Jr.: University of Michigan, Ann Arbor, MI 48109
William G. Henderson: University of Colorado, Aurora, CO 80045
Shukri F. Khuri: VA Healthcare System, West Roxbury, MA 02132

It is easier, and in some ways more valid, to measure the collective quality of an institution rather than that of an individual surgeon. This is because institutions are responsible for the functioning of important systems that influence results, whereas individual surgeons are not. An excellent surgeon practicing in an institution with poor anesthesia, nursing, or technology might well have poor results. Also, individual surgeons rarely operate on sufficient numbers of cases to generate statistical significance when comparisons are done, although this is much easier when evaluating institutional results. Donabedian, another pioneer in health services research, described how to measure institutional quality using a combination of structure, process, and outcome, all of which have unique attributes (2). We have described structure and process measurements of institutional quality in Chapter 6. This chapter will focus on how clinical outcomes might be used to characterize institutional surgical quality.

One way to analyze institutional quality is to query administrative data sets, which are large databases describing various aspects of medical care—for example, the Medical Provider Analysis and Review (MedPAR) database for Medicare patients. The advantage of administrative data is that it is relatively cheap and the data sets are very large. Thus, an investigator may inquire of the MedPAR database to characterize a single hospital's inpatient mortality rate or an entire state's inpatient mortality rate with relative ease. Although administrative data might in some circumstances be very helpful, these data sets have significant shortcomings. For example, they might suffer from "coding bias," in which discharge diagnoses describe not the most appropriate diagnosis but the diagnosis thought most likely to bring in maximal institutional revenue. Administrative data is collected retrospectively and in many cases by employees who are not medically sophisticated, which might lead to error. A lack of standardized definitions often confuses important issues. Administrative data fail to distinguish comorbid conditions from postoperative complications, a particular weakness in the analysis of surgical quality. Most importantly, the severity adjustment methodology suitable to administrative data might not be precise enough to make reliable conclusions.

The perceived limitations of administrative data led to the creation of a clinical outcomes reporting system known as the National Surgical Quality Improvement Program (NSQIP) (3–5). In 1986 there was a groundswell of opinion based on poor data or, worse, a series of anecdotes, that surgical care in the VA health-care system was inferior to that in the private sector. This opinion became a highly charged political issue and resulted in the passage of public law 99-166, which mandated that "the VA should report its surgical outcomes in comparison to the national average" and "the VA should report its surgical outcomes with risk adjustment…." Unfortunately, there was neither a national average nor a risk adjustment system. Recognizing that the question was unanswerable, Khuri et al. designed the National VA Surgical Risk Study (NVASRS), which developed a new

platform for data acquisition and analysis (6). This data-reporting system did not suffer from the described weaknesses in administrative data, and VA surgeons warmly received it. On the basis of data from 87,000 patients treated between 1991 and 1993, a risk-adjustment methodology was crafted and validated. In 1994, the NSQIP was created and applied to all 132 VAMC's performing surgery. For the first time, a clinical-outcomes methodology capable of monitoring and enhancing surgical clinical care was available. Subsequently this methodology has been applied successfully to nonfederal hospitals, as we will describe.

A comparison of administrative data sets and the NSQIP prospective data-collection methodology has been done. Using the VA Patient Treatment File (PTF), a large administrative data set, ICD-9CM codes for the preoperative risk variables used in NSQIP were found in only 45% of cases. Postoperative occurrences measured by NSQIP data collectors were found in only 41% of reviews. Sensitivity and positive predictive value of the administrative data were poor (7), averaging 0.175 and 0.186, respectively (Table 7-1). Sensitivity and positive predictive value should be equal to 0.90 to justify substituting ICD-0-CM codes for prospective NSQIP evaluations done by nurse coordinators. Even such dramatic clinical events as cerebrovascular accident (CVA) and myocardial infarction were not captured consistently in the PTF file. These data underscore the ability of the NSQIP system to accurately capture important preoperative and postoperative variables not found in administrative data.

TABLE 7-1

POSTOPERATIVE ADVERSE EVENTS IN 58 PAIRINGS OF NSQIP AND PTF DATA

	Sensitivity	Positive Predictive Value
Range:	0.000–0.740	0.000–0.560
Average:	0.175	0.186
	>0.550	>0.500
CVA	0.701	Post-op pulmonary
Myocardial Infarction	0.575	insufficiency 0.520

PTF, Patient Treatment File; CVA, cerebrovascular accident.

CRITICAL ELEMENTS IN THE COMPARATIVE EVALUATION OF SURGICAL QUALITY: NSQIP AS A MODEL USING CLINICAL OUTCOMES

Five critical elements are necessary to ensure fair and believable institutional comparisons of surgical quality using the outcomes approach. These elements have been incorporated into the NSQIP. The first element is the establishment of concrete endpoints. In surgery this is easier than in other disciplines because what is being measured is a very easily defined intervention: the operative procedure. In medical disciplines such a defined intervention is often not part of patient management. For example, control of blood pressure might involve multiple medications administered over a period of several months and either added or subtracted from the care plan. In surgery, the information of most interest—for example, mortality related to the operative procedure or the occurrence of a complication—is temporally more closely related to the intervention than in nonsurgical areas. A beneficial effect of antihypertensive therapy might not be evident for years, for example. Although some could argue the point, NSQIP chose a 30-day endpoint for the measurement of mortality and morbidity as a reasonable first step. A relatively short endpoint ensures better follow-up, and feedback, when it occurs, is fresh in the provider's mind. Conversely, the 30-day endpoint is long enough to allow for collection of events that occur outside the hospital and possibly at a different institution. Administrative data sets cannot ensure that a complication occurring after discharge will be captured because they include only inpatient data. Many patients experiencing a complication are not happy with the provider team and seek care elsewhere. A 30-day endpoint and efforts to contact patients individually at 30 days ensures that these complications, or mortality, are not lost to the system. The average 30-day follow-up in NSQIP is 97%.

A second important element of the NSQIP outcomes approach is the standardization of definitions and terms. This is hard work, but essential, and is often described as the "blocking and tackling" of outcomes measurement. Coming to agreement, particularly among doctors, takes time, and it is not a particularly exciting process. Nonetheless, a "comparative" evaluation of surgical results means nothing unless a precise and agreed-upon understanding of what is being measured exists. The NSQIP, in its evolution, spent years on this fundamental "blocking and tackling" aspect, and it is one of its most significant accomplishments. The result is a thick "data dictionary." To this day a "definitions committee" exists, meets regularly, irons out areas of controversy, and distributes its decisions to participating centers.

The importance of this level of detail is more easily appreciated by considering a single definition of a preoperative variable, "ETOH." Obviously alcoholism would be a significant variable to most clinicians. But what is it? How will nurse data collectors record a "yes" or "no" to this element in the absence of a strict definition? Is it two drinks a day in the week prior to surgery? Is it occasional binge drinking by a college sophomore? The definitions committee considered this issue and wrote the following:

ETOH:>2 drinks per day in the 2 weeks prior to admission. The patient admits to drinking >2 ounces of hard liquor or >2 12-oz cans of beer or >2 6-oz glasses of wine per day in the 2 weeks prior to admission. If the patient is a binge

drinker, divide out the number of drinks during the binge by the numbers of days of the binge, then apply the definition.

Regardless of whether one considers this alcoholism or not, the point is that all participants use the same definition, so that comparability means something.

The same process occurs for postoperative "occurrences" or complications. For example, how should renal dysfunction, an important complication, be defined? In the NSQIP lexicon two conditions are recognized.

"Progressive renal insufficiency" is the reduced capacity of the kidney to perform its function as evidenced by a rise in creatinine of >2 mg per day from the preoperative value, but with no requirement for dialysis. "Acute renal failure" applies to a patient who did not require dialysis preoperatively; there is worsening of renal dysfunction postoperatively, requiring hemodialysis ultrafiltration or peritoneal dialysis. TIP: If the patient refuses dialysis, still enter a 'yes' to this variable because he/she did require dialysis.

The definitions require a significant level of medical sophistication to interpret and record these elements accurately. A major source of confusion might potentially be introduced to the process if the data collector has little clinical background and is trying to make decisions retrospectively in the depths of the record room. The NSQIP architecture requires a nurse data collector with extensive training in NSQIP terminology. Tables 7-2 and 7-3 list the 30 preoperative variables and 22 postoperative "occurrences" that NSQIP recognizes.

These considerations bring up a third important element of the system for data collection: It is prospective rather than retrospective. Prospective data collection is important because it allows for "real-time" clarification of important management and outcome issues. Time and poor documentation often obscure something that happened a year

---

TABLE 7-2

THE 12 MOST PREDICTIVE PREOPERATIVE RISK FACTORS IN MORTALITY MODELS FOR NONCARDIAC SURGERY, IN ORDER

Serum albumin
ASA class
Disseminated cancer
Emergency operations
Age
BUN >40 mg/dL
DNR
Operation complexity score
SGOT >40 IU/mL
Weight loss >10% in 6 months
Functional status
WBC >11,000 mm^3

ASA, American Society of Anesthesiology; BUN, blood urea nitrogen; DNR, Do Not Resuscitate; SGOT, serum glutamic-oxaloacetic transferase; WBC, white blood cell.

TABLE 7-3

POSTOPERATIVE OCCURRENCES RECOGNIZED BY NSQIP

Wound Occurrences
Superficial incisional
Deep incisional
Organ space
Wound disruption

Respiratory Occurrences
Pneumonia
Unplanned intubation
Pulmonary embolism
On ventilator >48 hours

Urinary Tract Occurrences
Progressive renal insufficiency
Acute renal failure
Urinary tract infection

CNS Occurrences
CVA/stroke
Coma >24 hours
Peripheral nerve injury

Cardiac Occurrences
Cardiac arrest requiring CPR
Myocardial infarction

Other Occurrences
Bleeding >4 units RBCs
Graft/prosthesis/flap failure
DVT/ thrombophlebitis
Systemic sepsis
  SIRS
  Sepsis
  Septic shock

CVA, cerebrovascular accident; CPR, cardiopulmonary resuscitation; RBCs, red blood cells; DVT, deep venous thrombosis; SIRS, Systemic Inflammatory Response Syndrome.

previously. A prospective data-collection process, focused on discrete and well-defined elements, adds immeasurably to the accuracy of the data. Is there confusion about a postoperative complication? A page to the care team solves the problem because the case is ongoing and all are familiar with pertinent issues. Prospective data collection also sidesteps the important problem of "coding bias," the bane of administrative data sets. Coding bias refers to the institution's retrospective coding of case material to ensure maximum reimbursement rather than maximum accuracy.

A fourth important element of a quality reporting system involves the data collectors themselves. In the NSQIP these individuals are nurses who are sophisticated in the medical environment. Training of nurses involved in the process is critical, with documentation that the nurse data collector understands the critical distinctions made in the data dictionary. To this end, nurses in NSQIP undergo regular tests about this understanding, are graded, and are provided with feedback in areas that might be confusing to them. Interrater reliability measurements are done regularly. A team of two traveling experienced nurse coordinators visits NSQIP sites regularly to audit performance. The team selects 20 cases at random and compares the performance of the on-site nurse to the review by senior nurse coordinators. In this way there is a constant monitoring of the reliability of the data entered in the system.

The fifth critical element in a fair and believable quality system is a validated mechanism for risk adjustment (8,9). Try to make a quality determination about a hospital without risk adjustment, and the result is predictable: "Our patients are more complicated, sick, old, alcoholic, (and the latest) obese than yours." Because this might indeed be true, a risk-adjustment methodology that takes these factors into account, and thus levels the playing field, is critical. Importantly, the validity of the risk-adjustment methodology must be scrupulously addressed and its performance communicated to all involved. In this, trust is all-important.

To explain the risk-adjustment process, it is helpful to start with a "30,000-foot view." As was described, define and collect preoperative risk variables for each patient at each center. Determine and rank the ability of the preoperative variables to predict the collective endpoints (mortality and morbidity). On the basis of this assessment, construct a formula that best predicts the performance of all patients entered in the program. Once you establish this formula, you can apply it to an individual center's patients, using their respective preop variables so that an "expected" result for this specific set of patients is constructed in terms of 30-day mortality and morbidity. What actually happened is known, so you can express the two sets of results, observed and expected, in the form of a ratio, the O (observed) to E (expected) ratio. The observed-to-expected (O/E) ratio has become the accepted metric for outcomes results reporting.

This calculation brings up the question of which preoperative variables have been included. In the NSQIP, generic variables, potentially predictive of outcome and based on the literature, were chosen. Disease-specific and operative-specific variables were not included. Some otherwise important variables, such as EKG reports or chest x-ray reports, were not included because they could not be collected reliably at all sites.

Stepwise logistic regression models were used to develop the predictive models. Univariate t-tests or chi-square tests were first done to select variables that were related to 30-day mortality. These variables were then entered into stepwise logistic regression. The logistic regression model could then be applied to the data from each hospital to estimate the expected number of deaths from that hospital on the basis of the risk characteristics of its patients.

To test the predictive validity of the models, the samples were randomly divided into test and training samples. A C-index was then derived to reflect the predictability of the model in question. A C-index of 0.5 indicates no predictive value, whereas 1.0 indicates perfect predictive value. The models chosen in NSQIP show very high C-indices. New models are generated each reporting period, but the predictive variables, beta coefficients, and predictive validity have remained stable over many years. Table 7-2 shows the order of entry of most predictive preoperative risk variables in mortality models for noncardiac surgery.

We have shown in Table 7-4 an example of how logistic regression is used to calculate the probability of death for an individual patient and how the summed data for an institution results in an institutional O/E ratio (Table 7-5).

HOW RISK ADJUSTMENT INFLUENCES THE EVALUATION OF SURGICAL CARE QUALITY

One of the critical success factors of the NSQIP has been the support of participating surgeons. This support developed in part because surgeons trusted that valid risk adjustment would result in a fair comparative evaluation of surgical quality. In this regard, it is instructive to consider the evaluation of surgical care quality using both unadjusted and risk-adjusted institutional results. In Figure 7-1, unadjusted mortality rates are shown in the left panel and risk-adjusted rates for the same institutions are shown in the right panel. Institutions are ranked from 1 (best) to 44 (worst) in each panel. The crisscrossed lines indicate how perceptions about quality change with risk adjustment. Hospital 7, for example, is ranked relatively high in the nonadjusted panel but fares much worse when risk adjustment on its patient population is done. The conclusion, then, is that hospital 7 has a patient population that is significantly healthier than others and would have been expected to obtain excellent results but did not. In a separate review of 123 VA hospitals using this approach, Khuri et al. demonstrated that identification of

TABLE 7-4
CALCULATION OF O/E RATIOS

Following is an example of using the logistic regression model to predict the probability of death in a patient undergoing general surgery.

General Surgery: Probability (Death) $= \dfrac{e^{f(x)}}{1 + e^{f(x)}}$

Where $f(x) = -7.89 - (0.62 \times \text{albumin}) + (0.65 \times \text{ASA class})$
$+ (0.01 \times \text{BUN}) + (1.03 \times \text{disseminated cancer})$
$+ (1.01 \times \text{ascites}) + (0.03 \times \text{age}) + (0.56 \times \text{emergency})$

Patient #1: Albumin = 2.0 (3 SD below mean)
ASA = 4 (threat to life)
BUN + 102 (8 SD above mean)
Disseminated cancer = 0 (no)
Ascites = 1 (yes)
Age = 74
Emergency = 1 (yes)
$f(x) = -7.89 - 1.24 + 2.60 + 1.02 + 0.00 + 1.01 + 2.22 + 0.56 = -1.72$

$P(\text{Death}) = \dfrac{e^{-1.72}}{1 + e^{-1.72}} \quad = \quad \dfrac{.1791}{1 + .1791} = 15\%$

Patient #2: Albumin = 3.8 (average)
ASA = 1 (healthy)
BUN = 17 (average)
Disseminated cancer = 0 (no)
Ascites = 0 (no)
Age = 60 (average)
Emergency = 0 (no)
$f(x) = -7.89 - 2.36 + 0.65 + 0.17 + 0.00 + 0.00 + 1.80 + 0.00 = -7.63$

$P(\text{Death}) = \dfrac{e^{-7.63}}{1 + e^{-7.63}} \quad = \quad \dfrac{.0005}{1 + .0005} = 0.05\%$

BUN, blood urea nitrogen; ASA, American Society of Anesthesiology.

TABLE 7-5

HOW ARE THE O/E RATIOS CALCULATED FOR EACH INSTITUTION?

The observed-to-expected ratios are calculated for each institution as follows, using mortality as a hypothetical example. O/E ratios are not calculated unless there are a minimum of 50 cases that have been assessed in a subspecialty.

Patient No.	Actual Status P (death)	Alive = 0 Death = 1
1	0.15	1
2	0.0005	0
3	0.05	0
4	0.40	0
5	0.005	1
6	0.20	0
7	0.10	0
8	0.50	1
9	0.15	0
10	0.20	0
	Expected deaths	Observed deaths
	E = 1.8005	O = 3
	O/E RATIO = 3/1.8005 = 1.67	

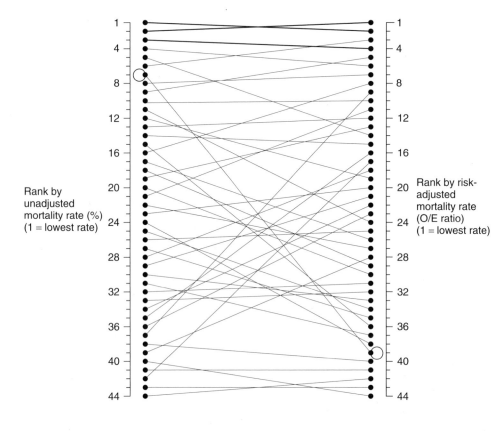

Figure 7-1 The left panel shows the best (1) to worst (44) unadjusted mortality rate. The right panel shows the best (1) to worst (44) hospitals ranked on the basis of observed-to-expected (O/E) mortality ratio. The rank of hospital 7 changed dramatically with risk adjustment.

Rank by unadjusted mortality rate (%) (1 = lowest rate)

Rank by risk-adjusted mortality rate (O/E ratio) (1 = lowest rate) high and low outliers by unadjusted mortality rates would have produced an incorrect "outlier" status (high or low) in 25 of 39 hospitals—an error rate of 64% (10).

RESULTS REPORTING USING THE O/E RATIO AT THE INSTITUTIONAL LEVEL

Having established an infrastructure that includes strict definitions, prospective data collection by trained nurse reviewers, and validated risk adjustment, it becomes possible to reliably rank the quality of care at different participating institutions. Figure 7-2 demonstrates how this comparative evaluation of quality is presented. "High" and "low" outliers are identified statistically by deviation from the expected O/E ratio of one. A "high" outlier hospital would be regarded as one that was experiencing more deaths and complications than would be expected on the basis of its patients' characteristics, and, conversely, a "low" outlier hospital would be regarded as demonstrating better results than would have been expected.

In order to show an actionable range of values, confidence intervals (CIs) of 90% were chosen for the mortality O/E ratio and 99% for morbidity, on the basis of the binomial distribution. When the CI includes the number 1, the observed and expected values are considered approximately equal. When the CI range is <1 (does not include 1), the institution is considered a "low" outlier. And, conversely, when the CI is >1 (does not include 1), the institution is considered a "high" outlier.

In the VA system, results are regularly reported for the combined surgical performance and for each of nine major subspecialties. Using this methodology, the department

TABLE 7-6
COMMUNICATION TO SERVICE CHIEFS

Communication Type	Performance
Commendation	Statistically significant "low outlier" in all operations model or two of four reporting periods
High-outlier status 1 (watch list)	Statistically significant "high outlier" for all operations model (and possibly some subspecialties) for most recent year
High-outlier status 2 (moderate concern)	Same as above, but for two reporting periods
High-outlier status 3 (serious concern)	Same as above, but for three reporting periods

leadership has at its disposal a reliable and continuous comparative evaluation of quality, which can be used for the patients' benefit.

At the national level, the NSQIP Executive Committee reviews performance of each institution annually. Institutions with "high" outlier status in mortality receive inquiries about results, with various levels of concern. Table 7-6 describes the warning system used to communicate concern to surgical chiefs. Service chiefs are asked to respond in writing about the institutional response to this concern and explain in detail what remedial steps they will implement. A level-2 concern requires a written explanation by the service chief to the Executive Committee. A level-3 concern mandates a site visit by members of the Executive Committee.

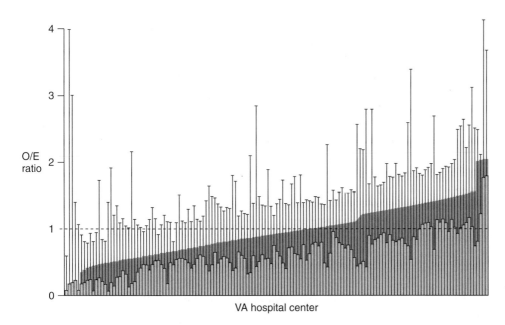

Figure 7-2   The y-axis shows the O/E ratio. On the x-axis, each bar represents a different VA hospital.

LINKING STRUCTURE AND PROCESS TO CLINICAL OUTCOME

The operant hypothesis in studies of surgical quality is that better outcomes reflect better institutional structure and process of care. Thus, an institution with a low-outlier O/E ratio would be assumed to have superior elements of structure, be they large operative volume, better nurse-staffing ratios, or technological resources, and true differences in process—for example, an increased use of perioperative beta-blockers to reduce the risk of postoperative myocardial infarction.

Relatively few surgical studies have focused on the validation of risk-adjusted outcomes by evaluating the associated structure and processes of care. The most prominent studies have centered on cardiac surgery. High-outlier and low-outlier hospitals were identified among hospitals performing cardiac surgery in New York State. Quality-of-care issues were identified by chart review in high-outlier hospitals significantly more often than in low-outlier hospitals (11). A review of administrative discharge data confirmed an association between a peer-review evaluation of care and risk-adjusted outcomes for cardiac surgery and angina but not for acute myocardial infarction or septicemia (12). Surgeons in six Northern New England medical centers identified associations between high-risk–associated mortality rates and structural and organizational aspects of a surgical practice, which include communications, aspects of decision-making training, and staff fatigue. More recently, the same group described associations between lower operative mortality and processes such as administration of aspirin, use of internal mammary grafts, and maintenance of a hematocrit over 24% during surgery (13).

The NSQIP has added importantly to this debate in two ways. First, the NSQIP added the evaluation of morbidity to the adverse outcomes possibly related to structure and process, in addition to mortality. Second, it structured an analysis by using site visits in which the site visiting team was blinded to the hospital's outlier status. This detailed and laborious experimental design validated that risk-adjusted outcomes have an important association with certain structures and processes of care (5).

Teams of reviewers (chief of surgery from a VA hospital, surgical nurse intensivist, and a member of the study team) were asked to evaluate the quality of a selected hospital using a structured protocol and scoring system. Seven dimensions of surgical care were considered: technology and equipment, technical competence of clinical staff, interface with clinical and support services, relationships with affiliated medical schools, monitoring of quality of care, communications, and coordination of work and leadership. Twenty carefully selected hospitals were evaluated. Hospitals were selected because of high-outlier O/E ratios for mortality ($n = 5$) and morbidity ($n = 5$), and for low-outlier O/E ratios for mortality ($n = 5$) and morbidity ($n = 5$). The examining teams had no knowledge of the hospital's outlier status, whether good or bad. The 2-day visit involved multiple interviews, tours of the OR recovery room and surgical nursing floors, "walk rounds" in the Surgical Intensive Care Unit (SICU), and many other areas.

When the study was completed, the site-review teams had correctly identified the outlier status of the examined hospital in 17 of 20 cases ($p < 0.05$). Low-outlier hospitals for mortality and morbidity were found to have significantly more equipment available in the SICU ($p < 0.05$). Scores for overall quality of care were higher for hospitals with low-outlier O/E ratios ($p < 0.05$), and technology was noted to be superior in low-outlier hospitals as well ($p < 0.001$).

In addition to the quantitative assessment, valuable information was gained from qualitative evaluation. For example, high-outlier hospitals used more per-diem nursing support (visitors, travelers) and tended to employ nurses with lower skill levels. Low-outlier hospitals demonstrated a high level of integration between VA faculty and faculty of the associated medical school and a close and functional relationship with internal medicine and cardiology. Low-outlier hospitals showed better use of information to develop quality improvement initiatives and had a closer and more developed interaction with nursing, manifested by frequent meetings and joint surgeon–nursing SICU rounds. The importance of good relationships and channels of communication was also noted for anesthesiology. Clinical supervision of surgical trainees was better in low-outlier hospitals. These quantitative and qualitative findings demonstrating a relationship between risk-adjusted outcomes and structure and process aspects of surgical care are important because they substantiate the use of risk-adjusted outcomes as a reasonable measure of quality, and they identify aspects of care that are associated with good results, many of which could be imported to high-outlier hospitals.

LINKING COORDINATION OF CARE TO CLINICAL OUTCOME: THE NSQIP EXPERIENCE

In the NSQIP system clinical outcomes are linked to process measures, as was described. A different question is whether clinical outcomes relate to care coordination, which is widely regarded as an important aspect of quality. For example, adverse events occurring in the hospital setting were strongly associated with failed or ineffective coordination among hospital staff (14). Coordination is a particularly important aspect of surgical quality because multiple interdependent units, including OR, ICU, recovery room, and patient care floors, and multiple interdependent groups of medical personnel, such as surgeons, nurses, anesthesiologists, and trainees, render care. An association between clinical outcomes and coordination of care enhances the validity of clinical outcomes as an important quality metric.

A recent study addressed this relationship between surgical care coordination and NSQIP outcome results (15). In this study coordination of care was considered in terms of programming and feedback. Programming refers to the clarification of work expectations, responsibilities, and activities prior to actual work. The development of clinical care guidelines would be a "programmed" aspect of care coordination. Feedback refers to communication between surgical services regarding performance—for example, results reporting to individuals or groups in routine mortality and morbidity conferences. Using 44 VA hospitals participating in the NSQIP, investigators surveyed hospital personnel with regard to levels of programming and feedback using a standardized survey instrument. Hospitals with measured high levels of programming and feedback showed statistically significant better clinical outcomes (lower O/E ratio) for morbidity, but not for mortality, as opposed to hospitals with the lowest levels of both programming and feedback. These data lend support to the idea that variables and outcomes measured in NSQIP are associated with coordination features of hospitals important in the prevention of postoperative morbidity and thus integral to quality.

MEASUREMENT AND QUALITY IMPROVEMENT

Mortality and morbidity rates have dropped dramatically in the decade since the NSQIP was instituted nationally in the VA system. Figures 7-3 and 7-4 show this important association.

But why did the results in the VA improve after initiation of the NSQIP quality measurement system? To be fair,

it is possible that the data-collection system simply recorded secular trends unrelated to NSQIP. Advances in anesthesia, technology, antibiotics, and improved patient selection could have been responsible. Only a randomized clinical trial on a hospital-by-hospital basis can authoritatively address the influence of NSQIP in improving the quality of surgical care, and such a study has not been done. Another possibility is that NSQIP affects quality by providing institutions with reliable results and providers are then motivated to improve, a "Hawthorne effect" in outcomes in the sense that something changes because it is being observed. Surgeons are competitive, and if they are told that they are not performing to expected levels (and believe the results), they will take whatever local action they believe to be effective. This can be seen as a passive effect of NSQIP. A third possibility is that improved results are subsequent to an active rather than passive role in quality improvement. For years NSQIP has examined the "best practices" in low-outlier hospitals and communicated this information to high-outlier hospitals. This more well-defined course of action seems logical and helpful, but the relative impact of any of the described possibilities cannot be absolutely known. Even if secular trends were responsible, it is important to note that the surgical community might not be aware that secular trends were causing surgical outcomes to improve in the absence of a reliable, nationally accepted data-collection system.

A concrete example of how the use of a national risk-adjusted data-collection and reporting system could improve patient care was recently reported (16). The NSQIP identified one VA as being a "high outlier" for morbidity in general surgery, and this information was communicated to the chief of surgery, who was otherwise

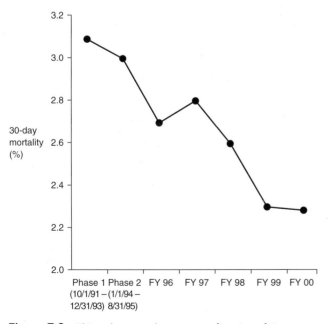

Figure 7-3   Thirty-day mortality rate as a function of time.

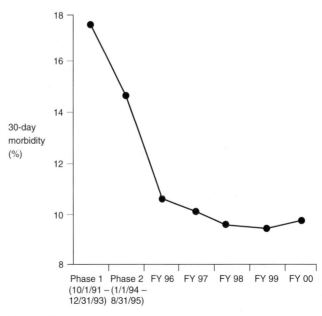

Figure 7-4   Thirty-day morbidity rate as a function of time.

unaware of a quality problem. Further, analysis of complications in general surgery reported to NSQIP was done. The data revealed a large number of wound infections as well as a seemingly high percentage of patients requiring prolonged ventilatory support. Each case with a complication reported by the NSQIP was then evaluated in detail. Cases with prolonged ventilatory support were judged to be explainable and consistent with good care, but the chief of surgery concluded that the incidence of wound complications was excessively high. A review of the surgical literature resulted in the creation of a "wound infection prevention protocol" based on an assessment of best practices. This protocol was subsequently implemented, with improved results. An analysis of practice patterns showed that surgical residents had been very aggressive about primary closure of contaminated wounds, based on the preference of previous surgeons, and relied upon careful inpatient inspection so that suspicious wounds could be opened promptly. The practice of surgery changed over time, length of stay (LOS) decreased, and wounds that would have otherwise been promptly opened presented to clinic with a wound infection. Thus, the reporting of quality data resulted in further analysis, process improvement, and improved results.

THE APPLICATION OF NSQIP TO THE PRIVATE SECTOR

The NSQIP has been an important contribution to the VA health-care delivery system, but the veteran population is in many important ways different from the "private sector" or patients in nonfederal hospitals. The VA population has far fewer women, less trauma, fewer emergency cases, and less hospital operative volume. An important evolutionary question for NSQIP was whether the same data-collection policies and procedures and the same risk-modeling techniques could be applied to different non-VA patient populations. The question is of obvious importance as strategy for a national surgical quality reporting system is discussed.

The question of applicability was addressed when three private-sector hospitals (University of Michigan, University of Kentucky, and Emory University) began collecting data on their patients using the NSQIP methodology in 1999. Over a one-year interval, they collected data on 2,747 patients, entered them in a website specifically created for this purpose, and analyzed them using the statistical risk-adjustment techniques used in the VA (17). When they applied the mortality model from the VA NSQIP to the non-VA patient population over the same interval, they obtained very high C-indices (0.934), indicating that the VA model predicted mortality in the non-VA patient population with a high degree of certainty. The C-indices for morbidity were somewhat lower (0.76) but still demonstrated important predictive value. Interestingly, in the morbidity model, the

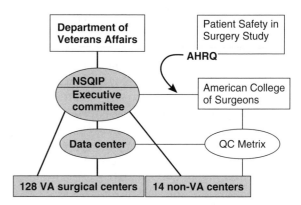

Figure 7-5 The relationship of Department of Veterans Affairs, the American College of Surgeons, and the NSQIP Executive Committee.

top five preoperative predictor variables were exactly the same in the VA and non-VA models (ASA class, contaminated wound, emergency class, abnormal albumin, complexity score).

This pilot data suggesting applicability to the private sector was then used to justify the creation of an expanded study group consisting of an additional 11 academic hospitals and four community hospitals. Funded by AHRQ, this group of 18 hospitals has participated in the Patient Safety in Surgery Study, an effort to measure the effect of a quality reporting system on overall mortality and morbidity. Although not completed, the accumulation of approximately 40,000 private-sector cases has allowed further comparisons to the VA model. These results have again documented convincingly that the NSQIP model can be used reliably in the private sector. The relationship of the Department of Veterans Affairs, The American College of Surgeons (a sponsor of the study), and the participating hospitals is shown in Figure 7-5. QC Metrix is a private data-collection and analytic unit created by NSQIP.

MAKING A BUSINESS CASE FOR QUALITY USING NSQIP

As NSQIP has moved into the private sector, the subject of cost has become more prominent. The use of clinical outcomes as a national measure of surgical quality has been criticized as being too expensive. Participating hospitals are required to hire a trained nurse reviewer whose only task is data collection and submission to NSQIP. When fringe benefits are included, a nurse salary might total $100,000 per year, depending on the region of the country. Licensing fees for the use of NSQIP methodology, the website, data reporting and analysis, and nurse education is estimated at ≈ $35,000. In this day of tightened belts in the health-care environment, $135,000 might seem too high a price for widespread implementation. A justification for this cost is needed.

One approach to justifying the investment in NSQIP is to evaluate the incidence and cost of surgical complications. Clearly, complications are expensive, but putting an actual dollar figure on a complication brings the subject into clearer focus. Preventive strategies can then be prioritized to the highest-cost complications. Preventing even a few of the costliest problems would justify the cost of data collection. Thomas et al. reviewed nonpsychiatric admissions to hospitals in Colorado and Utah in 1992 and found that the total cost of all adverse events was $661 million, which amounted to 4.8% of all health-care expenditures during that time period (18). Preventable operative complications accounted for 39% of costs, or $120 million. In another study, 66% of all adverse events were surgical and of these, 54% were preventable (19).

Although few would argue that preventing surgical complications would lower the cost of care, the NSQIP offers a mechanism that permits taking a more granular look at complications in a single hospital. This data would then be used, depending on the findings, to justify the $135,000 annual NSQIP outlay to hospital administrators. To do this, at our center we linked complications occurring in patients, as defined by NSQIP, to total costs using a proprietary cost-accounting software. We grouped surgical complications into four categories—respiratory, thromboembolic, cardiovascular, and infectious—for the analysis (20). Table 7-7 shows the results. Respiratory complications were by far the costliest postoperative problems, followed by thromboembolic, cardiovascular, and infectious. Because sick patients have more difficult operations and tend to get more complications, we used logistic regression analysis to adjust for procedure complexity and patient characteristics. Even then, the occurrence of a respiratory complication accounted for an additional $51,000 of cost to the institution.

If 54% of surgical complications are preventable, and the cost per complication is at this level, it is easy to argue that the prevention of only a few complications would justify the expense of NSQIP data collection. As mentioned earlier, the institution of NSQIP in the VA was associated with a 39% reduction in surgical morbidity, which supports this argument.

The business case for quality can also be made by considering the quality–cost relationship in a different way. The case is made that it is not quality alone, or cost alone, that is important but rather the value relationship,

$$\text{Value} = \frac{\text{Quality (NSQIP)}}{\text{Cost (TSI)}}$$

that is important. Previously, purchasers of health care have assumed, lacking good data, that quality was more or less equal among hospitals, so that purchasing decisions were made largely on the basis of cost. The NSQIP has the potential to put reliable numbers into the quality numerator, allowing purchasers to choose providers with the highest value, thus serving both employees and stockholders well.

NEXT STEPS IN THE EVOLUTION OF THE NSQIP

With strong backing from the American College of Surgeons and a successful pilot, a national effort to use risk-adjusted outcomes as measures of surgical quality is under way. Implementation of NSQIP in 150 private sector sites is envisaged over the course of 2 years. An Executive Committee will oversee NSQIP, and the ACS will administer it. For the first time a national risk-adjusted comparison of surgical quality will be available, including the VA, Department of Defense, and private-sector hospitals.

An additional step in the evolution of the NSQIP is decision support—that is, to get risk information to the care provider at the time that general strategy and the specific care plans are being outlined. Theoretically, this information will stimulate the surgeon to more consistently utilize national guidelines aimed at preventing complications. Considerable data exist to support the use of information technology to help in clinical decision support. A review of 68 controlled clinical trails found that two-thirds of physicians modified their behavior on the basis of decision support (21). Very few studies have focused on the surgical environment, however.

TABLE 7-7

FOUR COMPLICATION GROUPS

	Infectious	Cardiovascular	Respiratory	Thromboembolic
Unadjusted hospital costs (95% CI)	$8,209 ($5,566–$10,853)	$13,256 ($6,720–$19,799)	$54,430 ($51,770–$57,091)	$28,355 ($22,580–$34,130)
Adjusted for procedure complexity (95% CI)	$4,798 ($4,110–$5,486)	$13,330 ($11,579–$15,082)	$44,554 ($43,753–$45,356)	$15,727 ($14,004–$17,450)
Adjusted for complexity and patient characteristics (95%CI)	$2,207 ($1,301–$3,113)	$7,519 ($5,607–$9,437)	$51,409 ($49,868–$52,950)	$18,341 ($16,422–$20,259)

The NSQIP database is available to help in the decision support process. Over 1.2 million cases have now been entered into the NSQIP database. Models have been developed that stratify patients into risk categories for the occurrence of mortality or any of the 22 defined postoperative occurrences (22,23). The risk-stratification models can provide feedback to the surgeon electronically, indicating the level of risk assigned to major categories of complications. Those patients deemed "high-risk" might be further identified with a red flag "alert" mechanism. A link to accepted preventive guidelines would be provided. Because the involved electronic record keeping is relatively straightforward, surgeons using this technology would be able to see their practice patterns for the use of preventive practices in various risk categories and correlate this data with results. Likewise, the surgery chief would be able to view institutional conformance with clinical guidelines as data on surgical complications are reviewed.

A third evolutionary step in the development of the NSQIP is the addition of functional outcome data, in addition to mortality and morbidity. Health-services researchers, the medical community, and society at large are interested in the efficacy of surgical procedures, particularly on a risk-adjusted basis. In addition to cost data described previously, the functional data, for example, data from an SF-36 survey, can be put together with the more traditional elements of NSQIP to form an important backbone for future surgical research.

REFERENCES

1. Donabedian A. The end results of health care: Ernest Codman's contribution to quality assessment and beyond. *Milbank Q* 1989;67:233–256.
2. Donabedian A. *Exploration in quality assessment and monitoring*, Vol I. The Definition of Quality and Approaches to its Assessment. Ann Arbor, MI: Health Administration Press; 1980.
3. Khuri SF, Daley J, Henderson W, et al. Risk adjustment of the postoperative mortality rate for the comparative assessment of the quality of surgical care: results of the National Veterans Affairs Surgical Risk Study. *J Am Coll Surg* 1997;185:315–327.
4. Daley J, Khuri SF, Henderson W, et al. Risk adjustment of the postoperative morbidity rate for the comparative assessment of the quality of surgical care: results of the National Veterans Affairs Surgical Risk Study. *J Am Coll Surg* 1997;185:328–340.
5. Daley J, Forbes MG, Young GJ, et al. Validating risk-adjusted surgical outcomes: site visit assessment of process and structure. *J Am Coll Surg* 1997;185:341–351.
6. Khuri SF, Daley J, Henderson W, et al. The National Veterans Affairs Administration Surgical Risk Study: risk adjustment for the comparative assessment of the quality of surgical care. *J Am Coll Surg* 1995;180:519–531.
7. Best WR, Khuri SF, Phelen M. Identifying patient preoperative risk factors and postoperative adverse events in administrative databases: results of the Department of Veterans Affairs National Surgical Quality Improvement Program. *J Am Coll Surg* 2002; 194:257–266.
8. Iezzoni LI. *Risk adjustment for measuring health care outcomes*. Ann Arbor, MI: Health Administration Press; 1997.
9. Iezzoni LI. Using risk-adjusted outcomes to assess clinical practice: an overview of issues pertaining to risk adjustment. *Ann Thorac Surg* 1994;58:1822–1826.
10. Khuri SF, Daley J, Henderson W. The Department of Veterans Affairs' NSQIP: the first national, validated, outcome-based, risk-adjusted, and peer-controlled program for the measurement and enhancement of the quality of surgical care. *Ann Surg* 1998; 228:491–507.
11. Hannan EL, Kilburn H Jr., O'Donnell JF, et al. Adult open heart surgery in New York State. An analysis of risk factors and hospital mortality rates. *JAMA* 1990;264:2768–2774.
12. Thomas JW, Holloway JJ, Guire KE. Validating risk-adjusted mortality as an indicator of quality of care. *Inquiry* 1993;30: 6–22.
13. Peterson ED, DeLong ER, Jollis JG, et al. The effects of New York's bypass surgery provider profiling on access to care and patient outcomes in the elderly. *J Am Coll Cardiol* 1998; 32:993–999.
14. Andrews LB, Stocking C, Krizek T, et al. An alternative strategy for studying adverse events in medical care. *Lancet* 1997; 349:309–313.
15. Young GJ, Charns MP, Desai K, et al. Patterns of coordination and clinical outcomes: a study of surgical services. *Health Serv Res* 1998;33:1211–1236.
16. Neumayer L, Mastin M, Vanderhoof L, et al. Using the Veterans Administration national surgical quality improvement program to improve patient outcomes. *J Surg Res* 2000;88:58–61.
17. Fink AS, Campbell DA Jr., Mentzer RM Jr., et al. The national surgical quality improvement program in non-Veterans Administration hospitals: initial demonstration of feasibility. *Ann Surg* 2002;236:344–354.
18. Thomas EJ, Studdert DM, Newhouse JP, et al. Costs of medical injuries in Utah and Colorado. *Inquiry* 1999;36:255–264.
19. Gawande AA, Thomas EJ, Zinner MJ, et al. The incidence and nature of surgical adverse events in Colorado and Utah in 1992. *Surgery* 1999;126:66–75.
20. Dimick JB, Chen SL, Taheri PA, et al. Hospital costs associated with surgical complications: a report from the private sector NSQIP. *J Am Coll Surg* 2004:199;531–537.
21. Hunt DL, Haynes RB, Hanna SE, et al. Effects of computer based clinical decision support systems on physician performance and patient outcomes: a systematic review. *JAMA* 198;280: 1339–1346.

Management of
Surgical Complications

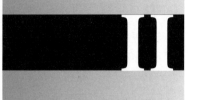

Assessment of

Perioperative Risk

8

Debabrata Mukherjee   *Kim A. Eagle*

■■■ **IDENTIFICATION OF RISK MARKERS 59**
Management of Specific Cardiovascular
    Conditions 60
Diagnostic Testing 62

■■■ **MODIFYING PREOPERATIVE RISK MARKERS 64**
Medical Therapy 65
Revascularization 66

■■■ **IDENTIFICATION OF POSTOPERATIVE COMPLICATIONS 67**

■■■ **MANAGEMENT OF COMPLICATIONS 67**

■■■ **CONCLUSION 67**

■■■ **REFERENCES 68**

In the United States approximately 25 million patients undergo noncardiac surgery every year. Of these, nearly 50,000 patients suffer perioperative myocardial infarction (MI), and cardiac events cause more than half of 40,000 perioperative deaths (1–3). Most perioperative cardiac morbidity and mortality is related to myocardial ischemia, congestive heart failure, or arrhythmias. Therefore, preoperative evaluation and management to reduce morbidity and mortality rates emphasize the detection, characterization, and treatment of coronary artery disease (CAD), left ventricular (LV) systolic dysfunction,

abnormal valve function, and significant arrhythmias. The purpose of preoperative evaluation is not to "clear" patients for surgery but to assess medical status and cardiac risks posed by the surgery planned and to recommend strategies to reduce risk. The preoperative evaluation has two goals: first, to identify patients at increased risk of an adverse perioperative cardiac event and, second, to modify cardiac risk to improve short-term and long-term clinical outcomes. This chapter reviews identification of risk markers preoperatively, opportunities for modifying risk, early identification of postoperative complications, and management of such complications. Its primary focus is on coronary artery and coronary heart disease because this problem dominates the clinical landscape.

IDENTIFICATION OF RISK MARKERS

The majority of patients at increased risk of adverse perioperative cardiac events can be identified using a simple bedside or office assessment. A careful history, physical examination, and review of the resting 12-lead electrocardiogram (ECG) are usually sufficient to allow stratification of most patients into low, intermediate, or high risk for an adverse perioperative cardiac event. Risk markers for adverse postoperative outcomes can be stratified as major, intermediate, and minor (Table 8-1) (4). Greater weight is given for active than for quiescent problems, and the severity of disease is used to modify its importance. Risk markers recognized as predictive of increased perioperative risk (4–7) include advanced age, poor functional capacity, and prior history or ECG evidence of CAD, congestive heart failure, arrhythmia, valvular heart

Debabrata Mukherjee: University of Kentucky, Lexington, KY 40536
Kim A. Eagle: University of Michigan, Ann Arbor, MI 48109

TABLE 8-1

CLINICAL PREDICTORS OF INCREASED PERIOPERATIVE CARDIOVASCULAR RISK

Major predictors
- Acute or recent myocardial infarction[a] with evidence of ischemia based on symptoms or noninvasive testing
- Unstable or severe[b] angina (Canadian class III or IV)
- Decompensated heart failure
- High-grade atrioventricular block
- Symptomatic ventricular arrhythmias with underlying heart disease
- Supraventricular arrhythmias with uncontrolled ventricular rate
- Severe valvular heart disease

Intermediate predictors
- Mild angina pectoris (class I or II)
- Prior MI by history or Q waves on ECG
- Compensated or prior heart failure
- Diabetes mellitus (particularly insulin-dependent)
- Renal insufficiency (creatinine ≥2.0 mg/dL)

Minor predictors
- Advanced age
- Abnormal ECG (left ventricular hypertrophy, left bundle branch block, ST –T abnormalities)
- Rhythm other than sinus (e.g., atrial fibrillation)
- Low functional capacity (inability to climb one flight of stairs with a bag of groceries)
- History of stroke
- Uncontrolled systemic hypertension

ECG, electrocardiogram.
[a]Recent myocardial infarction is defined as greater than 7 days but less than or equal to 1 month; acute myocardial infarction is within 7 days.
[b]May include stable angina in patients who are usually sedentary.
From Eagle KA, Berger PB, Calkins H, et al. ACC/AHA guideline update for perioperative cardiovascular evaluation for noncardiac surgery. *J Am Coll Cardiol* 2002;39:542–553, with permission.

disease, diabetes mellitus, uncontrolled systemic hypertension, renal insufficiency, and stroke.

Several features might be useful in the assessment of perioperative risk on physical examination. Patients with uncontrolled systemic hypertension should be identified and treated. Because congestive heart failure and valvular heart disease are associated with increased risk, physical findings suggestive of these diagnoses should be sought. The physical examination should include general appearance (cyanosis, pallor, dyspnea during conversation/minimal activity, Cheyne–Stokes respiration, poor nutritional status, obesity, skeletal deformities, tremor, and anxiety), blood pressure in arms, carotid pulses, extremity pulses, and ankle-brachial indices. Jugular venous pressure and positive hepatojugular reflex are reliable signs of volume overload in chronic heart failure, and pulmonary rales and chest x-ray evidence of pulmonary congestion correlate better with acute heart failure. Patients with aortic stenosis can be identified by a typical murmur and when accompanied by a diminished and delayed upstroke of the carotid or brachial pulse. Finally, the presence of carotid or other vascular bruits helps identify patients at increased risk of harboring occult CAD.

The type of surgery also has important implications for cardiac risk, and surgical procedures generally can be classified as having high, intermediate, and low cardiac risk on the basis of the likely degree and duration of hemodynamic stress during surgery and the potential correlation of the operation (e.g., vascular surgery) with concomitant coronary or other heart disease (Table 8-2). One can typically identify patients at very low clinical risk and patients at high clinical risk of an adverse perioperative cardiac event using the clinically available features described above. Patients at low clinical risk generally require no additional testing prior to noncardiac surgery. In patients undergoing elective noncardiac surgery in whom risk is determined to be intermediate or high, additional testing might be useful to better define risk (4). It is useful to employ a stepwise approach to the preoperative assessment of cardiac risk (Fig. 8-1).

Management of Specific Cardiovascular Conditions

Valvular Heart Disease

Severe aortic stenosis (valve area ≤1.0 cm^2) presents the greatest valve-associated cardiovascular risk for patients undergoing noncardiac surgery (4). The presence of fixed obstruction to LV outflow dramatically limits functional

TABLE 8-2

CARDIAC RISK STRATIFICATION FOR DIFFERENT TYPES OF SURGICAL PROCEDURES

High risk (Reported cardiac risk[a] >5%)
- Emergency major operations, particularly in the elderly
- Aortic, major vascular, and peripheral vascular surgery
- Extensive operations with large volume shifts or blood loss, or both

Intermediate risk (Reported cardiac risk <5%)
- Intraperitoneal or intrathoracic
- Carotid endarterectomy
- Head and neck surgery
- Orthopedic
- Prostate

Low risk[b] (Reported cardiac risk <1%)
- Endoscopic procedures
- Superficial biopsy
- Cataract
- Breast surgery

[a]Combined incidence of cardiac death and nonfatal myocardial infarction.
[b]Do not generally require further preoperative cardiac testing.
From Eagle KA, Berger PB, Calkins H, et al. ACC/AHA guideline update for perioperative cardiovascular evaluation for noncardiac surgery. *J Am Coll Cardiol* 2002;39:542–553, with permission.

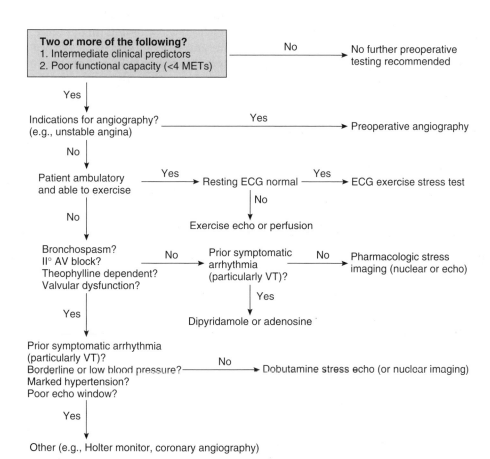

Figure 8-1 Supplemental preoperative evaluation: when and which test? a. Testing is only indicated if the results will impact care. b. Please refer to Table 8-1 for a list of clinical predictors and Table 8-2 for the definition of high-risk surgical procedures. c. Patients should be able to achieve more than or equal to 85% maximum predicted heart rate (MPHR). d. In the presence of left bundle branch block, vasodilator perfusion imaging is preferred. ECG, electrocardiogram; VT, ventricular tachycardia; METs, metabolic equivalents. (From Eagle KA, Berger PB, Calkins H, et al. ACC/AHA guideline update for perioperative cardiovascular evaluation for noncardiac surgery. *J Am Coll Cardiol* 2002;39:542–553, with permission.)

cardiac reserve and might be associated with intracavitary LV pressures in excess of 300 mm Hg. Accompanying LV hypertrophy predisposes the patient to diastolic dysfunction and pulmonary congestion. In general, aortic stenosis that is severe or symptomatic, or both, should be addressed prior to the patient's undergoing elective noncardiac surgery. In most cases aortic valve replacement is indicated as the definitive therapy of choice (8). If cardiac surgery is contraindicated, percutaneous aortic balloon valvotomy can be used to mitigate LV outflow obstruction, even if only as a temporizing measure. When neither surgery nor percutaneous aortic valvotomy is considered feasible, noncardiac surgery with careful hemodynamic assessment might still be appropriate, albeit with a heightened risk of perioperative death with a mortality risk of approximately 10% (9,10).

Mitral stenosis, when mild and asymptomatic, can usually be managed medically with heart rate control. Severe mitral stenosis should be corrected to prolong survival and patient complications, unrelated to the proposed noncardiac surgery, in accordance with American College of Cardiology (ACC)/American Heart Association (AHA) guidelines on management of vascular heart disease. In general, aortic and mitral regurgitation lesions are better tolerated perioperatively than stenotic lesions. Medical regimens for these individuals should be optimized preoperatively with diuretics and afterload reduction with vasodilators. Appropriate prophylaxis for bacterial endocarditis is indicated in patients with valvular heart disease and prosthetic heart valves. Appropriate perioperative antithrombotic therapy for patients with prosthetic heart valves is outlined in Table 8-3.

Cardiac Arrhythmias

In individuals with arrhythmias, a metabolic profile and the list of medications should be carefully reviewed and corrected. Even mild hypokalemia should be corrected in these individuals. Sustained or symptomatic ventricular arrhythmias should be treated with suppressive therapy. Patients with symptomatic bradyarrhythmias should be treated with temporary pacing and a permanent pacemaker implanted when indicated. If an individual already has a permanent pacemaker, this should be checked prior to surgery. Electrocautery should be minimized in patients who are totally pacemaker dependent, and pacemakers should be checked again after surgery to ensure that the settings are optimal. Typically, implanted defibrillators are turned off during surgery and turned back on afterward.

Hypertension

Mild to moderate hypertension should be managed with medical therapy and should be closely monitored during surgery. Individuals with severe hypertension (diastolic >110 mm) need control prior to surgery. For urgent surgery in patients with severe hypertension, intravenous agents might be used to achieve control of blood pressure. Abrupt withdrawal of β-blockers and clonidine should be avoided to prevent rebound hypertension.

Cardiomyopathy

Pulmonary artery catheters might be beneficial in patients with severe LV dysfunction. Close monitoring of the volume status, heart rate, and systemic vascular resistance is indicated in patients with hypertrophic cardiomyopathy. Intravascular volume depletion is poorly tolerated in these patients and might result in cardiogenic shock.

Diagnostic Testing

Routine laboratory tests such as serum creatinine, hemoglobin, platelet count, potassium level, liver profile, and

---

TABLE 8-3

ANTITHROMBOTIC THERAPY IN THE PERIOPERATIVE SETTING IN PATIENTS WITH PROSTHETIC HEART VALVES

- Very low risk surgery (dental work, superficial biopsy)
    - Briefly reduce the INR to low or subtherapeutic range and resume normal dose post-procedure

- High risk for thrombosis [recent (<1 year) thromboembolism, Bjork Shiley valve especially in mitral position, or ≥3 of the following risk factors: atrial fibrillation (A Fib), previous embolism, hypercoagulable condition, mechanical prosthesis, and LVEF <30%]
- Stop warfarin 72 hours prior to procedure
- Start heparin when INR ≤2.0
- Stop heparin 6 hours after the procedure
- Restart heparin within 24 hours and continue until INR ≥2.0

- Approach for patients between these two extremes
    - Physicians must assess the risk and benefit of reduced anticoagulation vs. perioperative heparin therapy

INR, international normalized ratio; LVEF, left ventricular ejection fraction.
From Eagle KA, Berger PB, Calkins H, et al. ACC/AHA guideline update for perioperative cardiovascular evaluation for noncardiac surgery. *J Am Coll Cardiol* 2002;39:542–553, with permission.

oxygen saturation are important in risk stratification. Arterial blood gas analysis is useful in patients with advanced pulmonary disease. A 12-lead ECG provides important prognostic information. Patients who are at low risk on the basis of history, physical examination, and routine laboratory tests might not need further evaluation. Noninvasive testing is primarily useful in intermediate-risk patients. The perioperative guidelines are straightforward about recommendations for patients about to undergo emergency surgery, the presence of prior cardiac revascularization, and the occurrence of major cardiac predictors. However, the majority of patients have either intermediate or minor clinical predictors of increased perioperative cardiovascular risk. Table 8-4 presents a shortcut approach to a large number of patients in whom the decision to recommend testing before surgery can be difficult. Essentially, if two of the three listed factors in Table 8-4 are true, we recommend consideration of the use of noninvasive cardiac testing as part of the pre-operative evaluation. In any patient with an intermediate clinical predictor, the presence of either a low functional capacity or high surgical risk should lead the physician to consider noninvasive testing. In the absence of intermediate clinical predictors, noninvasive testing should be considered when both the surgical risk is high and the functional capacity is low. Clinical predictors are defined in Table 8-1.

In most ambulatory patients the test of choice is exercise ECG testing, which can both provide an estimate of functional capacity and detect myocardial ischemia through changes in the ECG and hemodynamic response. The ability to exercise moderately beyond 4 to 5 metabolic equivalents (METs) without symptoms defines low risk. Patients who can achieve >85% of maximum predicted heart rate (MPHR) without EKG changes are at lowest risk. Patients with an abnormal EKG response at >70% of predicted heart rate are at intermediate risk and those with abnormal EKG response at <70% of predicted heart rate are at highest risk. It must be emphasized that although routine EKG stress testing has a sensitivity to identify one-vessel CAD of just 55% to 60%, its sensitivity for left main or advanced

three-vessel disease is far higher, in the 85% to 90% range. Thus, for the purposes of identifying the highest risk population, it is quite reasonable.

In patients with important abnormalities on their resting ECG [e.g., left bundle branch block (LBBB), LV hypertrophy with "strain" pattern, or digitalis effect], other techniques such as exercise echocardiography, exercise myocardial perfusion imaging, or pharmacological stress imaging might be indicated. Pharmacologic stress or perfusion imaging is indicated in patients undergoing orthopedic, neurosurgical, or vascular surgery who are unable to exercise or have LBBB/paced rhythm. The sensitivity and specificity of exercise thallium scans in the presence of LBBB are low, and overall diagnostic accuracy varies from 36% to 60% (11,12). In contrast, the use of vasodilator (dipyridamole/adenosine) nuclear stress testing in such patients has a sensitivity of 98%, a specificity of 84%, and a diagnostic accuracy of 88% to 92% (13–15). Thus, in patients with LBBB, dipyridamole or adenosine thallium imaging are the preferred methods.

In patients unable to perform adequate exercise, as with most patients with peripheral vascular disease (PVD), a nonexercise stress test should be used. In this regard, dipyridamole myocardial perfusion imaging testing and dobutamine echocardiography are the most commonly used tests. Intravenous dipyridamole should be avoided in patients with significant bronchospasm, critical carotid disease, or a condition that prevents their being withdrawn from theophylline preparations. Dobutamine should not be used as a stressor in patients with serious arrhythmias or severe hypertension or hypotension. For patients in whom echocardiographic image quality is likely to be poor, a myocardial perfusion study is more appropriate. If there is an additional question about valvular diseases, the echocardiographic stress test might be more useful. Often either stress perfusion or stress echocardiography is appropriate. In a meta-analysis of dobutamine stress echocardiography, ambulatory ECG, radionuclide ventriculography, and dipyridamole thallium scanning in predicting adverse

---

TABLE 8-4

GUIDE TO NONINVASIVE TESTING IN PREOPERATIVE PATIENTS IF ANY TWO FACTORS ARE PRESENT

1. Intermediate clinical predictors (Canadian class I or II angina, prior MI based on history or pathological Q waves, compensated or prior HF, or diabetes)
2. Poor functional capacity (<4 METs)
3. High surgical risk procedure (emergency major surgery[a], aortic repair or peripheral vascular, prolonged surgical procedures with large fluid shifts or blood loss)

MI, myocardial infarction; HF, heart failure; METs, metabolic equivalents.
[a]Emergency major operations might require immediately proceeding to surgery without sufficient time for noninvasive testing or preoperative interventions.
From Eagle KA, Berger PB, Calkins H, et al. ACC/AHA guideline update for perioperative cardiovascular evaluation for noncardiac surgery. *J Am Coll Cardiol* 2002;39:542–553, with permission.

cardiac outcome after vascular surgery, all tests had a similar predictive value, with overlapping confidence intervals (16). Another meta-analysis of 15 studies demonstrated that the prognostic value of noninvasive stress-imaging abnormalities for perioperative ischemic events is comparable between available techniques but that the accuracy varies with CAD prevalence (17). The expertise of the local laboratory in identifying advanced coronary disease is quite important in choosing the appropriate test.

Dipyridamole thallium stress testing to risk-stratify patients with suspected CAD is particularly effective before vascular surgery. Boucher et al. (18) reported on the utility of dipyridamole thallium imaging in the preoperative assessment of cardiac risk in patients with PVD. They evaluated 48 patients with suspected CAD before they underwent vascular surgery; 16 of these patients had thallium redistribution. All eight perioperative cardiac events occurred in patients who had preoperative thallium redistribution. Leppo et al. (19) performed dipyridamole thallium imaging in 100 consecutive patients admitted for elective peripheral vascular surgery and determined that the presence of thallium redistribution was the most significant predictor of serious nonfatal MI or cardiac death. The odds for a serious cardiac event were 23 times greater in a patient with thallium redistribution than in a patient without redistribution, strongly suggesting that myocardial imaging might be used as a primary screening test before elective vascular surgery (19). Many subsequent studies have confirmed the findings of these early papers. A meta-analysis by Shaw et al. (17) analyzed the results of 10 articles and 1994 vascular surgery candidates over a 9-year period. Cardiac death or nonfatal MI occurred in 1%, 7%, and 9% of patients with normal results, fixed defects, and reversible defects on thallium scans, respectively, demonstrating the utility of dipyridamole thallium scintigraphy for preoperative risk stratification.

The extent and severity of perfusion defects play a significant role in adverse perioperative events, as the more extensive the perfusion abnormalities or the finding of cavity dilation or thallium lung uptake, the worse the perioperative prognosis. Although the immediate purpose of preoperative examination is to assess the risk associated with the planned surgical procedure, the determination of long-term prognosis might be valuable in the overall management of a patient with known or suspected CAD. By using adenosine-sestamibi stress imaging, clinicians can assess both perfusion as well as regional and overall LV function. Thus, this form of nuclear cardiac imaging has largely superseded thallium imaging.

Dobutamine stress echocardiography has also been successfully used to identify patients at risk for cardiac complications of surgery, with very high negative predictive values. In a meta-analysis, patients with no dobutamine-induced wall-motion abnormalities had a very low event rate (0.4%), compared with a 23.4% event rate in patients who developed new wall-motion abnormalities during dobutamine infusion. Dobutamine stress echocardiography has also been shown to provide prognostic value for predicting late events after vascular surgery. Furthermore, like dipyridamole thallium imaging, the most useful role for stress echocardiography appears to be in patients at intermediate clinical risk.

For patients at high risk it might be appropriate to proceed with coronary angiography rather than perform a noninvasive test. For high-risk patients with contraindications to angiography or coronary revascularization, medical therapy with aggressive β-blockade might be the correct approach (20). In patients with unstable angina or evidence of residual ischemia after recent MI, direct coronary angiography might be indicated. In general, indications for preoperative coronary angiography are similar to those identified for the nonoperative setting (Table 8-5).

Combined Clinical and Scintigraphic Assessment

Although the sensitivity of dipyridamole thallium imaging for detecting patients at increased risk is excellent, one of its limitations for preoperative screening is its low specificity and positive predictive value. In order to improve the value of risk stratification, many reports have suggested utilization of the combination of clinical markers and noninvasive test results. Eagle et al. (20) first reported on using assessment of clinical markers (history of angina, MI, congestive heart failure, diabetes, and Q wave on ECG) and thallium redistribution to identify a low-risk subset of patients. The authors demonstrated that patients without any of these clinical markers did not require dipyridamole thallium testing. However, thallium redistribution had a significant predictive value in patients with 1 to 2 clinical risk factors. Within this group, two of 62 (3.2%; 95% CI, 0% to 8%) patients without thallium redistribution had events, compared with 16 events in 54 patients (29.6%; 95% CI, 16% to 44%) with thallium redistribution (20). L'Italien et al. (21) reported the results of a Bayesian model for perioperative risk assessment that combined clinical variables with dipyridamole thallium findings. This analysis examined the type of procedure, specific institutional complication rates, and other clinical factors in a sequential manner followed by the addition of the dipyridamole thallium findings. The addition of dipyridamole thallium data reclassified >80% of the moderate risk patients into low-risk (3%) and high-risk (19%) categories (p <0.0001) but provided no stratification for patients classified as low or high risk according to the clinical model.

MODIFYING PREOPERATIVE RISK MARKERS

CAD is responsible for the majority of life-threatening perioperative cardiac complications. Once recognized, specific therapy should be instituted to minimize the risk of

TABLE 8-5

AMERICAN COLLEGE OF CARDIOLOGY/AMERICAN HEART ASSOCIATION RECOMMENDATIONS REGARDING CORONARY ANGIOGRAPHY BEFORE/AFTER NONCARDIAC SURGERY

Class I: patients with suspected or known CAD (strongly recommended)
- Evidence for high risk of adverse outcome based on noninvasive test results
- Angina unresponsive to adequate medical therapy
- Unstable angina, particularly when facing intermediate-risk or high-risk noncardiac surgery
- Equivocal noninvasive test results in patients at high clinical risk undergoing high-risk surgery

Class IIa (weight of evidence/opinion is in favor of usefulness/efficacy)
- Multiple markers of intermediate clinical risk and planned vascular surgery (noninvasive testing should be considered first)
- Moderate to large ischemia on noninvasive testing but without high-risk features and lower LVEF
- Nondiagnostic noninvasive test results in patients of intermediate clinical risk undergoing high-risk noncardiac surgery
- Urgent noncardiac surgery while convalescing from acute MI

Class IIb (usefulness/efficacy is less well established by evidence/opinion)
- Perioperative MI
- Medically stabilized class III or IV angina and planned low-risk or minor surgery

Class III (contraindicated)
- Low-risk noncardiac surgery with known CAD and no high-risk results on noninvasive testing
- Asymptomatic after coronary revascularization with excellent exercise capacity (≥7 METs)
- Mild stable angina with good left ventricular function and no high-risk noninvasive test results
- Noncandidate for coronary revascularization owing to concomitant medical illness, severe left ventricular dysfunction (e.g., LVEF <0.20), or refusal to consider revascularization
- Candidate for liver, lung, or renal transplant >40 years old as part of evaluation for transplantation, unless noninvasive testing reveals high risk for adverse outcome

CAD, coronary artery disease; LVEF, left ventricular ejection fraction; MI, myocardial infarction; METs, metabolic equivalents.
From Eagle KA, Berger PB, Calkins H, et al. ACC/AHA guideline update for perioperative cardiovascular evaluation for noncardiac surgery. *J Am Coll Cardiol* 2002;39:542–553, with permission.

perioperative myocardial ischemia, MI, or death. Several studies have addressed the effect of anti-ischemic medical therapy on perioperative prognosis (22).

Medical Therapy

β-blockers

Several studies have evaluated the effectiveness of β-blockers in reducing perioperative cardiac risk. The first randomized, placebo-controlled study used atenolol in 200 high-risk patients scheduled to undergo noncardiac surgery, including vascular, orthopedic, intra-abdominal, and neurosurgical procedures (23). Atenolol was administered either intravenously or orally 2 days preoperatively and continued for 7 days postoperatively. The incidence of perioperative ischemia was significantly lower in the atenolol group than in the placebo group (23,24). There was no difference in the incidence of perioperative MI or death from cardiac causes, but the rate of event-free survival at 6 months was higher in the atenolol group.

Poldermans et al. studied the perioperative use of bisoprolol in elective major vascular surgery (25). Bisoprolol was started at least 7 days preoperatively, the dose adjusted to achieve a resting heart rate of <60 beats per minute and continued for 30 days postoperatively. The study was confined to patients who had at least one cardiac risk factor (a history of congestive heart failure, prior MI, diabetes, angina pectoris, heart failure, age >70 years, or poor functional status) and evidence of inducible myocardial ischemia on dobutamine echocardiography. Patients with extensive regional wall-motion abnormalities were excluded. Bisoprolol was associated with a 91% reduction in the perioperative risk of MI or death from cardiac causes from 34% to 4% in this high-risk population. Because of the selection criteria used in this trial, the efficacy of bisoprolol in the group at very highest risk—those in whom coronary revascularization or modification would be considered or for whom the surgical procedure might ultimately be cancelled—cannot be determined. The rate of events in the standard-care group of 34% suggests that all but the patients at highest risk were enrolled in the trial.

Urban et al. evaluated the role of prophylactic β-blockers in patients undergoing elective total knee arthroplasty (26). They preoperatively randomized 107 patients into two groups, control and β-blockers, who received postoperative esmolol infusions on the day of surgery and metoprolol for the next 48 hours to maintain a heart rate <80 bpm. The number of ischemic events (control, 50 minutes; β-blockers, 16 minutes) and total ischemic time (control, 709 minutes; β-blockers, 236 minutes) were significantly lower with esmolol compared to the control group. In this study prophylactic β adrenergic blockade administered after elective total knee arthroplasty was associated with a reduced prevalence and duration of postoperative myocardial ischemia detected with Holter monitoring (26). Thus, β-blockers have been demonstrated to be effective in reducing periprocedural complications in patients undergoing a wide range of surgical procedures.

Alpha 2-adrenergic Agonists

The effect of α 2-adrenergic agonists has also been studied in the perioperative period. Several small, randomized studies comparing clonidine with placebo failed to demonstrate that clonidine was effective in reducing the rates of MI and death from cardiac causes (16,27). Mivazerol, an intravenous α 2-adrenergic agonist administered by continuous infusion, was compared to placebo in patients with known coronary disease or risk factors for it who underwent major vascular or orthopedic procedures. Mivazerol was found to have no overall effect on the rates of cardiac complications (28). However, in the predefined subgroup of patients with known CAD who underwent major vascular surgery, mivazerol was associated with a significantly lower incidence of MI and death from cardiac causes. Some institutions in Europe use this agent, but it has not been available in the United States.

Calcium Channel Blockers and Nitrates

There are no large randomized trials of either nitrates or calcium channel antagonists in terms of reducing perioperative MI or cardiac death. Therefore, their use in the perioperative setting should mirror that in general cardiology practice. They are second-line agents to β-blockers for the control of angina or stress-induced ischemia. If a patient has required either or both to control ischemia, that drug should be continued perioperatively.

Statins

HMG CoA reductase inhibitors (statins) have been shown to reduce ischemic events, stroke, and cardiac death in patients with established atherosclerosis. Recently, in patients undergoing vascular surgery, several reports suggest statins might reduce perioperative coronary events (29). Because stains are known to reduce atherosclerotic plaque formation and growth and potentially stabilize plaques that have been pre-existent, it is not entirely surprising that they can reduce the risk of coronary plaque rupture and thrombosis during or after the stresses of vascular surgery. Further studies are needed to determine how long the statins must be given before a perioperative benefit can be realized.

Revascularization

Percutaneous Revascularization

No randomized trials of preoperative coronary revascularization have been performed, but several retrospective cohort studies have been published. Percutaneous coronary intervention (PCI) utilizing primarily balloon angioplasty has been evaluated in three studies of patients who were undergoing noncardiac surgery (30–32). The indications for PCI were not well described in the studies but most likely included the need to relieve symptomatic angina or reduce the perioperative risk of ischemia identified by noninvasive testing. All three studies had a low incidence of cardiac complications after noncardiac surgery, but no comparison groups were included.

One study used an administrative database of patients who were undergoing noncardiac surgery in Washington State. As compared with patients who did not undergo PCI preoperatively, those who did undergo the procedure had a lower incidence of perioperative cardiac complications (33). The benefit of revascularization was most apparent in the group that underwent PCI at least 90 days before noncardiac surgery. In contrast, when revascularization was performed within 90 days before noncardiac surgery, PCI was not associated with an improved outcome. This finding would suggest that PCI should not be used solely as a means of reducing perioperative risk. Coronary stents are now used in >80% of PCI, and use of stents during PCI presents unique challenges because of the risk of coronary thrombosis and bleeding during the initial recovery phase. In a cohort of 40 patients who received stents within 30 days of noncardiac surgery, all eight deaths and seven MIs, as well as eight of 11 bleeding episodes, occurred in patients who had undergone surgery within 14 days after stent placement (34). The complications appeared to be related to serious bleeding resulting from postprocedural anticoagulant therapy or to coronary thrombosis in those who did not receive 4 full weeks of antithrombotic therapy after stenting. In general, one should wait at least 2 weeks, and preferably 6 weeks, after coronary stenting to perform noncardiac surgery in order to allow complete endothelization and a full course of dual antiplatelet therapy to be given (35). Poststenting therapy currently includes a combination of aspirin and clopidogrel for at least 4 weeks, followed by aspirin for an indefinite period.

Coronary Artery Bypass Grafting

Coronary artery bypass grafting (CABG) has also been recommended to reduce the incidence of perioperative cardiac complications in highly selected patients. Evidence of a potential protective effect of preoperative CABG comes from follow-up studies of randomized trials and registries comparing medical and surgical therapy for CAD. The largest study to date included 3,368 noncardiac operations performed within a 10-year period among patients assigned to medical therapy or CABG in the Coronary Artery Surgery Study (36). Prior successful CABG had a cardio-protective effect among patients who underwent high-risk noncardiac surgery (abdominal, thoracic, vascular, or orthopedic surgery) (36). The perioperative mortality rate was nearly 50% lower in the group of patients who had undergone CABG than in those who received medical therapy (3.3% vs. 1.7%, $p <0.05$). There was no difference in the outcome of patients undergoing low-risk procedures such as breast or urologic surgery.

Fleisher et al. used Medicare claims data to assess 30-day and 1-year mortality after noncardiac surgery according to the use of cardiac testing and coronary interventions such as CABG and PCI within the year before noncardiac surgery (37). Preoperative revascularization significantly reduced the 1-year mortality rate for patients undergoing aortic surgery but had no effect on the mortality rate for those undergoing infrainguinal surgeries. Finally, an analysis of the Bypass Angioplasty Revascularization Investigation (BARI) evaluated the incidence of postoperative cardiac complications after noncardiac surgery among patients with multivessel coronary disease who were randomly assigned to undergo PCI or CABG for severe angina (38). At an average of 29 months after coronary revascularization, both groups had similar, low rates of postoperative MI or death from cardiac causes (1.6% in each group). These data suggest that prior successful coronary revascularization, when accompanied by careful follow-up and therapy for subsequent coronary symptoms or signs, is associated with a low rate of cardiac events after noncardiac surgery (38).

IDENTIFICATION OF POSTOPERATIVE COMPLICATIONS

In patients with known or suspected CAD, ECGs should be obtained at baseline, immediately after surgery, and on the first 2 days after surgery. Biomarkers such as CK-MB or troponin, or both, should be measured in high-risk patients after surgery and the following day. Current guidelines also recommend cardiac troponin measurements 24 hours postoperatively and on day 4 or hospital discharge (whichever comes first) in high-risk and intermediate-risk patients (4). The diagnosis of MI should be entertained when the typical cardiac biomarker profile is manifest in the immediate postoperative phase in combination with either symptom, suggesting myocardial ischemia or ECG changes of ischemia, or both. The possibility of perioperative ischemia or MI can then be estimated on the basis of the magnitude of biomarker elevation, new ECG abnormalities, hemodynamic instability, and quality and intensity of chest pain or other symptoms.

MANAGEMENT OF COMPLICATIONS

Despite optimal perioperative management, some patients will experience perioperative MI, which is associated with 40% to 70% mortality. The reason for the high mortality is multifactorial and largely related to substantial comorbidity in such patients. Patients who develop ST-elevation MI should be considered for urgent coronary reperfusion, whereas patients with non-ST-elevation MI should undergo risk stratification after initial stabilization with intensive medical therapy. Individuals who develop heart failure after surgery should be evaluated for the etiology of heart failure and treated on the basis of the precipitating or underlying cause. Immediate coronary angioplasty is feasible and beneficial in patients with ST-elevation MI. However, time to reperfusion is a critical determinant of outcome in acute MI, and any hope of benefiting patients who have a perioperative acute MI because of an acute coronary occlusion requires that revascularization be rapidly performed (i.e., within 12 hours of symptom onset). Because fibrinolytics are usually contraindicated in this circumstance and dual antiplatelet therapy might not be ideal either, balloon angioplasty without stenting often represents the best strategy.

Although immediate reperfusion therapy is an important therapy in acute ST-segment–elevation MI, the emphasis on reperfusion therapy should not detract from pharmacological therapy, which is also very important and has been shown to reduce adverse events in such patients, as well as in patients with non-ST-elevation acute coronary syndromes. Therapy with aspirin, a β-blocker, and often an ACE inhibitor, particularly for patients with low ejection fractions or anterior infarctions, should be administered where possible. Patients who sustain acute myocardial injury in the perioperative or postoperative period should receive careful medical evaluation for residual ischemia and overall LV function. In all cases the appropriate evaluation and management of complications and coronary risk factors such as angina, heart failure, hypertension, hyperlipidemia, cigarette smoking, diabetes (hyperglycemia), and other cardiac abnormalities should commence before hospital discharge. Most post-MI patients should also receive a statin at discharge.

CONCLUSION

Appropriate preoperative evaluation and therapy might significantly improve periprocedural and long-term outcomes. Successful management of high-risk patients requires an integrated "team" approach among surgeons, anesthesiologists, cardiologists, and generalists. In general, indications for further cardiac testing and revascularization are the same as in the nonoperative setting. In the absence of contraindications, β-blocker therapy should be considered in all patients at high risk for coronary events who are scheduled to undergo noncardiac surgery. For many patients, evaluation prior to noncardiac surgery might be the first comprehensive assessment of their short-term and long-term cardiac risk and provides an opportunity not only to decrease their immediate periprocedural risk but also to improve their long-term outcomes with appropriate evidence-based therapies. Early identification and appropriate management of postoperative complications is important and might prevent fatality.

REFERENCES

1. Mangano DT. Perioperative cardiac morbidity. *Anesthesiology* 1990;72:153–184.
2. National Center for Health Statistics. *Vital statistics of the United States: 1980*, Vol 2, Mortality (PHS) 85-1101. Hyattsville, MD: NCHS U.S. Public Health Service; 1985:2.
3. National Center for Health Statistics. *Vital statistics of the United States: 1988*, Vol 3, (PHS) 89-1232. Washington, DC: NCHS U.S. PHS; 1989:10–17, 66, 67, 100, 101.
4. Eagle KA, Berger PB, Calkins H, et al. ACC/AHA guideline update for perioperative cardiovascular evaluation for noncardiac surgery. *J Am Coll Cardiol* 2002;39:542–553.
5. Mukherjee D, Eagle KA. A common sense approach to perioperative evaluation. *Am Fam Physician* 2002;66:1824, 1826.
6. Mukherjee D, Eagle KA. Cardiac risk in noncardiac surgery. *Minerva Cardioangiol* 2002;50:607–619.
7. Mukherjee D, Eagle KA. Perioperative cardiac assessment for noncardiac surgery: eight steps to the best possible outcome. *Circulation* 2003;107:2771–2774.
8. Logeais Y, Langanay T, Roussin R, et al. Surgery for aortic stenosis in elderly patients. A study of surgical risk and predictive factors. *Circulation* 1994;90:2891–2898.
9. Raymer K, Yang H. Patients with aortic stenosis: cardiac complications in non-cardiac surgery. *Can J Anaesth* 1998;45:855–859.
10. Torsher LC, Shub C, Rettke SR, et al. Risk of patients with severe aortic stenosis undergoing noncardiac surgery. *Am J Cardiol* 1998;81:448–452.
11. DePuey EG, Guertler-Krawczynska E, Robbins WL. Thallium-201 SPECT in coronary artery disease patients with left bundle branch block. *J Nucl Med* 1988;29:1479–1485.
12. Larcos G, Gibbons RJ, Brown ML. Diagnostic accuracy of exercise thallium-201 single-photon emission computed tomography in patients with left bundle branch block. *Am J Cardiol* 1991; 68:756–760.
13. Rockett JF, Wood WC, Moinuddin M, et al. Intravenous dipyridamole thallium-201 SPECT imaging in patients with left bundle branch block. *Clin Nucl Med* 1990;15:401–407.
14. O'Keefe JH Jr, Bateman TM, Barnhart CS. Adenosine thallium-201 is superior to exercise thallium-201 for detecting coronary artery disease in patients with left bundle branch block. *J Am Coll Cardiol* 1993;21:1332–1338.
15. Hirzel HO, Senn M, Nuesch K, et al. Thallium-201 scintigraphy in complete left bundle branch block. *Am J Cardiol* 1984; 53:764–769.
16. Ellis JE, Drijvers G, Pedlow S, et al. Premedication with oral and transdermal clonidine provides safe and efficacious postoperative sympatholysis. *Anesth Analg* 1994;79:1133–1140.
17. Shaw LJ, Eagle KA, Gersh BJ, et al. Meta-analysis of intravenous dipyridamole-thallium-201 imaging (1985 to 1994) and dobutamine echocardiography (1991 to 1994) for risk stratification before vascular surgery. *J Am Coll Cardiol* 1996;27: 787–798.
18. Boucher CA, Brewster DC, Darling RC, et al. Determination of cardiac risk by dipyridamole-thallium imaging before peripheral vascular surgery. *N Engl J Med* 1985;312:389–394.
19. Leppo J, Plaja J, Gionet M, et al. Noninvasive evaluation of cardiac risk before elective vascular surgery. *J Am Coll Cardiol* 1987;9:269–276.
20. Eagle KA, Coley CM, Newell JB, et al. Combining clinical and thallium data optimizes preoperative assessment of cardiac risk before major vascular surgery. *Ann Intern Med* 1989;110: 859–866.
21. L'Italien GJ, Paul SD, Hendel RC, et al. Development and validation of a Bayesian model for perioperative cardiac risk assessment in a cohort of 1,081 vascular surgical candidates. *J Am Coll Cardiol* 1996;27:779–786.
22. Pasternack PF, Grossi EA, Baumann FG, et al. Beta blockade to decrease silent myocardial ischemia during peripheral vascular surgery. *Am J Surg* 1989;158:113–116.
23. Mangano DT, Layug EL, Wallace A, et al. Effect of atenolol on mortality and cardiovascular morbidity after noncardiac surgery. Multicenter study of perioperative ischemia research group. *N Engl J Med* 1996;335:1713–1720.
24. Wallace A, Layug B, Tateo I, et al. Prophylactic atenolol reduces postoperative myocardial ischemia. McSPI Research Group. *Anesthesiology* 1998;88:7–17.
25. Poldermans D, Boersma E, Bax JJ, et al. The effect of bisoprolol on perioperative mortality and myocardial infarction in high-risk patients undergoing vascular surgery. Dutch echocardiographic cardiac risk evaluation applying stress echocardiography study group. *N Engl J Med* 1999;341:1789–1794.
26. Urban MK, Markowitz SM, Gordon MA, et al. Postoperative prophylactic administration of beta-adrenergic blockers in patients at risk for myocardial ischemia. *Anesth Analg* 2000;90:1257–1261.
27. Stuhmeier KD, Mainzer B, Cierpka J, et al. Small, oral dose of clonidine reduces the incidence of intraoperative myocardial ischemia in patients having vascular surgery. *Anesthesiology* 1996;85:706–712.
28. Oliver MF, Goldman L, Julian DG, et al. Effect of mivazerol on perioperative cardiac complications during non-cardiac surgery in patients with coronary heart disease: the European Mivazerol Trial (EMIT). *Anesthesiology* 1999;91:951–961.
29. Poldermans D, Bax JJ, Kertai MD, et al. Statins are associated with a reduced incidence of perioperative mortality in patients undergoing major noncardiac vascular surgery. *Circulation* 2003;107:1848–1851.
30. Allen JR, Helling TS, Hartzler GO. Operative procedures not involving the heart after percutaneous transluminal coronary angioplasty. *Surg Gynecol Obstet* 1991;173:285–288.
31. Elmore JR, Hallett JW Jr, Gibbons RJ, et al. Myocardial revascularization before abdominal aortic aneurysmorrhaphy: effect of coronary angioplasty. *Mayo Clin Proc* 1993;68:637–641.
32. Gottlieb A, Banoub M, Sprung J, et al. Perioperative cardiovascular morbidity in patients with coronary artery disease undergoing vascular surgery after percutaneous transluminal coronary angioplasty. *J Cardiothorac Vasc Anesth* 1998;12:501–506.
33. Posner KL, Van Norman GA, Chan V. Adverse cardiac outcomes after noncardiac surgery in patients with prior percutaneous transluminal coronary angioplasty. *Anesth Analg* 1999;89: 553–560.
34. Kaluza GL, Joseph J, Lee JR, et al. Catastrophic outcomes of noncardiac surgery soon after coronary stenting. *J Am Coll Cardiol* 2000;35:1288–1294.
35. Wilson SH, Fasseas P, Orford JL, et al. Clinical outcome of patients undergoing non-cardiac surgery in the two months following coronary stenting. *J Am Coll Cardiol* 2003;42:234–240.
36. Eagle KA, Rihal CS, Mickel MC, et al. Cardiac risk of noncardiac surgery: influence of coronary disease and type of surgery in 3,368 operations. CASS investigators and University of Michigan heart care program. Coronary artery surgery study. *Circulation* 1997;96:1882–1887.
37. Fleisher LA, Eagle KA, Shaffer T, et al. Perioperative and long-term mortality rates after major vascular surgery: the relationship to preoperative testing in the Medicare population. *Anesth Analg* 1999;89:849–855.
38. Hassan SA, Hlatky MA, Boothroyd DB, et al. Outcomes of noncardiac surgery after coronary bypass surgery or coronary angioplasty in the Bypass Angioplasty Revascularization Investigation (BARI). *Am J Med* 2001;110:260–266.

Anesthesia Complications

Paul E. Kazanjian

9

■■■ INTRODUCTION 69

■■■ AIRWAY COMPLICATIONS 70

■■■ GENERAL ANESTHESIA 75
Potent Inhaled Anesthetics 75
Nitrous Oxide 76
Anesthesia Delivery Systems 76
Medications 77
Intraoperative Awareness 81

■■■ REGIONAL ANESTHESIA 81
Local Anesthetic Toxicity 81
Complications of Neuraxial Anesthesia 83

■■■ MISCELLANEOUS COMPLICATIONS
OF ANESTHESIA 87
Postoperative Nausea and Vomiting 87
Obesity and Morbid Obesity 88
Hypothermia 90
Hyperthermia 91
Anaphylactic and Anaphylactoid Reactions in the
    Perioperative Period 92
Positioning and Peripheral Nerve Injury 93
Ocular Injury 94

■■■ CONCLUSION 97

■■■ REFERENCES 97

INTRODUCTION

There are a wide variety of complications in anesthesiology, ranging from relatively frequent and minor adverse events to rare but disastrous outcomes, including brain damage and death. Anesthesiologists' expertise in management of the airway is crucial to the safe conduct of anesthesia care. Unfortunately, airway complications are a major source of serious morbidity and mortality. Anesthetic medications play a crucial role in rendering patients insensate, immobile, and unconscious, but they also account for a number of adverse effects and complications. Machines are used to administer drug infusions, ventilate the lungs, measure the blood pressure, and deliver volatile anesthetics and oxygen. Machines can break down or be misused, which sometimes results in patient injury. Like surgery, anesthesiology is a procedure-oriented field and some complications result from technical mishaps or untoward patient–device interactions.

Whole textbooks are devoted to the subject of complications in anesthesia, and this one chapter cannot cover the entire subject. This chapter serves as a starting point for surgeons interested in an introduction to the gamut of complications due to anesthesia. Also, the references at the end of this chapter are good resources for those interested in more information about individual types of anesthesia-related complications.

Throughout this chapter there are references to The American Society of Anesthesiologists Closed Claims Database. The Closed Claims Project was begun in 1984 in response to rising professional liability premiums. The intention was to identify anesthetic-related complications, improve patient safety, and improve the insurance problem for anesthesiologists. The project is an ongoing evaluation

Paul E. Kazanjian: University of Michigan, Ann Arbor, MI 48109 and in-depth analysis of nearly 6,000 closed claims from 35 professional liability insurance companies covering 60% of the anesthesiologists in the United States. Each case is described by a brief narrative summary describing the claim, patient information, surgical procedure and positioning, preanesthetic evaluation, anesthetic technique, events leading to the injury or claim, type and severity of injury, and the outcome of litigation. A physician reviews the case, rates the severity of injury, and determines the potential for prevention and appropriateness of anesthesia care. Claims are separated into two categories: damaging events and complications. The damaging event is the specific incident that leads to the complication, and the complication is the injury that a patient sustained. The findings are reported in the scientific literature, and a number of these articles have been referenced in this chapter. More information about the project and a complete bibliography are available on the ASA's Closed Claims Project website (1).

There are limitations to closed-claims analysis, including lack of data about the total population at risk for injury and nonrandom, retrospective data collection. For several reasons it is impossible to provide numerical estimates of risk or establish true incidence rates on the basis of closed-claims analysis. Not all adverse outcomes result in a malpractice claim, and 40% of practicing anesthesiologists are excluded from the analysis because their insurance companies do not participate in the Closed Claims Project. It is impossible to determine whether increases or decreases in cases over time represent actual changes in the rate of complications, a more or less litigious patient population, or both.

AIRWAY COMPLICATIONS

Management of the airway is a central activity of daily anesthetic practice, involving a variety of maneuvers and devices designed to support or maintain adequate oxygenation and ventilation when patients are incapable of doing so themselves. Techniques range from simple maneuvers to maintain airway patency during spontaneous ventilation to fiberoptic intubation of the trachea in patients who are difficult to intubate. Problems occurring during management of the airway are the most important cause of major anesthetic-related morbidity and mortality. In an analysis of closed claims in the American Society of Anesthesiologists Closed Claims Project, respiratory events are the single largest class of incidents leading to injury, accounting for 30% of claims in adults and 43% of claims in pediatric patients (2). Most of the adverse respiratory events were due to difficulty in managing the airway, including inadequate ventilation, esophageal intubation, and failure to intubate the trachea.

One of the most critical and potentially dangerous portions of an operation occurs at induction of, and emergence from, general anesthesia (GA). During induction of GA, the anesthetist transitions the patient from conscious and spontaneously breathing to unconscious and apneic. As a patient emerges from anesthesia, he or she passes through several stages of anesthesia, each of which has certain implications for management of the airway. Emergence from anesthesia is not an all-or-none phenomenon, and proper timing of endotracheal extubation is critical to avoid airway obstruction, aspiration, and hypoxemia. The attention of the entire operating room team should be focused on the patient, the anesthetist, and his or her assistant during these two phases of GA. Potentially life-threatening problems can develop quickly, in which case the anesthetist will require rapid, competent assistance. Emergent cricothyrotomy might be necessary, and the surgeon, regardless of his or her specialty, must be prepared to perform this life-saving technique at a moment's notice.

Oral intubation with an endotracheal tube (ETT) is usually performed after induction of anesthesia with a short-acting intravenous anesthetic such as thiopental or propofol. Alternatively, anesthesia can be induced by inhalation of nitrous oxide and steadily higher concentrations of a volatile anesthetic. Mask ventilation is established and anesthesia is maintained with an inhaled anesthetic, such as isoflurane. Muscle relaxants facilitate intubation by ablating reflexive resistance to laryngoscopy and intubation. Successful direct laryngoscopy and intubation then depend on patient characteristics, including adequate mouth opening, sufficient pharyngeal space, compliant submandibular tissue, and unimpaired atlantooccipital extension. If any one or more of these basic characteristics are abnormal, visualization and intubation might be difficult (3,4).

Induction of anesthesia, laryngoscopy, and tracheal intubation is stimulating and can be associated with marked hemodynamic changes, which can be of concern in certain subsets of patients, such as those with ischemic heart disease or intracranial aneurysm. The hemodynamic response depends on a variety of factors, such as the method of induction, the technique used for intubation, and the combination of anesthetic medications used to attenuate these responses. For example, a study comparing several induction regimens demonstrated that induction with thiopental alone resulted in undesirable hemodynamics (tachycardia and hypertension) and elevations of plasma catecholamines, whereas thiopental supplemented with fentanyl (6 μg per kg) attenuated this response (5). Barak et al. compared two methods of intubating anesthetized patients—direct laryngoscopy and fiberoptic bronchoscopy—and found that both methods resulted in similar hemodynamic changes (6). Heart rate and blood pressure increased after intubation but not during laryngoscopy or bronchoscopy.

There are alternatives to oral intubation with an ETT. For example, certain operations are best served by nasotracheal intubation. Many patients do not need tracheal intubation and mechanical ventilation during GA, and placement of a laryngotracheal mask airway (LMA) is sufficient. If tracheal intubation is required, there are alternatives to direct laryngoscopy under anesthesia. Awake intubation using fiberoptic technique, retrograde intubation, or surgical tracheostomy is an alternative method available for patients who are difficult to ventilate, difficult to intubate, or both (3,7–9).

A difficult airway is defined as a clinical situation in which an anesthesiologist experiences difficulty with face mask ventilation of the upper airway, difficulty with tracheal intubation, or both. If it is difficult or impossible to visualize the glottis despite proper positioning of the head and neck, laryngoscopy is difficult. Difficulty with an airway might be *anticipated* when preoperative evaluation reveals a history of, or physical exam suggestive of, difficult intubation. Although a number of complex clinical and radiographic factors that suggest potential difficulty with laryngoscopy and intubation have been described, most anesthesiologists rely on a more straightforward examination combined with clinical experience. Factors suggesting difficulty are a short muscular neck, a full set of teeth, a receding lower jaw, a high arched palate, a limited mouth opening, limited cervical extension, a chin-to-thyroid cartilage distance of <7 cm, and a Mallampati score of 3 or 4 (Table 9-1) (4). The Mallampati test classifies the ability to see the faucial pillars and uvula when the patient opens his or her mouth as wide as possible (10). When combined, the latter two criteria have a specificity of almost 98% (11,12).

At other times difficulty is *unanticipated* because there are no predisposing factors suggesting difficulty and intubation is expected to be uncomplicated. The latter situation can be especially problematic if it is difficult or impossible to *ventilate* the patient by mask after induction of anesthesia. The American Society of Anesthesiologists Task Force on Management of the Difficult Airway has developed and refined practice guidelines for managing these various clinical situations (8). The guidelines include an algorithm, which is reproduced in Figure 9-1. The practice guidelines and algorithm describe a set of strategies that might be executed in the acute situation of unfolding difficulty. A recent survey of anesthesiologists revealed that when confronted with a difficult airway scenario, most chose to approach the airway with direct laryngoscopy or fiberoptic techniques (13). All other methods were much less frequently used.

The lips, teeth, tongue, buccal mucosa, palate, and permanent dental appliances can be injured or damaged during laryngoscopy or by any one of a number of foreign objects (oral airway, bite block, ETT, laryngeal mask airway) placed in the airway during GA. Injury to the lips, both upper and lower, is common during intubation using a laryngoscope, especially when performed by inexperienced practitioners. Serious consequences are rare, and the injury can be treated conservatively. Dental injury requiring repair

TABLE 9-1

COMPONENTS OF THE PREOPERATIVE AIRWAY PHYSICAL EXAMINATION

Airway Examination Component	Nonreassuring Findings
Length of upper incisors	Relatively long
Relation of maxillary and mandibular incisors during normal jaw closure	Prominent "overbite" (maxillary incisors anterior to mandibular incisors)
Relation of maxillary and mandibular incisors during voluntary protrusion of mandible	Patient cannot bring mandibular incisors anterior to (mandible in front of) maxillary incisors
Interincisor distance (mouth opening)	<3 cm
Visibility of uvula	Not visible when tongue is protruded with patient in sitting position (e.g., Mallampati class >II)
Shape of palate	Highly arched or narrow
Compliance of mandibular space	Stiff, indurated, occupied by mass, or nonresilient
Thyromental distance	Less than three ordinary finger breadths
Length of neck	Short
Thickness of neck	Thick
Range of motion of head and neck	Patient cannot touch tip of chin to chest or cannot extend neck

From American Society of Anesthesiologists Task Force on Management of the Difficult Airway. Practice guidelines for management of the difficult airway: an updated report. *Anesthesiology* 2003;98(5):1269–1277, with permission.

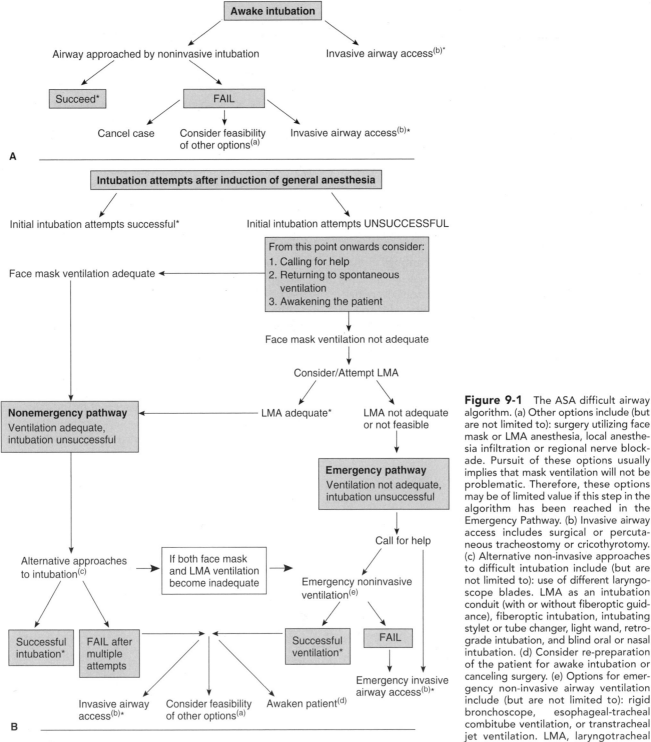

Figure 9-1 The ASA difficult airway algorithm. (a) Other options include (but are not limited to): surgery utilizing face mask or LMA anesthesia, local anesthesia infiltration or regional nerve blockade. Pursuit of these options usually implies that mask ventilation will not be problematic. Therefore, these options may be of limited value if this step in the algorithm has been reached in the Emergency Pathway. (b) Invasive airway access includes surgical or percutaneous tracheostomy or cricothyrotomy. (c) Alternative non-invasive approaches to difficult intubation include (but are not limited to): use of different laryngoscope blades. LMA as an intubation conduit (with or without fiberoptic guidance), fiberoptic intubation, intubating stylet or tube changer, light wand, retrograde intubation, and blind oral or nasal intubation. (d) Consider re-preparation of the patient for awake intubation or canceling surgery. (e) Options for emergency non-invasive airway ventilation include (but are not limited to): rigid bronchoscope, esophageal-tracheal combitube ventilation, or transtracheal jet ventilation. LMA, laryngotracheal mask airway.

*Confirm ventilation, tracheal intubation, or LMA placement with exhaled CO_2.

or extraction occurs in approximately 1 in 4,500 cases, and it usually involves the upper incisors (14). Preexisting poor dentition and difficulty intubating the patient increase the risk of damage to the teeth.

Tongue trauma and swelling can be the result of prolonged compression by an ETT, oral airway, or surgical retractor, or it can be the result of positioning the head in extreme flexion, especially when the patient is positioned head-up for posterior neurosurgical procedures. In contrast to other oral and dental injuries, injuries to the temporomandibular joint almost always occur in young, female, ASA physical status I and II patients, although patients with facial

TABLE 9-2

ASA PHYSICAL CLASSIFICATION

P1	A normal healthy patient
P2	A patient with mild systemic disease
P3	A patient with severe systemic disease
P4	A patient with severe systemic disease that is a constant threat to life
P5	A moribund patient who is not expected to survive without the operation
P6	A declared brain-dead patient whose organs are being removed for donor purposes

TABLE 9-3

CONDITIONS ASSOCIATED WITH ATLANTOAXIAL SUBLUXATION

Congenital	Down syndrome
	Odontoid anomalies
	Mucopolysaccharidoses
Acquired	Rheumatoid arthritis
	Still disease
	Ankylosing spondylitis
	Psoriatic arthritis
	Enteropathic arthritis (Crohn disease, ulcerative colitis)
	Reiter syndrome
	Trauma (odontoid fracture, ligamentous disruption)

From Crosby ET, Lui A. The adult cervical spine: implications for airway management. *Can J Anaesth* 1990;37(1):77–93, with permission.

skeletal abnormalities are also at risk (Table 9-2). The dislocated temporomandibular joint should be reduced immediately after the condition is recognized.

The topics of esophageal injury and laryngotracheal trauma are covered in Chapter 21 and in a recent review (15).

Improper manipulation of an unstable cervical spine might cause fracture or subluxation of the osseous components of the spine, resulting in cord compression and neurologic injury. Establishing a mask airway for ventilation and positioning the head and neck for intubation involves positioning the head and neck in the sniffing position by flexing the lower cervical spine and extending the occipital atlantoaxial complex. Most of motion during laryngoscopy and intubation in anesthetized, paralyzed patients with intact cervical spines occurs at the occiput-C1 junction (16). Theoretically, a person performing tracheal intubation can create or exacerbate a spinal cord injury, especially during difficult laryngoscopy, but there is little data to support this (17).

In the acute setting of a known or suspected spinal cord injury and a compromised airway, establishing an airway and supporting breathing takes precedence (17). Current Advanced Trauma Life Support guidelines recommend orotracheal intubation with manual in-line cervical spine stabilization, but the value of this and other stabilization maneuvers is unproven (16). In a study using cadavers, Lennarson et al. demonstrated that manual in-line stabilization did not prevent motion of the injured or intact cervical spine during laryngoscopy and intubation (16). Still, current teaching and guidelines advocate that all efforts should be made to minimize cervical spine motion during laryngoscopy and intubation. With careful technique, the risk of causing or worsening a spinal cord injury is low, regardless of the technique used to intubate the patient. During elective intubation the patient's anatomic configuration or halo cervical stabilization might suggest difficulty with direct laryngoscopy, and in these cases alternate techniques for intubation (fiberoptic) might be necessary.

A variety of conditions are associated with potential immobility or instability of the cervical spine, or both, such as Down syndrome, rheumatoid arthritis, ankylosing

spondylitis, and trauma (Table 9-3). High-risk rheumatoid patients are those with neck symptoms, advanced age, long-standing disease, erosive disease, and subcutaneous nodules. These patients should have lateral cervical spine x-rays performed in neutral position, flexion, and extension before GA.

Nasal intubation is a safe and useful technique when performed by experienced persons (Table 9-4). The most common complication is epistaxis, which is usually self-limited but which can be serious in anticoagulated patients or those patients with coagulopathy. Nasal bruising is also common, but frank mucosal tears, lacerations, and false submucosal passage are uncommon. Nasal intubation is potentially hazardous in certain conditions such as facial trauma and skull fracture in which inadvertent intubations of the cranium and orbit have been reported (19). The technique is generally contraindicated in these situations unless it is absolutely necessary and unless it is performed carefully with the assistance of fiberoptic bronchoscopy.

TABLE 9-4

INDICATIONS FOR NASAL INTUBATION

Head and neck surgery	Dental surgery
	Intraoral and oropharyngeal surgery
	Rigid laryngoscopy and microlaryngeal surgery
	Jaws wired or fixed shut at end of operation
General indications	Intraoral pathology including obstructive lesions
	Cervical spine instability or degenerative spine disease
	Obstructive sleep apnea

From Hall CE, Shutt LE. Nasotracheal intubation for head and neck surgery [comment]. *Anaesthesia* 2003;58(3):249–256, with permission.

The technique of nasal intubation has been recently and thoroughly reviewed (20). The authors emphasize several aspects of the technique in order to reduce the incidence of common complications, including careful preoperative assessment; preparation of the nasal mucosa with lubricating jellies and vasoconstrictors; selection of a supple, uncuffed tube; and careful insertion of a well-lubricated tube. Once the tube is beyond the nasopharynx, it can be guided into the trachea either blindly, under direct laryngoscopic visualization, or with the assistance of fiberoptic bronchoscopy. Once in place, the tube must be secured carefully to prevent inadvertent extubation and to avoid pressure on the nasal ala, which can cause tissue ischemia or necrosis.

Inadvertent intubation of the esophagus can occur when direct visualization of the glottis is difficult, but it can also occur when visualization is ideal. Esophageal intubation and ventilation of the stomach is of little consequence, *as long as the condition is rapidly recognized and corrected*. The presence of carbon dioxide (CO_2) in exhaled gases can be detected by end-tidal CO_2 monitoring and is the most accurate and reliable method of confirming proper placement of the ETT in the trachea. Clinical signs such as bilateral breath sounds, condensation in the ETT, chest wall movement, and absence of gastric sounds cannot be relied upon for confirmation because they are all potentially misleading. If the esophagus is intubated, the ETT should be left in place until the trachea is correctly intubated (12). Leaving the ETT in the esophagus helps protect the trachea from regurgitated gastric contents and helps identify the proper orifice for intubation.

One of the most common causes of intraoperative arterial oxygen desaturation in an otherwise healthy patient is bronchial intubation. An ETT that is placed too deeply will most likely intubate the right mainstem bronchus, resulting in hypoventilation of the left lung. Clinical evidence of this phenomenon (unilateral decreased breath sounds, increased inflation pressure, asymmetric chest expansion during inhalation) should be obvious. An otherwise normally placed ETT might migrate into a bronchus for a variety of reasons. A steep Trendelenburg position can force the abdomen, diaphragm, and chest organs to move cephalad toward the ETT. Flexion of the head will move the ETT deeper into the airway (21).

An endobronchial injury can be the result of misplaced ETTs, tube guides, tube changers, or properly placed double-lumen ETTs. Severe endobronchial injury almost always results in pneumothorax, which can rapidly progress to tension pneumothorax in patients receiving positive pressure ventilation (19).

The laryngeal mask airway is an invaluable tool for management of the airway in elective operations and certain emergency situations. In fact, the laryngeal mask airway has emerged as an important component of the difficult airway algorithm and is frequently successful in salvaging ventilation in patients who are difficult to intubate and difficult to

ventilate by face mask (22,23). Although many anesthesiologists and surgeons regard placement of an LMA as "less invasive" and less traumatic than direct laryngoscopy followed by endotracheal intubation, complications can occur with use of the LMA. In one review of airway complications in pediatric patients, the rate of complications was actually higher with the LMA than with endotracheal intubation, but they were clinically less significant (24). Complications with the LMA can be broadly divided into pharyngolaryngeal and neurovascular complications.

One disadvantage of the LMA is that it cannot provide complete protection against aspiration of gastric contents or secretions. The incidence of subclinical aspiration might be as high as 25%, but the incidence of serious aspiration appears to be much lower (19). The occurrence of mild hoarseness (12%), sore throat (10%), and dysphagia (4%) all appear to be related to malposition or excess cuff pressure. Pharyngeal abrasions and ulcers of the soft palate and uvula are usually associated with difficult placement of the device.

A variety of nerve injuries has been reported with use of the LMA, including lingual, recurrent laryngeal, and hypoglossal nerve damage (19). In general, serious nerve injuries seem to be related to neurovascular compression from excess pressure on pharyngeal structures. Excess pressure on adjacent structures might be a result of malposition of the device or excessive cuff inflation, especially in the presence of nitrous oxide. Thus, some injuries might be avoided by monitoring cuff pressure and keeping it at the lowest level that allows for adequate gas exchange. Malposition, however, might be hard to recognize because adequate ventilation might be possible even when the device is not properly seated. The only way to accurately confirm proper positioning is with fiberoptic examination of the glottis from within the LMA, but fiberoptic confirmation is not routinely performed (19).

Extubation is another critical phase (stage) in the conduct of GA, and it can be complicated by a variety of events including, but not limited to, aspiration, laryngospasm, negative-pressure pulmonary edema, and airway compression.

Tracheomalacia leading to tracheal collapse might produce upper airway obstruction following extubation. Tracheomalacia is usually secondary to thyroid goiter, in which the cartilaginous rings of the trachea are weakened or destroyed. In these cases removal of the goiter further compromises the trachea's structural integrity, and collapse can occur shortly after tracheal extubation. Reintubation is required. Subsequent treatment options are tracheostomy, tracheoplasty, or placement of external or internal tracheal support (25).

Laryngospasm is normally a protective reflex in which contraction of the intrinsic laryngeal muscles occludes the glottis. Usually, laryngospasm occurs to prevent aspiration of foreign material into the trachea and is mediated by the vagus nerve. The reflex can occur in response to the presence of airway irritants (secretions, blood, ETT) during a light plane of anesthesia. During this light plane of anesthesia, referred to as *stage II*, the level of anesthesia is insufficient to prevent the laryngospasm reflex but is too deep to allow a normal cough reflex (26). If laryngospasm occurs after tracheal extubation, upper airway obstruction might ensue. Laryngospasm is the most common cause of upper airway obstruction after tracheal extubation and is especially frequent in children after upper airway surgery (27). Ideally, all attempts should be made to avoid precipitating laryngospasm by removing potential irritants by thorough suctioning of the mouth and throat prior to extubation. Extubation should occur while the patient is deeply anesthetized or after the patient has passed out of stage II anesthesia and is following simple commands. Applying positive pressure during extubation can clear potentially irritating material from the cords. If laryngospasm develops, the precipitating irritating material should be removed while administering 100% oxygen by positive pressure ventilation. Occasionally, it is necessary to deepen the anesthesia or administer a small dose of succinylcholine to "break" the spasm, and sometimes reintubation is required.

Pulmonary edema might occur after acute upper airway tract obstruction, in which case it is termed *negative-pressure pulmonary edema*. The pulmonary edema occurs within minutes of the onset of airway obstruction, and radiologic findings demonstrate perihilar infiltrate with diffuse pulmonary edema. The pathogenesis of negative-pressure pulmonary edema is multifactorial, but the predominant mechanism is generation of markedly negative intrapleural pressures by forceful inspiration against an obstructed airway (28). The differential diagnosis includes acid aspiration, cardiogenic pulmonary edema, and iatrogenic volume overload, but the temporal relation of pulmonary edema to clinically obvious airway obstruction in an otherwise healthy patient strongly suggests negative-pressure pulmonary edema. The most frequent cause of airway obstruction leading to negative-pressure pulmonary edema is postextubation laryngospasm, but acute airway obstruction occurring anytime during management of the airway can be followed by negative-pressure pulmonary edema (29). The first priority in managing negative-pressure pulmonary edema is reestablishing a patent airway and assuring adequate oxygenation. Most cases resolve spontaneously without further complication, although some patients might require reintubation followed by a brief period of mechanical ventilation with positive end-expiratory pressure (28).

GENERAL ANESTHESIA

The term anesthesia signifies insensibility to surgical pain. Other components of anesthesia are amnesia, hypnosis (unconsciousness), muscle relaxation, inhibition of movement, and blunting of the autonomic response in response to noxious stimuli. A variety of drugs provides some or all of these components of anesthesia. The gamut of pharmacologic agents used in GA has been thoroughly reviewed elsewhere (30). Recent development of anesthetic medications has focused on those compounds with a rapid onset and recovery with minimal side effects and drug–drug interactions.

Potent Inhaled Anesthetics

Potent inhaled anesthetics (PIAs) are halogenated hydrocarbons and ether compounds that render patients amnestic and immobile to noxious stimuli. Current theories on the mechanisms of action of the PIAs have been recently reviewed (31). Their amnestic and hypnotic affects are mediated in the brain, but their action to inhibit movement in response to noxious stimuli is secondary to depression of spinal cord function. There are separate molecular targets for each of these actions. Although the volatile anesthetics can cause cardiopulmonary depression and death at concentrations near those that produce deep anesthesia, this is extremely rare, largely due to reliable gas delivery systems, agent analyzers, and hemodynamic monitors. Rather, adverse side effects are usually mild and include nausea, vomiting, and delirium.

The clinical effects of inhaled anesthetics, ranging from euphoria to profound cardiopulmonary depression, depend on the inhaled concentration. A number of scales are used to assess anesthetic potency and they are based on the relationship between alveolar concentration and a certain behavioral endpoint. The median alveolar concentration (MAC) is one of these scales and is defined as the median end-tidal concentration of inhaled anesthetic that ablates movement in response to surgical incision in 50% of the test population.

All the volatile anesthetics decrease blood pressure in a dose-dependent manner and all are myocardial depressants. The effects of halothane and enflurane are greater than isoflurane, sevoflurane, and desflurane in this regard. Halothane sensitizes the myocardium to the arrhythmogenic effects of epinephrine. Isoflurane and desflurane decrease blood pressure and peripheral vascular resistance while increasing heart rate. Animal studies suggest that isoflurane promotes "coronary steal" by dilating nondiseased coronary vessels and diverting blood flow to normal areas away from ischemic areas (32). Clinically, the effect is not apparent and, if factors affecting myocardial oxygen consumption are controlled, isoflurane anesthesia does not cause a greater incidence of ischemia than any other technique (33–35). In fact, there is growing evidence that isoflurane actually protects the myocardium, effectively limiting infarct size and improving functional recovery following myocardial ischemia through a mechanism similar to ischemic preconditioning (36).

PIAs are respiratory depressants and depress the normal response to hypercarbia in a dose-dependent manner. The

PIAs irritate the airways and might produce coughing or laryngospasm during inhalation induction of GA. Sevoflurane and halothane are the least irritating, and desflurane is the most irritating.

In a discussion of halothane-associated liver failure from 1970, halothane is regarded as close to an ideal anesthetic agent, despite many reports of halothane-induced hepatitis (37). Today this assessment is invalid because other agents are available that have a much better margin of safety. Halothane-associated liver damage presents as one of two clinical syndromes (38). Mild hepatic damage, moderately increased transaminase levels, occasional transient jaundice, and low morbidity characterize the first syndrome, which might have an incidence as high as 20%. The second syndrome is rare, occurs after repeated exposure to halothane, and is characterized by fulminant hepatic failure with high mortality. Even in 1970 an allergic type reaction was hypothesized despite halothane's relatively inert nature. Hepatotoxicity resulting in fulminant liver failure involves a humoral response that is directed toward hepatocyte cytochromes that have been altered by an oxidative reactive metabolite of halothane (39,40).

When the body metabolizes methoxyflurane, enflurane, and sevoflurane, fluoride ions are produced, which might be toxic to the kidneys, resulting in impairment of concentrating ability and acute renal failure. The metabolism of halothane, isoflurane, and desflurane does not produce significant levels of fluoride ions and there is little potential for nephrotoxicity with these compounds (40).

Sevoflurane reacts with the material in carbon dioxide absorbers to form a vinyl chloride called *Compound A*, which produces renal tubular necrosis in laboratory animals (40). Most human studies show that there is no clinical degradation in renal function even after prolonged exposure to low-flow sevoflurane anesthesia (41,42). In patients with impaired renal function, it would seem prudent to limit exposure to sevoflurane and use high fresh gas flow rates, which will "wash out" the compound from the anesthesia breathing circuit.

PIAs and nitrous oxide are known triggering agents for malignant hyperthermia (MH). Epinephrine, beta-adrenergic receptor agonists, and theophylline can cause arrhythmias in the presence of halothane. The myocardial depressant activity of inhaled anesthetics is increased in the presence of beta-blockers and calcium channel blockers.

Nitrous Oxide

Nitrous oxide is a relatively insoluble gas that is used primarily to supplement the PIAs in GA. It is used alone for analgesia in labor and outpatient procedures such as flexible sigmoidoscopy, colonoscopy, and dental procedures (43,44). The primary danger in using nitrous oxide is *hypoxia* that results from either using excess amounts of nitrous oxide or through diffusion. During recovery from anesthesia using nitrous oxide, large amounts of the gas

exit the blood and "flood" the alveoli, displacing alveolar oxygen and carbon dioxide. The patient can become hypoxic if supplemental oxygen is not provided along with adequate ventilatory support. The hypoxic ventilatory drive is blunted.

Nitrous oxide usually produces mild sympathetic stimulation when used with the PIAs, but it can cause profound cardiovascular depression when used in an anesthetic technique primarily based on opioids. It might also cause myocardial depression and hypotension in patients with coronary artery disease (45). Nitrous oxide raises pulmonary vascular resistance and might increase pulmonary artery pressure in patients with pulmonary hypertension.

Nitrous oxide inactivates vitamin B_{12}, which is an important component of two biochemical reactions. In the first reaction vitamin B_{12} acts as a cofactor in the formation of methionine, which is essential to DNA synthesis and to the maintenance of the myelin sheath in nerves. In the second reaction a form of vitamin B_{12} functions as a cofactor in a reaction that forms succinyl coenzyme A, which is important for lipid and carbohydrate synthesis via the Krebs cycle. Patients can develop megaloblastic anemia, bone marrow depression, and neurologic problems after either prolonged exposure to, or chronic inhalation of, nitrous oxide (46,47). Persons who have vitamin B_{12} deficiency from any cause, such as pernicious anemia, terminal ileum resection, or subtotal gastrectomy, are especially at risk of serious neurologic deterioration even after a single anesthetic with nitrous oxide. Neurologic manifestations are similar to vitamin B_{12} deficiency and might be reversed by vitamin B_{12} therapy (46). Patients who intentionally abuse the gas are also at risk of anemia and neurologic disease. Although nitrous oxide exposure is an occupational hazard to operating room personnel, the exact extent of the risk is not well established (48).

Nitrous oxide diffuses into gas-filled spaces in the body more quickly than nitrogen diffuses out. Thus, it can cause expansion of these spaces and cavities. Animal studies performed 40 years ago demonstrated that anesthesia with nitrous oxide caused expansion of air pockets within the pleural space (49). Bowel distension, tension pneumothorax, blindness after vitrectomy, venous air embolism, and hearing loss have all been reported to occur during, and have been attributed to, anesthesia with nitrous oxide (50–52). Interestingly, there is hardly any literature to support the contention that nitrous oxide definitely causes clinically significant bowel distention. In fact, one randomized trial comparing operative conditions with and without nitrous oxide for laparoscopic cholecystectomy failed to demonstrate any detectable difference (53).

Anesthesia Delivery Systems

The anesthesia machine comprises several components. At a minimum, the machine functions as a gas delivery system by providing a method of metering and delivering oxygen, dosing and delivering PIAs, and delivering controlled mechanical ventilation. In addition, the modern machine incorporates a wide variety of safety mechanisms, monitors, and alarms that are designed to alert the anesthetist to malfunction or operation that is outside normal parameters. A variety of physiologic monitors, computers, cabling, drug-delivery systems, suction devices, and other adjuvants might be attached to or incorporated into the machine.

The gas delivery system controls the flow of oxygen, air, and nitrous oxide from wall connections or gas cylinders. The vaporizers meter vapor from PIAs and blend the vapors with the fresh gas flow. The fresh gas flow enters the breathing circuit, which might or might not recirculate exhaled gases through a carbon dioxide scavenging system. During controlled ventilation, a mechanical ventilator controls delivery of gas to the patient. Thus, the gas delivery system in the anesthesia machine serves a critical function in delivering oxygen and anesthetic gases to the patient while also providing adequate ventilation and carbon dioxide removal.

Serious patient injuries, including death and brain injury, have resulted from misuse or failure of anesthesia gas delivery equipment. Other potential injuries are awareness, cardiovascular collapse, delayed recovery, and pneumothorax. In a study of closed claims the breathing circuit was the most common source of injury, followed by the vaporizers, ventilator, and the gas supply tank or line (54). Misconnect and disconnect of the breathing circuit were the most frequent initiating events. The two most common sites of disconnect were between the ETT and the circuit and between the ventilator and the breathing circuit. Half of the cases involved inadequate oxygenation as a result of disconnects, oxygen supply errors, and failures to turn on the ventilator. Misuse of equipment, defined as fault or error associated with the preparation, maintenance, or deployment of a medical device, was much more frequent than equipment failure.

Contemporary monitoring guidelines now mandate the use of devices to assure adequate oxygenation and ventilation. Some of the cases included in the analysis of closed claims occurred well before the widespread adoption of pulse oximetry and end-tidal carbon dioxide detection, and 53% of claims were judged to be preventable if pulse oximetry, capnography, or both had been used (54). Therefore, minimal monitoring should reduce the incidence of these events, if appropriately applied.

Medications

Intravenous Anesthetics, Sedatives

The ideal intravenous (IV) anesthetic should provide hypnosis, amnesia, and analgesia. In addition, it should have rapid onset, rapid elimination, and minimal or no side effects. Unfortunately, an ideal IV anesthetic does not exist, but several medications play an important role as adjuncts in balanced anesthesia. Several of the IV anesthetics are also used at lower doses for short-term or long-term sedation.

The barbiturates (thiopental, methohexital, and thiamylal) have a rapid and short action. They are some of the standard drugs used to induce anesthesia. They enhance and mimic the action of gamma amino butyric acid (GABA) at the GABA receptor in the central nervous system (CNS). The primary cardiovascular effect is venodilation and pooling of blood in the periphery. Blood pressure and cardiac output can drop because of decreased venous return (55). Hypotension can be severe in patients with impaired cardiac function, hypovolemia, adrenocortical insufficiency, uremia, or sepsis. The barbiturates are potent respiratory depressants; the degree of respiratory depression depends on the dose and rate of injection and presence of other medications. An induction dose that renders a patient unconscious will cause apnea. Smaller doses might leave the patient in a light plane of anesthesia and susceptible to laryngospasm, coughing, or bronchospasm during airway stimulation, such as placement of an oral airway or mask ventilation.

The barbiturates can cause serious tissue damage if the medication extravasates during IV injection or is accidentally injected intraarterially. Thiobarbiturates induce release of histamine from mast cells; an urticarial rash on the upper body and arms is common, but true anaphylactic reactions are unusual (56). Patients might experience delirium, prolonged somnolence and recovery, and headache after their anesthetic, especially if they are given high doses of barbiturates during short procedures. Barbiturates can precipitate acute abdominal pain, vomiting, tachycardia, hypertension, fever, confusion, seizures, paralysis, and even death in patients with various types of porphyria (57). In general, barbiturates are contraindicated in patients with porphyria, and several alternatives are available.

Benzodiazepines are a mainstay in contemporary anesthesia because of their hypnotic and amnestic properties combined with a low incidence of side effects. Midazolam is probably the most frequently used drug in the class. It causes a mild decrease in blood pressure, peripheral vascular resistance, and cardiac output when used alone. When midazolam is combined with other medications, especially the synthetic opioids, hypnosis, respiratory depression, and hypotension can be profound (58,59). The synergistic effect of midazolam and fentanyl or alfentanil has been exploited for induction of anesthesia in day surgery (60). Even when used for conscious sedation, midazolam alone can cause respiratory depression.

Etomidate is a substituted imidazole, like ketoconazole, that is used as an IV sedative-hypnotic to induce anesthesia. It can cause pain on injection, phlebitis, myoclonic movements, nausea, vomiting, and adrenocortical suppression. Nausea and vomiting are especially common (61). A major disadvantage of etomidate is its inhibition of cortisol and mineralocorticoid synthesis in the adrenal glands. This was first noted in the mid-1980s when increased mortality was reported in patients sedated with continuous infusions of etomidate (62). Both a single dose and continuous infusion of etomidate inhibit two mitochondrial cytochrome P450-dependent enzymes, which, in turn, inhibit adrenal steroid production (63,64). On the other hand, etomidate is generally associated with cardiovascular stability and preserved blood pressure during induction (65). Unfortunately, cardiovascular stability is not assured in all patients (66).

Propofol can cause pain on injection, cough, hiccups, involuntary skeletal muscle movements, and seizure-like episodes. Propofol causes less nausea and vomiting than thiopental. Like the barbiturates, propofol is a respiratory depressant and causes apnea with induction and decreased tidal volume with preserved respiratory rate during maintenance (67). Propofol usually causes a drop in blood pressure during induction of anesthesia because of vasodilation and decreased cardiac output from myocardial depression (68–70). In patients with coronary artery disease, propofol can cause cardiovascular depression and hypotension. Propofol is supplied as an aqueous emulsification of soybean oil, glycerol, and egg phosphatide, and it supports microbial growth at room temperature (71). Originally, propofol was preservative-free, but it now comes formulated with disodium edetate 0.005% as a microbial growth retardant. Epidemiologic studies have suggested that propofol, poor aseptic technique, and mishandling of this medication have contributed to postoperative infections, but there is considerable controversy over whether there is a true causal relationship (72–75). In response to these case reports, studies, and concerns, the manufacturer and the Food and Drug Administration (FDA) conducted an extensive education campaign and the package insert was changed. The insert now warns about the potential for infection and provides recommendations for proper methods to reduce this risk (76).

Recently, the term "propofol syndrome" has been used to describe a rare syndrome of cardiac failure, rhabdomyolysis, severe metabolic acidosis, and renal failure occurring in critically ill children and adults receiving high-dose, long-term propofol infusions (77). Apparently, propofol impairs free fatty acid utilization and mitochondrial activity, leading to an imbalance between energy demand and utilization. In some patients with critical illnesses, propofol, along with glucocorticoids and catecholamines, can lead to necrosis of cardiac and skeletal muscle.

Ketamine is a unique IV anesthetic because it provides sedation, amnesia, analgesia, and anesthesia. *In vivo*, ketamine increases heart rate, blood pressure, and pulmonary artery pressure by increasing sympathetic tone (78). Ketamine produces its sympathomimetic action through direct stimulation of CNS structures. Administration of ketamine can result in hypotension and myocardial depression in chronically ill patients with depleted catecholamine stores. Airway reflexes are usually maintained, but obstruction and apnea can occur. Oropharyngeal secretions can be

increased. Ketamine is a potent cerebral vasodilator that can increase the intracranial pressure. Ketamine is notorious for causing psychic disturbances and emergence delirium, which can occur in 15% to 30% of patients. These disturbances are described as extracorporeal (out-of-body) experiences, floating sensations, vivid dreams, and frank delirium (79). Administering benzodiazepines along with ketamine reduces the incidence of postanesthesia emergence reactions and adverse cardiovascular reactions.

Neuromuscular Blocking Agents

Muscle relaxation during anesthesia can be accomplished with a variety of methods and medications. Inhalational anesthesia works at the level of the spinal cord to inhibit movement to noxious stimulation. Local anesthetics are used during neuraxial blockade at the level of the spinal cord or peripherally with nerve blocks to block transmission along motor nerves, as well as sensory nerves. Finally, neuromuscular blocking drugs work at the level of the neuromuscular junction to interrupt transmission between the nerve ending and the muscle. Neuromuscular blocking drugs are indicated to facilitate endotracheal intubation and to decrease muscle tone during GA to improve surgical working conditions.

Neuromuscular blocking drugs have no intrinsic analgesic, hypnotic, or amnestic properties. These medications cause complete apnea and cessation of spontaneous breathing. Use of neuromuscular blocking drugs is indicated only if a means of artificial ventilation is available and feasible.

There are two major classes of muscle relaxants: depolarizing and nondepolarizing. Regardless of their classification, all muscle relaxants work by binding to, and interacting with, prejunctional and postjunctional nicotinic acetylcholine receptors at the neuromuscular junction. Neuromuscular blocking drugs also bind to rare extrajunctional nicotinic receptors, which are located on the muscle fibers away from the neuromuscular junction. Depolarizing muscle relaxants mimic acetylcholine at the postjunctional receptors, causing prolonged depolarization. Depolarization of the postjunctional receptors causes muscle contractions that are quickly replaced by flaccid paralysis, called *phase I block*. Only one depolarizer is in clinical use today, succinylcholine. It has a rapid onset and brief duration of action, making it a good drug in situations in which tracheal intubation must be performed rapidly after induction of anesthesia or where brief relaxation is desirable.

Succinylcholine generally causes an increase in the serum potassium of 0.5 to 1.0 mEq per L. There are certain pathologic conditions in which the rise in potassium can be much greater. In certain conditions, such as upper motor neuron disease (stroke, spinal cord injury), lower motor neuron disease, muscle disease (disuse atrophy, certain muscular dystrophies), muscle injury, and burns, there can be a proliferation of extrajunctional receptors. If succinylcholine is administered to a patient with one of these conditions, hyperkalemia can result from efflux of potassium through depolarized extrajunctional receptors. Schow et al. reviewed retrospectively the records from 40,000 anesthetics to evaluate the outcome following the administration of succinylcholine to hyperkalemic patients. They found no increased morbidity or mortality despite a consistent rise in the serum potassium (80). Thapa and Brull reviewed thoroughly the use of succinylcholine in the setting of renal failure and concluded that it could be used safely so long as the preoperative potassium level was within normal range, there was no neuropathy, and the dose of succinylcholine was not repeated (81).

Some patients do not metabolize succinylcholine normally and have a prolonged response to the drug. Four percent of patients have an abnormal gene that controls the quantity and quality of the enzyme that degrades succinylcholine, plasma cholinesterase. About 0.04% of patients are homozygous for this atypical gene and will have a prolonged neuromuscular block following administration of succinylcholine. Patients with severe liver disease and peripartum patients might also have decreased levels of plasma cholinesterase and prolonged blockade.

Patients who receive succinylcholine occasionally report postoperative myalgias and generalized muscle pain, which has been described as being similar to the pain experienced after intense physical exercise. The incidence of succinylcholine-induced myalgias is variously reported from 1.5% to 89% (82). It usually appears on the first postoperative day and is located in the neck, shoulders, and upper abdominal muscles. Although it would seem that intense fasciculations are the direct cause of myalgias, the exact etiology of the discomfort is unknown and probably complex (82). A number of strategies have been tried in efforts to reduce or abolish this adverse effect of succinylcholine, including pretreatment with lidocaine or a small-dose nondepolarizing neuromuscular blocking agent. A metaanalysis of a large number of studies revealed that the most effective therapy was pretreatment with 1.5 mg per kg of lidocaine (83).

Succinylcholine causes a mean intraocular pressure (IOP) increase of 4 to 7 mm Hg because of tonic contraction of extraocular muscles. Crying, Valsalva maneuvers, coughing, and cricoid pressure raise the IOP at least as much and perhaps more (84). Many anesthesiologists believe that succinylcholine is relatively contraindicated for induction in patients with open globe injury because of the fear of causing extrusion of vitreous contents (84). Yet there are no reports of eye damage after rapid-sequence induction of anesthesia with thiopental and succinylcholine. Furthermore, a variety of studies have compared the change in IOP after succinylcholine with other nondepolarizing muscle relaxants and have found little or no difference (85,86). A group of investigators developed a trauma model in the cat eye to investigate the effects of succinylcholine, and they found that the only

observable effect of succinylcholine administration was forward displacement of the lens and iris and that no intraocular content was lost in any case (87). Thus, the proscription against the use of succinylcholine in open globe emergencies appears to be based more on theoretical concerns than evidence. As one editorialist wrote, "The benefits (of succinylcholine) are real, the risks unproven"(88). The origin and history of this dogma has been reviewed recently (89).

Other side effects of succinylcholine are increased intracranial pressure, increased intragastric pressure, and bradycardia (90). Succinylcholine is a trigger of malignant hyperthermia in susceptible patients.

Unlike the depolarizers, a great number of nondepolarizing muscle relaxants are in clinical use, and more are being developed (91,92). Nondepolarizing muscle relaxants inhibit depolarization and muscle contraction by competitively antagonizing acetylcholine at the postjunctional receptors. Unlike succinylcholine, the administration of acetylcholinesterase inhibitors can reverse or antagonize neuromuscular blockade from nondepolarizers. The nondepolarizers vary in their onset and duration of action, metabolism, and side effect profiles (Table 9-5). One of the most dangerous consequences of use of nondepolarizing neuromuscular blockers is hypoventilation, hypercarbia, and hypoxemia following inadequate or incomplete antagonism (reversal). A variety of drugs and conditions result in prolonged blockade, including aminoglycosides (neomycin, streptomycin), clindamycin, hypermagnesemia, myasthenia gravis, and hypothermia. Combinations of different nondepolarizing neuromuscular blockers can be synergistic, resulting in unexpectedly prolonged blockade (93).

Both atracurium and cisatracurium are metabolized to a potentially toxic metabolite, laudanosine. Laudanosine crosses the blood–brain barrier and can cause excitement and seizure activity. In very high concentrations laudanosine can cause hypotension and bradycardia. Fortunately, accumulation of laudanosine and toxicity is extremely unlikely in standard clinical practice, especially in the case of cisatracurium (94). Laudanosine toxicity might be a concern in prolonged administration in intensive care units, especially in pediatric patients and those with liver and renal failure. Clinically, this has not been a significant problem.

Neuromuscular blocking drugs are used in critically ill patients for a variety of indications, such as facilitation of intubation and mechanical ventilation, control of increased intracranial pressure, reduction of muscle tone, and facilitation of diagnostic and therapeutic procedures. Unfortunately, use of these medications is associated with a number of complications, many of which are exactly the same as those seen in the operating room, such as skin breakdown, peripheral nerve injury, and corneal desiccation. Other complications are inadequate sedation and analgesia, inability to cough, thromboembolic complications from immobility, and inadequate ventilation in the event of disconnection of the ventilator circuit (95). One major complication of chronic use of these medications in

TABLE 9-5

CHARACTERISTICS OF COMMONLY USED NONDEPOLARIZING NEUROMUSCULAR BLOCKING AGENTS

Neuromuscular Blocking Agent	Class	Metabolism/ Elimination	Time to 25% Recovery from Intubating Dose (Minutes)	Characteristics	Notable Side Effects
Pancuronium	Aminosteroid	Renal	90–100	• Increased heart rate, blood pressure, cardiac output	• Cardiovascular effects may precipitate myocardial ischemia in patients with coronary artery disease
				• Vagolytic effect on cardiac muscarinic receptors	• Residual blockade
				• Sympathetic activation	
Vecuronium	Aminosteroid	Hepatic	40–50	• Structurally identical to pancuronium with exception of removal of one methyl group	• Free of cardiovascular side effects
		Active metabolite			• Residual blockade after prolonged infusion
Rocuronium	Aminosteroid	Renal, hepatic	40–45	• Rapid onset at ED95; alternative to succinyl-choline for rapid-sequence induction	• Anaphylactic reactions reported
		No active metabolites			• Recovery may be prolonged in the presence of hepatic and renal impairment
Atracurium	Benzylisoquinoline	Spontaneous degradation at physiologic pH and temperature (Hoffman elimination)	35–40	• Histamine release with intubating dose	• Facial flushing and hypotension with rapid injection
		Hydrolysis by nonspecific plasma esterases			• Laudanosine metabolite may cause cerebral excitation, seizures[a]
Cisatracurium	Benzylisoquinoline	Spontaneous degradation at physiologic pH and temperature (Hoffman elimination)	40–50	• No significant histamine release	• Free of cardiovascular side effects

[a]See text for details.
From Moore EW, Hunter JM. The new neuromuscular blocking agents: do they offer any advantages? *Br J Anaesth* 2001;87(6):912–925, with permission.

critically ill patients is the development of prolonged skeletal muscle weakness following discontinuance of neuromuscular blocker drugs. Prolonged neuromuscular weakness can be due to either alterations in pharmakinetics or functional defects in the motor unit (nerve, muscle, or neuromuscular junction) (96). Prolonged paralysis, muscle weakness, and ventilator dependence have been reported after the administration of aminosteroidal relaxants

(pancuronium, vecuronium) to patients who are receiving exogenous steroids or who have liver or renal failure (97,98). These conditions have also been reported after the administration of drugs of the benzylisoquinolinium class (atracurium, cisatracurium) (99,100). Resources are available that make specific recommendations about the indications, choice of drugs, dosage, and monitoring (95,96,101).

Analgesics

The opioid agonists are used as preoperative sedatives, as adjuncts to the PIAs in balanced anesthesia, as postoperative analgesics, and as adjuncts in neuraxial blockade. Morphine is the prototypical opioid agonist with analgesic properties (30). It also causes respiratory depression, apnea, nausea, and vomiting through CNS mechanisms. Histamine release accompanies morphine administration, which can cause significant vasodilation and hypotension, especially in hypovolemic patients. Large doses can cause sinus bradycardia. Morphine causes constipation, spasm of the sphincter of Oddi, and delayed gastric emptying.

Meperidine is structurally similar to atropine and can cause tachycardia, but it is otherwise well tolerated in healthy patients. Very large doses can cause clinically significant hypotension through decreased peripheral vascular resistance and decreased cardiac output. Meperidine also causes histamine release, like morphine (102). Unique to meperidine use are the side effects of serotonergic crisis and normeperidine toxicity. Normeperidine is a metabolite of meperidine that can cause CNS excitation and convulsions. Normeperidine has a long elimination half-life and can accumulate in renal failure. Postoperative neurotoxicity has been observed in patients receiving large doses of meperidine via patient-controlled anesthesia (103).

Fentanyl, sufentanil, alfentanil, and remifentanil are potent synthetic opioids that cause respiratory depression, apnea, and bradycardia (30). Large doses of the synthetic opioids can produce chest wall rigidity, which can be prevented by pretreatment with a nondepolarizing neuromuscular blocker. Remifentanil is unique because of its rapid elimination by plasma and tissue esterases, which allows this agent to be rapidly titrated via continuous IV infusion (104). Because of its rapid onset and brief duration of action, remifentanil is suited for cases in which noxious stimulation is intense but brief, such as diagnostic laryngoscopy.

Intraoperative Awareness

In a large survey of public attitudes toward preoperative assessment and risk, more respondents were concerned about memory loss and interoperative awareness than were concerned about death (105). Unfortunately, the incidence of intraoperative awareness is probably much higher than reported in the literature (0.2% to 1.0%) (106,107). Recollection, or recall, of intraoperative events underestimates awareness because not all patients who were aware of events during an operation can remember the fact afterward (108). When a forearm is isolated from exposure to muscle relaxants during anesthesia, arm movements can be used to assess perception and response to commands. Many studies have used this technique to establish that conscious perception can occur, with or without explicit memory formation, in an apparently anesthetized patient

(108,109). The incidence of awareness depends on the type of anesthesia, strength of stimulus, and the timing and method used to elicit recall. For example, cardiac surgery is associated with an incidence of awareness up to 23% (110). An incidence of 0.2% would suggest at least 30,000 cases of awareness per year in the United States; clearly, many patients share the same experiences as people in well-publicized cases in newspapers, television talk shows, and on the Internet. Awareness during GA can be a horrifying experience, and it can leave patients with a range of problems from temporary emotional distress to long-lasting post-traumatic stress disorder (111). This complication causes considerable distress for practitioners as well as for patients.

In closed-claims analysis, awareness accounted for 1.9% of 4,183 claims over >20 years, but the greatest proportion of claims occurred during the 1990s (112). Most claims involved women (77%), patients younger than age 60 (89%), ASA class I or II (68%), and elective surgery (87%). The authors used the term "awake paralysis" to describe inadvertent paralysis of an awake patient, and most of these cases were due to medication infusion errors or syringe swaps. Most claims were for "recall during anesthesia," which implied recall of events while receiving GA. These claims were associated with the absence of a volatile anesthetic (nitrous-narcotic-relaxant technique), female gender, obstetrics/gynecology operation, intraoperative opioid, and the use of neuromuscular blocking agents. Neuromuscular blocking agents, as a component of "balanced anesthesia," allow lower concentrations of volatile anesthetics to be used than would otherwise be necessary to prevent movement. Patient movement is a sign of inadequate anesthesia, and ablation of movement, along with using lower concentrations of volatiles, makes awareness a possible risk. A large, retrospective analysis of a database of anesthetic incident reports could not establish a cause of awareness in 16% of cases (113). Forty-four percent of cases were related to low inspired volatile anesthetic concentrations (or inadequate hypnosis) because of problems with vaporizers, breathing circuits, or agent monitors, prolonged attempts at intubation, or reduction in inspired volatile concentrations because of hemodynamic instability. The remaining 40% were caused by drug errors due to inattention, distraction, haste, or fatigue. Table 9-6 lists methods to reduce the incidence of awareness and steps to take in response to a case of awareness.

REGIONAL ANESTHESIA

Local Anesthetic Toxicity

Both anesthesiologists and surgeons frequently use local anesthetics in a wide variety of techniques. The efficacy of local anesthetics in providing anesthesia for local injection,

TABLE 9-6

INTRAOPERATIVE AWARENESS

Measures for Preventing Intraoperative Awareness [a]	Steps to Take Following a Complaint of Awareness During General Anesthesia [b]
• Consider amnestic agents for premedication (midazolam, scopolamine)	• Visit the patient as soon as possible, along with a witness
• Maintain and service anesthesia equipment regularly; check the anesthesia machine before each use, ensuring a correctly mounted vaporizer	• Document the patient's history and exact memory of events; keep a copy of the account
• Use an end-tidal agent monitor, with the low alarm set for a volatile concentration sufficient to prevent awareness	• Attempt to confirm the validity of the account, if necessary
• Use an adequate dose of induction agents; provide additional doses of hypnotic for repeated intubation attempts	• Provide the patient with a full explanation of the events
• Supplement nitrous/opiate technique with potent volatile agent	• Offer the patient follow-up, including psychological support, and document that this has been offered
• Supplement potent volatile agents with nitrous oxide and/or ensure adequate concentrations of volatile anesthetics	• Reassure the patient that he or she can have further general anesthetics with minimal risk of further episodes of awareness
• Be aware of the potential for awareness in hypovolemic patients with low concentrations of hypnotic; introduce these as soon as is practical	• If the cause of the awareness episode is not known, try to determine it
• Use muscle relaxants only when indicated; routinely use a peripheral nerve stimulator and ensure sufficient anesthesia until muscle strength returns	• Notify risk management and hospital administration
• When using total intravenous anesthesia, maintain a patent, secure intravenous line and periodically check the volume in the syringe to ensure the barrel is advancing	• Notify surgeon and primary care physician
• Clearly label all drug syringes immediately as they are drawn up; check this label carefully and do not rely on recognition of syringe size to confirm its contents; consider other methods of ensuring correct drug given	
• Mask auditory input	
• Consider use of depth of anesthesia monitor, if not routinely, then for selected cases	

[a]From Bergman IJ, Kluger MT, Short TG. Awareness during general anaesthesia: a review of 81 cases from the Anaesthetic Incident Monitoring Study. *Anaesthesia* 2002;57(6):549–556; Pitellie PH, Holmes MA, Domino KB. Awareness during anesthesia. In: Weber S, ed. *Anesthesia-related complications*. Philadelphia, PA: W.B. Saunders; 2002: 317–332, vii, with permission.
[b]From Bailey AR, Jones JG. Patients' memories of events during general anaesthesia. *Anaesthesia* 1997;52(5):460–476, with permission.

regional nerve blockade, central neuraxial blockade, and postoperative analgesia is clear. Unfortunately, local anesthetics can cause CNS or cardiovascular toxicity because of unintentional intravascular injection or administration of excessive amounts (Fig. 9-2). The incidence of systemic toxicity has decreased in recent years and is estimated to be between 7.5 and 20 per 10,000 cases (115). Both the CNS effects and cardiovascular effects are due to excess levels of local anesthetic in the blood.

High local anesthetic levels in the blood of the CNS initially result in excitation, which is due to blockade of neural inhibitory pathways in the amygdala (116). As blood levels rise, both inhibitory and excitatory pathways are inhibited, and excitation is followed by CNS depression. Early symptoms are light-headedness, dizziness, visual changes, and tinnitus. Shivering, muscle twitching, and tremors might precede generalized tonic-clonic seizures. Seizures can develop immediately if high blood levels are achieved rapidly, as in an intravascular injection into a

blood vessel supplying the brain. Hypoventilation, hypercarbia, and acidosis lower the seizure threshold, presumably through increased cerebral blood flow and increased uptake of local anesthetic in the brain.

Cardiovascular side effects are generally seen at higher blood levels than those that cause CNS toxicity (Fig. 9-3) (117). Cardiovascular toxicity is due to effects on both the vasculature and the heart. In the heart both electrical and mechanical activity is affected. Local anesthetics inhibit sodium channels, prolonging conduction time and depressing spontaneous pacemaker activity. There have been case reports of cardiac arrest with electrical standstill as a part of bupivacaine toxicity. Many of these cases were reported in young, healthy parturients receiving bupivacaine epidural anesthesia or analgesia, or both, for labor and were associated with difficult, prolonged, and occasionally futile resuscitation (115). Development and recovery from block differ between bupivacaine and lidocaine, helping explain the greater cardiac toxicity with bupivacaine (118). Lidocaine

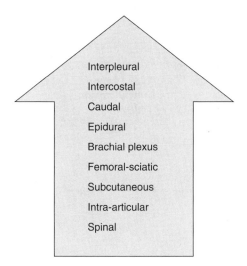

Interpleural

Intercostal

Caudal

Epidural

Brachial plexus

Femoral-sciatic

Subcutaneous

Intra-articular

Spinal

Figure 9-2 Ranking of peak blood levels of local anesthetics following a variety of regional blocks. (From Brown DL. Local anesthetic toxicity. In: Finucane BT, ed. *Complications of Regional Anesthesia*. Philadelphia: Churchill Livingstone; 1999, with permission.)

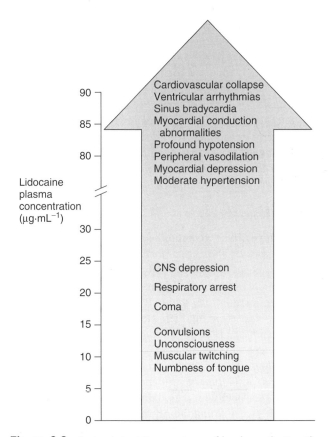

Lidocaine plasma concentration ($\mu g \cdot mL^{-1}$)

90 — Cardiovascular collapse
Ventricular arrhythmias
Sinus bradycardia
85 — Myocardial conduction
abnormalities
Profound hypotension
80 — Peripheral vasodilation
Myocardial depression
Moderate hypertension

30 —

25 — CNS depression

20 — Respiratory arrest

Coma

15 — Convulsions
Unconsciousness

10 — Muscular twitching
Numbness of tongue

5 —

0

Figure 9-3 Systemic toxicity symptoms of local anesthetics. The systemic symptoms associated with toxicity due to local anesthetics are represented on a scale corresponding to the approximate plasma lidocaine concentrations that produce the symptoms. In general, cardiovascular toxicity occurs at levels that are three times the levels that produce CNS toxicity. (From Brown DL. Local anesthetic toxicity. In: Finucane BT, ed. *Complications of Regional Anesthesia*. Philadelphia: Churchill Livingstone; 1999, with permission.)

blocks channels in a "fast-in, fast-out" fashion, allowing recovery of the sodium channel for a portion of the cardiac cycle. Bupivacaine, on the other hand, blocks sodium channels in a "slow-in, slow-out" manner at low concentrations and a in "fast-in, slow-out" manner at high concentrations. Thus, bupivacaine blocks the sodium channels throughout the cardiac cycle, leaving no opportunity for sodium channel recovery.

Clinically, tachycardia and hypertension accompany CNS toxicity. As blood levels of local anesthetics continue to rise, there is myocardial depression, hypertension, and decreased cardiac output. At even higher blood levels, peripheral vasodilation, profound hypotension, conduction abnormalities, sinus bradycardia, and ventricular arrhythmias lead to cardiovascular collapse. A number of factors influence cardiovascular toxicity. The ratio between doses that cause cardiovascular toxicity and CNS toxicity varies with each local anesthetic (119). For example, the cardiovascular toxicity to CNS toxicity ratio is lower with bupivacaine than for lidocaine. Hypoxemia and acidosis often accompany seizures and cardiovascular collapse and can potentiate local anesthetic-induced myocardial depression.

It is difficult to establish a maximal dose for each local anesthetic, even though such information is available in textbooks (Table 9-7) (120). For example, most local anesthetic-induced seizures are because of unintentional intravascular injection rather than uptake of excessive doses from regional blockade (121). Even a small amount of drug injected into an artery supplying the brain will cause seizures. The site of injection and the presence of vasoconstrictors also affect toxicity. In general, epinephrine decreases the peak plasma concentration of local anesthetic after it is injected, but the magnitude of this effect depends on both the local anesthetic and the site of injection (122). Finally, there are variations in the response of individual patients to different doses of local anesthetics.

The best treatment for local anesthetic toxicity is prevention. There are a number of methods to reduce the likelihood of unintentional intravascular injection, including aspiration after positioning the needle or catheter and adding epinephrine to the local anesthetic as an indicator of intravascular injection ("test dose") (115). The injection of relatively large volumes of local anesthetic should be done in increments, reducing the potential toxic dose if it is inadvertently injected intravascularly. CNS toxic responses are best treated with supplemental oxygen, benzodiazepines, or barbiturates and supportive measures; intubation and ventilation are rarely necessary. Cardiac toxicity might require aggressive and prolonged resuscitation measures and pharmacologic support.

Complications of Neuraxial Anesthesia

Neuraxial anesthesia (also known as *central neuraxial blockade*) includes spinal, epidural, and caudal techniques. These techniques involve deposition of local anesthetics, opioids, and/or other adjuvant medications in the spinal

TABLE 9-7

TOXICITY OF LOCAL ANESTHETICS

Drug	Maximum Dose	Equieffective Concentration	Toxic Plasma Concentration (µg/mL)
Lidocaine	4 mg/kg 300–500 mg	1% (10 mg/mL)	>5
Bupivacaine	2 mg/kg 175–200 mg	0.25% (2.5 mg/mL)	1.5

Note: A 1% solution contains 10 mg/mL.

canal, epidural space, or caudal epidural space. Various techniques might or might not utilize a catheter for prolonged or continuous drug administration.

Postdural Puncture Headache

Postdural puncture headache (PDPH), ocular disturbances, and auditory difficulties constitute a syndrome associated with cerebrospinal fluid leak and decreased intracranial pressure following dural puncture (123). This syndrome's most prominent and common symptom is bilateral, frontal, or occipital headache that is relieved when the patient is supine. Needle penetration of the dura results in a leak of cerebrospinal fluid, which leads to intracranial hypotension. Loss of cerebrospinal fluid allows the brain to drop caudad when the patient is upright and resulting in traction on the dura, which causes pain. The size of the defect and the incidence of headache is related to needle gauge, bevel design, orientation of the bevel, and angle of approach on insertion (124). Other factors that increase the incidence of PDPH are youth, female sex, pregnancy, dehydration, and prior history of the disorder (125). The use of small-gauge, noncutting spinal needles and refinement in technique have reduced the incidence of PDPH to 0.4% to 2% (126).

PDPH is usually benign and self-limited, but in severe cases the headache might be incapacitating and treatment is indicated. Many treatments have been proposed for PDPH, but the most effective by far is the epidural blood patch, which provides relief in 90% of patients after one patch (127,128). A second patch provides relief in another 8% of patients. The epidural blood patch is performed by aseptically transferring 8 to 15 mL of autologous blood to the epidural space at the level of the dural puncture. Magnetic resonance imaging of the lumbar region after a blood patch confirms that the hematoma causes a mass effect around the injection site that compresses the thecal sac (129). Mass effect was present at 30 minutes and 3 hours, but the clot had resolved by 7 hours. There was extensive extravasation of blood into the surrounding subcutaneous tissues, which might explain the most common side effect of blood patch, backache.

Backache

Transient minor backache is common after epidural (incidence of 30%) and spinal anesthesia (incidence of 21%) but is not necessarily causally related to the anesthetic technique (130). A prospective evaluation of women found that postpartum back pain was associated with antepartum back pain, greater weight, and younger age (131). The incidence was essentially the same (45%) in women who had received epidural anesthesias as in those who had not. An MRI study on volunteers demonstrated two potential sources for back pain in the lithotomy position: flattening of the lumbar lordosis, and added tension on the lumbosacral nerve roots (132). Serious, protracted back pain is rare after central neuraxial blockade and is most often due to trauma from needle insertion. Spinal or epidural needles might injure the intraspinous ligament, or patients might develop spasm of the paraspinous muscles. The abrupt, postoperative onset of back pain with a radicular component or neurologic signs might indicate the development of spinal hematoma. In that instance it warrants immediate investigation.

Urinary Retention

Postoperative urinary retention is common and is associated with all types of anesthesia and surgery (133). Difficulty in urinating can come from any number or combination of causes, including overdistention of the bladder, pain-induced reflex spasm of the urethral sphincters, trauma to the pelvic nerves or bladder, and pharmacologic effects. Urinary retention is more common in elderly men and in patients receiving opiates (134). In a large review of published studies of urinary retention in inguinal hernia surgery, the authors found that the incidence is lower with local anesthesia (0.4%) than with regional (2.4%) or general (3.0%) anesthesia (135). Spinal anesthesia rapidly eliminates the micturition reflex, which does not return until after motor and most sensory function has recovered. Patients should be monitored for return of bladder function, especially with long-acting local anesthetics. Urinary retention after epidural anesthesia seems to be related more to the epidural administration of opioids than to the local anesthetic.

Transient Neurologic Symptoms

Transient neurologic symptoms, consisting of a back pain or dysesthesia with bilateral radiation into the buttocks or legs, have been recently described as a complication of spinal anesthesia, especially when performed with lidocaine (123). Symptoms begin after total recovery from spinal anesthesia and within 24 hours of surgery. The incidence of this complication might be as high as 36%, depending on the type of surgery performed; the incidence is highest for procedures performed in the lithotomy position and lowest for those performed when the patient is supine (136). Incidence does not change with the concentration of lidocaine used in the spinal anesthetic (137). Although the exact etiology of transient neurologic symptoms is not known, it is thought that a toxic effect of local anesthetics is an important contributing factor and that local ischemia from nerve stretch might also contribute. The clinical implications are still unclear, but some practitioners avoid using lidocaine for spinal anesthetics, especially if the procedure will be performed in the lithotomy position (130).

Spinal Hematoma and Abscess

Paraplegia from spinal hematoma or epidural abscess, the most dreaded complications of neuraxial blockade, is rare (138). Meta-analysis of data from large retrospective studies suggests an incidence of spinal hematoma of 1:150,000 after epidural anesthesia and 1:220,000 after spinal anesthesia (139). In a comprehensive analysis of case reports between 1906 and 1994, Vandermeulen et al. found only 61 published cases of epidural hematoma or subdural hematoma, or both, involving central neuraxial blockade, and 42 of these occurred in patients who had a clotting disorder or who were using anticoagulants (138). Risk factors for hematoma formation following neuraxial blockade are full anticoagulation at the time of the procedure, coagulopathy (factor deficiency, thrombocytopenia, disseminated intravascular coagulopathy), and difficult needle or catheter placement (138). Epidural hematomas can occur spontaneously (the most common cause) or after diagnostic lumbar puncture followed by anticoagulation.

The most common site for hematoma formation is the epidural space, presumably because of traumatic disruption of the epidural venous plexus. Early symptoms are back pain or radicular pain, but muscle weakness might be the first complaint (138). Neurologic symptoms of lower extremity weakness and bowel and bladder dysfunction develop once enough blood has accumulated to create a mass effect and compress the spinal cord or nerve roots. Vigilance, regular neurologic assessment, and expeditious diagnostic studies are necessary to detect spinal hematoma early enough to avoid permanent neurologic damage. Recovery of neurologic function is possible if decompressive laminectomy is performed within 8 hours of the onset of paraplegia.

The reported incidence of epidural abscess in neuraxial anesthesia varies widely, depending on the study method, but it is generally low—between 1 in 2,000 and 1 in 5,000 catheters (140,141). Like spontaneous spinal hematoma, epidural abscess is more commonly reported from sources not related to epidural or spinal anesthesia. Abscess formation related to neuraxial blockade is believed to be due to introduction of bacteremic blood into the epidural space. Risk factors for infection and abscess formation are immunosuppression, bacteremia, caudal anesthesia, and breaks in aseptic technique. One recent survey of epidural abscesses found that half of incidents were associated with low molecular weight heparin therapy (141). In addition to back pain and neurologic symptoms, patients with epidural abscess usually present with fever, leukocytosis, meningeal signs, and signs of localized infection. Not surprisingly, *Staphylococcus aureus* was the most common etiologic agent in one large series (140). Once the diagnosis has been established, prompt therapy with antibiotics and surgical evacuation should be performed in order to maximize the likelihood of neurologic recovery.

Anticoagulation and Neuraxial Blockade

A number of large case series in a variety of operative settings have established the safety of systemic anticoagulation following neuraxial blockade in select patients using strict guidelines (126,142). In general, patients without preexisting coagulopathy can receive IV heparin 60 minutes following atraumatic insertion of an epidural catheter without significant risk of hematoma. On the other hand, there have been recent reports of spinal hematoma developing after spinal or epidural anesthesia in patients receiving low molecular weight heparin for perioperative thromboprophylaxis (139,143,144). Most of these cases involved epidural anesthesia, and some were related to removal of the epidural catheter while receiving heparin (145). The risk of fatal pulmonary embolus without prophylaxis is greater than the risk of spinal hematoma, but that does not mean that effective thromboprophylaxis takes precedence over, and excludes, regional anesthesia (146). A consensus from the American Society of Regional and Pain Medicine states that spinal or epidural anesthesia can be administered in the setting of heparinization or low molecular weight heparin administration so long as certain precautions are heeded (Table 9-8) (147).

Nerve Injury

Several large retrospective studies have confirmed that permanent injury to the spinal cord or nerve roots is uncommon (149). The most common neurologic complication of central blockade is damage to a nerve root from needle or catheter placement. Injury to the lumbosacral nerve root and the spinal cord made up 16% and 13% of closed claims related to nerve injuries, respectively, in the ASA's Closed Claims Project (150). In a prospective, multicenter study of serious complications of regional anesthesia, Auroy et al. found a low incidence of radiculopathy following spinal

TABLE 9-8

GUIDELINES FOR NEURAXIAL BLOCKADE IN THE SETTING OF ANTICOAGULATION

All	Systemic Heparinization	Low Molecular Weight Heparin
• Avoid neuraxial blockade in patients with coagulopathy	• Avoid neuraxial blockade in patients receiving antiplatelet medications	• Avoid neuraxial blockade in patients receiving both LMWH and antiplatelet medications
• Discontinue antiplatelet medications 7 days prior to operation	• Needle and/or catheter placement should occur at least 60 minutes prior to heparinization	• Withhold LMWH 12 to 24 hours prior to needle placement
• Discontinue oral anticoagulation 60 hours prior to operation	• Consider delaying or canceling surgery if needle or catheter placement is traumatic	• Delay the first postoperative dose of LMWH 12 to 24 hours following traumatic block
• Check coagulation profile (PT, aPTT, platelet count) prior to operation	• Monitor heparin affect and maintain within acceptable levels (1.5 to 2.0 times baseline)	• Postoperative twice-daily dosing: Indwelling catheters should be removed at least 2 hours prior to beginning postoperative LMWH thromboprophylaxis

• Use small-gauge needles and minimal catheter insertion depth (3–4 cm)
• Use a dilute local anesthetic solution for postoperative analgesia
• Regular neurological evaluation post-op
	• Remove catheter when heparin activity is low or completely reversed	• Postoperative once-daily dosing:
		  o Epidural catheters may be safely maintained
		  o The first dose should be administered 6 to 8 hours postoperatively and the second no sooner than 24 hours after the first dose
		  o Epidural catheters should be removed a minimum of 10 to 12 hours after the last dose of LMWH
		  o The first dose of LMWH can be administered 2 hours after epidural catheter removal

LMWH, Low Molecular Weight Heparin.
From Horlocker TT. Low molecular weight heparin and neuraxial anesthesia. *Thrombosis Res* 2001;101(1):141–154; Horlocker TT, Wedel DJ, Benzon H, et al. Regional anesthesia in the anticoagulated patient: defining the risks (the second ASRA Consensus Conference on Neuraxial Anesthesia and Anticoagulation). *Reg Anesth Pain Med* 2003;28(3):172–197; Tyagi A, Bhattacharya A. Central neuraxial blocks and anticoagulation: a review of current trends. *Eur J Anaesthesiol* 2002;19(5): 317–329, all with permission.

and epidural anesthesia (149). Needle insertion or drug injection was associated with pain or paresthesias in most cases. In contrast to the midline approach, the paramedian (oblique lateral) approach to the epidural and subarachnoid space directs the needle toward the dural cuff region of the nerve root, increasing the risk of injury.

Reynolds reported on a cluster of seven cases with persistent unilateral sensory loss, foot drop, and urinary symptoms (three patients) following spinal or combined spinal-epidural anesthesia. All had a painful lumbar puncture, and six had magnetic resonance imaging showing a syrinx in the conus. The authors pointed out that the termination of the conus is variable and emphasized the importance of performing the lumbar puncture at the correct level (151).

Spinal Cord Ischemia

The anterior spinal artery, which supplies the anterior portion of the spinal cord, has poor vertical anastomotic connections between radicular branches that supply it. The anterior spinal cord is susceptible to ischemic injury if the segmental blood supply is compromised through trauma.

A dense motor paralysis, variable sensory impairment, and preservation of position and vibratory sense characterize the anterior spinal artery syndrome. Injury to the anterior spinal artery has been reported with epidural catheter or needle placement, but surgical disruption of the blood supply or systemic hypotension is a much more likely cause (152).

Bradycardia, Hypotension, and Cardiac Arrest

Hypotension is common during neuraxial anesthesia and is better regarded as a side effect than a complication. Hypotension results from the preganglionic sympathetic block that reduces systemic vascular resistance and increases venodilation. Decreased venous return enhances vagal tone. High sympathectomy also results in bradycardia through blockade of the cardiac accelerator fibers, which arise from spinal levels T1 to T4. Decreased venous return, systemic hypotension, and bradycardia can reduce cardiac output. Moderate and severe bradycardia occurs in about 10% and 1% of neuraxial anesthetics, respectively, and can develop at any time during the anesthetic (153).

Risk factors for the development of hypotension and bradycardia during spinal and epidural anesthesia have been identified in large-scale prospective studies (Table 9-9) (154,155).

In the 1980s a review of closed insurance claims revealed a set of cases involving cardiac arrest during spinal anesthesia in otherwise healthy patients (156). The outcome in these cases was that most patients died or had severe neurologic injury. Further evaluation of these cases suggested that sedation and respiratory insufficiency might have contributed to the cardiac arrest. Cardiopulmonary resuscitation (CPR) in these witnessed cardiac arrests might have been ineffective because of sympathetic blockade during high spinal anesthesia and delayed administration of potent vasoconstrictors. In large, prospective surveys of complications of regional anesthesia, cardiac arrest during spinal anesthesia occurred with an incidence of 2.7 to 7.0 per 10,000 (149,157,158). The incidence of cardiac arrest during spinal anesthesia is higher than that seen with GA and epidural anesthesia. Survivors of cardiac arrest were younger and healthier, as measured by ASA classification. Sedation, respiratory insufficiency, and especially severe bradycardia have been implicated as major contributing factors to cardiac arrest. Studies in human volunteers given spinal anesthetics have shown that hypovolemia potentiates vagally mediated bradycardia and can even precipitate cardiac arrest (158). Other cases of bradycardia and cardiac arrest during spinal anesthesia have occurred after the addition of potent vasodilators such as sodium nitroprusside.

Studies in dogs show that spinal anesthesia suppresses the catecholamine response to cardiac arrest and reduces the coronary perfusion pressure that is obtained during cardiopulmonary resuscitation (159,160). The coronary perfusion pressure achieved during CPR in spinal anesthetized dogs was significantly below the threshold for predicting successful resuscitation, and relatively high doses (0.1 mg per kg) of epinephrine were required to restore coronary perfusion pressure (159). These studies help explain why CPR may be ineffective in patients suffering cardiac arrest during spinal anesthesia, and they suggest that high doses of vasopressors (epinephrine, norepinephrine, and/or vasopressin) might be required to restore coronary perfusion during CPR. In summary, severe bradycardia with hypotension should be treated rapidly with volume infusion, atropine, and vasopressors, preferably epinephrine (158). If cardiac arrest develops, CPR should be accompanied by early and aggressive administration of vasopressors.

Failed Block

Perhaps the most frequent complication of regional anesthesia is failure of the blockade. Entry into the epidural space is confirmed by tactile loss of resistance to pressure on the plunger of a syringe. This endpoint is subject to misinterpretation. Even with the visual clues of spinal technique (return of cerebrospinal fluid), failures occur in 4% to 17% of spinal anesthetics. The other extreme is total spinal anesthesia when an excessive dose of local anesthetic is delivered into the subarachnoid or subdural space. Patients are rendered apneic, unconscious, and hypotensive and require intubation, mechanical ventilation, and vasopressor support.

MISCELLANEOUS COMPLICATIONS OF ANESTHESIA

Postoperative Nausea and Vomiting

Postoperative nausea and vomiting (PONV) is anesthesiology's "big little problem," and a great deal of effort is focused on strategies to reduce the frequency of this complication. Nausea is an unpleasant sensation in the epigastrium

---

TABLE 9-9

RISK FACTORS FOR BRADYCARDIA AND HYPOTENSION DURING CENTRAL NEURAXIAL BLOCKADE

Technique	Risk Factors for Hypotension	Risk Factors for Bradycardia
Epidural anesthesia	• Epidural fentanyl • Increased spread of sensory blockade • Lack of tourniquet use • Use of carbonated lidocaine	• Female sex • Use of tourniquet
Spinal anesthesia	• Sensory block higher than the fifth thoracic dermatome • Age older than 40 years • Baseline systolic blood pressure <120 mm Hg • Use of combined spinal and general anesthesia • Dural puncture cephalad to the L2–L3 interspace • Addition of phenylephrine to the local anesthetic spinal block	• Baseline heart rate <60 bpm • ASA physical status I • Use of beta-adrenergic blocking agents • Sensory block higher than the fifth thoracic dermatome

that is associated with an urge to vomit, but vomiting is the forceful expulsion of gastric contents. The incidence of nausea and vomiting varies, depending on the patient population and setting, but generally affects 10% of patients in the postoperative anesthesia care unit and 30% of patients during the first 24 hours (161).

Vomiting is controlled by emetic centers that receive afferent input from many sources inside and outside the CNS. A major input is from the chemoreceptor trigger zone. Structures involved in vomiting are rich in dopaminergic, muscarinic, serotonergic, histaminic, and opioid receptors, which explains the basic approach of antagonizing various neurotransmitter receptors in order to control vomiting.

A multidisciplinary panel of experts recently published consensus guidelines on PONV based on a structured review of the medical literature (162). A great deal of useful information can be drawn from the conclusions reached by the expert panel and by other authors who have reviewed this topic (161). A variety of factors is suspected to influence the occurrence of PONV, including patient characteristics, site of surgery, duration of surgery, and type of anesthetic. A combination of factors contributes to the occurrence of nausea or vomiting, or both. For example, volatile anesthetics appear to be the most important cause of early vomiting in both children and adults, but late vomiting seems to be due to postoperative opioids (163). The guidelines stress identifying patients at high risk for PONV. Risk factors for PONV in adults are female sex, nonsmoking status, a history of PONV or motion sickness, duration of surgery, type of surgery (laparoscopy, ear–nose–throat, neurosurgery, breast, strabismus, laparotomy, plastic surgery), use of volatile anesthetics, use of nitrous oxide, and use of opioids.

Risk factors in children are similar to adults with the following differences. Vomiting is twice as frequent in children. The risk increases as children age but decreases after puberty, and sex differences are not seen before puberty.

Surprisingly, smoking protects against PONV, perhaps through increased clearance of anesthetic drugs due to enzyme induction (164). Apfel et al. have created a simplified risk score on the basis of identifying four primary risk factors: female sex, nonsmoking status, history of PONV, and opioid use (165). The incidence of PONV increases with the presence of one or more of these risk factors.

Strategies to reduce the baseline risk of PONV are listed in Table 9-10. There is no single "magic bullet," and the most effective strategy might be one that encompasses many or all of the methods listed. In certain high-risk patients a multimodal approach consisting of anxiolysis, hydration, supplemental oxygen, prophylactic antiemetics, total IV anesthesia without nitrous oxide, and ketorolac might be effective. The consensus guidelines suggest antiemetic therapy for prophylaxis in patients at moderate or high risk of PONV. There is no difference in the

TABLE 9-10

STRATEGIES TO REDUCE BASELINE RISK OF POSTOPERATIVE NAUSEA AND VOMITING

Use regional anesthesia instead of general anesthesia
Use propofol for induction and maintenance of anesthesia
Intraoperative supplemental oxygen
Adequate hydration
Avoid nitrous oxide
Avoid volatile anesthetics
Minimize intraoperative and postoperative opioids
Minimize or eliminate use of neostigmine

efficacy and safety profiles of the various serotonin (5-HT$_3$) receptor antagonists in the prophylaxis of PONV. These drugs have a favorable side effect profile; the most common problems are headache, constipation, and increased liver function tests. To be most effective, 5-HT$_3$ receptor antagonists, such as ondansetron, should be given at the end of surgery. Small doses of dexamethasone (2.5 to 5 mg) are effective in reducing PONV when given prior to induction of anesthesia. Although adverse events have not been reported in humans after a single bolus dose of dexamethasone, there is some evidence that a single dose can impair wound healing in rats (166). Droperidol is equally effective as ondansetron for prophylaxis of PONV and, like the 5-HT$_3$ receptor antagonists, is most effective when given at the end of surgery. The FDA has issued a "black box" warning that droperidol might cause death or life-threatening events associated with QT prolongation and torsade de pointes, but the warning is not well substantiated by the medical literature. The expert panel authoring the consensus guidelines expressed considerable concern about the validity of the FDA warning. Importantly, metoclopramide is not effective for PONV prophylaxis and has considerable side effects. Antiemetics should be given to patients who develop PONV and were not given prophylaxis or in whom prophylaxis failed. Treatment doses of the 5-HT$_3$ receptor antagonists are one quarter of those used for prophylaxis. In those patients failing prophylaxis, drugs used to treat PONV should be from a class other than the drugs used for prophylaxis. Interestingly, a small, subhypnotic dose of propofol (20 mg) is effective in treating PONV (167). An algorithm for managing PONV is presented in Figure 9-4.

Obesity and Morbid Obesity

Obesity has now reached epidemic proportions in the United States, and the lay press, as well as the medical literature, is addressing the health concerns of an obese population (168). The body mass index (BMI) is a measure of

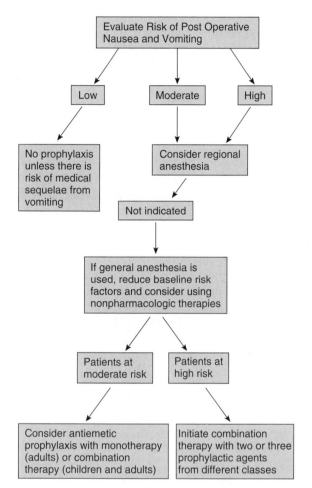

Figure 9-4 Algorithm for the management of postoperative nausea and vomiting. [From Gan TJ, Meyer T, Apfel CC, et al. Consensus guidelines for managing postoperative nausea and vomiting. *Anesthesia and Analgesia* 2003;97(1):62–71, with permission.]

the relationship between height and weight and it is calculated by the formula

$$BMI = \frac{\text{body weight (in kg)}}{\text{height}^2 \text{ (in meters)}}$$

A BMI of <25 kg per m² is normal, but a person with a BMI of 25 to 30 kg per m² is overweight. Persons with a BMI of >30, >35 and >55 kg per m² are considered obese, morbidly obese, and super morbidly obese, respectively, and have an increased risk of medical complications and increased mortality. Physiologic changes associated with obesity lead to an increased incidence of comorbid conditions, such as gallbladder disease, diabetes, hypertension, heart disease, osteoarthritis, and obstructive sleep apnea (169). Persons with a BMI >30 have an increased rate of mortality especially if they have an android (central or male) pattern of fat distribution or rapid weight gain after age 20.

Many of the pathophysiologic changes in obesity combine to increase the risk of complications during induction of anesthesia, maintenance of the airway, mask ventilation, intubation, and extubation. A fat face and cheeks, a fat, short neck, large tongue, excess pharyngeal tissue, restricted mouth opening, and large breasts can make mask ventilation and intubation difficult or impossible. Mask ventilation and intubation are also difficult in many patients with obstructive sleep apnea. Although only 5% of morbidly obese patients have obstructive sleep apnea, most patients with obstructive sleep apnea are obese (170). In obese patients with obstructive sleep apnea, the pharyngeal area is reduced because of deposition of fat in the pharyngeal tissues, and the airway is compressed externally by fat masses in the superficial neck area. All central depressants and muscle relaxants will promote pharyngeal collapse in obese patients with obstructive sleep apnea by diminishing the action of the pharyngeal dilator muscles. Thus, obese patients with or without obstructive sleep apnea are at risk of airway obstruction when given sedatives, anesthetics, or muscle relaxants. In a retrospective study of patients being surgically treated for obstructive sleep apnea, the complication rate was 13%. Seventy-seven percent of these complications were airway problems (171). Patients with problems during intubation were heavier, but patients experiencing problems following extubation had received more narcotic analgesia.

It is commonly believed that obese patients have increased intragastric volumes, increased intraabdominal pressures, increased incidence of hiatal hernia, and increased incidence of gastroesophageal reflux, all of which might put them at higher risk of gastric regurgitation and aspiration during mask ventilation, intubation, and extubation. Difficult mask ventilation can result in gastric insufflation, which further increases the risk of regurgitation and aspiration. Although the evidence for these risk factors is conflicting, many authors recommend taking routine precautions to prevent acid aspiration in obese patients (168).

In a large, multicenter study of adverse outcomes after GA, obesity was one of several predictors of severe respiratory outcomes (172). Obesity causes abnormalities of both lung volumes and gas exchange that are exacerbated by the supine position and anesthesia. Functional residual capacity (FRC) and expiratory reserve volume (ERV) are reduced so that tidal volume occurs at or below closing capacity, leading to closure of small airways, ventilation-perfusion mismatching, atelectasis, and arterial desaturation (168,173). Pelosi et al. studied the effects of BMI on respiratory function during anesthesia in 24 patients (eight normal weight patients, eight moderately obese patients, and eight morbidly obese patients) (173). With increasing BMI, there was an exponential decline in FRC, an exponential decline in compliance of the respiratory system, an increase in resistance, an exponential decline in the oxygenation index (Pa_{O_2}/PA_{O_2}), and an increase in the work of breathing

(173). Increased basal metabolic rate and high resting oxygen consumption, decreased FRC, and altered oxygenation work in combination to reduce the time it takes obese patients to desaturate during periods of hypoventilation or apnea. In general, obese patients desaturate rapidly after induction of anesthesia despite preoxygenation.

Morbidly obese patients can be difficult to ventilate and difficult to intubate. In addition, they are prone to rapid desaturation during apneic periods and they are at increased risk of acid aspiration. Therefore, many authorities recommend awake fiberoptic intubation for GA (168). Desaturation due to atelectasis during GA and mechanical ventilation is better treated with moderate levels of positive end-expiratory pressure than with excessive tidal volumes.

Obese patients are prone to hypertension, and obesity is recognized as an independent risk factor for ischemic heart disease, especially in patients with a central, android distribution of fat. Obesity-induced cardiomyopathy refers to a condition in which volume and pressure overload lead to heart failure, which is often biventricular. Increased blood volume and high cardiac output result in left ventricular enlargement and increased wall stress. Persistent, abnormally high wall stress promotes the development of eccentric hypertrophy, which results in LV systolic dysfunction, diastolic dysfunction, and clinical heart failure. Pulmonary hypertension secondary to obstructive sleep apnea can cause right ventricular enlargement, hypertrophy, and failure as well. In an autopsy study of morbidly obese patients who died of sudden cardiac death, 10 of 22 patients had dilated cardiomyopathy, six had severe coronary artery disease, and four had left ventricular hypertrophy without dilation (174).

Obese patients can present challenges with respect to IV access, patient positioning, monitoring, and regional anesthesia. For example, noninvasive blood pressure cuffs often do not fit properly even if they are large size, and it can be difficult or impossible to obtain an accurate blood pressure reading without direct arterial cannulation.

Independent of additional comorbid conditions, the physical state of obesity implies that patients are at increased risk of perioperative complications because of their excess weight and obese body habitus, although few studies are available to establish the precise impact of obesity on anesthesia and surgery (175). In a multivariate single-center study of 2,299 patients undergoing cardiac surgery, 25% of patients were obese and 13% were severely obese, and, with the exception of superficial wound infections and atrial dysrhythmias, obesity was an insignificant multivariate risk factor for adverse outcomes (176). In a similar study, Fasol et al. found that there was no difference in operative mortality between obese and nonobese cardiac surgery patients, but the former had higher rates of infection, sternal dehiscence, arrhythmias, and myocardial infarction (177). Choban and Flancbaum reviewed the literature for a number of elective surgical procedures and concluded that there was only a modest increase in perioperative complications and that these were mostly wound problems (175). Mortality was not increased and operative results were not adversely affected. On the other hand, obese patients had higher morbidity and mortality following trauma and burn surgery.

Hypothermia

Although the human thermoregulatory system normally maintains a core body temperature near 37°C, anesthesia and the patient's exposure to a cold environment often result in perioperative hypothermia. Hypothermia has been implicated as an important factor in numerous perioperative complications such as coagulopathy, surgical wound infection, and cardiac morbidity (178). A number of afferent receptors throughout the body terminate in the CNS, which normally responds to small variations in temperature to maintain thermal homeostasis within a narrow range. Besides obvious behavorial response to changes in temperature, effector responses to cold are vasoconstriction and shivering, and effector responses to warmth are cutaneous vasodilation and sweating. Normally, the threshold for response to warmth is maintained narrowly just 0.2°C above the response to cold. Thermoregulatory vasoconstriction and vasodilation occur in arteriovenous shunts located primarily in the fingers and toes.

General anesthesia and muscle relaxants abolish the behavioral response to perturbations in temperature, and they also prevent shivering (179). GA, opioids, and IV anesthetics lower the threshold for cold responses and widen the range of temperatures in which thermoregulatory responses are not triggered. Thus, anesthesia decreases the patient's response to cold and renders the patient poikilothermic over an extended range of temperatures (~4°C). During the first hour of GA, core temperature drops by 1° to 5°C because of redistribution of body heat from the core to the periphery secondary to opening of peripheral arteriovenous shunts. After the first hour temperature continues to decline because of loss of body heat in excess of metabolic production, although at a slower rate. Most heat is lost during this time through the skin by convection. The core temperature stops declining after 3 to 5 hours. This thermal plateau, or steady state, might be secondary to effective insulation or warming measures, or it might be due to intense thermoregulatory vasoconstriction in patients not well protected against heat loss.

Hypothermia affects patients given epidural or spinal anesthesia as well (179). Regional anesthesia blocks afferent and efferent neural components of the thermoregulatory response. Regional anesthesia also has a surprising central effect on thermoregulation, so that the CNS erroneously judges the skin temperature in blocked areas to be abnormally high. Undetected hypothermia is relatively common during spinal or epidural anesthesia because patients feel warmer and anesthetists seldom monitor temperature during regional anesthesia.

Hypothermia is used to protect the heart and CNS from potential periods of ischemia during cardiac surgery and neurosurgery. On the other hand, mild hypothermia reduces the resistance to wound infection by decreasing cutaneous blood flow and impairing immune function. Maintenance of normothermia has been shown to reduce the incidence of wound infections in patients undergoing colon resection (180). Hypothermia impairs platelet function and hinders activation of the coagulation cascade, resulting in coagulopathy, increased blood loss, and increased need for blood transfusion (181). Hypothermia increases the incidence of ventricular dysrhythmias and cardiac morbidity. Decreased metabolism and clearance of drugs can prolong postoperative recovery (178).

Normothermia is best maintained using a variety of measures to prevent heat loss and to actively warm the patient (178). Both cold blood and room-temperature IV fluid can significantly decrease body temperature and, when given in large amounts, these fluids should be warmed to prevent a further decline in temperature. Warming these fluids, however, will not actively increase a patient's body temperature. Skin is the major source of heat loss, and increasing the ambient temperature will reduce convective heat losses. Forced air warming blankets can also prevent convective losses. In addition, forced air warming is the most effective method of actively warming a patient. Despite some concerns about the increased turbulent airflow created by these warming devices, they do not appear to increase the risk of infections; in fact, these devices might reduce the incidence of wound infections (180). Skin is relatively vulnerable to injury from heat especially when pressure is applied to the skin. Circulating-water mattresses are relatively ineffective in warming the patient and can be a source of pressure-thermal injury. Patients at the extremes of age, patients who are debilitated, and those undergoing major operations might be especially at risk of burns from circulating-water mattresses (182).

Hyperthermia

There are numerous causes of perioperative hyperthermia, and increased body temperature might be due to iatrogenic causes or it might be secondary to any one of a number of diseases (183). A list of etiologies appears in Table 9-11. Iatrogenic intraoperative hyperthermia can occur during long procedures when the patient is completely covered by surgical drapes and the operative area is small. Excessive active warming can cause mild hyperthermia, especially in pediatric patients.

Malignant Hyperthermia

Malignant hyperthermia (MH) is a serious condition that develops in genetically predisposed patients who are exposed to certain "triggering agents," namely, the inhalational anesthetics and/or succinylcholine. Nonspecific signs and symptoms of MH are tachycardia, tachypnea, diaphoresis, and fever. More specific signs are skeletal muscle rigidity, myoglobinuria, myoglobinemia, hyperkalemia, hypercalcemia, and mixed acidosis (183). The most sensitive indicator of potential MH is an unanticipated increase (e.g., doubling or tripling) of the end-tidal CO_2 concentration while minute ventilation is kept constant. Although the exact cause of MH is not known, the pivotal role of increased intracellular calcium is well established (184). The consequences of increased intracellular calcium are activation of ATPases with depletion of

---

TABLE 9-11
DIFFERENTIAL DIAGNOSIS OF INTRAOPERATIVE HYPERTHERMIA

1. Iatrogenic causes
   (a) Active warming of patients (particularly pediatric patients)
   (b) Application of tourniquets to upper or lower extremities for prolonged periods (especially in children)
   (c) Injection of sclerosing solutions into arteriovenous malformations
   (d) Long procedures where patient is mostly covered with drapes

2. Hyperthermia secondary to diseases
   (a) Thyrotoxicosis and thyroid storm
   (b) Riley-Day syndrome (dopamine β-hydroxylase deficiency)
   (c) Osteogenesis imperfecta
   (d) Central nervous system dysfunction (status epilepticus, hypoxic encephalopathy)
   (e) Infectious agents (surgical manipulation of infected tissue, head trauma, prolonged surgery on urinary tract)

3. Drug-induced hyperthermia
   (a) Malignant hyperthermia
   (b) Neuroleptic malignant syndrome

ATP, actin–myosin interaction causing muscle contraction, consumption of glucose, glycogen, and oxygen, and generation of heat. As ATP is depleted, membrane integrity is compromised and potassium, myoglobin, creatine kinase, and tissue thromboplastin are released extracellularly. The treatment of MH is outlined in Table 9-12.

Anaphylactic and Anaphylactoid Reactions in the Perioperative Period

Unfortunately, allergic reactions are one of the major factors contributing to morbidity and mortality during anesthesia (185). Of the various types of allergic reactions, anaphylactic and anaphylactoid reactions are the most serious. This topic has been reviewed recently in the anesthesiology literature (186). Anaphylaxis is an immune-mediated allergic reaction and usually occurs on reexposure to a specific antigen, but it can occur on first exposure. The reaction involves (Ig)E-mediated release of proinflammatory mediators (histamine, prostacyclin, leukotrienes) from mast cells and basophils. Histamine acts on type 1 receptors to increase mucus production and heart rate and to cause flushing. Type 2 receptors are responsible for increasing vascular permeability, increasing gastric acid secretion, and airway mucus production. Prostaglandins and leukotriene receptors are present in bronchial smooth muscle, the skin, and the vascular bed. Activation of these receptors causes bronchoconstriction, cutaneous wheal, and increased vascular permeability. Anaphylactoid reactions are due to nonimmune release of inflammatory mediators and are clinically indistinguishable from anaphylactic reactions.

Anaphylaxis is an unanticipated, severe allergic reaction manifested by cardiovascular symptoms (tachycardia, hypotension, shock), cutaneous symptoms (urticaria, flushing, pruritus, angioedema), and respiratory symptoms (bronchospasm, wheezing, dyspnea, hypoxemia). In the patient covered by drapes and under GA, the early cutaneous signs might be overlooked and the diagnosis can be delayed or missed.

The most frequent class of anesthetic medications causing anaphylaxis is the muscle relaxants (187). Natural rubber latex is the second most common cause, followed by antibiotics and anesthetic induction agents. During cardiac surgery patients are exposed to large doses of a variety of antigenic medications, including heparin, protamine, and, occasionally, aprotinin. Yet antibiotics, muscle relaxants, and blood products account for most allergic reactions during cardiac cases (188). Table 9-13 reviews a number of medications used in the perioperative period and their allergic reactions.

Perhaps as many as 20% of intraoperative allergic reactions are due to latex. Natural rubber latex is a ubiquitous material found in a wide variety of medical products,

---

TABLE 9-12

SUGGESTED TREATMENT OF MALIGNANT HYPERTHERMIA

For consultation to help with patient management, call the MH Hotline: 1-800-MH-HYPER (1-800-644-9737) or 1-315-464-7079 if outside the US.

1. Call for experienced help.
2. Stop potent inhaled agents and succinylcholine.
3. Hyperventilate with 100% oxygen at two to three times the predicted minute ventilation.
4. Prepare and administer IV dantrolene 2.5 mg/kg. Repeat as often as necessary to control clinical signs of malignant hyperthermia.
5. Treat acidosis with sodium bicarbonate.
6. Avoid calcium channel blockers. Treat arrhythmias with other medications as needed.
7. Obtain blood gases, electrolytes, creatine kinase, blood and urine for myoglobin, coagulation profile. Measure creatine kinase every 6 hours until decreased. Follow coagulation profile to monitor for disseminate intravascular coagulation.
8. Treat hyperkalemia with glucose, insulin, and calcium.
9. Monitor core temperature and begin cooling measures, if hyperthermic (nasogastric lavage, rectal lavage and/or surface cooling). Avoid overcooling.
10. Continue intravenous dantrolene for at least 24 hours after control of the episode (approximately 1 mg/kg q 6 hours). Continue dantrolene administration for at least 36 hours after an event. Watch for recrudescence by monitoring in an ICU for at least 24 hours.
11. Ensure adequate urine output by hydration and diuretics.
12. Report patients who have had acute malignant hyperthermia episodes to the North American Malignant Hyperthermia Registry of the Malignant Hyperthermia Association of the United States: 1-412-692-5464.

TABLE 9-13

MEDICATIONS AND ALLERGIC REACTIONS

Local anesthetics	• Anaphylactic reactions to amide local anesthetics are extremely rare • True allergic reactions to esters account for <1% of reactions to local anesthetics • Allergic reactions are usually due to paraaminobenzoic acid metabolite of esters or methylparaben preservative
Muscle relaxants	• Muscle relaxants account for most anaphylactic reactions during anesthesia • Incidence: succinylcholine > benzylisoquoliniums > aminosteroids • Rocuronium: possible increased incidence when compared to other muscle relaxants • Benzylisoquinolinium compounds can cause direct mast cell degranulation
Opioids	• Allergic reactions to opioids are rare • Morphine causes nonimmunologic histamine release
Propofol	• Current evidence suggest that egg-allergic patients are not more likely to develop anaphylaxis
Inhaled anesthetics	• Immune-mediated hepatic injury
Aprotinin	• Antigenic, derived from bovine lung • 2.5% to 2.8% incidence of anaphylaxis on reexposure
Heparin	• Antigenic, derived from bovine or porcine intestine • Heparin induced thrombocytopenia is the most common nonanaphylactic reaction[a]
Protamine[b]	• Antigenic, derived from salmon sperm • Slightly increased risk on reexposure and in diabetic patients exposed to neutral protamine hagedorn or protamine zinc insulin • Increased risk in vasectomized patients and those with fish allergies is controversial
Vancomycin	• "Red man" syndrome of hypotension, pruritus, flushing and rash in 5% to 14%; due to nonimmunologic histamine release • Rare cases of (Ig)-E mediated hypersensitivity reactions
Penicillins, cephalosporins	• Penicillin accounts for 90% of all drug allergic reactions • Approximately 10% of patients who are allergic to penicillin are also allergic to cephalosporins
Isosulfan blue dye	• Approved for intraoperative lymphatic mapping and sentinel node biopsy procedures for breast cancer and melanoma • 1% to 2% incidence of allergic reactions including severe, anaphylactic reactions

[a] From Spinler SA, Dager W. Overview of heparin-induced thrombocytopenia. *Am J Health-Syst Pharm* 2003;60(5), S5-11, with permission.
[b] From Porsche R, Brenner Z. Allergy to protamine sulfate. *Heart Lung J Acute Crit Care* 1999;28(6):418–428; Cormack JG, Levy JH. Adverse reactions to protamine. *Coronary Artery Dis* 1993;4(5):420–425, with permission.

although latex-free alternatives are becoming more widely available. Expanding use of universal precautions has led to an increase in the use of gloves containing latex. This high demand for gloves resulted in the rapid manufacture of a product with increased protein content, which led to an increase in the incidence of latex anaphylaxis (192). Recent improvements in latex production and the increased use of low-protein, powder-free gloves have reduced the incidence of reactions. Not all reactions to latex are anaphylactic in nature. The most common reaction associated with latex is an irritant contact dermatitis that is probably due to the alkaline pH of latex gloves. Health care workers, patients with a history of multiple surgical procedures, spina bifida, atopic individuals, and those with fruit or food allergy (kiwi, chestnut, avocado, passion fruit, banana) are at increased risk of having a latex allergy. Parenteral or mucus

membrane exposure is most likely to lead to a severe reaction, but a reaction can develop in response to inhalation of airborne latex particles.

Avoiding latex-containing products is the only effective management option in most cases (192). Latex-allergic patients should be scheduled early in the day to reduce their exposure to aeroallergens. Prophylactic administration of steroids and antihistamines is not effective and is not recommended. Certain desensitization techniques might be effective in some cases.

Positioning and Peripheral Nerve Injury

A complete, thorough discussion of patient positioning is outside the scope of this chapter, and the reader is referred to textbooks and chapters dedicated to this subject. In most textbooks and chapters that cover positioning during surgery, most of the discussion is devoted to methods aimed at reducing postoperative complications of positioning. As pointed out in the ASA's practice advisory on prevention of perioperative peripheral neuropathies, there is scant evidence of a causal relation between intraoperative positioning and postoperative neuropathy (193).

Peripheral nerve injury can be caused by metabolic derangement, ischemia, excessive stretch, compression or pressure, direct trauma, or other unknown factors (194). Improper positioning of the patient is presumed to cause peripheral nerve injury through one or more of these mechanisms. Other causative factors have been associated with nerve injury, including automated blood pressure cuffs, subclinical diabetes, induced or prolonged hypotension, and stretch or compression during operative manipulation. Nerves with a preexisting injury are much more susceptible to permanent injury from a second, possibly subclinical, insult in the operating room. Patients might come to the operating room with a preexisting nerve injury from trauma or compressive syndromes, such as carpal tunnel syndrome or thoracic outlet syndrome.

Ulnar neuropathy represents one third of all nerve injuries reported in the Closed Claims Project. The ulnar nerve appears to be especially vulnerable to injury at the elbow as it courses near the medial epicondyle of the humerus (195). The cubital tunnel retinaculum can constrict the nerve, especially during flexion of the elbow. Yet it is disconcerting that several studies suggest that perioperative measures to protect the ulnar nerve from injury do not prevent postoperative ulnar neuropathy and that the cause of ulnar neuropathy might be beyond the anesthesiologist's control. In fact, most cases of ulnar neuropathy might not be related to positioning at all. In a large, retrospective study of ulnar nerve injuries following diagnostic and noncardiac surgical procedures, persistent ulnar neuropathies were identified in 414 cases, for an incidence of one per 2,729 patients (196). Seventy percent of the 414 patients with ulnar neuropathy were male, 9% had bilateral neuropathies, and many occurred even when precautions and padding were documented. Univariate analysis revealed the following risk factors: male gender, extremes of weight (BMI >37 or <24), and a hospital stay >14 days. No association was found with the duration of surgery, type of anesthetic, or patient position during surgery. Most cases presented >24 hours after the completion of the operation. Studies in normal conscious male volunteers reveal that patients might not perceive paresthesias of ulnar nerve compression even when somatosensory evoked potentials document impaired electrophysiologic function (195). Finally, ulnar neuropathy occurs in equal frequency in medical and surgical patients who are hospitalized for >2 days. Thus, patients, especially sedated and narcotized elderly men, who are in the supine position for a prolonged time might be vulnerable to ulnar neuropathy whether or not they have had an operation.

A variety of other complications of positioning is listed in Table 9-14.

Ocular Injury

Injury to the eye is a potentially disastrous complication. Ocular injury can occur during either ophthalmologic surgery or nonophthalmic surgery and can range from relatively minor corneal abrasion to permanent loss of vision. The broad category of ocular injury comprises various types of injuries, including corneal abrasion, vitreous loss and hemorrhage, and damage to the retina or visual pathway. The overall incidence of ocular injury appears to be low (0.06% to 0.17%) but might be greater in selected groups, such as patients undergoing operations with cardiopulmonary bypass (197,198). In a closed-claims analysis of eye injury associated with anesthesia, the most frequent complication resulting in a claim was corneal abrasion (199). Patient movement during ophthalmologic surgery resulting in blindness characterized the other subset of injury identified in the closed-claims analysis.

Corneal Abrasions

Risk factors for corneal abrasion are long surgical procedures, lateral positioning, operation on the head or neck, and GA (198). In most cases of corneal abrasion the exact mechanism of injury is unknown. Postulated mechanisms include prolonged exposure or contact with foreign bodies. GA reduces tear production, which predisposes the eye to desiccation, and GA impairs or obliterates protective behaviors and reflexes. Corneal abrasions can occur despite taping the eyelids closed and applying ointments. Injury prior to the placement of tapes has been described. After induction and prior to the placement of eye tapes, the patient is at risk of injury from a variety of foreign bodies, including wristwatch bands, name badges, stethoscopes, IV tubing, and monitoring cables. Exposure keratitis can still occur if the eyelids are not well approximated after taping. Likewise, inclusion of eyelashes under the eyelids during taping, or contact of the adhesive tape with the cornea, can lead to injury. Once the tapes are removed, the patient is once again at risk of corneal abrasion. During emergence, patients have been observed to injure their own eyes by reaching up to rub their face with an index finger that has a pulse oximeter on it. The anesthetist can also cause injury to the cornea at this time by dragging objects across the patient's face.

Damage to the Retina or Visual Pathway

The retina can be damaged through occlusion of the central retinal artery or its branches. Central retinal artery

TABLE 9-14

COMPLICATIONS OF VARIOUS PATIENT POSITIONS DURING OPERATIONS AND DIAGNOSTIC PROCEDURES

Position	Complications	Possible Mechanism	Potentially Protective Measures
Supine, head-down tilt	Decreased pulmonary compliance, increased work of breathing, increased inspiratory pressures, increased intracranial pressure, increased intracranial vascular congestion		
	Compression of subclavian neurovascular bundle or neurovascular structures emerging from the area of the scalene musculature	Shoulder brace malpositioned	Place shoulder brace over the acromioclavicular joint
Dorsal decubitus	Postural hypotension with head-elevated posture		Volume loading, vasopressors
	Pressure alopecia		Turn head frequently and/or use padded head support
	Pressure point reaction (heels, elbows, sacrum)	Prolonged pressure while immobile	Proper padding
	Brachial plexus injuries	Shoulder brace	Place shoulder brace over the acromioclavicular joint
		Lateral displacement of head Sternal retraction	Secure head in neutral position
	Long thoracic nerve dysfunction	Etiology and prevention unclear	
	Axillary trauma of the humeral head		Avoid excess abduction of the arm
	Radial nerve compression	Pressure from vertical bar of anesthesia screen, sternal retraction, excessive cycling of blood pressure cuff	Avoid prolonged pressure
			Avoid excessive cycling of automated blood pressure cuff
	Ulnar nerve at the elbow	See text	Use a padded armboard
			Arm abduction should be limited to 90 degrees in supine patients
			Position arm to decrease pressure on the postcondylar groove of the humerus
			Padded armboards and/or padding at the elbow may decrease the risk of upper extremity neuropathy
	Backache	Ligamentous relaxation during general and regional anesthesia	Maintain lumbar lordosis
			Place support under knees

(continued)

occlusion is thought to be due to direct pressure on the globe, emboli, or low perfusion pressure. Visual loss is usually unilateral and permanent. Ischemic optic neuropathy results from damage to, or impairment of, the circulatory supply to the optic nerve. The etiology of ischemic optic neuritis is unknown, but it has been associated with large blood loss, hypotension, anemia, the prone position, and preexisting cardiovascular disease. Visual impairment is bilateral and might improve with time in some cases.

TABLE 9-14
(continued)

Position	Complications	Possible Mechanism	Potentially Protective Measures
Lateral decubitus	Ocular injury (corneal abrasion, displacement of lens, retinal ischemia)	Direct contact	Protect (tape) eyes before turning
		Pressure on eye	Avoid direct pressure to eyes
		Systemic hypotension	
	Ear injury	Dependent ear folded or compressed	Palpate ear to check padding
	Neck pain	Excessive lateral flexion, ventral flexion, extension or rotation	Secure head in neutral position
	Suprascapular injury	Ventral circumduction of the dependent shoulder	Supporting pad under the thorax just caudad to the axilla
	Long thoracic nerve syndrome		
	Compartment syndrome of down-side upper extremity	Mediad compression or circumduction of down-side shoulder	Supporting pad under the thorax just caudad to the axilla
	Aseptic necrosis of the up-side femoral head	Pressure compression of arterial blood supply	Place restraining tapes across up-side on the soft tissue between head of femur and iliac crest
Ventral decubitus (prone)	Ocular injury (corneal abrasion, displacement of lens, retinal ischemia)	Direct contact	Protect (tape) eyes before turning
		Pressure on eye	Avoid direct pressure to eyes
		Systemic hypotension	
	Neck pain	Lateral rotation of head	Keep head secured in sagittal plane
	Ulnar and radial nerve injuries	See text	See supine position
	Thoracic outlet syndrome (severe pain)	Compression of brachial plexus and subclavian vessels near first rib	Avoid overhead arm position in patients with preoperative signs and symptoms of thoracic outlet syndrome
Head-elevated	Postural hypotension		Volume loading, vasopressors, decrease inhaled anesthetics, change patient position incrementally
	Air embolism	Incised vein above the level of the heart	
	Pneumocephalus	Air trapped in superior regions of cranium	
	Midcervical tetraplegia	Marked flexion of neck with stretching of spinal cord compromising its vasculature in midcervical area	
	Edema of face, tongue (macroglossia), and neck	Venous and lymphatic obstruction by prolonged neck flexion	

The incidence of visual loss due to ischemic optic neuritis is low, and most information is derived from analysis of case reports and closed claims (197,199). In July 1999 the Postoperative Visual Loss Registry was established to collect and analyze information on closed-claims cases of visual loss (200). Most cases in this analysis have ophthalmologic diagnoses of central retinal artery occlusion and ischemic optic neuritis and are associated with spine surgery (67%), followed by cardiopulmonary bypass procedures (10%). Interestingly, the analysis has revealed strong evidence that ischemic optic neuritis occurs in the absence of direct pressure on the globe, in contrast to a commonly held perception.

CONCLUSION

Most anesthesiologists would like to believe that the delivery of anesthesia is relatively safe and that recent advances in monitoring, pharmacology, anesthesia delivery systems, resident training, and information technology have made surgeons' practice even safer. Despite significant biases and limitations, the Closed Claims Project has provided information that suggests that anesthesia care is becoming safer. Studies based on the Closed Claims Project have influenced anesthetic practice and have stimulated research in problem areas (201). For example, the Closed Claims Project has identified that three damaging events account for nearly half of all claims of injury: respiratory system events, cardiovascular system events, and problems with equipment. The three most common complications or injuries are death (30%), brain damage (12%), and nerve damage (18%). Thus, management strategies directed at these few areas of clinical practice might have large results on decreasing injury leading to claims. Cheney et al. found that respiratory events accounted for a third of claims and that 85% of these claims involved brain damage or death (202). Most of these adverse events were due to inadequate ventilation, esophageal intubation, and difficult tracheal intubation. Furthermore, most of these claims were thought to be preventable by pulse oximetry and capnography monitoring. Partly on the basis of these findings, the ASA formulated new standards for perioperative monitoring that stress the use of pulse oximetry and capnography, and the ASA created practice guidelines for management of the difficult airway. Although the Closed Claims Project cannot determine whether the actual incidence of severe injuries is decreasing, trends in outcomes suggest that this is so (201).

The administration of anesthesia invokes remarkable physiologic changes that are sometimes subtle but often profound. The neurologic system is greatly affected, either regionally or globally. The state of anesthesia and the effects of the medications used to block the response to noxious stimuli likewise affect the cardiovascular and respiratory systems. Anesthesia converts a relatively hardy, independent, and resilient person into a patient who is dependent, vulnerable, and barely a few moments away from jeopardy, damage, or demise. Modern anesthetic practice has made the process seem routine, but with each anesthetic there is a risk of complications or adverse outcome. Unfortunately, every surgeon will become familiar with some of the more common adverse events and might have a brush with some of the rare ones as well. It is hoped that the increasing complexity of surgical operations,

presence of multiple comorbid conditions, and advancing age of the patient population will not negate the beneficial impact of improvements in anesthesia safety.

REFERENCES

1. Posner K. ASA Closed Claims Project. 2004. http://depts.washington.edu/asaccp/
2. Caplan RA, Posner KL, Ward RJ, et al. Adverse respiratory events in anesthesia: a closed claims analysis. *Anesthesiology* 1990;72(5): 828–833.
3. Behringer EC. Approaches to managing the upper airway. *Anesthesiol Clin North Am* 2002;20(4):813–832, vi.
4. Rose DK, Cohen MM. The airway: problems and predictions in 18,500 patients [comment]. *Can J Anaesth* 1994;41(5 Pt 1): 372–383.
5. Chraemmer-Jorgensen B, Hertel S, Strom J, et al. Catecholamine response to laryngoscopy and intubation. The influence of three different drug combinations commonly used for induction of anaesthesia [comment]. *Anaesthesia* 1992;47(9):750–756.
6. Barak M, Ziser A, Greenberg A, et al. Hemodynamic and catecholamine response to tracheal intubation: direct laryngoscopy compared with fiberoptic intubation. *J Clin Anesth* 2003;15(2): 132–136.
7. American Society of Anesthesiologists Task Force on Management of the Difficult Airway. Practice guidelines for management of the difficult airway, a report. *Anesthesiology* 1993; 78(3): 597–602.
8. American Society of Anesthesiologists Task Force on Management of the Difficult Airway. Practice guidelines for management of the difficult airway: an updated report. *Anesthesiology* 2003;98(5): 1269–1277.
9. Stern Y, Spitzer T. Retrograde intubation of the trachea. *J Laryngol Otol* 1991;105(9):746–747.
10. Mallampati SR, Gatt SP, Gugino LD, et al. A clinical sign to predict difficult tracheal intubation: a prospective study. *Can Anaesth Soc J* 1985;32(4):429–434.
11. Frerk CM. Predicting difficult intubation [comment]. *Anaesthesia* 1991;46(12):1005–1008.
12. Hagberg C, Boin MH. Management of the airway: complications. In: Benumof JL, Saidman LJ, eds. *Anesthesia and perioperative complications*, 2nd ed. St. Louis, MO: Mosby; 1999:3–24.
13. Rosenblatt W, Wagner P, Ovassapian A, et al. Practice patterns in managing the difficult airway by anesthesiologists in the United States. *Anesth Analg* 1998;87(1):153–157.
14. Warner ME, Benenfeld SM, Warner MA, et al. Perianesthetic dental injuries: frequency, outcomes, and risk factors. *Anesthesiology* 1999;90(5):1302–1305.
15. Loh KS, Irish JC. Traumatic complications of intubation and other airway management procedures. In: Bogetz MS, ed. *The upper airway and anesthesia*. Philadelphia, PA: W.B. Saunders; 2002:953–969.
16. Lennarson PJ, Smith D, Todd MM, et al. Segmental cervical spine motion during orotracheal intubation of the intact and injured spine with and without external stabilization. *J Neurosurg* 2000; 92(Suppl. 2):201–206.
17. Dutton RP. Anesthetic management of spinal cord injury: clinical practice and future initiatives. *Int Anesthesiol Clin* 2002;40(3): 103–120.
18. Crosby ET, Lui A. The adult cervical spine: implications for airway management. *Can J Anaesth* 1990;37(1):77–93.
19. Weber S. Traumatic complications of airway management. In: Weber S, ed. *Anesthesia-related complications*. Philadelphia, PA: W.B. Saunders; 2002:265–274, v–vi.
20. Hall CE, Shutt LE. Nasotracheal intubation for head and neck surgery [comment]. *Anaesthesia* 2003;58(3):249–256.
21. Conrardy PA, Goodman LR, Lainge F, et al. Alteration of endotracheal tube position. Flexion and extension of the neck. *Crit Care Med* 1976;4(1):7–12.
22. Parmet J, Colonna-Romano P, Horrow J, et al. The laryngeal mask airway reliably provides rescue ventilation in cases of

unanticipated difficult tracheal intubation along with difficult mask ventilation. *Anesth Analg* 1998;87(3):661–665.

23. Benumof JL. Laryngeal mask airway and the ASA difficult airway algorithm [comment]. *Anesthesiology* 1996;84(3):686–699.

24. Bordet F, Allaouchiche B, Lansiaux S, et al. Risk factors for airway complications during general anaesthesia in paediatric patients. *Paediat Anaesth* 2002;12(9):762–769.

25. Geelhoed GW. Tracheomalacia from compressing goiter: management after thyroidectomy. *Surgery* 1988;104(6):1100–1108.

26. Rex MA. A review of the structural and functional basis of laryngospasm and a discussion of the nerve pathways involved in the reflex and its clinical significance in man and animals. *Br J Anaesth* 1970;42(10):891–899.

27. Hartley M, Vaughan RS. Problems associated with tracheal extubation [comment]. *Br J Anaesth* 1993;71(4):561–568.

28. Lang SA, Duncan PG, Shephard DA, et al. Pulmonary oedema associated with airway obstruction [comment]. *Can J Anaesth* 1990;37(2):210–218.

29. Deepika K, Kenaan CA, Barrocas AM, et al. Negative pressure pulmonary edema after acute upper airway obstruction. *J Clin Anesth* 1997;9(5):403–408.

30. Hug CC Jr. New perspectives on anesthetic agents [Review] [64 refs]. *Am J Surg* 1988;156(5):406–415.

31. Campagna JA, Miller KW, Forman SA. Mechanisms of actions of inhaled anesthetics. *N Engl J Med* 2003;348(21):2110–2124.

32. Buffington CW, Romson JL, Levine A, et al. Isoflurane induces coronary steal in a canine model of chronic coronary occlusion. *Anesthesiology* 1987;66(3):280–292.

33. Tuman KJ, McCarthy RJ, Spiess BD, et al. Does choice of anesthetic agent significantly affect outcome after coronary artery surgery? *Anesthesiology* 1989;70(2):189–198.

34. Cason BA, Verrier ED, London MJ, et al. Effects of isoflurane and halothane on coronary vascular resistance and collateral myocardial blood flow: their capacity to induce coronary steal. *Anesthesiology* 1987;67(5):665–675.

35. Pulley DD, Kirvassilis GV, Kelermenos N, et al. Regional and global myocardial circulatory and metabolic effects of isoflurane and halothane in patients with steal-prone coronary anatomy. *Anesthesiology* 1991;75(5):756–766.

36. Agnew NM, Pennefather SH, Russell GN. Isoflurane and coronary heart disease [comment]. *Anaesthesia* 2002;57(4):338–347.

37. Aach R. Halothane and liver failure. *JAMA* 1970;211(13):2145–2147.

38. Elliott RH, Strunin L. Hepatotoxicity of volatile anaesthetics. *Br J Anaesth* 1993;70(3):339–348.

39. Hubbard AK, Roth TP, Gandolfi AJ, et al. Halothane hepatitis patients generate an antibody response toward a covalently bound metabolite of halothane. *Anesthesiology* 1988;68(5):791–796.

40. Kenna JG, Jones RM. The organ toxicity of inhaled anesthetics. *Anesth Analg* 1995;81(Suppl. 6):S51–S66.

41. Conzen PF, Kharasch ED, Czerner SF, et al. Low-flow sevoflurane compared with low-flow isoflurane anesthesia in patients with stable renal insufficiency [comment]. *Anesthesiology* 2002;97(3):578–584.

42. Kharasch ED, Frink EJ, Jr., Artru A, et al. Long-duration low-flow sevoflurane and isoflurane effects on postoperative renal and hepatic function. *Anesth Analg* 2001;93(6):1511–1520.

43. Forbes GM, Collins BJ. Nitrous oxide for colonoscopy: a randomized controlled study [comment]. *Gastrointestinal Endosc* 2000;51(3):271–277.

44. Harding TA, Gibson JA. The use of inhaled nitrous oxide for flexible sigmoidoscopy: a placebo-controlled trial. *Endoscopy* 2000;32(6):457–460.

45. Eisele JH, Reitan JA, Massumi RA, et al. Myocardial performance and N$_2$O analgesia in coronary-artery disease. *Anesthesiology* 1976;44(1):16–20.

46. Flippo TS, Holder WD Jr. Neurologic degeneration associated with nitrous oxide anesthesia in patients with vitamin B12 deficiency. *Arch Surg.* 1993;128(12):1391–1395.

47. Louis-Ferdinand RT. Myelotoxic, neurotoxic and reproductive adverse effects of nitrous oxide. *Adverse Drug React Toxicol Rev* 1994;13(4):193–206.

48. Suruda A. Health effects of anesthetic gases. *Occupat Med* 1997;12(4):627–634.

49. Eger EI 2nd, Saidman LJ. Hazards of nitrous oxide anesthesia in bowel obstruction and pneumothorax. *Anesthesiology* 1965;26(1):61–66.

50. Ohryn M. Tympanic membrane rupture following general anesthesia with nitrous oxide: a case report. *AANA J* 1995;63(1):42–44.

51. Seaberg RR, Freeman WR, Goldbaum MH, et al. Permanent postoperative vision loss associated with expansion of intraocular gas in the presence of a nitrous oxide-containing anesthetic. *Anesthesiology* 2002;97(5):1309–1310.

52. Astrom S, Kjellgren D, Monestam E, et al. Nitrous oxide anesthesia and intravitreal gastamponade. *Acta Anaesthesiol Scand* 2003;47(3):361–362.

53. Taylor E, Feinstein R, White PF, et al. Anesthesia for laparoscopic cholecystectomy. Is nitrous oxide contraindicated? *Anesthesiology* 1992;76(4):541–543.

54. Caplan RA, Vistica MF, Posner KL, et al. Adverse anesthetic outcomes arising from gas delivery equipment: a closed claims analysis [comment]. *Anesthesiology* 1997;87(4):741–748.

55. Anagnostou JM, Stoelting RK. Complications of drugs used in anesthesia. In: Benumof JL, Saidman LJ, eds. *Anesthesia and perioperative complications.* St. Louis, MO: Mosby; 1999:161–191.

56. Hirshman CA, Edelstein RA, Ebertz JM, et al. Thiobarbiturate-induced histamine release in human skin mast cells. *Anesthesiology* 1985;63(4):353–356.

57. Harrison GG, Meissner PN, Hift RJ. Anaesthesia for the porphyric patient [comment]. *Anaesthesia* 1993;48(5):417–421.

58. Ben-Shlomo I, abd-el-Khalim H, Ezry J, et al. Midazolam acts synergistically with fentanyl for induction of anaesthesia. *Br J Anaesth* 1990;64(1):45–47.

59. Heikkila H, Jalonen J, Arola M, et al. Midazolam as adjunct to high-dose fentanyl anaesthesia for coronary artery bypass grafting operation. *Acta Anaesthesiol Scand* 1984;28(6):683–689.

60. Vinik HR, Bradley EL Jr, Kissin I. Midazolam-alfentanil synergism for anesthetic induction in patients. *Anesth Analg* 1989;69(2):213–217.

61. Zacharias M, Dundee JW, Clarke RS, et al. Effect of preanaesthetic medication on etomidate. *Br J Anaesth* 1979;51(2):127–133.

62. Wagner RL, White PF, Kan PB, et al. Inhibition of adrenal steroidogenesis by the anesthetic etomidate. *N Engl J Med* 1984;310(22):1415–1421.

63. Wagner RL, White PF. Etomidate inhibits adrenocortical function in surgical patients. *Anesthesiology* 1984;61(6):647–651.

64. Crozier TA, Beck D, Schlaeger M, et al. Endocrinological changes following etomidate, midazolam, or methohexital for minor surgery. *Anesthesiology* 1987;66(5):628–635.

65. Gooding JM, Corssen G. Effect of etomidate on the cardiovascular system. *Anesth Analg* 1977;56(5):717–719.

66. Price ML, Millar B, Grounds M, et al. Changes in cardiac index and estimated systemic vascular resistance during induction of anaesthesia with thiopentone, methohexitone, propofol and etomidate [comment]. *Br J Anaesth* 1992;69(2):172–176.

67. Goodman NW, Black AM, Carter JA. Some ventilatory effects of propofol as sole anaesthetic agent. *Br J Anaesth* 1987;59(12):1497–1503.

68. Lepage JY, Pinaud ML, Helias JH, et al. Left ventricular performance during propofol or methohexital anesthesia: isotopic and invasive cardiac monitoring. *Anesth Analg* 1991;73(1):3–9.

69. Claeys MA, Gepts E, Camu F. Haemodynamic changes during anaesthesia induced and maintained with propofol. *Br J Anaesth* 1988;60(1):3–9.

70. Prys-Roberts C, Davies JR, Calverley RK, et al. Haemodynamic effects of infusions of diisopropyl phenol (ICI 35 868) during nitrous oxide anaesthesia in man. *Br J Anaesth* 1983;55(2):105–111.

71. Sosis MB, Braverman B. Growth of *Staphylococcus aureus* in four intravenous anesthetics. *Anesth Analg* 1993;77(4):766–768.

72. Bennett SN, McNeil MM, Bland LA, et al. Postoperative infections traced to contamination of an intravenous anesthetic, propofol [comment]. *N Engl J Med* 1995;333(3):147–154.

73. Veber B, Gachot B, Bedos JP, et al. Severe sepsis after intravenous injection of contaminated propofol. *Anesthesiology* 1994;80(3):712–713.

74. Nichols RL, Smith JW. Bacterial contamination of an anesthetic agent [comment]. *N Engl J Med* 1995;333(3):184–185.

75. Bach A, Geiss HK. Propofol and postoperative infections [comment]. *N Engl J Med* 1995;333(22):1505–1506; discussion 1507.

76. Sklar GE. Propofol and postoperative infections. *Ann Pharmacother* 1997;31(12):1521–1523.

77. Vasile B, Rasulo F, Candiani A, et al. The pathophysiology of propofol infusion syndrome: a simple name for a complex syndrome. *Intensive Care Med* 2003;29(9):1417–1425.

78. Gooding JM, Dimick AR, Tavakoli M, et al. A physiologic analysis of cardiopulmonary responses to ketamine anesthesia in noncardiac patients. *Anesth Analg* 1977;56(6):813–816.

79. White PF, Way WL, Trevor AJ. Ketamine—its pharmacology and therapeutic uses. *Anesthesiology* 1982;56(2):119–136.

80. Schow AJ, Lubarsky DA, Olson RP, et al. Can succinylcholine be used safely in hyperkalemic patients? *Anesth Analg* 2002;95(1):119–122.

81. Thapa S, Brull SJ. Succinylcholine-induced hyperkalemia in patients with renal failure: an old question revisited. *Anesth Analg* 2000;91(1):237–241.

82. Wong SF, Chung F. Succinylcholine-associated postoperative myalgia [comment]. *Anaesthesia* 2000;55(2):144–152.

83. Pace NL. The best prophylaxis for succinylcholine myalgias: extension of a previous meta-analysis. *Anesth Analg* 1993;77(5):1080–1081.

84. Cunningham AJ, Barry P. Intraocular pressure—physiology and implications for anaesthetic management. *Can Anaesth Soc J* 1986;33(2):195–208.

85. Mitra S, Gombar KK, Gombar S. The effect of rocuronium on intraocular pressure: a comparison with succinylcholine. *Eur J Anaesthesiol* 2001;18(12):836–838.

86. Zimmerman AA, Funk KJ, Tidwell JL. Propofol and alfentanil prevent the increase in intraocular pressure caused by succinylcholine and endotracheal intubation during a rapid sequence induction of anesthesia. *Anesth Analg* 1996;83(4):814–817.

87. Moreno RJ, Kloess P, Carlson DW. Effect of succinylcholine on the intraocular contents of open globes [comment]. *Ophthalmology* 1991;98(5):636–638.

88. McGoldrick KE. The open globe: is an alternative to succinylcholine necessary? [comment] *J Clin Anesth* 1993;5(1):1–4.

89. Vachon CA, Warner DO, Bacon DR. Succinylcholine and the open globe. Tracing the teaching. *Anesthesiology* 2003;99(1):220–223.

90. Cook DR. Can succinylcholine be abandoned? *Anesth Analg* 2000;90(Suppl. 5):S24–S28.

91. Sparr HJ, Beaufort TM, Fuchs-Buder T. Newer neuromuscular blocking agents: how do they compare with established agents? *Drugs* 2001;61(7):919–942.

92. Moore EW, Hunter JM. The new neuromuscular blocking agents: do they offer any advantages? *Br J Anaesth* 2001;87(6):912–925.

93. Cammu G. Interactions of neuromuscular blocking drugs. *Acta Anaesthesiol Belgica* 2001;52(4):357–363.

94. Fodale V, Santamaria LB. Laudanosine, an atracurium and cisatracurium metabolite. *Eur J Anaesthesiol* 2002;19(7):466–473.

95. Murphy GS, Vender JS. Neuromuscular-blocking drugs. Use and misuse in the intensive care unit. *Crit Care Clin* 2001; 17(4):925–942.

96. Prielipp RC, Coursin DB, Wood KE, et al. Complications associated with sedative and neuromuscular blocking drugs in critically ill patients. *Crit Care Clin* 1995;11(4):983–1003.

97. Douglass JA, Tuxen DV, Horne M, et al. Myopathy in severe asthma. *Am Rev Respirat Dis* 1992;146(2):517–519.

98. Segredo V, Caldwell JE, Matthay MA, et al. Persistent paralysis in critically ill patients after long-term administration of vecuronium. *N Engl J Med* 1992;327(8):524–528.

99. Coursin DB, Prielipp RC. Prolonged paralysis with atracurium infusion. *Crit Care Med* 1995;23(6):1155–1157.

100. Prielipp RC, Coursin DB, Scuderi PE, et al. Comparison of the infusion requirements and recovery profiles of vecuronium and cisatracurium 51W89 in intensive care unit patients. *Anesth Analg* 1995;81(1):3–12.

101. Murray MJ, Cowen J, DeBlock H, et al. Clinical practice guidelines for sustained neuromuscular blockade in the adult critically ill patient. *Crit Care Med* 2002;30(1):142–156.

102. Flacke JW, Flacke WE, Bloor BC, et al. Histamine release by four narcotics: a double-blind study in humans. *Anesth Analg* 1987;66(8):723–730.

103. Simopoulos TT, Smith HS, Peeters-Asdourian C, et al. Use of meperidine in patient-controlled analgesia and the development of a normeperidine toxic reaction. *Arch Surg* 2002;137(1):84–88.

104. Michelsen LG, Hug CC, Jr. The pharmacokinetics of remifentanil. *J Clin Anesth* 1996;8(8):679–682.

105. Matthey P, Finucane BT, Finegan BA, et al. The attitude of the general public towards preoperative assessment and risks associated with general anesthesia. *Can J Anaesth* 2001;48(4):333–339.

106. Kerssens C, Klein J, Bonke B. Awareness: Monitoring versus remembering what happened. *Anesthesiology* 2003;99(3):570–575.

107. Sandin RH, Enlund G, Samuelsson P, et al. Awareness during anaesthesia: a prospective case study. *Lancet* 2000;355(9205):707–711.

108. Bailey AR, Jones JG. Patients' memories of events during general anaesthesia. *Anaesthesia* 1997;52(5):460–476.

109. Russell IF. Midazolam-alfentanil: an anaesthetic? An investigation using the isolated forearm technique. *Br J Anaesth* 1993;70(1):42–46.

110. Tempe DK, Siddiquie RA. Awareness during cardiac surgery. *J Cardiothorac Vasc Anesth* 1999;13(2):214–219.

111. Osterman JE, Hopper J, Heran WJ, et al. Awareness under anesthesia and the development of posttraumatic stress disorder. *Gen Hosp Psychiat* 2001;23(4):198–204.

112. Domino KB, Posner KL, Caplan RA, et al. Awareness during anesthesia: a closed claims analysis. *Anesthesiology* 1999;90(4):1053–1061.

113. Bergman IJ, Kluger MT, Short TG. Awareness during general anaesthesia: a review of 81 cases from the Anaesthetic Incident Monitoring Study. *Anaesthesia* 2002;57(6):549–556.

114. Pitellie PH, Holmes MA, Domino KB. Awareness during anesthesia. In: Weber S, ed. *Anesthesia-related complications*. Philadelphia, PA: W.B. Saunders; 2002:317–332, vii.

115. Mulroy MF. Systemic toxicity and cardiotoxicity from local anesthetics: incidence and preventive measures. *Reg Anesth Pain Med* 2002;27(6):556–561.

116. Liu PL, Feldman HS, Giasi R, et al. Comparative CNS toxicity of lidocaine, etidocaine, bupivacaine, and tetracaine in awake dogs following rapid intravenous administration. *Anesth Analg* 1983;62(4):375–379.

117. Covino BG. Toxicity of local anesthetic agents. *Acta Anaesthesiol Belgica* 1988;39(3 Suppl. 2):159–164.

118. Clarkson CW, Hondeghem LM. Mechanism for bupivacaine depression of cardiac conduction: fast block of sodium channels during the action potential with slow recovery from block during diastole. *Anesthesiology* 1985;62(4):396–405.

119. Morishima HO, Pedersen H, Finster M, et al. Bupivacaine toxicity in pregnant and nonpregnant ewes. *Anesthesiology* 1985;63(2):134–139.

120. Scott DB. Maximum recommended doses of local anaesthetic drugs. *Br J Anaesth* 1989;63(4):373–374.

121. Brown D, Ransom D, Hall J, et al. Regional anesthesia and local anesthetic-induced systemic toxicity: seizure frequency and accompanying cardiovascular changes. *Anesth Analg* 1995;81(2):321–328.

122. Braid DP, Scott DB. Effect of adrenaline on the systemic absorption of local anaesthetic drugs. *Acta Anaesthesiol Scand*, Suppl. 1966;23:334–346.

123. Liu SS, McDonald SB. Current issues in spinal anesthesia [comment]. *Anesthesiology* 2001;94(5):888–906.

124. Lambert DH, Hurley RJ, Hertwig L, et al. Role of needle gauge and tip configuration in the production of lumbar puncture headache. *Reg Anesth* 1997;22(1):66–72.

125. Lybecker H, Moller JT, May O, et al. Incidence and prediction of postdural puncture headache. A prospective study of 1021 spinal anesthesias. *Anesth Analg* 1990;70(4):389–394.

126. Gerancher JC, Liu SS. Complications of neuraxial (spinal/epidural/caudal) anesthesia. In: Benumof JL, ed. *Anesthesia and perioperative complications*, 2nd ed. St. Louis, MO: Mosby; 1999:50–65.

127. Vercauteren MP, Hoffmann VH, Mertens E, et al. Seven-year review of requests for epidural blood patches for headache after dural puncture: referral patterns and the effectiveness of blood patches. *Eur J Anaesthesiol* 1999;16(5):298–303.

128. Safa-Tisseront V, Thormann F, Malassine P, et al. Effectiveness of epidural blood patch in the management of post-dural puncture headache [comment]. *Anesthesiology* 2001;95(2):334–339.

129. Beards SC, Jackson A, Griffiths AG, et al. Magnetic resonance imaging of extradural blood patches: appearances from 30 min to 18 h [comment]. *Br J Anaesth* 1993;71(2):182–188.

130. Gupta S, Tarkkila P, Finucane BT. Complications of central neural blockade. In: Finucane BT, ed. *Complications of regional anesthesia*. Philadelphia, PA: Churchill Livingstone; 1999:184–212.

131. Breen TW, Ransil BJ, Groves PA, et al. Factors associated with back pain after childbirth. *Anesthesiology* 1994;81(1):29–34.

132. Hirabayashi Y, Igarashi T, Suzuki H, et al. Mechanical effects of leg position on vertebral structures examined by magnetic resonance imaging. *Reg Anesth Pain Med* 2002;27(4):429–432.

133. Pertek JP, Haberer JP. Effets de l'anesthesie sur la miction et retention aigue d'urine postoperatoire [Effects of anesthesia on postoperative micturition and urinary retention]. *Ann Franc Anesth Reanimat* 1995;14(4):340–351.

134. Petros JG, Rimm EB, Robillard RJ. Factors influencing urinary tract retention after elective open cholecystectomy. *Surg Gynecol Obstet* 1992;174(6):497–500.

135. Jensen P, Mikkelsen T, Kehlet H. Postherniorrhaphy urinary retention—effect of local, regional, and general anesthesia: A review. *Reg Anesth Pain Med* 2002;27(6):612–617.

136. Pollock JE. Transient neurologic symptoms: etiology, risk factors, and management [comment]. *Reg Anesth Pain Med* 2002;27(6):581–586.

137. Pollock JE, Liu SS, Neal JM, et al. Dilution of spinal lidocaine does not alter the incidence of transient neurologic symptoms. *Anesthesiology* 1999;90(2):445–450.

138. Vandermeulen EP, Van Aken H, Vermylen J. Anticoagulants and spinal-epidural anesthesia [comment]. *Anesth Analg* 1994;79(6):1165–1177.

139. Horlocker TT. Low molecular weight heparin and neuraxial anesthesia. *Thrombosis Res* 2001;101(1):141–154.

140. Kindler CH, Seeberger MD, Staender SE. Epidural abscess complicating epidural anesthesia and analgesia. An analysis of the literature [comment]. *Acta Anaesthesiol Scand* 1998;42(6):614–620.

141. Wang LP, Hauerberg J, Schmidt JF. Incidence of spinal epidural abscess after epidural analgesia: a national 1-year survey. *Anesthesiology* 1999;91(6):1928–1936.

142. Canto M, Casas A, Sanchez MJ, et al. Thoracic epidurals in heart valve surgery: neurologic risk evaluation. *J Cardiothorac Vasc Anesth* 2002;16(6):723–726.

143. Wysowski DK, Talarico L, Bacsanyi J, et al. Spinal and epidural hematoma and low-molecular-weight heparin. *N Engl J Med* 1998;338(24):1774–1775.

144. Lumpkin MM. FDA public health advisory. *Anesthesiology* 1998;88(2):27A–28A.

145. Horlocker T, Heit J. Low molecular weight heparin: biochemistry, pharmacology, perioperative prophylaxis regimens, and guidelines for regional anesthetic management. *Anesth Analg* 1997;85(4):874–885.

146. Bergqvist D, Wu CL, Neal JM. Anticoagulation and neuraxial regional anesthesia: perspectives. *Reg Anesth Pain Med* 2003;28(3):163–166.

147. Horlocker TT, Wedel DJ, Benzon H, et al. Regional anesthesia in the anticoagulated patient: defining the risks (the second ASRA Consensus Conference on Neuraxial Anesthesia and Anticoagulation). *Reg Anesth Pain Med* 2003;28(3):172–197.

148. Tyagi A, Bhattacharya A. Central neuraxial blocks and anticoagulation: a review of current trends. *Eur J Anaesthesiol* 2002;19(5):317–329.

149. Auroy Y, Narchi P, Messiah A, et al. Serious complications related to regional anesthesia: results of a prospective survey in France [comment]. *Anesthesiology* 1997;87(3):479–486.

150. Cheney FW, Domino KB, Caplan RA, et al. Nerve injury associated with anesthesia: a closed claims analysis. *Anesthesiology* 1999;90(4):1062–1069.

151. Reynolds F. Damage to the conus medullaris following spinal anaesthesia [comment]. *Anaesthesia* 2001;56(3):238–247.

152. Ben-David B, Rawa R. Complications of neuraxial blockade. In: Weber S, ed. *Anesthesia-related complications*. Philadelphia, PA: W.B. Saunders; 2002:669–694.

153. Lesser JB, Sanborn KV, Valskys R, et al. Severe bradycardia during spinal and epidural anesthesia recorded by an anesthesia information management system. *Anesthesiology* 2003;99(4):859–866.

154. Carpenter RL, Caplan RA, Brown DL, et al. Incidence and risk factors for side effects of spinal anesthesia [comment]. *Anesthesiology* 1992;76(6):906–916.

155. Curatolo M, Scaramozzino P, Venuti F, et al. Factors associated with hypotension and bradycardia after epidural blockade. *Anesth Analg* 1996;83(5):1033–1040.

156. Caplan RA, Ward RJ, Posner K, et al. Unexpected cardiac arrest during spinal anesthesia: a closed claims analysis of predisposing factors [comment]. *Anesthesiology* 1988;68(1):5–11.

157. Auroy Y, Benhamou D, Bargues L, et al. Major complications of regional anesthesia in France: the SOS Regional Anesthesia Hotline Service [comment]. *Anesthesiology* 2002;97(5):1274–1280.

158. Pollard JB. Cardiac arrest during spinal anesthesia: common mechanisms and strategies for prevention. *Anesth Analg* 2001;92(1):252–256.

159. Rosenberg J, Wahr J, Sung C, et al. Coronary perfusion pressure during cardiopulmonary resuscitation after spinal anesthesia in dogs. *Anesth Analg* 1996;82(1):84–87.

160. Rosenberg JM, Wortsman J, Wahr JA, et al. Impaired neuroendocrine response mediates refractoriness to cardiopulmonary resuscitation in spinal anesthesia. *Crit Care Med* 1998;26(3):533–537.

161. Watcha MF. Postoperative nausea and emesis. In: Weber S, ed. *Anesthesia-related complications*. Philadelphia, PA: W.B. Saunders; 2002:709–722.

162. Gan TJ, Meyer T, Apfel CC, et al. Consensus guidelines for managing postoperative nausea and vomiting. *Anesth Analg* 2003;97(1):62–71.

163. Apfel CC, Kranke P, Katz MH, et al. Volatile anaesthetics may be the main cause of early but not delayed postoperative vomiting: a randomized controlled trial of factorial design [comment]. *Br J Anaesth* 2002;88(5):659–668.

164. Sweeney BP. Editorial II: Why does smoking protect against PONV? *Br J Anaesth* 2002;89(6):810–813.

165. Apfel CC, Laara E, Koivuranta M, et al. A simplified risk score for predicting postoperative nausea and vomiting: conclusions from cross-validations between two centers. *Anesthesiology* 1999;91(3):693–700.

166. Durmus M, Karaaslan E, Ozturk E, et al. The effects of single-dose dexamethasone on wound healing in rats. *Anesth Analg* 2003;97(5):1377–1380.

167. Gan TJ, El-Molem H, Ray J, et al. Patient-controlled antiemesis: a randomized, double-blind comparison of two doses of propofol versus placebo. *Anesthesiology* 1999;90(6):1564–1570.

168. Adams JP, Murphy PG. Obesity in anaesthesia and intensive care. *Br J Anaesth* 2000;85(1):91–108.

169. Bray GA. Risks of obesity. *Primary Care Clin Office Pract* 2003;30(2):281–299, v–vi.

170. Benumof JL. Obstructive sleep apnea in the adult obese patient: implications for airway management. *J Clin Anesth* 2001;13(2):144–156.

171. Esclamado RM, Glenn MG, McCulloch TM, et al. Perioperative complications and risk factors in the surgical treatment of obstructive sleep apnea syndrome. *Laryngoscope* 1989;99(11):1125–1129.

172. Forrest JB, Rehder K, Cahalan MK, et al. Multicenter study of general anesthesia. III. Predictors of severe perioperative adverse outcomes [comment] [erratum appears in *Anesthesiology* 1992;77(1):222]. *Anesthesiology* 1992;76(1):3–15.

173. Pelosi P, Croci M, Ravagnan I, et al. The effects of body mass on lung volumes, respiratory mechanics, and gas exchange during general anesthesia. *Anesth Analg* 1998;87(3):654–660.

174. Duflou J, Virmani R, Rabin I, et al. Sudden death as a result of heart disease in morbid obesity. *Am Heart J* 1995;130(2):306–313.

175. Choban PS, Flancbaum L. The impact of obesity on surgical outcomes: a review. *J Am Coll Surg* 1997;185(6):593–603.

176. Moulton MJ, Creswell LL, Mackey ME, et al. Obesity is not a risk factor for significant adverse outcomes after cardiac surgery. *Circulation* 1996;94(Suppl. 9):II87–II92.

177. Fasol R, Schindler M, Schumacher B, et al. The influence of obesity on perioperative morbidity: retrospective study of 502 aorto-coronary bypass operations. *Thorac Cardiovasc Surg* 1992;40(3):126–129.

178. Sessler DI. Complications and treatment of mild hypothermia. *Anesthesiology* 2001;95(2):531–543.

179. Sessler DI. Mild perioperative hypothermia. *N Engl J Med* 1997;336(24):1730–1737.

180. Kurz A, Sessler DI, Lenhardt R, et al. Perioperative normothermia to reduce the incidence of surgical-wound infection and shorten hospitalization. *N Engl J Med* 1996; 334(19): 1209–1216.

181. Winkler M, Akca O, Birkenberg B, et al. Aggressive warming reduces blood loss during hip arthroplasty. *Anesth Analg* 2000;91(4):978–984.

182. Cheney FW, Posner KL, Caplan RA, et al. Burns from warming devices in anesthesia. A closed claims analysis [comment]. *Anesthesiology* 1994;80(4):806–810.

183. Rosenberg H, Frank SM. Causes and consequences of hypothermia and hyperthermia. In: Benumof JL, Saidman LJ, eds. *Anesthesia and perioperative complications*, 2nd ed. St. Louis, MO: Mosby; 1999:338–356.

184. MacLennan DH, Phillips MS. Malignant hyperthermia. *Science* 1992;256(5058):789–794.

185. Fasting S, Gisvold SE. Serious intraoperative problems—a five-year review of 83,844 anesthetics [Problemes peroperatoires graves—une revue de 83 844 anesthesies sur cinq ans]. *Can J Anaesth* 2002;49(6):545–553.

186. Hepner DL, Castells MC. Anaphylaxis during the perioperative period. *Anesth Analg* 2003;97(5):1381–1395.

187. Laxenaire MC, Mertes PM. Groupe d'Etudes des Reactions Anaphylactoides Peranesthesiques. Anaphylaxis during anaesthesia. Results of a two-year survey in France. *Br J Anaesth* 2001;87(4):549–558.

188. Ford S, Kam P, Baldo B, et al. Anaphylactic or anaphylactoid reactions in patients undergoing cardiac surgery. *J Cardiothorac Vasc Anesth* 2001;15(6):684–688.

189. Spinler SA, Dager W. Overview of heparin-induced thrombocytopenia. *Am J Health-Syst Pharm* 2003;60(5), S5–11.

190. Porsche R, Brenner Z. Allergy to protamine sulfate. *Heart Lung J Acute Crit Care* 1999;28(6):418–428.

191. Cormack JG, Levy JH. Adverse reactions to protamine. *Coronary Artery Dis* 1993;4(5):420–425.

192. Hepner DL, Castells MC. Latex allergy: an update. *Anesth Analg* 2003;96(4):1219–1229.

193. Practice advisory for the prevention of perioperative peripheral neuropathies: a report by the American Society of Anesthesiologists Task Force on Prevention of Perioperative Peripheral Neuropathies. *Anesthesiology* 2000;92(4):1168–1182.

194. Warner MA. Perioperative neuropathies. *Mayo Clin Proc* 1998; 73(6):567–574.

195. Prielipp RC, Morell RC, Butterworth J. Ulnar nerve injury and perioperative arm positioning. In: Weber S, ed. *Anesthesia-related complications*. Philadelphia, PA: W.B. Saunders;2002:351–365, vii–viii.

196. Warner MA, Warner ME, Martin JT. Ulnar neuropathy. Incidence, outcome, and risk factors in sedated or anesthetized patients [comment]. *Anesthesiology* 1994;81(6):1332–1340.

197. Roth S, Gillesberg I, eds. *Injuries to the visual system and other sense organs*, 2nd ed. St. Louis, MO: Mosby; 1999.

198. Roth S, Thisted RA, Erickson JP, et al. Eye injuries after nonocular surgery. A study of 60,965 anesthetics from 1988 to 1992. *Anesthesiology* 1996;85(5):1020–1027.

199. Gild WM, Posner KL, Caplan RA, et al. Eye injuries associated with anesthesia. A closed claims analysis [comment]. *Anesthesiology* 1992;76(2):204–208.

200. Lee LA. ASA postoperative visual loss registry: preliminary analysis of factors associated with spine operations. *ASA Newslett* 2003;67(6):7–8.

201. Lee LA, Domino KB. The Closed Claims Project. Has it influenced anesthetic practice and outcome? In: Weber S, ed. *Anesthesia-related complications*. Philadelphia, PA: W.B. Saunders; 2002:247–263.

202. Cheney FW, Posner KL, Caplan RA. Adverse respiratory events infrequently leading to malpractice suits. A closed claims analysis. *Anesthesiology* 1991;75(6):932–939.

Complications of Wound Healing

10

Michael G. Franz

■■■ **NORMAL WOUND HEALING 102**
Hemostasis 103
Inflammation 103
Fibroproliferation and Remodeling 104
The Lag Phase 106

■■■ **PREOPERATIVE RISK FACTORS FOR WOUND COMPLICATIONS 107**
Contamination and Infection 107
Tissue Hypoperfusion 107
Malnutrition 108
Chronic Disease 108
Pharmacologic Agents 108
Genetic Defects 109
Atypical Wounds 109

■■■ **MODIFICATION OF PREOPERATIVE RISK FACTORS 109**
Minimize Contamination 109
Antibiotics 109
Resuscitation 109
Wound Closure Technique 109
Nutrient Supplementation 110

■■■ **IDENTIFICATION OF POSTOPERATIVE WOUND COMPLICATIONS 110**
Wound Infections 110
Dehiscence 111
Neoplasms 111
Hypertrophic Scars and Keloids 111

■■■ **MANAGEMENT OF WOUND COMPLICATIONS 111**
Wound Dressings 111
Antibiotics 111
Wound Adjuvants 112
Debridement 112
Scar Revision 113

■■■ **REFERENCES 113**

Wound healing failure is the mechanism of many surgical complications. Deficient tissue repair leads to anastomotic leaks and fascial dehiscences, while overabundant tissue repair occurs in keloids and luminal strictures. Dysregulated wound healing, therefore, is a common cause of poor surgical outcomes. Although wounds are most frequently understood to mean injuries to the skin, practicing surgeons appreciate the importance of wounds and wounding to all types of tissue. The cellular and molecular pathways by which all types of injured tissues heal share common integrated components. Consequently, a basic understanding of the biologic components of tissue repair is necessary to prevent or correct the complications of wound healing.

NORMAL WOUND HEALING

A wound initially is tissue that has lost normal structure and functions as the result of internal or external forces. Wound healing is the sequence of cellular and molecular events activated at the time of injury resulting in a time-dependent

Michael G. Franz: University of Michigan, Ann Arbor, MI 48109

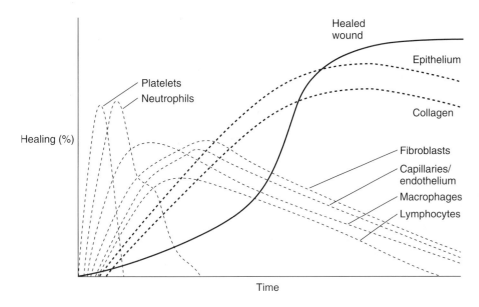

Figure 10-1 Successful acute wound healing requires the coordinated activation of cellular and molecular repair pathways beginning at the moment of injury. Each component must then be integrated into a continuum during the host response. Clinically, it is the rate of recovery in breaking strength that often determines the outcome of an acute wound.

pattern of tissue repair (1). The integration of each component pathway along the continuum of the host response to injury results in complete wound healing (Fig. 10-1). Classically, the phases of wound healing are described as hemostasis, inflammation, fibroproliferation, and remodeling (maturation).

Hemostasis

The composition of damaged tissue changes continuously during wound maturation and remodeling of the newly synthesized matrix. The dynamic process involves complex molecular and cellular interactions during which the initial fibrin-rich clot is transformed into a collagen-rich scar. Before a wound can heal it must stop bleeding. Therefore, the earliest phase of wound healing following injury is characterized by the deposition of fibrinogen, a soluble plasma protein synthesized by the liver and secreted into the systemic circulation. Fibrinogen extravasates from disrupted blood vessels and fills the gap of the wound. The coagulation cascade is activated and sustained through thrombin-mediated cleavage of fibrinogen, leading to the formation of fibrin monomers that polymerize into an insoluble fibrin clot to prevent further bleeding. The fibrin network also establishes the provisional matrix that allows migration of monocytes, fibroblasts, and endothelial cells into the wound. Fibroblasts within the fibrin clot synthesize collagen, and the fibrin matrix is progressively degraded and replaced with a collagen-rich scar (2). Fibrinogen has also been reported to induce angiogenesis. Other mediators activated during hemostasis such as platelet-derived growth factor (PDGF) and thrombin peptides have overlapping regulatory effects on many of the cellular elements of early tissue repair, such as fibroblasts and endothelial cells (3).

Inflammation

The cellular and humoral inflammatory phase is induced next, and an immune barrier is established against pathologic microorganisms. It is well known that a wound out of bacterial balance will not heal (4). The redundancy of the signals for the wound inflammatory response and wound healing is beginning to be described. Necrotic tissue locally releases cellular breakdown products capable of maintaining and amplifying the early inflammatory response following injury. Eicosanoids, 20-carbon metabolites of arachidonic acid derived from cell-membrane fatty acids, function as primary mediators in the wound healing scheme. Macrophages are tissue leukocytes fundamental to the inflammatory response following injury, which provides an abundant reservoir of potent tissue growth factors necessary for repair, such as transforming growth factor-β(TGF-β) The intensity of the early inflammatory response is greater in adult wound healing, in which protection against microbial insult supports tissue repair. During fetal wound healing up to midgestation, the intensity of this tissue inflammatory response is blunted. This might in part be due to immaturity of the cellular immune system and reduced growth factor production (5). The blunted immediate tissue inflammatory response *in utero* is one potential explanation for the phenomenon of scarless fetal healing.

Over the past decade, the free radical nitric oxide (NO) has emerged as a fundamental signaling molecule for many biologic processes (6,7). NO has proven especially important in physiologic responses important to surgeons, such as following traumatic injury and during sepsis. NO level and activity is central to the regulation of vascular tone during shock and is equally important as a metabolite that can establish a host barrier against microorganism invasion.

NO is synthesized by one of three isoforms of nitric oxide synthase (NOS). Inducible NOS (iNOS) is upregulated following tissue injury. Most data suggest that local NO production promotes normal wound healing. NOS inhibitors delay the healing of acute excisional wounds, while supplemental NO provided via molecular donors accelerates acute wound healing. The recovery of incisional wound breaking strength is also delayed following NOS blockade. Knockout mice missing the iNOS gene exhibit marked impairment of acute healing that can be reversed by iNOS gene transfer. It appears that NO contributes to acute tissue repair by promoting collagen synthesis and angiogenesis (8).

Once bleeding is controlled, the increased permeability of vessels adjacent to the injury facilitates the migration of inflammatory cells into the wound. Polymorphonuclear leukocytes (neutrophils) are the predominant initial inflammatory cell population to enter the wound site. The rise in wound neutrophil number begins almost immediately following injury and peaks by postinjury day 2. The primary function of acute wound neutrophils appears to be phagocytosis of invading microbes and release of cytochemoattractants to further propagate the cellular inflammatory response. In neutrophil depleted animal models it has been shown that neutrophils are not mandatory for the progression of normal tissue repair (3). However, it is also well known that if a wound infection develops, healing will be delayed. In patients with chronic granulomatous disease in which an absence of the enzyme NADPH-oxidase occurs, the intracellular killing of bacteria and fungi within neutrophils is impaired. This defect results in chronic infections, which retard the repair process.

Following burns, there is delayed tissue necrosis secondary to vascular occlusion caused by thrombi deposition in the vascular bed surrounding the burn wound. The absence of blood flow through these vessels results in extended tissue necrosis and an increase in the wound surface area. Preventing the infiltration of circulating neutrophils into a burn wound using blocking antibodies directed against neutrophil surface antigens has been shown in animal models to prevent the development of secondary burn necrosis. Observations such as these demonstrate that a balance between wound benefit and wound detriment exists and that excessive neutrophil-derived factors such as oxygen radicals can actually impede tissue repair.

Circulating monocytes enter the wound in a second wave of inflammatory cells within 24 hours after the appearance of neutrophils (1). Monocytes terminally differentiate into tissue macrophages upon exiting the vasculature and entering the wound site. Macrophages are clearing houses for many important molecular signals for the propagation of the wound repair process, such as oxygen free radicals, inflammatory cytokines, and tissue growth factors. Tissue macrophages also have the capacity to undergo cell division within the wound site and, like the neutrophils, can clear the wound of contaminating microbes as well as nonviable tissue. Macrophage synthesis and release of tissue growth factors is a predominant signal mechanism for the initiation of the proliferative phase of the repair process. Macrophage-derived growth factors promote the migration of synthetic cells into the wound site and the production of a new connective tissue matrix (1). The regulated progression from a controlled tissue inflammatory response to an efficient fibroplastic phase is required for normal healing.

Fibroproliferation and Remodeling

Once hemostasis is achieved, ongoing injury has ceased, and an immune barrier is in place, wound healing trajectories shift toward fibroplasia and tissue repair. In adults the mechanism of tissue repair favors the rapid establishment of mechanical integrity over structural and functional tissue regeneration. Scar tissue replaces normal tissue following injury and is often a source of subsequent wound complications. Tissue regeneration following injury occurs only in select adult structures, such as the liver, or in relatively small surface area epidermal wounds. Over time, wound matrix cell number diminishes and collagen bundles are increasingly organized during remodeling. This final phase of wound healing can continue for years until a maximum wound strength plateau is finally reached.

The proliferative phase of acute tissue repair begins with the arrival of fibroblasts into the wound site on about postinjury day 2 or 3. Fibroblasts work to replace the fibrin-based provisional matrix established during the inflammatory or lag phase of tissue repair with a collagen-rich granulation tissue that is characteristic of the proliferative phase. Fibroblasts also synthesize and release glycosaminoglycans and proteoglycans that are important components of the extracellular matrix of granulation tissue. Simultaneously, vascular regeneration (angiogenesis) is occurring, using the maturing matrix as a scaffold. The newly formed vascular conduits supply nutrient building blocks to the cellular elements of the granulation tissue. In dermal wounds, overlying epidermal cells begin to migrate across the tissue defect at about this time to restore the skin's epithelial barrier function. Although inflammatory cells provide the initial defense against microbial invasion following injury, surface coverage ultimately provides this protection.

The migration and proliferation of fibroblasts into the acute wound is in large part regulated by potent tissue growth factors such as PDGF, TGF-β, and basic fibroblast growth factor (bFGF) (9). Fibroblasts begin to migrate into the wound as soon as 2 days following injury. After 4 days, fibroblasts are the major cell type in the developing granulation tissue. At first the wound fibroblast number increases via migration from adjacent unwounded tissue, but soon the wound fibroblast population rapidly increases via cell proliferation. The acute wound fibroblast density is maximized between 7 and 14 days after injury and is under the potent influence of wound growth factor levels. Activated tissue macrophages are a primary source for the various growth factors, including TGF-β, transforming growth factor-α (TGF-α), and bFGF. As acute tissue repair proceeds and macrophage number decreases, other cells in the wound such as fibroblasts, endothelial cells, and keratinocytes begin to synthesize and secrete growth factors. Fibroblasts secrete bFGF, TGF-β, PDGF, insulin-like growth factor (IGF-I), and keratinocyte growth factor (KGF). Endothelial cells produce vascular endothelial growth factor (VEGF), bFGF, and PDGF. Keratinocytes synthesize TGF-β, TGF-α, and KGF. These growth factors together stimulate continued acute wound cellular proliferation, production of extracellular matrix proteins and glycoproteins, and angiogenesis.

Fibroblasts require a scaffold or matrix to specifically bind to and move across in order to enter the acute wound environment and initiate tissue repair. Extracellular hyaluronic acid promotes cell migration and proliferation early in the repair process (10,11). Soon after, a falling hyaluronic acid concentration in the acute wound and rising chondroitin sulfate levels inhibit fibroblast migration and proliferation and induce fibroblast differentiation and mature connective tissue synthesis. Unlike unwounded dermal fibroblasts, granulation tissue fibroblasts organize intracellular actin molecules into polymers, a feature of many migrating cell types.

When acute wound fibroblasts reach a high density and cell-cell contact inhibition occurs, the polymerized intracellular actin chains condense into cytoplasmic stress fibers that have been shown to contain α-smooth muscle actin. These wound fibroblasts staining for α-smooth muscle actin are named myofibroblasts (11,12). It is controversial whether myofibroblast contraction is the dominant mechanism by which the healing acute wound undergoes subsequent contraction. It has been shown both *in vivo* and *in vitro* that myofibroblasts might not be necessary for wounds to contract (13). Other studies have shown that cell-traction forces on the wound matrix generated by activated fibroblasts through the action of cytoplasmic fine actin filaments are responsible for wound contraction. The myofibroblast might be a terminally differentiated fibroblast preparing for apoptosis (programmed cell death) rather than a central cell type necessary for wound contraction.

Collagen is the major protein component of wound connective tissue. Modifications of the chemical composition of collagen determine its biologic function. Fourteen isoforms of collagen, each the product of a unique gene, have been described (14). The connective tissue collagens are all helical in structure, with the distinctive repeating tripeptide sequence of glycine-X-Y, with the Y position usually occupied by proline or hydroxyproline. Glycine and proline amino acids are required for mature collagen molecules to assume tertiary triple helical structure. Different isoforms of collagen are expressed in different tissues and tissue locations at various times during healing. Type I collagen is the predominant type in bone and tendon. Type III and type I collagens are present in more elastic soft tissues, such as blood vessels, dermis, and fascia. Unwounded dermis contains approximately 80% type I collagen and 20% type III collagen. Acute wound granulation tissue, in contrast, expresses twice as much type III collagen. Type III collagen is considered "immature" and is less cross-linked than mature type I collagen, with a lower resulting tensile strength.

Normal collagen synthesis and secretion requires hydroxylation of lysine and proline residues. The cofactors necessary for enzymatic collagen hydroxylation are ferrous iron, molecular oxygen, α-ketoglutarate, and vitamin C. Impaired wound healing results from deficiencies in any of these cofactors, as during tissue hypoxia or with diets low in vitamin C. After synthesizing and releasing collagen, wound fibroblasts work to organize new extracellular collagen molecules into fibers oriented between specialized cellular clefts. Fibrillar collagen is made even more insoluble through the covalent cross-linking of collagen peptides located at the nonhelical ends of the molecule. The interstitial enzyme lysyl oxidase catalyzes this important action (15).

The organization of collagen bundles in the acute wound and in unwounded dermis is different. Collagen fiber bundles are arranged in a basket-weave pattern in unwounded dermis, while in acute wound granulation tissue mature collagen fibers are oriented in overlapping arrays parallel to the wound surface and usually along lines of maximum tension. The parallel array arrangement of granulation tissue collagen and of mature scar contributes to the abnormal rigidity of scar tissue.

The delivery of nutrient synthetic components is required for acute wound healing to progress. Initially, there is no vascular supply to the wound center and the appearance of new, viable tissue is limited to wound margins that are in contact with uninjured tissue. The formation of new blood vessels in acute granulation tissue (angiogenesis) occurs by a budding or sprouting mechanism from intact vessels at the wound borders. The development of vascular outgrowths requires endothelial cell proliferation. Numerous tissue growth factors, such as VEGF and bFGF, play central regulatory roles in neovascularization and subsequent tissue repair (16). Macrophages are necessary for wound neovascularization.

The acute granulation tissue that replaces the fibrin-based provisional matrix is a transitional tissue, and when it matures it usually produces scar. Acute wound granulation tissue is the result of the processes of inflammation, fibroplasia, angiogenesis, and extracellular matrix synthesis. It is characterized by a high density of capillaries, fibroblasts, macrophages, and loosely organized thin collagen fibril bundles. The metabolic activity of acute granulation tissue is high as rapid cell proliferation proceeds synchronously with high-level protein synthesis as well as lactate and CO_2 production.

When the wound defect is filled and as time passes, the maturing granulation tissue undergoes remodeling. The density of macrophages and fibroblasts is reduced. Fibroblast and myofibroblast terminal differentiation and subsequent apoptosis is the mechanism by which maturing wound fibroblast number is reduced. After skin healing the epidermis of the resultant scar differs from uninjured skin because it lacks the rete pegs that normally anchor into the underlying connective tissue matrix. There is also no regeneration of lost subepidermal appendages such as hair follicles or sweat glands following skin healing. Eventually, angiogenesis diminishes, wound blood flow falls, and metabolic activity slows.

Fibroblasts then further consolidate thin collagen fiber bundles into thick collagen cables. There is a change in scar tissue collagen composition as the 30% level of type III collagen present in acute granulation tissue drops to approximately 10% in mature scar (17). Finally, wound contraction occurs. Fibroblasts pack collagen fibers as a contractile unit. Cells and matrix generated within the wound site produce force vectors directed to achieve a further reduction in wound volume. As wound contraction proceeds, the injured tissue is replaced by uninjured surrounding tissue.

The Lag Phase

Recruiting the cellular and molecular elements of tissue repair into the wound site takes time. The "lag phase" of wound healing is defined as the earliest period of time following wounding when hemostasis, inflammation, and early fibroplasias are induced. It is during the lag phase of wound healing that acute wounds are most vulnerable to mechanical failure (dehiscence). The wound tensile strength is 0% to 30% of its maximum value during the first 7 days following wounding. This interval is the time during which patients are increasing wound loads.

Epithelialization involves the proliferation and migration of epithelial cells. The process completes wound coverage over a bed of granulation tissue or over a partial thickness injury to an epithelialized structure like the skin or gastrointestinal (GI) mucosa. Repair epithelial cells are derived from the wound periphery from uninjured epithelium or from specialized subepithelial structures like hair follicles and sweat glands in the skin. In incisions this distance is very short and the establishment of epithelial coverage should be complete within days. Epithelialization contributes nothing to the gain in wound breaking strength—an important process that is slow to initiate and continues for long after the wound has been resurfaced. Following acute dermal injury, such as burns, the early closure of an open wound by epithelialization initiates the wound remodeling process within the underlying granulation tissue. Numerous models have described the molecular signaling that occurs between regenerating epithelial structures and the underlying supporting mesenchymal tissue. Early wound surface coverage reduces the likelihood of disabling hypertrophic scar formation and improves the overall cosmetic result. When the wound surface area is small, regenerative reepithelialization might occur with little or no scar formation.

Contraction is a metabolically active mechanism by which wound volume is mechanically diminished. Although the mechanism of wound contraction is complex, it appears to involve tractional forces generated by repair fibroblasts transmitted to the wound extracellular matrix via cellular adhesion molecules (13). The early wound matrix is composed in large part by collagen, fibrin, fibronectin, and vitronectin. Intracellular fibroblast cytoskeletal polymerization, an energy requiring process, is the source of the tractional forces. Some evidence also suggests that terminally differentiated wound fibroblasts, called *myofibroblasts*, are involved. These cells express cytoplasmic smooth muscle actin and are contractile.

Wound failure occurs when there is an abnormality in the magnitude or duration of the sequential components of tissue repair. Inadequate hemostasis due to platelet dysfunction or poor technique results in hematoma formation with ensuing mechanical disruption of the provisional wound matrix. Delayed or deficient inflammatory responses increase the risk of wound contamination or infection. A *prolonged* inflammatory response due to foreign material delays the progression of tissue repair into the fibroproliferative phase in which rapid gains in breaking strength and wound contraction should occur. Impaired fibroblast activation in turn impedes the establishment of

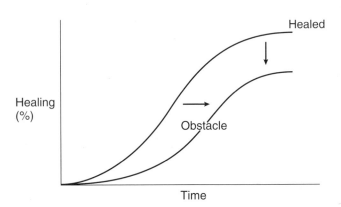

Figure 10-2 Wound healing failure occurs when an obstacle to normal repair pathways results in an abnormality in the magnitude or duration of the sequential components of tissue repair. The impediment to normal wound healing might be biologic or mechanical in origin and might derive from the wounded host or from external forces.

the early wound matrix and synthesis of immature scar. Epithelialization requires an underlying functional bed of granulation tissue. Obstacles to normal wound healing therefore shift the wound healing trajectory and result in wound complications (Fig. 10-2).

PREOPERATIVE RISK FACTORS FOR WOUND COMPLICATIONS

Contamination and Infection

The risk factors for surgical wound complications can be broadly categorized as local or systemic wound healing impediments (Table 10-1). The most common local risk factor is wound contamination. The risk for wound contamination and infection can be predicted by categorizing surgical wounds according to clinical circumstances. In increasing order of risk for wound infection they are operating in (i) a clean field (ii) a clean-contaminated field (iii) a contaminated field and (iv) an infected or dirty field (Table 10-2). A clean operative field minimizes wound bacterial exposure by operating upon otherwise normal and healthy soft tissue usually breeching only the skin. The bacterial organisms normally colonizing skin surfaces are predominantly Gram-positive *Staphylococcus* and *Streptococcus* species. Following standard operative field sterile preparation, expected wound infection rates in this setting are 1% to 3% (18,19). Examples include breast biopsies and inguinal hernia repair. An operation is classified clean-contaminated if an organ that is colonized with high numbers of potentially pathologic bacteria is breeched. Common examples are colorectal and pulmonary resections. In this setting expected wound infection rates are reduced to 10% with appropriate preoperative preparation and prophylaxis. A procedure is classified as contaminated if high-level, uncontrolled bacterial contamination occurs, especially when associated with local tissue injury. Examples of these procedures include repair of gunshot wounds of the colon or severe burn injuries. Wound infection rates in these settings are 33% to 60% (18).

Necrotic tissue exacerbates defective wound repair. Bacteria use necrotic debris as a nutrient source, increasing the likelihood of invasive wound infection. Metabolites of cell-membrane arachidonic acid released from dying cells are toxic to adjacent normal cells. Necrotic debris within the wound also establishes a mechanical barrier against the influx of wound repair cells, such as fibroblasts and keratinocytes. Tissue proteases released by necrotic cells degrade wound growth factors, preventing the initiation of growth factor-dependent repair pathways.

Tissue Hypoperfusion

Operating during periods of shock increases the risk of surgical wound failure. Wound infection and dehiscence rates increase threefold when operating during profound hypotension and acidosis (20). Tissue perfusion is impaired as a consequence of other disorders, including peripheral vascular disease, edema, hypothermia, vasospastic disease, and venous hypertension. Irradiated tissue is also hypoperfused as the result of microangiopathy. Previously irradiated tissue might be especially susceptible to wound necrosis given its reduced capillary blood supply and increased fibrosis, which results in an abnormal wound inflammatory response.

Reduced capillary perfusion results in a low tissue oxygen tension, which is associated with collagen defects and increased wound infections (21). Severe ischemia and hypoxia can directly inhibit other wound healing processes such as angiogenesis and epithelialization. Transcutaneous

TABLE 10-1
IMPEDIMENTS TO WOUND HEALING

Systemic	Local
Malnutrition	Contamination
Chronic diseases	Trauma
Pharmacologic agents	Tissue hypoperfusion
Shock	Irradiation
Age	Neoplasm
Genetic repair defects	Factitious wounding

TABLE 10-2
RISK FOR WOUND CONTAMINATION AND INFECTION ACCORDING TO CLINICAL CIRCUMSTANCES

Wound Classification	Examples	Risk for Wound Infection (%)
Dirty-infected	Infected traumatic wound with necrotic debris	60
Contaminated	Gunshot wound to left colon	33
Clean-contaminated	Elective colon resection	5
Clean	Breast biopsy or hernia repair	1

tissue oxygen monitors provide a clinically available means for measuring wound oxygen levels. Chronic wounds like pressure ulcers and diabetic foot ulcers do not heal when tissue oxygen levels fall below 30 mm Hg.

Malnutrition

Patients who are severely malnourished or actively catabolic, as during the systemic inflammatory response syndrome, demonstrate impaired healing (22). The deleterious effects of malnutrition are expressed in each of the phases of wound healing. An altered inflammatory response might result from the effects of malnutrition on immune function. Animals fed protein-free diets develop reduced levels of fibronectin and complement, both important chemotactic factors for fibroblasts and macrophages. Decreased polymorphonuclear leukocyte activity against fungi and bacteria has been measured in children suffering kwashiorkor protein deficiency (23). Prolonged protein malnutrition limits collagen synthesis, fibroblast proliferation, and neovascularization.

Although nutritional status is difficult to measure in most clinical settings, a serum albumin <3 g per dL increases the risk of wound infection and incisional hernia formation. A large Veterans Administration cooperative study of perioperative risk factors found that a low preoperative serum albumin level was the single most significant variable for predicting surgical morbidity (20). Wound infection and acute wound failure were among the most commonly observed complications. Protein synthesis and cell division are stimulated at wound sites, and an abundant supply of amino acids is necessary to sustain repair. Fatty acid deficiencies are known to cause delayed dermal healing. Cancer cachexia is associated with profound delays in wound repair. Elevated circulating cytokine levels, such as tumor necrosis factor-α, contribute through disturbances in the normal wound inflammatory response.

Micronutrient deficiency can also impair wound healing. Vitamin A is a cofactor for normal cell differentiation and epithelial keratinization. Vitamin C is critical for strength gain in healing wounds, catalyzing the hydroxylation of proline and lysine residues during collagen cross-linking. Vitamin K is required for the synthesis of several coagulation proteins, including prothrombin. Deficiencies are therefore associated with excessive bleeding from wounded tissue and abnormal provisional matrix formation. Trace mineral deficiencies can develop in surgical patients, especially those treated with prolonged parenteral nutrition and in patients with chronic conditions such as alcoholism, GI disorders, and diabetes. Zinc acts as a cofactor to many enzymatic reactions involved in DNA synthesis, protein synthesis, mitosis, and cellular proliferation. Reduced zinc levels result in delayed epithelialization and fibroblast proliferation. Iron is a cofactor in collagen synthesis, and low iron levels indirectly impair healing because of reduced oxygen transport.

Chronic Disease

Underlying disease in the injured host can complicate wound healing. Diabetes mellitus is known to delay the closure of dermal foot ulcers, but it is not clear that incisional healing is delayed in diabetics. Diabetics are more susceptible to wound infection because of impaired neutrophil chemotaxis and phagocytosis. The clean wound infection rate is higher in diabetic patients (11%) than in the general patient population (24).

Increasing patient age is not a consistent risk factor for global wound healing complications. There appears to be a minor defect in epidermal-dermal repair that is the result of changes in tissue extracellular matrix structure and resultant elasticity of aged skin, but this does not appear to effect myofascial, GI, or vascular repair. In specific models increased host age is associated with impaired wound healing. Fibroblast proliferation and activity are diminished and collagen production and wound contraction are slowed (23). Tissue repair observed in the elderly is often complicated by an increased incidence of comorbid conditions and polypharmacy.

Immunodeficiency states have been associated with delayed wound healing. In the presence of an impaired immune defense, wound bacterial loads might rise to uncontrolled levels and delay healing trajectories. Although polymorphonuclear leukocytes are not absolutely required for wound healing, the absence or reduction in wound macrophage number or activity leads to significant impairment of tissue repair (1).

Acute and chronic liver diseases are associated with delays in wound healing. In animal models acute jaundice caused a 25% to 50% reduction in abdominal incision bursting strength after 1 week (1). Long-standing jaundice had less of an inhibitory effect on healing incisions. Clinically, increased fascial dehiscence has been reported following laparotomy performed in jaundiced patients, especially those with malignant causes for jaundice. Acute wound failure rates of 60% have been observed in small series.

Pharmacologic Agents

Cytotoxic and metabolically active pharmacologic agents should always be considered when managing a wound. The active cellular components of wound healing, like macrophages, fibroblasts, and epithelial cells, are targets for undesirable inhibitory side effects. Although there are not many class one data sets proving the impairment of tissue repair by most pharmacologic agents, clinical experience and pharmacologic mechanisms should alert all clinicians managing wounds to the possibility of drug-induced wound complications.

It is not clear that corticosteroid use delays most soft tissue repair following surgical wounding. Category II evidence suggests that epidermal repair is delayed, but there is no solid evidence that myofascial or GI healing is impaired (25). Steroids have been shown to inhibit fibroblast function *in vitro*. Although the recovery of dermal tensile strength is delayed in rodents treated with corticosteroids at the time of incision, the effects of corticosteroids on human clinical wound healing have not been well studied. Mechanistically, it is likely that corticosteroids impair tissue repair through their inhibitory effects on inflammation and structural gene expression. The inhibitory effect of cortisone on skin wound strength in rodents is negated if vitamin A is given concurrently. No data are available on the treatment of patients on steroids with vitamin A prior to surgical wounding, although empirical therapy might be reasonable.

Cytotoxic agents can induce profound delays in wound repair by inhibiting cell proliferation, DNA, and protein synthesis. Chemotherapeutic drugs might suppress the normal wound inflammatory response as well as inhibit fibroblast proliferation and collagen deposition. Clinically, it is usual to delay administration of an antineoplastic agent in a postoperative cancer patient until the acute wound healing phases are completed because of concern for adverse drug effects on wound healing (usually 3 to 6 weeks).

Genetic Defects

The classic genetic disorder with an abnormal wound healing phenotype is the Ehlers-Danlos syndrome. Variable penetrance of the defective structural protein genes might cause subtle clinical presentations. There are at least 12 distinct subtypes of Ehlers-Danlos, and although it is infrequent, encountering such a patient occurs in most surgical careers. Ehlers-Danlos syndrome is often associated with fragile skin, weakened scar and wound disruption, spontaneous aneurysms in major blood vessels, and bleeding disorders. A careful personal and family history as well as physical exam should alert the observant surgeon to these disorders. Other frequently encountered patients with disordered wound healing include Marfan syndrome patients. Newer genetic and biochemical evidence suggests that spontaneous abdominal aortic aneurysm patients might also express abnormal content or collagen protease activity contributing to both arterial wall weakness and defective wound healing. Abdominal aortic aneurysm patients are commonly encountered in surgical practices. Once a clinical diagnosis associated with defective tissue repair is made, great care must be exercised in wound closure and management since there are no known methods for correcting the defective biochemical pathways.

Atypical Wounds

Wound malignancy should always be considered and a biopsy performed in any open wound that is difficult to debride and fails to heal. In a difficult-to-heal wound, factitious injury or recurrent trauma should be considered.

MODIFICATION OF PREOPERATIVE RISK FACTORS

Minimize Contamination

Minimization of microbial wound contamination lowers the incidence of wound infection and wound failure. Antiseptic preparation of the surgical site is known to reduce the incidence of wound infection following clean cases. In the case of GI surgery, preoperative luminal mechanical and antibiotic preparation reduces exposure to enteric bacteria and lowers wound infection rates (18). Sharp debridement of necrotic tissue from acute and chronic wounds increases the incidence of complete wound healing (4). In the case of gross wound contamination, the wound should be copiously irrigated at the time of the operation and all foreign material removed.

Antibiotics

Therapeutic tissue antibiotic levels at the surgical site during incision reduce the incidence of wound infection following clean and clean-contaminated cases. This requires that a bolus dose of the appropriate antibiotic be given just prior to the time of wounding. Antibiotics with a spectrum of coverage for Gram-positive skin organisms are indicated for clean cases (e.g., first-generation cephalosporin). An antibiotic class with broader Gram-negative coverage is indicated for clean-contaminated GI cases (e.g., second-generation cephalosporin). It is not clear that antibiotic administration following grossly contaminated traumatic injuries lowers the incidence of postoperative wound infections. Because of the high incidence of wound infection following contaminated cases, antibiotics are typically begun empirically.

Resuscitation

Transcutaneous oxygen tension is the optimal method for measuring nutritive skin perfusion and has a direct correlation with the success of dermal healing. Molecular oxygen is necessary for mature collagen formation, and optimized collagen fibril cross-linking fails as tissue oxygen pressure (P_{O_2}) levels fall below 40 mm Hg. Periwound P_{O_2} <30 mm Hg implies there might be insufficient oxygen for healing. Below 10 mm Hg, oxygen is deficient and growth factors have little chance of inducing healing mechanisms for these wounds. In most models hyperbaric oxygen (HBO) therapy has been found to improve wound oxygen delivery and to induce angiogenesis in ischemic wounds (21).

Wound Closure Technique

Primary wound closure is defined as the surgical closure of a wound within several hours after the wound is made. Primary wound closure results in low infection and wound failure rates for clean and clean-contaminated wounds. Whenever possible, incisions should be placed in lines of minimal tension to prevent hypertrophic scarring. This is especially true in locations of cosmetic importance such as the face. For example, on the forehead the lines of minimal tension are transverse, so that a transverse incision will heal with a thinner and finer scar-line than a perpendicular, vertical incision.

Following gross wound contamination, secondary closure ("healing by secondary intent") will reduce wound infection rates. Secondary intention occurs in an open, full-thickness wound that heals by the host biologic mechanisms of epithelialization, contraction, collagen deposition, and granulation tissue formation. Although better than wound infection, the drawback of this approach is that open wounds require more nursing care and result in a worse cosmetic result.

Delayed primary closure provides an alternative. This technique involves leaving a contaminated wound open with moist dressing changes until bacterial balance is achieved. When quantitative wound culture levels fall to $\leq 10^5$ colony forming units per gram of wound tissue, the wound healing success rate following closure approaches that of primary closure (1). Delayed primary closure also provides the time necessary for the cellular and molecular elements of tissue repair to enter the wound prior to wound closure. Delayed primary closure is usually performed 24 hours to several days following injury.

Tertiary wound closure involves the transfer of viable autologous tissue from a distant site to the wound. Partial thickness skin grafting is a frequently used example. The technique can accelerate epithelialization when wound contraction has stopped or there is a large surface area of granulation tissue.

The choice of suture material does not significantly affect wound healing. In principle, the suture should provide approximation of the injured tissue and maintain bursting strength until wound mechanics recover. A very rapidly absorbed suture material would therefore be appropriate for a low load wound repair in which wound tensile strength rapidly recovers, such as following corneal keratotomy. In contrast, wound closure following abdominal wall laparotomy requires a stout suture material that maintains its mechanical integrity for the 6 to 12 weeks necessary for recovery of maximal wound bursting strength. Class 2 and 3 data suggest that braided suture materials are associated with higher suture abscess rates, especially when used in contaminated wounds. Bacteria lodge within the interstices of braided suture and escape wound immune cell phagocytosis.

Acute wound failure is most often due to suture pulling through adjacent tissue and not suture fracture or knot slippage (25). Tissue failure occurs in the biochemically active zone adjacent to the acute wound edge in which proteases activated during normal tissue repair result in a loss of native tissue integrity. This is especially true for GI anastomoses in which a fall in wound tensile strength has been measured during the first 3 days following repair (26–30). The breakdown of the tissue matrix adjacent to the wound appears to be part of the mechanism for mobilizing the many cellular elements of acute tissue repair.

Nutrient Supplementation

Preoperative nutritional repletion has been shown to improve surgical wound outcomes only in cases of severe malnutrition (31). In fact, some studies suggest that aggressive preoperative nutritional supplementation increases wound complications and surgical morbidity and mortality, especially in oncology patients. The additional procedures required for peripheral and enteral access as well as delays in surgical therapy contribute to the disappointing results of aggressive preoperative attempts at nutritional therapy.

IDENTIFICATION OF POSTOPERATIVE WOUND COMPLICATIONS

A healing wound should remain structurally and functionally intact and display no signs of inflammation. There should be no intense redness, warmth, swelling, or pain (rubor, calor, tumor, and dolor). Progressive fibroplasia should result in a prominent midwound "healing ridge" (Fig. 10-3).

Wound Infections

A wound infection exists when $>10^5$ invasive organisms per gram of wound tissue or any level of β hemolytic streptococcus are present. This manifests clinically as wound cellulitis, drainage, odor, and/or pain.

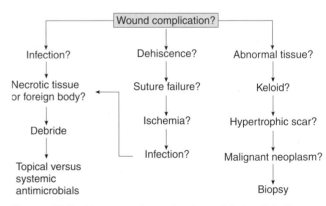

Figure 10-3 Most wound complications might be clinically categorized as infections, mechanical failure (dehiscence), or abnormal tissue (neoplasia). A systematic approach to wound complications can guide accurate diagnosis and therapy.

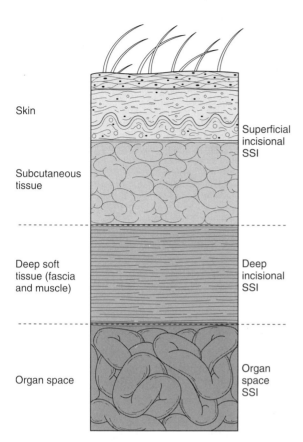

Skin

Subcutaneous
tissue

Deep soft
tissue (fascia
and muscle)

Organ space

Superficial
incisional
SSI

Deep
incisional
SSI

Organ
space
SSI

Figure 10-4 The accurate diagnosis and therapy of wound infections requires precise anatomical localization. Tracking of uncontrolled soft tissue infections along fascial planes might progress to myonecrosis, as in Fournier gangrene. The development of bullae in the skin surrounding a wound should always raise concern for an invasive wound infection. Wound tissue biopsies provide the most definitive diagnosis of wound infection. SSI, surgical site infection.

Accurate diagnosis of wound infections requires precise anatomical localization (Fig. 10-4). Complicated deep wound infections might progress to fasciitis or myonecrosis, as in Fournier gangrene. Surrounding skin bullae should always raise concern for an invasive wound infection, as should unexplained fevers occurring near the fifth postoperative day. If the clinical presentation is confusing or if empiric therapy fails, wound biopsy for histology and quantitative wound cultures provide the most definitive diagnosis of wound infection. Surface wound cultures might suggest a pathogenic organism and guide antimicrobial therapy, but a wound infection is not defined until tissue invasion occurs with associated tissue inflammation (32).

Dehiscence

Acute wound failure can present as mechanical wound separation or dehiscence. Dermal wound separation worsens cosmetic results but is unlikely to cause significant harm. Abdominal wall, GI, and vascular anastomosis wound failure can have life-threatening outcomes and will be discussed

in later chapters. Wound dehiscence occurs when the distractive forces exerted perpendicular to a wound edge exceed the recovery of wound mechanical properties (33).

Neoplasms

Malignancy should be considered in a nonhealing wound and a biopsy performed in any open area that is difficult to debride and is failing to heal.

Hypertrophic Scars and Keloids

Hypertrophic scars are raised and often inflamed but confined to the area of the original wound. Most will resolve slowly over 1 to 2 years without surgical intervention. There is some evidence that steroid derivative injections (triamcinolone) can inhibit the prolonged inflammatory phase of scar formation and induce remodeling. Keloids, in contrast, extend beyond the boundaries of the original wound and do not regress spontaneously. Keloids tend to recur following excision, and excision alone is rarely adequate therapy to prevent recurrence. Intralesional steroid therapy has shown benefit. Any steroid therapy must be used with close surveillance to avoid tissue atrophy and skin depigmentation. Antihistamine therapy might improve the burning and itching often associated with keloids and might help to avoid cyclical attempts at surgical excision.

MANAGEMENT OF WOUND COMPLICATIONS

Wound Dressings

Most wound complications can be managed nonoperatively. Appropriately dressing and protecting a wound can reduce the incidence of wound complications. Basic wound healing studies and clinical research have confirmed that wound healing is optimized in a moist environment (34). The ideal wound dressing therefore should protect a wound against desiccation (hydrophobic dressing). In addition, dressings should keep a wound clean, protect against wound trauma, absorb exudates, and minimize wound pain (Fig. 10-5).

Specific types of wounds have unique requirements for optimized tissue repair. Pressure ulcers need off-loading to improve capillary perfusion of the wound and surrounding skin and to minimize traumatic shear forces. Venous stasis ulcers heal best when lower extremity sequential compression is used, in part to improve capillary perfusion and tissue oxygen delivery (35).

Antibiotics

Antibiotic chemotherapy improves outcomes for the treatment of wound infections. Therapeutic wound and

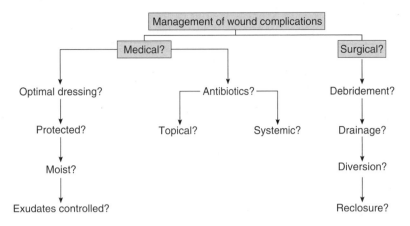

Figure 10-5 The management of wound complications might apply nonoperative and operative principles. The optimum dressing protects the wound from repeat trauma and maintains a moist wound environment. Topical antibiotic therapy might be effective when the infection is confined to the wound, especially when wound blood supply is compromised. Surgical therapy is fundamental to the successful management of complicated wounds.

periwound tissue levels are required for antimicrobial efficacy. For antibiotic therapy to be successful, a wound must first be adequately prepared. This most commonly means debridement of necrotic tissue and the excision of foreign material.

Therapeutic wound tissue antibiotic levels can be achieved both locally and systemically. Often, infected nonhealing wounds are hypoperfused, limiting the delivery of systemically administered antibiotics. Burn eschars, venous stasis ulcers, and pressure ulcers are common examples. In these settings topically applied antimicrobials such as silver sulfadiazine and sulfamylon preparations might be efficacious. Systemically applied antibiotics will improve wound healing rates only if minimum inhibitory concentrations are reached in the wounded and infected tissue. Regardless of the route of wound antibiotic therapy, the anti-infectives used will be most effective if directed to the organisms infecting the wound. This can be achieved by performing quantitative wound cultures. In general, first-generation penicillins and cephalosporins provide a spectrum of coverage for most Gram-positive skin surface organisms, while second-generation and third-generation cephalosporins and modified, later-generation penicillins increase Gram-negative and enteric coverage at the expense of anti Gram-positive activity.

Wound Adjuvants

The high prevalence of nonhealing wounds has stimulated the development of novel adjuvants designed to improve wound-healing outcomes. Vacuum assisted wound closure can improve closure rates. The most common design allows maintenance of a moist wound environment, drainage of wound exudates, and continuous negative pressure to the open wound surface. This arrangement has been shown to accelerate the appearance of repair fibroblasts in the wound and to improve wound perfusion (36). HBO therapy has also been shown to improve the healing rates of difficult wounds. When transcutaneous tissue oxygen levels of >30 mm Hg are

achieved, reported wound closure rates have been accelerated by 50% (21).

Debridement

A skin wound should be reopened when wound infection is suspected or if surrounding cellulitis does not respond to antibiotics. This allows a quantitative wound culture to be performed for more accurate diagnosis. In addition, an open wound can be debrided with moist gauze dressing changes several times a day. Dressing debridement lowers wound bacterial counts directly and by removing from the wound necrotic tissue that acts as a nutrient supply for invasive organisms.

Necrotic wounds might need more aggressive surgical intervention. Necrotic wound tissue is by definition without a blood supply and will not heal. Necrotic tissue should therefore always be debrided from wounds. The most reliable way to debride any wound is sharply using standard surgical principles. Necrotic tissue should be excised back to healthy appearing soft tissue with obvious blood supply. All foreign material like asphalt or retained sutures should also be debrided from a nonhealing wound. Debridement might be limited by extension to a nonhealing surface or structure such as tendon sheath or bone. In these cases a viable tissue transfer might be indicated. Chemical enzymatic wound debridement is efficacious when surgical debridement is not available, but it remains a second-line alternative to complete surgical excision. Protease compounds of papain and collagenases are often applied. Chemical debridement is effective only for the removal of necrotic soft tissue and biofilms. Enzymatic treatment cannot replace surgical debridement of complicating foreign materials.

Seromas and hematomas can impede wound healing. These fluid collections mechanically distract wound edges and reduce capillary perfusion. Wound fluid collections also increase the risk of wound infection. Whenever possible, wound seromas or hematomas that are not spontaneously resolving or that are associated with a wound complication like infection or dehiscence should be aspirated or drained through the open incision. If the wound fluid collection is associated with a nearby implanted device, it might be best to attempt needle aspiration of the fluid collection under sterile conditions to minimize the risk of a foreign body infection.

Scar Revision

Scars resulting in poor cosmetic results can be surgically revised. The broad goal of scar revision is to reorient the scar into lines of tension so that the dimension of the scar is oriented into lines of relaxation. The techniques most often used for dermal scars are Z-plasties or W-plasties. Stricture-plasties of GI strictures apply the same principles in an effort to redirect scar forces.

REFERENCES

1. Robson MC, Steed DL, Franz MG. Wound healing: biologic features and approaches to maximize healing trajectories. *Curr Probl Surg* 2001;38(2):77–89.
2. Henry G, Garner WL. Inflammatory mediators in wound healing. *Surg Clin North Am* 2003;83:491–497.
3. Clark RAF. *The molecular and cellular biology of wound repair*, 2nd ed. New York: Plenum Publishing; 1995.
4. Robson MC, Hill DP, Woodske ME, et al. Wound healing trajectories as predictors of effectiveness of therapeutic agents. *Arch Surg* 2000;135:773–777.
5. Ferguson MW, Whitby DJ, Shah M, et al. Scar formation: the spectral nature of fetal and adult wound repair. *Plast Reconstr Surg* 1996;97:854–860.
6. Tzeng E, Billiar TR. Nitric oxide and the surgical patient: identifying therapeutic targets. *Arch Surg* 1997;132:977–982.
7. Yamasaki K, Edington HD, McClosky C, et al. Reversal of impaired wound repair in iNOS-deficient mice by topical adenoviral-mediated iNOS gene transfer. *J Clin Invest* 1998;101:967–971.
8. Leibovich SJ, Polverini PJ, Fong TW, et al. Production of angiogenic activity by human monocytes requires an L-arginine/nitric oxide synthase-dependent effector mechanism. *Proc Natl Acad Sci USA* 1994;91:4190–4194.
9. Rappolee DA, Mark D, Banda MJ, et al. Wound macrophages express TGF-α and other growth-factors in vivo: analysis by mRNA phenotyping. *Science* 1988;241:708–712.
10. Pajulo OT, Pulkki KJ, Lertola KK, et al. Hyaluronic acid in incision wound fluid: a clinical study with the Cellstick device in children. *Wound Repair Regen* 2001;9(3):200–204.
11. Gosiewska A, Yi CF, Brown LJ, et al. Differential expression and regulation of extracellular matrix-associated genes in fetal and neonatal fibroblasts. *Wound Repair Regen* 2001;9(3):213–222.
12. Morgan CJ, Pledger WJ. Fibroblast proliferation. In: Cohen IH, Diegelmann RF, Lindblad WJ, eds. *Wound healing: biochemical and clinical aspects*. Philadelphia, PA: WB Saunders; 1992:63–76.
13. Ballas CB, Davison JM. Delayed wound healing in aged rats is associated with increased collagen gel remodeling and contraction by skin fibroblasts, not with differences in apoptotic or myofibroblast cell populations. *Wound Repair Regen* 2001;9(3):223–237.
14. Prockop DJ, Kivirikko KI, Tuderman L, et al. The biosynthesis of collagen and its disorders. *N Engl J Med* 1979;301:13–23.
15. Jorgensen LN, Kellehave F, Karlsmark T, et al. Reduced collagen accumulation after major surgery. *Br J Surg* 1996;83:1591–1594.
16. Robson MC, Mustoe TA, Hunt TK. The future of recombinant growth factors in wound healing. *Am J Surg* 1998;176 (Suppl.2A):80–82.
17. Friedman DW, Boyd CD, Norton P, et al. Increases in type III collagen gene expression and protein synthesis in patients with inguinal hernias. *Ann Surg* 1993;218:754–760.
18. Culver DH. Surgical wound infection rates by wound class, operative procedure and patient risk index. *Am J Med* 1991;91(Suppl. 3B):152–157S.
19. Horan TC, Gaynes RP, Martone WJ, et al. CDC definitions of nosocomial surgical site infections, 1992: a modification of CDC definitions of surgical wound infections. *Am J Infect Control* 1992;20:271–274.
20. Best WR, Khuri SF, Phelan M, et al. Identifying patient preoperative risk factors and postoperative adverse events in administrative databases: results from the Department of Veterans Affairs National Surgical Quality Improvement Program. *J Am Coll Surg* 2002;194(3):257–266.
21. Hunt TK. Physiology in wound healing. In: Clowes GHA, ed. *Trauma, sepsis and shock: the physiological basis of therapy*. New York: Marcel Dekker Inc; 1988:443–471.
22. Demling RH, DeSanti L. The stress response to injury and infection: the role of nutritional support. *Wounds* 2000;12:3.
23. Leaper DJ, Gottrup F. Surgical wounds. In: Leaper DJ, Harding KG, eds. *Wounds: biology and management*. Oxford: Oxford University Press; 1998:23–40.
24. Gibbons GW. Lower extremity bypass in patients with diabetic foot ulcers. *Surg Clin North Am* 2003;83:659–669.
25. Carlson MA. Acute wound failure. Wound healing. *Surg Clin North Am* 2001;77(3):607–635.
26. Folli S, Morgagni P, Bazzocchi F, et al. An alternative repair technique for anastamotic leakage after total gastrectomy. *J Am Coll Surg* 2000;190(6):757–759.
27. Vignali A, Fazio WV, Lavery I, et al. Factors associated with the occurrence of leaks in stapled rectal anastamosis: review of 1,014 cases. *J Am Coll Surg* 1997;185:105–113.
28. Irvin TT, Hunt TK. Pathogenesis and prevention of disruption of colonic anastamoses in traumatized rats. *Br J Surg* 1974;61:437–439.
29. Tadros T, Wobbes T, Hendriks T. Blood transfusion impairs the healing of experimental intestinal anastamoses. *Ann Surg* 1992;215:276–281.
30. Tani T, Tsutamoto Y, Eguchi Y, et al. Protease inhibitor reduces loss of tensile strength in rat anastamosis with peritonitis. *J Surg Res* 2000;88:135–141.
31. Williams JG, Barbul A. Nutrition and wound healing. *Surg Clin North Am* 2003;83:571–596.
32. Robson MC, Shaw RC, Heggers JP. The reclosure of postoperative incisional abscesses based on bacterial quantification of the wound. *Ann Surg* 1970;171:279.
33. DuBay DA, Franz MG. Acute wound healing: the biology of acute wound failure. *Surg Clin North Am* 2003;83:463–481.
34. Bolton L, Pirone L, Chen J. Dressings' effects on wound healing. *Wounds* 1990;2:126–134.
35. Macdonald JM, Sims N, Mayrovitz HN. Lymphedema, lipedema and the open wound: the role of compression therapy. *Surg Clin North Am* 2003;83:639–658.
36. Lionelli GT, Lawrence WT. Wound dressings. *Surg Clin North Am* 2003;83:631–633.

Surgical Site Infections

11

Gerard M. Doherty

▬▬ **CLASSIFICATION AND RISK OF SURGICAL SITE INFECTION 114**

Classifications 114

Risk of Infection 116

National Nosocomial Infection Surveillance 116

Microbiology of Surgical Site Infection 118

Specific Risk Factors 118

▬▬ **PREVENTION OF SURGICAL SITE INFECTION 118**

Tissue Oxygenation 119

Bowel Preparation 120

Treatment of Remote Infections 120

Skin Preparation 120

Operating Room Environment 121

Operating Room Personnel 121

Antibiotic Prophylaxis 122

Operative Care 123

Incision Care 123

▬▬ **TREATMENT OF SURGICAL SITE INFECTION 123**

▬▬ **SUMMARY 124**

▬▬ **REFERENCES 124**

Surgical site infections (SSIs) are potential complications of all operative interventions. In order to minimize the risk of SSI for any procedure, the surgeon must understand the risk of infection and the available interventions for preventing it,

Gerard M. Doherty: University of Michigan, Ann Arbor, MI 48109

as well as the management options available if one does occur. The prevention methods include optimizing the patient's health and tissue perfusion preoperatively and postoperatively, minimizing wound contamination by careful sterile techniques, avoiding residual devitalized tissues by careful operative technique, and, finally, administering prophylactic antimicrobials appropriate to the infectious risk in the most advantageous doses and timing. Treatment methods include drainage of infected fluid collections, removal of devitalized tissue, elimination of sources of contamination, and appropriately selected antibiotics.

CLASSIFICATION AND RISK OF SURGICAL SITE INFECTION

Classifications

The consistent discussion of SSIs requires standardized definitions for both the presence of infection and the risk of infection. Only with the definition of these two issues can the actual institutional occurrence of an infection be rationally interpreted. SSIs are commonly discussed and classified according to their sites and the level of contamination associated with the procedure.

Sites

The Centers for Disease Control (CDC) has developed standardized surveillance criteria for defining SSIs (1–3). According to these criteria SSIs are defined as being either incisional or organ space. The incisional infections are further divided into either superficial incisional or deep incisional SSIs (Fig. 11-1). Superficial incisional site infections

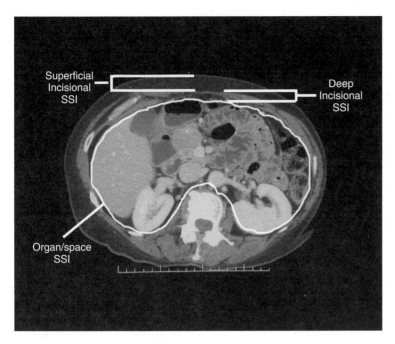

Figure 11-1 Surgical site infection depth classification: The classification of SSI on the basis of the infection's deepest extent. Superficial incisional infections involve only the skin and subcutaneous tissues. Extension into the fascia or muscular layers of the body wall is deep incisional wound infection. Involvement of the solid or hollow viscous organs or their surrounding potential spaces inside the body wall are organ/space infections.

include only the skin and subcutaneous tissues. This is the most common type of wound infection. Less common, and also often requiring more invasive management, are deep incisional SSIs. These infections involve the deep soft tissue such as fascia and muscle of the abdominal wall. Organ space infections involve either the solid or hollow organs themselves or the potential spaces surrounding them. Examples of this include intraperitoneal abscess, hepatic abscess, and retroperitoneal abscess. The CDC mandates the use of these descriptors to characterize SSIs in its National Nosocomial Infection

Surveillance (NNIS) system (1). This system has been used since 1970 to report trends in nosocomial infections in US acute care hospitals. These definitions must be carefully followed in order to provide interpretable and comparable results.

Contamination

SSIs can also be characterized based on the extent of contamination of the procedure (4). The descriptive surgical wound classification scheme (Table 11-1) is used to help

TABLE 11-1

SURGICAL WOUND CLASS

Class	Description
Clean	Uninfected operative wound without inflammation or entry into the respiratory, alimentary, genital, or urinary tracts.
Clean-contaminated	Uninfected operative wound through which the respiratory, alimentary, genital or urinary tracts are entered in a controlled fashion without unusual contamination. Specific examples include operations on the biliary tree, appendix, vagina, and oropharynx if no unusual contamination or evidence of gross infection occurs.
Contaminated	Operations with major breaks in sterile technique, gross spillage from the alimentary tract or acute, nonpurulent inflammation. Also includes open, fresh, traumatic wounds.
Dirty-infected	Operations into fields that are contaminated by existing clinical infection or alimentary contents from perforated viscus. Also includes traumatic wounds that are older and contain retained devitalized tissue.

characterize the inoculum of infectious agent that affects the risk of a patient developing infection. Wounds are classified along a spectrum from clean to dirty or infected wounds. The risk of wound infection increases as the level of bacterial contamination of the wound increases.

Risk of Infection

For surgical infection to occur there must be microbial contamination of the surgical site. However, not all microbial contamination results in SSI; also, the same bacterial inoculum does not always result in SSI. There are a variety of modifying features in addition to the dose and virulence of the wound contaminants (Fig. 11-2).

Features of the bacteria that can affect the occurrence of SSI include the dose of the bacterial inoculum. If a surgical site is contaminated with >100,000 microorganisms per gram of tissue, the risk of SSI is high (5,6). However, the dose of microorganisms can be much lower if the bacteria contain or produce toxins that increase their ability to invade a host, produce damage within the host, or survive in the host tissue (7,8). Some bacterial surfaces inhibit phagocytosis, particularly with polysaccharide capsules, which limit an important early host defense system. Other bacteria might produce potent exotoxins that disrupt cell membranes or intracellular metabolism and can thus invade tissues and limit an effective host response. Still

other bacterial species produce a glycocalyx and associated extracellular component (slime) that physically shields the bacteria from the host immune system and inhibits the binding and penetration of antimicrobial drugs. Each of these factors specific to the bacteria can modify the dose necessary for a wound contaminant to produce an SSI.

Other features of the wound and the host can produce a relative resistance or lack of resistance to SSI. In particular, the presence of devitalized tissue or foreign body within a contaminated wound can increase the risk of SSI by limiting the ability of the host responses to clear the bacterial inoculum. In addition, the status of the host immune system can change the host resistance to infection (9,10). If the native immune system is suppressed by medications, chronic illness, hyperglycemia, or nutritional deficiency, a smaller dose of bacterial contamination might still produce an infection. Alternatively, the addition of antibiotic agents to the wound environment might enhance the host immune system's ability to respond to wound contaminants (4).

The goal of understanding the relationship between the dose of wound contaminants, the presence of devitalized tissue or foreign bodies, and the host resistance to infection is to be able to modify each of these factors to limit the occurrence of SSI (4). Efforts to eliminate or diminish the wound contamination include skin preparation, bowel preparation, and incision care for the patient. This is also the motivation for operating room cleanliness and sterile technique. Operative technique, operative strategy choices regarding foreign body use, and the use of laparoscopy can alter the presence of devitalized tissue or foreign bodies within the wound and might thus limit the risk of SSI. Finally, careful attention to the host resistance to infection and the appropriate use of antimicrobial prophylactic drugs might alter this component of the SSI balance. Thus, the careful consideration of these issues is important to minimizing the risk of this complication.

National Nosocomial Infection Surveillance

The NNIS system was established in 1970 in selected hospitals within the United States (1). These hospitals began routinely reporting their nosocomial infection surveillance data to a national database. Over 300 acute care adult or children's hospitals participate; their identities are confidential. The NNIS data are collected according to standardized protocols and include separate components for adult and pediatric intensive care unit infection rates, high-risk nursery infection rates, and surgical infection rates. The SSI statistics are mainly contained within this third component.

The NNIS surgical patient surveillance data are categorized according to the procedures performed. Records for every patient include information on risk factors such as wound class, duration of operation, American Society of Anesthesiologists (ASA) score, and the use of laparoscopy or endoscopy to perform the procedure. These data are then

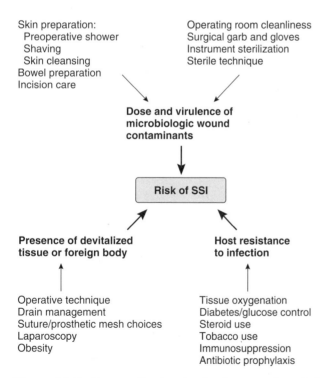

Figure 11-2 Factors affecting the development of surgical site infections. A variety of host, contaminating organism, and treatment factors affect the development of SSI. SSI, surgical site infection.

combined to create risk index categories. The risk index category is calculated by counting the number of risk factors that the patient has. The risk factors are an ASA score ≥3, a duration of operation greater than the 75th percentile for that procedure, or a wound class of contaminated or dirty. There are nominally four risk index categories for SSIs representing patients who have zero, one, two, or three of the risk factors. However, if two risk index categories were similar, then those two categories are combined into a single category (Table 11-2). For example, in Table 11-2, although there are four separate risk categories for colon operations,

in the small bowel category there are only three reported risk index categories, as 2 and 3 are combined into 2,3. For other data sets, there were insufficient patients in some categories to perform statistical analysis, and so those risk index categories are not reported.

The data in Table 11-2 represent the 1992 to 2003 mean infection rate per 100 procedures for all hospitals (1). The data are then separated by percentile of hospitals to demonstrate the spread in infection rate across institutions. These data provide very reliable and well-defined information regarding SSI rates for commonly performed

TABLE 11-2

PERCENTILE DISTRIBUTIONS OF HOSPITAL RISK OF SSI BY PROCEDURE AND NNIS RISK INDEX

Procedure	NNIS Risk Index	No. of Hospitals	Mean Rate[a]	Mean Rate for Percentile of Hospitals				
				10%	25%	50%	75%	90%
Cardiac	1	109	1.50	0	0.44	1.14	1.74	2.79
Cardiac	2,3	85	2.21	0	0	1.28	3.01	4.93
CABG[b]	0	30	1.18	0	0	0.88	2.20	3.23
CABG[b]	1	182	3.45	1.41	2.19	3.28	4.30	6.11
CABG[b]	2	173	5.51	2.27	3.68	5.42	7.66	10.00
Thoracic	0	21	0.36	0	0	0	0	0.88
Thoracic	1	36	1.02	0	0	0	1.49	2.73
Thoracic	2,3	21	2.48	0	0	1.45	3.57	5.89
Laparoscopic Appendectomy	0	21	0.73	0	0	0	0.80	1.62
Appendectomy	0	47	1.33	0	0	1.08	2.08	3.53
Appendectomy	1	58	2.77	0	1.36	2.36	4.00	5.78
Appendectomy	2	36	4.76	0	0	2.94	5.41	7.77
Laparoscopic Cholecystectomy	0	86	0.44	0	0	0	0.51	1.17
Cholecystectomy	0	90	0.68	0	0	0.39	1.15	2.44
Cholecystectomy	1	73	1.76	0	0	1.38	3.25	5.22
Cholecystectomy	2	46	3.28	0	0.30	3.21	4.65	6.83
Colon	0	94	4.00	0	2.00	3.51	4.94	6.42
Colon	1	102	5.64	2.22	3.59	5.18	6.94	8.55
Colon	2	81	8.55	3.85	5.65	8.99	11.62	17.19
Colon	3	27	11.53	1.84	7.65	13.19	16.33	23.41
Gastric	0	28	2.63	0	0	2.22	4.48	6.76
Gastric	1	47	4.83	0.49	2.05	4.20	8.07	9.41
Gastric	2	30	8.82	1.69	4.34	8.06	13.66	22.22
Small bowel	0	24	5.17	0	1.49	4.48	6.38	10.13
Small bowel	1	34	7.49	2.2	4.23	7.02	8.44	12.35
Small bowel	2,3	27	9.23	5.11	6.39	8.11	13.23	16.67
Herniorrhaphy	0	48	0.79	0	0	0.54	1.77	2.42
Herniorrhaphy	1	52	2.08	0	0.66	1.82	3.19	5.88
Herniorrhaphy	2,3	26	4.40	0	0	3.70	5.16	6.33
Mastectomy	0	58	1.01	0	0	0.73	1.59	3.09
Mastectomy	1	52	2.20	0	0.56	2.16	3.33	6.43
Splenectomy	0,1,2,3	20	2.93	0	0	3.26	4.55	6.04
Vascular	0	67	0.91	0	0	0	1.71	3.03
Vascular	1	106	1.73	0	0.78	1.54	2.54	3.79
Vascular	2,3	100	4.42	0.99	2.88	4.76	6.60	8.61

[a]per 100 procedures.
[b]Coronary artery bypass graft, includes vein harvest site.
From National Nosocomial Infections Surveillance (NNIS). System report, data summary from January 1992 through June 2003, issued August 2003.
Am J Infect Control 2003;31:481–498, with permission.

procedures across the United States, which allows bench-marking and comparison of hospital infection rates. Hospital infection rates can be compared to these only if the data is collected completely and in accordance with the CDC definitions. If these definitions are followed, the demonstration of a high rate of infection for some procedure might help to identify an area that should be investigated further, as it might indicate some specific or systemic problem within the institution that is creating a discrepancy. Similarly, a rate substantially lower than the national benchmark data might indicate either an exceptional level of practice or a failure to detect infections by the surveillance program that is in place. The institution of some hospital infection control program to define these rates, such as the NNIS system, is an important component of quality systems-based patient care.

Microbiology of Surgical Site Infection

The microbiology of SSIs has not changed significantly during the last decade (1,4,11). The most commonly isolated pathogens include *Staphylococcus aureus*, coagulase-negative staphylococci, enterococcus species, and *Escherichia coli*. However, there has been an increasing incidence of SSIs caused by antibiotic resistant pathogens, such as methicillin resistant *S. aureus* (11). This increased proportion of SSIs caused by resistant pathogens might be due to the increased and widespread use of broad spectrum antibiotics.

Most SSIs are caused by pathogens that are identified on the patient's skin (Table 11-3). Thus most operations can be complicated by infection with *S. aureus* or coagulase-negative *Staphylococcus*. However, a violation of the respiratory or gastrointestinal (GI) tract or other sites that are colonized with bacteria might lead to infection with specific organisms. Examples of this include Gram-negative bacilli, anaerobic bacteria, or enterococci that might complicate operations on the GI tract. Operations that traverse the oropharyngeal mucosa might contaminate the wound with oropharyngeal anaerobic bacteria, which can cause infections in these wounds.

Knowledge of the specific pathogen that is likely to cause SSIs is necessary in order to appropriately select prophylactic antimicrobial therapy for those patients at risk.

Specific Risk Factors

Effect of Laparoscopy on Risk

One of the important features in the risk of SSI is the use of laparoscopy to perform the procedure (1,4). Laparoscopy might be expected to decrease the risk of SSI because of decreased tissue trauma, decreased dead space in the subcutaneous tissue that might provide a site for SSI, and more limited tissue trauma overall. In fact, the NNIS data appeared to bear this out (1). The use of the laparoscope to

do similar procedures significantly decreases the occurrence of SSI. This advantage might be offset if the laparoscopic procedure takes significantly longer (>75th percentile for that procedure). In general, the decreased tissue trauma for laparoscopy appears to have a beneficial affect on the SSI risk. For cholecystectomy and colon operations, the use of a laparoscope for the procedure subtracts one point from the risk index category. For appendectomy and gastric operations, the laparoscopic improvement in risk only occurred if the patient had no other risk factors, and so a separate category of laparoscopic cholecystectomy and colon operations with a zero score was created.

Tobacco Use

The use of tobacco might increase the risk of SSI by delaying primary wound healing (12–14). This has been clearly demonstrated for sternal or mediastinal SSIs after cardiac surgery. It is not known whether short-term smoking cessation alters this risk.

Diabetes

The contribution of diabetes to SSI risk is controversial only because there are often other confounding variables in diabetic patients undergoing operations. These might include the presence of vascular disease and obesity. However, some data suggest a relationship between increasing levels of hemoglobin A1C, increased glucose levels, and the presence of diabetes with SSI risk (9). It is not clear that tighter perioperative glucose control will alter the risk of SSI, although data regarding phagocytic properties of the host immune system would suggest that hyperglycemia impairs this important early host defense mechanism.

Steroid Use

Patients receiving steroids or other immunosuppressive drugs are predisposed to developing SSI (10). Patients who are on long-term steroids for Crohn disease or chronic immunosuppression following solid organ transplantation have a higher risk of SSI (15). There is limited opportunity to alter this post-transplantation immunosuppression in patients in whom immunosuppression is necessary. However, recognition of the increased risk might allow increased attention to other factors predisposing or protecting from SSI.

PREVENTION OF SURGICAL SITE INFECTION

The prevention, or minimization of risk, of SSI requires knowledge of all the risk factors for infection and the modification of each of these as much as possible. Although discussion of the prevention of SSI is often

TABLE 11-3

LIKELY SURGICAL SITE INFECTION PATHOGENS AND PROPHYLACTIC ANTIBIOTIC OPTIONS

Procedure Site	Pathogen	Antibiotic Prophylaxis[a,b]	
		First Choice	Second Choice

Breast
Abdominal wall hernia
Vascular
Placement of grafts,
  prostheses, or
  other foreign material
	S. aureus
	Coagulase-negative staphylococcus
		Cefazolin 1 g IV, single dose	Clindamycin 600 mg IV, or
			Vancomycin 1 g IV

Noncardiac thoracic	S. aureus Coagulase-negative staphylococcus Streptococcus pneumoniae Gram-negative bacilli	Cefazolin 1 g IV, single dose	Clindamycin 600 mg IV, or Vancomycin 1 g IV
Biliary tract[c] Pancreas Small bowel Appendix Colon and rectum[d]	S. aureus Gram-negative bacilli Anaerobes Enterococci	Cefotetan 1 g IV, single dose or Ampicillin/sulbactam 1.5 g IV	Clindamycin 600 mg and Gentamicin 2 mg/kg IV
Liver transplant	S. aureus Gram-negative bacilli Anaerobes Enterococci	Ampicillin/sulbactam 3 g IV; then 1.5 g every 3 hours intra- operatively	Levofloxacin 500 mg IV
Kidney transplant	S. aureus Coagulase-negative staphylococcus Gram-negative bacilli Anaerobes Enterococci	Cefazolin 1 g, single dose	Levofloxacin 500 mg IV
Esophagus Stomach Duodenum	S. aureus Gram-negative bacilli Streptococci Oropharyngeal anaerobes (peptostreptococci)	Cefazolin 1 g, single dose	Clindamycin 600 mg IV, or Vancomycin 1 g IV

Head and neck (with
  entry through
  oropharyngeal
  mucosa)
	S. aureus
	Streptococci
	Oropharyngeal anaerobes
	  (peptostreptococci)
		Cefazolin 1 g, single dose
		or
		Ampicillin/sulbactam 1.5 g IV
			Clindamycin 600 mg and
			Gentamicin 2 mg/kg IV

[a]Prophylactic antibiotics should be administered within 60 minutes before incision. Antibiotic infusions (vancomycin or fluoroquinolones) should be completed within 60 minutes of incision.
[b]For most procedures a single dose of antibiotics is adequate. One additional intraoperative dose should be given after 3 hours, if the operative procedure requires more than 3 hours.
[c]Laparoscopic cholecystectomy has a lower incidence of SSI than open procedures, and antibiotic prophylaxis is not necessary.
[d]Mechanical and antibiotic bowel preparation prior to operation; the mechanical portion of the preparation is controversial and may be omitted (see text). Oral neomycin sulfate 1 g and erythromycin base 1 g is given after the mechanical preparation is complete, at 19, 18, and 9 hours prior to operation.
From Mangram AJ et al. Guideline for prevention of surgical site infection, 1999. *Am J Infect Control* 1999;27:97-132 (www.cdc.gov/ncidod/hip; non-copyright-protected government document); Surgical Infection Prevention Guidelines, Centers for Medicare and Medicaid Services, National Quality Improvement Projects (http://www.medqic.org/content/nationalpriorities/topics/projectdes.jsp?topicID=461) University of Michigan Pharmacy and Therapeutics Committee, Antimicrobial Subcommittee Guidelines (draft, 2004), with permission.

focused on antimicrobial prophylaxis timing and choices, other important factors must be considered.

Tissue Oxygenation

Prospective data have demonstrated that decreased tissue oxygenation is associated with increased risk of SSI. This effect is explainable on the basis of the need for oxygen radical production in the early phases of host defense against bacteria contaminants. A variety of perioperative issues can affect the level of tissue oxygenation. Hypothermia triggers peripheral vasoconstriction, which decreases tissue oxygenation. In addition, relative dehydration and pain with peripheral vasoconstriction also contribute to decreased tissue oxygenation. Thus, to optimize peripheral tissue oxygenation and to try to minimize the risk of SSI, adequate pain control, adequate or superadequate intravascular hydration, and maintenance of normal body temperature are all important, as is adequate supplemental oxygen delivery. Resuscitation with colloid might be as effective as resuscitation with crystalloid solutions for the maintenance of intravascular volume and peripheral tissue oxygenation. Delivery of supplemental oxygen also decreases the incidence of wound infection. In a prospective randomized trial, colorectal surgery patients who received supplemental oxygen ($FIO_2 = 0.8$) had a lower infection rate than those who did not ($FIO_2 = 0.3$), with actual rates of 5.2% and 11.2%, respectively (16). This was correlated with an increased subcutaneous tissue oxygen partial pressure. In addition, supplemental crystalloid to maintain high intravascular volume and, presumably, perfusion (16 to 18 mL/kg/h) increased the subcutaneous tissue oxygen partial pressure. Tissue oxygenation was also improved in patients randomly assigned to more aggressive control of postoperative pain (17,18).

Bowel Preparation

For operations that will open the colon through the mucosa, mechanical preparation of the bowel and alteration of its flora with oral antibiotics have been used for many years to try to decrease the risk of SSI. The utility of mechanical preparation of the bowel in association with the reduction of intraluminal bowel flora is not clear. Three recent meta-analyses of the available randomized clinical trials fail to support the hypothesis that mechanical bowel preparation decreases infectious complications (19–21). In fact, each shows that the risk of anastomotic leakage is significantly increased after mechanical bowel preparation for elective colon or rectal operations. The standard bowel preparation with antibiotics includes neomycin and erythromycin base delivered prior to operation (Table 11-3). In contrast to the mechanical preparation, the use of oral antibiotics plus intravenous antibiotics has been consistently superior to intravenous antibiotics alone, in both individual randomized trials and meta-analysis of the available data (22,23). In addition, patients should have adequate tissue levels of effective antimicrobial agents delivered intravenously in the standard prophylactic regimen, as the tissue levels correlate with the risk of SSI (22).

Treatment of Remote Infections

Patients with infections remote from the site of planned operation should have these treated preoperatively. Most infections result in some circulating microbial load and some immune impairment of the patient. The creation of a new operative wound with its devitalized tissue and potential foreign body creates another site where this infection might be harbored. Thus it is important and generally recommended that remote sites of infection be adequately treated or that at least treatment be begun prior to creating new wounds.

Skin Preparation

Skin preparation is performed to try and decrease the bacterial wound contaminant at the time of operation. The preparation of the skin involves several steps that might each contribute to an optimal outcome.

Preoperative Shower

A preoperative antiseptic shower or bath can decrease skin microbial counts. However, in spite of the demonstration of the decrease in skin microbial counts and trends toward decreased SSI rates, preoperative showers do not definitively reduce SSI rates (24,25). Gross contamination of the skin should be cleansed prior to bringing the patient into the operating room environment.

Hair Removal

Removal of hair from the surgical site is controversial. It has been a habit in the United States to remove the hair from the surgical site prior to operation because of concern about contamination. However, studies have demonstrated that removal of the hair by shaving the night before operation is associated with a higher risk of infection than shaving or clipping the hair immediately prior to the operation (26). In addition, depilatories appear to have a lower infection rate than shaving or clipping, but they have some significant hypersensitivity reaction rates (27). Some studies demonstrate that preoperative hair removal by any means has a higher risk of infection than no hair removal at all. It is clear that if the hair is to be removed, it should be clipped in as atraumatic a fashion as possible immediately prior to the operation (27–30). Alternatively, removing no hair at all appears acceptable (31).

Operating Room Skin Preparation

The preparation of the skin in the operating room is designed to remove as much of the bacterial load as possible from the operative site prior to incision (4). The skin should be free of gross contamination prior to the initiation of the skin preparation. The antiseptic is applied in concentric circles beginning at the area of the proposed incision and working out to the periphery of the field. The area prepared should be wide and should include room to extend the incision, place drains, or create new incisions if necessary. A variety of antiseptic agents can be used to decrease the bacterial counts on the skin. These include povidone iodine, chlorhexidine, and alcohol-containing products as the most frequently utilized agents.

Operating Room Environment

The operating room is designed as a sterile environment to try to minimize the contamination of the operative wound by environmental bacteria. For this reason the operating suite has features designed to limit the available bacteria.

Ventilation

Room air can contain bacteria-laden dust, lint, exfoliated skin, or respiratory droplets. To try to limit this, operating rooms are maintained at a positive pressure relative to corridors and adjacent areas (32). This prevents airflow from less clean areas into the operating rooms. The ventilation systems for the operating room should have at least two filter beds in series and be designed to produce a minimum of 15 air changes per hour (33). This helps to clear any airborne contamination created by personnel in the room.

The amount of airborne contamination in the room is affected by the number of people moving around in the room as well as the number of times that the door to the room is opened. Limitation of these activities to only those necessary is important.

Additional mechanisms to try to decrease the airborne contamination in operating rooms can include the use of laminar airflow designs. This moves particle-free air over the aseptic operating field at a uniform velocity, sweeping away any particles in its path (32). These systems have been studied only in orthopedic procedures in which there does seem to be some small but real further decrease in SSI risk beyond the use of other efforts. Another strategy that has been used is intraoperative ultraviolet radiation to try to sterilize the air within the operating room; this does not appear to decrease overall SSI risk based on prospective data (4).

Room Surfaces

The surfaces in the operating room (including tables, floors, walls, ceilings, and lights) must be cleansed routinely in order to reestablish a clean environment for each operation (4). No data support routine disinfection of these surfaces between operations in the absence of gross contamination or visible soiling. If such contamination does occur, a disinfectant agent should be used prior to the next operation (34). Wet vacuuming of the floor with a hospital disinfectant should be performed routinely after the last operation of the day or night. No data support the use of special disinfectant procedures or periodic closing of an operating room if a dirty operation has been performed. Sticky mats on the floor at the entrance to operating rooms do not reduce the number of organisms on shoes, stretcher wheels, or flat surfaces in the operating room and do not reduce the incidence of SSI (4).

Instrument Sterilization

Surgical instruments should be sterilized prior to use to limit the introduction of bacteria into the wounds. Surgical instruments can be sterilized by steam under pressure, dry heat, or ethylene oxide (35). The quality of sterilization must be routinely monitored in order to insure adequate elimination of microbial contamination. A biological indicator must be used for microbial monitoring of steam autoclave performance.

Flash sterilization of surgical instruments is the use of rapid steam sterilization for immediate instrument use (4,36). This immediate sterilization is often used during an operation for instruments that have not been sterilized or that have been dropped or otherwise contaminated during the procedure. Flash sterilization is not recommended for routine sterilization because it does not allow for timely biological indicators to monitor the sterilizer's performance. These approaches also typically use minimal sterilization cycle parameters designed to sterilize the instruments in the shortest time. Flash sterilization should generally not be used as an alternative to purchasing additional instrument sets or merely to save time between operations (4). In addition, flash sterilization is not recommended for implantable devices because of the potential for serious infection. Thus all surgical instruments should be conventionally sterilized prior to routine use, and flash sterilization should be limited to the truly urgent or emergent need for sterilization or resterilization of equipment.

Operating Room Personnel

Specific rituals in the operating room are established to protect the patient from contamination by bacteria carried by the health care workers and also to protect the health care workers from contaminants carried by the patient. Attention to these activities is important to maintain a safe environment.

Surgical Scrub

Members of the surgical team who are directly involved in the operation and the handling of the sterile instruments used in the field must perform some surgical scrub prior to covering with surgical gown and gloves. The purpose of the surgical scrub is to decrease or eliminate bacteria from the hands and arms to limit the possibility of transmission to the operative wound (37). Currently in the United States most surgical personnel skin preparation is done using either povidone iodine solutions or chlorhexidine gluconate solution (38). Outside the United States the use of alcohol-based agents is the standard, although this is gaining use in the United States (39). Any one of these approaches appears to have the capability of decreasing the hand bacterial colony counts (38,40). It is important that, whatever skin preparation is selected, it be used in accordance with its instructions to obtain optimal effect.

Scrubbing technique, the duration of the scrub, and the techniques used for drying and gloving can all affect the colony counts on the hands (37). Recent data show that a shorter (e.g., 2-minute) hand preparation is as effective as the traditional 10-minute hand scrub to reduce bacterial colony counts (41,42). It is also clear that the initial scrub of an operating day should include thorough cleaning underneath the fingernails, as this is a site of entrapped bacterial load.

Surgical Garb and Gloves

Operating room personnel typically wear a work uniform that includes scrub pants, shirts, or dress (43,44). The hospital frequently maintains and launders these. There are no studies that evaluate the wearing or handling of the scrub suit as it relates to SSI risk. However, Occupational Safety and Health Administration (OSHA) regulations require that soiled or contaminated scrub suits be changed for the protection of the wearer. Many institutions have policies regarding the laundering of the scrub suits and the wearing of the suits outside the operating room or outside the facility (43). No data support any particular policies.

Similarly, surgical masks have been worn to try to limit bacteria from the operative personnel from contaminating the air in the operating room (43). However, the efficacy of this is unproven. The main benefit of the surgical mask might be in protecting the wearer from exposure to blood or body fluids that might splash during the procedure. In addition, OSHA regulations require not only that the mask be worn to protect the wearer but also that eye protection be worn to protect the eyes from splashes (34). For patients with special infectious risks, more densely filtering masks might be useful to protect the health care personnel from exposure to tuberculosis, for example.

Surgical personnel wear surgical caps and hoods in order to decrease the contamination of the field by hair or dead skin from the scalp (43). These are inexpensive methods that appear to be effective in preventing this problem. SSI outbreaks have been traced to bacteria carried in the hair.

Shoe covers do not decrease the risk of SSI or decrease the bacteria counts on the operating room floor (43). However, OSHA regulations recommend shoe covers whenever gross contamination of the wearer is likely (34).

Sterile Gloves and Gown

After the surgical scrub the operating room personnel who will be in direct contact with the operating room field don a surgical gown and sterile gloves (37,44). These are worn to minimize transmission of microorganisms from the hands and arms of team members to the patient, as well as to prevent contamination of the team members with the patient's blood and body fluids (34). If the glove is punctured or torn, it should be changed promptly. Wearing two pairs of gloves decreases the incidence of health care worker contact with patients' blood or body fluids when compared to wearing only a single pair of gloves (45). Similarly, the sterile gown creates a barrier between the surgical field and the health care worker's arms and torso. The role of the gowns is also to protect the health care workers from exposure to the patient's blood and body fluids.

Antibiotic Prophylaxis

Antibiotic prophylaxis is best delivered as a very short course of effective antimicrobial agent just prior to operative incision. This course is not attempting to sterilize tissues, but if timed correctly it can decrease the dose of wound contaminant experienced by the patient. It is important to provide the antimicrobial shortly before incision so that effective concentrations are obtained at the incision site.

Four important principles might maximize the effectiveness of an antimicrobial prophylaxis plan (4). First, the chosen agent must be used for every patient in whom there is data that the use of antimicrobial prophylaxis is effective or for those procedures after which an infection would be a catastrophic event. Second, the chosen antibiotic agent should ideally be safe, inexpensive, and bactericidal for the likely microbiologic wound contaminants for the planned operation. Third, the course of antibiotics should be very brief but timed to provide a bactericidal concentration of drug in the serum and tissues at the moment of incision and through the operation. Fourth, the therapeutic levels of the antimicrobial agent should be maintained until just a few hours following the closure of the incision. Continuation of antibiotics beyond that time is not necessary and does not further decrease the wound infection rate.

The selection of antimicrobial agents can be guided by the likely infections that can occur with the procedure (Table 11-3). The options listed in the table are commonly recommended but are not exclusively effective. Any antibiotic choices and regimens that conform to the principles noted above should be useful.

For procedures that have very low rates of SSI, antimicrobial prophylaxis might not be useful. Examples of these procedures include clean operations in areas of high resistance to infection, such as thyroid operations, parathyroid operations, and simple hernia operations. However, the alteration of the host immune defenses, the utilization of foreign body for some procedures, or the presence of other risk factors might increase the risk of SSI to the extent that prophylactic antibiotics could be useful. For most of these situations sufficient prospective data to make firm recommendations on the basis of level 1 evidence do not exist.

Operative Care

The proper operative technique and care of the patient is an often neglected area of potential benefit in protecting the patient from SSI. The technique of operation should be designed to minimize the length of operation, limit the operative procedure to the task at hand, minimize the amount of dead space and devitalized tissue created during the operation, as well as to limit the amount of contamination in the wound (4). All these issues should decrease the risk of SSI.

Drains/Dead Space Management

A particularly vexing issue can be the management of dead space within the abdomen, chest, or subcutaneous tissues (46,47). These areas where devitalized tissue or fluid might accumulate can be fertile sites for bacterial growth and the creation of a SSI. If possible, the operative strategy should include a way to obliterate such dead space. This can at times be done by allowing other normal tissues to collapse into this area. Alternatively, it might require the placement of closed suction drains in order to evacuate the fluid that would otherwise collect there. Evacuation of this fluid temporarily might allow the normal healing tissues to become adherent and eliminate this potential dead space. The use of closed suction drains rather than open drains is preferable (46,47). Open drains allow bacteria to enter the surgical site more easily and thus increase the bacterial load and potential for infection.

Tissue Handling

Proper operative technique includes gentle handling of the tissues and avoids the creation of devitalized tissue in the wound. Clean dissection of the planes, when possible, and debridement of devitalized tissue is important to diminishing the potential for postoperative SSI. Although this phenomenon is extraordinarily difficult to study prospectively, in retrospective analysis the presence of devitalized tissue in a wound greatly increases the risk of perioperative wound infection (48).

Incision Care

The care of the postoperative incision varies depending on the type of closure applied. The principle is to minimize the contamination that might enter the surgical site through the incision (4). If the incision has been closed with a nonocclusive technique, such as sutures, skin tapes, or staples, then a sterile dressing should cover the wound for 24 to 48 hours. Beyond 48 hours, a primarily healing wound is most likely sealed to the outside environment and further contamination should not occur. Other wound closure strategies might avoid the need for the postoperative dressing by sealing the wound at the completion of the operation. For instance, the use of occlusive surgical glue dressings avoids the need for this step.

TREATMENT OF SURGICAL SITE INFECTION

Once SSIs occur, their treatment consists of two aspects. These are the drainage of infected tissues or fluids from the wound and the provision of appropriate antimicrobial therapy (49,50).

Superficial incisional wound infections may occasionally be treated by antimicrobial therapy alone (51,52). If the incision has erythema surrounding it and no evidence of swelling or fluid collection, antibiotic therapy might be effective. However, often skin and subcutaneous infections involve devitalized tissue and fluid collection. In this case the best treatment is opening the affected portion of the wound and draining out the infected fluid (51,52). A very short course of antibiotics might be then necessary to decrease the surrounding cellulitis. Once the erythema has resolved, antimicrobial therapy is generally not necessary. These infections are typically from skin flora, such as *S. aureus* and coagulase-negative *Staphylococcus*. The same antibiotics that are useful in the prophylaxis against these infections are generally useful for their treatment (Table 11-3).

For deep incisional wound infections, wound opening and debridement of the affected tissue is nearly always necessary. Antibiotics alone are inadequate at effectively treating these infections. The precise approach depends on the site of the infection. For common abdominal wound infections, opening of the skin and subcutaneous tissue and debridement of the underlying affected muscle and fascia is often necessary (51). This debridement may be carried out acutely by sharp debridement or more chronically by serial dressing changes to the open wound (53). Antimicrobial therapy should again be provided acutely for the appropriate bacteria likely to be involved. Long-term antibiotic therapy is not generally necessary once the surrounding skin erythema has resolved. Persistent infection in the wound is more likely due to persistent devitalized tissue or foreign body rather than to inadequate antimicrobial therapy.

Management of organ space infections is typically now approached by percutaneous catheter drainage of the site of infection, with concomitant appropriate antimicrobial therapy (54). Again, the specific approach depends on the site of infection. For the most intraperitoneal abscesses, localization by computed tomography or ultrasound examination can then help guide percutaneous placement of a drainage catheter. The catheter drainage is intended to completely empty the cavity of fluid and to attempt to have the surrounding normal tissues obliterate the potential space (49,51). If the infected fluid or tissue cannot be removed through a catheter, open drainage and debridement might be necessary. Again, appropriate antimicrobial therapy should be delivered until the patient has clear evidence of resolving systemic infection, including fever and leukocytosis. However, the persistence of these findings is more likely due to undrained or undetected sites of infection rather than to inadequate antimicrobial therapy.

The management of SSIs complicated by tissue loss, foreign bodies, and infection of chronically damaged or poorly vascularized tissue (sternal infections, infections in irradiated tissues, or infections in areas after multiple procedures) might require creative approaches to supply normal, vascularized tissue to the area in order to clear the infection and heal the wound. This might require pedicled or free tissue transfer from other sites in the patient in order to achieve wound coverage and healing. Experience and sound surgical judgment are necessary for consistent success in these difficult situations.

SUMMARY

SSIs can complicate nearly every operative intervention. Knowledge of the risk of infection, the microbiology of likely infections, and the effective preventive measures is necessary to minimize the potential for this complication in any individual patient.

REFERENCES

1. National Nosocomial Infections Surveillance (NNIS). System report, data summary from January 1992 through June 2003, issued August 2003. *Am J Infect Control* 2003;31:481–498.
2. Horan TC, Emori TG. Definitions of key terms used in the NNIS System. *Am J Infect Control* 1997;25:112–116.
3. Horan TC, Gaynes RP, Martone WJ, et al. CDC definitions of nosocomial surgical site infections, 1992: a modification of CDC definitions of surgical wound infections. *Infect Control Hosp Epidemiol* 1992;13:606–608.
4. Mangram AJ, Horan TC, Pearson ML, et al. Guideline for prevention of surgical site infection, 1999. Centers for Disease Control and Prevention (CDC) Hospital Infection Control Practices Advisory Committee. *Am J Infect Control* 1999;27:97–132.
5. Krizek TJ, Robson MC. Evolution of quantitative bacteriology in wound management. *Am J Surg* 1975;130:579–584.
6. Krizek TJ, Robson MC. Biology of surgical infection. *Surg Clin North Am* 1261;55:1261–1267.
7. Henderson B, Poole S, Wilson M. Microbial/host interactions in health and disease: who controls the cytokine network? [Review]. *Immunopharmacology* 1996;35(1):1–21.
8. Henderson B, Poole S, Wilson M. Bacterial modulins: a novel class of virulence factors which cause host tissue pathology by inducing cytokine synthesis [Review]. *Microbiol Rev* 1996;60(2):316–341.
9. Latham R, Lancaster AD, Covington JF, et al. The association of diabetes and glucose control with surgical-site infections among cardiothoracic surgery patients [see comment]. *Infect Control Hosp Epidemiol* 2001;22:607–612.
10. Gil-Egea MJ, Pi-Sunyer MT, Verdaguer A, et al. Surgical wound infections: prospective study of 4,468 clean wounds. *Infect Control* 1987;8:277–280.
11. Schaberg DR, Culver DH, Gaynes RP. Major trends in the microbial etiology of nosocomial infection. *Am J Med* 1991;91:16.
12. Holley DT, Toursarkissian B, Vasconez HC, et al. The ramifications of immediate reconstruction in the management of breast cancer. *Am Surg* 1995;61:60–65.
13. Beitsch P, Balch C. Operative morbidity and risk factor assessment in melanoma patients undergoing inguinal lymph node dissection. *Am J Surg* 1992;164:462–465.
14. Nagachinta T, Stephens M, Reitz B, et al. Risk factors for surgical-wound infection following cardiac surgery. *J Infect Dis* 1987;156:967–973.
15. Post S, Betzler M, von Ditfurth B, et al. Risks of intestinal anastomoses in Crohn's disease. *Ann Surg* 1991;213:37–42.
16. Greif R, Akca O, Horn EP, et al, Outcomes Research Group. Supplemental perioperative oxygen to reduce the incidence of surgical-wound infection [see comment]. *N Engl J Med* 2000;342:161–167.
17. Akca O, Melischek M, Scheck T, et al. Postoperative pain and subcutaneous oxygen tension. *Lancet* 1999;354:41–42.
18. Arkilic CF, Taguchi A, Sharma N, et al. Supplemental perioperative fluid administration increases tissue oxygen pressure [see comment]. *Surgery* 2003;133:49–55.
19. Slim K, Vicaut E, Panis Y, et al. Meta-analysis of randomized clinical trials of colorectal surgery with or without mechanical bowel preparation. *Br J Surg* 2004;91:1125–1130.
20. Bucher P, Mermillod B, Morel P, et al. Does mechanical bowel preparation have a role in preventing postoperative complications in elective colorectal surgery? *Swiss Med Wkly* 2004;134:69–74.
21. Guenaga KF, Matos D, Castro AA, et al. Mechanical bowel preparation for elective colorectal surgery. *Cochrane Database of Syst Rev* 2003;2:CD001544.
22. Zelenitsky SA, Ariano RE, Harding GK, et al. Antibiotic pharmacodynamics in surgical prophylaxis: an association between intraoperative antibiotic concentrations and efficacy. *Antimicrob Agents Chemother* 2002;46:3026–3030.
23. Lewis RT. Oral versus systemic antibiotic prophylaxis in elective colon surgery: a randomized study and meta-analysis send a message from the 1990s. *Can J Surg* 2002;45:173–180.
24. Hayek LJ, Emerson JM, Gardner AM. A placebo-controlled trial of the effect of two preoperative baths or showers with chlorhexidine detergent on postoperative wound infection rates. *J Hosp Infect* 1987;10:165–172.
25. Paulson DS. Efficacy evaluation of a 4% chlorhexidine gluconate as a full-body shower wash. *Am J Infect Control* 1993;21:205–209.
26. Cruse PJ, Foord R. The epidemiology of wound infection. A 10-year prospective study of 62,939 wounds. *Surg Clin North Am* 1980;60:27–40.
27. Seropian R, Reynolds BM. Wound infections after preoperative depilatory versus razor preparation. *Am J Surg* 1971;121:251–254.
28. Hamilton HW, Hamilton KR, Lone FJ. Preoperative hair removal. *Can J Surg* 1977;20:269–271,274–265.
29. Ko W, Lazenby WD, Zelano JA, et al. Effects of shaving methods and intraoperative irrigation on suppurative mediastinitis after bypass operations. *Ann Thorac Surg* 1992;53:301–305.
30. Moro ML, Carrieri MP, Tozzi AE et al, Italian PRINOS Study Group. Risk factors for surgical wound infections in clean surgery: a multicenter study. *Ann Ital Chir* 1996;67:13–19.
31. Winston KR. Hair and neurosurgery [see comment]. *Neurosurgery* 1992;31:320–329.
32. Chow TT, Yang XY. Ventilation performance in operating theatres against airborne infection: review of research activities and practical guidance. *J Hosp Infect* 2004;56:85–92.
33. American Institute of Architects. *Guidelines for design and construction of hospital and health care facilities.* Washington, DC: American Institute of Architects Press; 1996.
34. Occupational Safety and Health Administration. Anonymous Occupational exposure to bloodborne pathogens—OSHA. Final rule. *Fed Reg* 1991;56:64004–64182.
35. Association of periOperative Registered Nurses. Recommended practices for cleaning and caring for surgical instruments and powered equipment. *AORN J* 2002;75:627–630.
36. Bolding B. Flash sterilization (steam). *Can Oper Room Nurs J* 2003;21:31–33.

37. Association of periOperative Registered Nurses Recommended Practices. C. Recommended practices for surgical hand antisepsis/hand scrubs. *AORN J*, 2004;79:416–418.
38. Paulson DS. Comparative evaluation of five surgical hand scrub preparations. *AORN J* 1994;60:246.
39. Gruendemann BJ, Bjerke NB. Is it time for brushless scrubbing with an alcohol-based agent? *AORN J* 2001;74:859–873.
40. Larson EL, Aiello AE, Heilman JM, et al. Comparison of different regimens for surgical hand preparation. *AORN J* 2001;73:412–414.
41. O'Shaughnessy M, O'Malley VP, Corbett G, et al. Optimum duration of surgical scrub-time. *Br J Surg* 1991;78:685–686.
42. Deshmukh N, Kramer JW, Kjellberg SI. A comparison of 5-minute povidone-iodine scrub and 1-minute povidone-iodine scrub followed by alcohol foam. *Mil Med* 1998;163:145–147.
43. Association of Operating Room Nurses. Anonymous recommended practices for surgical attire. *AORN J* 1998;68:1048–1052.
44. Association of periOperative Registered Nurses. Recommended practices for selection and use of surgical gowns and drapes. *AORN J* 2003;77:206–210.
45. Twomey CL. Double gloving: a risk reduction strategy. *Jt Comm J Qual Saf* 2003;29:369–378.
46. Dougherty SH, Simmons RL. The biology and practice of surgical drains. Part II. *Curr Probl Surg* 1992;29:633–730.
47. Dougherty SH, Simmons RL. The biology and practice of surgical drains. Part 1. *Curr Probl Surg* 1992;29:559–623.
48. Weigelt JA, Haley RW, Seibert B. Factors which influence the risk of wound infection in trauma patients. *J Trauma-Inj Infect Crit Care* 1987;27:774–781.
49. Fry DE. The economic costs of surgical site infection. *Surg Infect* 2002;3(Suppl. 1):S37–S43.
50. Colizza S, Rossi S. Antibiotic prophylaxis and treatment of surgical abdominal sepsis. *J Chemother* 2001;13(Spec No. 1):193–201.
51. Pollock AV. The treatment of infected wounds. [Review]. *Acta Chir Scand* 1990;156:505–513.
52. Rogers PN, Wright IH. Postoperative intra-abdominal sepsis. *Br J Surg* 1987;74:973–975.
53. Thomas S. Alginate dressings in surgery and wound management: Part 3. *J Wound Care* 2000;9:163–166.
54. Fry DE. Noninvasive imaging tests in the diagnosis and treatment of intra-abdominal abscesses in the postoperative patient. *Surg Clin North Am* 1994;74:693–709.

Septic Shock

12

Stewart C. Wang

■■ **PATHOPHYSIOLOGY 127**

■■ **EVALUATION 127**
History 128
Clinical Assessment 128
Laboratory Studies 128

■■ **MANAGEMENT 129**
Shock 129
Fluids 129
Vasopressors 129
Early Goal-directed Supportive Therapy 131
Human Activated Protein C 131
Corticosteroids 131

■■ **COMPLICATIONS OF SEPTIC SHOCK 132**
Pulmonary 132
Renal 132
Hematologic 132
Endocrine 132
Gastrointestinal and Hepatic 133
Neurologic 133
Multiple-organ Failure 133

■■ **REFERENCES 133**

Septic shock is defined as sepsis with hypotension despite adequate fluid resuscitation combined with perfusion abnormalities that might include, but are not limited to, lactic acidosis, oliguria, or an acute alteration in mental status. Hypotension is defined as a systolic blood pressure of <90 mm Hg or a reduction of ≥40 mm Hg from baseline in the absence of other causes for the fall in blood pressure. Patients who require inotropic or vasopressor support despite adequate fluid resuscitation are in septic shock (1–3).

Septic shock is part of the spectrum of clinical responses to infection that begins with sepsis and progresses toward severe sepsis and then organ dysfunction and septic shock. Sepsis is the systemic response to infection and is defined as the presence of a systemic inflammatory response together with definitive evidence of infection. Infection is defined as a microbial phenomenon characterized by an inflammatory response to the presence of microorganisms or the invasion of normally sterile host tissue by those organisms. Systemic inflammatory response syndrome (SIRS) is a widespread inflammatory response to a variety of severe clinical insults. It is manifested by the occurrence of two or more of the following: (a) temperature >38°C or <36°C, (b) heart rate >90 beats per minute, (c) respiratory rate >20 breaths per minute or Pa_{CO_2} <32 mm Hg, and (d) WBC >12,000 per mm^3 or <4000 per mm^3, or immature (band) forms accounting for >10% of the neutrophils present. Septic shock is to be differentiated from severe sepsis. Severe sepsis is sepsis associated with organ dysfunction, hypoperfusion, or hypotension. When hypotension persists in a septic patient despite adequate fluid resuscitation, septic shock is present.

Each year in the United States >650,000 cases of sepsis are diagnosed, with >100,000 deaths (4,5). From an analysis of six million hospital discharge records, the incidence of severe sepsis is an estimated 2% of all hospital admissions and three cases per 1,000 population. Data gathered from 22 intensive care units (ICUs) around Paris

Stewart C. Wang: University of Michigan, Ann Arbor, MI 48109 between 1993 and 2000 (6) showed that septic shock accounted for >8% of all ICU admissions. The observed mortality rate for septic shock was 60%.

PATHOPHYSIOLOGY

Over the past 5 years, the molecular mechanisms underlying the host immune response to infection have begun to be deciphered. The negative and destructive features of the septic response are the systemic manifestations of what is otherwise a positive and beneficial local inflammatory response to tissue injury. Severe sepsis leading to shock develops because of a dysregulation in host responses, such that the mechanisms initially recruited to fight infection produce life-threatening tissue damage and death (7).

Infection starts with the invasion and proliferation of microorganisms. This is rapidly followed by host monocyte/macrophage recognition of specific microbial products by a family of "pattern-recognition receptors" that include the Toll-like receptors (TLRs). Lipopolysaccharide (LPS or endotoxin) is a component of the cell wall of Gram-negative bacteria and is recognized by TLR-4. TLR-2 recognizes peptidoglycan and lipoteichoic acid from Gram-positive bacteria and zymosan from yeast. Other members of the TLR family specifically recognize flagellin, CpG-rich bacterial DNA, and bacterial lipopeptides (8). Monocyte expressed class II major histocompatibility complex molecules and the $V\beta$ domains of the T-cell receptor bind bacterial exotoxins (9).

In addition to the above-described receptor systems found on immune cells, humoral pathways are also important for the recognition of microbial pathogens. The complement system recognizes pathogen-associated molecular patterns on bacteria and fungi, leading to complement activation and the generation of the C5b-C9 membrane attack complex, as well as C3a and C5a peptide mediators of inflammation and phagocyte recruitment. The plasma kallikrein–kinin system is activated by negatively charged surfaces and produces an array of soluble mediators with neutrophil-activating and chemotactic properties. Kininogen and bradykinin which induces vascular permeability are part of the induced cascade.

In response to different pathogen products, the cells of the immune system produce microbicidal agents and soluble mediators in an effort to eliminate the invading pathogen and to initiate an adaptive immune response. The soluble mediators produced are proinflammatory cytokines, chemokines, prostanoids, as well as reactive oxygen and nitrogen species (7). Elevated circulating levels of these mediators lead to progressive endothelial dysfunction and microvascular injury. Macrophage-produced cytokines induce endothelial cell expression of adhesion markers that in turn mediate neutrophil attachment, recruitment, and persistence at inflammatory sites.

Activated leukocytes, as well as bacterial products themselves, also activate the coagulation cascade. Tissue factor is released in response to proinflammatory cytokines such as TNF-α and IL-1 and leads to the formation of thrombin and fibrin clots. Concurrently, many endogenous fibrinolytic mechanisms are impaired because of the release of plasminogen-activator inhibitor-1, production of thrombin-activatable fibrinolysis inhibitor, and decreased conversion of protein C to the serine protease-activated protein C. Activated protein C exerts important antithrombotic activities by inactivating factors Va and VIIIa, which limits thrombin generation and reduces its procoagulant and antifibrinolytic properties. Activation of protein C normally occurs by thrombin bound to endothelial thrombomodulin, but thrombomodulin expression becomes markedly impaired with progressive endothelial dysfunction. Altered local coagulation and progressive microvascular thrombosis, in conjunction with hypotension, lead to tissue hypoperfusion and shock.

Sepsis can be thought of as a process comprised of two major components, infectious and inflammatory. The clinical inflammatory response extends from infection to sepsis, severe sepsis, and septic shock, and clinical outcome progressively worsens with advancing stages. In a large study examining the natural history of patients with SIRS, 48% were found to have infections: 26% had sepsis only, 18% developed severe sepsis, and 4% developed septic shock (10). Bacteremia was increased with the severity of the clinical response. Positive blood cultures were found in 17% of patients with sepsis and in 69% of patients with septic shock.

Patients with sepsis have a decreased mortality rate only compared with patients with severe sepsis or septic shock (11–13). The mortality rate from septic shock is between 35% and 40% in the month following onset of septic shock. The mortality from hypovolemic shock varies greatly and depends on the etiology as well as the rapidity with which it is recognized and treated (14).

EVALUATION

Shock is the physiologic condition in which there is inadequate oxygen delivery. This leads to cellular hypoxia and disruption of necessary biochemical processes with resultant tissue and organ dysfunction. In the early phases, these alterations can be reversed, but they rapidly become irreversible, leading to cell death, end-organ damage, multiple organ failure (MOF), and death. Shock is broadly divided into three categories: (a) hypovolemic, (b) cardiogenic, and (c) distributive.

Hypovolemic shock results from inadequate intravascular volume and decreased cardiac preload that lead to decreased cardiac output (CO) and end-organ perfusion. Hypovolemic shock is generally due to either loss of blood or fluid. Blood loss can be secondary to trauma, GI bleeding, ruptured aortic aneurysm, or other causes. Fluid loss can be due to intestinal obstruction, pancreatitis, burns, diarrhea, as well as other causes.

Cardiogenic shock is due to failure of the heart as a pump. The four major causes of cardiogenic shock are arrhythmias, cardiomyopathies, mechanical abnormalities, and obstructive disorders. Arrhythmias such as atrial fibrillation can suppress CO by disrupting normal coordination of atrial and ventricular filling and pumping. Bradyarrhythmias and heart block can markedly decrease CO and end-organ perfusion. Cardiomyopathies, whether due to ischemic, viral infection, or other reasons, can cause severe deficits in myocardial contractility and CO. Mechanical causes of pump failure are valvular insufficiency or chordae tendineae rupture. Obstructive causes such as pericardial tamponade, massive pulmonary embolism, and tension pneumothorax can also disrupt the heart's ability to function as a pump.

Abnormally low systemic vascular resistance causes distributive shock and can be due to a variety of causes. Septic shock is generally classified within the distributive shock category, although it can present with components of the other two categories. Aside from septic shock, other types of distributive shock are neurogenic shock after central nervous system (CNS) or spinal cord injury, Addisonian crisis, myxedema coma, anaphylaxis, as well as drug or toxin reactions.

History

Patients presenting with septic shock might be in such dire condition as to be unable to provide a clear history. Nonetheless, it is important to elicit a history of current and recent complaints from the patient or the patient's family. Preexisting conditions such as diabetes, malignancy, and immunosuppression are important to consider. Current medication regimens as well as recent alterations in medication might provide important clues about the patient's underlying pathophysiology. In surgical patients presenting with shock, a detailed surgical history is essential. This surgical history must include not only a list of past and planned surgical procedures but also the underlying pathology requiring surgical intervention.

The nature, extent, and outcome of recent surgical procedures and the patient's perioperative course must be taken into consideration as they might shed considerable light on why the patient is presenting with shock. Was the operation elective or emergent? Which body cavities were opened? Was it a clean, contaminated, or dirty operation? Was a hollow viscus opened? Is there an anastamosis? What is the patient's underlying condition? Where are the locations of the patient's symptoms? What is the nature of the patient's complaints? To which organ systems are the complaints most attributable? The differential diagnosis for a patient presenting with septic shock following recent emergency operation for colonic perforation would differ greatly from that of a patient presenting with septic shock one year after lung transplantation.

Clinical Assessment

The physical examination should focus on rapid assessment of the patient's current clinical condition, differentiating the different types of shock and determining the etiology of the patient's shock. Patients presenting with shock must be continuously monitored in an ICU setting. For patients in shock, arterial catheterization provides a more accurate measure of blood pressure than noninvasive techniques.

Clinical signs of decreased global perfusion are oliguria, delayed capillary refill, cool skin, and decreased level of consciousness in addition to hypotension. Although elevated lactate levels can be due to causes other than septic shock, efforts to normalize lactate levels by means of hemodynamic optimization should be considered (15). The prognostic value of blood lactate concentration has been established in septic shock patients (16,17). Gastric tonometry has been shown to be a predictor of multiorgan dysfunction syndrome and mortality in patients with septic shock (18,19). However, resuscitation of critically ill patients on the basis of gastric tonometry failed to significantly improve outcome (20).

Hemodynamic measurements can be made in septic shock patients using pulmonary artery catheterization. Parameters such as CO, pulmonary artery occlusion pressure, and systemic vascular resistance can be useful in differentiating septic shock from other forms of shock. Pulmonary artery catheterization can also provide useful information about the adequacy of fluid resuscitation, the effectiveness of vasopressors and inotropes, as well as the effect of mechanical ventilatory support on hemodynamics (21). However, pulmonary artery catheterization is frequently associated with inaccurate measurements (22) and one retrospective analysis suggested worsened clinical outcome with pulmonary artery catheterization (23). At this time there is no conclusive clinical evidence about the utility and potential benefit of pulmonary artery catheterization in septic shock.

Laboratory Studies

Laboratory tests are helpful to assess the patient's condition and evidence of organ dysfunction as well as response to treatment. They can help identify the etiology of the patient's shock. Basic tests are arterial blood gas, lactate level, complete blood count (CBC) with differential, basic chemistries, amylase and lipase, liver function tests, cardiac enzymes, coagulation profile, fibrinogen, and fibrin split products. A urinalysis and toxicology screen might also provide helpful information. Cosyntropin challenge or cortisol levels can be used to detect adrenal insufficiency.

It is essential to identify the causative microbial pathogen and the sites of infection. Although sepsis and septic shock can result from infections at many sites, the most common sites are the lungs, abdomen, urinary tract, and skin (24). Blood, sputum, and urine cultures can be helpful in identifying the source of sepsis. For patients in shock, a chest x-ray and electrocardiogram are essential for basic assessment of the cardiopulmonary system. Plain or contrast radiographs and radionuclide studies can be used to determine the presence of surgical complications such as visceral perforation or obstruction and anastamotic disruption. Computed tomography or magnetic resonance imaging scans might help detect the presence of infectious foci or fluid collections.

MANAGEMENT

The essential steps in the management of septic shock are the same as those used to treat patients with mild or moderate sepsis: (a) resuscitation, (b) diagnosis of the infectious focus, (c) antibiotic therapy, and (d) infectious source control. Because of the severity of the disease process, these steps must be undertaken concurrently (Fig. 12-1). We discuss identification of the infectious foci and institution of the appropriate antibiotic treatment and source control in greater detail in Chapter 11, hence the current focus will be on resuscitative measures for septic shock.

Shock

Shock is a medical emergency and must be treated immediately. As with any critical patient, treatment must first address the ABCs—the patient's airway, breathing, and circulation. First, the airway must be assessed and supported. Patients in septic shock might have a depressed level of consciousness or encephalopathy and require intubation for airway protection. Second, ventilation and oxygenation should be assessed and supported as necessary with supplemental oxygen or mechanical ventilation if indicated. Third, circulatory function is assessed and supported with volume expansion and vasopressors as necessary. By definition, patients in septic shock have circulatory failure, and prompt treatment is necessary to avoid multiple organ dysfunction.

Fluids

The hypotension observed in septic shock is multifactorial in origin. Sepsis can cause myocardial depression and decreased vasomotor tone. In addition, there might be significant loss of plasma volume into the interstitial space, resulting in severe intravascular hypovolemia. Intravascular volume should be restored rapidly using boluses with careful assessment of the patient's physiologic status before and after each bolus. This volume resuscitation should be repeated in expeditious fashion until blood pressure and tissue perfusion are returned to normal and tissue hypoxia is corrected. Volume expansion in patients with septic shock must be aggressive, with careful monitoring of the patient to determine the endpoint of fluid resuscitation. When invasive monitoring is available, fluid resuscitation should be given until a central venous pressure of 8 to 14 mm Hg or pulmonary artery occlusive pressure of 14 to 18 mm Hg is achieved. The patient's respiratory status must be monitored closely during this resuscitation as patients with septic shock have increased pulmonary capillary leak, which in the setting of increased filling pressures can lead to impaired oxygenation. The appearance of crackles on lung auscultation or a decrease in arterial oxygen saturation suggests that adequate fluid resuscitation has been achieved.

Volume expansion can be carried out using either crystalloid or colloid solutions. A large number of clinical studies have compared colloid with crystalloid resuscitation, but there is no clear evidence that one has significant clinical benefit over the other (25–27). Of course, a given volume of colloid results in greater expansion of the intravascular volume than does an equal volume of crystalloid. The cost of volume resuscitation using colloid is also significantly greater than that using crystalloid.

Vasopressors

Once intravascular volume has been adequately expanded with fluid resuscitation, the continued presence of hypotension indicates the need for vasopressors and inotropic agents. Sepsis can cause decreased vasomotor tone and vasopressors can be used to counteract these effects if necessary to restore normal blood pressure, perfusion, and oxygenation once intravascular volume has been adequately restored. Expansion of intravascular volume is preferred as the first line of intervention as long as it increases CO and blood pressure without seriously impairing gas exchange (11). However, vasopressor therapy might also be needed prior to adequate intravascular volume expansion to maintain perfusion in the presence of life-threatening hypotension.

There are a variety of vasopressors with differing effects on cardiac and peripheral vascular activity, as well as differing levels of α-adrenergic and β-adrenergic agonistic activity. The vasopressors that have been used for the treatment of septic shock are dopamine, norepinephrine, phenylephrine, epinephrine, and vasopressin. Dopamine and epinephrine are more likely to cause tachycardia than norepinephrine and phenylephrine. Dopamine and norepinephrine both raise blood pressure and CO; however, dopamine has a greater effect on raising CO than norepinephrine (28). Although all the pressors mentioned have been used to treat septic shock, recent reports suggest a trend toward the preferred use of norepinephrine. Several studies have found norepinephrine to be more effective

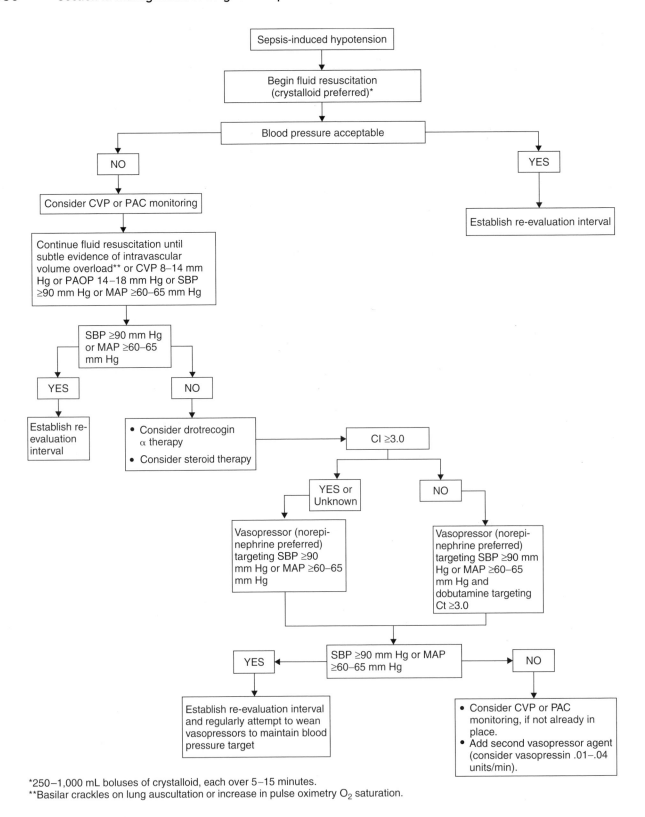

Figure 12-1 Flow diagram for management of septic shock. CVP, central venous pressure; PAC, pulmonary artery catheter; SBP, systolic blood pressure; MAP, mean arterial pressure. (From Dellinger RP. Cardiovascular management of septic shock. *Crit Care Med* 2003;31:951, with permission.)

than dopamine in refractory septic shock (29,30). In a prospective study of 97 patients in septic shock, mortality was decreased in patients treated with norepinephrine (62% mortality) compared with patients treated with either epinephrine or high-dose dopamine (82% mortality) (31). Potential advantages of norepinephrine over dopamine are less tachycardia and no interference with the hypothalamic pituitary axis (32,33). The typical intravenous dose range for norepinephrine is 1 to 30 μg per minute.

Vasopressin has recently been reported to be effective in the treatment of hypotension in septic shock. Plasma levels of vasopressin have been found to be inappropriately low in patients with septic shock (34), perhaps due to exhaustion of neurohypophyseal stores from prolonged stimulation or impairment of baroreflex-mediated stimulation of vasopressin release (35–37). Vasopressin therapy to restore normal circulating levels has been shown to be effective in reversing hypotension in septic patients, enabling withdrawal of other vasopressors (38–41). The intravenous dosing of vasopressin should be limited to 0.01 to 0.04 units per minute as higher doses increase the risk of splanchnic and coronary artery ischemia as well as lead to decreases in CO (35).

Sepsis can also cause myocardial depression with decreased global contractility. A number of mediators upregulated during sepsis, such as tumor necrosis factor-α, interleukin-1, and nitric oxide, are known to depress myocardial contractility (15,42). Septic patients have been demonstrated to have reduced ejection fraction and biventricular dilation (43,44). In the presence of severe myocardial depression and inadequate CO in septic shock, dobutamine therapy can be added. In the presence of hypotension, vasopressors must be administered in addition to the dobutamine. Dobutamine increases myocardial contractility by stimulating β_1-adrenergic receptors. The typical dose range for dobutamine is 5 to 15 μg/kg/min.

Early Goal-directed Supportive Therapy

A recent prospective study randomized 263 patients presenting with septic shock to either standard control therapy or to early goal-directed therapy (45). Standard therapy consisted of volume resuscitation targeting a central venous pressure of 8 to 12 mm Hg, followed by vasopressor therapy to maintain a mean arterial pressure of 65 mm Hg. Early goal-directed therapy added measurement of central venous oxyhemoglobin saturation (CVo$_2$ sat). Following volume administration and vasopressor support as in the standard treatment group, additional therapy was based on the CVo$_2$ saturation. If the CVo$_2$ saturation was <70%, blood was transfused to achieve a hematocrit of 30%. If CVo$_2$ saturation remained <70% following the transfusion, dobutamine was added to a maximum of 20 μg/kg/min in an attempt to achieve a CVo$_2$ saturation of 70%. In-hospital mortality in the early goal-directed

therapy group was 30.5%, significantly lower than the observed mortality rate of 46.5% in the standard therapy group (45). This approach of monitoring the oxygen supply–demand relationship during therapy of septic shock appears promising; additional trials are forthcoming.

Human Activated Protein C

In 2001 the results of a multicenter trial using recombinant human activated protein C (drotrecogin alfa, Xigris) for the treatment of septic shock were published. 1,690 patients were randomly assigned to receive a 96-hour infusion of drotrecogin alfa or placebo, beginning within 24 hours of presentation with known or suspected severe infection and evidence of shock (46). A significant improvement in 28-day mortality rate was noted in the drotrecogin-treated group (24.7% vs. 30.8%). Treatment was found to be of greatest benefit in the most acutely ill subset of patients with an APACHE II score ≥25. Drotrecogin alfa treatment was found to be associated with more rapid recovery of cardiac and pulmonary function (47), as well as lower incidence of multiple-organ dysfunction. However, treatment was also associated with increased incidence of bleeding complications, such as fatal intracranial hemorrhage. The U.S. Food and Drug Administration (FDA) subsequently approved drotrecogin alfa for treatment of adults with septic shock. The estimated cost is >$6,000 per treatment course at the suggested dosing regimen of 24 μg/kg/hr for 96 hours. The cost–benefit ratio of drotrecogin alfa treatment has been examined. The cost per year of life saved with treatment is $24,000 to $27,000 for the most acutely ill patients with APACHE II scores ≥25. Former smokers and less acutely ill patients (APACHE II <25) received significantly less benefit from drotrecogin alfa treatment (48,49).

Corticosteroids

There have been a large number of clinical trials examining corticosteroid therapy for sepsis and septic shock. Significant shortcomings of these trials are inconsistent patient inclusion criteria, differing drug dosing regimens, and variable definitions for sepsis and septic shock. The majority of early studies used high-dose steroids for short durations, usually 1 day (50).

More recent studies have utilized physiologic stress-dose corticosteroids for longer durations. In one recent prospective study patients with septic shock requiring catecholamines for >48 hours were randomly assigned to receive corticosteroid (hydrocortisone 100 mg IV TID for 5 days) or placebo; 68% of the 22 patients receiving corticosteroid therapy were weaned off vasopressors within 7 days as opposed to 21% of 19 patients receiving placebo (51). Despite the shorter duration of catecholamine dependence, no significant improvement in mortality was observed.

Subsequently, a larger trial of 300 adults with septic shock was conducted, comparing a 7-day course of treatment with hydrocortisone (50 mg IV every 6 hours) and fludrocortisone (50 mg every day) or placebo (52). The majority (76%) of the study subjects had evidence of adrenal insufficiency as demonstrated by an increase of ≤9 μg per dL in plasma cortisol following cosyntropin challenge (250 μg) (53). It was among these patients with evidence of adrenal insufficiency that a treatment benefit was noted. The benefits were significantly decreased 28-day mortality (53% vs. 63%) and resolution of vasopressor dependence (57% vs. 40%). There was no observed increase in the incidence of adverse events.

COMPLICATIONS OF SEPTIC SHOCK

Septic shock is an extremely severe complication of many disease processes and operations in surgical patients, carrying with it a very high mortality rate. If treatment is successful and the patient survives, the most common resultant complications are failure of individual organ systems or MOF.

Pulmonary

The lungs are the organ system most susceptible to injury from septic shock. Acute lung failure in the setting of surgery and sepsis is known as *acute respiratory distress syndrome*, or ARDS. Despite advances in mechanical ventilatory assistance and supportive care, the mortality rate for ARDS remains high. Mortality is greater for ARDS because of sepsis than for other causes such as multiple trauma, fat embolism, and gastric aspiration (54). A higher incidence of ARDS is present in patients with septic shock as a result of pulmonary rather than nonpulmonary infection (55,56).

Mechanical ventilation is an essential component of ARDS treatment. Over the past decade much attention has focused on limiting the adverse effects of mechanical ventilation, which are ventilator-induced lung injury, barotrauma or volutrauma, atelecto-trauma, and biotrauma (57–59). Mechanical ventilation in ARDS might exacerbate lung injury by alveolar overdistension or repetitive alveolar recruitment-derecruitment, thereby increasing alveolar capillary permeability and inflammatory mediator release (60). Recent trials using lower tidal volumes to minimize this damage have shown an improvement in survival (61).

Renal

Renal dysfunction is commonly observed in patients with septic shock. Hypoperfusion secondary to intravascular volume depletion or vasopressors, altered intravascular coagulation, and nephrotoxicity from drugs such as aminoglycosides are just some of the contributing factors

in patients with septic shock. The development of oliguric acute renal failure places additional stress on other failing organ systems and significantly increases the mortality rate of critically ill patients. Renal replacement therapy with intermittent hemodialysis is the standard treatment. A recent prospective trial compared daily dialysis with alternate-day dialysis and showed a significant reduction in mortality (28% vs. 46%) in critically ill patients, most of whom were septic. Patients receiving daily hemodialysis had better control of uremia, fewer hypotensive episodes, and more rapid resolution of acute renal failure (62).

A large number of soluble mediators with overlapping and synergistic biologic effects are released during septic shock. Because multiple interventions based on blocking a single mediator have failed to show clinical efficacy, direct removal of inflammatory mediators from the circulation is intuitively attractive (57). This strategy might interrupt the inflammatory cascade and attenuate septic shock and MOF (63). Although a few preliminary trails have shown some benefit (64), multiple randomized controlled trials using continuous hemofiltration or plasma filtration in septic patients have shown no improvement either in hemodynamics or outcome (65–67).

Hematologic

Bacterial products can directly activate the coagulation cascade. Proinflammatory cytokines such as TNF-α, IL-1β, and IL-6 that are released during the host response to infection also activate coagulation and enhance formation of thrombin and fibrin clot (68,69). Circulating mediators also cause endothelial cell damage and expression of adhesion markers. All these processes lead to the unbalancing of normal intravascular coagulation and can result in disseminated intravascular coagulation. Sepsis causes depletion of antithrombotic proteins such as activated protein C, and treatment with activated protein C has improved mortality and outcome in patients with septic shock.

The severe systemic inflammatory response incited by infection leads subsequently to a compensatory anti-inflammatory response in the host. During the time when this latter anti-inflammatory response predominates, the host immune system is less responsive and microbial pathogens might be able to establish new sites of infection.

Endocrine

Recent studies have reported that patients with severe sepsis might develop either relative adrenal insufficiency or SIRS-induced glucocorticoid receptor resistance (70,71). Adrenal insufficiency can be diagnosed with a short corticotrophin stimulation test, and treatment of nonresponders has been effective in reversing septic shock. Plasma levels of vasopressin have been found to be inappropriately low in patients with septic shock (34), and vasopressin therapy to restore normal circulating levels has been shown to be effective in reversing hypotension in septic patients (39–41).

Septic patients commonly develop hyperglycemia and insulin resistance, which increases the risk of complications such as severe infections, critical illness polyneuropathy, MOF, and death (72, 73). A recent prospective, randomized, controlled trial examined the effect of intensive insulin therapy to normalize blood glucose in critically ill patients (74). There was significant mortality reduction in the intensive treatment group in which blood glucose was maintained between 4.4 and 6.1 mmol per L compared to the conventional treatment group in which blood glucose was maintained between 10.0 and 11.1 mmol per L. Both in-hospital deaths and ICU length of stay were improved by intensive insulin therapy. Of note, the greatest reduction in mortality occurred from deaths due to MOF with a septic focus.

Gastrointestinal and Hepatic

Gastrointestinal ileus and malabsorption are frequently observed in patients with septic shock, and malnutrition is commonly found in these patients as well. Recent studies have shown improved outcome with early initiation of enteral feedings as well as the superiority of enteral feedings over TPN (75,76). Early jejunal feedings might help maintain the normal bacterial microflora and the GI tract's barrier function, thereby minimizing bacterial and endotoxin translocation (77). The rate of septic complications was lower in patients treated with early jejunal feeding compared with conventional parenteral nutrition (78). The addition of glutamine to enteral and parenteral feeds might improve immune cell function and also preserve intestinal morphology, thereby preserving intestinal barrier function (79,80).

Septic patients being treated with antibiotics are at risk for development of pseudomembranous colitis. Low perfusion might also lead to intestinal ischemia or pancreatitis. Septic patients are at increased risk of stress gastritis and ulceration. Gastric pH should be monitored and controlled.

Cholestatic jaundice is also frequently observed in severely septic patients. Bilirubin can become elevated above 20 mg per dL. Parenteral nutrition can cause fatty infiltration of the liver and also contribute to the cholestatic jaundice. Provision of nutritional support via enteral rather than parenteral feedings can decrease this complication. Cholestasis and hypoperfusion from septic shock might contribute to the development of acalculous cholecystitis, which must be treated promptly.

Neurologic

The nervous system is an active participant in the systemic response to sepsis. Recent experimental studies have shown that afferent vagal nerve stimulation during sepsis increases the secretion of corticotrophin-releasing hormone, adrenocorticotropic hormone (ACTH), and cortisol (81). In a mouse model of endotoxemia, vagal nerve stimulation prevented the onset of shock in animals following vagotomy (82). Systemic sepsis commonly produces brain dysfunction, sepsis-associated encephalopathy, which can vary from a transient, reversible encephalopathy to irreversible brain damage. The encephalopathy in the acute phase clinically resembles many metabolic encephalopathies: a diffuse disturbance in cerebral function with sparing of the brain stem. The severity of the encephalopathy, as reflected in progressive EEG abnormalities, often precedes, and then parallels, dysfunction in other organs (83).

Multiple-organ Failure

The incidence of MOF or dysfunction varies depending on the definition and classification scheme used (84). The most commonly used MOF score is that of Knaus et al., which uses objective definitions for five-organ system failures (85). They reported in 1985 that a single-organ system failure was associated with 40% mortality, two-organ system failures were associated with 60% mortality, and three or more organ system failures lasting >3 days were associated with 98% mortality (85). MOF is often the final complication of critical illness and is the leading cause of death in patients admitted to an ICU (84,86,87).

Severe sepsis and septic shock are the most common causes of MOF (86). Although outcome following the onset of MOF has improved slightly in the last several decades and new therapies appear to hold promise, prevention remains the optimal way to treat MOF. Rapid, adequate volume resuscitation as well as aggressive support of dysfunctioning organ systems is critical. These measures together with appropriate antibiotic coverage, control of the infectious source, adequate nutrition, and aggressive pulmonary management are important for reversing the downward physiologic spiral that leads from septic shock to MOF and death.

REFERENCES

1. American College of Chest Physicians/Society of Critical Care Medicine. Consensus conference: definitions for sepsis and organ failure and guidelines for the use of innovative therapies in sepsis. *Crit Care Med* 1992;20:864.
2. Balk RA. Severe sepsis and septic shock. Definitions, epidemiology, and clinical manifestations. *Crit Care Clin* 2000;16(2): 179–192.
3. Levy, MM, et al. 2001 SCCM/ESICM/ACCP/ATS/SIS international sepsis definitions conference. *Crit Care Med* 2003;31(4): 1250–1256.
4. Martin GS, et al. The epidemiology of sepsis in the United States from 1979 through 2000. *N Engl J Med* 2003;348(16): 1546–1554.
5. Angus DC, et al. Epidemiology of severe sepsis in the United States: analysis of incidence, outcome, and associated costs of care. *Crit Care Med* 2001;29(7):1303–1310.
6. Annane D, et al. Current epidemiology of septic shock: the CUB-Rea network. *Am J Respir Crit Care Med* 2003;168(2):165–172.

7. Lolis E, Bucala R. Therapeutic approaches to innate immunity: severe sepsis and septic shock. *Nat Rev* 2003;2:635–645.

8. Aderem A, Ulevitch RJ. Toll-like receptors in the induction of the innate immune response. *Nature* 2000;406(6797):782–787.

9. Papageorgiou AC, Acharya KR. Microbial superantigens: from structure to function. *Trends Microbiol* 2000;8(8):369–375.

10. Brun-Buisson C, Doyon F, Carlet J, French bacteremia-sepsis study group. Bacteremia and severe sepsis in adults: a multicenter prospective survey in ICUs and wards of 24 hospitals. *Am J Respir Crit Care Med* 1996;154(3 Pt 1):617–624.

11. Bone RC, et al. A controlled clinical trial of high-dose methylprednisolone in the treatment of severe sepsis and septic shock. *N Engl J Med* 1987;317(11):653–658.

12. Dhainaut JF et al, CPD571 Sepsis Study Group. CDP571, a humanized antibody to human tumor necrosis factor-alpha: safety, pharmacokinetics, immune response, and influence of the antibody on cytokine concentrations in patients with septic shock. *Crit Care Med* 1995;23(9):1461–1469.

13. Bone RC et al, The E5 Sepsis Study Group. A second large controlled clinical study of E5, a monoclonal antibody to endotoxin: results of a prospective, multicenter, randomized, controlled trial. *Crit Care Med* 1995;23(6):994–1006.

14. Shoemaker WC. Temporal physiologic patterns of shock and circulatory dysfunction based on early descriptions by invasive and noninvasive monitoring. *New Horiz* 1996;4(2):300–318.

15. Ruokonen E, Parviainen I, Uusaro A. Treatment of impaired perfusion in septic shock. *Ann Med* 2002;34(7-8):590–597.

16. Friedman G, et al. Combined measurements of blood lactate concentrations and gastric intramucosal pH in patients with severe sepsis. *Crit Care Med* 1995;23(7):1184–1193.

17. Vincent JL, et al. Serial lactate determinations during circulatory shock. *Crit Care Med* 1983;11(6):449–451.

18. Maynard N, et al. Assessment of splanchnic oxygenation by gastric tonometry in patients with acute circulatory failure. *JAMA* 1993; 270(10):1203–1210.

19. Marik PE. Gastric intramucosal pH. A better predictor of multiorgan dysfunction syndrome and death than oxygen-derived variables in patients with sepsis. *Chest* 1993;104(1):225–229.

20. Gomersall CD, et al. Resuscitation of critically ill patients based on the results of gastric tonometry: a prospective, randomized, controlled trial. *Crit Care Med* 2000;28(3):607–614.

21. Mimoz O, et al. Pulmonary artery catheterization in critically ill patients: a prospective analysis of outcome changes associated with catheter-prompted changes in therapy. *Crit Care Med* 1994; 22(4):573–579.

22. Squara P, Bennett D, Perret C. Pulmonary artery catheter: does the problem lie in the users? *Chest* 2002;121(6):2009–2015.

23. Connors AF Jr, et al. The effectiveness of right heart catheterization in the initial care of critically ill patients. SUPPORT Investigators. *JAMA* 1996;276(11):889–897.

24. Vincent JL, De Backer D. Pathophysiology of septic shock. *Adv Sepsis* 2001;1:87–92.

25. Choi PT, et al. Crystalloids vs. colloids in fluid resuscitation: a systematic review. *Crit Care Med* 1999;27(1):200–210.

26. Schierhout G, Roberts I. Fluid resuscitation with colloid or crystalloid solutions in critically ill patients: a systematic review of randomised trials. *Br Med J* 1998;316(7136):961–964.

27. Cook D, Guyatt G. Colloid use for fluid resuscitation: evidence and spin. *Ann Intern Med* 2001;135:205–208.

28. Dellinger RP. Cardiovascular management of septic shock. *Crit Care Med* 2003;31(3):946–955.

29. Martin C, et al. Norepinephrine or dopamine for the treatment of hyperdynamic septic shock? *Chest* 1993;103(6):1826–1831.

30. Meadows D, et al. Reversal of intractable septic shock with norepinephrine therapy. *Crit Care Med* 1988;16(7):663–666.

31. Martin C, et al. Effect of norepinephrine on the outcome of septic shock. *Crit Care Med* 2000;28:2758–2765.

32. LeDoux D, et al. Effects of perfusion pressure on tissue perfusion in septic shock. *Crit Care Med* 2000;28(8):2729–2732.

33. Van den Berghe G, de Zegher F. Anterior pituitary function during critical illness and dopamine treatment. *Crit Care Med* 1996; 24(9):1580–1590.

34. Landry DW, et al. Vasopressin deficiency contributes to the vasodilation of septic shock. *Circulation* 1997;95(5):1122–1125.

35. Holmes CL, et al. Physiology of vasopressin relevant to management of septic shock. *Chest* 2001;120(3):989–1002.

36. Sharshar T, et al. Depletion of neurohypophyseal content of vasopressin in septic shock. *Crit Care Med* 2002;30(3):497–500.

37. Reid IA. Role of vasopressin deficiency in the vasodilation of septic shock. *Circulation* 1997;95(5):1108–1110.

38. Morales D, et al. Reversal by vasopressin of intractable hypotension in the late phase of hemorrhagic shock. *Circulation* 1999; 100(3):226–229.

39. Argenziano M, et al. A prospective randomized trial of arginine vasopressin in the treatment of vasodilatory shock after left ventricular assist device placement. *Circulation* 1997;96(9 Suppl): 286–290.

40. Dunser MW, et al. The effects of vasopressin on systemic hemodynamics in catecholamine-resistant septic and postcardiotomy shock: a retrospective analysis. *Anesth Analg* 2001;93(1):7–13.

41. Malay MB, et al. Low-dose vasopressin in the treatment of vasodilatory septic shock. *J Trauma* 1999;47(4):699–703; discussion 703–705.

42. Kumar A, et al. Tumor necrosis factor alpha and interleukin 1beta are responsible for in vitro myocardial cell depression induced by human septic shock serum. *J Exp Med* 1996;183(3): 949–958.

43. Parker MM, Ognibene FP, Parrillo JE. Reversible depression of myocardial function in septic shock confirmed by a load-independent measure of ventricular performance. *Clin Res* 1990; 38:340A.

44. Parker MM, Suffredini AF, Natanson C. Responses of left ventricular function in survivors and nonsurvivors of septic shock. *J Crit Care* 1989;4:19–25.

45. Rivers E, et al. Early goal-directed therapy in the treatment of severe sepsis and septic shock. *N Engl J Med* 2001;345(19): 1368–1377.

46. Bernard GR, et al. Efficacy and safety of recombinant human activated protein C for severe sepsis. *N Engl J Med* 2001;344(10): 699–709.

47. Vincent JL, et al. Effects of drotrecogin alfa (activated) on organ dysfunction in the PROWESS trial. *Crit Care Med* 2003;31(3): 834–840.

48. Manns BJ, et al. An economic evaluation of activated protein C treatment for severe sepsis. *N Engl J Med* 2002;347(13): 993–1000.

49. Angus DC, et al. Cost-effectiveness of drotrecogin alfa (activated) in the treatment of severe sepsis. *Crit Care Med* 2003;31(1):1–11.

50. Lefering R, Neugebauer EA. Steroid controversy in sepsis and septic shock: a meta-analysis. *Crit Care Med* 1995;23(7): 1294–1303.

51. Bollaert PE, et al. Reversal of late septic shock with supraphysiologic doses of hydrocortisone. *Crit Care Med* 1998;26(4): 645–650.

52. Annane D, et al. Effect of treatment with low doses of hydrocortisone and fludrocortisone on mortality in patients with septic shock. *JAMA* 2002;288(7):862–871.

53. Annane D, et al. A 3-level prognostic classification in septic shock based on cortisol levels and cortisol response to corticotropin. *JAMA* 2000;283(8):1038–1045.

54. Sloane PJ, et al. A multicenter registry of patients with acute respiratory distress syndrome. Physiology and outcome. *Am Rev Respir Dis* 1992;146(2):419–426.

55. Hyers TM. Prediction of survival and mortality in patients with adult respiratory distress syndrome. *New Horiz* 1993;1(4): 466–470.

56. Luce JM. Acute lung injury and the acute respiratory distress syndrome. *Crit Care Med* 1998;26(2):369–376.

57. Sharma S, Kumar A. Septic shock, multiple organ failure, and acute respiratory distress syndrome. *Curr Opin Pulm Med* 2003;9(3):199–209.

58. Dreyfuss D, et al. Intermittent positive-pressure hyperventilation with high inflation pressures produces pulmonary microvascular injury in rats. *Am Rev Respir Dis* 1985;132(4):880–884.

59. Tremblay L, et al. Injurious ventilatory strategies increase cytokines and c-fos m-RNA expression in an isolated rat lung model. *J Clin Invest* 1997;99(5):944–952.

60. Ranieri VM, et al. Effect of mechanical ventilation on inflammatory mediators in patients with acute respiratory distress syndrome: a randomized controlled trial. *JAMA* 1999;282(1): 54–61.

61. Network TARDS. Ventilation with lower tidal volumes as compared with traditional tidal volumes for acute lung injury and the acute respiratory distress syndrome. *N Engl J Med* 2000; 342:1301–1308.

62. Schiffl H, Lang SM, Fischer R. Daily hemodialysis and the outcome of acute renal failure. *N Engl J Med* 2002;346(5):305–310.

63. Pinsky MR, et al. Serum cytokine levels in human septic shock. Relation to multiple-system organ failure and mortality. *Chest* 1993;103(2):565–575.

64. Ronco C, et al. A pilot study of coupled plasma filtration with adsorption in septic shock. *Crit Care Med* 2002;30(6): 1250–1255.

65. John S, et al. Effects of continuous haemofiltration vs intermittent haemodialysis on systemic haemodynamics and splanchnic regional perfusion in septic shock patients: a prospective, randomized clinical trial. *Nephrol Dial Transplant* 2001;16(2): 320–327.

66. Cole L, et al. A phase II randomized, controlled trial of continuous hemofiltration in sepsis. *Crit Care Med* 2002;30(1):100–106.

67. Reeves JH et al, Plasmafiltration in sepsis study group. Continuous plasmafiltration in sepsis syndrome. *Crit Care Med* 1999;27(10): 2096–2104.

68. Esmon CT, Taylor FB Jr., Snow TR. Inflammation and coagulation: linked processes potentially regulated through a common pathway mediated by protein C. *Thromb Haemost* 1991;66(1): 160–165.

69. Yan SB, Grinnell BW. Recombinant human protein C, protein S, and thrombomodulin as antithrombotics. *Perspect Drug Discov* Res 1993;1:503–520.

70. Lamberts SW, Bruining HA, de Jong FH. Corticosteroid therapy in severe illness. *N Engl J Med* 1997;337(18):1285–1292.

71. Annane D, et al. Impaired pressor sensitivity to noradrenaline in septic shock patients with and without impaired adrenal function reserve. *Br J Clin Pharmacol* 1998;46(6):589–597.

72. Wolfe RR, et al. Effect of severe burn injury on substrate cycling by glucose and fatty acids. *N Engl J Med* 1987;317(7):403–408.

73. McCowen KC, Malhotra A, Bistrian BR. Stress-induced hyperglycemia. *Crit Care Clin* 2001;17(1):107–124.

74. van den Berghe G, et al. Intensive insulin therapy in critically ill patients. *N Engl J Med* 2001;345(19):1359–1367.

75. Heyland DK, Cook DJ, Guyatt GH. Enteral nutrition in the critically ill patient: a critical review of the evidence. *Intensive Care Med* 1993;19(8):435–442.

76. Heyland DK. Nutritional support in critically ill patients. A critical review of the evidence. *Crit Care Clin* 1998;14(3): 423–440.

77. Nakad A, et al. Is early enteral nutrition in acute pancreatitis dangerous? About 20 patients fed by an endoscopically placed nasogastrojejunal tube. *Pancreas* 1998;17(2):187–193.

78. Olah A, et al. Randomized clinical trial of specific lactobacillus and fibre supplement to early enteral nutrition in patients with acute pancreatitis. *Br J Surg* 2002;89(9):1103–1107.

79. Griffiths RD, Jones C, Palmer TE. Six-month outcome of critically ill patients given glutamine-supplemented parenteral nutrition. *Nutrition* 1997;13(4):295–302.

80. Griffiths RD, et al. Infection, multiple organ failure, and survival in the intensive care unit: influence of glutamine-supplemented parenteral nutrition on acquired infection. *Nutrition* 2002;18 (7-8):546–552.

81. Gaykema RP, Dijkstra I, Tilders FJ. Subdiaphragmatic vagotomy suppresses endotoxin-induced activation of hypothalamic corticotropin-releasing hormone neurons and ACTH secretion. *Endocrinology* 1995;136:4717.

82. Borovikova LV, et al. Vagus nerve stimulation attenuates the systemic inflammatory response to endotoxin. *Nature* 2000;405: 458–462.

83. Wilson JX, Young GB. Progress in clinical neurosciences: sepsis-associated encephalopathy: evolving concepts. *Can J Neurol Sci* 2003;30:98–105.

84. Baue AE, Durham R, Faist E. Systemic inflammatory response syndrome (SIRS), multiple organ dysfunction syndrome (MODS), multiple organ failure (MOF): are we winning the battle? *Shock* 1998;10:79–89.

85. Knaus WA, et al. Prognosis in acute organ-system failure. *Ann Surg* 1985;202:685–693.

86. Beal AL, Cerra FB. Multiple organ failure syndrome in the 1990s. Systemic inflammatory response and organ dysfunction. *JAMA* 1994;271:226–233.

87. Wenzel RP. Treating sepsis. *N Engl J Med* 2002;347:966–968.

Hypovolemic Shock

13

Saman Arbabi

■ INTRODUCTION AND ETIOLOGY 136

■ DIAGNOSIS OF HYPOVOLEMIC SHOCK 137
Pitfalls in Diagnosis 139
Monitoring 139

■ TREATMENT 139
Choice of Resuscitation Fluid 140
Endpoints for Fluid Resuscitation 141

■ REFERENCES 142

INTRODUCTION AND ETIOLOGY

Shock is defined as inadequate oxygen delivery to tissue. Oxygen delivery to tissue should meet or exceed the body's oxygen demand or requirement (1). Oxygen delivery is dependent on cardiac output, hemoglobin concentration, and arterial oxygen saturation. Cardiac output, in turn, depends on preload, afterload, and contractility. Hypovolemic shock is inadequate delivery of oxygen due to low intravascular volume or preload. In addition, if hypovolemic shock is due to hemorrhage, there could be a decrease in hemoglobin concentration, which further decreases oxygen delivery.

The etiology for hypovolemic shock can be separated into two groups: with or without total body fluid depletion (Table 13-1). Hemorrhage, gastrointestinal (GI) losses, renal losses, and skin losses are associated with total body fluid depletion (2). In this classification, bleeding into a body cavity, such as intra-abdominal and retroperitoneal bleeding, or bleeding from closed pelvic and extremity fractures is considered total body fluid loss. In an adult, significant amounts of blood can be lost in these cavities without any external hemorrhage. For example, closed fractures of the femur or hip might be associated with a blood loss >2 liters (3). Pelvic fractures can result in the loss of several liters of blood into the retroperitoneum (4). A majority of blunt trauma patients with pelvic fracture and shock have multiple potential sources of hemorrhage (4,5). Although the severity and pattern of pelvic fractures might predict a population at risk for massive hemorrhage, these indices cannot be used to exclude significant pelvic bleeding in individual patients (4–6). Most blunt trauma patients undergo abdominopelvic CT scan as part of their workup, and a recent retrospective cohort has demonstrated a high correlation between pelvic hemorrhage volume from pelvic CT scans and the need for pelvic angiography/embolization and transfusion (4). Use of pelvic hemorrhage volume as a guideline for treatment has not yet been tested in a prospective study.

The GI tract secretes 3 to 6 liters of fluid, all of which is reabsorbed except for a small amount lost in the stool (2,7). Intractable vomiting, small bowel obstruction, diarrhea, ileostomy dysfunction, and fistulas might

Saman Arbabi: University of Michigan, Ann Arbor, MI 48109

TABLE 13-1
ETIOLOGIES OF HYPOVOLEMIC SHOCK

A With total body fluid depletion
1) Hemorrhage
   (a) External
   (b) Internal
      (i) GI tract hemorrhage
      (ii) Thoracic, retroperitoneal, pelvic, intra-abdominal bleeding
      (iii) Closed long bone fractures
2) Gastrointestinal tract losses
3) Renal losses
4) Skin losses
5) Open wound losses
6) Burns

B Without total body fluid depletion
1) Redistribution of the intravascular fluid to the interstitial or intracellular space
   (a) Injury and tissue edema due to trauma, burn, or recent operation
   (b) Inflammation such as pancreatitis
   (c) Anaphylaxis
2) Decreased preload due to increased intravascular capacity (Distributive shock)
   (a) Toxins
   (b) Drugs

impair this reabsorption. Most of these etiologies are also associated with electrolyte disturbances and malnutrition. Vomiting can induce metabolic alkalosis, hypokalemia, hypochloremia, and hypovolemia. Renal compensation for hypovolemia is associated with reabsorption of sodium in exchange for hydrogen and potassium ions, which further aggravates electrolyte disturbances. Diarrhea is associated with hypokalemia and acidosis, in part because of bicarbonate loss (8,9). Elderly patients who have received a bowel-prep before operation might have significant hypovolemia from fluid losses in the GI tract and liquid stool. GI bleeding is a special case with a combination of bleeding and GI tract fluid loss. Hypovolemia should be considered in patients with melena, hematemesis, and guaiac positive stool.

The causes for hypovolemic shock without total body fluid depletion can be divided into two groups: (i) redistribution of the intravascular fluid to the interstitial or intracellular space and (ii) decrease in preload due to increased intravascular capacity. Redistribution of fluid might happen in tissue injury due to trauma or burn, recent operation, anaphylaxis, or inflammatory processes such as pancreatitis. Although the patient might have increased total body fluid, intravascular volume is low, making the patient hypovolemic. This is a common cause of low urine output in the first 24 hours after major surgery. Signs or symptoms of shock should alert the clinician to consider other causes, such as bleeding or cardiac etiology. Hypovolemia from fluid redistribution is occasionally difficult to diagnose. Physical examination might

demonstrate significant tissue and pulmonary edema, and distinguishing this from congestive heart failure might be difficult. As discussed later in this chapter, direct measurement of cardiac preload might help with diagnosis.

Increased intravascular capacity in response to drugs and toxins might also induce hypovolemic shock without actual fluid loss from the intravascular space. Some clinicians consider this group as a separate category called *distributive shock*. Additionally, hypovolemic shock overlaps with other shock classifications. Although septic shock is classically defined separately, in part some of the hemodynamic derangement of septic shock is due to low intravascular volume from fluid redistribution and vasodilatation. Moreover, decreases in preload due to increased capacity from spinal cord injuries are usually classified as neurogenic shock rather than hypovolemic shock.

DIAGNOSIS OF HYPOVOLEMIC SHOCK

Hypovolemic shock is a clinical diagnosis. Obtaining an accurate history is extremely important. A history of thoracoabdominal trauma, external bleeding, long bone or pelvic fracture, GI hemorrhage, vomiting, diarrhea, lack of fluid intake, excessive heat, diuretic use, excessive thirst, or polyuria might aid in the diagnosis and etiology of hypovolemic shock. Other etiologies should be considered, especially in patients with a history of recent invasive procedures. It would be a tragedy if reversible causes such as tension pneumothorax or cardiac tamponade were misdiagnosed as hypovolemic shock.

Physical signs of hypovolemic shock are due to decreased organ perfusion. Since stroke volume is dependent on preload, afterload, and contractility, a decrease in preload will induce a decrease in cardiac output and circulating volume. This decrease will initiate a cascade of neuroendocrine responses (7). By increasing heart rate, the body attempts to compensate for decreasing stroke volume. Tachycardia is a prominent symptom of hypovolemic shock when fluid losses approach or exceed 15% of intravascular volume (1).

$$(\text{Stroke Volume}) \times (\text{Heart rate}) = \text{Cardiac output (CO)}$$

Ohm's Law states that changes in pressure are directly proportional to flow and resistance. Therefore, in hypovolemic patients who have decreased cardiac output (flow), systemic blood pressure might be maintained if there is an appropriate increase in systemic vascular resistance (SVR).

$$(\text{CO}) \times (\text{SVR}) \propto (\text{Mean Arterial Pressure–Central Venous Pressure})$$

The increase in SVR is due to a selective increase in the resistance in arteries and arterioles that supply various organs. This alteration is a compensatory mechanism that maintains blood flow to vital organs such as the heart and brain. Increased SVR restricts blood flow to "nonvital" organs such as the skin and skeletal muscle; thus patients with hypovolemic shock present with cool and clammy skin. This redistribution of blood will shunt oxygen delivery to high metabolic demand organs, such as the heart and brain, rather than to tissue with low metabolic demand, such as skin (7). This process partly accounts for an increase in oxygen extraction ratio and a decrease in mixed venous saturation (7,10).

The effect of fluid loss on acid-base balance depends on etiology. Upper GI losses due to vomiting might be associated with hypochloremic metabolic alkalosis. Diarrhea or pancreatic fluid losses are associated with bicarbonate loss and metabolic acidosis. In hemorrhagic shock, decreased oxygen delivery to the tissue will shift the balance to anaerobic metabolism with increased lactic acid production and metabolic acidosis.

Table 13-2 demonstrates stages of hypovolemia (1,3,7). Compensatory mechanisms allow a large loss of fluid to occur before blood pressure is affected. In previously healthy patients, hypovolemia of up to 15% blood volume loss is associated with minimal blood pressure changes (3). The first change seen in the systemic blood pressure is a decrease in pulse pressure, the difference between systolic and diastolic blood pressure. The increased SVR in response to decreased preload will predominately increase the diastolic component with a decrease in pulse pressure. Beyond 30%, blood volume loss is associated with a fall in systolic blood pressure and with tachycardia, tachypnea, and mental status changes. This degree of fluid loss requires immediate intervention. Delay might induce ischemic changes and subsequent ischemia-reperfusion injury and worse outcomes (3,7).

Urine output has been used traditionally to assess circulating volume status. In the hypovolemic patient a complex of neuroendocrine responses increases urine concentration and decreases urine volume with avidity to sodium and water (11). Hourly urine output of 0.5 mL per kg for adults and 1 mL per kg for children is thought to be adequate (12). Although low urine output is seen in hypovolemic shock, it is not a specific or sensitive measure. Septic, cardiogenic, and hepatic shock are also associated with oliguria. Oliguria might also be due to renal or postrenal causes. Postrenal causes of oliguria such as urinary tract or catheter obstruction should be considered.

Any decrease in glomerular filtration rate will cause increases in blood urea nitrogen (BUN) and creatinine. Since creatinine is produced by skeletal muscle and is not reabsorbed by the renal tubules, it is a more reliable representative of renal function than BUN (2). The normal ratio of BUN to plasma creatinine is 10:15 (2). Since there is an increase in urea absorption with hypovolemia, the BUN/creatinine ratio is elevated above 20 (13).

Fractional excretion of sodium (FE_{Na}) can be used to distinguish renal from prerenal causes of oliguria. This calculation is based on concentration of sodium (Na) and creatinine (Cr) in both plasma and urine (14).

$$FE_{Na}\% = [\text{Urine Na}]\,[\text{Plasma Cr}]/[\text{Urine Cr}][\text{Plasma Na}] \times 100$$

Prerenal states are associated with significant reabsorption of sodium with FE_{Na} <1% (15). In contrast, FE_{Na} is >1% in acute tubular necrosis (ATN), since damaged tubules are not able to absorb sodium. A urinalysis might also help to distinguish between ATN and hypovolemia. Although ATN is associated with abnormal levels

TABLE 13-2

CLASSIFICATION OF HYPOVOLEMIC SHOCK

	Class I	Class II	Class III	Class IV
Circulating volume loss %	>15	15–30	>30–40	>40
Heart rate (bpm)	<100	Tachycardia	Tachycardia	Marked tachycardia
Pulse pressure	Normal	Narrowed	Narrowed	Unobtainable or very narrow
Systolic blood pressure	Normal	Minimal decrease	Decrease	Significant decrease
Hourly urine output	≥0.5 cc/kg	≤0.5 cc/kg	<0.5 cc/kg	Minimal
Mental status	Normal	Anxious	Confused and anxious	Markedly depressed or lethargic

of protein and cells, urinalysis is normal in hypovolemia. The presence of ATN does not exclude hypovolemia, and they might coexist. In addition, FE_{Na} in patients who receive diuretics might be inaccurate.

Conversely, high urine output does not exclude hypovolemia. Hypovolemia in the presence of osmotic diuretics as seen in hyperglycemia, diabetes insipidus, or acute alcohol intoxication might be associated with normal or high urine output. Urine output data should be judged in light of other clinical findings.

Pitfalls in Diagnosis

Tachycardia, low pulse pressure, low blood pressure, low urine output, mental status changes, and cold extremities are some of the physical signs of hypovolemic shock. There are many diagnostic pitfalls in clinical assessment of hypovolemic shock (16). Intensive care unit (ICU) patients might have hypovolemic shock with increased interstitial fluid. Distinguishing hypovolemic shock from cardiogenic and septic shock might be difficult, especially in the elderly. Tachycardia is a common symptom of other causes, such as pain, sepsis, and cardiogenic shock. Elderly people and patients who use β-adrenergic and calcium channel blockers might have a normal heart rate in the presence of hypovolemia (7). Low urine output might be due to renal or postrenal causes. Conversely, high urine output might be due to osmotic diuretics or the inability of the kidney to concentrate urine. As already discussed, blood pressure changes might be late signs of hypovolemia. In pediatric patients hypotension is a late and ominous sign (14).

Monitoring

Direct measurement of cardiac preload or left ventricular (LV) filling pressure might assist with the diagnosis of hypovolemic shock. The goal is to estimate the LV end-diastolic pressure (LVEDP). The most commonly used measures of preload are central venous pressure (CVP), determined by a central venous catheter, and pulmonary capillary wedge pressure (PCWP), measured by pulmonary artery catheter. One measures PCWP by inflating a balloon in the pulmonary artery and creating a continuous column of blood to the left atrium. PCWP reflects left atrial pressure, which is an approximation of LVEDP. CVP is a measure of right atrial pressure that estimates right ventricle end-diastolic pressure. CVP is a poor predictor of LVEDP in patients with increased pulmonary artery resistance, chronic obstructive pulmonary disease, right heart failure, and valvular abnormalities (17–20).

Normal PCWP is 6 to 12 mm Hg. These values are of limited use in the ICU patient who might have increased intrathoracic pressure, positive pressure ventilation, abnormal LV compliance, and mitral valve abnormalities (7). Values <10 mm Hg are associated with low preload and hypovolemia. In the compromised patient the PCWP may

be increased up to 18 mm Hg to improve the Frank-Starling curve and increase cardiac output.

PCWP and CVP might be poor predictors of LV preload in patients who have high intrathoracic pressure. Intubated patients with a high positive end-expiratory pressure (PEEP), PEEP $\geq$10 cm H_2O, present a common problem. Since lung stiffness is different in each patient, the transmission of alveolar pressure to pulmonary vessels varies. Several methods have been proposed to adjust for PEEP in PCWP and CVP measurements (17), but none has been uniformly accepted. Another preload measurement is right ventricular end-diastolic volume (RVEDV), which is measured by a modified pulmonary artery catheter. Multiple studies have demonstrated RVEDV index to be superior to PCWP in cardiac preload measurements, especially in patients with increased thoracic pressure (18,19). At higher PEEP values, cardiac index correlates significantly better with RVEDV index than PCWP or CVP (20,21). The optimum RVEDV index range is between 80 to 160 mL per m^2, with the mean in the 120 to 140 mL per m^2 range (21).

Although pulmonary artery catheter use is an established technique in the surgical ICU, no randomized studies demonstrate survival benefit. Pulmonary artery catheters should be used only as an adjunct to thorough clinical assessment. Indiscriminate or inappropriate use of pulmonary artery catheters might be associated with complications without significant benefit to the patient (22–24). ICU specialists are continuously looking for more accurate or less invasive methods of measuring intravascular volume status, such as the esophageal Doppler monitor. In this technique, a small-caliber Doppler ultrasound is placed in the esophagus via the oral or nasal route, measuring Doppler waveform to estimate preload and cardiac function (25). Although some of these newer methods have shown promise, more studies are needed to define their efficacy and limitations.

TREATMENT

In shock, the treatment goal is to establish adequate tissue perfusion rapidly and safely. Although in the case of hypovolemic shock the main problem is low intravascular volume, airway control and breathing come first. Assessment of any patient in shock requires rapid evaluation with appropriate maneuvers to obtain a secure airway and adequate breathing.

Sources of hemorrhage must be controlled. In GI bleeding this might include upper or lower GI tract evaluation with maneuvers to stop bleeding. Operative intervention and control of hemorrhage is the mainstay therapy for trauma patients. The timing of fluid resuscitation in penetrating trauma remains controversial. Some authors have suggested delay of IV resuscitation until the bleeding source is under control (26–28). They have proposed that aggressive fluid resuscitation in patients with uncontrolled bleeding source might increase blood pressure, with disruption of natural homeostatic mechanism such as thrombus formation, with subsequent increase in bleeding, necessitating more resuscitation (29,30). This vicious circle might induce hypothermia and dilution of clotting factors. A randomized clinical trial demonstrated improved survival in patients with penetrating torso injuries with delayed fluid resuscitation until operative intervention (28). This study involved patients who were rapidly transported with a short scene-to-operating room time. The findings of this study should not be generalized to trauma patients in rural areas with long transport time, blunt mechanisms of injury, or head trauma. Although most surgeons agree that transport to a trauma center should not be delayed, most of them have not adopted a strategy of withholding fluid resuscitation, and further research is required.

Fluid resuscitation is the cornerstone of treatment for hypovolemic shock. In class III and IV hypovolemic shock patients with hypotension, vasoactive drugs are used only as a stopgap measure until adequate resuscitation restores organ perfusion and blood pressure. Two of the most commonly used drugs are norepinephrine and dopamine (31,32). At low doses dopamine increases cardiac output via β-adrenergic effects, and at high doses dopamine increases SVR and mean arterial blood pressure via α_1-adrenergic effects. In septic shock, most recent studies demonstrate a more favorable hemodynamic profile and renal blood flow with norepinephrine versus dopamine (31,32). Norepinephrine has α- and β_1-adrenergic effects and increases SVR and blood pressure without a drop in cardiac output. Phenylephrine is another vasoactive drug that has α_1-adrenergic effects, which increases mean arterial blood pressure by increasing SVR and afterload. This drug might have some benefits in patients with tachycardia, since phenylephrine does not increase the heart rate; however, an increase in afterload might further decrease cardiac output and increase strain on the myocardium. Dobutamine is a β-agonist that might worsen hypotension in hypovolemic patients, since its β_2 properties cause vasodilatation (7,33). In hypovolemic patients, use of any of these agents should be limited and temporary until adequate fluid resuscitation is achieved.

Resuscitation should be initiated with large-bore intravenous lines (16-gauge or larger). In burned patients, 2 to 4 mL of Ringer lactate is recommended for each percent total body surface area (TBSA) burn per kilogram body weight (12). Therefore, a 70 kg man who has 10% TBSA burn should receive 1,400 to 2,800 mL of fluid. Half of this amount should be given in the first 8 hours and the rest in the next 16 hours. Burn patients with inhalation injury might require significantly more fluid resuscitation. Conversely, a patient who has clinical signs of adequate resuscitation might not require all the fluid recommended in the guideline.

Trauma patients are usually given a 2-liter fluid challenge or 20 cc per kg fluid bolus. For class III and IV hemorrhagic shock, blood transfusion is necessary (3). In most patients symptoms of hypovolemia are seen after at least 10% to 15% of the intravascular volume has been lost. Therefore, resuscitation with <500 mL of isotonic fluid in surgical adult patients is not advised.

Choice of Resuscitation Fluid

The choice of fluid resuscitation has become one of the most controversial topics in critical care. There are three basic choices: blood and blood products, colloids, and crystalloids. The blood substitutes are not currently clinically available and are not discussed here.

Red cell transfusion to normalize blood counts offers several theoretical advantages. Increased hemoglobin concentration will increase oxygen capacity and might increase oxygen delivery to tissue. Red blood cell transfusions are an efficient means of resuscitation, since blood cells will remain in the intravascular space. In patients with active bleeding, blood cell transfusion is appropriate. There is a debate over blood cell transfusion in critically ill patients without an active source of hemorrhage. If it is available, there is no question that autologous fresh blood is the best resuscitation fluid. However, readily available blood bank red blood cells are neither autologous nor fresh. Storage of blood impairs red blood cell deformability and flow in the microcirculation (34). This consideration might partly explain findings from multiple studies that demonstrate the inability of red blood cell transfusion to improve tissue hypoxia (34–38). In addition, it is well known that allogeneic blood transfusion is immunosuppressive. Blood transfusions were used in the past to increase the success rate of renal transplants. Blood transfusions are associated with an increase rate of cancer recurrence and nosocomial infections (39–41). Some believe that the residual leukocytes present in the allogeneic blood products are responsible for this immunomodulatory effect. Studies with leukocyte-depleted blood products or leukoreduction products are in clinical trial (42). There is also a small risk for transmission of viral infection such as hepatitis C and HIV.

A recent prospective randomized study demonstrated that a restrictive strategy of red-cell transfusion (hemoglobin concentration maintained at 7.0 to 9.0 g per dL) might be superior to a liberal transfusion strategy (hemoglobin concentration maintained at 10.0 to 12.0 g per dL) in critically ill patients, with the possible exception of patients with acute myocardial infarction and unstable angina (43). Use of other blood products such as fresh frozen plasma (FFP) is indicated for coagulation factor deficiencies. Using FFP for massive resuscitation without evidence of coagulation factor deficiency is controversial (44).

Theoretically, the use of colloids in resuscitation of hypovolemic patients is associated with preservation of plasma osmotic pressure, more efficient plasma volume expansion, and decreased tissue and pulmonary edema. However, clinical studies have not demonstrated a significant improvement in patient outcomes with colloid resuscitation (45,46). The three most commonly used colloids are albumin, Hetastarch, and Dextran-70. The use of Dextran-70 has been limited because of its association with anaphylactic reaction and antithrombotic effect (47). In addition to a colloid effect, albumin has been promoted as a free radical and toxin scavenger. Resuscitation with 25% albumin attenuates lung injury in rat models, in part due to its antioxidant property (48). Nevertheless, several clinical studies have not demonstrated any beneficial effect in using albumin (49,50). The Cochrane Group published a meta-analysis comparing albumin to crystalloid resuscitation with an overall increased mortality associated with albumin (51). The use of a mixed and heterogeneous population of patients was a significant limitation of this study (46). The controversy in the use of albumin in resuscitation will only be resolved with further well-designed clinical studies.

Crystalloids have been the mainstay for treatment of hypovolemia. A number of solutions are available, with normal saline and Ringer solution being the most commonly used. Normal saline (0.9% NaCl) has 154 mEq of both sodium and chloride and has a slightly higher osmolarity than plasma. Use of normal saline has been associated with hyperchloremic acidosis, which has limited the benefit of this solution (52).

Hypertonic saline resuscitation (7.5% NaCl) has been promoted for efficient intravascular volume resuscitation, rapid restoration of blood pressure and cardiac output with improved cerebral perfusion, and potential for expanding circulating volume by reabsorption of fluid from interstitial space (53,54). Hypertonic saline might decrease the required volume resuscitation with decreased tissue edema, a property that was thought to be beneficial in trauma patients, especially with head injury (55). Initial studies demonstrated the safety of hypertonic saline resuscitation with a trend in improved outcomes of head injury patients or patients requiring surgery (56,57). More recently, hypertonic saline has been viewed as a fluid with significant modulation of systemic inflammatory response secondary to reperfusion injury, which might be beneficial in patients with shock (58). Early hypertonic saline administration might attenuate innate immune response to injury, such as macrophage, neutrophil, and endothelial cell activation, and decrease the risk for future organ dysfunction syndrome (59–62). Hypertonic saline directly activates endothelial cells to produce prostacyclin, which decreases vascular resistance and improves microvascular circulation (60). Clinical trials are in progress to evaluate the outcome of patients in shock following blunt traumatic injury who are randomized to receive 250 mL of 7.5% hypertonic saline/6% dextran followed by Ringer solution versus Ringer solution alone (63). Currently, hypertonic saline is not routinely used and further research is required to define the timing, the amount, and the patient population that might benefit from hypertonic saline resuscitation (64).

Ringer solution is the solution used by most surgeons for resuscitation of hypovolemic patients. It is physiologically balanced with electrolyte properties most similar to plasma, with 130 mEq Na^+, 4 mEq of both K^+ and Ca^{2+}, 109 mEq of Cl^- and 28 mEq of HCO_3. Owing to the presence of potassium, Ringer solution should not be given to patients with hyperkalemia or renal failure. It has been routinely used for massive resuscitation for trauma and burn patients. Recent studies have demonstrated a potential association between Ringer solution resuscitation and modulation of leukocyte function (65,66). Most commercially available Ringer solutions are a racemic mixture of D and L stereoisomers. Although the L-isomer is associated with low toxicity, the D-isomer, which is normally only produced by GI flora, has been associated with clinical toxicity and potentially harmful changes in leukocyte function (65,67). Although further studies of the effect of Ringer solution resuscitation in surgical patients are in progress, it remains a clinically acceptable solution for resuscitation of surgical patients.

Endpoints for Fluid Resuscitation

The ultimate endpoint for fluid resuscitation is achieving adequate tissue perfusion. Many clinical indicators have been used, including resolution of tachycardia, acidosis, and improved mental status, extremity perfusion, and urine output. The primary endpoint in critically ill patients who have pulmonary artery catheters remains elusive. There are studies regarding optimal values of cardiac index, mixed oxygen venous saturation, and oxygen delivery index (68,69). Investigators have demonstrated that critically injured patients who achieved a supranormal oxygen delivery index of at least 600 mL/min/m^2 had higher survival rates (70). Further studies have not supported a set oxygen delivery index as an endpoint for resuscitation (68). The endpoint for fluid resuscitation remains a clinical judgment that might be guided by physiological parameters, laboratory values such as pH, and pulmonary artery catheter values such as oxygen delivery index and mixed venous oxygen saturation.

In summary, rapid identification and treatment of hypovolemic shock is vital to the successful outcome of surgical patients. Hypovolemic shock is a clinical diagnosis based on the patient history and on physiological and laboratory parameters. Selective use of invasive monitoring, such as pulmonary artery catheterization, with appropriate interpretation of data, can aid in the diagnosis and treatment. Although fluid resuscitation is the cornerstone of management, the best form of fluid resuscitation has yet to be identified.

REFERENCES

1. Buchman TG, Jacobsohn E. Shock. In: Greenfield LJ, Mulholland MW, Oldham KT, Zelenock GB, Lillemoe KD, eds. *Surgery: scientific principal and practice*. Philadelphia: Lippincott; 2001:202–217.
2. Post TW, Rose BD. Clinical manifestations and diagnosis of volume depletion. UpToDate, Inc. Available at: http://www.utdol.com/application/topic.asp?file=pc_neph/6291&type=A&selectedTitle=2~19.
3. American College of Surgeons. *Advance trauma life support: instructor manual*, 6th ed. Chicago, IL: American College of Surgeons; 1997.
4. Blackmore CC, Jurkovich GJ, Linnau KF, et al. Assessment of volume of hemorrhage and outcome from pelvic fracture. *Arch Surg* 2003;138(5):504–508; discussion 508–509.
5. Poole GV, Ward EF, Muakkassa FF, et al. Pelvic fracture from major blunt trauma. Outcome is determined by associated injuries. *Ann Surg* 1991;213(6):532–538; discussion 538–539.
6. Cryer HM, Miller FB, Evers BM, et al. Pelvic fracture classification: correlation with hemorrhage. *J Trauma* 1988;28(7): 973–980.
7. Groeneveld ABJ. Hypovolemic shock. In: Parrillo JE, Dellinger RP, eds. *Critical care medicine*, 2nd ed. St. Louis: Mosby; 2002:465–500.
8. Assadi F, Copelovitch L. Simplified treatment strategies to fluid therapy in diarrhea. *Pediatr Nephrol* 2003;18(11):1152–1156.
9. Sack DA, Sack RB, Nair GB, et al. Cholera. *Lancet* 2004; 363(9404):223–233.
10. Schlichtig R, Kramer DJ, Pinsky MR. Flow redistribution during progressive hemorrhage is a determinant of critical O2 delivery. *J Appl Physiol* 1991;70(1):169–178.
11. Rose B, Post TW. *Clinical physiology of acid-base and electrolyte disorders*. New York: McGraw-Hill; 2001.
12. American Burn Association. *Advance burn life support course: provider manual*. Chicago, IL: American Burn Association; 2001.
13. Dossetor JB. Creatininemia versus uremia. The relative significance of blood urea nitrogen and serum creatinine concentrations in azotemia. *Ann Intern Med* 1966;65(6):1287–1299.
14. Magnuson DK. Neonatal and pediatric physiology. In: Greenfield LJ, Mulholland MW, Oldham KT, Zelenock GB, Lillemoe KD, eds. *Surgery: scientific principal and practice*, 3rd ed. Lippincott Williams & Wilkins; 2001:1901–1931.
15. Miller TR, Anderson RJ, Linas SL, et al. Urinary diagnostic indices in acute renal failure: a prospective study. *Ann Intern Med* 1978;89(1):47–50.
16. Cohn JN. Blood pressure measurement in shock. Mechanism of inaccuracy in auscultatory and palpatory methods. *JAMA* 1967; 199(13):118–122.
17. Teboul JL, Pinsky MR, Mercat A, et al. Estimating cardiac filling pressure in mechanically ventilated patients with hyperinflation. *Crit Care Med* 2000;28(11):3631–3636.
18. Diebel LN, Myers T, Dulchavsky S. Effects of increasing airway pressure and PEEP on the assessment of cardiac preload. *J Trauma* 1997;42(4):585–90; discussion 590–1.
19. Luecke T, Roth H, Herrmann P, et al. Assessment of cardiac preload and left ventricular function under increasing levels of positive end-expiratory pressure. *Intensive Care Med* 2004;30(1): 119–126.
20. Cheatham ML, Nelson LD, Chang MC, et al. Right ventricular end-diastolic volume index as a predictor of preload status in patients on positive end-expiratory pressure. *Crit Care Med* 1998;26(11):1801–1806.
21. Durham R, Neunaber K, Vogler G, et al. Right ventricular end-diastolic volume as a measure of preload. *J Trauma* 1995;39(2): 218–223; discussion 223–214.
22. Sandham JD, Hull RD, Brant RF. et al. A randomized, controlled trial of the use of pulmonary-artery catheters in high-risk surgical patients. *N Engl J Med* 2003;348(1):5–14.
23. Bernard GR, Sopko G, Cerra F. et al. Pulmonary artery catheterization and clinical outcomes: national heart, lung, and blood institute and food and drug administration workshop report. Consensus statement. *JAMA* 2000;283(19):2568–2572.
24. Robin ED. The cult of the Swan-Ganz catheter. Overuse and abuse of pulmonary flow catheters. *Ann Intern Med* 1985; 103(3):445–449.
25. Seoudi HM, Perkal MF, Hanrahan A, et al. The esophageal Doppler monitor in mechanically ventilated surgical patients: does it work? *J Trauma* 2003;55(4):720–725; discussion 725–726.
26. Baskett PJ. ABC of major trauma. Management of hypovolaemic shock. *BMJ* 1990;300(6737):1453–1457.
27. Capone AC, Safar P, Stezoski W, et al. Improved outcome with fluid restriction in treatment of uncontrolled hemorrhagic shock. *J Am Coll Surg* 1995;180(1):49–56.
28. Bickell WH, Wall MJ Jr, Pepe PE, et al. Immediate versus delayed fluid resuscitation for hypotensive patients with penetrating torso injuries. *N Engl J Med* 1994;331(17):1105–1109.
29. Silbergleit R, Satz W, McNamara RM, et al. Effect of permissive hypotension in continuous uncontrolled intra-abdominal hemorrhage. *Acad Emerg Med* 1996;3(10):922–926.
30. Solomonov E, Hirsh M, Yahiya A, et al. The effect of vigorous fluid resuscitation in uncontrolled hemorrhagic shock after massive splenic injury. *Crit Care Med* 2000;28(3):749–754.
31. Marik PE, Mohedin M. The contrasting effects of dopamine and norepinephrine on systemic and splanchnic oxygen utilization in hyperdynamic sepsis. *JAMA* 1994;272(17):1354–1357.
32. Bellomo R, Kellum JA, Wisniewski SR, et al. Effects of norepinephrine on the renal vasculature in normal and endotoxemic dogs. *Am J Respir Crit Care Med* 1999;159(4 Pt 1):1186–1192.
33. Shoemaker WC, Appel PL, Kram HB. Measurement of tissue perfusion by oxygen transport patterns in experimental shock and in high-risk surgical patients. *Intensive Care Med* 1990;16(Suppl. 2): S135–S144.
34. McCrossan L, Masterson G. Blood transfusion in critical illness. *Br J Anaesth* 2002;88(1):6–9.
35. Steffes CP, Bender JS, Levison MA. Blood transfusion and oxygen consumption in surgical sepsis. *Crit Care Med* 1991;19(4): 512–517.
36. Marik PE, Sibbald WJ. Effect of stored-blood transfusion on oxygen delivery in patients with sepsis. *JAMA* 1993;269(23): 3024–3029.
37. Lorente JA, Landin L, De Pablo R, et al. Effects of blood transfusion on oxygen transport variables in severe sepsis. *Crit Care Med* 1993;21(9):1312–1318.
38. Conrad SA, Dietrich KA, Hebert CA, et al. Effect of red cell transfusion on oxygen consumption following fluid resuscitation in septic shock. *Circ Shock* 1990;31(4):419–429.
39. Blumberg N, Heal JM. Immunomodulation by blood transfusion: an evolving scientific and clinical challenge. *Am J Med* 1996;101(3):299–308.
40. Taylor RW, Manganaro L, O'Brien J, et al. Impact of allogenic packed red blood cell transfusion on nosocomial infection rates in the critically ill patient. *Crit Care Med* 2002;30(10): 2249–2254.
41. Gazmuri RJ, Shakeri SA. Blood transfusion and the risk of nosocomial infection: an underreported complication? *Crit Care Med* 2002;30(10):2389–2391.
42. Nathens A. Effect of leukoreduction on infection risk in trauma. NIH. Available at: http://crisp.cit.nih.gov/crisp/CRISP_LIB.getdoc?textkey=6617894&p_grant_num=5R01GM066117-02&p_query=&ticket=7244112&p_audit_session_id=32302045&p_keywords=. Accessed February 3, 2004.
43. Hebert PC, Wells G, Blajchman MA, et al. A multicenter, randomized, controlled clinical trial of transfusion requirements in critical care. Transfusion requirements in critical care investigators, Canadian critical care trials group. *N Engl J Med* 1999; 340(6):409–417.
44. Contreras M, Ala FA, Greaves M, et al. Guidelines for the use of fresh frozen plasma. British committee for standards in haematology, working party of the blood transfusion task force. *Transfus Med* 1992;2(1):57–63.
45. Tranbaugh RF, Lewis FR. Crystalloid versus colloid for fluid resuscitation of hypovolemic patients. *Adv Shock Res* 1983; 9:203–216.
46. Boldt J. The good, the bad, and the ugly: should we completely banish human albumin from our intensive care units? *Anesth Analg* 2000;91(4):887–895.
47. Waters LM, Christensen MA, Sato RM. Hetastarch: an alternative colloid in burn shock management. *J Emerg Nurs* 1990; 16(4):279–287.

48. Powers KA, Kapus A, Khadaroo RG, et al. Twenty-five percent albumin prevents lung injury following shock/resuscitation. *Crit Care Med* 2003;31(9):2355–2363.

49. Ferguson ND, Stewart TE, Etchells EE. Human albumin administration in critically ill patients. *Intensive Care Med* 1999;25(3):323–325.

50. Schierhout G, Roberts I. Fluid resuscitation with colloid or crystalloid solutions in critically ill patients: a systematic review of randomised trials. *Br Med J* 1998;316(7136):961–964.

51. Cochrane Injuries Group Albumin Reviewers. Human albumin administration in critically ill patients: systematic review of randomised controlled trials. *Br Med J* 1998;317(7153):235–240.

52. Waters JH, Gottlieb A, Schoenwald P, et al. Normal saline versus lactated Ringer's solution for intraoperative fluid management in patients undergoing abdominal aortic aneurysm repair: an outcome study. *Anesth Analg* 2001;93(4):817–822.

53. Rocha-e-Silva M, Negraes GA, Soares AM, et al. Hypertonic resuscitation from severe hemorrhagic shock: patterns of regional circulation. *Circ Shock* 1986;19(2):165–175.

54. Gemma M, Cozzi S, Piccoli S, et al. Hypertonic saline fluid therapy following brain stem trauma. *J Neurosurg Anesthesiol* 1996;8(2):137–141.

55. Young WF, Rosenwasser RH, Vasthare US, et al. Preservation of post-compression spinal cord function by infusion of hypertonic saline. *J Neurosurg Anesthesiol* 1994;6(2):122–127.

56. Vassar MJ, Perry CA, Gannaway WL, et al. 7.5% sodium chloride/dextran for resuscitation of trauma patients undergoing helicopter transport. *Arch Surg* 1991;126(9):1065–1072.

57. Mattox KL, Maningas PA, Moore EE, et al. Prehospital hypertonic saline/dextran infusion for post-traumatic hypotension. The U.S.A. multicenter trial. *Ann Surg* 1991;213(5):482–491.

58. Junger WG, Coimbra R, Liu FC, et al. Hypertonic saline resuscitation: a tool to modulate immune function in trauma patients? *Shock* 1997;8(4):235–241.

59. Coimbra R, Hoyt DB, Junger WG, et al. Hypertonic saline resuscitation decreases susceptibility to sepsis after hemorrhagic shock. *J Trauma* 1997;42(4):602–606; discussion 606–607.

60. Arbabi S, Garcia I, Bauer G, et al. Hypertonic saline induces prostacyclin production via extracellular signal-regulated kinase (ERK) activation. *J Surg Res* 1999;83(2):141–146.

61. Arbabi S, Rosengart MR, Garcia I, et al. Hypertonic saline solution induces prostacyclin production by increasing cyclooxygenase-2 expression. *Surgery* 2000;128(2):198–205.

62. Cuschieri J, Gourlay D, Garcia I, et al. Hypertonic preconditioning inhibits macrophage responsiveness to endotoxin. *J Immunol* 2002;168(3):1389–1396.

63. Bulger EM. The Effect of Hypertonic Resuscitation for Blunt Trauma. NIH. Available at: http://crisp.cit.nih.gov/crisp/ CRISP_LIB.getdoc?textkey=6595669&p_grant_num=1R01HL07323301&p_query=&ticket=7339989&p_audit_session_id=33255274&p_keywords=. Accessed 2/12/2004, 2004.

64. Pruitt BA Jr. Does hypertonic burn resuscitation make a difference? *Crit Care Med* 2000;28(1):277–278.

65. Koustova E, Stanton K, Gushchin V, et al. Effects of lactated Ringer's solutions on human leukocytes. *J Trauma* 2002;52(5):872–878.

66. Koustova E, Rhee P, Hancock T, et al. Ketone and pyruvate Ringer's solutions decrease pulmonary apoptosis in a rat model of severe hemorrhagic shock and resuscitation. *Surgery* 2003;134(2):267–274.

67. Veech RL, Fowler RC. Cerebral dysfunction and respiratory alkalosis during peritoneal dialysis with D-lactate-containing dialysis fluids. *Am J Med* 1987;82(3):572–574.

68. Velmahos GC, Demetriades D, Shoemaker WC, et al. Endpoints of resuscitation of critically injured patients: normal or supranormal? A prospective randomized trial. *Ann Surg* 2000;232(3):409–418.

69. McKinley BA, Kozar RA, Cocanour CS, et al. Normal versus supranormal oxygen delivery goals in shock resuscitation: the response is the same. *J Trauma* 2002;53(5):825–832.

70. Shoemaker WC. Monitoring and therapy for young trauma patients. *Crit Care Med* 1994;22(4):548–549.

Fluid and Electrolyte Abnormalities

14

Bradley D. Freeman

■■■ **INTRODUCTION 144**

■■■ **FLUID COMPARTMENTS 144**

■■■ **CRYSTALLOIDS 145**
Types of Crystalloid Solutions 145
Indications for Crystalloid Solution Use 145

■■■ **COLLOIDS 146**
Hypertonic Saline 148

■■■ **CONCLUSION 148**

■■■ **REFERENCES 148**

INTRODUCTION

Intravenous fluid therapy is integral to the practice of surgery. For many patients, such as those undergoing minor procedures or only briefly requiring parenteral hydration, intravenous fluid prescription is uncomplicated. In contrast, for patients who have undergone complex operations, sustained major trauma, or possess significant comorbidities, meticulous attention to fluid therapy is essential to avoiding serious electrolyte disturbance and other adverse results. Further, because of the substantial range in acquisition costs of currently available intravenous fluid preparations coupled with an environment increasingly focused on cost containment, economic considerations are becoming a

Bradley D. Freeman: Washington University School of Medicine, St. Louis, MO 63110

greater part of surgical decision-making in this area. This chapter's purpose is to focus on basic aspects of fluid management, to discuss potential complications and electrolyte derangements associated with commonly used intravenous fluids, and to review recent literature examining the relative risks and benefits of selected therapies. The ultimate goal of this analysis is to promote an approach to intravenous fluid management that is evidence-based and cost-effective.

FLUID COMPARTMENTS

Knowledge of body fluid compartment distribution is essential both to understanding the physiologic changes that occur following surgery or injury and to guiding intravenous fluid use. Total body water equals roughly 60% of lean body weight, is slightly higher in men, is most concentrated in skeletal muscle, and declines steadily with age. Total body water can be divided into two major compartments: an intracellular fluid compartment, comprising 60% of the total body water compartment (40% of lean body weight), and an extracellular fluid compartment, comprising 40% of the total body water compartment (20% of lean body weight). The extracellular fluid space is further subdivided into an intravascular compartment (equaling roughly 10% of total body water or 25% of the extracellular fluid space) and an extravascular or interstitial compartment (roughly 30% of the total body water or 75% of the extracellular fluid space). Surgeons speak frequently of "third space" fluid losses or "fluid third spacing."

The third fluid space is extracellular fluid that is neither intravascular nor interstitial and is not immediately physiologically connected to these compartments. The third fluid space represents a patient's nonspecific response to acute injury (e.g., surgery, infection, or trauma), with the magnitude and duration of third space fluid accumulation proportional to the degree of the inciting insult and the time course of its resolution. Third space fluid accumulation must be taken into account when prescribing intravenous fluids either for maintenance therapy or for resuscitation.

CRYSTALLOIDS

Types of Crystalloid Solutions

Commonly used intravenous fluids are divided into two categories, crystalloids and colloids. Crystalloids contain sodium as their osmotically active particle and distribute throughout the entire extracellular space in such a way that approximately 25% to 30% of the infused volume remains in the intravascular compartment (1). The predominant effect of crystalloid administration is to expand the interstitial, not the intravascular, space (2). Although a variety of crystalloid solutions are available, the prototypes are 0.9% NaCl (normal saline) and lactated Ringer solution. Normal saline contains Na^+ and Cl^- at concentrations slightly greater than that found in plasma; lactated Ringer solution contains these constituents as well as K^+, Ca^{2+}, and a HCO_3^- source at near physiologic levels. With minor exceptions, normal saline and lactated Ringer solution can be used interchangeably, and few complications are specifically associated with these formulations. Lactated Ringer solution should not be used in patients with hyperkalemia. Further, the Ca^{2+} present in lactated Ringer can bind certain drugs, diminishing bioavailability, as well as chelate citrate present in packed red blood cells, promoting coagulation (2). For this reason lactated Ringer solution is contraindicated as a diluent for blood (2). The lactate in lactated Ringer solution does not interfere with serum lactate measurements (1). Most commonly used crystalloid solutions are derivatives of either lactated Ringer solution or normal saline.

Dextrose is a common additive to crystalloids. The original intent of incorporating dextrose into intravenous fluids was to provide a source of nonprotein calories, thus potentially diminishing protein catabolism. A 5% dextrose solution provides approximately 170 kcal per liter. Although the clinical benefit of this protein sparing effect is unproven, the use of dextrose containing fluids is essential in the perioperative management of fasting diabetics to decrease the likelihood of ketosis (3). These solutions are likewise useful as a source of free water replacement in patients who are unable to tolerate oral hydration. Solutions containing only 5% dextrose are not effective volume expanders because only 10% of the infused volume remains within the intravascular space (1). Dextrose solutions have some potential adverse effects. Dextrose adds an additional osmotic load to crystalloid solutions. In situations in which glucose utilization is impaired, such as critical illness, the infused glucose might accumulate and create an osmotic effect that can promote dehydration (2). Further, dextrose infusions might theoretically result in increased CO_2 and lactate production (4,5). This latter concern is of uncertain clinical importance in most surgical patients.

Indications for Crystalloid Solution Use

Crystalloids are used in several situations, most commonly as a maintenance fluid. Maintenance fluids must replace approximately 75 mEq of Na^+ lost daily and provide approximately 40 to 50 mEq per day of K^+ (6). Because of the large body stores and limited daily losses of Ca^{2+} and Mg^{2+}, maintenance replacement of these elements is unnecessary in patients who require a short course of intravenous therapy (6). For the patient with intact renal and cardiopulmonary function, a common maintenance fluid prescription is dextrose 5%/0.45% NaCl with supplemental KCl (20 mEq per L) or lactated Ringer solution with 5% dextrose (D5LR) infused at 1 to 2 mL/kg/hr. The presence of acute or chronic organ dysfunction requires modification of the volume or composition of fluid infused. For most general surgical patients requiring short courses of intravenous therapy, such as those awaiting resolution of postoperative ileus, it is not necessary to determine serum electrolyte concentrations on a daily basis.

Findings of a recent study examining the effect of postoperative fluid management on postsurgical ileus might cause reexamination of current practice in use of maintenance therapy. In a small prospective trial, Lobo et al. randomized patients following elective colon surgery to receive either standard fluid therapy (defined as volume exceeding 3 L per day and sodium load of 154 mEq per day or greater) or fluid restriction (fluid volume not exceeding 2 L per day and sodium load not exceeding 77 mEq per day) (7). Gastric emptying, studied on the fourth postoperative day, was significantly delayed in patients receiving standard fluid therapy compared to patients managed with fluid restriction. Likewise, patients receiving standard fluid therapy had slower resolution of ileus and longer hospital lengths of stay. The mechanism underlying these findings is unclear but was postulated to be due to development of bowel wall edema secondary to hypoalbuminemia or sodium excess. This small study has not been replicated, and the findings might not be generalizable to the larger general surgical population.

A second indication for crystalloid use is as replacement therapy in the setting of either preexisting or ongoing fluid losses or electrolyte disturbances. The nature or source of fluid loss might lead to electrolyte abnormalities and dictate the composition of the intravenous fluid to be used. Although a detailed discussion of all conceivable electrolyte abnormalities occurring in general surgical patients is beyond the scope of this chapter, two commonly encountered scenarios merit mention. The most common electrolyte abnormality observed in general surgical patients is hypokalemic, hypochloremic metabolic alkalosis resulting from loss of gastric secretions via nasogastric tubes. This electrolyte abnormality is a chloride responsive alkalosis; accordingly, its correction requires administration of a Cl^- source in addition to supplemental K^+, usually normal saline with supplemental KCl. For patients who have substantial nasogastric losses (>1 L per day), serum electrolytes should be determined daily and this abnormality should be anticipated and corrected accordingly. A second electrolyte disturbance frequently encountered in surgical practice is metabolic acidosis secondary to high HCO_3^- loss, such as occurs in the presence of proximal small bowel enterocutaneous fistula. Lactated Ringer solution, because it contains a HCO_3^- source, is the appropriate replacement fluid in this setting.

A third indication for crystalloid use is resuscitation. Crystalloids are appropriate as a first line treatment of shock, regardless of etiology, and have the advantages of being inexpensive, readily available, and reaction-free. Excessive crystalloid administration might result in peripheral and pulmonary edema, and may occur before intravascular volume is completely restored. Indicators of adequate resuscitation, such as central venous pressure, pulmonary capillary wedge pressure, or end organ function, should guide the volume of crystalloid administered, as well as the need for other means of hemodynamic support, such as packed red blood cell transfusion or vasopressor administration [8]. Debate continues on the relative advantages and disadvantages of crystalloids for this indication.

COLLOIDS

Colloids contain a large molecular weight molecule that does not readily cross the capillary membrane as the principal osmotically active substance [1]. Colloid infusions have the effect of primarily expanding the intravascular space [2]. In contrast to crystalloids that have a number of potential uses, the primary indication for colloid administration is acute volume expansion.

The prototypical colloid solutions are albumin preparations. Albumin is the most abundant protein in plasma, accounting for as much as 85% of colloid osmotic pressure. Human serum albumin is commercially available in an isotonic diluent as both a 5% solution (50 g per L) and a 25% solution (250 g per L). These products are heat-treated and pose no risk for viral transmission [1]. Administration of 5% albumin preparations expands the intravascular space by roughly 50% of the volume infused. In contrast, administration of 25% albumin preparations expands intravascular volume by an amount equaling four- to fivefold the volume infused due to shift of interstitial fluid into the intravascular space. Twenty-five percent albumin solutions are administered in small volumes (50 to 100 mL); because the accompanying sodium load is small, these preparations are also known as "salt poor albumin."

Twenty-five percent albumin solutions should not be administered to patients who are hypovolemic.

A number of other colloid solutions are available for clinical use. Hydroxyethyl starch is a synthetic colloid with an average molecular weight of 69 kdal, making it comparable physically to albumin [9]. Hydroxyethyl starch is available as a 6% solution in isotonic saline, which has an oncotic effect equivalent to a 5% albumin solution. Hydroxyethyl starch is slightly more potent as a volume expander than albumin (achieving an effective volume expansion of 30% greater than the volume infused). However, because the osmotic effect dissipates within 24 hours, volume expansion is relatively short-lived. Hydroxyethyl starch molecules are cleaved by amylases present in blood, parenchymal tissue, and the reticular endothelial system [9]. Cleavage causes mild hyperamylasemia but does not indicate pancreatitis. Similarly, hydroxyethyl starch infusion produces prolongation of the activated partial thromboplastin time that does not appear to be associated with clinically significant bleeding. Hydroxyethyl starch is used for volumes of infusion not to exceed 1,500 mL per day, though infusions of larger volumes in a 24-hour period appear well tolerated [1]. Hydroxyethyl starch should be administered with caution in individuals with significant coagulopathy or bleeding diathesis [1].

Dextrans are glucose polymers that are available in two preparations: 10% dextran 40 and 6% dextran 70, with molecular weights of 40 kdal and 70 kdal respectively [1]. Small dextran particles are rapidly renally excreted, while dextran molecules larger than 55 kdal possess half-lives of several days. Because of its significantly longer half-life, dextran 70 is more commonly used for volume expansion. A 6% dextran solution in an isotonic diluent is roughly comparable to a 6% hetastarch solution in capacity for volume expansion. The principal disadvantage of dextran solutions is coagulopathy. Dextran produces a dose-related reduction in platelet function and fibrin clot tensile strength, as well as an increase in fibrinolytic activity [1]. It is recommended that dextran infusions be limited to 20 mL/kg/d or 1.5 g/kg/d [1]. Dextrans are not widely used in the United States as a resuscitation fluid but are frequently used as an anticoagulant.

The major drawback to colloid use is cost. Relative to crystalloids, colloids cost seven times as much to achieve the same degree of volume expansion. Further, in addition to the adverse effects noted, colloids are associated with a very small risk of hypersensitivity (an incidence of 0.085% of infusions or less, depending on the preparation) [9].

Is Colloid Administration of Benefit for Resuscitation?

Debates on the potential advantages and disadvantages of crystalloid or colloid administration have largely centered on the relative efficiencies of these two classes of agents to achieve volume expansion, and, by extension, the effects of these relative volumes on clinically significant endpoints, such as development of acute lung injury and mortality.

The volume of crystalloid required for resuscitation can be as much as 12-fold greater than the volume of colloid solution required to reach the same hemodynamic endpoint (1). Given the unique biological profile of albumin (e.g., antioxidant, free radical scavenger, and drug transporter), coupled with the observation that hypoalbuminemia is associated with adverse outcomes in a number of disease states, there might be additional rationale for the use of albumin preparations as a resuscitation fluid (10,11). Despite 5 decades of experience with albumin use and reports from dozens of clinical trials, enrolling thousands of patients and examining the effects of albumin administration as well as the use of other colloids, little or no consensus exists on the relative merits of these agents.

The most recent information regarding the benefits or risks of colloid therapy in resuscitation is provided by several systematic literature analyses. (Fig. 14-1). In 1998 the Cochrane Group published a meta-analysis of 30 controlled trials enrolling over 1,400 patients in which albumin (or plasma protein fraction) infusion was compared to either crystalloid infusion or no specific treatment (12). Although there was no overall effect of colloids on survival in the setting of hypovolemia [relative risk of mortality with 95% confidence intervals (RR [95% CI]=146[0.97−2.22])], in two subgroups, patients with burns and hypoalbuminemia,

albumin administration was associated with an increased mortality risk [RR (95% CI)=2.40(1.11−5.19) and 1.69(1.07−2.67), respectively] (12). Following publication of this report, albumin use in the United Kingdom declined dramatically (13). Subsequently, Choi et al. reported a meta-analysis of 17 studies enrolling approximately 800 patients that compared infusion of isotonic crystalloids to albumin and other colloids (14). Although there was no difference comparing treatment groups with respect to the primary endpoints of mortality, pulmonary edema, or hospital length of stay, colloid infusion appeared to adversely effect survival in the subgroup of trauma patients (14). In addition, Wilkes et al. reported a meta-analysis of 55 trials enrolling 3,500 patients comparing crystalloid to albumin therapy. This analysis again demonstrated no statistically significant difference in overall mortality [RR (95% CI)= 1.11(0.95−1.28)] (10,15). Similar analyses have examined trials that compared crystalloid resuscitation to either dextran or hetastarch, with no discernable benefit for either class of colloid (16).

Meta-analyses are exploratory and hypothesis-generating, and they should not be considered a substitute for appropriately designed and controlled clinical trials (17). Nonetheless, these and other techniques of secondary data analysis are useful for summarizing large numbers of clinical

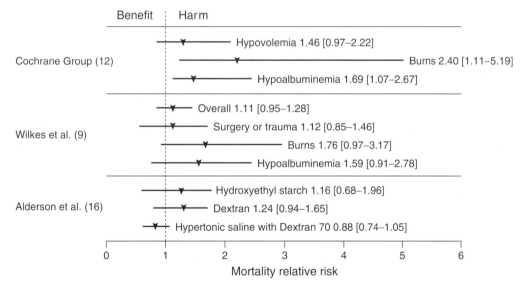

Figure 14-1 Meta-analyses of clinical studies comparing crystalloid and colloid resuscitation. Plots of point estimates of relative risk of mortality (triangle) with 95% confidence intervals (horizontal lines) for all patients and selective subgroups from metaanalyses of trials comparing crystalloids and colloids as a resuscitative strategy. Relative risk of 1 is consistent with no effect on mortality (vertical line), relative risk <1 is consistent with beneficial effect of colloid use relative to crystalloid use, and relative risk >1 is consistent with a harmful effect of colloid use relative to crystalloid use. Although many of the 95% confidence intervals include 1, the relative risk point estimates exceed 1 for many trials, consistent with an adverse effect on survival with colloid use. It is estimated that a trial enrolling approximately 6,000 patients would be necessary to convincingly demonstrate the effect of colloids as a resuscitation fluid. (From Wilkes MM, Navickis RJ. Patient survival after human albumin administration. *Ann Intern Med* 2001;135:149–164; Cochrane Injuries Group Albumin Reviewers. Human albumin administration in critically ill patients: systematic review of randomized controlled trials. *Br Med J* 1998;317:235–240; Cook DJ, Guyatt G. Colloid use for fluid resuscitation: evidence and spin. *Ann Intern Med* 2001;135:205–208; Alderson P, Schierhout G, Roberts I, et al. Colloids versus crystalloids for fluid resuscitation in critically ill patients. *The Cochrane Library* 2003;4, with permission.)

trials and for reconciling the results of conflicting reports. The studies cited raise interesting and potentially important questions on the safety and efficacy of colloid preparations as a resuscitation fluid (10,12,14). On the basis of the existing literature, if colloid preparations have a clinically important effect on survival, either positive or negative, that effect is small (e.g., <10% difference in mortality) and would require a study enrolling nearly 6,000 patients to demonstrate (15). In the absence of unequivocal clinical evidence and given the costs of most colloid preparations relative to crystalloids, it is difficult to recommend their routine use as a resuscitation fluid. These agents are licensed and approved for a variety of indications; whether they are likewise beneficial in these settings has not been convincingly demonstrated.

Hypertonic Saline

Hypertonic saline is a very efficient volume expander. For each milliliter of hypertonic saline infused, approximately 7 milliliters of free water is drawn into the extracellular space (1). The intravascular hypertonic benefit dissipates within 15 minutes as a result of equilibration between the intravascular and interstitial compartments. To achieve a more sustained effect, hypertonic saline is typically coinfused with a colloid. Most clinical trials have used dextran 70. Hypertonic saline infusion might be of theoretical benefit in patients following head trauma. By increasing systemic blood pressure, hypertonic saline improves cerebral blood flow. Unlike other crystalloids, hypertonicity antagonizes the development of cerebral edema and intracranial hypertension and might result in improvement of cerebral perfusion pressure (18). There have been several prospective, randomized evaluations to determine the feasibility of hypertonic saline as a prehospital resuscitation strategy. None of these studies showed a convincing benefit of hypertonic saline use (19–21). Similar findings were reported in a secondary data analysis, which involved 17 trials enrolling 869 patients (18) (Fig. 14-1). Given that the trials analyzed were small, included heterogeneous patient populations, and were of variable quality, the possibility that hypertonic saline might be of benefit could not be excluded (18). This hypothesis requires testing in an adequately powered prospective trial. At present this agent is not recommended for routine use. There has been recent renewed interest in hypertonic saline because of in vitro data suggesting that this agent might both favorably modulate the inflammatory response and enhance microcirculatory perfusion (22–24). Whether these observations will translate into clinical efficacy in selected settings, such as septic shock, awaits validation.

CONCLUSION

Despite a history of more than 150 years, intravenous fluid therapy continues to be an area of debate and investigation (25). This chapter has attempted an evidence-based approach to guide prescription of representative commercially available intravenous fluids. With the exceptions noted, the predominant crystalloid solutions (e.g., lactated Ringer solution or 0.9% NaCl) and their respective derivatives might be used interchangeably as maintenance therapy and resuscitation fluids. Use of these agents as replacement fluids should be individualized to the clinical situation. The bulk of clinical evidence does not suggest that colloid solutions provide benefit over crystalloids as a resuscitation strategy. However, given the heterogeneity of the studies published to date, both with respect to populations of patients enrolled and quality, one cannot rule out that colloid resuscitation might be of benefit in selected circumstances. As evidenced by recent *in vitro* investigations of hypertonic saline, future uses of intravenous fluids might possess therapeutic value beyond volume and electrolyte replenishment.

REFERENCES

1. Rainey TG, Read CA. Pharmacology of colloids and crystalloids. In: Chernow B, ed. *The pharmacological approach to the critically ill patient*. Baltimore, MD: Williams & Wilkins; 1994:272–290.
2. Marino PL. Colloid and crystalloid resuscitation. In: Marino PL, ed. *The ICU book*, 2nd ed. Baltimore, MD: Williams & Wilkins; 1998:228–241.
3. Jonasson O. Surgical aspects of diabetes mellitus. In: Sabiston DC, Lyerly HK, eds. *Textbook of surgery*, 15th ed. Philadelphia, PA: WB Saunders; 1997:176–185.
4. Degoute CS, Ray MJ, Manchon M, et al. Intraoperative glucose infusion and blood lactate: endocrine and metabolic relationships during abdominal aortic surgery. *Anesthesiology* 1989;71: 355–361.
5. Talpers SS, Romberger DJ, Bunce SB, et al. Nutritionally associated increased carbon dioxide production. *Chest* 1992;102: 551–555.
6. O' Flaherty D, Giesecke AH. Crystalloid fluid therapy. In: Nimmo WS, Rombotham DJ, Smith G, eds. *Anaesthesia*. London: Blackwell Scientific Publications; 1994: 554–567.
7. Lobo DN, Bostock KA, Neal KR, et al. Effect of salt and water balance on recovery of gastrointestinal function after elective colonic resection: a randomized controlled trial. *Lancet* 2002; 359:1812–1818.
8. Freeman BD, Natanson C. Hypotension, shock, and multiple organ failure. In: Wachter RM, Goldman L, Hollander H, eds. *Hospital medicine*. Baltimore, MD: Lippincott Williams & Wilkins; 2000:123–132.
9. Ratner LE, Smith GW. Intraoperative fluid management. *Surg Clin North Am* 1993;73:229–241.
10. Wilkes MM, Navickis RJ. Patient survival after human albumin administration. *Ann Intern Med* 2001;135:149–164.
11. Goldwasser P, Feldman J. Association of serum albumin and mortality risk. *J Clin Epidemiol* 1997;50:693–703.
12. Cochrane Injuries Group Albumin Reviewers. Human albumin administration in critically ill patients: systematic review of randomized controlled trials. *Br Med J* 1998;317:235–240.
13. Roberts I, Edwards P, McLelland B. More on albumin. Use of human albumin in UK fell substantially when systematic review was published. *Br Med J* 1999;318:1214–1215.
14. Choi PTL, Yip G, Quinonez LG, et al. Crystalloids vs. colloids in fluid resuscitation: a systematic review. *Crit Care Med* 1999;27: 200–210.
15. Cook DJ, Guyatt G. Colloid use for fluid resuscitation: evidence and spin. *Ann Intern Med* 2001;135:205–208.
16. Alderson P, Schierhout G, Roberts I, et al. Colloids versus crystalloids for fluid resuscitation in critically ill patients. *The Cochrane Library* 2003;4.

17. Freeman BD, Gerstenberger EP, Banks S. Using secondary data in statistical analysis. In: Gallin JI, ed. *Principles and practice of clinical research*. San Diego, CA: Academic Press; 2002: 251–257.

18. Bunn F, Robert I, Tasker R, et al. Hypertonic versus isotonic crystalloid for fluid resuscitation in critically ill patients (Cochrane Review). *The Cochrane Library* 2003.

19. Mattox KL, Maningas PA, Moore EE, et al. Prehospital hypertonic saline/dextran infusion for post-traumatic hypotension. *Ann Surg* 1991;213:482–491.

20. Vassar MJ, Fischer RP, O'Brien PE, et al. A multicenter trial of resuscitation of injured patients with 7.5% sodium chloride. *Arch Surg* 1993;128:1003–1013.

21. Wade CE, Kramer GC, Grady JJ, et al. Efficacy of hypertonic 7.5% saline and 6% dextran-70 in treating trauma: a meta-analysis of controlled clinical trials. *Surgery* 1997;122: 609–616.

22. Gushchin V, Alam HB, Rhee P, et al. cDNA profiling in leukocytes exposed to hypertonic resuscitation fluids. *J Am Coll Surg* 2003;197:426–432.

23. Shields CJ, O'Sullivan AW, Wang JH, et al. Hypertonic saline enhances host response to bacterial challenge by augmenting receptor-independent neutrophil intracellular superoxide formation. *Ann Surg* 2003;238:249–257.

24. Pascual JL, Khwaja KA, Chaudhury P, et al. Hypertonic saline and the microcirculation. *J Trauma* 2003;54:S133–S140.

25. Cosnett JE. The origins of intravenous fluid therapy. *Lancet* 1989;333:768–771.

Acute Renal Failure

15

Kareem D. Husain   Craig M. Coopersmith

■■■ DEFINITION AND EPIDEMIOLOGY 150

■■■ PERIOPERATIVE RISK 151

■■■ DIAGNOSIS AND CLASSIFICATION 152

■■■ PREVENTION 152

    Maintenance of Intravascular Blood Volume 152
    Prevention of Contrast-induced Nephropathy 153
    Dopamine and Dopamine Agonists 154
    Loop Diuretics 154
    Other Agents 154

■■■ MANAGEMENT 155

■■■ SUMMARY 155

■■■ REFERENCES 156

DEFINITION AND EPIDEMIOLOGY

Acute renal failure (ARF) is commonly recognized as an abrupt loss and sustained decline in glomerular filtration rate (GFR) leading to the accumulation of nitrogenous wastes and other toxins. Proposed definitions of ARF include (a) acute increase in serum creatinine of 0.5 mg per dL if the baseline level is <2.5 mg per dL or an increase in creatinine by >20% if the baseline level is >2.5 mg per dL, (b) an increase in serum creatinine of 50% over baseline, a reduction in the calculated creatinine clearance of 50%, or a decrease in renal function resulting in the need for dialysis, and (c) an elevation in the serum creatinine concentration of 1.5 mg/dL/d with urine output <410 mL per day and no preexisting chronic dialysis (1–3).

ARF develops in 2% to 7% of hospitalized patients, an incidence that has remained stable for the last 20 years. Approximately 0.5% of hospitalized patients eventually require dialysis for this condition. Surgery is a common cause of ARF and accounts for 20% to 50% of all hospital-acquired cases, making it the second most common cause of hospital-acquired ARF. The overall incidence of postoperative ARF is 1.2%, but it ranges from 0% to 31% depending on the procedure performed. Thoracoabdominal aneurysm repair, suprarenal or emergency abdominal aortic aneurysm repair, cardiac surgery, hepatic transplant, and operation in the presence of obstructive jaundice result in the highest risk of postoperative renal failure. In addition, 2% of patients receiving radiocontrast dye for CT scans or angiography develop ARF.

The need for dialysis after postoperative ARF depends on the renal failure's severity and duration. Absolute indications for dialysis include severe hyperkalemia, acidosis, and volume overload. Uremia is a relative indication. The need for dialysis markedly changes survival in ARF. A prospective randomized trial of over 40,000 Veterans Administration patients undergoing cardiac surgery demonstrated a 30-day mortality of 64% in patients with ARF requiring dialysis compared to 4% mortality in patients without ARF (3).

Although most people who develop ARF in the postoperative setting recover at least some of their renal function, up to 17% require chronic dialysis. Mortality from ARF ranges from 10% to 20% in mild cases to 40% to 60% in more severe cases (an increase in serum creatinine of

Kareem D. Husain: Barnes-Jewish Hospital, St. Louis, MO 63110
Craig M. Coopersmith: Washington University School of Medicine, St. Louis, MO 63110

>3.0 mg per dL and requirement of renal replacement therapy) to 70% to 90% in the cases requiring intensive care unit (ICU) treatment.

The economic cost of ARF is significant as well. One study of patients undergoing esophageal or hepatic resection in which 2.6% of patients developed ARF estimated the added cost of this complication to be >$25,000 per patient (4).

PERIOPERATIVE RISK

Perioperative risk factors associated with the development of ARF are summarized in Table 15-1. Preexisting renal insufficiency and diabetes markedly increase a patient's risk of developing ARF in the postoperative setting. Aminoglycoside antibiotics, radiocontrast dye, arterial thromboembolism, and cardiovascular surgery disproportionately increase the risk of ARF developing in patients with preexisting renal insufficiency. In addition, diabetics have a 7% reported incidence of ARF following general surgical procedures, and this value increases to 20% to 30% in diabetic patients with concomitant infection, peripheral vascular disease, and/or peripheral neuropathy (2). Diabetics also have a 10-fold greater risk of deteriorating renal function in the presence of hypovolemia. Both patients with preexisting renal insufficiency and diabetes mellitus are particularly susceptible to toxic reactions to radiocontrast dye.

TABLE 15-1

PERIOPERATIVE RISK FACTORS ASSOCIATED WITH ARF

Preexisting renal insufficiency
Diabetes mellitus
Increased age
Male gender
Use of nephrotoxic drugs and agents
Sepsis
Hyperbilirubinemia/jaundice
Left ventricular dysfunction
Increased intraabdominal pressure (IAP)
Chronic disease
    COPD
    Coronary artery disease
    Peripheral vascular disease
    Hypertension
    Cirrhosis
    Cerebral vascular disease
    Renal disease
Type of operation
    Cardiac
    Biliary
    Relief of obstructive jaundice
    Thoracoabdominal
    Liver transplant

Hypertension, peripheral vascular disease, preexisting cardiovascular and respiratory disease, cirrhosis, massive blood transfusion, an ejection fraction of <35% or cardiac index <1.7 L/min/m^2, and male gender are all risk factors for developing ARF.

The elderly are especially susceptible to ARF because of the aging kidney's loss of functional reserve and inability to withstand acute insults. Since GFR decreases with age, elderly patients are more susceptible to volume depletion secondary to an aged kidney's inability to conserve salt and maximally concentrate urine.

Sepsis also increases the risk of ARF in the perioperative setting. The incidence of ARF is 16% in septic surgical ICU patients, compared to 1% to 7% in nonseptic ICU patients (5). ARF usually occurs 3 days after the onset of sepsis and is associated with an increase in both morbidity and mortality.

One underrecognized risk factor for perioperative ARF is elevated intra-abdominal pressure. Elevated intra-abdominal pressure can lead to abdominal compartment syndrome, which might cause total renal failure in addition to a number of other life-threatening abnormalities. Either acute or chronic factors can contribute to elevated intra-abdominal pressure, but the devastating effects of abdominal compartment syndrome are typically seen when elevations in intra-abdominal pressure are acute (6). Although trauma and intraoperative or postoperative hemorrhage remain the most common etiologies of abdominal compartment syndrome, the number of entities that are known to cause this disorder is rapidly expanding and includes tight abdominal closures, compression by burn eschars, pancreatitis, and as a complication of ascites formation, endoscopy, percutaneous tracheostomy, mesenteric revascularization, and pneumothorax tracking into the abdominal cavity. Normal intra-abdominal pressure is 0 to 12 mm Hg (average 6 mm Hg), and renal pathophysiology is not related to abdominal pressure at this level. Renal abnormalities might be detectable when abdominal pressure reaches 15 to 20 mm Hg. Between 20 and 35 mm Hg, no clear guidelines exist on when a patient has abdominal compartment syndrome, other than the general definition that a patient has the syndrome when the patient's intra-abdominal pressure is high enough to cause organ dysfunction. In the acute setting, when abdominal pressures are greater than 35 mm Hg, patients frequently have anuria, and abdominal decompression is emergently indicated as a life-saving measure.

Although iatrogenic injury to the renal collecting system during an operation cannot always be avoided, its incidence can be minimized with careful preoperative planning and intraoperative technique. Any patient whose ureters are expected to be difficult to identify during laparotomy should have ureteral stents placed preoperatively. Intraoperative identification of the ureters must also be performed during any case in which dissection or electrocautery, or both, could result in their inadvertent division.

DIAGNOSIS AND CLASSIFICATION

An accurate assessment of the etiology of ARF is crucial to prevent further worsening of renal function and to treat reversible causes. A thorough history (including recent medications and exposure to radiocontrast dye), physical examination, and proper diagnostic testing will lead to the best clinical management of these patients. Initial laboratory measurements should include a basic metabolic profile, urine electrolytes with calculation of a fractional excretion of sodium (FE_{Na}), urinalysis, and measurement of urine osmolality.

ARF may be classified by etiology or amount of urine made per day. For diagnostic and therapeutic purposes, ARF is divided into prerenal (12% to 60% of cases), intrarenal (20% to 80% of cases), and postrenal (1% to 10% of cases) causes. Diagnostic laboratory findings in ARF are summarized in Table 15-2. Although the calculated FE_{Na} is often used to determine the category of ARF, with a value <1% usually signifying a prerenal cause, contrast-induced nephropathy and sepsis can also be associated with a low FE_{Na}.

The differential diagnosis of common causes of prerenal, intrarenal and postrenal failure in the surgical patient is listed in Table 15-3. Because obstruction can lead to postrenal ARF, assessment of Foley catheter patency should always accompany the examination of an oliguric patient. If warranted by the clinical situation, a renal ultrasound should be obtained since hydronephrosis might be a sign of postrenal ARF.

Patients with ARF can also be subdivided into those with nonoliguric (urine output >400 mL per day), oliguric (urine output <400 mL per day), and anuric renal failure (urine output <50 mL per day). Patients with nonoliguric renal failure have a better prognosis, although there is no evidence that "converting" oliguric ARF to nonoliguric ARF with diuretics improves outcome.

PREVENTION

Despite decades of research in how to prevent ARF, very few interventions have been reproducibly successful. An overview of interventions that have been proposed or studied, or both, to prevent ARF are listed in Table 15-4.

Maintenance of Intravascular Blood Volume

The single most important way to prevent perioperative ARF is to maintain adequate intravascular volume. Depending on the clinical situation, this may range from aggressive fluid administration with isotonic crystalloids or colloids to keeping the patient on maintenance fluids to balance the patient's insensible losses. When the patient has an adequate cardiac function, euvolemia ensures sufficient renal blood flow, reduces vasoconstrictive stimuli, and improves urine flow.

It is essential to determine whether the cause of renal insufficiency is prerenal hypoperfusion or an intrinsic event such as acute tubular necrosis (ATN) because prerenal ARF is completely reversible if renal perfusion and glomerular filtration pressure are restored rapidly. Assessment of intravascular volume status is based on physical examination, urine output, laboratory values, and, potentially, invasive monitoring. Depending on the severity of hypovolemia, the patient might present along a spectrum from subtle signs to cardiovascular collapse. The simplest way to examine volume status is by urine output. A hydrated patient without a Foley catheter in place should void at least once every 8 hours and make 0.5 mL/kg/hr (280 mL per shift in a 70 kg person). If urine output appears inadequate, placement of a Foley catheter will aid in monitoring urine volume. Two common clinical scenarios that result in seemingly adequate urine output despite intravascular hypovolemia are hyperglycemia (an obligate osmotic diuresis can begin with glucose levels >180 mg per dL) and recent diuretic administration. Patients with elevated blood glucose or those who receive diuretics intraoperatively therefore require special attention to their volume status since they can become markedly intravascularly depleted and yet still appear to have adequate urine output.

Oliguria in the postoperative period usually reflects hypovolemia. In addition to maintenance fluids and replacement of blood loss, intraoperative insensible losses

TABLE 15-2

DIAGNOSIS OF ARF

Condition	BUN/Cr Ratio	Urinalysis	FE_{Na}	Urine Na	Urine Osmolality
Prerenal ARF	>20 mg/dL	Hyaline casts, trace or no proteinuria	<1%	<10 mEq/L	>500 mOsm
Intrarenal ARF	10–15 mg/dL	RBCs±WBCs, tubular epithelial cells, myoglobinuria, eosinophiluria, proteinuria	>1–3%	>20 mEq/L	250–350 mOsm
Postrenal ARF	10–15 mg/dL	Normal±hematuria, cellular debris	>1–3%		<350 mOsm

FE_{Na}, fractional excretion of sodium.

TABLE 15-3

ACUTE RENAL FAILURE IN THE SURGICAL SETTING

Prerenal ARF (renal hypoperfusion)
    Hypovolemia/trauma
    GI losses
    Hypotension
    Cardiac failure
    Sepsis
    Arterial vasoconstriction/obstruction
    ACE inhibitors
    NSAIDs
    Abdominal compartment syndrome
Intrarenal ARF
    Pharmacological agents
        Aminoglycoside antibiotics
        Radiocontrast dye
        Amphotericin B
        Cyclosporins
        Cisplatin
        NSAIDs
        Low molecular weight dextran
    Myoglobinuria (rhabdomyolysis)
    Pyelonephritis
    Preexisting renal disease
    Gram-negative endotoxin
    Hemoglobinuria (hemolysis)
    Uric acid
    Bilirubinemia
Postrenal ARF
    Ureteral obstruction or injury (stones, surgery, trauma)
    Urethral obstruction or injury (BPH, malignancy, trauma)
    Bladder dysfunction or injury (anesthesia, neural injury, obstruction)

ARF, acute renal failure; GI, gastrointestinal; ACE, angiotensin-converting enzyme; NSAIDs, nonsteroidal anti-inflammatory drugs; BPH, benign prostatic hyperplasia.

TABLE 15-4

PREVENTIVE MEASURES FOR MINIMIZING PERIOPERATIVE ARF

Definitely helpful
Aggressive maintenance of intravascular volume with appropriate fluid administration
Avoidance of nephrotoxic agents

Likely helpful
Acetylcysteine for contrast-induced nephropathy

Possibly helpful
Hemofiltration for patients with serum creatinine >2.0 mg/dL for contrast-induced nephropathy
Fenoldopam after aortic or cardiac surgery
Operative avoidance of ischemic injury
Sodium bicarbonate for contrast-induced nephropathy
Mannitol for rhabdomyolysis

Unlikely to be helpful
Loop diuretics
Adenosine antagonists

Not helpful
"Renal dose" dopamine
Atrial natriuretic peptide
Calcium channel blockers
Insulin-like growth factor-1

might be estimated to be 1 to 3 mL/kg/hr for a small incision, 3 to 7 mL/kg/hr for a medium incision, and 9 to 11 mL/kg/hr for a large incision. Although the anesthesiologist should perform adequate fluid resuscitation intraoperatively, the surgeon must verify each patient's fluid balance in the immediate postoperative period and administer additional fluid if necessary. Nearly all patients with oliguria in the perioperative period are able to tolerate two boluses of 500 mL of isotonic crystalloid solution or a single bolus of 500 mL of a colloid. Special care should be given to patients with a severely decreased left ventricular ejection fraction, patients who are dependent on high dose diuretic preoperatively, and patients whose operation would not be expected to result in postoperative hypovolemia.

In patients who do not respond to initial fluid boluses, the physician must decide whether to administer additional fluid boluses or to obtain additional monitoring. No universal guidelines can dictate what constitutes a "reasonable" amount of fluid administration before pursuing additional monitoring. However, patients with larger incisions and longer operations might require more fluid than an average surgical patient, and younger patients generally tolerate fluid overload better than older ones. For patients in whom additional information is needed to estimate intravascular volume, central venous pressure (CVP) provides a useful reflection of right heart filling pressures. In cases in which the CVP is a poor estimate of left heart filling volumes (as occurs with significant valvular disease or pulmonary hypertension), a Swan-Ganz catheter or esophageal echocardiogram might be useful. In general, there is a paucity of convincing evidence that these devices prevent renal failure or improve outcomes, although maintaining intravascular volume according to CVP or wedge pressure reduces the incidence of postoperative ARF in thoracoabdominal aortic aneurysm repair. In the unusual state that a poor cardiac output limits renal blood flow, inotropic agents might be necessary as an adjuvant to proper fluid administration.

Prevention of Contrast-induced Nephropathy

Contrast-induced nephropathy accounts for 10% of ARF in hospitalized patients. Although nephropathy induced by radiocontrast dye is uncommon in patients with normal renal function, its incidence increases to 5% in patients with mild renal insufficiency and to 50% in those with severe renal dysfunction and diabetes.

Acetylcysteine, a glutathione precursor and oxygen free-radical scavenger, has been extensively studied for prevention of contrast-induced nephropathy. Results vary somewhat, but the preponderance of evidence suggests that acetylcysteine combined with adequate hydration leads to a smaller rise in serum creatinine than hydration alone, regardless of whether contrast is given for a CT scan or for angiography. A meta-analysis of seven recent trials with over 800 patients shows this improvement is not related to the amount of radiocontrast dye given nor to the degree of renal insufficiency before the dye load is given (7). Although doses vary slightly between studies, a common dosage of acetylcysteine is 600 mg given orally twice a day for 24 hours prior to administration of radiocontrast, followed by the same dose for 1 day following procedure.

Although dye-induced ATN is rarely significant enough to require hemodialysis, patients with higher baseline serum creatinine have a greater chance of requiring renal replacement therapy after receiving radiocontrast. Although acetylcysteine appears to prevent a rise in creatinine after radiocontrast, there is no convincing evidence that it alters the need for dialysis. Patients with a baseline creatinine of >2.0 mg per dL who receive hemofiltration 4 to 8 hours before and 18 to 24 hours after dye load for coronary angiography appear to have a decreased need for longer-term dialysis after radiocontrast. In a recent study of 114 patients who met these criteria, 25% of control patients (hydration alone) required dialysis compared to 3% of patients treated with prophylactic hemofiltration (8). The relevance of this study to ARF in the perioperative period remains to be demonstrated.

A single study has also recently been published comparing the efficacy of hydration with sodium bicarbonate to hydration with sodium chloride for the prevention of contrast-induced nephropathy (9). In this single center trial of 119 patients, the incidence of contrast-induced nephropathy was 13.6% in patients receiving sodium chloride but only 1.7% in patients who received a sodium bicarbonate bolus of 3 mL per kg over 1 hour before contrast and 1 mL/kg/hr for 6 hours after contrast. No patient in either group required dialysis. Similar to n-acetylcysteine, sodium bicarbonate is postulated to work as a free-radical scavenger. There are no data on the efficacy of combining n-acetylcysteine with sodium bicarbonate hydration, nor are there data on the use of this agent in the perioperative period.

Dopamine and Dopamine Agonists

Low-dose ("renal dose," 1 to 3 µg/kg/min) dopamine has been studied for over 30 years and is still widely used by many practitioners. Although numerous theoretical benefits of low-dose dopamine exist, it is an ineffective agent in preventing ARF. Although low-dose dopamine is frequently successful in improving urinary output, it does not alter mortality, need for dialysis, or onset of ARF. A recent prospective randomized trial of this agent in patients with the systemic inflammatory response syndrome and oliguria (10), as well as a recent meta-analysis of 24 studies

involving over 1,000 patients, demonstrate this (11). Because low-dose dopamine might worsen splanchnic oxygenation, impair GI function, impair endocrine and immunologic systems, and blunt ventilatory drive while not preventing ARF, dialysis, or mortality, this strategy should not be used in clinical practice.

Dopamine agonists have also received a great deal of attention in the management of ARF. Like dopamine, the selective dopamine-1 agonist fenoldopam mesylate has been shown to increase renal blood flow, urine output, and sodium excretion. In multiple small prospective trials, fenoldopam decreased the risk of postoperative ARF following abdominal aortic aneurysm repair and coronary artery bypass (1), but it does not prevent further renal deterioration in patients with chronic renal insufficiency receiving radiocontrast (12). Large-scale trials are necessary to determine if fenoldopam should be used in high-risk patients for the prevention of ARF.

Loop Diuretics

Loop diuretics such as furosemide are commonly used in the setting of developing ARF since they frequently "convert" oliguric renal failure into nonoliguric failure, and nonoliguric failure is associated with improved outcomes. However, few data support the notion that loop diuretics change outcome. A recent retrospective study of 552 patients with ARF in the ICU (not all surgical patients) demonstrated a 68% increased risk of in-hospital mortality and a 77% increase in odds of death or nonrecovery of renal function in patients treated with diuretics (13). In addition, three small randomized trials (including one following cardiac surgery) demonstrated that diuretics do not change mortality or the need for dialysis. On the basis of these data, diuretic usage cannot be recommended for perioperative ARF.

Other Agents

Adenosine antagonists might protect patients from renal ischemia due to a decrease in oxygen delivery to the renal medulla. The administration of theophylline in patients receiving radiocontrast slightly lessens the reduction in GFR. Additionally, aminophylline administration to patients following major abdominal surgery causes an increase in renal sodium and osmolar clearance and diuresis. Further studies are required to assess adenosine antagonists as potential therapeutic tools for ARF.

In vascular surgery, ischemia/reperfusion injury commonly occurs, and perioperative procedures can be used to bypass areas of surgical manipulation and maintain perfusion of vital organs. In general, such strategies are not beneficial, but they might have a role in patients with renal and/or abdominal occlusive vascular disease who might otherwise have little or no perfusion to the kidneys for a significant time during operation.

Atrial natriuretic peptide, insulin-like growth factor, and calcium blockers have all been proposed as potential renoprotective agents in surgical patients. Although preclinical and small studies were promising to varied degrees with each agent, no benefit or potential harm is evident in larger trials and none of these is currently recommended for clinical use.

MANAGEMENT

Management of ARF is generally supportive. Adequate intravascular volume and cardiac output must be maintained, as inadequate renal perfusion can worsen ARF. For patients with severe ARF, renal replacement is the definitive therapeutic intervention. Absolute indications for dialysis include symptomatic volume overload that cannot be managed with fluid restriction or diuretic usage, or both, electrolyte abnormalities (most commonly hyperkalemia), and severe acidosis. Symptomatic uremia associated with a blood urea nitrogen level >100 mg per dL represents a relative indication. Renal replacement can take the form of intermittent hemodialysis or continuous renal replacement therapy. Continuous renal replacement requires lower flows in the dialysis circuit and causes less hemodynamic instability than intermittent dialysis and can be especially useful for hypotensive patients. Outcomes have not been documented to be different between intermittent and continuous hemodialysis. A recently published prospective, randomized trial of surgical and medical ICU patients demonstrated improved survival with daily hemodialysis compared to hemodialysis every other day (14). Subsequent concerns have been raised about dialysis clearance in this study's control group, and the benefit of daily dialysis remains unproven.

Temporary dialysis in perioperative patients with ARF is typically initiated through a large bore, double lumen central venous catheter. The preferred site is the right internal jugular vein, which yields consistent flow rates and is technically simple (note: this is one of the few instances that this anatomic site is preferred over the subclavian vein for vascular access, secondary to the increased risk of infection in catheters placed in the internal jugular vein). Complications of dialysis catheters are similar to those seen with the placement of any central venous catheter. Immediate complications include pneumothorax, arterial cannulation, bleeding, and air embolism. A common delayed complication is catheter-related bloodstream infection. Catheter-related bloodstream infection is manifested by fever, leukocytosis, and hypotension in severe cases, and although this complication can occur at any time the risk of infection increases the longer the vascular access device is in place. If no other source of infection is apparent, the catheter should be removed and two sets of blood cultures should be drawn.

The patient should also be started on broad-spectrum antibiotics until culture results are known. The decision to remove or keep a dialysis catheter in a septic patient with another possible source of infection must be made on an individual basis. Another frequent complication of dialysis access is thrombosis of the vessel in which the catheter has been placed. Thrombosis is frequently clinically silent but can have significant implications for long-term dialysis access if a patient's renal failure does not resolve.

Patients with chronic renal failure should be dialyzed through their previously placed arteriovenous fistula (or much less commonly their peritoneal dialysis catheter). Although surgery at another site should not affect continuation of dialysis per se, perioperative hypotension increases the risk of thrombosis of a previously patent fistula and should be avoided if possible.

One cause of renal failure that occurs disproportionately in the trauma surgery population is rhabdomyolysis. The treatment of ARF due to rhabdomyolysis, as with other forms of renal failure, is supportive, with emphasis placed on maintenance of intravascular volume. Because renal damage results from the mechanical obstruction of tubules by myoglobin, there are theoretical advantages to enforcing diuresis (with adequate intravascular volume). Mannitol, an osmotic diuretic that does not enter cells and is freely filtered and not reabsorbed by the tubules, not only flushes necrotic tubular debris from nephrons but also has free-radical scavenging properties. The evidence supporting mannitol is based on experimental animal studies and retrospective clinical studies, and there is no clear evidence demonstrating its efficacy in preventing or treating ARF in rhabdomyolysis. Maintaining an alkaline (pH >6.5) urine has also been advocated in the treatment of rhabdomyolysis to decrease the toxicity of myoglobin to renal tubules. There is no clear evidence in patients to determine the efficacy of alkalinizing the urine.

SUMMARY

Although ARF is relatively common in the perioperative setting, especially in high-risk patients, few proven interventions prevent its occurrence. Maintenance of adequate intravascular volume and avoidance of nephrotoxic agents are clearly beneficial. In patients with some degree of renal insufficiency who require a dye load for either a CT scan or angiography, acetylcysteine is likely more effective than hydration alone in preventing a rise in creatinine, although whether this prevents the need for dialysis in high-risk patients is uncertain, and hydration with sodium bicarbonate might be more effective than with sodium chloride. Many pharmacologic therapies that have been proposed to prevent ARF are either unproven or are clearly not helpful. Low-dose dopamine has been conclusively shown to have no role in preventing ARF, and the use of diuretics to convert oliguric ATN to nonoliguric ATN should be discouraged. Treatment of ARF is supportive, with maintenance of adequate vascular volume playing an important role. Either intermittent or continuous hemodialysis is appropriate for patients who need renal replacement therapy, depending on the patient's hemodynamic status.

REFERENCES

1. Singri N, Ahya SN, Levin ML. Acute renal failure. *JAMA* 2003; 289(6):747–751.
2. Carmichael P, Carmichael AR. Acute renal failure in the surgical setting. *ANZ J Surg* 2003;73(3):144–153.
3. Chertow GM, Lazarus JM, Christiansen CL, et al. Preoperative renal risk stratification. *Circulation* 1997;95(4):878–884.
4. Dimick JB, Pronovost PJ, Cowan JA, et al. Complications and costs after high-risk surgery: where should we focus quality improvement initiatives? *J Am Coll Surg* 2003;196(5):671–678.
5. Hoste EA, Lameire NH, Vanholder RC, et al. Acute renal failure in patients with sepsis in a surgical ICU: predictive factors, incidence, comorbidity, and outcome. *J Am Soc Nephrol* 2003;14(4): 1022–1030.
6. Saggi BH, Sugerman HJ, Ivatury RR, et al. Abdominal compartment syndrome. *J Trauma* 1998;45(3):597–609.
7. Birck R, Krzossok S, Markowetz F, et al. Acetylcysteine for prevention of contrast nephropathy: meta-analysis. *Lancet* 2003; 362(9384):598–603.
8. Marenzi G, Marana I, Lauri G, et al. The prevention of radiocontrast-agent-induced nephropathy by hemofiltration. *N Engl J Med* 2003;349(14):1333–1340.
9. Merten GJ, Burgess WP, Gray LV, et al. Prevention of contrast-induced nephropathy with sodium bicarbonate. *JAMA* 2004;291: 2328–2334.
10. Bellomo R, Chapman M, Finfer S, et al. Australian and New Zealand Intensive Care Society (ANZICS) Clinical Trials Group. Low-dose dopamine in patients with early renal dysfunction: a placebo-controlled randomised trial. *Ann Intern Med* 2000; 356(9248):2139–2143.
11. Kellum JA, Decker M. Use of dopamine in acute renal failure: a meta-analysis. *Crit Care Med* 2001;29(8):1526–1531.
12. Stone GW, McCullough PA, Tumlin JA, et al. Fenoldopam mesylate for the prevention of contrast-induced nephropathy: a randomized controlled trial. *JAMA* 2003;290(17):2284–2291.
13. Mehta RL, Pascual MT, Soroko S, et al. Diuretics, mortality, and nonrecovery of renal function in acute renal failure. *JAMA* 2002; 288(20):2547–2553.
14. Schiffl H, Lang SM, Fischer R. Daily hemodialysis and the outcome of acute renal failure. *N Engl J Med* 2002;346(5):305–310.

Pulmonary Complications

16

Mark R. Hemmila

■ **INTRODUCTION** 157

■ **PREOPERATIVE PULMONARY FUNCTION** 157
Preoperative Assessment 159

■ **ACUTE PULMONARY COMPROMISE** 160
Loss of Airway 160
Tension Pneumothorax 161

■ **SMOKE INHALATION AND BURNS** 161
Smoke Inhalation 161
Carbon Monoxide Poisoning 162

■ **ASPIRATION PNEUMONIA** 163
Chemical Pneumonitis 163
Bacterial Pneumonia 164
Mechanical Obstruction 164

■ **NOSOCOMIAL PNEUMONIA** 164
Risk Factors, Etiology, and Prevention 164
Diagnosis and Treatment 165

■ **ACUTE RESPIRATORY DISTRESS SYNDROME** 166
Permissive Hypercapnia 167
Intratracheal Pulmonary Ventilation 167
Pressure Control and Inverse Ratio Ventilation 169
Open Lung Approach 169
Prone Positioning 170
Corticosteroids 170
Extracorporeal Life Support 170

■ **REFERENCES** 171

Mark R. Hemmila: University of Michigan, Ann Arbor, MI 48109

INTRODUCTION

The fire of life is maintained by the oxidation of metabolic substrates and the production of carbon dioxide. This creates the kinetic energy that sustains all bodily functions. As a vital organ, the lungs serve a dual role in allowing the absorption of oxygen gas into the body and the excretion of carbon dioxide to the atmosphere. For surgical patients undergoing elective or emergent operation, safe airway management and maintenance of optimal pulmonary function are paramount to successful perioperative care. Pulmonary complications can occur on multiple levels and at varying rates of clinical urgency. The successful clinician lives by the rule that "chance favors the prepared mind" and is ever vigilant for compromise in a patient's pulmonary function.

Pulmonary complications span a wide range of different etiologies but have a similar result in that they affect either oxygenation or ventilation of the patient. The following is a discussion of risk for pulmonary complications, diagnosis, and management of life-threatening pulmonary problems. The pathogenesis, clinical presentation, prevention, and treatment of severe pulmonary insufficiency will be covered. Basic management of mechanical ventilation in the surgical patient with acute lung injury will also be described, along with novel strategies to manage patients with severe acute respiratory distress syndrome (ARDS).

PREOPERATIVE PULMONARY FUNCTION

Preoperative assessment of respiratory status and identification of high-risk patients is of critical importance in preventing pulmonary complications in surgery patients.

TABLE 16-1

RISK FACTORS FOR DEVELOPING POSTOPERATIVE PULMONARY COMPLICATIONS

Definite risk factors
Chronic obstructive lung disease
Cessation of smoking less than 8 weeks prior to surgery
Current smoking history
Poor general health status, defined as ASA class >2
Serum albumin <3 g/dL
BUN >30 mg/dL
Surgery lasting >3 hours
Use of pancuronium as a neuromuscular blocker

Probable risk factors
General anesthesia
Emergency surgery
$PaCO_2$ >45 mm Hg

Possible risk factors
Current upper respiratory tract infection
Abnormal chest x-ray
Age >70 years

From Smetana GW. Evaluation of preoperative pulmonary risk. UpToDate 11.3 available online at: http://www.utdol.com. Accessed December 28, 2003, with permission.

Several potential factors increase the risk of developing pulmonary complications during or following surgery, as outlined in Table 16-1. A respiratory complication is defined as any pulmonary abnormality that produces identifiable disease or dysfunction that is clinically significant and impairs a patient's clinical course (1–4). Important examples of clinically significant pulmonary complications include atelectasis, pneumonia, respiratory failure with prolonged mechanical ventilation, exacerbation of underlying chronic lung disease, and bronchospasm (4). Patient-related risk factors that increase the risk of postoperative pulmonary complications are smoking, poor general health status, metabolic abnormalities, and chronic obstructive pulmonary disease (COPD) (4).

Smoking is a known and repeatedly demonstrated risk factor for postoperative pulmonary complications. Smoking increases the relative risk of pulmonary complications among all patients who smoke as compared to nonsmokers by an odds ratio (OR) of 1.4 to 4.3 (5–7). This increased risk among smokers extends to those without chronic lung disease (5). In a prospective study of 200 patients who underwent coronary artery bypass surgery, there was a lower risk of pulmonary complications in patients who stopped smoking at least 8 weeks prior to surgery than in current smokers (14.5% vs. 33%) (8). Ironically, patients who ceased smoking less than 8 weeks before surgery had an increased risk of pulmonary complications compared to current smokers (57.1% vs. 33%). Patients who stopped smoking for more than 6 months had rates similar to those who never smoked (11.1% vs. 11.9%).

General health status is an excellent determinant of overall fitness for surgical intervention and is an important predictor of pulmonary risk. The Goldman cardiac risk index can predict pulmonary as well as cardiac complications (9–11). The commonly used American Society of Anesthesiologists (ASA) classification, which evaluates overall risk of perioperative mortality, has been shown to be an effective predictor of postoperative respiratory complications (12,13). An ASA class of 2 or greater places the patient at a 1.5-fold to 3.2-fold increased risk for pulmonary complications from thoracic or abdominal surgery (4). Poor exercise tolerance is a strong identifier of patients at risk for pulmonary complications. For patients over 65, the inability to complete 2 minutes of stationary bicycle exercise, sufficient to raise the heart rate to greater than 99 beats per minute, was the strongest predictor of pulmonary complications in a multivariate analysis of patients undergoing abdominal or noncardiac thoracic surgery (11).

The National Veterans Administration Surgical Quality Improvement Program is a multiinstitutional study that has prospectively collected data on surgical outcomes and comorbidities. The program relates this data to observed versus expected morbidity and mortality ratios using risk adjusted indices. A multifactorial risk index model for predicting postoperative respiratory failure in men after major noncardiac surgery was created from this study (Table 16-2) (14). Two

TABLE 16-2

POSTOPERATIVE RESPIRATORY FAILURE RISK INDEX

Preoperative Predictor	Point Value
Type of surgery	
Abdominal aortic aneurysm	27
Thoracic	21
Neurosurgery, upper abdominal, or peripheral vascular	14
Neck	11
Emergency surgery	11
Albumin (<3 g/dL)	9
BUN (>30 mg/dL)	8
Partially or fully dependent functional status	7
History of COPD	6
Age (years)	
≥70	6
60–69	4

Class	Point Total	Predicted Probability of Pulmonary Failure
1	≤10	0.5%
2	11–19	2.2%
3	20–27	5.0%
4	28–40	11.6%
5	>40	30.5%

From Arozullah AM, Daley J, Henderson WG, et al. Multifactorial risk index for predicting postoperative respiratory failure in men after major noncardiac surgery. *Ann Surg* 2000;232:250, with permission.

metabolic abnormalities associated with a significant risk for pulmonary complications were identified. A serum albumin of <3 gm per dL was associated with a 2.5-fold increase, and blood urea nitrogen (BUN) >30 mg per dL had a 2.3-fold increase in pulmonary complications following major noncardiac surgery. In addition, types of surgery with an increased risk and an odds ratio (OR) >2 for pulmonary complications included abdominal aortic aneurysm, thoracic, peripheral vascular, upper abdomen, neurological, neck, and emergency surgery.

Chronic lung disease is the most important patient-related risk factor for postoperative pulmonary complications. Unadjusted relative risks of postoperative complications for patients with COPD range from 2.7 to 6.0 (4,15). Patients with severe COPD are up to six times more likely to have a postoperative pulmonary complication than patients without COPD (15). In a case control study of 164 patients undergoing abdominal surgery, patients with abnormal findings on lung examination consistent with COPD had an OR of 5.8 for pulmonary complications (10). Medical treatment of patients with symptomatic COPD should be optimized prior to elective general surgery. The use of bronchodilators, physical therapy, antibiotics, smoking cessation, and in selected cases systemic corticosteroids can reduce the risk of postoperative complications in patients with COPD (4). Patients with COPD have an increased risk for pulmonary complications, but there is no exact level of impaired pulmonary function below which all surgery is contraindicated. In a study of 12 very high-risk surgical patients who all had an FEV1 <1 L, only 3 of 15 surgeries were associated with postoperative complications, and there were no deaths in these patients (16).

Age and obesity are two common risk factors that have been assumed to be associated with increased risk for pulmonary complications. However, when data are analyzed to account for coexisting medical conditions, both of these risk factors are not always independently predictive of increased pulmonary risk. The risk of surgical mortality is fairly similar for all age groups when stratified by ASA class (17). A multivariate analysis for postoperative respiratory failure identified age >60 years as a minor risk factor (14). Patients aged 60 to 69 had an OR of 1.51, and patients aged >70 had an OR of 1.91 for pulmonary complications.

A review of ten published series of bariatric surgery patients showed a 3.9% incidence of pneumonia and postoperative atelectasis, which is similar to the general population (18). Prospective studies show that body mass index >25 kg per m^2 is an independent risk factor for postoperative pulmonary complications (7,19). Published discrepancies exist because the literature does not always distinguish between obesity and comorbid conditions associated with obesity that can contribute to increased pulmonary risk. A large review of six studies with 4,526 patients showed that the risk for pulmonary complications was identical for obese and nonobese patients

undergoing abdominal or thoracic surgery (4). In summary, the increase in risk for pulmonary complications from age or obesity is small and is probably more directly related to preexisting comorbidities associated with these two conditions.

Preoperative Assessment

Patient history and physical examination are the classic starting points for evaluating preoperative pulmonary risk. Identification of findings in the patient history, such as exercise intolerance, dyspnea on exertion, wheezing, cigarette smoking, cough, and sputum production, might indicate a need for more detailed evaluation of pulmonary function. Physical examination should focus on detecting hypoventilation in weak or debilitated patients and hyperinflation in patients with chronic pulmonary disease. Wheezing, rales, or rhonchi on auscultation should trigger further examination. Physical evidence of cardiac insufficiency, obesity, cyanosis, tobacco use, and poor oral hygiene should be considered a relative indication for pulmonary function assessment.

A chest x-ray is part of the complete evaluation of any patient with abnormalities discovered on history or physical examination. Chest x-ray should also be routine for any patient scheduled to undergo thoracotomy and for all patients 40 years or older. Performance of a maximal respiratory inhalation and exhalation maneuver in the clinic can be revealing. The ability to climb two flights of stairs at a constant pace without dyspnea is a reasonable screening tool for detecting patients with respiratory, cardiac, or joint disease. Some patients might be too obese, weak, sedentary, or debilitated to complete this test. Inability to succeed at this test should prompt further investigation into overall fitness for elective operation, and corrective measures might need to be instituted.

Much confusion and debate exists over the benefit of preoperative pulmonary function testing (PFT). Often these tests confirm what is already clinically evident based on history and physical examination without adding substantially to the clinical estimate of pulmonary risk. A subset of patients with reversible pulmonary disease on spirometry might benefit from aggressive correction with bronchodilators and antiinflammatory medications. A 1990 American College of Physicians (ACP) consensus statement on preoperative PFT offered the following recommendations for formal spirometry (20):

- Coronary artery bypass surgery or upper abdominal surgery with a history of tobacco smoking or dyspnea
- Lower abdominal surgery if there is uncharacterized pulmonary disease with anticipated prolonged or extensive surgery
- Head and neck or orthopedic surgery with uncharacterized pulmonary disease
- Lung resection

These guidelines are very liberal and can lead to more preoperative spirometry testing than necessary. The following is a more objective approach (21) based on recent literature:

- Obtain PFTs for patients with COPD or asthma if clinical evaluation cannot determine whether the patient is at his or her best baseline and that bronchoconstriction is optimally reduced. Testing might identify patients who will benefit from more aggressive preoperative medical management.
- Obtain PFTs for patients with dyspnea or exercise intolerance that is unexplained after clinical evaluation.
- PFTs should not be ordered routinely prior to abdominal surgery or other high-risk surgeries.
- PFTs should not be used as the primary factor to deny surgery.

A preoperative arterial blood gas analysis identifies patients with hypercapnia. No data suggest that carbon dioxide retention increases pulmonary risk beyond that already established on the basis of clinical risk factors recognized on history and physical examination. Patients with a $Paco_2$ >45 mm Hg usually have severe COPD, which is an already identified risk factor associated with a potential sixfold increase in risk for pulmonary complications. Preoperative arterial blood gas values serve primarily as a baseline for postoperative comparison and for decisions about postoperative ventilation rather than as a screening test for adequacy of pulmonary function (22). The ACP recommends preoperative arterial blood gas analysis in the following patients (20):

- Patients scheduled to undergo coronary artery bypass surgery or upper abdominal surgery with a history of tobacco use or dyspnea
- All patients undergoing formal lung resection

There is no role for preoperative arterial blood gas analysis alone to identify high-risk patients or to deny surgery.

ACUTE PULMONARY COMPROMISE

In the awake, alert, and conversive patient patency and protection of the airway is a given. During major operations the airway is usually orotracheally intubated with a cuffed tube that provides a secure conduit for flow of respiratory gases. Many surgical patients are at risk for acute pulmonary compromise during the immediate perioperative period. A surgical patient can experience acute compromise in his or her respiratory status for several reasons.

Loss of Airway

Patients who have undergone neck operations such as parathyroidectomy, thyroidectomy, or carotid endarterectomy are at risk for postoperative airway compromise.

Hoarseness and stridor in the first 48 hours after operation can be caused by vocal cord edema from intubation, possible recurrent laryngeal nerve injury, or wound hematoma. Symptoms of hypoxia such as restlessness, irritability, and somnolence all might occur in the postoperative patient for a variety of reasons but should heighten suspicion for a respiratory problem as part of the differential diagnosis. Prompt physical examination of the patient helps to sort out the etiology and severity of airway compromise. Pulse oximetry should be performed on all patients with respiratory difficulties. Patients with obvious neck swelling and compromise due to wound hematoma should have their wounds opened immediately, and appropriate clinical measures should be taken, including evacuation, reestablishment of hemostasis, endotracheal intubation, and possible tracheostomy. The latter can be performed at the bedside if necessary (23).

Vocal cord edema can be distinguished from recurrent laryngeal nerve injury by indirect laryngoscopy using a flexible fiberoptic nasopharyngoscope. Mild to moderate vocal cord edema can be managed with humidification of the inspired air and close airway monitoring. More severe cases might require treatment with steroids such as dexamethasone 10 mg IV every 6 to 12 hours or even tracheostomy performed in the operating room. The use of steroids is controversial and has only been proven beneficial in prospective randomized clinical trials of neonates and children under 5 years old who were administered dexamethasone 0.25 to 0.5 mg per kg IV prior to planned extubation (24,25). Dexamethasone treated patients had fewer episodes of stridor and reintubation compared to the control group who did not get steroids. However, when a dangerous degree of airway compromise has developed, as evidenced by nasal flaring, subcostal retraction, and use of accessory muscles, the patient should be prepared for immediate tracheostomy. Oral tracheal intubation might be extremely difficult or impossible in this situation and should be attempted only once, if at all, prior to tracheostomy.

Damage to the recurrent laryngeal nerve can lead to acute airway compromise. Clinical evidence of a unilateral recurrent laryngeal injury is suggested by a weak, whispery voice (Table 16-3). Voice changes might also be accompanied by difficulty with complete glottic closure during coughing or Valsalva maneuver. Inability to close the glottis might be exacerbated with combined injury to the external branch of the superior laryngeal nerve and the recurrent laryngeal nerve. In isolated recurrent laryngeal nerve injury, the intact external branch of the superior laryngeal nerve innervates the cricothyroid muscle to maintain full adduction of the ipsilateral vocal cord. When the superior laryngeal nerve is also damaged, full adduction and glottic closure is not possible, and the vocal cord is paralyzed in the intermediate position away from the midline. In most instances of isolated recurrent laryngeal nerve injury, the contralateral vocal cord will move across the midline over a few weeks time to abut the paralyzed cord. This produces a

TABLE 16-3

SIGNS AND SYMPTOMS OF LARYNGEAL NERVE INJURY

	Voice	Glottic Closure	Airway
Recurrent			
Unilateral	Weak	Weak	Good
Bilateral	Normal	Adequate	Poor
External branch, Superior recurrent			
Unilateral	Lowered	Weakened	Good
Bilateral	Lowered	Loss of reflex	Good
Combined injury			
Unilateral	Weak	Poor	Good
Bilateral	Weak	Weak	Adequate

From Newsome HH Jr. Complications of thyroid surgery. In: Greenfield LG, ed. *Complications in surgery and trauma*, 2nd ed. Philadelphia: J.B. Lippincott Company; 1990:654, with permission.

relatively normal voice. Therefore, it is imperative to exclude occult recurrent laryngeal nerve injury by performing indirect laryngoscopy prior to neck operation in any patient who has had previous neck surgery, regardless of the quality of the patient's voice (23).

If both recurrent laryngeal nerves are rendered nonfunctional, the vocal cords will become paralyzed in the fully adducted position. This might lead to acute respiratory compromise. The patient will experience difficulty with inspiration, and severe stridor is usually evident. Paradoxically, the voice might be normal during this crisis as the vocal cords are apposed in the midline. Immediate treatment of bilateral recurrent laryngeal nerve injury involves reintubation or tracheostomy. Some patients will have a temporary loss of function that recovers over the next few weeks (23).

Tension Pneumothorax

Tension pneumothorax occurs when air enters the potential space between the parietal and visceral pleura of the chest and becomes trapped. The affected lung collapses and subsequently mediastinal shift occurs. Shift in the mediastinum leads to kinking of the superior and inferior vena cava with concomitant impairment in venous return and cardiac output. Ventilation of the contralateral lung is also diminished, and high peak airway pressures can be observed. Common causes of tension pneumothorax include traumatic injury, spontaneous rupture of a pneumocele, laparoscopy with operation at the esophageal hiatus, and mechanical ventilation with positive end-expiratory pressure (PEEP) (26).

Diagnosis of a tension pneumothorax requires timely clinical assessment. Signs and symptoms that are consistent with tension pneumothorax include the following: severe respiratory distress, hypotension, unilateral absence of breath sounds, neck vein distention, tracheal deviation,

chest wall crepitus, and cyanosis. Waiting for a confirmatory chest x-ray in the setting of a tension pneumothorax will most certainly result in a fatal outcome. Treatment is based on the clinical examination. The pleural space should be decompressed with a large bore angiocatheter (12 to 14) inserted through the chest wall into the second intercostal space in the midclavicular line. This will convert the tension pneumothorax to a simple pneumothorax. Chest decompression should be immediately followed by insertion of a thoracostomy tube to reexpand the collapsed lung. Patients who are not intubated and undergo bilateral needle thoracostomies require immediate or simultaneous airway intubation and positive-pressure ventilation.

SMOKE INHALATION AND BURNS

Fires in confined spaces can have devastating consequences, as evidenced by the recent mass casualty event resulting in approximately 100 deaths at a West Warwick, RI nightclub in the winter of 2003. Most deaths from a fire scene are due to smoke inhalation injury rather than from cutaneous burns and associated complications (27,28). The presence of inhalation injury in association with a burn increases the overall mortality rate and often results in significant pulmonary complications (29). In a patient with a >40% total body surface area burn, the presence of inhalation injury increases mortality from 3% to 27%. The same patient has over 95% mortality if he or she is older than 60.

Smoke Inhalation

Smoke inhalation leads to injury by four mechanisms: direct thermal injury to the airways, hypoxia, exposure of the bronchopulmonary system to toxins, and pulmonary absorption of systemic toxins. Smoke tends to be dry and therefore has a low specific heat even at high temperatures. Thermal injuries tend to be limited to the airway above the glottis, including the nasopharynx, oropharynx, and larynx (30). Thermal injuries to the lower respiratory tract are unusual and occur in situations in which the smoke contains superheated particles or steam (31). Injury to the upper airway mucosa from heat produces erythema, ulceration, and edema. Heat damage to the pharynx can cause edema severe enough to lead to obstruction of the airway. Upper airway edema usually occurs during the first 24 hours after thermal injury, but it can be delayed in unresuscitated patients until fluid administration is under way. When present, edema usually resolves in 2 to 5 days (32). Diagnosis depends on the history and surveillance physical examination for signs and symptoms of smoke exposure. Symptoms such as dyspnea, stridor, and cyanosis should prompt early control of the airway by endotracheal intubation. Securing of the endotracheal tube in a burn patient is of paramount importance as a dislodged tube might be impossible to replace because of upper airway edema.

Hypoxia is primarily a result of consumption of oxygen by the fire that drives down the F_{IO_2} of the ambient air that the victim breathes. Severe hypoxia leads to a critical reduction in the level of oxygen delivery to the organs beyond which the body cannot compensate, eventually resulting in death by asphyxiation. Hypoxemia can potentiate the toxicity of inhaled carbon monoxide and hydrogen cyanide (33). Hypoxemia can also result in an increase in respiratory rate and minute ventilation, thereby markedly increasing the amount of smoke subsequently inhaled and worsening exposure to systemic and bronchopulmonary toxins (30).

Small particles and toxic gases in smoke can reach the distal airways and alveoli. These compounds result in an acute inflammatory reaction initially mediated by neutrophils (33). Symptoms might include persistent coughing, bronchorrhea, dyspnea, and wheezing. Physiologic changes triggered by the inflammatory cascade can result in worsened ventilation/perfusion (V/Q) matching and increased susceptibility to pulmonary infections. Severe cases can progress to ARDS. Bronchoscopy in these patients will reveal erythema, edema, and ulcerations of the airways, often in conjunction with carbonaceous sputum (30).

Carbon Monoxide Poisoning

Carbon monoxide gas in smoke can be systemically absorbed across the lung and have potentially fatal consequences. Carbon monoxide binds to hemoglobin with an affinity 200 times greater than oxygen (27). If a sufficient amount of circulating hemoglobin is bound to carbon monoxide, tissue hypoxia and cell death will occur. The most immediate threat is to oxygen-sensitive organs such as the brain. Carboxyhemoglobin (HbCO) levels of 40% to 60% cause obtundation and loss of consciousness. Levels of 20% to 40% cause central nervous system dysfunction of varying degrees. Interestingly, HbCO levels of 5% to 10% are found in smokers and in people in urban areas who are exposed to heavy traffic, but these levels of carbon monoxide absorption are rarely symptomatic (27).

The diagnosis of carbon monoxide poisoning is based on compatible history and physical examination. Symptoms and signs are relatively nonspecific and can include headache, nausea, malaise, altered cognition, dyspnea, angina, seizures, cardiac arrhythmias, congestive heart failure, and coma (34). Elevated HbCO levels might cause a cherry-red appearance of the skin. This physical finding is present in only half of patients with severe carbon monoxide poisoning (27). In carbon monoxide poisoning the blood's oxygen content is reduced, but the amount of oxygen dissolved in the plasma is unaffected by the hemoglobin-bound carbon monoxide. Arterial blood gas analysis will appear normal except for the HbCO level, which requires a cooximeter for measurement. HbCO levels correlate poorly with the extent of poisoning (Table 16-4), and do not predict delayed neurologic sequelae. Neurologic deficits, particularly loss of consciousness, worsen prognosis (35).

Placing the patient with carbon monoxide poisoning on 100% oxygen reduces the half life of carbon monoxide in the blood from 4 hours for patients on room air to 1 hour. All patients with elevated HbCO levels should receive 100% oxygen until levels of <10% are reached. Given limited availability and the absence of proven benefit within the medical literature, hyperbaric oxygen (HBO) is considered optional. Transfer to a burn center should not usually be delayed in favor of HBO treatment for carbon monoxide poisoning (34).

All patients with suspected carbon monoxide poisoning or inhalational injury should initially receive humidified 100% oxygen by face mask. Additional evidence must be sought on history and physical examination to confirm suspected inhalational injury. Confinement to fire in a closed space, breathing of large quantities of smoke or noxious fumes, singed facial hair, facial burns, perioral soot, carbonaceous sputum, hoarseness, stridor, and impaired consciousness are all signs and symptoms that might warrant further investigation into the possibility of inhalational injury and trigger potential intervention. An arterial blood gas analysis should be performed and cooximetry obtained to evaluate the level of HbCO in the bloodstream. Patients

TABLE 16-4

SIGNS AND SYMPTOMS OF CARBON MONOXIDE POISONING

Level of Carboxyhemoglobin (%HbCO)	Signs and Symptoms
<20	None, headache, confusion
20–40	Disorientation, fatigue, nausea, visual disturbances
40–60	Hallucination, combativeness, coma, shock
>60	Death

From Demling RH. Burn care in the immediate resuscitation period. In: Wilmore DW, Cheung LY, Harken AH, et al., ed. *ACS surgery: principles and practice.* 2003 ed. New York: WebMD Inc., 2003:52, with permission.

with a high suspicion for inhalation injury or evidence of severe carbon monoxide poisoning should undergo elective orotracheal intubation to secure the airway. In equivocal cases the use of flexible fiberoptic nasopharyngeal endoscopy might reveal upper airway erythema and soft tissue edema that can progress to airway compromise if left untreated.

If severe injury to the tracheobronchial tree has occurred, the necrotic epithelium of the airways will begin sloughing around postinjury day 3 to 4 (33,36). This increase in secretions places the patient at risk for airway compromise from obstruction, development of atelectasis, and onset of bacterial pneumonia. Impairment of pulmonary host defense mechanisms, such as mucociliary clearance, function of alveolar macrophages, and recruitment of polymorphonuclear leukocytes can also increase the risk for pneumonia (37). Management of the patient in this clinical phase is largely supportive and involves chest physical therapy, postural drainage, and bronchoscopy if necessary to control secretions. Antibiotics should only be used empirically when bacterial pneumonia is suspected and continued only subsequent to confirmatory sputum or quantitative bronchoalveolar lavage culture.

ASPIRATION PNEUMONIA

Aspiration pneumonia is a pulmonary complication that occurs following abnormal entry of fluid, particulate matter, or gastrointestinal (GI) secretions into the respiratory tract. Two physiologic requirements are usually necessary to produce aspiration pneumonia. First, there must be a compromise in the normal upper airway defenses that protect the distal respiratory tree from exposure to noxious substances. This can consist of loss of glottic closure, inhibition of cough reflex, and failure of clearance mechanisms, all of which are commonly found in the obtunded or anesthetized patient. Second, an inoculation of the lower airways with deleterious fluid or particulate matter must occur. This inoculum can be detrimental to pulmonary function from direct toxic effect, stimulation of an inflammatory process due to a large bacterial bolus, or creation of airway obstruction from a sufficient volume of particulate matter (38).

Aspiration pneumonia should be distinguished from pneumonia itself. Community acquired or nosocomial pneumonia commonly occurs following small volume aspiration of microorganisms found in the oral cavity or nasopharynx. The organisms that typically produce pneumonia, such as Staphylococcus aureus, Streptococcus pneumoniae, Haemophilus influenzae, and Gram-negative bacilli, are all considered virulent bacteria, and only a small inoculum is required. Aspiration pneumonia is a term reserved for pulmonary infection and/or pneumonitis caused by altered clearance mechanisms of less virulent, primarily anaerobic bacteria that constitute the normal flora of a patient susceptible to aspiration. Conditions

TABLE 16-5
CONDITIONS THAT PREDISPOSE TO ASPIRATION PNEUMONIA

Reduced consciousness
  Diminished cough reflex
  Compromised glottic closure

Neurologic insult
  Dysphagia

Disorders of the upper GI tract
  Esophageal disease
  Surgery of upper airway or esophagus
  Gastroesophageal reflux

Mechanical Disruption of Glottic Closure or Esophageal Sphincter
  Endotracheal intubation
  Bronchoscopy
  Upper endoscopy
  Nasoenteric intubation

Other
  Pharyngeal anesthesia
  Protracted vomiting
  Recumbent position

found in surgical patients that predispose them to aspiration pneumonia are listed in Table 16-5.

Chemical Pneumonitis

Aspiration of gastric and oropharyngeal contents can lead to pulmonary complications from three mechanisms: chemical pneumonitis, bacterial infection, and mechanical obstruction. The aspiration of 1 to 3 mL per kg of gastric contents with a pH ≤ 2.5 leads to rapid pneumonitis characterized by atelectasis, peribronchial hemorrhage, pulmonary edema, and damage to bronchial epithelial cells (39–41). An intense inflammatory response occurs, and within 4 hours the alveoli are filled with marginated polymorphonuclear leukocytes and fibrin. The lung parenchyma eventually becomes grossly edematous and hemorrhagic with loss of alveoli and consolidation. Patients usually follow one of three scenarios after aspiration of gastric contents: (a) rapid progressive respiratory failure resulting in death within 24 hours (12%), (b) prompt resolution over 4 to 5 days (62%), or (c) initial improvement followed by development of nosocomial bacterial pneumonia (26%) (42).

The diagnosis of chemical pneumonitis following aspiration is presumptive and is based on clinical suspicion and features such as abrupt onset of severe respiratory symptoms with significant dyspnea, low-grade fever, cyanosis, diffuse crackles on auscultation, severe hypoxemia, and infiltrates on chest x-ray involving dependent lung segments. Treatment is largely supportive and centers on the provision of oxygen, protection of the airway, and tracheal suctioning. The acid material is rapidly neutralized in the lung, and damage is already well established by the time a physician or other health care professional becomes aware of the aspiration event. Animal studies have demonstrated therapeutic benefit from positive-pressure ventilation, intravenous administration of high molecular weight colloids, and infusion of sodium nitroprusside into the pulmonary artery (PA) (43–46). However, recommendations on the use of the latter two therapies in the treatment of human patients remain indeterminate. The immediate use of corticosteroids to treat chemical pneumonitis following gastric aspiration is unsupported (47); however, there is a role for this drug in the treatment of unresolving ARDS should it develop over the ensuing days (48).

Bacterial Pneumonia

Bacterial pneumonia following aspiration is usually caused by organisms that commonly reside in the upper airways or stomach. These bacteria are less virulent and are primarily anaerobes that reside in the gingival creases. Compared to community-acquired pneumonia, onset is quite slow, with patients manifesting cough, fever, purulent sputum, and dyspnea evolving over a period of several days or weeks rather than hours (38). The absence of rigors is characteristic of nonpyogenic pneumonia since patients with aspiration pneumonia from anaerobes almost never have shaking chills. Many patients with aspiration pneumonia do not present acutely with infection. Instead, they present late with complications characterized by suppuration and necrosis within the lung (49–51). Lung abscesses, necrotizing pneumonia, or empyema all represent delayed presentations of untreated aspiration pneumonia.

Antibiotics are the most important component of treatment for aspiration pneumonia associated with bacterial infection. Clindamycin is currently the preferred drug for anaerobic infections above the diaphragm, including pulmonary infections (38,52). Alternative regimens include amoxicillin-clavulanate, piperacillin-tazobactam, and penicillin combined with metronidazole. When nosocomial pneumonia is suspected, companion aerobic bacteria, particularly Gram-negative bacilli or Staphylococcus aureus, are more important than anaerobes. Therapy should therefore be directed at these virulent organisms.

Mechanical Obstruction

Aspiration can flood the lung with fluid and particulate matter. These materials might not be intrinsically toxic to the lung, but they can cause acute airway obstruction. Fluids that can be aspirated that are not toxic to the lung are saline, barium, most ingested fluids, including water, and gastric contents with a pH >2.5. Patients who are at risk for mechanical obstruction are those who cannot protect their airways or cough secondary to neurologic deficit or impaired consciousness. The obvious treatment is tracheal suctioning and prevention. The most important preemptive measure in hospitalized patients is to keep the patient in the semiupright or upright position (53–55).

Solid objects such as peanuts, vegetable particles, small parts, and teeth can become aspirated and lodged in the airway (38). Foreign body aspiration is more common among young children, and plant products are problematic because they cannot be visualized on chest x-ray. For large objects that become lodged in the larynx or trachea, sudden respiratory distress with cyanosis, stridor, and aphonia can ensue. Treatment consists of the Heimlich maneuver with firm rapid pressure applied to the upper abdomen in an attempt to force the diaphragm upward, generating enough pressure to dislodge the particle. Smaller particles will become lodged in the more distal portions of the tracheal-bronchial tree. These patients present with cough, and chest x-ray demonstrates atelectasis or obstructive emphysema with cardiac shift and elevated diaphragm. Unilateral wheezing might be appreciated if there is partial obstruction. The primary intervention is therapeutic rigid or fiberoptic bronchoscopy performed in the operating room (56).

NOSOCOMIAL PNEUMONIA

Nosocomial pneumonia is defined as pneumonia occurring 48 hours after admission to the hospital and excluding any infection that is present or incubating at the time of admission (57). Ventilator-associated pneumonia is a specific form of nosocomial pneumonia that refers to the development of bacterial pneumonia in patients with acute respiratory failure who have been receiving mechanical ventilation for over 48 hours (58). Patients in the surgical intensive care unit (ICU) have higher rates of nosocomial pneumonia than in the medical ICU (59). Data from the National Nosocomial Infection Surveillance system shows that the four types of ICUs with the highest incidence of ventilator-associated pneumonia all care for surgical patients and are the burn, neurosurgical, trauma, and surgical ICUs, respectively (60).

Risk Factors, Etiology, and Prevention

The leading risk factor for nosocomial pneumonia is mechanical ventilation. Endotracheal intubation increases the risk of nosocomial pneumonia between sixfold and 21-fold (61). Other significant risk factors for nosocomial pneumonia identified on multivariate analysis include the following: age >70 years, chronic lung disease, depressed consciousness, large volume aspiration, thoracic surgery, frequent ventilator circuit changes, presence of intracranial pressure monitor, presence of nasogastric tube, H-2 blocker or antacid therapy, transport from the ICU to diagnostic or therapeutic procedures, previous exposure to antibiotics, reintubation, hospitalization during the fall or winter, and mechanical ventilation for ARDS (62). Gastric pH might have a significant role in risk for nosocomial pneumonia. A randomized controlled trial (RCT) compared three strategies of stress ulcer prophylaxis (ranitidine, antacid, and sucralfate) (63). The incidence of ventilator-associated pneumonia was significantly lower with sucralfate (5%) than with antacids (16%) and ranitidine (21%). Supine positioning can predispose patients to microaspiration and development of nosocomial pneumonia. A randomized trial of positioning in 90 intubated patients was terminated early when interim analysis revealed a significantly lower incidence of nosocomial pneumonia in the semirecumbent versus supine patients (5% vs. 23%) (55).

Nosocomial pneumonias are frequently polymicrobial, with Gram-negative bacilli as the predominant organism in over 60% of infections (61). Six of the seven most frequently identified pathogens on culture for nosocomial pneumonia are Gram-negative bacilli: (a) *Pseudomonas aeruginosa* (17%), (b) *Staphylococcus aureus* (16%), (c) *Enterobacter* species (11%), (d) *Klebsiella* species (7%), (e) *Escherichia coli* (6%), (f) *Haemophilus influenzae* (6%), and (g) *Serratia marcescens* (5%) (62). Each separate ICU has its own intrinsic flora and might have other virulent bacterial organisms that are high in prevalence for nosocomial pneumonia, such as *Acinetobacter* species and *Streptococcus pneumoniae*. It is of critical importance to know the offending pathogens in the ICU in which one practices when choosing empiric antibiotic therapy for patients with suspected nosocomial pneumonia.

Diagnosis and Treatment

Accurate diagnosis of pneumonia remains elusive. Clinical signs and symptoms suggestive of pneumonia include new or progressive infiltrate on chest x-ray, fever, white blood cell (WBC) count greater than 10,000 per mm^3, purulent sputum, and increasing oxygen requirements (64). Presence of positive findings for three or more of these signs and symptoms should trigger the obtaining of a sputum sample for Gram stain and confirmatory bacterial culture followed by empiric administration of antibiotics. Tracheal aspirate, protected specimen brush, or bronchoalveolar lavage can be used to obtain sputum samples for culture. Quantitative bronchoscopic specimens are more accurate in confirming the diagnosis but have the disadvantage of being time-consuming and expensive. A prospective randomized clinical study evaluated whether an invasive test using protected brush specimens or bronchoalveolar lavage was superior to clinical criteria in 431 patients with suspicion of ventilator-associated pneumonia (65). Patients who underwent invasive testing had a significantly lower 14-day mortality rate (16% vs. 26%). This survival advantage remained at day 28 and was also associated with an increase in antibiotic-free days as well as a lower mean number of antibiotics administered. Operator variability and differences between ICUs make it difficult to universally replicate and

apply these results. Also, the threshold for a positive quantitative bronchoalveolar lavage culture varies between 10^4 and 10^5 cfu per mL in published studies. However, there is a definite trend in the literature toward utilizing bronchoalveolar lavage to improve the accuracy of pneumonia diagnosis and to decrease pneumonia treatment costs through the reduction of false-positive cultures (64,66,67).

Because definitive diagnosis is difficult, many patients are incorrectly suspected of having pneumonia. This error can lead to overtreatment from empiric antibiotic therapy with all of its risks for superinfection and antibiotic toxicity. Conversely, it has been established that inadequate antibiotic therapy significantly affects mortality from infections and is an important independent predictor of hospital mortality with an OR of 4.27 (68,69). Inadequate initial antibiotic selection is associated with a significant increase in ventilator-associated pneumonia mortality (37% vs. 15.4%) compared to adequate initial therapy (70). The choice of proper antibiotic treatment for nosocomial pneumonia should be guided by recent antibiotic therapy, the indigenous bacterial flora of the hospital and ICU, the presence of underlying diseases, the type of patient (e.g., trauma, burn, general surgery), and the available culture data. The type of patient impacts heavily on the organism that is the most likely culprit for nosocomial pneumonia—for example, trauma patients: aspiration, oral flora type organisms; burn patients: *Staphylococcus aureus*; general surgery patients: virulent Gram-negative bacilli. In the absence of positive microbial culture data, patients with three of the five clinical signs and symptoms of pneumonia should be placed on empiric antibiotic therapy.

Three questions are vital in choosing the appropriate empiric antibiotic therapy for each individual hospital, ICU, and patient (71):

- Is the patient at risk for methicillin-resistant *Staphylococcus aureus* (MRSA)?
- Is *Acinetobacter baumannii* a problem in the institution?
- Is the patient at risk for *Pseudomonas aeruginosa* infection?

At a bare minimum, the empiric antibiotic regimen chosen should have activity against *Enterobacter* species, *Klebsiella* species, *E. coli*, *Proteus* species, *Serratia marcescens*, *Haemophilus influenzae*, methicillin-sensitive *Staphylococcus aureus*, and *Streptococcus pneumoniae* (62). Patients who have aspirated, who have underlying medical conditions such as recent abdominal surgery, coma, head trauma, diabetes mellitus, renal failure, or COPD, are being treated with steroids or antibiotics, or who have a prolonged ICU stay might require additional coverage for anaerobes, MRSA, and Legionella. Coverage for *Pseudomonas aeruginosa* and antibiotic-resistant Gram-negative bacilli such as *Acinetobacter baumannii* should also be considered in critically ill patients receiving antibiotics prior to the onset of pneumonia and in institutions in which these bacteria are common pathogens.

If MRSA is a frequent nosocomial pathogen in the institution, vancomycin will be a necessary first choice for empiric *Staphylococcal* coverage, but it should be discontinued if MRSA is not isolated on culture. The literature supports empiric monotherapy with third-generation cephalosporins with antipseudomonal activity, but caution is suggested as monotherapy has been associated with the development of resistant strains in documented cases of *Pseudomonas aeruginosa* infection (62). Combination therapy is associated with a survival benefit compared to monotherapy in patients with pseudomonal pneumonia and bacteremia (72).

A current empiric antibiotic strategy for nosocomial pneumonia employed in our surgical, trauma, and burn ICU follows:

- Patients suspected of having nosocomial pneumonia are identified by having three of five clinical criteria for pneumonia (new or progressive infiltrate on chest x-ray, fever, elevated WBC count >10,000 per mm^3, purulent sputum, and increasing oxygen requirements).
- Perform quantitative bronchoalveolar lavage.
- Initiate empiric antibiotic therapy with one of the following antibiotic combinations based on patient's medical comorbidities:

  - Piperacillin/tazobactam with gentamicin
  - Piperacillin/tazobactam with levofloxacin
  - Levofloxacin with gentamicin.

- Add Vancomycin if patient is at risk for MRSA.
- If the quantitative bronchoalveolar lavage culture results are >10^4 cfu per mL, continue antibiotics and tailor coverage based on organism and sensitivities.
- If the quantitative bronchoalveolar lavage culture results are <10^4 cfu per mL, discontinue antibiotic therapy.

Previously, experts have recommended long courses (14 to 21 days) of antibiotic treatment for nosocomial pneumonia. Recent prospective randomized studies on this subject have begun to challenge this dogma. In a large European study of 401 patients diagnosed with ventilator-associated pneumonia by quantitative bronchoalveolar lavage culture, 197 patients were randomly assigned to receive 8 days of antibiotic therapy, and 204 to receive 15 days of antibiotic treatment (73). Primary outcome measures were mortality, recurrence of pneumonia, and antibiotic-free days. Patients treated for 8 days had no excess mortality (18.8% vs. 17.2%). It has been our practice to treat chromosomally mediated resistance-prone bacteria such as *Acinetobacter* species, *Pseudomonas aeruginosa*, *Enterobacter* species, *Serratia* species, and *Citrobacter* species for a minimum of 10 days. *Pseudomonas aeruginosa*, *Enterobacter* species, and *Acinetobacter* species are known to be highly resistant and therefore receive double coverage with two antibiotics. *Staphylococcus aureus* pneumonia is treated for a minimum of 14 days. Patients suspected of having anaerobic bacterial pneumonia should also be placed on clindamycin or flagyl empirically. The selection of empiric antibiotic therapy must take into account patient data and should be institution-specific.

ACUTE RESPIRATORY DISTRESS SYNDROME (ARDS)

ARDS refers to patients with acute and progressive respiratory disease of a noncardiac nature, in association with diffuse, bilateral pulmonary infiltrates demonstrated on chest x-rays, and with hypoxemia (74). Acute lung injury and its more severe form, known as ARDS, are clinical syndromes pathologically characterized by acute and persistent pulmonary inflammation with increased vascular permeability. In 1994, the American-European Consensus Conference on ARDS established written clinical definitions of acute lung injury and ARDS, which are listed in Table 16-6 (75). In recent years significant advances in understanding of the pathophysiology of ARDS and lung injury have been made, leading to prospective randomized clinical trials and attempts to improve therapy on the basis of scientific knowledge. Despite these recent advances, the mortality from severe ARDS remains high—between 40% and 60% in both adults and children (74,76).

The pathophysiology of ARDS is complex but can be summarized as massive capillary leak that is the result of an excessive inflammatory response in the host's lung tissue. ARDS has a rapid onset over 4 to 48 hours and can persist for days to weeks. ARDS progresses through four distinct clinical phases. Phase one is the initial prodrome that is characterized by dyspnea, tachypnea, and a respiratory alkalosis with a normal PaO_2. This phase is driven by inflammatory mediators and activation of inflammatory cells such as alveolar macrophages. Phase two is marked by the onset of lung injury in the first 24 hours. This

---

TABLE 16-6

DEFINITION OF ACUTE LUNG INJURY AND ARDS

Acute lung injury
   Acute onset of pulmonary failure
   PaO_2/FiO_2 ratio <300 mm Hg[a]
   Bilateral infiltrates on chest x-ray
   PCWP <18 mm Hg

ARDS
   All of criteria for acute lung injury
   PaO_2/FiO_2 ratio <200 mm Hg[a]

---

[a]Regardless of the level of positive end-expiratory pressure (PEEP). From Bernard GR, Artigas A, Brigham KL, et al. The consensus committee report of the American-European consensus conference on ARDS: definitions, mechanisms, relevant outcomes and clinical trial coordination. *Intensive Care Med* 1994;20:225–232, with permission.

results in the clinical findings of hypoxemia and radiographic evidence of scattered pulmonary infiltrates bilaterally. During this time, increased pulmonary capillary permeability leads to interstitial edema, neutrophil margination, and an interstitial inflammatory response. This process ultimately causes a severe loss of alveolar units in the patient. The third phase results in progressive lung injury. Injury is evidenced by increased shunt fraction and severe hypoxemia. The pulmonary parenchyma undergoes microvascular thrombosis, redistribution of pulmonary blood flow, and increasing edema of the alveolar capillary membranes. During the fourth and final phase, the inflammatory response switches from acute to chronic and is associated with ongoing inflammation and pulmonary fibrosis. Macrophages and progressive interstitial fibrosis that can become irreversible dominates the inflammatory response (77,78).

Basic scientific advances have improved our understanding of the pathophysiology of ARDS, and therapeutic options are emerging to treat the excessive inflammatory response of early ARDS and the irreversible fibroproliferative response of late ARDS (77). Identification of risk factors for ARDS has allowed early implementation of alternative ventilator strategies to reduce iatrogenic lung injury and exacerbation of pulmonary failure in surgical patients at increased risk. Treatment of ARDS is focused on eliminating the inciting source, utilizing protective ventilator strategies to minimize ventilator-induced lung injury, avoidance of additional organ failure, pharmacologic intervention to reduce lung inflammation and fibrosis, and provision of adequate nutrition. Failing all other therapies, extracorporeal life support (ECLS) may be employed in rare circumstances for severe ARDS patients.

The diagnosis of ARDS is based on findings of acute onset of severe hypoxemia (Pao_2 <200 mm Hg) and bilateral infiltrates on chest x-ray (Fig. 16-1) in the absence of pulmonary edema. In some clinical situations it might become necessary to place a Swan-Ganz catheter into the pulmonary artery (PA) to verify that the pulmonary capillary wedge pressure (PCWP) is <18 mm Hg in order to rule out pulmonary edema as the etiology of acute respiratory failure. The presence of a PCWP <18 mm Hg favors acute lung injury or ARDS over hemodynamic pulmonary edema. However, an elevated PCWP does not exclude ARDS. If pulmonary infiltrates on chest x-ray and hypoxemia do not improve within 24 to 48 hours following normalization of PCWP, acute lung injury or ARDS has most likely occurred simultaneously with hemodynamic pulmonary edema (79).

Permissive Hypercapnia

Management of mechanical ventilation for patients with ARDS involves understanding how to minimize and prevent ventilator-induced lung injury. Webb and Tierney (80) first demonstrated ventilator-induced lung injury in animals in 1974, when they revealed the detrimental effects of ventilation at a peak inspiratory pressure of 45 cm H_2O in rats. Subsequently, investigators have documented an increase in pulmonary edema and histopathology in rats ventilated at a peak inspiratory pressure of 45 cm H_2O for only 5 to 20 minutes (81). Healthy sheep, when mechanically ventilated at a peak inspiratory pressure as low as 30 to 40 cm H_2O, showed an increase in wet-to-dry lung weight, deterioration in gas exchange, an increase in the surface tension of lung lavage fluid, and lung lesions consistent with ARDS (82).

To avoid ventilator-induced lung injury, clinicians have applied the concept of permissive hypercapnia, in which arterial carbon dioxide is allowed to rise to levels as high as 120 mm Hg while the blood pH is maintained above 7.1 to 7.2 by the intravenous administration of buffer solutions (83). Mortality in adults was reduced to 26% compared to the expected mortality of 53% based on an Acute Physiology and Chronic Health Evaluation (APACHE) II score when low-volume, pressure-limited ventilation with permissive hypercapnia was applied to patients with ARDS (84). When implementing permissive hypercapnia, the progressive rise in $Paco_2$ should not exceed 10 mm Hg per hour and only rarely should the maximum level exceed 80 to 100 mm Hg. Patients might require heavy sedation and even chemical paralysis to overcome the hypercapnic respiratory drive and avoid discomfort. Potential deleterious effects of hypercapnia include elevation in intracranial pressure in patients with brain injury, mild hypertension, increased cardiac output, and increased pulmonary vascular resistance (77).

Intratracheal Pulmonary Ventilation

A potential technique to avoid hypercapnia with low tidal volume (V_T) ventilation is to flush out the carbon dioxide residing in the dead space with tracheal gas insufflation. Intratracheal pulmonary ventilation uses a continuous flow of ventilator gas through a reverse thrust catheter positioned at the distal end of the endotracheal tube to reduce physiologic dead space (Fig. 16-2) (85). The technique of intratracheal pulmonary ventilation effectively reverses the flow of fresh gas at the tip of the endotracheal tube and entrains gas exiting the lungs by the Venturi effect. Thus, during the expiratory phase, fresh gas is continuously introduced at the level of the carina, reducing the anatomic dead space and augmenting CO_2 removal. During inspiration, the exhalation valve on the ventilator closes and the gas flows prograde, inducing a V_T ventilation of the lung. In animal studies intratracheal pulmonary ventilation has been shown to reduce anatomic dead space, enhance ventilation of small lungs, and facilitate the removal of CO_2 while maintaining low airway pressures (86).

Intratracheal pulmonary ventilation can maintain reasonable levels of ventilation in normal animals at peak inspiratory pressure levels one-half to one-third those required during conventional mechanical ventilation (12).

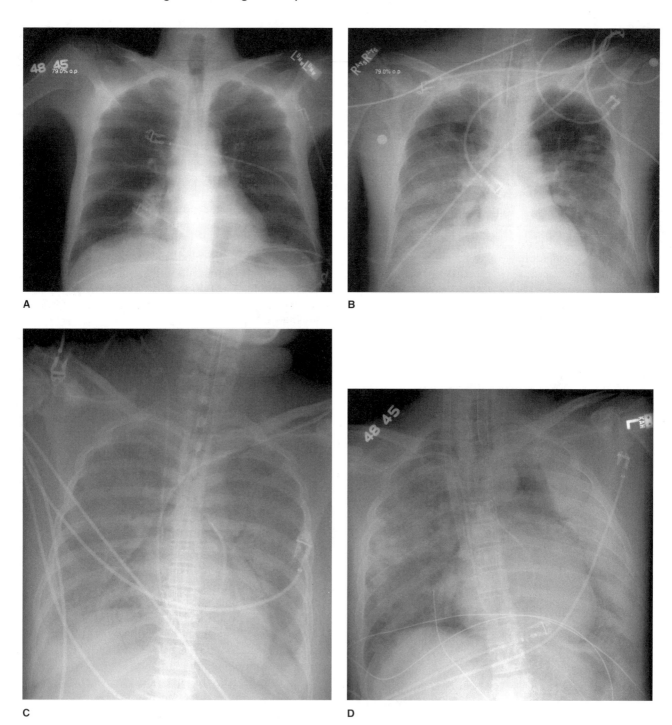

Figure 16-1 Common radiologic features of ARDS. All chest x-rays are portable anteroposterior projection. **A:** 40-year-old man with diabetic ketoacidosis and right lower lobe infiltrate from Streptococcal pneumonia. **B:** The same man 1 day later with severe bilateral blossoming of pulmonary infiltrates. **C:** 49-year-old woman with Staphylococcal sepsis and bilateral ground glass pulmonary infiltrates. Note the presence of air bronchograms. **D:** 36-year-old man with Blastomycosis pneumonia and dense patchy infiltrates bilaterally. This patient required ECLS for 16 days and was discharged to rehabilitation on hospital day 32.

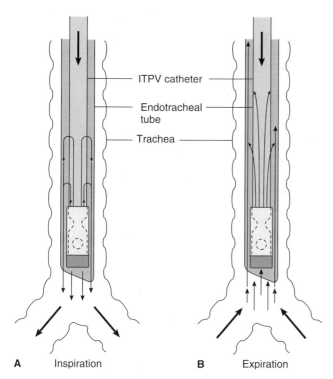

Figure 16-2 Reverse thruster catheter used to perform intra-tracheal pulmonary ventilation. **A:** During inspiration, the exhalation valve on the ventilator is closed and gas flows prograde, filling the lung with a tidal volume. **B:** During expiration, the valve on the ventilator is open and gas flows retrograde, entraining and replacing the gas in the anatomic dead space. ITPV, intratracheal pulmonary ventilation. (From Hemmila MR, Hirschl RB. Advances in ventilatory support of the pediatric surgical patient. *Curr Opin Pediatr* 1999;11:245, with permission.)

Use of intratracheal pulmonary ventilation in five neonatal and pediatric patients with uncontrollable hypercarbia was associated with a reduction in the $PaCO_2$ from 100 ± 29 mm Hg to 47 ± 25 mm Hg within 4 to 6 hours of initiation of therapy (87). Intratracheal pulmonary ventilation is a very promising new ventilation technique, and results of clinical studies evaluating its efficacy compared to conventional volume ventilation or pressure control ventilation are eagerly awaited.

Pressure Control and Inverse Ratio Ventilation

Conventional ventilation involves volume cycling with V_Ts in the 10 to 15 mL per kg range. An alternative mode of ventilation used in ARDS patients is pressure control ventilation. In this mode the target peak and plateau airway pressure is kept <40 cm H_2O by feedback servo regulation of the ventilator flow rate. The pressure versus time curve for a breath in pressure control ventilation resembles a square wave in which a uniform pressure is generated throughout the inspiratory cycle. This results in noticeably smaller V_Ts (4 to 8 mL per kg) with each breath and possible hypercapnia, especially in stiff noncompliant lungs. The V_T generated will vary considerably with changes in compliance, and rapid decreases in compliance can lead to inadequate ventilation. Use of pressure control ventilation allows tight control of airway pressures, minimization of barotrauma, and enhanced recruitment of collapsed alveoli throughout the inspiratory cycle.

The normal inspiratory to expiratory ratio is 1:3 or 1:4. By lengthening the time of the inspiratory phase, one increases the time available for gas exchange and potentially inflates collapsed alveoli. In some instances it is necessary to invert this ratio so that more time is spent during inspiration than expiration—so-called inverse ratio ventilation. Inverse ratio ventilation allows for less time for recruited alveoli to collapse during expiration. As long as there is adequate time for CO_2 clearance, mean airway pressure is monitored, and the patient is appropriately sedated to overcome the unnatural breathing pattern provided by this mode of ventilation, it can be a safe and effective way of increasing oxygenation and recruiting functional residual capacity (FRC) in severe respiratory failure. Pressure control ventilation and pressure control-inverse ratio ventilation are standard techniques used in neonatal mechanical ventilation.

Open Lung Approach

One of the more common means of recruiting collapsed alveoli and increasing FRC is to use PEEP. By not allowing all the pressure in the lung to escape during expiration, alveoli that are unstable and prone to collapse cannot do so. This technique can be thought of as holding the lung partially open so that the next breath is not starting from total collapse in a noncompliant lung. The optimal level of PEEP to use in ARDS patients is difficult to determine, but evidence is emerging to suggest that optimal recruitment and maintenance of lung volume occurs when PEEP is set at a value that matches or exceeds the lower inflection point (P_{flex}) on the inspiratory static pressure-volume curve (88). A single breath compliance curve with V_T plotted against static airway pressure will demonstrate two inflection points. The lower one represents the theoretical critical opening pressure of most alveoli available for recruitment, and the upper point represents the loss of elastic properties of the lung secondary to overdistension (77).

The combination of PEEP to recruit FRC and pressure control ventilation to minimize barotrauma has been termed the "open lung approach" (89,90). This strategy involves maintaining the PEEP above the lower inflection point of the pressure-volume curve, keeping the V_T <6 mL per kg, avoiding static airway pressures >40 cm H_2O, utilizing permissive hypercapnia, and the stepwise use of pressure-limited modes of ventilation (89). A recent study showed an improved survival at 28 days (62% vs. 29%), a higher rate of weaning from mechanical ventilation, and a lower rate of barotrauma in the patient group that received the protective lung strategy or "open lung approach" compared to controls (90). There was, however, no difference in the in-hospital mortality for these patients. The low 28-day survival in the control group has raised questions about this trial's validity. More recently, the NIH ARDSNET research group published the results of a prospective randomized trial of low V_Ts (6 mL per kg) compared to traditional V_Ts (12 mL per kg) for mechanical ventilation in ARDS (91). This trial was stopped early after the enrollment of 861 patients because the mortality was significantly lower in the group treated with lower V_Ts than in the group with traditional V_Ts (31% vs. 40%). The mean plateau pressures were 25 ± 6 and 33 ± 8 cm H_2O, respectively. A reduction of 25% in the mortality of these patients with lower V_Ts offers strong evidence for a protective lung strategy approach to mechanical ventilation in patients with ARDS.

Prone Positioning

Patient positioning can have a sometimes dramatic effect on oxygenation and ventilation in severe ARDS. Changing patient position to prone or steep lateral decubitus positions can improve the distribution of perfusion to ventilated lung regions leading to improvement in oxygenation (92,93). Prone positioning in ARDS patients can improve oxygenation in 60% to 70% of patients (94). A multicenter randomized trial of conventional treatment versus placing patients in a prone position for 6 or more hours daily for 10 days was conducted on patients with acute lung injury or ARDS (94). The mortality rate did not differ for the prone versus conventional positioning group at any point during the study, with up to 6 months follow-up. The mean increase in the PaO_2 to FIO_2 ratio was greater in the prone than supine group (63 ± 67 vs. 45 ± 68). There was no difference between the two groups in the incidence of complications related to positioning. The mean PaO_2 of 85 to 88 mm Hg and mean PaO_2/FIO_2 ratio of 125 to 129 are still quite high for patients with severe ARDS, and therefore these patients might not have been likely to benefit considerably by the prone intervention in terms of mortality.

Prone postioning is labor-intensive and complicated. The mains risks are extubation and pressure sores. However, a trained and dedicated nursing staff that is aware of potential benefits in critically ill patients with severe pulmonary failure can safely perform the technique. Prone positioning is a crucial tool for keeping patients with severe respiratory failure off extracorporeal life support and for lung recruitment in patients on extracorporeal life support. Prone postioning is not used until PaO_2 and PaO_2/FIO_2 ratio are significantly below 100. The technique involves alternating prone with supine postioning every 6 hours using appropriate cushioning of the dependent portions of the body. Patients will often experience an initial worsening in respiratory status with each change in position, but this passes quickly in the first 15 to 30 minutes to eventual improvement in oxygenation and ventilation, with 70% of the overall improvement occurring in the first hour of pronation (94).

Corticosteroids

Recent studies have suggested a benefit for the use of corticosteroids in refractory disease, or the late, fibroproliferative stage of ARDS (77). The mechanism of action for the steroid effect on the fibroproliferative response seems to involve modulation of macrophage and fibroblast activity that can lead to irreversible pulmonary fibrosis. Investigators conducted an RCT of steroid administration in late ARDS (48). There were 24 patients in the study; 16 were treated with methylprednisolone and eight were randomized to placebo. Four of the eight control patients crossed over to the steroid arm for failure to improve. The dose administered was 2 mg/kg/day in divided doses, starting 7 days after the diagnosis of ARDS and continuing for 32 days total. There were significant reductions in lung injury and organ failure scores and an improvement in the PaO_2/FIO_2 ratio. Hospital associated mortality was 12% for the treatment group and 62% for the control group; however, only four patients remained in the placebo group because of patient crossover during the study.

Extracorporeal Life Support

The technique of ECLS for patients with severe ARDS involves a veno-venous or veno-arterial life support circuit with a membrane oxygenator to temporarily take over the

TABLE 16-7

OUTCOME IN ARDS WITH ECLS

| | | Severe ARDS Survival | |
Author	Year	Conventional Rx	ECLS Rx
Zapol	1979	8%	10%
Gattinoni	1986	—	49%
Brunet	1993	—	50%
Morris	1994	42%	33%
Macha	1996	—	39%
Kolla	1997	—	54%
Peek	1997	—	66%
Lewandowski	1997	—	55%
Ullrich	1999	—	62%
ELSO Registry	2003	—	52%

From Barlett RH. Extracorporeal life support in the management of severe respiratory failure. *Clin Chest Med* 2000;21(3):555-61, with permission.

function of the lung with regards to oxygenation and ventilation. While on ECLS, mechanical ventilator settings are adjusted to minimize ventilator-induced lung injury and to maximize the recruitment of FRC. Use of ECLS for severe ARDS in neonates is of proven benefit (95,96), but for adult patients the technique remains controversial. Although ECLS has failed to have a demonstrated survival advantage for adults in prospective randomized clinical trials, considerable data support its ability to salvage severe ARDS patients failing all other means of respiratory support (Table 16-7). The University of Michigan experience with ECLS has yielded survival to hospital discharge rates of 85% in neonates, 74% in children, and 52% in adults with severe ARDS (97). The treatment program for adults involves an algorithm that aims to normalize body physiology, aggressively recruit FRC and minimize barotrauma (Table 16-8). This algorithm used in 141 patients with respiratory failure referred for consideration of ECLS yielded a survival rate of 62% in patients with severe ARDS (median initial PaO_2/FiO_2 ratio of 66) (98).

The primary circumstance for use of ECLS in patients with severe respiratory failure is when, after optimal ventilator and medical management, the risk of dying from ARDS is considered to be >80% (Table 16-9). This requirement translates to an alveoli-arterial oxygen gradient >600 mm Hg or a PaO_2/FiO_2 ratio of <70 on 100% oxygen. Patients should also have a transpulmonary shunt fraction >30% despite maximal conventional therapy. Adult patients are typically cannulated percutaneously with large 21 to 23 Fr catheters for drainage and infusion of blood. Anticoagulation is necessary and is titrated to a level of 180 seconds as measured by whole blood activated clotting time. ECLS allows for a decreasing of mechanical ventilator settings to nondamaging "rest" levels while maintaining

TABLE 16-8

ALGORITHM FOR TREATMENT OF SEVERE ARDS

Mechanical ventilator
  Pressure control mode
  Limit PIP to 35–40 cm H_2O
  Best PEEP
  Titrate FiO_2 for SaO_2 >90 and SvO_2 >70
  Inverse I:E ratio

Monitors
  Continuous cardiac output Swan-Ganz catheter
  Arterial line

Treatments
  Prone positioning
  Transfuse to Hct 40–45
  Diuresis to dry weight (furosemide drip or CVVH)
  Chemical sedation and paralysis
  Full nutrition
  Cooling

TABLE 16-9

ADULT ECLS CRITERIA

Indications	Contraindications

• Duration of ventilation
  —<5-7 days, 7-10 days only if ventilated with high pressures for <7 days
• Compliance
  —<0.5 mL/cm H_2O/kg
• Oxygenation
  — PaO_2/FiO_2 <100
  — Shunt >30%
	• Prolonged conventional mechanical ventilation
	• Poor neurologic status
	• Incurable disease
	
	• Age >70 years
	• PA pressures >$\frac{2}{3}$ systemic blood pressure
	• Unresolved surgical issues

FRC recruitment measures. Once native lung function has improved, the patient is trialed off of ECLS at moderate ventilator settings that allow for potential increases in therapy—for example, FiO_2 0.5 to 0.6. If the trial off of ECLS is successful, the cannulas are removed and recovery continues. Patients who can be successfully decannulated from ECLS have an 86% chance of being discharged from the hospital alive and of going on to complete recovery (97).

REFERENCES

1. Kroenke K, Lawrence VA, Theroux JF, et al. Operative risk in patients with severe obstructive pulmonary disease. *Arch Intern Med* 1992;152:967–971.
2. Pedersen T, Eliasen K, Henriksen E. A prospective study of risk factors and cardiopulmonary complications associated with anaesthesia and surgery: risk indicators of cardiopulmonary morbidity. *Acta Anaesthesiol Scand* 1990;34:144–155.
3. Gracey DR, Divertie MB, Didier EP. Preoperative pulmonary preparation of patients with chronic obstructive pulmonary disease: a prospective study. *Chest* 1979;76:123–129.
4. Smetana GW. Preoperative pulmonary evaluation. *N Engl J Med* 1999;340:937–944.
5. Wightman JA. A prospective survey of the incidence of postoperative pulmonary complications. *Br J Surg* 1968;55:85–91.
6. Morton HJV. Tobacco smoking and pulmonary complications after surgery. *Lancet* 1944;1:368–370.
7. Brooks-Brunn JA. Predictors of postoperative pulmonary complications following abdominal surgery. *Chest* 1997;111:564–571.
8. Warner MA, Offord KP, Warner ME, et al. Role of preoperative cessation of smoking and other factors in postoperative pulmonary complications: a blinded prospective study of coronary artery bypass patients. *Mayo Clin Proc* 1989;64:609–616.
9. Goldman L, Caldera DL, Nussbaum SR, et al. Multifactorial index of cardiac risk in noncardiac surgical procedures. *N Engl J Med* 1977;297:845–850.
10. Lawrence VA, Dhanda R, Hilsenbeck SG, et al. Risk of pulmonary complications after elective abdominal surgery. *Chest* 1996;110:744–750.
11. Gerson MC, Hurst JM, Hertzberg VS, et al. Prediction of cardiac and pulmonary complications related to elective abdominal and noncardiac thoracic surgery in geriatric patients. *Am J Med* 1990;88:101–107.
12. Wong D, Weber EC, Schell MJ, et al. Factors associated with postoperative pulmonary complications in patients with severe

chronic obstructive pulmonary disease. *Anesth Analg* 1995; 80:276–284.

13. Warner DO, Warner MA, Barnes RD, et al. Perioperative respiratory complications in patients with asthma. *Anesthesiology* 1996; 85:460–467.

14. Arozullah AM, Daley J, Henderson WG, et al. Multifactorial risk index for predicting postoperative respiratory failure in men after major noncardiac surgery. *Ann Surg* 2000;232:242–253.

15. Kroenke K, Lawrence VA, Theroux JF, et al. Postoperative complications after thoracic and major abdominal surgery in patients with and without obstructive lung disease. *Chest* 1993;104: 1445–1451.

16. Milledge JS, Nunn JF. Criteria of fitness for anaesthesia in patients with chronic obstructive lung disease. *Br Med J* 1975; 3:670–673.

17. Thomas DR, Ritchie CS. Preoperative assessment of older adults. *J Am Geriatr Soc* 1995;43:811–821.

18. Pasulka PS, Bistian BR, Benotti PN, et al. The risks of surgery in obese patients. *Ann Intern Med* 1986;104:540–546.

19. Hall JC, Tarala MD, Hall JL, et al. A multivariate analysis of the risk of pulmonary complications after laparotomy. *Chest* 1991; 99:923–927.

20. American College of Physicians. Preoperative pulmonary function testing. *Ann Intern Med* 1990;112:793–794.

21. Smetana GW. Evaluation of preoperative pulmonary risk. UpToDate 11.3 available online at: http://www.utdol.com. Accessed December 28, 2003.

22. Bartlett RH, Rich PB. Pulmonary insufficiency. In: Wilmore DW, Cheung LY, Harken AH et al., eds. *ACS surgery: principles and practice*, 2003 ed. New York: WebMD Inc; 2003: 1047–1057.

23. Newsome HH Jr. Complications of thyroid surgery. In: Greenfield LG, ed. *Complications in surgery and trauma*, 2nd ed. Philadelphia, PA: JB Lippincott Co; 1990:649–659.

24. Couser RJ, Ferrara TB, Falde B, et al. Effectiveness of dexamethasone in preventing extubation failure in preterm infants at increased risk for airway edema. *J Pediatr* 1992;121:591–596.

25. Anene O, Meert KL, Uy H, et al. Dexamethasone for the prevention of postextubation airway obstruction: a prospective, randomized, double-blind, placebo-controlled trial. *Crit Care Med* 1996;24:1666–1669.

26. Pryor JP, Schwab CW, Peitzman AB. Thoracic injury. In: Peitzman AB, Rhodes M, Schwab CW et al., eds. *The trauma manual*, 2nd ed. Philadelphia, PA: Lippincott Williams & Wilkins; 2002:203–223.

27. Chapter 2: Airway management and smoke inhalation injury. In: *Advanced burn life support course: provider's manual*. Chicago, IL: American Burn Association; 2003:25–31.

28. Levine MS, Radford EP. Fire victims: medical outcomes and demographic characteristics. *Am J Public Health* 1977;67:1077–1080.

29. Ryan CM, Schoenfeld DA, Thorpe WP, et al. Objective estimates of the probability of death from burn injuries. *N Engl J Med* 1998;338:362–366.

30. Haponik EF, Crapo RO, Herndon DN, et al. Smoke inhalation. *Am Rev Respir Dis* 1988;138:1060–1063.

31. Weiss SM, Lakshminarayan S. Acute inhalation injury. *Clin Chest Med* 1994;15:103–116.

32. Heimbach DM, Waeckerle JF. Inhalation injuries. *Ann Emerg Med* 1988;17:1316–1320.

33. Demling R. Smoke inhalation injury. *New Horiz* 1993;1:422–484.

34. Mandel J, Schellenberg J, Hales CA Smoke inhalation. UpToDate 11.3 available online at: http://www.utdol.com. Accessed December 10, 2003.

35. Seger D, Welch L. Carbon monoxide controversies: neuropsychologic testing, mechanisms of toxicity, and hyperbaric oxygen. *Ann Emerg Med* 1994;24:242–248.

36. Demling RH. Smoke inhalation injury. In: Shoemaker WC, Ayres SM, Genvik A et al., eds. *Textbook of critical care*, 3rd ed. Philadelphia, PA: WB Saunders; 1995:1506–1516.

37. Herlihy JP, Vermeulen PM, Joseph PM, et al. Impaired alveolar macrophage function in smoke inhalation injury. *J Cell Physiol* 1995;163:1–8.

38. Bartlett JG. Aspiration pneumonia. UpToDate 11.3 available online at: http://www.utdol.com. Accessed December 10, 2003.

39. Greenfield LJ, Singleton RP, McCaffree DR, et al. Pulmonary effects of experimental graded aspiration of hydrochloric acid. *Ann Surg* 1969;170:74–86.

40. Fisk RL, Symes JF, Aldrige LL, et al. The pathophysiology and experimental therapy of acid pneumonitis in ex vivo lungs. *Chest* 1970;57:364–370.

41. Cameron JL, Caldini P, Toung JK, et al. Aspiration pneumonia: physiologic data following experimental aspiration. *Surgery* 1973;72:238–245.

42. Bynum LJ, Pierce AK. Pulmonary aspiration of gastric contents. *Am Rev Respir Dis* 1976;114:1129–1136.

43. Broe PJ, Toung TJ, Permutt S, et al. Aspiration pneumonia: treatment with pulmonary vasodilators. *Surgery* 1983;94:95–99.

44. Cameron JL, Sebor J, Anderson PR, et al. Aspiration pneumonia: results of treatment by positive-pressure ventilation in dogs. *J Surg Res* 1968;8:447–457.

45. Peitzman AB, Shires GT III, Illner HK, et al. Pulmonary acid injury: effects of positive end-expiratory pressure and crystalloid vs. colloid fluid resuscitation. *Arch Surg* 1982;117:662–668.

46. Toung TJ, Cameron JL, Kimera T, et al. Aspiration pneumonia: treatment with osmotically active agents. *Surgery* 1981;89: 588–593.

47. Wolfe JE, Bone RC, Ruth WE. Effects of corticosteroids in the treatment of patients with gastric aspiration. *Am J Med* 1977;63: 719–722.

48. Meduri GU, Headley AS, Golden E, et al. Effect of prolonged methylprednisolone therapy in unresolving acute respiratory distress syndrome. *JAMA* 1998;280:159–165.

49. Bartlett JG. Anaerobic bacterial infections of the lung and pleural space. *Clin Infect Dis* 1993;4:S248–S255.

50. Finegold SM. Aspiration pneumonia. *Rev Infect Dis* 1991; 13(Suppl 9):S737–S742.

51. Bartlett JG. Anaerobic bacterial pneumonitis. *Am Rev Respir Dis* 1979;119:19–23.

52. Gilbert DN, Moellering RC Jr., Sande MA, eds. *The sanford guide to antimicrobial therapy*, 32nd ed. Hyde Park: Antimicrobial Therapy, Inc.; 2002.

53. Torres A, Serra-Batlles J, Ros E, et al. Pulmonary aspiration of gastric contents in patients receiving mechanical ventilation: the effect of body position. *Ann Intern Med* 1992;116:540–543.

54. Orozco-Levi M, Torres A, Ferrer M, et al. Semirecumbent position protects from pulmonary aspiration but not completely from gastroesophageal reflux in mechanically ventilated patients. *Am J Respir Crit Care Med* 1995;152:1387–1390.

55. Drakulovic M, Torres A, Bauer TT, et al. Supine body position as a risk factor for nosocomial pneumonia in mechanically ventilated patients: a randomized trial. *Lancet* 1999;354:1851–1858.

56. Zavala DC, Rhodes ML. Foreign body removal: a new role for the fiberoptic bronchoscope. *Ann Otol Rhinol Laryngol* 1975;84: 650–656.

57. Goodman L. Postoperative chest radiograph: I. Alterations after abdominal surgery. *Am J Roentgenol* 1980;132:533–541.

58. Pingleton S, Fagon J, Pfeifer MP, et al. Patient selection for clinical investigation of ventilator-associated pneumonia: criteria for evaluating diagnostic techniques. *Chest* 1992;102:553S–556S.

59. Cunnion KM, Weber DJ, Broadhead WE, et al. Risk factors for nosocomial pneumonia: comparing adult critical-care populations. *Am J Respir Crit Care Med* 1996;153:158–162.

60. National Nosocomial Infections Surveillance (NNIS) Report, data summary from October 1986-April 1997, issued May 1997. A report from the NNIS system. *Am J Infect Control* 1997;25: 477–487.

61. Centers for Disease Control and Prevention. Guideline for prevention of nosocomial pneumonia. *Respir Care* 1994;39: 1191–1198.

62. Galil K, Zaleznik DF. Nosicomial pneumonia. UpToDate 11.3 available online at: http://www.utdol.com. Accessed February 17, 2003.

63. Prod'hom G, Leuenberger P, Koerfer J, et al. Nosocomial pneumonia in mechanically ventilated patients receiving antiacid, ranitidine, or sucralfate. *Ann Intern Med* 1994;120:653–662.

64. Wahl WL, Franklin GA, Brandt MM, et al. Does bronchoalveolar lavage enhance our ability to treat ventilator-associated pneumonia in a trauma-burn intensive care unit? *J Trauma* 2003;54: 633–639.

65. Fagon JY, Chastre J, Wolff M, et al. Invasive and noninvasive strategies for management of suspected ventilator-associated

pneumonia. A randomized trial. *Ann Intern Med* 2000;132: 621–630.

66. Croce MA, Fabian TC, Schurr MJ, et al. Using bronchoalveolar lavage to distinguish nosocomial pneumonia from systemic inflammatory response syndrome: a prospective analysis. *J Trauma* 1995;39:1134–1140.

67. Croce MA, Fabian TC, Wadde-Smith L, et al. Utility of Gram's stain and efficacy of quantitative culture for posttraumatic pneumonia. *Ann Surg* 1998;227:743–751.

68. Meduri GU, Johanson WG Jr. International consensus conference: clinical investigation of ventilator-associated pneumonia. Introduction. *Chest* 1992;102:551S–552S.

69. Kollef MH, Sherman G, Ward S, et al. Inadequate antimicrobial treatment of infections: a risk factor for hospital mortality among critically ill patients. *Chest* 1999;115:462–474.

70. Rello J, Gallego M, Mariscal D, et al. The value of routine microbial investigation in ventilator-associated pneumonia. *Am J Respir Crit Care Med* 1997;156:196–200.

71. Rello J, Diaz E. Pneumonia in the intensive care unit. *Crit Care Med* 2003;31:2544–2551.

72. Hilf M, Yu VL, Sharp J, et al. Antibiotic therapy for pseudomonas aeruginosa bacteremia: outcome correlations in a prospective study of 200 patients. *Am J Med* 1989;87:540–546.

73. Chastre J, Wolff M, Fagon JY, et al. Comparison of 8 vs 15 days of antibiotic therapy for ventilator-associated pneumonia in adults: a randomized trial *JAMA* 2003;290:2588–2598.

74. Hemmila MR, Hirschl RB. Advances in ventilatory support of the pediatric surgical patient. *Curr Opin Pediatr* 1999;11:241–248.

75. Bernard GR, Artigas A, Brigham KL, et al. The consensus committee report of the American-European consensus conference on ARDS: definitions, mechanisms, relevant outcomes and clinical trial coordination. *Intensive Care Med* 1994;20:225–232.

76. Beaufils F, Mercier JC, Farnoux C, et al. Acute respiratory distress syndrome in children. *Curr Opin Pediatr* 1997;9:207–212.

77. Bulger EM, Jurkovich GJ, Gentilello LM, et al. Current clinical options for the treatment and management of acute respiratory distress syndrome. *J Trauma* 2000;48:562–572.

78. Demling RH. Pulmonary dysfunction. In: Wilmore DW, Cheung LY, Harken AH, et al., eds. *ACS surgery principles and practice 2003*. New York: WebMD Inc.; 2003:1433–1453.

79. Hansen-Flaschen J, Siegel MD. Acute respiratory distress syndrome: definition; diagnosis; and etiology. *UpToDate* 2003; 11.3:1–8.

80. Webb HH, Tierney DF. Experimental pulmonary edema due to intermittent positive pressure ventilation with high inflation pressures. Protection by positive end-expiratory pressure. *Am Rev Respir Dis* 1974;110:556–565.

81. Dreyfuss D, Basset G, Soler P, et al. Intermittent positive-pressure hyperventilation with high inflation pressures produces pulmonary microvascular injury in rats. *Am Rev Respir Dis* 1985;132:880–884.

82. Tsuno K, Prato P, Kolobow T. Acute lung injury from mechanical ventilation at moderately high airway pressures. *J of Appl Physiol* 1990;69:956–961.

83. Hickling KG, Henderson SJ, Jackson R. Low mortality associated with low volume pressure limited ventilation with permissive hypercapnia in severe adult respiratory distress syndrome. *Intensive Care Med* 1990;16:372–377.

84. Hickling KG, Walsh J, Henderson S, et al. Low mortality rate in adult respiratory distress syndrome using low-volume, pressure-limited ventilation with permissive hypercapnia: a prospective study. *Crit Care Med* 1994;22:1568–1578.

85. Kolobow T, Powers T, Mandava S, et al. Intratracheal pulmonary ventilation (ITPV): control of positive end-expiratory pressure at the level of the carina through the use of a novel ITPV catheter design. *Anesth Analg* 1994;78:455–461.

86. Schnitzer JJ, Thompson JE, Hedrick HL, et al. High-frequency intratracheal pulmonary ventilation: improved gas exchange at lower airway pressures. *J Pediatr Surg* 1997;32:203–206.

87. Makhoul IR, Bar-Joseph G, Blazer S, et al. Intratracheal pulmonary ventilation in premature infants and children with intractable hypercapnia. *ASAIO* 1998;44:82–88.

88. Artigas A, Bernard GR, Carlet J, et al. The American-European consensus conference on ARDS, part 2: ventilatory, pharmacologic, supportive therapy, study design strategies and issues related to recovery and remodeling. *Intensive Care Med* 1998; 24:378–398.

89. Amato MB, Barbas CS, Medieros DM, et al. Beneficial effects of the "open lung approach" with low distending pressures in acute respiratory distress syndrome: a prospective randomized study on mechanical ventilation. *Am J Respir Crit Care Med* 1995; 152:1835–1846.

90. Amato MB, Barbas CS, Medieros DM, et al. Effect of a protective-ventilation strategy on mortality in the acute respiratory distress syndrome. *N Engl J Med* 1998;338:347–354.

91. The Acute Respiratory Distress Syndrome Network. Ventilation with lower tidal volumes as compared with traditional tidal volumes for acute lung injury and the acute respiratory distress syndrome. *N Engl J Med* 2000;342:1301–1308.

92. Piehl MA, Brown RS. Use of extreme position changes in acute respiratory failure. *Crit Care Med* 1976;4:13–14.

93. Douglas WW, Rehder K, Beynen FM, et al. Improved oxygenation in patients with acute respiratory failure: the prone position. *Am Rev Respir Dis* 1977;115:559–566.

94. Gattinoni L, Tognoni G, Pesenti A, et al. Effect of prone positioning on the survival of patients with acute respiratory failure. *N Engl J Med* 2001;345:568–573.

95. Bartlett RH, Roloff DW, Cornell RG, et al. Extracorporeal circulation in neonatal respiratory failure: a prospective randomized study. *Pediatrics* 1985;76:479–487.

96. UK Collaborative ECMO Trial Group. UK collaborative randomized trial of neonatal extracorporeal membrane oxygenation. *Lancet* 1996;348:75–82.

97. Extracorporeal Life Support Organization. Annual ECMO Registry Report. July 2003.

98. Rich PB, Awad SS, Kolla S, et al. An approach to the treatment of severe adult respiratory failure. *J Crit Care* 1998;13:26–36.

Cardiac Complications

17

Wendy L. Wahl

▰▰▰ **INTRODUCTION 174**

▰▰▰ **PREOPERATIVE EVALUATION 175**
Type of Operation 175
Clinical Risk Factors and Cardiac Risk Indices 175

▰▰▰ **NONINVASIVE AND INVASIVE CARDIAC TESTING 176**
Electrocardiogram 176
Exercise and Nuclear Stress Testing 177
Cardiac Catheterization 177
Preoperative Testing Recommendations 177

▰▰▰ **PREOPERATIVE INTERVENTIONS 177**
Coronary Artery Bypass Grafting 177
β-blockers 177
Other Adrenergic Blocking Agents 179

▰▰▰ **OPERATIVE MONITORING 180**

▰▰▰ **POSTOPERATIVE COMPLICATIONS 180**
Heart Failure 180
Myocardial Infarction and Ischemia 181
Arrhythmias 182

▰▰▰ **SUMMARY 182**

▰▰▰ **REFERENCES 182**

Wendy L. Wahl: University of Michigan, Ann Arbor, MI 48109

INTRODUCTION

Every year, over 25 million patients in the United States undergo noncardiac operations (1). One million of these patients will have coronary artery disease (CAD), an estimated 2 to 3 million more will have cardiac risk factors, and more than 4 million will be 65 or older (1). As the population continues to age, the number of annual surgical procedures will rise. Approximately one million surgical patients will sustain perioperative cardiac complications including death, congestive heart failure (CHF), and myocardial infarction (MI) per year. For patients over 40, the overall risk of perioperative cardiac complications is less than 5% (2), but it varies among patients depending on clinical risk factors for CAD and the type of surgical procedure. Patients over 75, those with a history of cardiovascular disease or CHF, and those undergoing a vascular surgical procedure carry much higher associated risks (3). Surgery-specific and clinical factors that allow for cardiac risk stratification should be routinely assessed to guide preoperative risk determination and appropriate evaluation. The costs and risks of an invasive evaluation, such as a coronary angiogram, are prohibitive if done for all patients. Non-invasive testing would also be cost-prohibitive if performed on every preoperative patient. To minimize risks and maximize benefits to patients undergoing noncardiac procedures, the American College of Physicians in 1997 (4–6) and the American College of Cardiology with the American Heart Association (AHA) in 2002 published guidelines for the assessment and management of cardiac risk (7).

PREOPERATIVE EVALUATION

Type of Operation

The type of surgery planned is an important cardiac risk factor. In a study of patients with known CAD treated with medical therapy, 3,368 patients underwent noncardiac surgery. "High-risk" procedures involving the abdominal cavity, thoracic cavity, head and neck, or suprainguinal vascular surgery carried an overall perioperative MI rate of 2.7% and a death rate of 3.3% for those treated medically for CAD. These rates compare to an MI rate of 0.8 and mortality rate of 1.0 for those with no identified CAD (8). Major vascular surgery was associated with an 8.5% risk of perioperative MI and a mortality rate of 3.3%. In patients undergoing orthopedic, breast, skin, or transurethral prostatectomy procedures, the combined cardiac event rate was less than 1% and not different for those with or without preexisting cardiac disease (8). The associated cardiac risk for the various operative procedures might depend on a number of factors. Larger fluid or blood losses and fluid shifts are more likely in extensive intrathoracic or intraabdominal procedures. Major chest or abdominal procedures are also associated with a higher likelihood of prolonged mechanical ventilation, which might increase cardiac stress. Patients undergoing major vascular operations are more likely to have generalized atherosclerosis with CAD (8,9).

Clinical Risk Factors and Cardiac Risk Indices

Many risk stratification indices have been formulated to quantify cardiac risk for patients with cardiovascular disease. CAD manifested by angina or MI heralds an increased risk for cardiac complications. In addition to CAD, many other determinants, such as age, cardiac rhythm, history of heart failure or cerebrovascular disease, creatinine ≥ 2 mg per dL, and diabetes, have been used to adjust for cardiac risk (2,6,7,10). Despite the variation in the factors included in the cardiac risk indices, all provide similar predictions of cardiac risk (11).

The original Goldman cardiac risk index, which studied 1,001 patients aged 40 or older, identified nine independent factors and assigned points to each one (Table 17-1). Patients were stratified according to the total number of points into four risk groups. Those patients with the lowest risk score (0 to 5 points) had a less than 1% chance of a cardiac event. Patients with moderate points (6 to 12 points or 13 to 25 points) had a cardiac complication rate of 9%, whereas 78% of patients with ≥ 26 points developed a major cardiac complication. The Goldman index does have limitations, especially in those who fall into the intermediate risk group where risk estimates might be too low. The index was developed at a single medical center and might reflect institutional bias. The data set on which the index was based is from the 1970s and might not reflect current practices in surgery, medicine, or anesthesia. Finally, there

TABLE 17-1

GOLDMAN CARDIAC RISK INDEX: INDEPENDENT CORRELATES OF PERIOPERATIVE CARDIAC EVENTS

Points	Factor
11	Preoperative S_3 gallop or jugular venous distension
10	Myocardial infarction in the prior 6 months
7	Atrial premature contractions or rhythm other than sinus on preoperative electrocardiogram
7	Greater than five premature ventricular beats per minute at any time prior to operation
5	Age older than 70 years
4	Emergency operation
3	Intraperitoneal, intrathoracic, or aortic operation
3	Significant valvular aortic stenosis
3	Presence of one or more signs of poor medical condition, including: serum potassium <3 or serum bicarbonate <20 mEq/L, creatinine >3 mg/dL, pO_2 <60 or pCO_2 >50 mm Hg, chronic liver disease, or bedridden status from noncardiac causes

From Goldman L, Caldera DL, Nussbaum SR, et al. Multifactorial index of cardiac risk in noncardiac surgical procedures. *N Engl J Med* 1977; 297:845, with permission.

were very few vascular patients included in the original index data set (2). Despite these limitations, other studies have confirmed the original findings of Goldman et al. (Table 17-2) (12).

Both Goldman and, later, Detsky et al. modified the original Goldman index. To simplify the calculation of risk, Goldman et al. developed a revised index that based cardiac risk on six independent predictors of cardiac complications. The revised Goldman cardiac risk index studied cardiac morbidity and mortality associated with 2,893 patients undergoing elective noncardiac procedures and was later validated in 1,422 patients (10). The rate of

TABLE 17-2

ESTIMATION OF CARDIAC RISK FROM STUDIES USING THE GOLDMAN INDEX

Goldman Risk Class	Percent Cardiac Morbidity/Mortality
Class I (0 to 5 points)	1.3
Class II (6 to 12 points)	4.7
Class III (13 to 25 points)	15.3
Class IV (>25 points)	56

From Bronson D, Halperin A, Marwick T. Evaluating cardiac risk in noncardiac surgery patients. *Cleve Clin J Med* 1995;62:391, with permission.

cardiac complications was 0.4%, 0.9%, 7%, and 11% for patients with 0, 1, 2, or 3 or more predictive factors, respectively. The revised Goldman risk factors are: history of heart failure, history of cerebrovascular disease, preoperative serum creatinine more than 2 mg per dL, preoperative need for insulin, history of ischemic heart disease (including MI, positive exercise stress test, abnormal Q waves on electrocardiogram [ECG], ongoing use of nitrates, current angina, or chest pain believed to be from ischemia), and an operative procedure that is intraperitoneal, intrathoracic, or nonperipheral vascular surgery (10).

Detsky et al. modification added angina and pulmonary edema to the original Goldman index. A high number of points were given for patients with recent pulmonary edema, unstable angina 3 months prior to surgery, and angina at rest or with minimal activity (6). Similar to the Goldman index, patients at the lower end of the intermediate risk group might have an underestimation of cardiac risk. Both indices might not be accurate in predicting risk for vascular surgery patients (13).

To improve estimation of cardiac risk in vascular surgery patients, Eagle et al. identified five clinical and two dipyridamole-thallium test predictors of postoperative cardiac events. The five clinical predictors and two dipyridamole-thallium predictors were derived through logistic regression analysis of 254 consecutive patients undergoing nuclear cardiology imaging prior to vascular operations (Table 17-3) (14). The correlation between the clinical and nuclear cardiology test predictors and cardiac events of ischemic pulmonary edema, MI, or cardiac death are listed in Table 17-4. Validation of Eagle's criteria was provided by a later prospective study of 517 abdominal aortic surgery patients. Vanzetto et al. found that the addition of thallium imaging in the intermediate risk group improved the predictive power, where those with two to four risk factors had

TABLE 17-4

CORRELATION BETWEEN EAGLE CRITERIA AND POSTOPERATIVE ISCHEMIC EVENTS IN VASCULAR SURGERY PATIENTS

Number of Predictors	Thallium Redistribution	Percent Cardiac Events
Initial Logistic Regression Model: Vascular Surgery Patients[a]		
0	—	3.1
1 or 2	None	3.2
1 or 2	Present	29.6
3 or more	—	50
Prospective Validation: Abdominal Aortic Surgery Patients[b]		
0	—	2.4
1	—	4
2 to 4	None	0
2 to 4	Present	13
≥5	None	3
≥5	Present	32

[a]From Eagle KA, Coley CM, Newell JB, et al. Combining clinical and thallium data optimizes preoperative assessment of cardiac risk before major vascular surgery. *Ann Intern Med* 1989;110:859, with permission.
[b]From Vanzetto G, Machecourt J, Blendea D, et al. Additive value of thallium single-photon emission computed tomography myocardial imaging for prediction of perioperative events in clinically selected high cardiac risk patients having abdominal aortic surgery. *Am J. Cardiol* 1996;77:143, with permission.

a 13% risk of death or MI with positive imaging compared to a 0% risk with a normal study. Even in the high-risk group with five or more predictors, a negative thallium test was associated with a 3% risk of a cardiac event compared to a 32% risk for a positive test (15).

NONINVASIVE AND INVASIVE CARDIAC TESTING

Electrocardiogram

ECG remains an essential screening tool in preoperative evaluation. In some studies the absence of preoperative and immediate postoperative (first 24 to 48 hours) ischemic ST-segment depression on ECG in intermediate risk vascular surgery patients predicted a low risk for perioperative cardiac events (16,17). Patients with left bundle branch block, left ventricular hypertrophy with a strain pattern, or digitalis effect were not studied, however, which limits the applicability of these findings to all patients. Other ECG abnormalities (MI pattern or arrhythmia) are included in preoperative risk assessment indices and

TABLE 17-3

EAGLE CRITERIA FOR ASSESSING CARDIAC RISK IN VASCULAR SURGERY PATIENTS

Clinical Predictors

Age older than 70 years
Diabetes mellitus requiring therapy other than diet modification
Ventricular ectopy requiring therapy
History of angina
Q waves on electrocardiogram

Dipyrimadole-Thallium Test Predictors

Electrocardiogram changes during or after dipyridamole infusion
Evidence of thallium redistribution

From Eagle KA, Coley CM, Newell JB, et al. Combining clinical and thallium data optimizes preoperative assessment of cardiac risk before major vascular surgery. *Ann Intern Med* 1989;110:859, with permission.

warrant further investigation on the basis of the rest of the preoperative risk factors.

Exercise and Nuclear Stress Testing

Exercise stress testing without myocardial imaging remains a cornerstone for determining functional status and for detecting cardiac ischemia. There are several limitations to the use of exercise stress testing in preoperative patients. The sensitivity of exercise testing is suboptimal if patients do not perform to maximal exercise levels. An abnormal ECG might preclude exercise stress testing. Many patients cannot reach their target heart rate because of limitations from arthritis or fractures, pain from claudication, pulmonary disease, or other medical conditions. Patients who are unable to tolerate exercise to at least 85% of predicted maximal heart rate carry a 24% associated risk of perioperative cardiac events even without ischemic ECG changes (18,19).

For patients who cannot tolerate exercise stress testing or who have suboptimal results, preoperative dipyridamole-thallium imaging can help stratify intermediate risk patients. Many studies report higher perioperative cardiac complications in intermediate risk patients with thallium defects on imaging relative to those without thallium defects. In one study of vascular surgery patients with an intermediate cardiac risk by Goldman criteria treated with medical management for CAD, 23% with fixed thallium defects, 33% with reversible thallium defects, and 4% with no defects sustained cardiac events (20). The number and extent of cardiac segments with reversible thallium defects also correlate with an adverse cardiac event. More than one reversible thallium defect carries a higher perioperative cardiac risk (21).

Dobutamine stress echocardiography is another accepted noninvasive imaging tool that provides information about resting and stress systolic heart function. This technique has proven useful in preoperative evaluation of vascular surgery patients with three or more clinical risk factors for postoperative cardiac events. In this patient subset, for patients taking a β-blocker who had stress-induced ischemia on dobutamine echocardiography, the incidence of cardiac events in the first 30 postoperative days was 10.6% compared to 2% for those without ischemia (22).

Measurement of left ventricular ejection fraction (LVEF) might enhance the predictive capacity of nuclear cardiac imaging. In a single study using transthoracic echo for LVEF measurement, patients with an ejection fraction greater than 50% with an abnormal thallium image had no cardiac complications. In the group with a LVEF of less than 50% and an abnormal thallium study, 55% had a cardiac complication (23).

Cardiac Catheterization

In a study of 878 patients, 96% of patients without diabetes, angina, MI, and CHF had no evidence of severe CAD when evaluated by coronary arteriography (24). Additionally, no studies show that coronary angiography findings predict cardiac complications after operation. Because coronary angiography bears the procedural risks of death and stroke, catheterization is recommended only for those being independently considered for cardiac revascularization rather than for risk stratification in noncardiac procedures.

Preoperative Testing Recommendations

For patients with intermediate risk based on the discussed cardiac risk indices, noninvasive testing allows for improved prediction of cardiac risk. The published guidelines for further testing include the use of ECG, noninvasive left ventricular function measurements, and either exercise or pharmacologic stress testing.

The algorithm is outlined in Table 17-5 (7). The task force outlined a stepwise progression for preoperative cardiac evaluation that incorporates clinical risk factors, type of surgery, and cardiac testing.

PREOPERATIVE INTERVENTIONS

Coronary Artery Bypass Grafting

For patients with severe CAD documented by coronary arteriography, revascularization reduces postoperative death after major noncardiac operations (8,25,26). The cardiac death rate dropped from 3.3% to 1.7% and the MI rate decreased from 2.7% to 0.8% for those treated with coronary artery bypass grafting (CABG) versus medical management, respectively (8). The advantage was most pronounced in patients evaluated for later vascular surgery procedures, where there was a significant long-term survival benefit in those treated with CABG rather than medical therapy. This benefit was greatest in vascular surgery patients with three-vessel CAD. For patients undergoing low-risk noncardiac procedures (breast, urologic, orthopedic, or skin), the risk of a cardiac event was low (<1.0%) and was not altered by prior CABG (8).

β-blockers

In addition to coronary arteriography with potential stenting, angioplasty, or even CABG, a number of medical interventions have decreased postoperative cardiac events. Several studies have reported the effectiveness of β-blockers in reduction of postoperative ischemic events. The use of β-blockers is reported as a major process to improve patient safety (27) but is not formally included in preoperative published guidelines (4,7). In a review of all recent prospective randomized studies looking at perioperative cardiac events after β-blockade (28), five of six studies demonstrated an improvement in cardiac and all-cause mortality (22,29–32). The improvement in

TABLE 17-5

AMERICAN COLLEGE OF CARDIOLOGY/AMERICAN HEART ASSOCIATION TASK FORCE RECOMMENDATIONS FOR PREOPERATIVE CARDIAC ASSESSMENT FOR NONCARDIAC SURGERY

Step 1. Perform emergent surgery, all other procedures go to step 2.

Step 2. If the patient has no signs or symptoms of ongoing cardiac ischemia and has undergone coronary revascularization within the last 5 years proceed to surgery, if not, go to step 3.

Step 3. If a coronary arteriogram or stress test was performed within the last 2 years with favorable results and the patient has no new or changed symptoms, proceed to surgery. Otherwise go to step 4.

Step 4. For patients with major predictors of cardiac complications (unstable coronary disease, decompensated CHF, ongoing arrhythmia, severe valvular disease) surgery should be delayed or canceled if possible. Patients should undergo maximization of medical management and strong consideration for coronary angiography to direct subsequent care. Otherwise go to step 5.

Step 5. For those with intermediate clinical predictors (mild angina, prior MI, history of compensated CHF, diabetes mellitus, or renal insufficiency) undergoing a low-risk surgical procedure (endoscopy, skin, ophthalmologic procedures, or breast surgery) proceed to operation. For those with minimal risk factors and good functional capacity (can climb a flight of stairs, walk on level ground at 4 mph, run a short distance, scrub a floor, or play a game of golf) proceed to operation. Otherwise go to step 6.

Step 6. For those with intermediate risk factors undergoing vascular surgery, for those with intermediate risk factors and poor functional capacity or those with minimal risk factors but poor functional capacity, further noninvasive testing is recommended. If noninvasive testing supports a low-risk status, proceed to surgery. Otherwise perform cardiac arteriography to guide further therapy. Patients who are not operative candidates for coronary revascularization should either proceed to operation with maximal medical management and perioperative monitoring or be considered for alternative surgical strategies.

From Eagle KA, Berger PB, Calkins H, et al. ACC/AHA guideline update for perioperative cardiovascular evaluation for noncardiac surgery—executive summary: a report of the American College of Cardiology/American Heart Association Task Force on Practice Guidelines (Committee to Update the 1996 Guidelines on perioperative cardiovascular evaluation for noncardiac surgery). *J Am Coll Cardiol* 2002;39:542–553, with permission.

mortality was most prominent for patients at high risk (22). The only study reporting no benefit with β-blockers included patients with a low baseline risk of cardiac events and a target heart rate of less than 80 beats per minute (33). Although the other studies used different β-blockers at varying doses and schedules, the endpoint was to provide preoperative β-blockade to a goal heart rate of 70 beats per minute. The applicability of β-blocker use in all patients is limited by the lack of data on type of surgical procedures performed and a wide variation of preexisting cardiac risk in study patients (28).

Mangano et al. found no difference for in-hospital mortality in male, β-blocked patients undergoing major noncardiac surgery at a Veterans Administration hospital (29). Interestingly, there was a relative reduction in all-cause mortality that continued to at least 2 years after operation. The difference in mortality, which appeared postoperatively within 8 months, was attributed to a reduction in cardiac events. The mortality risk reduction at 1 year was 67% and 48% at 2 years (29). The treatment group results might have been biased by the concomitant use of angiotensin-converting enzyme (ACE) inhibitors and because the group was more likely to remain on a β-blocker postoperatively. After adjusting for these differences in multivariate models, the difference in mortality was still supported. Recommendations for the use of perioperative β-blockers and a revised cardiac risk index are listed in Table 17-6.

Poldermans et al. found a larger benefit from β-blockade in vascular surgery patients with documented ischemia on dobutamine echocardiography. The β-blocker group had a 90% reduction in cardiac death or MI at 30 days (34). The differences in benefits from β-blockers can be partially ascribed to the baseline cardiac risk of the patient population, where those with the highest benefit are most at risk.

In patients undergoing low-risk procedures or patients with low cardiac risk, the effectiveness of β-blockers is not clear (23). There are risks to β-blockade, which include bradycardia in about one-quarter of patients, of which half require atropine therapy perioperatively (30). Another study using a nonselective β-blocker in major thoracic operations reported a higher incidence of bradycardia, hypotension, and a trend toward more pulmonary edema (35). An additional risk of long-term β-blocker therapy is the risk of increased adrenergic activity if β-blocker therapy is held or stopped perioperatively. A prospective observational study in patients on long-term β-blockers found a higher rate of MI in those who had β-blockers discontinued immediately after surgery (36). The effect was not seen in other trials that used a shorter duration of β-blockade (30,31). The optimal duration of therapy for patients receiving β-blockade perioperatively deserves further investigation.

Studies that support benefit with β-blockers used a β_1-selective β-blocker. Nonselective agents such as propranolol have more adverse pulmonary side effects, with more bronchospasm and pulmonary edema (35). In studies using a β_1-selective β-blocker, the beneficial effect appears to be class-dependent rather than drug-dependent. Although the optimal dosing for perioperative β-blockade remains unclear, the positive effect of targeted heart rate control of $\leq$70 beats per minute is generally accepted. The

TABLE 17-6

CRITERIA FOR USE OF PERIOPERATIVE β-BLOCKADE

Minor Clinical Criteria

For patients with two or more of the following criteria, use beta-blockers:

Age ≥65 years
Hypertension
Current smoker
Serum cholesterol of ≥240 mg/dL
Diabetes mellitus not requiring insulin therapy

Revised Cardiac Risk Index Criteria

For patients with any of the following criteria, use beta-blockers:

High-risk noncardiac operation (intraperitoneal, intrathoracic, or suprainguinal vascular procedure)
Ischemic heart disease, defined by one or more of the following:
    History of myocardial infarction
    History of or current angina
    Ongoing used of sublingual nitroglycerine
    Positive exercise stress test
    Q waves on ECG
    Chest pain in patients after PTCA or CABG
Cerebrovascular occlusive disease, defined as:
    History of transient ischemic attack
    History of cerebrovascular accident
Diabetes mellitus requiring insulin therapy
Chronic renal insufficiency with baseline creatinine of ≥2.0 mg/dL

From Mangano DT, Layug EL, Wallace A, et al. Multicenter Study of Perioperative Ischemia Research Group. Effect of atenolol on mortality and cardiovascular morbidity after noncardiac surgery: multicenter study of perioperative ischemia research group. *N Engl J Med* 1996;35:1713–1720; From Boersma E, Poldermans D, Bax JJ, et al. Predictors of cardiac events after major vascular surgery: role of clinical characteristic, dobutamine echocardiography, and β-blocker therapy. *JAMA* 2001;285:1865–1873, with permission.

safest conclusion derived from recent perioperative β-blocker studies suggests starting β-blockers up to 1 month prior to surgery and continuing through the hospitalization. Longer therapy is reasonable if medical follow-up is available (28). There is evidence that β-blocker therapy is underutilized in many patients who have appropriate indications for use (37–39). β-blockade is recommended for long-term use in heart failure patients and reduces perioperative mortality. For heart failure patients, dosing requires close monitoring and is not titrated to heart rate (40,41).

With the effectiveness of β-blockade, some authors question whether further risk stratification is still necessary (42). With the benefit of β-blockade in high-risk patients [5 or more points in the revised cardiac risk index of Lee et al. (10)], the cardiac event rate was 14%. In light of this, a recommendation for further noninvasive testing is still made for any patient with an estimated

cardiac complication risk of 3.4% or higher (28). After review of the current literature on perioperative cardiac complications in patients treated with β-blockers, Auerbach and Goldman made several clinical recommendations (28). For patients deemed at lowest risk, with an estimated cardiac event rate of less than 1% without β-blockers, it is unlikely that β-blockade will provide additional benefit. In highest-risk patients (those with a revised cardiac index of 3 or greater), additional risk stratification with either noninvasive or invasive testing is warranted, in addition to β-blockers. Wherever feasible, oral β-blockers should be started preoperatively and adjusted for heart rate control. Oral β-blockers should be resumed as soon as possible postoperatively with intravenous forms used until oral medications are tolerated (Table 17-7) (28).

Other Adrenergic Blocking Agents

Patients receiving selective α_2 receptor blockade might have improved outcomes. Clonidine decreases blood pressure and heart rate and lowers norepinephrine levels in

TABLE 17-7

PERIOPERATIVE β-BLOCKERS AND DOSING REGIMENS

Outpatient or Posthospital Admission

If not on β-blockers and patient has more than minimal risk:
    Atenolol 50–100 mg orally every day until surgery or
    Bisoprolol 5–10 mg every day
        Start up to 30 days prior to surgery
        Titrate to heart rate ≤65 bpm

Patient on long-term β-blockers:
    Continue present therapy
    Titrate dose to heart rate of ≤65 bpm

Immediate Perioperative Period

Atenolol, 5–10 mg intravenously, to reach target heart rate before anesthetic induction, whether on preoperative β-blockers or not.

Postoperative period
    Patient not able to take oral medication and hemodynamically stable:
        Atenolol, 5–10 mg intravenously, twice daily to target heart rate
    Patient unstable (labile hemodynamics or high bleeding risk):
        Esmolol, 500 mcg/kg intravenously for 1 minute, then infuse at 50–200 mcg/kg/min to target heart rate
    Patient on oral medications:
        When transitioning to oral, overlap first oral dose with intravenous dose to maintain target heart rate
        Resume perioperative β-blocker at previous dose, titrate as necessary to target heart rate

From Auerbach AD, Goldman L. β-Blockers and reduction of cardiac events in noncardiac surgery. *JAMA* 2002;287:1435–1444, with permission.

surgical patients—all factors that decrease myocardial ischemia. In one study looking at vascular surgery patients treated with clonidine, there were fewer cardiac ischemic events (43). In another study, α_2-antagonists decrease post-ganglionic noradrenaline availability and spinal efferent sympathetic output with a lowered incidence of perioperative ischemia (44). In a large European randomized trial, patients having noncardiac surgery did not have lower all-cause mortality or MI after treatment with mivazerol. In a subgroup analysis, cardiac deaths were lower in the treated group (45). Currently, mivazerol is not available in the United States.

OPERATIVE MONITORING

All forms of anesthesia induce cardiovascular effects. Inhaled anesthetics decrease mean arterial pressure in a dose-dependent manner through vasodilation, with a decrease in cardiac output secondary to myocardial depression and reduced sympathetic tone. Epidural anesthesia can induce hypotension and a secondary rise in venous capacitance with reduced left ventricular preload. Inadvertent intravenous administration of lidocaine or bupivicaine can cause arrhythmias and cardiovascular collapse (46). Most episodes of cardiac ischemia, however, occur in the absence of major hemodynamic changes, with only a small rise in heart rate. Silent ischemia might be due to coronary vasoconstriction related to reduced myocardial oxygenation or thrombosis (47).

For patients with decreased LVEF, significant valvular disease, recent MI, or unstable angina, clinicians often employ perioperative invasive cardiac monitoring with a pulmonary artery catheter (PAC) (48). Some physicians recommend preoperative placement of a PAC to improve hemodynamics through preload maximization and inotropes (49,50). Despite these practices, few data support that either preoperative or intraoperative PAC use improves outcomes. The best prospective study on PAC use looked at patients aged 60 or older undergoing major urgent or elective surgery. The mortality rate for those with a PAC was 7.8% compared to 7.7% for those without a PAC. The 60-day mortality was not different between groups. The incidence of postoperative heart failure was the same at 12.9% versus 11.2%, respectively. The pulmonary embolism rate was higher in those with a PAC (0.9 versus 0%) (51). These findings were confirmed in a prospective study of 4,059 patients having major noncardiac surgery (52).

For vascular surgery patients, one small prospective randomized study of patients having arterial limb salvage procedures had improved outcomes with PAC use (53). In the same study, of 1,065 patients undergoing suprainguinal vascular procedures, PAC use did not demonstrate the same benefits (53). A metaanalysis of all randomized studies involving vascular surgery patients did not reveal a benefit

from PAC use (54). In 1,094 CABG patients who were randomized to either a central venous catheter or PAC, no differences in ICU stay, death rate, postoperative MI, or other noncardiac complications were found (55). Despite this data, PAC's are used in most centers performing cardiac surgery (51,56).

In a 1997 consensus statement endorsed by five critical care societies that reviewed the PAC literature, little or no benefit for PAC use was seen in patients undergoing cardiac, low-risk aortic, or neurosurgical procedures, nor was there a benefit in those age 65 years or older (57). On the basis of nonrandomized reports and expert opinion, PAC use for high-risk vascular surgery and aortic valve surgery was supported. In summary, there is little evidence in support of routine use of PAC in most operative patients.

POSTOPERATIVE COMPLICATIONS

Heart Failure

Heart failure is the most common cardiac complication occurring after noncardiac surgery. Overall, 1% to 6% of patients develop heart failure after major surgery. The risk is higher for patients with known CAD, valvular disease, or known congestive heart failure where 6% to 25% develop postoperative heart failure (2,17). Postoperative pulmonary edema can occur from causes other than heart failure and should be distinguished from CHF. Negative pressure pulmonary edema in young, healthy adults who have laryngospasm might occur in up to 0.1% of anesthetic cases (58). The mechanism is poorly understood, but recovery is excellent. Postoperative pulmonary edema might also be seen after pneumonectomy (59), lateral decubitus positioning (60), lung transplantation (61), or cocaine use (62).

Preoperative identification of heart failure is an independent predictor of worsened cardiac outcome after major surgery in most cardiac risk indices, as previously discussed. Once heart failure is identified postoperatively, treatment is similar to medical management for nonsurgical cases. Patients identified with heart failure should be assessed for new or unstable cardiac ischemia. This assessment might be difficult since most postoperative MIs present atypically, where pain is often not a key symptom. If cardiac ischemia is suspected, electrocardiography, cardiac monitoring, and cardiac enzyme measurements should be performed. Postoperative patients with heart failure, but not cardiac ischemia, have the same outcome as nonsurgical patients with heart failure. In a study of 444 patients with cardiac risk factors, 17% had cardiac events in the immediate postoperative period. Eight of these patients had active ischemia, and 30 had heart failure without ischemia. Only patients who had active postoperative ischemia had worsened outcomes in follow-up at 2 years (17).

The preoperative and postoperative management of heart failure includes assessment of myocardial ischemia. Swan-Ganz catheter measurements, if available, suggest heart failure if the pulmonary artery wedge pressure is ≥18 mm Hg. In myocardial ischemia these measurements might be misleading if a wedge pressure is measured after the ischemia has resolved and the transient ventricular dysfunction has cleared. Plasma brain natriuretic peptide (BNP) can distinguish between heart failure and lung disease with a fair degree of accuracy for patients presenting with dyspnea. BNP concentrations are much higher in heart failure patients than in patients with primary lung disease or dysfunction. A BNP value of >100 pg per mL diagnosed heart failure with a sensitivity of 90% and a specificity of 74% (63). The role of BNP in postoperative patients has not been studied.

Supplemental oxygen, morphine sulfate, and diuretics should be started once the diagnosis is made. Morphine sulfate decreases central sympathetic outflow with arteriolar and venous dilation and subsequent lowered cardiac filling pressures. At a dose of 2 to 4 mg intravenously, repeated every 15 minutes as necessary, the work of breathing is also decreased (64).

Diuretic therapy should be started to decrease preload. Furosemide is the most common diuretic used for acute CHF. An initial dose of 40 mg leads to a peak diuresis at 30 minutes after intravenous administration. After furosemide injection in acute pulmonary edema, there is an initial venodilation with decreased pulmonary congestion. This effect is seen prior to diuresis and is attributed to a prostaglandin effect (65).

Patients with the preoperative diagnosis of heart failure might already be receiving an ACE inhibitor or β-blocker. Perioperative ACE inhibitor use might be associated with perioperative hypotension through blunting of the renin-angiotensin system response to surgical stress. Vascular surgery patients who continued ACE inhibitors through the perioperative period had more episodes of intraoperative hypotension than those who discontinued the medication 12 to 24 hours preoperatively (66). A second study in CABG patients reported similar findings for hypotension but also found significant problems with postoperative hypertension requiring therapy (67). For patients on ACE inhibitors for hypertension, it is reasonable to continue treatment until the time of surgery. For patients with heart failure, particularly with baseline low blood pressure, holding the ACE inhibitor might induce less intraoperative hypotension. The benefits and risks should be considered and the patient carefully monitored in terms of fluid status and hemodynamics.

β-blocker use perioperatively does improve outcomes for patients with heart failure. Ideally, β-blockade should be started as far as a month in advance of operation and the drug titrated to effect. For nonoperative patients developing heart failure, β-blockers improve outcomes and are recommended (68,69). For postsurgical patients who are not on β-blockers, no studies address starting β-blocker therapy immediately after surgery.

Myocardial Infarction and Ischemia

Patients with known cardiac risk factors are more likely to have perioperative ischemic events. For male patients over 40 undergoing noncardiac procedures, 4.1% with known CAD and 0.8% of those with vascular disease, but no CAD, had an MI (3). Intraoperative two-lead ECG monitoring is routine for all patients. Intraoperative ischemia detected by two-lead ECG monitoring was associated with all perioperative cardiac events in a study of male patients undergoing noncardiac surgery (70). The addition of 12-lead ECG or transesophageal echocardiography (TEE) was of little incremental value in detecting intraoperative ischemia in noncardiac surgery patients (70). In a group of 200 high-risk male patients the highest incidence of ischemia was documented postoperatively rather than intraoperatively (71).

The diagnosis of perioperative MI can be difficult since skeletal muscle injury is unavoidable in many operative procedures. Creatine kinase (CK) and its isoforms might be unreliable in the face of operative muscle injury. The isoenzyme form of CK, MB, constitutes a lower percentage of the total CK in skeletal muscle than heart muscle. Despite this, the following conditions make the use of CK-MB for MI diagnosis less accurate: myocardial injury after cardiopulmonary resuscitation, cardioversion, defibrillation, cardiac and noncardiac operations, blunt chest trauma with possible cardiac injury, hypothyroidism, renal failure, and cocaine use (72–76).

Cardiac troponins I and T are cardiac regulatory proteins that control calcium-mediated actin and myosin interactions. Cardiac troponin levels generally start to rise 4 to 6 hours after an MI, and up to 12 hours is necessary to detect all elevations (72,77). In one study comparing echocardiographic wall motion abnormalities with elevated cardiac enzymes, all patients with a perioperative MI had elevated serum troponin levels. For patients without new echocardiographic abnormalities, 19% had CK elevations but only 1% had a rise in troponin levels (77).

For patients with documented acute MI in the postoperative period, few data specific to the postoperative period are available. The initial goal of therapy is to relieve ischemic chest pain through the use of intravenous nitroglycerin and morphine sulfate as necessary (78). Antithrombotic therapy with aspirin should be started unless there is a contraindication. Reperfusion therapy is strongly recommended with primary percutaneous coronary intervention (PCI) or thrombolysis. PCI is preferred over thrombolysis therapy. If PCI is not contraindicated in the postoperative setting, the time to maximal benefit is 2 to 3 hours from the time of presentation. These interventions might not be feasible for surgical patients in the immediate postoperative period due to potential bleeding complications. Active bleeding, systolic blood pressure over 175 mm Hg, trauma, or drug allergy are contraindications to thrombolytic therapy (78).

Other drug therapies are also recommended. Antiplatelet therapy with aspirin is indicated in all patients with acute MI in the absence of an absolute contraindication (78). In a review of 15 trials of antiplatelet therapy, patients with an acute MI had a 30% reduction in cardiovascular events (79). As soon as feasible, the patient should chew 160 mg to 325 mg of aspirin for a rapid antiplatelet effect. Transrectal aspirin can be given in patients who are not taking oral medications. β-blockers should be started unless there is a contraindication, such as hypotension or bradycardia. Intravenous atenolol or metoprolol should be titrated to a goal heart rate of less than 70 beats per minute. β-blockade in the presence of acute MI is associated with up to a 40% reduction in mortality in those with ST elevation in the post-thrombolytic era. Prior to thrombolytics, β-blockers provided a 10% to 15% decrease in mortality (80,81). Since many postoperative patients cannot undergo thrombolysis because of bleeding risks, the latter risk reduction might be more reflective of surgical results.

Arrhythmias

Although postoperative arrhythmias are most common after cardiac surgery, arrhythmias can occur after any surgical procedure and are more common in patients with preoperative cardiac risk factors. Atrial fibrillation complicates 10% to 40% of CABG procedures and up to 60% of valve replacement operations (82). When a rapid heart rhythm is detected, evaluation of the patient for signs and symptoms of cardiovascular instability are paramount. Signs and symptoms of hypotension, heart failure or pulmonary congestion, shock, decreased consciousness, and acute MI require immediate cardioversion (83). For stable patients the emphasis should be diagnosis of the specific rhythm disturbance and identification of patients with poor LVEF (83). The AHA, in conjunction with the International Liaison Committee on Resuscitation, developed an algorithm and guidelines for the management of tachyarrhythmias. The four categories of tachycardia are: atrial fibrillation and flutter, narrow-complex tachycardias, wide-complex tachycardias of unknown type, and stable monomorphic or polymorphic ventricular tachycardia (83).

Atrial fibrillation should be treated with medications that slow the ventricular rate by inhibiting conduction through the atrioventricular node. Regardless of the duration of atrial fibrillation, either a β-blocker or calcium channel blocker should be given. Digoxin is an alternative agent, but it has a slower onset of action. If these therapies are unsuccessful in slowing ventricular response or are contraindicated, amiodarone is indicated (84–86). In select patients with a duration of less than 48 hours, cardioversion might be indicated. For patients who do not convert to sinus rhythm, anticoagulation with coumadin is recommended to prevent embolic complications (83).

Narrow-complex tachycardias include junctional, atrial, and paroxysmal supraventricular tachycardias. If a specific diagnosis cannot be made on careful inspection of a 12-lead ECG, vagal maneuvers or adenosine might be helpful in slowing the rate for rhythm identification (87). True junctional tachycardias might be due to digitalis toxicity and should be investigated. Exogenous cathecolamines and theophylline might induce junctional and atrial tachycardias as well. These rhythms can be treated with calcium channel blockers or β-blockers in the absence of poor left ventricular function (83).

Wide-complex tachycardias require careful inspection to determine the etiology. On a 12-lead ECG, atrioventricular dissociation might be a helpful marker. Although adenosine might differentiate narrow-complex rhythms, adenosine might be harmful in patients with a ventricular rhythm and might increase accessory pathway conduction and induce hypotension (87).

Ventricular tachycardia is often an unstable, life-threatening rhythm. In the face of a rate >150 beats/minute, hypotension, or mental status changes, defibrillation is necessary. Further pharmacologic therapy should be based on the QT interval on a baseline ECG. Patients with QT prolongation might have a congenital form that can be treated with lidocaine, β-blockers, and overdrive pacing (83,88). Acute QT prolongation is treated with withdrawal of the causative agent, if known, and correction of any electrolyte abnormalities. Further drug therapies include magnesium (especially for a torsades de pointes rhythm), overdrive pacing, phenytoin, and lidocaine (89). Polymorphic ventricular tachycardia without QT prolongation is most often secondary to ischemia, and aggressive treatment is warranted. Evaluation for acute MI should be started and treated as appropriate. For stable monomorphic ventricular tachycardia, pharmacologic therapy includes procainamide, amiodarone, and lidocaine (88,90).

SUMMARY

Cardiac complications after surgical procedures are fairly common. Cardiac events can be reduced by preoperative risk assessment, cardiac testing, and implementation of either surgical or percutaneous coronary revascularization or medical management. Although postoperative cardiac outcomes have improved with advances in technology and medical management, as the population continues to age in the United States, the number of patients with coronary artery risk factors is expected to increase.

REFERENCES

1. Massie MB, Mangano DR. Risk stratification for noncardiac surgery; how (and why)? *Circulation* 1993;87:1752–1755.
2. Goldman L, Caldera DL, Nussbaum SR, et al. Multifactorial index of cardiac risk in noncardiac surgical procedures. *N Engl J Med* 1977;297:845–850.

3. Ashton CM, Peterson NJ, Wray NP, et al. The incidence of perioperative myocardial infarction in men undergoing noncardiac surgery. *Ann Intern Med* 1993;118:504–510.

4. American College of Physicians. Guidelines for assessing and managing the perioperative risk from coronary artery disease associated with major noncardiac surgery. *Ann Intern Med* 1997;127:309–312.

5. Palda VA, Detsky AS. Clinical guideline, part II. Perioperative assessment and management of risk from coronary artery disease. *Ann Intern Med* 1997;127:313–328.

6. Detsky AS, Abrams HB, Forbath N, et al. Cardiac assessment for patients undergoing noncardiac surgery. *Arch Intern Med* 1986;146:2131–2134.

7. Eagle KA, Berger PB, Calkins H, et al. ACC/AHA guideline update for perioperative cardiovascular evaluation for noncardiac surgery—executive summary: a report of the American College of Cardiology/American Heart Association Task Force on Practice Guidelines (Committee to update the 1996 guidelines on perioperative cardiovascular evaluation for noncardiac surgery). *J Am Coll Cardiol* 2002;39:542–553.

8. Eagle KA, Rihal CS, Mickel MC, et al for the CASS Investigators and the University of Michigan Heart Care Program. Cardiac risk of noncardiac surgery: influence of coronary disease and type of surgery in 3,368 operations. *Circulation* 1997;96:1882–1887.

9. Criqui MH, Langer RD, Fronek A, et al. Mortality over a period of 10 years in patients with peripheral arterial disease. *N Engl J Med* 1992;326:381–386.

10. Lee TH, Marcantonio ER, Mangione CM, et al. Derivation and prospective validation of a simple index for predication of cardiac risk of major noncardiac surgery. *Circulation* 1999;100:1043–1049.

11. Gilbert K, Larocque BJ, Patrick LT. Prospective evaluation of cardiac risk indices for patients undergoing noncardiac surgery. *Ann Intern Med* 2000;133:356–359.

12. Bronson D, Halperin A, Marwick T. Evaluating cardiac risk in noncardiac surgery patients. *Cleve Clin J Med* 1995;62:391–400.

13. Younis LT, Miller DD, Chaitman BR. Preoperative strategies to assess cardiac risk before noncardiac surgery. *Clin Cardiol* 1995;18:447–454.

14. Eagle KA, Coley CM, Newell JB, et al. Combining clinical and thallium data optimizes preoperative assessment of cardiac risk before major vascular surgery. *Ann Intern Med* 1989;110:859–866.

15. Vanzetto G, Machecourt J, Blendea D, et al. Additive value of thallium single-photon emission computed tomography myocardial imaging for prediction of perioperative events in clinically selected high cardiac risk patients having abdominal aortic surgery. *Am J Cardiol* 1996;77:143–148.

16. Raby KE, Barry J, Creager MA, et al. Detection and significance of intraoperative myocardial ischemia in peripheral vascular surgery. *JAMA* 1992;268:222–227.

17. Mangano DT, Browner WS, Hollenberg M et al, The Study of Perioperative Ischemia Research Group. Association of perioperative myocardial ischemia with cardiac morbidity and mortality in men undergoing noncardiac surgery. *N Engl J Med* 1990;323:1781–1788.

18. McPhail N, Calvin JE, Shariatmadar A, et al. The use of preoperative exercise testing to predict cardiac complications after arterial reconstruction. *J Vasc Surg* 1988;7:60–68.

19. Gerson MC, Hurst JM, Hertzberg VS, et al. Cardiac prognosis in noncardiac geriatric surgery. *Ann Intern Med* 1985;103:832–837.

20. Stratmann HG, Younis LT, Wittry MD, et al. Dipyridamole technetium 99m sestamibi myocardial tomography for preoperative cardiac risk stratification before major or minor nonvascular surgery. *Am Heart J* 1996;132:536–541.

21. Brown KA, Rowen M. Extent of jeopardized viable myocardium determined by myocardial perfusion imaging best predicts perioperative cardiac events in patients undergoing noncardiac surgery. *J Am Coll Cardiol* 1993;21:325.

22. Kontos MC, Brath LK, Akosah KO, et al. Cardiac complications in noncardiac surgery: relative value of resting two-dimensional echocardiography and dipyridamole thallium imaging. *Am Heart J* 1996;132:559–566.

23. Boersma E, Poldermans D, Bax JJ, et al. Predictors of cardiac events after major vascular surgery: role of clinical characteristic,

24. Paul SD, Eagle KA, Kuntz KM, et al. Concordance of preoperative clinical risk with angiographic severity of coronary artery disease inpatients undergoing vascular surgery. *Circulation* 1996;94:1561–1566.

25. Rihal CS, Eagle KA, Mickel MC, et al. Surgical therapy for coronary artery disease among patients with combined coronary artery and peripheral vascular disease. *Circulation* 1995;91:46–53.

26. Domanski M, Ellis S, Eagle KA. Does preoperative coronary revascularization before noncardiac surgery reduce the risk of coronary events in patients with known coronary artery disease? *Am J Cardiol* 1995;75:829–831.

27. Shojania KG, Duncan BW, McDonald KM, et al. *Making health care safer: a critical review of patient safety practices: evidence report/technology assessment no. 43*, Rockville, MD: Agency for Healthcare Research and Quality; 2001:Publication 01-E058.

28. Auerbach AD, Goldman L. β-Blockers and reduction of cardiac events in noncardiac surgery. *JAMA* 2002;287:1435–1444.

29. Mangano DT, Layug EL, Wallace A et al, Multicenter Study of Perioperative Ischemia Research Group. Effect of atenolol on mortality and cardiovascular morbidity after noncardiac surgery: multicenter study of perioperative ischemia research group. *N Engl J Med* 1996;35:1713–1720.

30. Stone JG, Foex P, Sear JW, et al. Myocardial ischemia in untreated hypertensive patients: effect of a single small oral dose of a beta-adrenergic blocking agent. *Anesthesiology* 1988;68:495–500.

31. Raby KE, Brull SJ, Timimi F, et al. The effect of heart rate control on myocardial ischemia among high-risk patients after vascular surgery. *Anesth Analg* 1999;88:477–482.

32. Wallace A, Layug B, Tateo I et al, McSPI Research Group. Prophylactic atenolol reduces postoperative myocardial ischemia. *Anesthesiology* 1998;88:7–17.

33. Urban MK, Markowitz SM, Gordon MA, et al. Postoperative prophylactic administration of beta-adrenergic blockers in patients at risk for myocardial ischemia. *Anesth Analg* 2000;90:1257–1261.

34. Poldermans D, Boersma E, Bax JJ, et al. The effect of bisoprolol on perioperative mortality and myocardial infarction in high-risk patients undergoing vascular surgery. *N Engl J Med* 1999;341:1789–1794.

35. Bayliff CD, Massel DR, Inculet RI, et al. Propranolol for the prevention of postoperative arrhythmia after general thoracic surgery. *Ann Thorac Surg* 1999;67:182–186.

36. Shammash JB, Trost JC, Gold JM, et al. Perioperative beta-blocker withdrawal and mortality in vascular surgery patients. *Am Heart J* 2001;141:148–153.

37. Krumholz HM, Radford MJ, Wang Y, et al. National use and effectiveness of beta-blockers for the treatment of elderly patients after acute myocardial infarction: national cooperative cardiovascular project. *JAMA* 1998;280:623–629.

38. White CM. Prevention of suboptimal beta-blocker treatment in patients with myocardial infarction. *Pharmacotherapy* 1999;33:1063–1072.

39. Wang TJ, Stafford RS. National patterns and predictors of beta-blocker use in patients with coronary artery disease. *Arch Intern Med* 1998;158:1901–1906.

40. Packer M. Current role of beta-adrenergic blockers in management of chronic heart failure. *Am J Med* 2001;110:81S–94S.

41. Heart Failure Society of America. HFSA guidelines for management of patients with heart failure caused by ventricular systolic dysfunction: pharmacological approaches. *Pharmacotherapy* 2000;20:495–522.

42. Litwack RS, Gilligan DM, DeGruttola V. Beta-blockade for patients undergoing vascular surgery. *N Engl J Med* 2000;342:1052–1053.

43. Stuhmeier KD, Mainzer B, Cierpka J, et al. Small, oral dose of clonidine reduces incidence of intraoperative myocardial ischemia in patients having vascular surgery. *Anesthesiology* 1996;85:706–712.

44. Fox K, Dargie HJ, de Bono DP, et al. Effect of an alpha(2) antagonist (miverazol) on limiting myocardial ischaemia in stable angina. *Heart* 1999;82:383–385.

45. Oliver MF, Goldman L, Julian DG et al. The European Mivazerol Trial Group. Effect of mivazerol on perioperative cardiac complications during non-cardiac surgery in patients with coronary

artery disease: the European Mivazerol Trial Group. *Anesthesiology* 1999;91:951–961.

46. Albright GA. Cardiac arrest following regional anesthesia with etidocaine or bupivicaine. *Anesthesiology* 1979;51:285–287.

47. Rosenfeld BA, Beattie C, Christopherson R et al, Perioperative Ischemia Randomized Anesthesia Trial Study Group. The effects of different anesthetic regimens on fibrinolysis and the development of postoperative arterial thrombosis. *Anesthesiology* 1993; 79:435–443.

48. Sola JE, Bender JS. Use of the pulmonary artery catheter to reduce operative complications. *Surg Clin North Am* 1993;73:253–264.

49. Shoemaker WC, Kram HB, Appel PL, et al. The efficacy of central venous and pulmonary artery catheters and therapy based upon them in reducing mortality and morbidity. *Arch Surg* 1990;125: 1332–1337.

50. Shoemaker WC, Appel PL, Kram HB, et al. Prospective trial of supranormal values of survivors as therapeutic goals in high-risk surgical patients. *Chest* 1988;94:1176–1186.

51. Sandham JD, Hull RD, Brant RF, et al. A randomized, controlled trial of the use of pulmonary-artery catheters in high-risk surgical patients. *N Engl J Med* 2003;348:5–14.

52. Polanczyk CA, Rohde LE, Goldman L, et al. Right heart catheterization and cardiac complications in patients undergoing noncardiac surgery: an observational study. *JAMA* 2001;286:309–314.

53. Berlauk JF, Abrams JH, Gilmour IJ, et al. Preoperative optimization of cardiovascular hemodynamics improves outcome in peripheral vascular surgery. A prospective, randomized clinical trial. *Ann Surg* 1991;214:289–297.

54. Barone JE, Tucker JB, Rassias D, et al. Routine perioperative pulmonary artery catheterization has no effect on rate of complications in vascular surgery: a meta-analysis. *Am Surg* 2001;67: 674–679.

55. Tuman KJ, McCarthy RJ, Spiess BE, et al. Effect of pulmonary artery catheterization on outcome in patients undergoing coronary artery surgery. *Anesthesiology* 1989;70:199–206.

56. Leibowitz AB, Beilin Y. Pulmonary artery catheters and outcome in the perioperative period. *New Horiz* 1997;5:214–221.

57. Pulmonary artery consensus conference: consensus statement. *Crit Care Med* 1997;25:910–925.

58. McConkey PP. Postobstructive pulmonary oedema-a case series and review. *Anaesth Intensive Care* 2000;28:72–76.

59. Waller DA, Gebitekin C, Saunders NR, et al. Noncardiogenic pulmonary edema complicating lung resection. *Ann Thorac Surg* 1993;55:140–143.

60. Snoy FJ, Woodside JT. Unilateral pulmonary edema (down lung syndrome) following urological operation. *J Urol* 1984;132: 776–777.

61. Ablett MJ, Grainger AJ, Keir MJ, et al. The correlation of the radiologic extent of lung transplantation edema with pulmonary oxygenation. *Am J Roentgenol* 1998;171:587–589.

62. Singh PP, Dimich I, Shamsi A. Intraoperative pulmonary oedema in a young cocaine smoker. *Can J Anaesth* 1994;41:961–964.

63. Morrison LK, Harrison A, Krishnaswamy P, et al. Utility of a rapid B-natriuretic peptide assay in differentiating congestive heart failure from lung disease in patients presenting with dyspnea. *J Am Coll Cardiol* 2002;39:202–209.

64. Pur-Shahriari AA, Mills RA, Hoppin FG, et al. Comparison of chronic and acute effects of morphine sulfate on cardiovascular function. *Am J Cardiol* 1967;20:654–659.

65. Dikshit K, Vyden JK, Forrester JS, et al. Renal and extrarenal hemodynamic effects of furosemide in congestive heart failure after myocardial infarction. *N Engl J Med* 1973;288:1087–1090.

66. Coriat P, Richer C, Dourake T, et al. Influence of chronic angiotensin-converting enzyme inhibition on anesthetic induction. *Anesthesiology* 1994;81:299–307.

67. Pigott DW, Nagle C, Allman K, et al. Effect of omitting regular ACE inhibitor medication before cardiac surgery on haemodynamic variables and vasoactive drug requirements. *Br J Anaesth* 1999;83:715–720.

68. Hjalmarson A, Goldstein S, Fagerberg B, et al. Merit-hf Study Group. Effects of controlled-release metoprolol on total mortality, hospitalizations, and well-being in patients with heart failure: the metoprolol cr/xl randomized intervention trial in congestive heart failure (merit-hf). *JAMA* 2000;283:1295–1302.

69. Packer M, Coats AJ, Fowler ME, et al. Effect of carvediolol on survival in severe chronic heart failure. *N Engl J Med* 2001; 344:1651–1658.

70. Eisenberg MJ, London MJ, Browner WE, et al. The Study of Perioperative Ischemia Research Group. Monitoring for myocardial ischemia during noncardiac surgery. A technology assessment of transesophageal echocardiography and 12-lead electrocardiography. *JAMA* 1992;8:210–216.

71. Mangano DT. The Study of Perioperative Ischemia (SPI) Research Group. Characteristics of electrocardiographic ischemia in high-risk patients undergoing surgery. *J Electrocardiol* 1990; 23:20–27.

72. Adams JE III, Bodor GS, Davila-Roman VG, et al. Cardiac troponin I: a marker with high specificity for cardiac injury. *Circulation* 1993;88:101–106.

73. Adams JE III, Davila-Roman VG, Bessey PQ, et al. Improved detection of cardiac contusion with cardiac troponin I. *Am Heart J* 1996;131:308–312.

74. Hollander JE, Levitt MA, Young GP, et al. Effect of recent cocaine use on the specificity of cardiac markers for diagnosis of acute myocardial infarction. *Am Heart J* 1998;135:245–252.

75. Hochberg MC, Koppes GM, Edwards CQ, et al. Hypothyroidism presenting as a polymyositis-like syndrome. *Arthritis Rheum* 1976;19:1363–1366.

76. Jaffe AS, Ritter C, Meltzer V, et al. Unmasking artifactual increases in creatine kinase isoenzymes in patients with renal failure. *J Lab Clin Med* 1984;104:193–202.

77. Adams JE III, Sicard GA, Allen BT, et al. Diagnosis of perioperative myocardial infarction with measurement of cardiac troponin I. *N Engl J Med* 1994;330:670–674.

78. Ryan TJ, Antman EM, Brooks NH, et al. 1999 Update: ACC/AHA guidelines for the management of patients with acute myocardial infarction: executive summary and recommendations. A report of the American college of cardiology/American heart association task force on practical guidelines (committee on management of acute myocardial infarction). *Circulation* 1999;100:1016–1030.

79. Antithrombotic Trialists' Collaboration. Collaborative meta-analysis of randomised trials of antiplatelet therapy for prevention of death, myocardial infarction, and stroke in high-risk patients. *Br Med J* 2002;324:71–87.

80. First International Study of Infarct Survival Collaborative Group. Randomised trial of intravenous atenolol among 16027 cases of suspected acute myocardial infarction: ISIS-1. *Lancet* 1986;2:57–66.

81. Roberts R, Rogers WJ, Mueller HS, et al. Immediate versus deferred beta-blockade following thrombolytic therapy in patients with acute myocardial infarction. Results of the thrombolysis in myocardial infarction (TIMI) II-B study. *Circulation* 1991;83:422–437.

82. Maisel WH, Rawn JD, Stevenson WG. Atrial fibrillation after cardiac surgery. *Ann Intern Med* 2001;135:1061–1073.

83. The American Heart Association in collaboration with the International Liaison Committee on Resuscitation. Guidelines 2000 for cardiopulmonary resuscitation and emergency cardiovascular care. Part 6; advanced cardiovascular life support: 7D: the tachycardia algorithms. *Circulation* 2000;102:I158–I165.

84. Farshi R, Kistner D, Sarma JSM, et al. Ventricular rate control in chronic atrial fibrillation during daily activity and programmed exercise: a crossover open-label study of five drug regimens. *J Am Coll Cardiol* 1999;33:304–310.

85. Platia EV, Michelson EL, Porterfield JK, et al. Esmolol versus verapamil in the acute treatment of atrial fibrillation or atrial flutter. *Am J Cardiol* 1989;63:925–929.

86. Ellenbogen KA, Dias VC, Cardello FP, et al. Safety and efficacy of intravenous diltiazem in atrial fibrillation or atrial flutter. *Am J Cardiol* 1995;75:45–49.

87. Camm AJ, Garratt CJ. Adenosine and supraventricular tachycardia. *N Engl J Med* 1991;325:1621–1629.

88. Griffith MJ, Linker NJ, Garratt CJ, et al. Relative efficacy and safety of intravenous drugs for termination of sustained ventricular tachycardia. *Lancet* 1990;336:670–673.

89. Tzivoni D, Keren A, Cohen AM, et al. Magnesium therapy for torsades de pointes. *Am J Cardiol* 1984;53:528–530.

90. Naccarelli GV, Jalal S. Intravenous amiodarone, another option in the acute management of sustained ventricular tachyarrhythmias. *Circulation* 1995;92:3154–3155.

Abnormalities in Coagulation

18

Alvin H. Schmaier

■ INTRODUCTION 185

■ ASSESSING RISK FOR BLEEDING
IN PROSPECTIVE SURGICAL PATIENTS 185

■ DETERMINING THE DIAGNOSIS OF A BLEEDING
SURGICAL PATIENT IN THE OPERATING ROOM
OR RECOVERY ROOM 188
Anticoagulation 188
Disseminated Intravascular Coagulation 190
Liver Disease 190
Vitamin K Deficiency 191
Massive Transfusion 191
Managing Massive Bleeding 191

■ ASSESSING RISK AND PREVENTION FOR
THROMBOSIS IN THE SURGICAL PATIENT 192
Arterial Thrombosis 192
Venous Thrombosis 192
Therapy for Thrombosis and Its Prevention 194

■ SUMMARY 194

■ REFERENCES 194

INTRODUCTION

Bleeding or thrombosis can be a serious complication associated with surgery, whether elective or emergent. When

Alvin H. Schmaier: University of Michigan, Ann Arbor, MI 48109

approaching the proposed surgical patient, one needs to address a few critical items to exclude the possibility of abnormal bleeding and increased risk for thrombosis, independent of possible complications that can arise during the procedure. The purpose of this chapter is threefold: (i) to provide a concise and thorough approach to assessing bleeding risk in the prospective surgical patient, (ii) to provide a practical and thorough differential diagnosis of causes of surgical bleeding and thrombosis, and (iii) to suggest general and specific means to manage or prevent the various bleeding and clotting situations that occur in these patients.

ASSESSING RISK FOR BLEEDING IN PROSPECTIVE SURGICAL PATIENTS

Bleeding or thrombosis is the ill consequence of a loss in the delicate balance among hemostasis (clot formation), fibrinolysis (clot lysis), and anticoagulation (regulation) of the various plasma proteins and cells in the intravascular compartment. For the last 40 years, the blood coagulation system has been represented as a cascade of proteolytic reactions leading to clot formation. This concept really describes blood coagulation that occurs in a test tube and not physiologic hemostasis. A current hypothesis is that the blood coagulation, fibrinolysis, and anticoagulant systems are an interacting group of proteins that amplify the activation and inhibition of one another (Fig. 18-1) (1,2). In this hypothesis of physiologic hemostasis, factor VIIa-tissue factor (TF-VIIa) activates factor IX to factor IXa. This pathway dominates because a protein called tissue factor pathway inhibitor (TFPI) blocks activation of factor X by TF-VIIa. Factor IXa (IXa) in the presence of factor VIIIa (VIIIa)

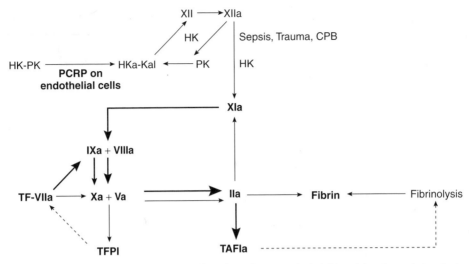

Figure 18-1 Physiologic hemostasis. Physiologic hemostasis is initiated by tissue factor-factor VIIa (TF-VIIa) activating factor IX. The plasma protein tissue factor pathway inhibitor (TFPI) blocks factor VIIa-TF from directly activating factor X *in vivo*. Factor IXa in the presence of factor VIIIa (IXa + VIIIa) activates factor X to factor Xa. Factor Xa in the presence of factor Va (Xa + Va) then activates prothrombin to thrombin (IIa). Formed thrombin (IIa) can clot fibrinogen to make fibrin, and naturally occurring fibrinolytic mechanisms will dissolve this clot. If the need to generate thrombin is great, the initially formed thrombin will also activate factor XI to factor XIa (XIa). Formed factor XIa then amplifies factor IX activation, leading to amplified thrombin formation (IIa). Increased thrombin formation also results in the activation of a thrombin activable fibrinolysis inhibitor (TAFIa, carboxypeptidase U) that inhibits the natural fibrinolytic mechanism. Independent of the tissue factor-factor VIIa mechanism for blood coagulation, activation of factor XII (XII) in sepsis, trauma, or cardiopulmonary bypass results in reciprocal activation with prekallikrein (PK) and subsequent High molecular weight kininogen (HK) activation of more factor XII to factor XIIa (XIIa), which can then result in factor XI activation. This latter mechanism for factor XI activation is pathophysiologic, not physiologic. Physiologic activation of PK on endothelial cells by the enzyme prolylcarboxypeptidase (PRCP) results in plasma kallikrein formation and, subsequently, factor XII activation. However, this pathway does not lead to factor XI activation.

activates factor X to factor Xa (Xa), which in the presence of factor Va (Va) activates prothrombin (II) to thrombin (IIa). A little thrombin can proteolyze fibrinogen to make a fibrin clot. However, this same thrombin can activate factor XI to factor XIa (XIa) to amplify more thrombin activation through factors IXa and VIIIa and, subsequently, factors Xa and Va (Fig. 18-1). More thrombin formation can also activate a fibrinolysis inhibitor, thrombin activable fibrinolysis inhibitor (TAFIa, a.k.a. carboxypeptidase U) that makes fibrin more resistant to fibrinolysis (Fig. 18-1). Inhibitors to each of the coagulation and fibrinolysis enzymes additionally regulate this system. Under physiologic circumstances factor XIIa is not an activator of factor XI. *In vivo*, plasma prekallikrein (PK) of the plasma kallikrein/kinin system is the first enzyme to be activated to plasma kallikrein by an endothelial cell-associated enzyme called prolylcarboxypeptidase (PRCP) (Fig. 18-1). Formed plasma kallikrein then activates factor XII to an active enzyme. This system does not contribute to physiologic hemostasis because deficiencies of each of these proteins are not associated with bleeding. However, in disease or injury such as that seen after sepsis, trauma, and cardiopulmonary bypass, formed factor XIIa activates factor XI, increasing thrombin formation as well (Fig. 18-1).

Although there is an elegant understanding of physiologic hemostasis, the clinician needs to make management decisions based on current clinical test availability. The current means to assess bleeding risk in the prospective surgery patient is by history and simple laboratory tests (Table 18-1) (3). Thrombosis risk should be assessed by the extent of the patient's ambulatory ability as well as the nature of the proposed surgery. At present, no good laboratory assays prospectively predict thrombosis risk. The physician should ask if

TABLE 18-1

PREOPERATIVE VARIABLES TO ASSESS BLEEDING AND CLOTTING RISK

History
    Patient history of bleeding at surgery, trauma, tooth extractions
    Family history of bleeding at surgery, trauma, tooth extractions
    Medication history: antiplatelet agents, NSAIDS, anticoagulants

Laboratory
    Complete blood count including platelet count
    Activated partial thromboplastin time (APTT)
    Prothrombin time (PT)

there have been prior operations, injuries, or tooth extractions, and, if so, if there has been abnormal bleeding requiring additional care, transfusions, or a revisit to the physician or hospital, for either the patient or an immediate family member. Furthermore, the surgeon needs to take a thorough medication history. The common use of aspirin and other platelet inhibitors, as well as anti-inflammatory drugs that can interfere with platelet function, should be known. A positive answer to any one of these questions puts the patient into a higher risk category. Alternatively, thrombosis risk is assessed by prior history and the ambulatory nature of the patient. As will be discussed below, the nature of the surgical procedure contributes to the risk for thrombosis.

The clinical laboratory provides a great deal of information to assess bleeding risk in a patient preparing for surgery. There is controversy regarding the cost-effective approach to assess bleeding risk. The activated partial thromboplastin time (APTT) is the most global screening assay for a coagulation protein defect, but it will not pick up the rare (1/500,000 to 1/1,000,000) patient with factor VII deficiency. Alternatively, the prothrombin time (PT), if abnormal, is probably a better predictor of bleeding at the time of surgery than the APTT, if abnormal. The bleeding time has been shown not to predict abnormal surgical bleeding. However, a patient who has a bleeding disorder, but who is on no medications and has a normal APTT and PT, may have von Willebrand disease or a platelet function disorder that may be recognized only by a bleeding time rather than by sophisticated, costly specialized laboratory studies. The following will be a description of what the tests measure. The decision to use all or a portion of these tests for screening to determine risk for bleeding must rest in the hands of the clinician based on the history of the patient and the family.

The screening tests of the APTT and PT measure specific portions of the coagulation protein system (Fig. 18-2, Table 18-2). Knowing the results of these assays provides

major diagnostic power to predict the potential cause for bleeding in a prospective surgical patient. The differential diagnosis of an isolated prolonged APTT depends on whether or not the patient has a bleeding history. If there is a bleeding history, factor VIII (VIII) deficiency is nine times more common than factor IX (IX) deficiency. Both occur almost exclusively in males since they are sex-linked. These individuals have a lifelong bleeding history. Spontaneous inhibitors to VIII can arise in elderly patients and individuals postpartum, with a connective tissue disorder, or with a B cell malignancy. Factor XI (XI) deficiency is much less common, and 50% of the patients are Jewish with an Eastern European background. Alternatively, if there is no bleeding history, but the APTT alone is prolonged, the most likely cause for the prolonged APTT is a lupus anticoagulant. A lupus anticoagulant in general is the most likely cause for a prolonged APTT. Other causes of long APTT that are not associated with bleeding include factor XII (XII), PK, or high

TABLE 18-2

DIFFERENTIAL DIAGNOSIS OF ABNORMAL SCREENING TESTS FOR BLEEDING DISORDERS

Abnormal activated partial thromboplastin time (APTT) alone
  Associated with bleeding: VIII, IX, XI defects
  Not associated with bleeding: XII, prekallikrein (PK), high molecular weight kininogen (HK), lupus anticoagulants

Abnormal prothrombin time (PT) alone
  VII defects

Combined abnormal APTT and PT
  Medical conditions: anticoagulants, DIC, liver disease, vitamin K deficiency, massive transfusion
  Rarely dysfibrinogenemias, factors X, V, and II defects

Long bleeding time alone
  Normal platelet count: von Willebrand disease or a platelet function defect (congenital or acquired—usually medication)
  Low platelet count

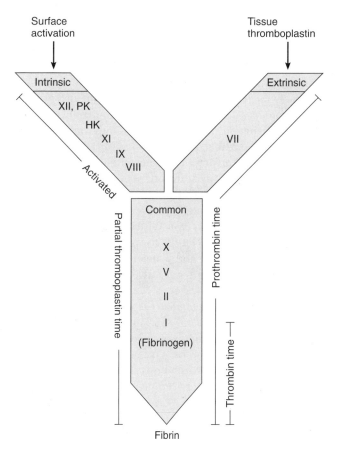

Figure 18-2 Description of common coagulation blood tests and what proteins these tests measure. The activated partial thromboplastin time (APTT) measures the functional integrity of all the proteins of the so-called "Intrinsic" and "Common" pathways of the coagulation system. These proteins include factor XII (XII), prekallikrein (PK), high molecular weight kininogen (HK), factors XI, IX, VIII, X, V, II (thrombin), and I (fibrinogen). The prothrombin time (PT) measures the functional integrity of the proteins of the so-called extrinsic pathway [factor VII (VII)] and the proteins of the common pathway. The thrombin clotting time only measures the functional integrity of fibrinogen.

molecular weight kininogen (HK) deficiencies (Fig. 18-2, Table 18-2). These last three protein defects are quite rare.

An isolated abnormal PT is commonly associated with a factor VII (VII) deficiency. This is quite uncommon but is associated with abnormal bleeding at operation. Depending on the reagents that are used for coagulation tests at an institution, an isolated abnormal PT can also occur with a dysfibrinogenemia and factor X, V, and II deficiencies.

When the APTT and PT are both prolonged, the physician must consider a number of medical conditions. The most common causes of combined prolonged APTT and PT are anticoagulation, disseminated intravascular coagulation (DIC), liver disease, vitamin K deficiency, and massive transfusions. Each of these entities will be discussed in more detail in the next section of this chapter. Once these medical conditions are excluded, only rare coagulation protein defects or deficiencies should be considered. The most common cause of an abnormal coagulation protein defect yielding a prolonged PT and APTT is an abnormal fibrinogen (dysfibrinogenemia). Dysfibrinogenemias are most commonly seen in patients with liver disease, from any cause. Much less common is deficiency or inhibitors to factors X, V, and II (prothrombin). True deficiencies of each of these three proteins are probably incompatible with normal fetal gestation and parturition. Even the extremely rare patient who appears to be fully deficient in these proteins actually has a small amount of the protein of interest being produced. More commonly, one sees antibodies to factors V that arise spontaneously and antibodies to factor II and X arising in patients with lupus and malignancy, respectively. In addition, acquired factor X deficiency arises in patients with amyloidosis.

Finally, a bleeding patient with a normal PT, APTT, and platelet count may have von Willebrand disease or, less commonly, a true platelet function defect. Patients with von Willebrand disease and platelet function defects have easy bruisability of soft tissues. If the patient is not on a medication that can interfere, a classic template bleeding time can be useful to recognize the possibility of either of these disorders. If abnormal, specialized testing can be performed to make the diagnosis of a deficiency, a defect in von Willebrand factor, or a platelet function defect. Independent of the bleeding time, there is still no universally accepted alternative screening test for potential bleeding disorders due to von Willebrand factor or platelet function defects. Finally, all patients with a reduction of their platelet count below 100,000/µL are at increased risk of bleeding at the time of surgery.

DETERMINING THE DIAGNOSIS OF A BLEEDING SURGICAL PATIENT IN THE OPERATING ROOM OR RECOVERY ROOM

One of the most challenging aspects of consultative medicine is the emergent assessment of the bleeding patient in the OR or recovery room. As a hemostasis consultant, one's role is to be certain to detect any cause of bleeding due to some medical factor(s) that can be corrected by means other than additional surgery. Although acute, the approach to these patients is the same as assessing risk for bleeding in the preoperative evaluation. The first issue regards the documentation of the preoperative variables examined prior to surgery. For example, patients with a long medication list could be on anticoagulants [e.g., low molecular weight heparin, aspirin, clopidogrel (Plavix)] that do not necessarily prolong screening coagulation tests but increase a patient's risk of perioperative bleeding. Thus, the surgeon needs to be aware of prior medication history and its possible role in surgical bleeding. After the medications are reviewed, the assessment for other specific acquired bleeding states proceeds.

As mentioned in the previous section, acquired bleeding states are usually due to anticoagulation, DIC, liver disease, vitamin K deficiency, or massive transfusion (Table 18-3) (4,5). Usually, each of these conditions is associated with a prolonged PT and APTT. Each of these conditions will be discussed as to diagnosis and immediate means to specifically treat them.

Anticoagulation

Anticoagulant and antiplatelet agents suffuse medical practice today allowing for interventional procedures as well as preventing thrombosis. Some of these agents do not markedly prolong the blood coagulation times, and thus their presence in the patient would not necessarily be recognized unless appreciated upon a careful review of a patient's medication list. The surgeon must be aware of these agents and their pharmacokinetics in preparing the

---

TABLE 18-3

ACQUIRED SURGICAL BLEEDING

Anticoagulation
  Antifibrin agents:
    Unfractionated heparin (standard heparin)
    Low molecular weight heparin
    Fondaparinux (Arixtra)
    Warfarin
    Direct thrombin inhibitors: hirudin (Refludan, Lepirudin), argatroban, bivalirudin (Angiomax)

  Antiplatelet agents:
    Aspirin
    Clopidogrel
    Glycoprotein IIb/IIIa antagonists (tirofiban, eptifibatide, abciximab)

Disseminated intravascular coagulation—acute

Liver disease

Vitamin K deficiency

Massive transfusion

patient for surgery. In this section only currently approved drugs will be discussed (Table 18-3). In general, anticoagulants can be classified into two groups: antifibrin agents and antiplatelet agents. Antifibrin agents can be subclassified into nonspecific inhibitors and specific inhibitors. The nonspecific anticoagulants consist of unfractionated heparin and warfarin. These agents at their usual therapeutic dose prolong the PT and the APTT. Unfractionated heparin (standard heparin) has a short half-life (1 to 2 hours), allowing for normalization of bleeding risk within 4 hours after its infusion is stopped. With the exception of CPB surgery usage, surgery patients on unfractionated heparin need be delayed only 4 hours after stopping the drug before beginning the procedure. Individuals on unfractionated heparin who start to bleed need only red blood cell (RBC) and plasma support (see the discussion below on the effect of massive transfusion) for the duration of time they are at risk. Usually, sufficient drug is metabolized within hours to prevent the need for additional therapy. Protamine sulfate is almost never needed to correct abnormal bleeding in an individual on heparin.

Warfarin therapy, however, presents different challenges. Normally it takes at least 5 days to fully anticoagulate a patient with warfarin. The delay arises because the drug needs to inhibit and alter the synthesis of four coagulation protein zymogens (proenzymes) before its anticoagulation effect is achieved. Since these targets have variable half-lives (4 hours to 5 days), it takes at least 5 days before a full anticoagulation effect is achieved. Thus, the patient on warfarin at the time of surgery also needs 5 days to correct its anticoagulation effect. Patients on warfarin should have this medication stopped at least 1 week before having elective surgery. Current practice is to anticoagulate the patient with low molecular weight heparin up to the time of operation, if necessary, on the basis of the risk of thrombosis. Postoperatively, the patient may need to be treated with at least 5 days of parenteral low molecular weight heparin if the risk of early anticoagulation is warranted by the risk of thrombosis until the reinstituted warfarin therapy can become effective as an anticoagulant again. If surgery is emergent and the patient is on warfarin, there are a few options. In general, a patient fully anticoagulated on warfarin has only about 5% to 15% normal coagulant activity of coagulation factors II, VII, IX, and X. Further, the remaining 85% to 95% of these factors is synthesized abnormally and thus acts as a coagulation protein inhibitor, potentiating the risk of bleeding. Since normal hemostasis requires effective coagulation factor levels to be at least 50%, these patients would require about 80% or more of their plasma volume to be replaced. In a 70-kg person, plasma volume is 60% of blood volume ($\sim$7% of body weight) or $\sim$3 L plasma (or 12 units of fresh frozen plasma) to be instantly given to the patient to correct the patient's hemostatic defect. Most patients and blood banks cannot tolerate a replacement prescription like this. Thus, surgery should be avoided if possible in a patient fully anticoagulated with warfarin. However, if therapy is needed in

such a patient (e.g., an intracerebral hemorrhage in a patient on warfarin), there are a few options. One option is to exchange the whole body plasma by plasmapheresis. Another is to acutely replenish the patient with a vitamin K factor concentrate, if available (6). Third would be acute replacement with factor VIIa concentration (7,8). This latter therapy will be discussed in more detail below because it is considered state of the art.

In addition to the above nonspecific anticoagulants, several new antifibrin agents are specifically directed to coagulation factors Xa and thrombin (IIa). All the low molecular weight heparins and fondaparinux are mostly directed to factor Xa and not thrombin. At doses that are therapeutic for the treatment for deep vein thrombosis (DVT) these agents, in various individuals, will not or will only slightly prolong the screening tests of the PT and APTT. Therefore, these assays cannot be used to exclude the possibility that these agents are present in the patient. Although the PT and APTT are not markedly prolonged after low molecular weight heparin or fondaparinux administration, the risk of bleeding in patients treated with these agents is similar to that of unfractionated heparin. If hemorrhage occurs, there is no immediate antidote, although recombinant factor VIIa infusion could be used (see below). Low molecular weight heparins may have longer half-lives (2 to 4.5 hours) than unfractionated heparin; the half-life depends on the preparation. Fondaparinux has an 18-hour half-life, so if bleeding occurs while on this agent, support has to be given for this longer period of time. Both low molecular weight heparin and fondaparinux are excreted renally. Therefore, patients with renal dysfunction have longer clearance times. Also, both agents are stored in adipose tissue, allowing for anticoagulant accumulation in obese patients. Both of these latter factors can be associated with abnormal bleeding as a result of drug levels higher than anticipated.

The direct thrombin inhibitors, hirudin, argatroban, and bivalirudin, are antifibrin agents that interact specifically with the thrombin active site, exosite I, or both. All will prolong the screening tests for coagulation disorders. If renal and liver functions are normal, hirudin or bivalirudin and argatroban are eliminated in 0.4 to 2 hours, respectively. Thus, if a patient is on these drugs, only a short time needs to pass before the patient can go to surgery. Further, support for abnormal bleeding will be brief. Alternatively, renal failure can markedly delay the clearance of hirudin, making this recombinant, foreign protein impossible to eliminate. In cases of severe renal failure even with a normal blood urea nitrogen (BUN) and creatinine on continuous venovenous hemofiltration (CVVH), hirudin can become virtually impossible to eliminate. Great care is essential to choose to use this drug in dynamic clinical situations.

In addition to the above list of antifibrin agents, antiplatelet agents are increasingly being used in clinical medicine (Table 18-3). These agents do not influence the PT and APTT, but they will prolong the bleeding time. Aspirin, a platelet cyclooxygenase I and II inhibitor, has become ubiquitous in the management of coronary artery disease. A single 80 mg tablet of aspirin will interfere with platelet function for all platelets present at the instant when the agent was taken. Thus, after aspirin administration the patient's platelet function will not become normal until the entire platelet pool has been resynthesized (10 to 12 days). Patients taking aspirin may require platelet transfusions if bleeding complicates planned or emergent operation. Clopidogrel (Plavix) is a platelet ADP $P2Y_{12}$ receptor antagonist. It too is an irreversible platelet inhibitor. Patients on clopidogrel should stop taking the agent before elective surgery. Vitamin E is a protein kinase C inhibitor that interferes with platelet function. Some patients on vitamin E will also have abnormal bleeding at the time of surgery. Last, the glycoprotein IIb/IIIa ($\alpha_{2b}\beta_3$ integrin) antagonists are used to inhibit platelets in the acute coronary syndrome. Although tirofiban or eptifibatide are rapidly excreted when its infusion is stopped, the monoclonal antibody glycoprotein IIb/IIIa antagonist abciximab can remain in the circulation for 15 days, with the potential to cause hemorrhage.

Disseminated Intravascular Coagulation

DIC is a clinicopathologic condition that arises in patients because of sepsis, malignancy, obstetrical complications at the time of surgery, and massive tissue injury. In the surgery patient, DIC is usually not a preoperative variable, except with the obstetrical catastrophes, for consideration for surgery. Rather, it is a complication that occurs during surgery or in the postoperative period. DIC during surgery can occur in a number of operative conditions. Surgeries for prostate cancer and in the brain have been associated with acute DIC. In circulatory arrest operations on the arch of the aorta or main pulmonary arteries, DIC is a frequent complication due to the chilling of the patient and tissue destruction. Abruptio placenta and placenta previa are associated with acute hemorrhagic DIC, whereas retained dead fetus is associated with a DIC that is not hemorrhagic but prothrombotic. DIC can also occur in the postoperative period because of sepsis. DIC with sepsis is most commonly seen with gram-negative infections, but it can occur with gram-positive infections and, in the immunosuppressed patient, with fungemia.

The diagnosis of DIC is the combined evidence of laboratory testing in an appropriate clinical setting. Finding a prolonged PT and APTT with a reduced fibrinogen and platelet count usually indicates DIC in the hospitalized patient until proven otherwise (9). The diagnosis of DIC is made by the presence of a confirmatory test that shows the simultaneous presence of thrombin and plasmin formation. Currently, the D-Dimer assay is the confirmatory test that, if positive, shows that both thrombin and plasmin have been formed. The D-Dimer measures plasmin-cleaved, insoluble, cross-linked fibrin that originally arose from thrombin cleavage of fibrinogen. D-Dimer assays are characteristic for DIC

but not pathognomonic. D-Dimer assays can be positive in individuals with resolving large vessel thrombosis and soft tissue hematomas, entities that can also occur in surgery patients.

Management of DIC begins with the recognition of the syndrome and the treatment of the underlying disease. Treatment of abruptio placenta, placenta previa, or retained dead fetus is removal of the inciting etiology by surgical means. DIC associated with sepsis is first treated with removal of the inciting infectious focus with antibiotics or, if appropriate, surgical means. Once the inciting cause is appreciated and any specific therapy applied, general medical therapy can be provided for the DIC. Most cases of DIC associated with surgery are hemorrhagic coagulopathies resulting in consumption of coagulation factors and platelets. Thus, therapy should be directed toward replacement of missing coagulation factors or platelets, or both. Each platelet transfusion is bathed in fresh plasma. Therefore, platelet infusion also provides some plasma replacement and additional replacement with fresh frozen plasma may not be necessary. The purpose of fresh frozen plasma replacement is not only to replace the consumed coagulation proteins but also to provide plasma protease inhibitors—for example, antithrombin, $\alpha_2$antiplasmin, C1 esterase inhibitor, and so on—that reduce the degree of active proteolytic reactions occurring in the plasma. If the fibrinogen levels are low—that is, <150 mg per dL—specific replacement is with cryoprecipitate. If the patient has sepsis, adjunctive therapy with activated protein C concentrate is also indicated at present. If known, this therapy works best in patients not heterozygous for Factor V Leiden. The entire purpose of therapy is to support the patient so that the underlying condition can be brought under control. Anticoagulant therapy has little role in most of these patients, except in individuals with acryl cyanosis and digital ischemia where small doses of heparin (4 to 5 U per kg constant infusion without a bolus) may ameliorate the prothrombotic nature of the inciting etiology. Heparin (unfractionated heparin or low molecular weight heparin) should be used only if there is an endpoint in a limited disease state that needs to be achieved.

Liver Disease

It is important for surgeons to know if a proposed patient has liver disease. In addition to the anesthesia risk, most coagulation proteins and inhibitors are made in the liver. Thus, these patients have an increased risk of bleeding. Patients with serious liver disease have prolonged PT and APTTs. Not only is synthesis of these proteins reduced, but also those proteins made are often abnormal, functioning as inhibitors to normal coagulation proteins. As in patients on warfarin, replacement therapy with fresh frozen plasma is not completely feasible because too much replacement is usually needed. Also, depending on the protein's half-life (e.g., that of factor VII is only 3 to 4 hours), it is not practical to keep up with replacement needs over long periods. In addition to reduction in synthesis of coagulation proteins and inhibitors in patients with liver disease, liver disease itself results in abnormal anatomy, such as portal hypertension that increases a patient's risk of bleeding from esophageal varices, gastritis, and hemorrhoids. Furthermore, portal hypertension results in hypersplenism and thrombocytopenia and granulocytopenia. In general, PK is one of the first proteins to be decreased in liver disease and fibrinogen is one of the last. Abnormal fibrinogens (dysfibrinogenemias) are very common in patients with liver disease. All the vitamin K–dependent proteins (factors II, VII, IX, and X, proteins C, S, and Z) decrease in liver disease. Factors VIII and V also decrease. Moreover, antithrombin and other serpin plasma protein inhibitors also decrease in liver disease. Thus these patients have reduced procoagulants and anticoagulants, adjusting the baseline for hemostasis at level other than that seen in normals.

Preoperative management of patients with liver disease requires thinking about a number of variables. All these patients should be given vitamin K to be certain that they are not deficient. If the procedure is short, coverage during the procedure with fresh frozen plasma may be sufficient. However, its duration may be too short to be effective. If a patient is mostly deficient in fibrinogen (i.e, <100 mg per dL) or if the fibrinogen functions abnormally, cryoprecipitate infusion is appropriate. In these patients cryoprecipitate infusion may be sufficient. Alternatively, if the patient has a decrease in all factors and is thrombocytopenic, the most global means to treat such a patient is with platelet transfusions, aiming to keep the platelet count >100,000 per μL throughout the operative procedure and during the first 24 hours postop, subsequently tapering off slowly. Finally, if all fails, recombinant factor VIIa infusion at 40 to 60 μg per kg as a single IV bolus acutely can be used to control a bleeding diathesis.

Vitamin K Deficiency

Vitamin K, a lipid soluble vitamin, is provided by dietary intake of leafy green vegetables and by synthesis of intestinal flora. The body has 1-month stores. In the surgical patient, vitamin K deficiency is mostly seen in the very ill patient on antibiotics who has subsisted on parenteral nutrition. Not infrequently, IV fluids are not supplemented with vitamin K. After 4 to 6 weeks of parenteral nutrition and antibiotic treatment, the patient becomes vitamin K deficient. Vitamin K deficiency can also be seen in patients who have anatomic bypass of the small intestine, malabsorption, biliary tract obstruction, and, rarely, reduced dietary intake. For example, alcoholics are often vitamin K deficient. Warfarin also interferes with two enzymes necessary for vitamin K utilization. Vitamin K

has a critical role in the γ-carboxylation reaction of glutamic acid residues, γ-carboxyglutamic acid, of the so-called vitamin K–dependent coagulation proteins, factors II, VII, IX, and X, and proteins C, S, and Z. This reaction on certain amino acids on the amino terminus of these proteins is critical for these proteins to bind to cells and phospholipids so that they can participate in physiologic coagulation reactions. Vitamin K usually is replaced through oral therapy. However, if necessary, parenteral replacement can be performed. Intramuscular, rather than intravenous, is the preferred, safe route of administration.

Massive Transfusion

Bleeding complications from massive transfusion itself can occur as result of the extent of anticoagulant being poured into the patient when there are lots of transfusions in a short period of time. Ten percent of the volume of each unit of packed RBCs, platelets, and fresh frozen plasma consists of acid-citrate-dextrose anticoagulant. This anticoagulant chelates plasma divalent cations, such as calcium, magnesium, and zinc, such that they cannot participate in the blood protein coagulation reactions. If in a 24-hour period, 1.5 times the patient's blood volume is transfused, the accumulation of the citrate anticoagulant can be massive, producing anticoagulation itself and an acquired coagulopathy. For example, in a 70-kg man, 7% of body weight, or 4.9 kg or liters, is the blood volume. If this individual received 1.5 times his blood volume, he was transfused 7.35 L of blood products, of which 0.735 L or 735 mL was anticoagulant alone. Thus the anticoagulant volume and dilution of his endogenous plasma from all the transfusions conspire to lead to an anticoagulated state. Such a situation occurs in the operating room when there is vigorous RBC replacement. In most circumstances, this problem can be avoided by linking one unit of fresh frozen plasma to every four to six units of RBC transfusion. In addition, one ampule of calcium should be administered for every four to six units of transfused RBCs and one unit of fresh frozen plasma to overcome the anticoagulant effect of the sodium citrate.

Managing Massive Bleeding

There are times in the operating room when bleeding occurs and appropriate therapy has been instituted but the surgeon still believes that hemostasis has not been achieved in a sufficiently timely manner. In these critical situations, an immediate, short-term means to get a handle on the hemorrhage is the use of intravenous infusion of recombinant factor VIIa (rVIIa) (10,11). Recombinant VIIa infusion directly activates IX or X, or both, to lead to thrombin formation. In essence, the infusion makes the patient prothrombotic. This fact carries a real risk of inducing thrombosis in the coronary and cerebral circulation.

However, life-threatening bleeding in the OR may mandate its use. Although the literature provides a wide range of dosing that can be used, our experience tells us that a more conservative dosage from 40 to 60 μg per kg is often sufficient to achieve hemostasis safely in most patients with an acute hemorrhage not immediately controllable by more traditional means. FVIIa therapy works best in individuals who have been repleted with coagulation proteins in fresh frozen plasma. rFVIIa is expensive, and if it is going to work, it will do so by single intravenous infusion. If hemorrhage is not controlled by a second infusion of the agent, causes for bleeding other than a medical hemostatic defect must be sought.

ASSESSING RISK AND PREVENTION FOR THROMBOSIS IN THE SURGICAL PATIENT

Although bleeding in any patient is dramatic and anxiety-provoking to the surgical staff, thrombosis is a silent cause of morbidity and mortality. More surgical patients die of thrombotic complications resulting from surgery than from bleeding. It is incumbent upon the physician to be knowledgeable about the risks for thrombosis that occur in the surgical patient. The best treatment for thrombosis is thrombosis prevention. In general, venous thrombosis occurs in an area of low flow and consists of an initial platelet thrombus followed by an accumulation of red cells in a fibrin mesh. Alternatively, arterial thrombus is mostly platelet-rich, occurring in areas of high blood flow. Both venous and arterial thrombosis have known risk factors for this condition (12).

Arterial Thrombosis

It is beyond this chapter's scope to fully discuss the risk factors for myocardial infarction (MI) and stroke. However, we do know of certain protein risk factors that contribute to arterial thrombosis. In particular, elevation of homocysteine and antiphospholipid antibodies contribute to risk of both arterial and venous thrombosis. Each will be discussed in the section below on venous thrombosis. One weak factor for increased risk for arterial thrombosis is the elevation of lipoprotein(a) [Lp(a)]. Lp(a) consists of low density lipoprotein (LDL) and apolipoprotein(a). Apolipoprotein(a) has 98% sequence identity to kringle 4 of plasminogen, the portion of plasminogen that binds to cells and phospholipids, the place where clinically significant thrombolysis occurs. Therefore, Lp(a) is both atherogenic and prothrombotic.

Venous Thrombosis

Risk factors for venous thrombosis in the surgical patient are numerous. After 2 weeks of bed rest, there is a 20%

likelihood for thrombosis in a 20-year-old individual, but a 60% likelihood for thrombosis in a 60-year-old patient. Obese patients are more likely to have a thrombosis complication than lean patients. A preoperative ambulatory patient has a lower risk for thrombosis than a bed-ridden individual. Further, a patient with a stroke is more likely to have a thrombosis in the paretic limb than in the non-paretic limb. The surgical patient with cardiac disease is more thrombus prone than if there was no cardiac disease. Young women on oral contraceptives put to bed rest will have more risk for thrombosis than if they were not on contraceptives. Surgery, itself, promotes thrombosis. The degree of risk depends on the nature of the surgery and the amount of time the patient is under anesthesia. For example, orthopedic surgery (hip, knee) is associated with actual flexing and occlusion of the femoral and popliteal veins, respectively. The incidence of DVT is 35% to 40% and 50%, respectively. In abdominothoracic surgery the risk for thrombosis is 14% to 35%. In urologic surgery the risk for a DVT is 7% for a transurethral resection but 35% for a suprapubic prostatectomy. Similarly, in gynecologic surgery a vaginal hysterectomy has a 7% risk for thrombosis but a total abdominal hysterectomy has a 27% risk. Last, surgical patients with malignancy have a higher risk for thrombosis as a result of the malignancy itself. This risk can manifest itself years before the clinical presentation of the cancer.

In addition to these situational risk factors for thrombosis, there are now a number of recognized protein defects that increase the risk for thrombosis in surgical patients (Table 18-4). The importance of recognizing these conditions preoperatively is that in affected patients special attention to thrombosis risk at the time of surgery and postoperatively may temper the risk. By far the most common molecular defect associated with thrombosis is the factor V Leiden nucleotide polymorphism (G to A mutation at base pair 1691 of coagulation factor V) that results in a protein that is resistant to activated protein C inactivation (i.e., activated protein C resistance) (13,14). The factor V Leiden defect is the most common inherited

---

TABLE 18-4

PROTEIN BASIS FOR INCREASED THROMBOSIS RISK

Factor V Leiden (activates protein C resistance)
Elevated homocysteine
Prothrombin 20210
Protein C deficiency or defect
Protein S deficiency or defect
Dysfibrinogenemias
Antithrombin
Dysplasminogenemias

cause for thrombosis in western populations, approaching 20% of unselected cases and 40% of cases with family histories (15). Further, it is associated with other prothrombotic risk factors. Factor V Leiden is considered a low risk factor for thrombosis. However, when combined with other risk factors or when individuals with the defect are put at high risk for thrombosis situations, it can summate with the other entities, increasing thrombosis risk. Some data suggests that patients with the factor V Leiden defect may have early graft closure after coronary artery bypass surgery.

Homocysteine elevation ($\sim$10%) is the next most common entity associated with increased risk for thrombosis. Homocysteine levels of 11 or more is a risk factor for cardiovascular disease. Elevated homocysteine injures endothelial cells, producing free radicals, and thus interferes with the thromboprotective mechanism on vascular endothelium and promotes atherosclerosis. Patients who have elevations in homocysteine should be treated with oral folate. The third most common risk factor for increased thrombosis risk is a gene mutation in prothrombin, prothrombin 20210 ($\sim$6%). This polymorphism in the 3′ untranslated region of the prothrombin gene produces increased amounts of a normal prothrombin, thus tipping the balance toward a prothrombotic state. Like factor V Leiden, both elevations of homocysteine and the prothrombin 20210 mutation are weak isolated risk factors for thrombosis. However, with surgery their importance increases.

More serious, but less common, protein defects associated with thrombosis are protein C and S deficiencies (Table 18-4). These protein defects interfere with the major anticoagulant function of the protein C and S systems. Together, patients with these combined defects constitute about 4% to 5% of instances with thrombosis. Patients with these protein defects and a history of thrombosis may require lifelong anticoagulation. Abnormal fibrinogens (dysfibrinogens) are a heterogenous group of disorders, some of which have increased risk for thrombosis. Antithrombin deficiency or defects carries a very serious prothrombotic risk. Fortunately, these patients are quite rare and constitute <1% of all patients seen with thrombosis. Recognition of this defect in a patient with thrombosis requires lifelong anticoagulation. Finally, abnormal plasminogens (dysplasminogenemia) are rare risk factors for thrombosis.

In addition to the molecular/protein defects that increase a patient's risk for thrombosis, certain medical conditions are also associated with thrombosis. The surgeon needs to be aware of these conditions as well so that special precautions can be made to protect these patients from thrombosis at the time of elective or emergent surgery (Table 18-5). As mentioned above, DIC can be associated with thrombosis. If DIC occurs in a patient with malignancy, special effort is necessary to prevent the venous thrombosis that can occur in these individuals. The best prevention for thrombosis in the cancer patient is

TABLE 18-5

MEDICAL/HEMATOLOGIC CONDITIONS ASSOCIATED WITH INCREASED RISK FOR THROMBOSIS

Disseminated intravascular coagulation (DIC)
Heparin-induced thrombocytopenia and thrombosis syndrome (HITTS)
Antiphospholipid syndrome
Thrombotic thrombocytopenic purpura (TTP)
Hemolytic uremic syndrome (HUS)
Myeloprolifreative disorders

prophylaxis with low molecular weight heparin (16). Another medical condition predisposing to thrombosis is heparin-induced thrombocytopenia and thrombosis syndrome (HITTS). This entity is most commonly seen in patients who have had cardiopulmonary bypass surgery. A very high percentage of patients after CPB will have antibodies to heparin. Also, about 1% and 2.5% of patients who get DVT prophylaxis with low molecular weight heparin or unfractionated heparin, respectively, will develop HITTS anywhere from 3 to 14 days after completion of therapy. Any patient who presents with new thrombosis postop and who received prophylactic heparin therapy has to be considered to have HITTS until proven otherwise. When recognized, these patients are treated with withdrawal of the heparin and anticoagulation with an alternative anticoagulant such as argatroban, hirudin, or bivalirudin.

Antiphospholipid antibody syndrome is another entity that increases thrombosis risk in surgical patients. These patients can have both arterial and venous thrombosis. The condition is recognized by evidence of antiphospholipid antibodies as determined by measuring anticardiolipin antibodies, elevation of β_2 glycoprotein I, and studies for lupus anticoagulants. Antiphospholipid antibodies interfere with the anticoagulant nature of annexin II, preventing it from getting to endothelial cell membranes to reduce thrombin formation. Patients with antiphospholipid antibodies are prone to thrombosis and, thus, care needs to be addressed to prevent it from occurring. The rare hematologic conditions of thrombotic thrombocytopenic purpura (TTP), a deficiency or antibody to the von Willebrand factor cleaving enzyme, ADAMTS13 (a disintegrin and metalloproteases with a thrombospondin-1-like domain), and hemolytic uremic syndrome (HUS) because of Shiga toxin from E. coli 0157:H7, present with severe thrombocytopenia and a microangiopathic hemolytic anemia. These patients are usually excluded from surgical intervention. Last, myeloproliferative disorders such as polycythemia vera and essential thrombocytosis are conditions with elevated platelet counts and a high increased risk for thrombosis.

Prior to surgery, efforts should be made to reduce the elevated platelet count as well as to be generous in prophylaxis for thrombosis.

Therapy for Thrombosis and Its Prevention

The best therapy for thrombosis in the patient who is at increased risk is its prevention. In a trial of 4,121 patients undergoing major surgical procedures, the use of low dose unfractionated heparin resulted in a reduction of DVT to only 7.7% of patients versus 24.6% of patients in the untreated control group (17). This landmark study established the need for DVT prophylaxis in the surgical patient. It is beyond this chapter's scope to discuss the pros and cons of subcutaneous heparin or low molecular weight heparin versus compression stockings to prevent postoperative DVT in surgical patients. Both approaches have merit. In preparation for surgery, patients on anticoagulants should have their oral anticoagulant, warfarin, stopped 7 days before surgery. In its place, subcutaneous low molecular weight heparin should be administered up to 12 to 24 hours prior to surgery. Likewise, as soon as the surgeon determines that the risk for postoperative bleeding has passed, subcutaneous low molecular weight heparin should be started on the patient with increased thrombosis risk. If DVT arises in the postoperative patient, therapy should proceed based on current treatment protocols for all DVT patients (18). The use of vena cava umbrellas should be reserved for the rare patient who cannot tolerate full anticoagulation (e.g., active GI bleed) in the postoperative period.

SUMMARY

Evaluation of the surgery patient for bleeding and thrombosis risk follows from the same kind of evaluation of any patient for bleeding and thrombosis. Current diagnostic tools are good for assessing bleeding risk; thrombosis risk, on the other hand, requires a good knowledge of the patient's history as well as the nature of the surgical situation the patient will experience. Much information is available to guide the surgeon in diagnosis and therapy. As in all situations, attention to history and laboratory assays makes a difference in providing care to patients.

REFERENCES

1. Schmaier AH. Principles of hemostasis. In: Schmaier AH, Petruzzelli LM, eds. *Hematology for the medical student.* Baltimore, MD: Lippincott, Williams & Wilkins; 2003:71–77.
2. Meijers JCM, Tekelenburg WL, Bouma BN, et al. High levels of coagulation factor XI as a risk factor for venous thrombosis. *N Engl J Med* 2000;342:696–701.
3. Schmaier AH. Approach to the bleeding patient. In: Schmaier AH, Petruzzelli LM, eds. *Hematology for the medical student.* Baltimore, MD: Lippincott, Williams & Wilkins; 2003:79–83.
4. Schmaier AH. Acquired disorders of blood coagulation. In: Humes HD, ed. *Kelley's textbook of internal medicine,* 4th ed. Philadelphia, PA: Lippincott, Williams & Wilkins; 2000: 1718–1723.
5. Schmaier AH. Acquired bleeding disorder. In: Schmaier AH, Petruzzelli LM, eds. *Hematology for the medical student.* Philadelphia, PA: Lippincott, Williams & Wilkins; 2003:99–104.
6. Boulis NM, Bobek MP, Schmaier AH, et al. Use of factor IX complex in warfarin-related intracranial hemorrhage. *Neurosurgery* 1999;45:1113–1118.
7. Deveras RAE, Kessler CM. Reversal of warfarin-induced excessive anticoagulation with recombinant human factor VIIa concentrate. *Ann Intern Med* 2002;137:884–888.
8. Lin J, Hanigan WC, Tarantino M, et al. The use of recombinant activated factor VII to reverse warfarin-induced anticoagulation in patients with hemorrhage in the central nervous system: preliminary findings. *J Neurosurg* 2003;98:737–740.
9. Colman RW, Robboy SJ, Minna JD. Disseminated intravascular coagulation (DIC): an approach. *Am J Med* 1972;52:679–689.
10. Midathada MV, Mehta P, Waner M, et al. Recombinant factor VIIa in the treatment of bleeding. *Am J Clin Path* 2004;121: 124–137.
11. Bijsterveld NR, Moons AH, Boekholdt M, et al. Ability of recombinant factor VIIa to reverse the anticoagulant effect of the pentasaccharide Fondaparinux in healthy volunteers. *Circulation* 2002;106:2550–2554.
12. Schmaier AH. Evaluation of thrombosis. In: Schmaier AH, Petruzzelli LM, eds. *Hematology for the medical student.* Philadelphia, PA: Lippincott, Williams & Wilkins; 2003: 121–126.
13. Svensson PJ, Dahlback B. Resistance to activated protein C as a basis for venous thrombosis. *N Engl J Med* 1994;330:517–522.
14. Greengard JS, Eichinger S, Griffin JH, et al. Brief report: variability of thrombosis among homozygous siblings with resistance to activated protein C due to an Arg-Gln mutation in the gene for factor V. *N Engl J Med* 1994;331:1559–1562.
15. Bavikatty NR, Killeen AA, Akel N, et al. Association of the prothrombin G20210A mutation with Factor V Leiden in a midwestern American population. *Am J Clin Path* 2000;114:272–275.
16. Lee AY, Levine MN, Baker RI, et al. Randomized comparison of low molecular-weight heparin versus a coumarin for the prevention of recurrent venous thromboembolism in patients with cancer. *N Engl J Med* 2003;349:146–153.
17. Kakkar VV, Corrigan TP, Fossard DP, et al., International Multicentre Trial Group. Prevention of fatal postoperative pulmonary embolism by low doses of heparin. *The Lancet* 1975; II:46–51.
18. Bates SM, Ginsberg JS. Treatment of deep-vein thrombosis. *N Engl J Med* 2004;351:268–277.

Complications

of Nutritional Support

19

Daniel H. Teitelbaum   Imad F. Btaiche   Saleem Islam

■ **PARENTERAL NUTRITION 195**

■ **INDICATIONS FOR PARENTERAL NUTRITION IN SURGICAL PATIENTS 196**
Indications 196
Indications for Preoperative Nutrition 196
Indications for Postoperative Nutrition 196

■ **COMPLICATIONS OF NUTRITIONAL ASSESSMENT AND MONITORING 196**

■ **COMPLICATIONS OF MALNUTRITION 197**
Kwashiorkor and Marasmus 197
Complications of Malnutrition 197
Efficacy of Correcting Malnutrition 197

■ **METABOLIC COMPLICATIONS OF PARENTERAL NUTRITION 198**
Hyperglycemia 198
Hypoglycemia 199
Hyperlipidemia 199
Respiratory Decompensation 200
Refeeding Syndrome 200
Electrolyte Abnormalities 201
Acid-base Disturbances 203
Liver Complications 203

■ **COMPLICATIONS OF DELIVERY 204**
Parenteral 204
Enteral Nutrition 207

■ **SUMMARY 208**

■ **REFERENCES 208**

Daniel H. Teitelbaum and Imad F. Btaiche: University of Michigan, Ann Arbor, MI 48109

Saleem Islam: University of Mississippi Medical School, Jackson, MS 39216

Nutritional support can be provided by intravenous (parenteral) or gastrointestinal (enteral) delivery of nutrients. In general, enteral nutrition is less complicated and preferable. However, the development of parenteral nutrition (PN) within the last 4 decades has allowed critical nutritional support for many patients.

PARENTERAL NUTRITION

PN is the administration of complete and balanced nutrition via the intravenous route to support anabolism and weight maintenance or gain when the gastrointestinal tract cannot or should not be used. Adequate nutrition is essential for patient recovery, and PN is a life-saving therapy in patients with intestinal failure. Conversely, a lack of adequate nutrition may lead to a decline in wound healing and possibly an increase in perioperative complications. However, PN can be associated with many complications, including metabolic, infectious, and technical. Aside from the delivery of PN, good nutritional care requires careful assessment of the patient's nutritional status and a determination of which patients should, or should not, receive PN.

INDICATIONS FOR PARENTERAL NUTRITION IN SURGICAL PATIENTS

Indications

PN is indicated when the gastrointestinal tract cannot be fully used. This includes patients with significant peritonitis, lack of adequate intestinal length, or a malabsorptive state. Additionally, patients with specific gastrointestinal disorders, including intractable diarrhea, protracted vomiting, enterocolitis, motility disorders, inflammatory bowel disease, enteric fistulae with high output, and bowel obstruction may require parenteral feedings for a prolonged time.

Indications for Preoperative Nutrition

In adults, provision of enteral feedings preoperatively for 2 to 3 weeks may reduce postoperative wound infections, anastomotic leakage, hepatic and renal failure, and length of hospital stay (1). Data for PN support is much less clear. The first definitive study to approach this question was the VA cooperative study, which examined a large number of malnourished patients who needed major abdominal or thoracic operations (2). Patients were randomized to preoperative PN (along with a short course of postoperative PN) versus surgery without any PN. Surprisingly, those patients who received PN had higher rates of infectious complications, including pneumonias, urinary tract infections, and wound infections. The only patients with proven benefit from perioperative PN were the ones who had severe malnutrition. A meta-analysis of patients receiving PN in the perioperative period showed that PN was associated with a 10% increase in the absolute rate of postoperative complications (3). This finding was confirmed by a more recent meta-analysis of critically ill adults, which demonstrated only a marginal benefit of preoperative PN in mildly or moderately malnourished patients (4). A benefit of preoperative PN was noted only in those patients who were severely malnourished. The cause of these increased infections has not been definitively determined. However, these studies have had a dramatic affect in reducing the aggressive use of PN in surgical patients, confining the preoperative use to those patients with severe malnutrition.

Indications for Postoperative Nutrition

Use of aggressive postoperative nutritional support is even more controversial (5). In adults, the provision of enteral nutrients may reduce the rate of sepsis and may lower costs. However, enteral intolerance can limit one's ability to achieve complete nutritional support (6). These data suggest that, when indicated, postoperative nutrition should be started early, utilizing a combination of PN and EN until the gastrointestinal tract fully recovers. The effect of PN on postoperative healing is also unclear as many

studies are contradictory. Because results in the area of postoperative nutritional support are not clear, aggressive postoperative feedings are recommended only in those patients who can receive enteral nutrition without complication. Postoperative PN should be restricted to those patients who will not start enteral nutrition for at least 7 to 10 days (7).

COMPLICATIONS OF NUTRITIONAL ASSESSMENT AND MONITORING

As stated above, many patients who require operative intervention suffer from malnutrition due either to a variety of feeding disorders or to the underlying disease process for which they will need surgery. Nutritional assessment is a critical aspect of the initial evaluation of all surgical patients, and the incidence of malnutrition in surgical patients has been well documented in several reviews. In one review by Mullen et al., 95% of all surgical patients had one abnormal nutritional parameter and 35% had three indicators of malnutrition (8). In addition to adults, pediatric surgical patients may also be at risk for malnutrition. Cameron et al. showed that the prevalence of chronic malnutrition was similarly high at 65% and the incidence increased to 80% in those who were cardiac surgical infants (9). Clearly, recognizing and categorizing the severity of the malnourished state is the best way to determine which patient will require perioperative nutrition support. Recognition and correction of malnutrition prior to elective surgery may eliminate or reduce the rates of surgical morbidity and mortality. Although a significantly malnourished patient can easily be identified, those patients with mild to moderate malnutrition are frequently difficult to identify. Classically, indicators of malnutrition have relied on biochemical and physical parameters. These have included measurements of albumin and morphometric measurements, including triceps skin fold and forearm circumferences. Hypoalbuminemia has long been considered an index of protein depletion and has been shown to be associated with an increased rate of postoperative mortality (10). Unfortunately, low albumin levels are not a good indicator of nutritional status and may lead to a misleading classification of the nutritional status (11). A more reliable modality to define malnutrition is the use of a baseline subjective global assessment (SGA). Such an assessment is easy to obtain and has a high degree of reliability with regard to the determination of degree of malnutrition (12). An SGA consists of a history and physical examination and should include an evaluation of weight loss (>10% for severe malnutrition), anorexia, or vomiting, as well as physical evidence of muscle wasting. Patients at particular risk for malnutrition include those with large open wounds with the concomitant loss of protein and increased metabolic needs, extensive burns, blunt trauma, and sepsis.

COMPLICATIONS OF MALNUTRITION

Kwashiorkor and Marasmus

Classically, malnutrition has been divided into two basic forms, protein-calorie malnutrition—or marasmus—and protein deficiency—or kwashiorkor (Table 19-1). Although these processes are most prevalent in third-world countries, the conditions may be manifested in hospitalized patients. The most common clinical example of a marasmic patient is one who has been taking in an inadequate diet for several weeks to months. A common example would be a nursing home patient who has a depressed mental condition. Such a patient, if admitted and deprived of any nutritional support, will begin to utilize remaining somatic muscle to support gluconeogenesis. In this case the patient will develop a mixed picture of an acute kwashiorkor state over a baseline state of marasmus. The outcome of such patients is notoriously poor (13). Common settings in which such conditions can occur are in the septic, burned, or traumatized patient. These patients may lose as much as 30 g of nitrogen per day, the equivalent of 2.5 lb of wet muscle weight loss daily. Along with this loss of muscle mass will be a number of adverse complications which directly affect the outcome of surgical patients.

Complications of Malnutrition

Impaired healing can result from severe states of malnutrition and potentially lead to disruption of intestinal anastomoses as well as wound dehiscence and infection. Previous studies have shown decreased tensile strength of intestinal anastomoses in malnourished rats, which could be prevented by PN repletion. An effort should be made, when possible, to minimize impaired wound healing by preoperatively repleting patients who are *severely* undernourished and by preventing postoperative starvation. Zinc, vitamin C (ascorbic acid), and vitamin A deficiencies may also lead to impaired wound healing and should be prevented. Malnutrition may also lead to an increased risk of respiratory difficulties, such as atelectasis and pneumonia, secondary to decreased strength of respiratory muscles and the inability to cough. The lack of muscle strength probably decreases the patient's forced vital capacity and tidal volume and, therefore, prolongs the need for intubation and mechanical ventilation with their associated complications of pneumothorax, tracheal-innominate artery erosion, tracheal stenosis, and sepsis. Although immediate total parenteral nutrition (TPN) is not indicated, for those who do not take enteral intake for 7 to 10 days PN should be initiated. Several investigators have found a marked increase in septic complications in malnourished patients (14). Undernutrition alone results in depressed T-lymphocyte numbers and function (15). Impaired leukocyte function could increase the risk of pneumonia. Recent studies suggest that severe malnutrition can cause breakdown of the intestinal mucosal barrier to bacteria with bacterial translocation from the gut lumen to the portal venous system (16,17). Neutropenia has also been noted with copper deficiency, and impaired neutrophil chemotaxis and phagocytosis have also been found with phosphate deficiency. Impaired body defenses will increase the risk of pneumonia, wound infections, and intracavitary abscesses.

Efficacy of Correcting Malnutrition

It is important to note that although pneumonia and respiratory failure are major causes of death for persons who are starved, there is little evidence that nutritional repletion improves pulmonary function and prevents pneumonia (18). One of the best controlled studies that suggests that early nutritional support may help surgical patients is from Sandstrom et al. (19). In this study patients were

TABLE 19-1

COMPARISON OF MARSMUS AND KWASHIORKOR

Disease	Clinical Setting	Time to Develop	Clinical Features	Laboratory	Clinical Course	Mortality
Marasmus	↓ Calorie intake	Months or years	Starved appearance, weight <80% of UBW, TSF <3 mm, MAMC <15 cm	Possible normal albumin and transferrin	Reasonably preserved responsiveness to short-term stress	Low, unless related to underlying disease
Kwashiorkor	↓ Protein intake during stress	Weeks	Well-nourished appearance, easy hair pluckability, edema	Low albumin and transferrin	Poor wound healing, decubitus ulcers, skin breakdown	High

UBW, usual body weight; TSF, triceps skin fold; MAMC, midarm muscle circumference.
From Khalidi N, Btaiche IF, Kovacevich DS, eds. *The parenteral and enteral nutrition manual*, 8th ed. Ann Arbor, MI: The University of Michigan Hospitals and Health Centers, 2003, with permission.

randomized to receive postoperative PN versus dextrose. Those patients who did not initiate enteral intake prior to 14 days and who were randomized to receive only dextrose had a 10-fold higher mortality and a twofold higher rate of sepsis. Based on meta-analyses, correction of malnutrition is indicated in only severely malnourished surgical patients (2). Overly aggressive use of PN may lead to a much higher incidence of complications. In fact, meta-analysis of the routine use of postoperative PN support suggests that it is associated with a 10% increase in complications (3). Although PN has numerous associated complications, enteral nutrition is associated with several complications as well. In a detailed meta-analysis comparing enteral to PN, no advantage was noted between the two modalities of delivering nutrition other than that the cost of enteral nutrition was ten times lower (20).

METABOLIC COMPLICATIONS OF PARENTERAL NUTRITION

Just as malnutrition may lead to a number of problems with perioperative morbidity, use of PN may be equally or more deleterious. Thus, use of PN requires an extensive understanding of indications of PN, knowledge of proper prescribing, and careful monitoring.

Hyperglycemia

Hyperglycemia is the most common complication associated with PN. Dextrose infusion rate and the patient's underlying conditions determine carbohydrate tolerance. Dextrose oxidation is reduced under stress, such as in critically ill and surgical patients (21). Predisposing factors to hyperglycemia also include sepsis, multiorgan failure, diabetes, acute pancreatitis, and drug therapy that alters glucose metabolism (e.g., corticosteroids, tacrolimus, catecholamine vasopressors).

Stress-induced hyperglycemia is the result of increased endogenous glucose production in response to increased release of counterregulatory hormones and cytokines that stimulate glycogenolysis and gluconeogenesis. In stressed patients elevated insulin levels fail, however, to suppress gluconeogenesis or to increase cellular glucose uptake, which results in hyperglycemia. In a small study group ($n = 5$) of low stress postoperative adult patients, dextrose infusion rates up to 7 mg/kg/minute were tolerated (22). However, data from hypermetabolic adult burn patients showed a maximum tolerable glucose infusion rate of 5 mg/kg/minute (23). Even lower rates at ≤4 mg/kg/minute in stressed adult patients are better tolerated. In a retrospective review of 102 nondiabetic adult patients who received PN, hyperglycemia occurred in 49% of patients with dextrose infusion rates of >5 mg/kg/minute and 11% of patients developed hyperglycemia with dextrose infusion rates

between 4.1 and 5 mg/kg/minute. None of the patients who received dextrose infusions at ≤4 mg/kg/minute had hyperglycemia (24).

Hyperglycemia, if left untreated, can result in serious complications, including fluid and electrolyte imbalances, hyperglycemic hyperosmolar nonketotic coma, and increased infectious risk (see Table 19-2). *In vitro* and animal studies have shown that hyperglycemia can impair neutrophil chemotaxis and adhesion, reduce phagocytosis, and inhibit complement fixation (25,26). Poorly controlled diabetics have shown impaired polymorphonuclear leucocyte function (27) and reduced bactericidal activity (28), with phagocytic function improving with glycemic control (29). Notably, hyperglycemia has been shown to increase the risk for nosocomial and wound infections in surgical diabetic patients (30,31).

Hyperglycemia has been defined as serum glucose concentrations >200 mg per dL (32), and serum glucose concentrations of 150 to 200 mg per dL have been long considered acceptable in stressed patients (33). However, recent data from surgical intensive care patients show that tighter glucose control may be more beneficial in reducing patient morbidity and mortality (34). Van den Berghe et al. conducted a prospective, randomized, controlled study to evaluate the outcomes of intensive and conventional insulin therapy in 1,548 adult surgical intensive care unit (ICU) patients. Patients were randomized to receive intensive insulin therapy with a goal of serum glucose concentrations of 80 to 110 mg per dL or a conventional insulin therapy to maintain serum glucose concentrations between 180 and 200 mg per dL when serum glucose levels were exceeding 220 mg per dL. Study results showed that patients in the intensive insulin group had a 43% reduction in mortality, a 46% reduction in sepsis, and a 35% reduction in need for prolonged antibiotic therapy, as compared to the conventional insulin treatment group. Patients in the intensive insulin group also had reduced acute renal failure and ventilator dependency. Benefits of intensive insulin therapy on reducing mortality were notable in the long-stay ICU patients (>5 days) (34). A follow-up multivariate

TABLE 19-2

CONSEQUENCES OF OVERFEEDING

Source of Overfeeding	Consequences
Total calories	Hepatic steatosis; cholestasis
Dextrose	Hyperglycemia; hypertriglyceridemia; hepatic steatosis; hypercapnia; increased infection risk
Lipid emulsions	Hyperlipidemia; hypertriglyceridemia; hepatic steatosis

logistic regression analysis of results showed that benefits derived from intensive insulin therapy were the result of normoglycemia rather than the insulin dose. Also, a direct correlation was found between blood glucose concentrations and hospital mortality. In the long-stay patients the cumulative hospital mortality was 15% in patients with mean blood glucose concentrations <110 mg per dL, about 27% in those with mean blood glucose concentrations between 110 and 150 mg per dL, and 40% in patients with mean blood glucose concentrations >150 mg per dL (35). These data suggest that even small reductions in blood glucose may have a significant effect on improving patient outcome.

In order to avoid hyperglycemia and allow physiologic adaptation to dextrose infusion, dextrose infusion rate in adult PN patients should be started at ≤2 mg/kg/minute as a continuous infusion. The rate can be thereafter advanced to goal over the next few days based on caloric needs and glucose tolerance to a maximum of 4 mg/kg/minute. Dextrose infusion rate should be kept at ≤2 mg/kg/minute in patients requiring insulin until glucose control is achieved. In obese patients the dextrose infusion rate should be calculated based on the adjusted ideal body weight since adipose tissue is not a metabolically active tissue (36). Caloric distribution in PN is best maintained at 50% to 60% from dextrose, 20% to 30% from lipids, and 10% to 20% from proteins. If hyperglycemia occurs, a portion of the dextrose may be substituted with lipids until glucose control is achieved without exceeding 60% of the total daily calories from lipids.

Serum glucose concentrations up to 200 mg per dL can be managed with a sliding scale regimen of subcutaneous regular insulin. If a patient is receiving PN, 70% of the average sliding scale insulin dose used can be added to the PN solution and the insulin dose can be adjusted thereafter. However, the normal serum glucose target between 80 and 110 mg per dL proposed by the van den Berghe et al. study necessitates the use of an insulin drip for the control of severe hyperglycemia (34). This allows titration of the insulin dose based on serum glucose concentrations and provides a safe and effective method of glycemic control (37). Such tight control of glucose should be confined to the ICU setting. Although exogenous insulin increases cellular glucose uptake and normalizes blood glucose levels, insulin does not increase glucose oxidation. As such, little benefit is derived from excessive dextrose infusion at a rate that exceeds the body's glucose oxidative capacity. Instead, excess dextrose is converted to fat, which results in hypertriglyceridemia and fatty liver (hepatic steatosis).

In order to provide adequate calories and avoid overfeeding, critically ill patients should ideally have their energy expenditure measured using indirect calorimetry on an average of two to three times weekly instead of relying on caloric estimates (38). However, data from indirect calorimetric measurements should be interpreted in relation to specific patient factors. Matching caloric intake to energy expenditure is not always possible. In fact, attempting to adjust the carbohydrate and lipid calories to match the high-energy expenditure during severe hypermetabolism would likely meet with intolerance and metabolic complications. In select patients, heavier sedation, better pain control, or wound treatment may be of benefit in reducing energy expenditure. Recent studies have shown that the use of the β-adrenergic blocker propranolol in burn (39) and head injury (40) patients may attenuate hypermetabolism and possibly reduce catabolism.

Hypoglycemia

Although such symptoms of hypoglycemia as diaphoresis, confusion, and agitation have been reported when TPN is abruptly terminated, hypoglycemia is rarely observed in adults, although it is more common in children. Nevertheless, 10% dextrose should always be administered after any interruption of TPN. If one has additional time, the rate of TPN administration should be reduced by one-half for 60 minutes prior to turning the administration completely off. Such a routine should be standard for patients on cycled PN.

Hyperlipidemia

Hyperlipidemia in patients receiving PN usually manifests in increased serum triglyceride levels, although other alterations in the plasma lipid profile may also occur. Hypertriglyceridemia associated with PN is mainly the result of excessive fat synthesis from dextrose overfeeding, the result of excessive lipid infusion, or a result of impaired lipid clearance (41). Severe hypertriglyceridemia (serum triglyceride concentrations >1,000 mg per dL) may precipitate acute pancreatitis (42).

Dextrose overfeeding (see Table 19-2), not excess lipid infusion, is the main cause of hypertriglyceridemia in patients receiving PN. One-third of glucose is normally converted to fat during lipogenesis. However, the amount of fat generated can be higher with dextrose overfeeding, with formed fat being deposited in the liver or transported from the liver as triglyceride-rich very low-density lipoproteins (VLDL) (43). In patients receiving PN, several factors cause reduction in lipid emulsion clearance, including sepsis, multiorgan failure (44), obesity, diabetes (45), liver disease (46), renal failure (47), pancreatitis (48), and medications that alter fat metabolism (e.g., cyclosporine, sirolimus, corticosteroids). Propofol, a sedative agent formulated in a 10% lipid emulsion that is commonly used in the ICU, can also cause a dose-dependent elevation in serum triglyceride concentrations (49).

Intravenous lipid emulsions currently marketed in the United States are composed of long-chain triglycerides (LCTs). LCT-based lipid emulsions are available in 10%, 20%, and 30% emulsions that provide 1.1, 2, and 3 kcal per mL, respectively. Following infusion, the lipoprotein lipase (LPL) enzyme hydrolyzes lipid particles in the bloodstream to release fatty acids. The liver lipase enzyme metabolizes lipid remnants in the liver to generate VLDL and low-density lipoproteins (LDLs). Normally, about 80% of lipids are cleared in 1 hour. However, lipid emulsion clearance is reduced in critically ill patients as a result of stress-induced reduction in LPL activity (50).

The differences in the phospholipid-to-triglyceride (PL/TG) ratio in the various lipid emulsion formulations are the basis for clearance differences between the lipid formulations. The PL/TG ratio of the 10%, 20%, and 30% lipid emulsion is 0.12, 0.06, and 0.04, respectively. This translates to two and three times higher phospholipid amounts in the 10% compared to the 20% and 30% lipid emulsions, respectively. Excess phospholipids in the 10% emulsion is believed to result in the formation of abnormal lipoprotein X particles. Lipoprotein X is a large particle made predominantly from phospholipids and cholesterol and has a long half-life of 2 to 4 days (51). Lipoprotein X that appears in the blood of patients with the infusion of the 10% lipid emulsions is believed to cause hyperlipidemia by competing for metabolism with the infused lipid emulsion particles (52). A 5-day infusion of the 10% emulsion to postoperative trauma patients resulted in increased plasma phospholipids and cholesterol levels. This was not, however, observed with the infusion of the 20% lipid emulsion (53). Others have made such observations (54–56). Although the difference has not been shown to alter the clinical course of patients, higher concentrations of lipid emulsions are desirable in critically ill surgical patients (57). The 30% lipid emulsion is FDA-approved for infusion in total nutrient admixtures (TNA: admixture of amino acids, dextrose, and lipid emulsions in one solution) and is most advantageous in patients with fluid restriction due to its higher caloric concentration.

In acutely ill patients receiving PN, serum triglyceride concentrations should be monitored at baseline once lipid goal is achieved and then once weekly thereafter. If hypertriglyceridemia occurs, dextrose overfeeding should be ruled out first and the dextrose load should be reduced if needed. Reducing the lipid dose may be necessary once hypertriglyceridemia does not improve following the reduction of the dextrose amount. Lipid emulsions should preferably be infused continuously over 24 hours to improve their clearance (58).

Another etiology of hypertriglyceridemia is carnitine deficiency. This state is particularly prevalent in premature patients. Daily lipid infusion should be withheld when the patient's serum is lipemic or when serum triglyceride concentrations are >400 mg per dL. In such cases the lipid emulsion dose should be given only two to three times weekly. In order to prevent essential fatty acid deficiency, linoleic acid should provide 3% to 4% of daily caloric intake. Practically, providing 300 mL of the 20% lipid

emulsion twice weekly is sufficient to prevent essential fatty acid deficiency in adults.

Fatty acid deficiency is extremely uncommon as long as some supplementation of the PN contains lipids. Nevertheless, withdrawal of lipids will be manifested by skin changes, anemia, thrombocytopenia, and a fatty liver.

Respiratory Decompensation

Hypercapnia in PN patients can be the result of carbohydrate overfeeding with a subsequent excess production of carbon dioxide (CO_2). The respiratory quotient (RQ) ($RQ = VCO_2/VO_2$) for carbohydrate, protein, and fat is 1, 0.8, and 0.7, respectively, with carbohydrate oxidation generating the most CO_2 production. Normally, energy-mixed substrates yield a RQ around 0.85 (59). A RQ >1 indicates overfeeding and lipogenesis (60). Dextrose infusion rates exceeding 4 mg/kg/minute in critically–ill patients will typically result in an increase in the RQ that is >1 (61).

The increased respiratory workload associated with the generation of excess CO_2 production may exacerbate or result in acute respiratory acidosis, respiratory insufficiency, and prolongation of ventilator dependence (62). These deleterious effects may occur within hours of dextrose overfeeding, especially in cachectic patients and in those with limited pulmonary reserve (63). In PN patients, keeping dextrose infusion rates ≤4 mg/kg/minute and reducing the total caloric delivery will result in lower CO_2 production (58). Although an RQ >1 may reflect excess carbohydrate feeding, an RQ <1 does not, however, exclude overfeeding. This is the case of hypermetabolic patients where oxygen consumption and minute ventilation increase with increased CO_2 production (64).

Refeeding Syndrome

Refeeding syndrome describes the fluid and electrolyte disturbances, vitamin deficiencies, and glucose intolerance that occur in severely malnourished patients upon rapid initiation of feeding (oral, enteral, or parenteral). Metabolic derangements of the refeeding syndrome can result in cardiac, pulmonary, renal, and neuromuscular complications. Patients at high risk for refeeding syndrome include those with chronic starvation, severe weight loss, chronic alcoholism, anorexia nervosa, and malabsorption syndromes (65,66).

Hypophosphatemia, hypokalemia, and hypomagnesemia (see section below) are the three most common and potentially severe electrolyte disturbances that may occur during the refeeding syndrome. Potassium, magnesium, and organic phosphates are primarily intracellular ions and are cofactors in macronutrient metabolism. As a result of significant weight loss, total body stores of these electrolytes become depleted. However, their serum concentrations may appear normal at first due to their extracellular shift to maintain homeostasis. As a result of anabolism that occurs with feeding initiation following starvation, these electrolytes are redistributed intracellularly, which results in their decreased serum concentrations (67). With rapid initiation of carbohydrate feeding, insulin secretion is stimulated, which shifts phosphorus and potassium intracellularly. Phosphorus demands are also increased for the synthesis of the high-energy phosphates such as adenosine triphosphate (ATP), 2,3-diphosphoglycerate (2,3-DGP), and glycerol-3-phosphate dehydrogenase (G-3PD). With limited phosphorus availability in starved patients, the increased phosphorus demand results in severe hypophosphatemia (68,69). A key to preventing the refeeding syndrome is to first identify patients at highest risk. Once identified, nutrient delivery, especially carbohydrates, should be started at low amounts and then advanced slowly to caloric goal over 3 to 5 days. Empiric supplementation of phosphorus, potassium, and magnesium can also be started before feeding is initiated. Providing additional vitamin supplementation to cachectic patients with additional thiamine of 100 mg per day and folic acid of 1 mg per day is recommended.

Electrolyte Abnormalities

These issues occur more commonly with intravenous support. Deficiency or excess of any of the electrolytes may happen—the most frequent problems are those with sodium, potassium, phosphorus, and magnesium.

Sodium

By far the commonest problem encountered is hyponatremia, typically resulting from the administration of hypotonic solutions. This is usually observed with TPN; however, excess free water enterally may also lead to lower serum sodium. If the sodium levels drop below 125 mmol per dL, neurologic symptoms can occur and it is imperative to replete the deficiency over a period of time to avoid central pontine myelinolysis (70). Preventing hyponatremia and other common electrolyte aberrancies is possible with daily labs when starting support intravenously and adjusting nutrient delivery as needed. When a steady state is reached, labs can be done three times a week and then weekly to monthly in chronic patients. In the event of any significant change in the composition or clinical situations, such as excess emesis and diarrhea, one should check the labs more frequently.

Conversely, hypernatremia is the result of dehydration due to either inadequate free water (either enteral or parenteral) or excess losses (emesis, stoma output, diarrhea, sweating). Again, neurolgic symptoms may occur, especially when the serum level exceeds 160 mmol per dL. In this case the free water deficit is calculated and replaced over a 24- to 48-hour period to prevent complications

(70,71). The formula for repleting free water is:

$$\textit{Free water deficit (L)} \simeq 0.6 \times \textit{body weight (kg)} \times [1-(140/\textit{serum sodium})]$$

Potassium

Hypokalemia can happen when there are excess losses or inadequate provision. This anion is a very important component in electrical conduction and has a profound effect on muscle function, including cardiac muscle. As a patient on TPN becomes anabolic and begins to synthesize new protein, an obligatory requirement exists for intracellular potassium. Therefore, intravenous potassium is administered at 2 to 4 mEq/kg/day in infants and small children or at 40 mEq/L/day in older children and adults. Higher doses may be required in the early phase of refeeding; the need can be determined by monitoring the patient's serum potassium concentration. Replacement may be more rapid in the case in which central venous access is available. Continuous EKG monitoring is advised during rapid infusion. One may anticipate excess losses when there is emesis or diarrhea or when the patient is on diuretics. In these cases prophylactic potassium supplementation should be provided to avoid hypokalemia and the level should be monitored more frequently. Hyperkalemia occurs less frequently and may be due to an error in constituting the TPN. Patients receiving TPN may develop an elevated serum potassium level if they are not significantly anabolic and are unable to fully utilize the administered potassium. Other causes of hyperkalemia include decreased renal function, metabolic acidosis, tissue necrosis, and systemic sepsis. Potassium should be reduced or withheld from the PN solution until the underlying problem is resolved. In situations in which there may be concurrent potassium administration, TPN sources of potassium need to be reduced.

Vitamins and Trace Elements

Vitamin deficiencies, especially of water-soluble vitamins, occur in malnourished patients. Dextrose infusion increases thiamine demands since thiamine is a cofactor in the intermediate carbohydrate metabolism. Thiamine deficiency has resulted in Wernicke encephalopathy (72) and lactic acidosis (73). PN supplementation with trace elements is critical as a number of deficiencies may result with them (see Tables 19-3 and 19-4).

Phosphate and Magnesium

Magnesium and phosphate, as well as potassium, are required during an anabolic state and during protein synthesis. Phosphate and magnesium abnormalities are usually noted shortly after initiation of nutritional support. This is due to a rapid production of ATP from depleted

TABLE 19-3

REQUIREMENTS AND CLINICAL CHARACTERISTICS OF SOME GENERALLY RECOGNIZED MICRONUTRIENTS

Nutrient	Adult RDAs	Signs of Deficiency	Laboratory Assay	Adult Dose for Oral Supplementation
Iron	1–15 mg	Pallor, fatigue, microcytic anemia	Fe:TIBC ratio, ferritin	320 mg ferrous sulfate twice daily for 1 month
Iodine	150 μg	Goiter, hypothyroidism	Urine iodine	Potassium iodide
Zinc	12–15 mg	Acrodermatitis enteropathica, growth retardation, hair loss, delayed wound healing	Serum and urine zinc	20–40 mg per day zinc sulfate
Copper	1.5–3 mg	Hypochromic anemia not responsive to iron, neutropenia, steely hair	Serum copper, ceruloplasmin	2–3 mg per day cupric sulfate
Manganese	2–5 mg	Scaly dermatitis, retarded hair and nail growth, Increased PT not responsive to vitamin K, hypercalcemia, hyperphosphatemia	Urinary N-methyl nicotinamide	2–5 mg per day elemental manganese
Chromium	50–200 μg	Neuropathy, high free fatty acids, glucose intolerance not responsive to insulin	Glucose tolerance test	200 μg per day
Selenium	50–70 μg	Cardiomyopathy, muscle pain, weakness, macrocytosis, skin and hair depigmentation, glucose intolerance	REC glutathione peroxidase	70 μg per day

From Khalidi N, Btaiche IF, Kovacevich DS, eds. *The parenteral and enteral nutrition manual*, 8th ed. Ann Arbor, MI: The University of Michigan Hospitals and Health Centers, 2003, with permission.

stores, which uses up the available phosphate stores and shifts it intracellularly (see the section above entitled "Refeeding Syndrome"). It is important to be cognizant of this phenomenon and check serum phosphate levels frequently after starting enteral or PN in a severely malnourished patient. Conditions leading to hypokalemia may also cause hypomagnesemia (e.g., renal losses and anabolic state), and it is not possible to replete potassium without magnesium as well. Hypomagnesemia may cause a functional ileus, hyperreflexia, and seizures. Clinical features of phosphate and magnesium abnormalities depend on the level of deficiency. Severe hypophosphatemia has resulted in respiratory, neuromuscular, hematologic complications, and even death in cachectic patients following aggressive

TABLE 19-4

VITAMIN DEFICIENCIES/TOXICITIES WITH CLINICAL CHARACTERISTICS

Vitamin	Deficiency	Toxicity
A	Dry skin, hyperkeratosis, dry conjunctiva	Hepatomegaly, muscle pain, malaise, opthalmoplegia, fever, icterus, rash, pseudotumor cerebri
B$_1$ (thiamine)	Beriberi, encephalopathy, heart failure, confusion, decreased tendon reflexes, acidosis	None
B$_2$ (riboflavin)	Angular stomatitis, cheilosis, atrophy of lingual papillae, glossitis, magenta tongue	Photohemolysis in premature infants
B$_6$ (pyridoxine)	Personality changes, irritability, depression, filiform hypertrophy of lingual papillae, aphthous stomatitis, nasolabial seborrhea, forehead rash	Sensory neuropathy, degeneration of sensory root ganglia
B$_{12}$	Megaloblastic anemia, neurologic symptoms, sore tongue, weakness, neuropsychiatric manifestations	None
K	Elevated prothrombin time	None

PN initiation without adequate phosphorus supplementation (67,74). Hypophosphatemia can also manifest as paresthesias, weakness, and convulsions within a few days of PN initiation (75). Severe hypokalemia can cause cardiac, neuromuscular, gastrointestinal, metabolic, and renal dysfunction. Similarly, hypomagnesemia can have cardiac, neuromuscular, and gastrointestinal effects. Since hypokalemia and hypomagnesemia can coexist, successful correction of hypokalemia depends on normalizing serum magnesium concentrations.

Acid-base Disturbances

Acid-base disturbances in adult patients receiving PN are primarily related to the underlying patient conditions instead of the PN components. However, excess acetate in PN can lead to metabolic alkalosis (76), and excess chloride can cause metabolic acidosis (77). Acid-base disorders are managed primarily by correcting the underlying problem. However, altering the chloride-to-acetate ratio in PN may be useful in correcting minor acid-base abnormalities. Acetate is converted *in vivo* at a one-to-one molar ratio to bicarbonate. As such, diarrhea and enterocutaneous fistula losses resulting in a bicarbonate deficit can be adjusted by increasing the acetate sources (as sodium or potassium) in PN. Conversely, in patients with high gastric suctioning, increasing the chloride salts (as sodium or potassium) in PN can compensate for loss of gastric hydrochloric acid.

Liver Complications

A transient elevation of liver enzymes is common within 1 to 2 weeks of PN initiation, but liver enzymes will return to normal following PN cessation (78). However, prolonged PN can lead to more severe liver toxicities, including steatosis, steatohepatitis, cholestasis, and cholelithiasis.

Hepatic steatosis describes fat accumulation in the hepatocytes when liver lipid accumulation exceeds its removal (79). Steatohepatitis describes an advanced stage of severe hepatic inflammation that can rapidly progress to liver fibrosis and cirrhosis (80). Patients with hepatic steatosis are usually asymptomatic, and liver enzymes correlate poorly with the degree of fatty infiltration (81). Steatosis should be ruled out when hepatomegaly, malaise, and abdominal discomfort occur. Although hepatic steatosis in PN patients is primarily the result of dextrose overfeeding (82), other factors, such as lipid overfeeding (83), deficiencies of carnitine (84), choline (78), and essential fatty acids, may also contribute (85).

Excess calories and imbalance in the carbohydrate-to-lipid ratio in PN can lead to hepatic steatosis (86). Patients who receive dextrose infusions have a much greater tendency (53%) to develop hepatic steatosis compared to only 17% of those who receive a mixed lipid and dextrose solution (30% and 70% of nonprotein calories from lipids

and dextrose, respectively) (87). Also, patients who received lipid-free PN developed fatty liver, possibly as a result of essential fatty acid deficiency, and steatosis resolved following lipid supplementation (88). In rare instances of fat overfeeding, fat overload syndrome characterized by hypertriglyceridemia, fatty liver, hepatosplenomegaly, coagulopathy, fever, and multiorgan dysfunction have been described (89).

Avoiding carbohydrate and total calorie overfeeding and providing a balanced PN are essential to prevent hepatic steatosis. Up to one-third of total calories can be provided from lipids, while carbohydrate calories should provide no more than 60% of total calories and the remaining calories should come from proteins.

Carnitine deficiency has been proposed as a cause of hepatic steatosis. Carnitine is an amine that transports LCTs into the mitochondria for oxidation and is not a normal supplement of PN. Carnitine deficiency has been proposed to cause liver fat accumulation (90). However, carnitine deficiency is primarily described in premature infants and is extremely rare in adults. The role of carnitine in enhancing fat clearance and preventing hepatic steatosis remains questionable. The correlation between plasma and tissue carnitine levels is uncertain; patients may have normal plasma carnitine levels and still develop hypertriglyceridemia.

The role of choline deficiency in hepatic steatosis is also unclear. Choline is a quaternary amine that is ubiquitous in diet. It is also derived *in vivo* from methionine metabolism. Deficiency of phosphatidylcholine, a byproduct of choline and a component of lipoprotein synthesis, has been proposed to cause abnormal lipoprotein production and to promote triglyceride accumulation in the liver (91). Although methionine is provided from amino acids in PN, choline deficiency may still occur as intravenous methionine is metabolized differently than with enteral administration (92). Limited data are available about the effects of choline supplementation on reversing steatosis in PN patients (93). A pilot study of home PN patients with hepatic steatosis showed that intravenous choline chloride supplementation at 2 g per day in PN for up to 24 weeks was safe and effective in reducing the degree of hepatic steatosis (94). More research, however, is needed to clarify the role of choline in liver disease and before routine choline supplementation to PN can be recommended.

PN-associated cholelithiasis is the result of decreased gallbladder contractility during fasting. In the absence of oral intake or enteral stimulation, there is decreased secretion of cholecystokinin (CCK), a peptide hormone secreted in the duodenum in response to meals to induce gallbladder contractility (95). Fasting PN patients have been observed to have a distended gallbladder and absence of gallbladder contractions, a finding not observed in enterally fed patients (96). As a result of bile stasis, bile accumulation in the biliary tract facilitates cholesterol gallstone formation (97) and calcium biliru-binate precipitation in the form of sludge (98). Biliary sludge, gallstones, and hyperviscous and tenacious bile were recovered during gallbladder surgery to relieve refractory cholestasis in PN-dependent patients (99, 100). Patients with short bowel syndrome are especially at increased risk for cholelithiasis and biliary sludge (101). This is due to impaired bile flow, disrupted bile enterohepatic cycling, and canalicular accumulation of toxic bile acids, such as lithocholic acid (102). Although use of cholecystokinin-octapeptide has been suggested in patients receiving a prolonged course of PN, results have been mixed at best (103,104), and a recent study has failed to show efficacy in preventing cholelithiasis in neonates (105).

PN-associated cholestasis (PNAC) occurs primarily in infancy and is less common in older children and adults (106,107). Predisposing factors to PNAC include duration of PN, prematurity, overfeeding, short bowel, bowel rest, and sepsis (108,109). More recently, PNAC has been described in a number of adult patients on long-term PN (110). The etiology of PNAC is unknown. Bowel rest leads to increased intestinal permeability, alteration in gut hormone secretion, reduction in bile flow, decreased bile salt excretion, bacterial overgrowth, bacterial and endotoxin translocation from the gut, and impaired intestinal immunologic mechanisms (111,112). All these factors may contribute to the development of PNAC. Limited data have also implicated the naturally derived phytosterols in the extracted oil of the lipid emulsions in causing liver injury, but their effects remain uncertain (113). Most recently, a derangement in the expression of bile canalicular transport proteins has been shown in a rodent model of PN (114). These transport proteins are responsible for the production of bile within the canalicular space, and a loss of this function may well be a major mechanism in the development of PNAC. Liver function tests in patients with PNAC may show increased serum liver transaminases, alkaline phosphatase, bilirubin, and gamma glutamyl transferase concentrations (115). However, a rise in serum conjugated bilirubin concentration >2 mg per dL is considered the most commonly accepted marker of cholestasis. Jaundice occurs with advanced cholestasis (116).

PNAC is reversible if PN is discontinued before irreversible liver damage occurs. Because of the detrimental effects of bowel rest, early initiation of enteral or oral feedings and weaning PN is the best way to prevent PNAC. In addition, it is essential to avoid overfeeding, use balanced sources of calories, cycle PN, and avoid and promptly treat sepsis.

Pharmacologic measures have been used to prevent PNAC, improve bile flow, provide symptomatic relief of cholestasis, and reduce the toxic insults to the liver. Unfortunately, little evidence has shown definitive efficacy. Ursodeoxycholic acid has been shown to improve bile flow and reduce the clinical signs and symptoms of cholestasis;

however, a prospective study in infants (the group most prone to PNAC) failed to demonstrate drug efficacy (117). Cholecystokinin-octapeptide (sincalide) was used in infants to induce gallbladder contraction and improve bile flow (118). Use of cholecytokinin, however, has not been shown to be effective in preventing PNAC in a recently performed controlled trial (119). Treatment of bacterial overgrowth with oral antibiotics (e.g., metronidazole, gentamicin, neomycin) during prolonged bowel rest may be beneficial in reducing bacterial translocation across the intestinal wall and possibly prevent their potential hepatotoxic effects (120). Short bowel syndrome patients with end-stage liver disease may benefit from combined liver and bowel transplantation. Early referral of short bowel syndrome patients at high risk for liver complications for bowel transplantation may possibly become a viable life-saving option before irreversible liver damage occurs (121).

COMPLICATIONS OF DELIVERY

Delivery systems depend on the route of nutritional support—parenteral or enteral. Additionally, there are a limited number of broad categories of these delivery problems, including mechanical, infectious, and thrombotic complications for the intravenous route and mechanical and infectious for the enteral route (Tables 19-5 and 19-6).

Parenteral

Mechanical

Although delivery of PN may be performed via the peripheral route, it has several limitations, including osmolarity-induced thrombosis, which limits the concentration of dextrose to 12.5%, thus limiting the total number of calories via this route. PN via the central route is thus the preferred route. Central venous access is usually obtained via a

---

TABLE 19-5

POTENTIAL COMPLICATIONS OF CENTRAL ACCESS

Pneumothorax
Hemothorax
Subclavian artery/vein injury
Cardiac injury/arrhythmias
Carotid artery injury
Catheter malposition
Catheter embolism
Thromboembolism
Thoracic duct injury
Lung injury
Nerve injury
Air embolism

percutaneous route to the internal jugular or subclavian or the common femoral veins. More commonly, access may be obtained by peripherally inserted central catheters (PICC lines) (122). Needle injury to the vein or an adjacent artery is rare but does occur, especially in unskilled hands (123). Malposition of the catheter can lead to problems as well. This includes cardiac injury, pericardial effusion and tamponade, and arrhythmias. Additionally, if the catheter is not located centrally, these hypertonic solutions can result in thrombotic issues. Malpositioning occurs frequently with subclavian access with the catheter tip ending in the ipsilateral jugular vein or the contralateral innominate. Therefore, it is mandatory to check the catheter position radiographically before usage—either with fluoroscopy or static images. Pneumothorax occurs in 1% to 2% of cases of central venous line insertion; this

TABLE 19-6

POTENTIAL COMPLICATIONS OF ENTERAL FEEDING AND PREVENTIVE INTERVENTIONS

Complication	Possible Reasons	Suggested Treatment
GASTROINTESTINAL		
Diarrhea (6–8 loose, watery stools per day)	Osmotic overload	• Review medications for hypertonic elixirs, sorbitol-containing oral liquid medications, and antacids • Dilute elixirs and change to nonsorbitol-containing oral liquid medications • Provide continuous feeding rather than bolus • May require judicious use of antidiarrheal medication
	Lactose intolerance	• Change formula to lactose-free • Monitor lactose intake if also taking oral diet
	Contaminated formula	• Change bag and tubing every 24 hours
	Nervous tension	• Promote restful environment
	Bacterial overgrowth; oral medications	• Review oral medications, especially for antibiotics and H_2 receptor antagonists for possible side effects
	Low residue feedings	• Use of fiber-enriched formula may be helpful
Nausea	Volume overload	• Decrease total volume/flow rate
Vomiting	Obstruction, delayed gastric emptying, drug-induced	• Rule out obstruction • Evaluate medication profile
Cramping	Intolerance due to rapid administration	• Decrease total volume/flow rate
Delayed gastric emptying	Diabetes, gastric surgery, trauma, sepsis	• Check gastric residuals every 4 hours and return up to 200 mL into the stomach • If residuals > twice the hourly rate, hold tube feeding for 1 hour and recheck • May also consider small bowel feeding
Constipation	Insufficient fluid intake	• Increase fluid intake
	Decreased bowel mobility	• Increase physical activity as tolerated
	Low residue feedings	• Use of fiber-enriched formula may be helpful
METABOLIC		
Altered glucose, electrolyte, LFTs, and renal function tests	Excess or insufficient administration; prolonged administration of tube feeding containing low sodium; excessive free water	Monitor glucose, especially in diabetics and in elderly • Sudden glucose intolerance may indicate sepsis • Measure electrolytes and input and outputs • Weigh regularly • Reassess appropriateness of feeding formula • Reduce free water requirements
Dehydration	Insufficient free water	• Increase fluid intake • Administer additional free water each day based on body weight • Monitor input and output
	Diarrhea	• See gastrointestinal complications
	Hyperglycemia	• Monitor glucose, especially in elderly and diabetic patients
Overhydration	Excess fluid administration; renal failure	• Decrease volume of fluid administered • Monitor input and output • Reassess appropriateness of feeding formula; switch to a calorie dense formula

(continued)

TABLE 19-6

(continued)

Complication	Possible Reasons	Suggested Treatment
MECHANICAL		
Dislodged tube	Confused patient	• Restrain patient, bridle tube, or place permanent feeding tube
Obstructed tube	Inadequate flushing	• Flush tubes with 5–30 mL every 4 hours, after checking gastric residuals, after each medication, and before reconnecting
	Incompatible medications	• Administer medication individually; do not add medications to feeding bag
	Tablets	• Crush medications well or use liquid forms • Have patient take tablet orally, if possible • Suggested treatment: instill in tube a mixture of one crushed tablet of Viokase with one crushed tablet of sodium bicarbonate dissolved in 5 mL of warm water; clamp tube for 5–10 minutes, then gently flush tube
Aspiration	Rapid administration of feeding	• Decrease administration flow rate • Check residuals every 4 hours • Hold tube feeding if residuals > twice the hourly rate; in adults hold for a maximum amount of 150 mL
	Incorrect patient position	• Raise head of bed at least 30° during continuous feeding and 1 hour after and during bolus feedings
	Tube malposition	• Confirm placement with low upright chest x-ray • Be aware that a feeding tube can come into the pharynx with coughing or other activity; if in doubt, check by aspiration, insufflation, or x-ray

From Khalidi N, Btaiche IF, Kovacevich DS, eds. The *parenteral and enteral nutrition manual*, 8th ed. Ann Arbor, MI: The University of Michigan Hospitals and Health Centers, 2003, with permission.

usually occurs in the setting of obtaining subclavian access and less commonly with the internal jugular vein. This is due to transgression of the pleural space and puncture of lung apex (124). Another complication of malpositioning is the pinch-off syndrome (125,126). In this condition a catheter placed into the subclavian is pinched between the first rib and clavicle due to it being inserted too medially. It may manifest itself as catheter occlusion depending on body position or as the inability to aspirate blood. If clinically suspected, it should be confirmed by chest radiography and removed with insertion of a more laterally placed device. Failure to replace such a line may lead to catheter disruption and embolous of the distal end. The details of proper central venous access insertion are beyond the scope of this section, but Table 19-5 contains a list of the potential complications.

Infectious

Infectious complications associated with TPN range from 7% to 27% (127). If proper sterile and aseptic techniques are not used while obtaining central access, acute line infections can occur. It is vital to perform placement with gown, gloves, and mask. This is especially true when performing tunneled line access for prolonged nutritional support. Care must be taken when accessing these lines as well. Use of central venous

lines (CVLs) for multiple drugs and blood draws, as well as TPN, has been shown to increase infectious complications (128,129). In fact, when a formal protocol for catheter insertion and care is instituted, a dramatic reduction in catheter infections can be seen. In one prospective study the rate of catheter infections declined from 11.3/1,000 catheter days to 1.6/1,000 catheter days over the 4-year period in which these methods were used (130). It appears that multiple central venous lumens may predispose patients to a higher risk of infection, but this association is not proven (131). PICC lines did not have a significantly lower incidence of infection; however, PICC lines have been associated with higher rates of thrombophlebitis (132).

Catheter infections may occur from one of three sources: insertion site, the hub, or seeded via the bloodstream. The hub has often been considered the most common source of central line infections, and great care must be used to protect this site when gaining access to these lines (133). Infections secondary to bacteria from around the entrance site include skin contaminants such as staphylococci or streptococci (134). These organisms can colonize the fibrin sleeve that develops around the catheter tip and start proliferating. Other infections are a result of seeding from other foci, such as bacterial translocation, and may be Gram-negative or enteric in nature (135). One of the most common sources of CVL infections is from the hub itself. In one study, the majority of CVL infections was due to an infected hub, with negative skin cultures (133). Although tunneling of the catheter was initially thought to reduce the rate of CVL infections, this does not appear to reduce infection rates (136).

Fungal infections are dreaded problems, as they are associated with higher mortality, especially in immunocompromised adults (137). In general, a positive fungal culture will require line removal as they are otherwise recalcitrant to therapy (138). Attempts to clear a fungal infection are only occasionally successful and often result in death. For most bacterial infections, if the patient is clinically not in septic shock, treating through the line with antibiotics is appropriate (139,140). This applies to silastic catheters; temporary polyvinyl chloride lines, however, must be removed. In general, bacterial infections will clear from a silastic catheter 80% to 90% after the first infection and less frequently with subsequent infections (141). Lack of clearance requires removal of the catheter. Treatment failure is much more frequently seen in the presence of abscess, immunocompromised status, and the organisms *Pseudomonas aeruginosa* and *Candida albicans*. Data from a series of pediatric patients with short bowel syndrome suggest that these populations are at highest risk for catheter infections (142,143). Patients who manifest with a catheter infection along the subcutaneous track require catheter removal, as antibiotics are generally ineffective in these cases.

The usual workup of a patient on PN who develops an acute, unexplained fever should include a blood culture. The diagnosis of a catheter infection can be made on a single positive culture, and matching peripheral and central cultures are no longer necessary (144). Empiric antibiotic therapy may be used if the patient appears septic. Most fevers are due to some other source; however, if fever persists, a line change over a wire (for temporary lines) with culture of the catheter tip should be performed. Newer catheters that are impregnated with antibiotics may reduce the incidence of infections (145).

Thrombotic

Chronic indwelling central catheters are associated with development of thrombi. These may present acutely with ipsilateral limb swelling and inability to infuse solutions. Fortunately, they rarely lead to a pulmonary embolism. Treatment by catheter removal and replacement in an alternate site is usually sufficient. Unfortunately, in patients who have long-term dependence on PN, this may lead to loss of access sites and, with no access, loss of nutrition. Some advocate the use of anticoagulation therapy in low doses (e.g., warfarin or urokinase) to prevent these complications, with some success (146,147). The catheter itself may also become occluded due to thrombosis. Such problems may be treated with intracatheter lytic therapy. Catheters that have been in place for longer periods of time may also suffer occlusion from calcium deposits or lipid

deposits, which may respond to dilute infusion of hydrochloric acid or ethanol (148).

Enteral Nutrition

Similar to parenteral administration, enteral delivery of nutrition is associated with a wide number of complications (Table 19-6).

Mechanical

Enteral nutritional support is usually obtained by some form of access to the gastrointestinal tract. For relatively short-term support, temporary tubes via the nose or mouth are used. These tubes can irritate and damage the mucosa of the nasal passage, causing rhinorrhea, epistaxis, and a blockage of the sinuses, leading to sinusitis. A well-described source of fevers of unknown origin in a patient with a long-standing nasoenteric tube is a maxillary sinusitis. This is best treated by removal of the tube, nasal decongestant sprays, and occasional drainage of the sinus. Occasionally, if the feeding tube is not secured appropriately, the cartilage of the anterior nares may be damaged. Inflammation around the eustachian tubes in the nasopharynx may lead to otitis media. To avoid these problems, the newer enteral feeding tubes are smaller and less rigid; however, these smaller tubes may carry an increased risk of being positioned in the tracheobronchial tree, especially in an obtunded or sedated patient (149). In order to identify this problem before damage occurs, one must obtain radiologic confirmation of the tube position prior to initiating feeds. Auscultatory confirmation alone, though a helpful adjunct, is not adequate.

In certain patients with gastric emptying problems or reflux, postpyloric tubes are used. These are placed via the nares and have weighted tips that allow them to be carried past the pylorus into the duodenum with peristaltic action (150). These tubes must be marked after confirming placement as they may be dislodged. Occasional complications noted with these tubes have been damage to the esophagus or stomach with gastritis and perforations. These occur more often with the more rigid tubes. Acute gastric distention may also occur, especially in patients receiving nasogastric bolus feeding or with gastroparesis. This can lead to vomiting and aspiration (see the next section) as well as perforation of the stomach. Additionally, acute distention of the stomach may cause hypotension from a vagal response. To avoid this, the stomach should be aspirated periodically to ensure that it is emptying. Occasionally, one may require using medications to enhance gastric motility or a change to a postpyloric tube.

Long-term enteral access is usually obtained surgically. Access can be either to the stomach or to the jejunum, depending on the patient's specific needs. Technical complications from the operation may occur. These tubes may also be malpositioned and dislodged, requiring replacement. In the past 20 years most enteral feeding tubes have been placed using minimally invasive techniques [percutaneous endoscopic gastrostomy (PEG) or laparoscopic] (151,152). Early dislodgement of a PEG may cause the stomach to pull away from the abdominal wall and lead to peritonitis (152). After 3 months the stomach is generally well adhered to the abdominal wall. When these tubes become dislodged, especially in children, the access hole shrinks down fairly rapidly, often within a few hours. The caregivers and patients must be instructed to take immediate action to replace the tube if this occurs.

Infectious

Aspiration is the most feared complication from enteral nutrition (153). This can result from either a primary tube malposition in the tracheobronchial tree or from reflux/emesis and aspiration. Aspiration of stomach contents may be particularly harmful as the acid leads to severe pneumonitis and a capillary leak into the alveoli, causing the adult respiratory distress syndrome (ARDS). Although enteral feedings are clearly less expensive than TPN, complications are not dissimilar between the two groups. In a recent meta-analysis examining complications by these two routes, complication rates were the same in both groups (20). Although postpyloric feedings have been advocated in the early postoperative period (6), this may not have as great an advantage as initially perceived. In fact, the incidence of aspiration is not significantly different between patients receiving postgastric or intragastric feedings (154,155). In cases where gastric acid secretion has been controlled with histamine receptor blocking drugs or proton pump inhibitors, the stomach contents become colonized with Gram-negative bacteria and aspiration of this would potentially lead to a bacterial pneumonia. These complications significantly prolong hospital and intensive care stays, may lead to mortality, and certainly lead to increased health care costs. Thus, taking precautions to avoid them should be part of routine and protocol driven care.

As mentioned previously, sinusitis and otitis media can occur in patients with nasal tubes. Sinusitis is more common and is seen almost universally with these tubes. It may present as unexplained fevers in patients or with nasal discharge. Using smaller caliber tubes has decreased but not eliminated this problem. CT scan of the head is frequently used to make this diagnosis. Treatment consists of changing the tube to the other side, nasal spray, and antibiotics. If longer term nutritional support is deemed necessary, consideration should be given for surgical access.

SUMMARY

Advances in nutritional science over the last 4 decades have improved the care of countless patients. The management of nutrition can have complications, however, in the provision of too much or too little of any nutrient or supplement, as well as mechanical or infectious complications of the delivery mechanism. Knowledge of these complications is critical to proper planning and patient management.

REFERENCES

1. Kudsk K, Croce M, Favian T, et al. Enteral versus parenteral feeding. Effects on septic morbidity after blunt and penetrating abdominal trauma. *Ann Surg* 1992;215(5):503–511.
2. Group TVATPNCS. Perioperative total parenteral nutrition in surgical patients. *N Engl J Med* 1991;325(8):525–532.
3. Klein S, Kinney J, Jeejeebhoy K, et al. Nutrition support in clinical practice: review of published data and recommendations for future research directions. *J Parenter Enteral Nutr* 1997;21: 133–156.
4. Heyland DK, MacDonald S, Keefe L, et al. Total parenteral nutrition in the critically ill patient: a meta-analysis. *JAMA* 1998; 280(23):2013–2019.
5. Minard G, Kudsk KA. Postoperative nutrition in surgery for major trauma [Review] [28 refs]. *Curr Opin Clin Nutr Metab Care* 1998;1(1):35–39.
6. Boulanger BR, Brennemann FD, Rizoli SB, et al. Insertion of a transpyloric feeding tube during laparotomy in the critically injured: rationale and plea for routine use. *Injury* 1995;26(3): 177–180.
7. August D, Teitelbaum DH. Guidelines for the use of parenteral and enteral nutrition in adult and pediatric patients. *J Parenter Enteral Nutr* 2002;26(1):1SA–137SA.
8. Mullen JL, Buzby GP, Waldman MT. Prediction of operative morbidity and mortality by preoperative nutritional assessment. *Surg Forum* 1979;30:80.
9. Cameron JW, Rosenthal A, Olson AD. Malnutrition in hospitalized children with congenital heart disease. *Arch Pediatr Adolesc Med* 1995;149(10):1098–1102.
10. Merritt RJ, Blackburn GL. Nutritional assessment and metabolic response to illness of the hospitalized child. In: Suskind RM, ed. *Textbook of pediatric nutrition.* New York: Raven Press, 1981: 285–307.
11. Baker J, Detsky A, Wesson D. Nutritional assessment: a comparison of clinical judgment and objective measurements. *N Engl J Med* 1982;306:969–972.
12. Detsky JM, Baker JP, O'Rourke K, et al. Perioperative parenteral nutrition: a meta-analysis. *Ann Intern Med* 1987;107:195–203.
13. Bistrian BR. Nutritional assessment and therapy of protein-calorie malnutrition in the hospital. *J Am Diet Assoc* 1977;71(4): 393–397.
14. Bistrian BR. Interaction of nutrition and infection in the hospital setting. *Am J Clin Nutr* 1977;30(8):1228–1235.
15. Keenan RA, Moldawer LL, Yang RD, et al. An altered response by peripheral leukocytes to synthesize or release leukocyte endogenous mediator in critically ill, protein-malnourished patients. *J Lab Clin Med* 1982;100(6):844–857.
16. Reynolds JV, O'Farrelly C, Feighery C, et al. Impaired gut barrier function in malnourished patients. *Br J Surg* 1996;83(9): 1288–1291.
17. Wiren M, Soderholm JD, Lindgren J, et al. Effects of starvation and bowel resection on paracellular permeability in rat small-bowel mucosa *in vitro. Scand J Gastroenterol* 1999;34(2): 156–162.
18. Torosian MH. Perioperative nutrition support for patients undergoing gastrointestinal surgery: critical analysis and recommendations. *World J Surg* 1999;23(6):565–569.
19. Sandstrom R, Drott C, Hyltander A, et al. The effect of postoperative intravenous feeding (TPN) on outcome following major surgery evaluated in a randomized study. *Ann Surg* 1993;217(2): 185–195.
20. Braunschweig C, Levy P, Sheean P, et al. Enteral compared with parenteral nutrition: a meta-analysis. *Am J Clin Nutr* 2001; 74(4):534–542.

21. Bjerke HS, Shabot MM. Glucose intolerance in critically ill surgical patients: relationship to total parenteral nutrition and severity of illness. *Am Surg* 1992;58:728–731.

22. Wolfe RR, O'Donnell TF, Stone MD, et al. Investigation of factors determining the optimal glucose infusion rate in total parenteral nutrition. *Metabolism* 1980;29:892–900.

23. Burke JF, Wolfe RR, Mullany CJ, et al. Glucose requirements following burn injury. *Ann Surg* 1979;190:274–285.

24. Rosmarin DK, Wardlaw GM, Mirtallo J. Hyperglycemia associated with high, continuous infusion rates of total parenteral nutrition dextrose. *Nutr Clin Pract* 1996;11:151–156.

25. Hostetter MK. Perspectives in diabetes: handicaps to host defense: effects of hyperglycemia on C3 and *Candida albicans*. *Diabetes* 1990;39:271–275.

26. Van Oss CJ, Border JR. Influence of intermittent hyperglycemic glucose levels on the phagocytosis of microorganisms by human granulocytes *in vitro*. *Immunol Commun* 1978;7:669–676.

27. Kjersem H, Hilsted J, Madsbad S, et al. Polymorphonuclear leucocyte dysfunction during short term metabolic changes from normo- to hyperglycemia in type 1 (insulin dependent) diabetic patients. *Infection* 1988;16:215–221.

28. Rayfield EJ, Ault MJ, Keusch GT, et al. Infection and diabetes: the case for glucose control. *Am J Med* 1982;72:439–450.

29. Bagdade JD, Nielson KL, Bulger RJ. Reversible abnormalities in phagocytic function in poorly controlled diabetic patients. *Am J Med Sci* 1972;263:451–456.

30. Pomposelli JJ, Baxter JK, Babineau TJ, et al. Early postoperative glucose control predicts nosocomial infection rate in diabetic patients. *J Parenter Enteral Nutr* 1998;22:77–81.

31. Furnay AP, Zerr KJ, Grunkemeier GL, et al. Continuous intravenous insulin infusion reduces the incidence of deep sternal wound infection in diabetic patients after cardiac surgical procedures. *Ann Thorac Surg* 1999;67:352–362.

32. McCowen KC, Malhotra A, Bistrian BR. Stress-induced hyperglycemia. *Crit Care Clin* 2001;17:107–124.

33. Golden SH, Peart-Vigilance C, Kao WH, et al. Perioperative glycemic control and the risk of infectious complications in a cohort of adults with diabetes. *Diabetes Care* 1999;22:1408–1414.

34. van den Berghe G, Wouters PJ, Weekers F, et al. Intensive insulin therapy in critically ill patients. *N Engl J Med* 2001;345(19):1359–1367.

35. Van Den Berghe G, Wouters PJ, Bouillon R, et al. Outcome benefit of intensive insulin therapy in the critically ill: insulin dose versus glycemic control. *Crit Care Med* 2003;31:359–366.

36. Amato P, Keating KP, Quercia RA, et al. Formulaic methods of estimating caloric requirements in mechanically ventilated obese patients: a reappraisal. *Nutr Clin Pract* 1995;10:229.

37. Brown G, Dodek P. Intravenous insulin nomogram improves blood glucose control in the critically ill. *Crit Care Med* 2001;29:1714–1719.

38. Hunter DC, Jaksic T, Lewis D, et al. Resting energy expenditure in the critically ill: estimations versus measurements. *Br J Surg* 1988;75:875–878.

39. Herndon DN, Hart DW, Wolf SE, et al. Reversal of catabolism by β-blockade after severe burns. *N Engl J Med* 2001;345:1223–1229.

40. Chiolero RL, Breitenstein E, Thorin D, et al. Effects of propranolol on resting metabolic rate after severe head injury. *Crit Care Med* 1989;17:328–334.

41. Jeejeebhoy KN, Anderson GH, Nakhooda AF, et al. Metabolic studies in total parenteral nutrition with lipid in man. Comparison with glucose. *J Clin Invest* 1976;57:125–136.

42. Cameron JL, Capuzzi DM, Zuidema GD, et al. Acute pancreatitis with hyperlipemia: evidence of persistence defect in lipid metabolism. *Am J Med* 1974;56:482–487.

43. Aarsland A, Chinkes D, Wolfe RR. Hepatic and whole-body fat synthesis in humans during carbohydrate overfeeding. *Am J Clin Nutr* 1997;65:1774–1782.

44. Samra JS, Summers LK, Frayn KN. Sepsis and fat metabolism. *Br J Surg* 1996;83:1186–1196.

45. Garber AJ, Vinik A, Creeps SR. Detection and management of lipid disorders in diabetic patients. *Diabetes Care* 1992;15:1068–1073.

46. Muscaritoli M, Cangiano C, Cascino A, et al. Exogenous lipid clearance in compensated liver cirrhosis. *J Parenter Enteral Nutr* 1986;10:599–603.

47. Attman PO, Samuellson O, Alaupovic P. Diagnosis and classification of dyslipidemia in renal disease. *Blood Purif* 1996;14:49–57.

48. Carmen JL. Lipid abnormalities and acute pancreatitis. *Hosp Pract* 1977;12:95–101.

49. Eddleston JM, Shelly MP. The effect on serum lipid concentrations of a prolonged infusion of propofol. Hypertriglyceridaemia associated with propofol administration. *Intensive Care Med* 1991;17:424–426.

50. Tsuguhiko T, Mashima Y, Yamamori H, et al. Intravenous intralipid 10% vs 20% hyperlipidemia, and increase in lipoprotein X in humans. *Nutrition* 1992;8:155–160.

51. Messing B, Peynet J, Poupon J, et al. Effect of fat-emulsion phospholipids on serum lipoprotein profile during 1 mo of cyclic total parenteral nutrition. *Am J Clin Nutr* 1990;52:1094–1100.

52. Carpentier YA. Intravascular metabolism of fat emulsions. *Clin Nutr* 1989;8:115–125.

53. Roulet M, Wiesel PH, Pilet M, et al. Effects of intravenously infused egg phospholipids on lipid and lipoprotein metabolism in postoperative trauma. *J Parenter Enteral Nutr* 1993;17:107–112.

54. Haumont D, Richelle M, Deckelbaum RJ, et al. Effect of liposomal content of lipid emulsions on plasma lipid concentrations in low birth weight infants receiving parenteral nutrition. *J Pediatr* 1992;121:759–763.

55. Kalfarentzos F, Kokkinis K, Leukaditi K, et al. Comparison between two fat emulsions: intralipid 30 percent vs intralipid 10 percent in critically ill patients. *Clin Nutr* 1998;17:31–34.

56. Nordenstrom J, Thorne A. Comparative studies on a new concentrated fat emulsion: intralipid 30% vs. 20%. *Clin Nutr* 1993;12:160–167.

57. Druml W, Fischer M, Ratheiser K, et al. Use of intravenous lipids in critically ill patients with sepsis without and with hepatic failure. *J Parenter Enteral Nutr* 1998;22:217–223.

58. Abbott WC, Grakauskas AM, Bistrian BR, et al. Metabolic and respiratory effects of continuous and discontinuous lipid infusions. Occurrence in excess of resting energy expenditure. *Arch Surg* 1984;119:1367–1371.

59. Ireton-Jones CS, Turner WWJ. The use of respiratory quotient to determine the efficacy of nutrition support regimens. *J Am Diet Assoc* 1987;87:180–183.

60. Elia M, Livesey G. Theory and validity of indirect calorimetry during net lipid synthesis. *Am J Clin Nutr* 1988;47:591–607.

61. Guenst JM, Nelson LD. Predictors of total parenteral nutrition-induced lipogenesis. *Chest* 1994;105:553–559.

62. Covelli HD, Black JW, Olsen MS, et al. Respiratory failure precipitated by high carbohydrate loads. *Ann Intern Med* 1981;95:579–581.

63. Aguilaniu B, Goldstein-Shapses S, Pajon A, et al. Muscle protein degradation in severely malnourished patients with COPD subject to short-term TPN. *J Parenter Enteral Nutr* 1992;16:248–254.

64. Rodriguez JL, Askanazi J, Weissman C, et al. Ventilatory and metabolic effects of glucose infusions. *Chest* 1985;88:512–518.

65. Solomon SM, Kirby DF. The refeeding syndrome: a review. *J Parenter Enteral Nutr* 1990;14:90–97.

66. Brooks MJ, Melnik G. The refeeding syndrome: an approach to understanding its complications and preventing its occurrence. *Pharmacotherapy* 1995;15:713–726.

67. Nesbakken R, Reinlie S. Magnesium and phosphorus: the electrolytes of energy metabolism. *Acta Anaesthesiol Scand* 1985;29:60–64.

68. O'Connor LR, Wheeler WS, Bethune JE. Effect of hypophosphatemia on myocardial performance in man. *N Engl J Med* 1977;297:901–903.

69. Lichtman MA, Miller DR, Cohen J, et al. Reduced red cell glycolysis, 2, 3 diphosphoglycerate and adenosine triphosphate concentration, and increased hemoglobin-oxygen affinity caused by hypophosphatemia. *Ann Intern Med* 1971;74:562–568.

70. Luckey A, Parsa C. Fluid and electrolytes in the aged. *Arch Surg* 2003;138:1055–1060.

71. Beaty L, Pemberton D. *Treatment of water, electrolyte, and acid-base disorders in the surgical patient.* New York: McGraw-Hill, 1994.

72. Baughman FA, Papp JP. Wernike's encephalopathy with intravenous hyperalimentation: remarks on similarities between Wernike's encephalopathy and the phosphate depletion syndrome. *Mt Sinai J Med* 1976;43:48–52.

73. Kitamura K, Takahashi T, Tanaka H, et al. Two cases of thiamine deficiency-induced lactic acidosis during total parenteral nutrition. *Tohoku J Exp Med* 1993;171:129–133.

74. Weinsier RL, Krumdieck CL. Death resulting from overzealous total parenteral nutrition: the refeeding syndrome revisited. *Am J Clin Nutr* 1980;34:393–399.

75. Silvis SE, Paragas PD. Paresthesias, weakness, seizures, and hypophosphatemia in patients receiving hyperalimentation. *Gastroenterology* 1972;62:513–520.

76. Eliahou HE, Feng PH, Weinberg U, et al. Acetate and bicarbonate in the correction of uraemic acidosis. *Br Med J* 1970;4:399–401.

77. Richards CE, Drayton M, Jenkins H, et al. Effect of different chloride infusion rates on plasma base excess during neonatal parenteral nutrition. *Acta Paediatrica* 1993;82:678–682.

78. Sheldon GF, Petersen SR, Snaders R. Hepatic dysfunction during hyperalimentation. *Arch Surg* 1978;113(4):504–508.

79. Zamir O, Nussbaum MS, Bhadra S, et al. Effect of enteral feeding on hepatic steatosis induced by total parenteral nutrition. *J Parenter Enteral Nutr* 1994;18:20–25.

80. Powell EE, Cooksley WGE, Hanson R, et al. The natural history of nonalcoholic steatohepatitis: a follow-up study of forty-two patients for up to 21 years. *Hepatology* 1990;11:74–80.

81. Sax HC, Bower RH. Hepatic complications of total parenteral nutrition. *J Parenter Enteral Nutr* 1988;12(6):615–618.

82. Lowry SF, Brennan MF. Abnormal liver function during parenteral nutrition: relation to infusion excess. *J Surg Res* 1979; 26:300–307.

83. Nussbaum MS, Fischer JE. Pathogenesis of hepatic steatosis during total parenteral nutrition. *Surg Annu* 1991;23(Pt 2):1–11.

84. Palombo JD, Schnure F, Bistrian BR. et al. Improvement of liver function tests by administration of L-carnitine to a carnitine-deficient patient receiving home parenteral nutrition: a case report. *J Parenter Enteral Nutr* 1987;11:88–92.

85. Richardson TJ, Sgoutas D. Essential fatty acid deficiency in four adult patients during total parenteral nutrition. *Am J Clin Nutr* 1975;28:258–263.

86. Campos AC, Oler A, Meguid MM, et al. Liver biochemical and histological changes with graded amounts of total parenteral nutrition. *Arch Surg* 1990;125:447–450.

87. Zagara G, Locati L. Role of total parenteral nutrition in determining liver insufficiency in patients with cranial injuries. Glucose vs glucose + lipids. *Minerva Anestesiol* 1989;55(12):509–512.

88. Reif S, Tano M, Oliverio R, et al. Total parenteral nutrition-induced steatosis: reversal by parenteral lipid infusions. *J Parenter Enteral Nutr* 1991;15:102–104.

89. Heyman MB, Storch S, Ament ME. The fat overload syndrome. Report of a case and literature review. *Am J Dis Child* 1981;135: 628–630.

90. Tao RC, Peck GK, Yoshimura NN. Effect of carnitine on liver fat and nitrogen balance in intravenously fed growing rats. *J Nutr* 1981;111:171–177.

91. Yao ZM, Vance DE. The active synthesis of phosphatidylcholine is required for very low density lipoprotein secretion from rat hepatocytes. *J Biol Chem* 1988;263:2998–3004.

92. Buchman AL. Choline deficiency during parenteral nutrition in humans. *Nutr Clin Pract* 2003;18:353–358.

93. Buchman AL, Dubin M, Jenden D, et al. Lecithin increases plasma free choline and decreases hepatic steatosis in long-term parenteral nutrition patients. *Gastroenterology* 1992;102(4 pt 1): 1363–1370.

94. Buchman AL, Ament M, Sohel M, et al. Choline deficiency causes reversible hepatic abnormalities in patients receiving parenteral nutrition: proof of a human choline requirement: a placebo-controlled trial. *J Parenter Enteral Nutr* 2001;25:260–268.

95. Roslyn JJ, DenBesten L, Pitt HA, et al. Resident research award. Effects of cholecystokinin on gallbladder stasis and cholesterol gallstone formation. *J Surg Res* 1981;30(3):200–204.

96. Jawaheer G, Pierro A, Lloyd DA, et al. Gall bladder contractility in neonates: effects of parenteral and enteral feeding [published erratum appears in *Arch Dis Child Fetal Neonatal Ed* 1995 Nov;73(3):F198]. *Arch Dis Child Fetal Neonatal Ed* 1995;72(3): F200–F202.

97. Gurll NJ, Meyer PD, DenBesten L. The effect of cholesterol crystals on gallbladder function in cholelithiasis. *Surg Forum* 1977;28:412–413.

98. Allen B, Bernhoft R, Blanckaert N, et al. Sludge is calcium bilirubinate associated with bile stasis. *Am J Surg* 1981;141:51–56.

99. Cooper A, Ross AJ, O'Neill JAJ, et al. Resolution of intractable cholestasis associated with total parenteral nutrition following biliary irrigation. *J Pediatr Surg* 1985;20(6):772–774.

100. Rintala R, Lindahl H, Pohjavuori M, et al. Surgical treatment of intractable cholestasis associated with total parenteral nutrition in premature infants. *J Pediatr Surg* 1993;28(5):716–719.

101. Caniano DA, Starr J, Ginn-Pease ME. Extensive short-bowel syndrome in neonates: outcome in the 1980s. *Surgery* 1989;105: 119–124.

102. Hofmann AF. Defective biliary secretion during total parenteral nutrition: probable mechanisms and possible solutions. *J Pediatr Gastroenterol Nutr* 1995;20(4):376–390.

103. Teitelbaum D, Han-Markey T, Drongowski R, et al. Use of cholecystokinin to prevent the development of parenteral nutrition-associated cholestasis. *J Paren Enter Nutr* 1997;21(2):100–103.

104. Sitzman JV, Pitt HA, Steinborn PA, et al. Cholecystokinin prevents parenteral nutrition induced biliary sludge in humans. *Surg Gynecol Obstet* 1990;170(1):25–31.

105. Tsai S, Strouse P, Drongowski R, et al. Use of Cholecystokinin-octapeptide to prevent TPN-associated gallstone disease. *J Pediatr Surg* 2005;40:263–267.

106. Beath SV, Davies P, Papadopoulou A, et al. Parenteral nutrition-related cholestasis in postsurgical neonates: multivariate analysis of risk factors. *J Pediatr Surg* 1996;31(4):604–606.

107. Teitelbaum DH, Tracy T. Parenteral nutrition-associated cholestasis. *Semin Pediatr Surg* 2001;10(2):72–80.

108. Teitelbaum DH. Parenteral nutrition-associated cholestasis. *Curr Opin Pediatr* 1997;9:270–275.

109. Btaiche IF, Khalidi N. Parenteral nutrition-associated liver complications in children. *Pharmacotherapy* 2002;22:188–211.

110. Cavicchi M, Beau P, Crenn P, et al. Prevalence of liver disease and contributing factors in patients receiving home parenteral nutrition for permanent intestinal failure. *Ann Intern Med* 2000; 132(7):525–532.

111. Yang H, Finaly R, Teitelbaum DH. Alteration in epithelial permeability and ion transport in a mouse model of total parenteral nutrition. *Crit Care Med* 2003;31(4):1118–1125.

112. Kiristioglu I, Antony P, Fan Y, et al. Total parenteral nutrition-associated changes in mouse intestinal intraepithelial lymphocytes. *Dig Dis Sci* 2002;47(5):1147–1157.

113. Iyer K, Spitz L, Clayton P. New insight into mechanisms of parenteral nutrition–associated cholestasis: role of plant sterols. *J Pediatr Surg* 1998;33(1):1–6.

114. Tazuke Y, Drongowski RA, Btaiche I, et al. Effects of lipid administration on liver apoptotic signals in a mouse model of total parenteral nutrition (TPN). *Pediatr Surg Int* 2004;20(4):224–228.

115. Beale EF, Nelson RM, Bucciarelli RL, et al. Intrahepatic cholestasis associated with parenteral nutrition in premature infants. *Pediatrics* 1979;64(3):342–347.

116. Vileisis RA, Inwood RJ, Hunt CE. Prospective controlled study of parenteral nutrition-associated cholestatic jaundice: effect of protein intake. *J Pediatr* 1980;96(5):893–897.

117. Heubi JE, Wiechmann DA, Creutzinger V, et al. Tauroursodeoxycholic acid (TUDCA) in the prevention of total parenteral nutrition-associated liver disease. [see comment]. *J Pediatr* 2002;141(2):237–242.

118. Teitelbaum DH, Han-Markey T, Drongowski RA, et al. Use of cholecystokinin to prevent the development of parenteral nutrition-associated cholestasis. *J Parenter Enteral Nutr* 1997;21(2): 100–103.

119. Teitelbaum DH, Tracy TJ, Aouthmany M, et al. Use of cholecystokinin-octapeptide for the prevention of parenteral nutrition-associated cholestasis. *Pediatrics* 2005 (*in press*).

120. Capron JP, Gineston JL, Herve MA, et al. Metronidazole in prevention of cholestasis associated with total parenteral nutrition. *Lancet* 1983;1(8322):446–447.

121. Teitelbaum D, Drongowski R, Spivak D. Rapid development of hyperbilirubinemia in infants with the short bowel syndrome as

a correlate to mortality: possible indication for early small bowel transplantation. *Trans Proc* 1996;28(5):2677–2678.

122. Correia M, Guimaraes J, de Mattos L, et al. Peripheral parenteral nutrition: an option for patients with an indication for short-term parenteral nutrition. *Nutr Hosp* 2004;19(1):14–18.

123. Foley MJ. Radiologic placement of long-term central venous peripheral access system ports (PAS Port): results in 150 patients. *J Vasc Interv Radiol* 1995;6(2):255–262.

124. Domino K, Bowdle T, Posner K. Injuries and liability related to central vascular catheters: a closed claims analysis. *Anesthesiology* 2004;100(6):1411–1418.

125. Andris DA, Krzywda EA, Schulte W, et al. Pinch-off syndrome: a rare etiology for central venous catheter occlusion. *J Parenter Enteral Nutr* 1994;18(6):531–533.

126. Hinke DH, Zandt-Stastny DA, Goodman LR, et al. Pinch-off syndrome: a complication of implantable subclavian venous access devices. *Radiology* 1990;177(2):353–356.

127. Lane R, Matthay M. Central line infections. *Curr Opin Crit Care* 2002;8:441–448.

128. Faubion WC, Wesley JR, Khalidi N, et al. Total parenteral nutrition catheter sepsis: impact of the team approach. *J Parenter Enteral Nutr* 1986;10(6):642–645.

129. Reed CR, Sessler CN, Glauser FL, et al. Central venous catheter infections: concepts and controversies. *Intensive Care Med* 1995; 21(2):177–183.

130. Berenholtz SM, Pronovost PJ, Lipsett PA, et al. Eliminating catheter-related bloodstream infections in the intensive care unit. *Crit Care Med* 2004;32(10):2014–2020.

131. Dezfulian C, Lavelle J, Nallamothu B, et al. Rates of infection for single-lumen versus multilumen central venous catheters: a meta-analysis. *Crit Care Med* 2003;31(9):2385–2390.

132. Cowl C, Weinstock J, Al-Jurf A. Complications and cost associated with parenteral nutrition delivered to hospitalized patients through either subclavian or peripherally-inserted central catheters. *Clin Nutr* 2000;19:237–243.

133. Sitges-Serra A, Puig P, Linares J, et al. Hub colonization as the initial step in an outbreak of catheter-related sepsis due to coagulase negative staphylococci during parenteral nutrition. *J Parenter Enteral Nutr* 1984;8(6):668–672.

134. King DR, Komer M, Hoffman J, et al. Broviac catheter sepsis: the natural history of an iatrogenic infection. *J Pediatr Surg* 1985; 20(6):728–733.

135. Kurkchubasche AG, Smith SD, Rowe MI. Catheter sepsis in short-bowel syndrome. *Arch Surg* 1992;127:21–25.

136. Sitges-Serra A, Linares J. Tunnels do not protect against venous-catheter-related sepsis [letter]. *Lancet* 1984;1(8374): 459–460.

137. Lecciones JA, Lee JW, Navano EE, et al. Vascular catheter associated fungemia: analysis of 155 episodes. *Clin Infect Dis* 1992;14:875.

138. Widmer AF. Management of catheter-related bacteremia and fungemia in patients on total parenteral nutrition. *Nutrition* 1997;13(Suppl. 4):18S–25S.

139. Mermel LA. Prevention of catheter-related infections. *Ann Intern Med* 2000;132:391–402.

140. O'Grady NP, Alexander M, Dellinger EP, et al. Guidelines for the prevention of intravascular catheter-related infections. Centers for Disease Control and Prevention. *Morb Mortal Wkly Rep* 2002; 51(RR-10):1–29.

141. Krzywda EA, Andris DA, Edmiston CE. Catheter infections: diagnosis, etiology, treatment and prevention. *Nutr Clin Practice* 1999;14:178.

142. Johnson PR, Decker MD, Edwards KM, et al. Frequency of broviac catheter infections in pediatric oncology patients. *J Infect Dis* 1986;154(4):570–578.

143. Coran AG, Spivak D, Teitelbaum DH. An analysis of the morbidity and mortality of short-bowel syndrome in the pediatric age group. *Eur J Pediatr Surg* 1999;9(4):228–230.

144. Hospital Infection Control Advisory Committee CfDCaP. Guidelines for prevention of intravascular-device related infections. *Infect Control Hosp Epidemiol* 1996;17:438.

145. Attar A, Messing B. Evidence-based prevention of catheter infection during parenteral nutrition. [see comment]. *Curr Opin Clin Nutr Metab Care* 2001;4(3):211–218.

146. Andrew M, Marzinotto V, Pencharz P, et al. A cross-sectional study of catheter-related thrombosis in children receiving total parenteral nutrition at home. *J Pediatr* 1995;126(3):358–363.

147. Klerk C, Smorenburg S, Buller H. Thrombosis prophylaxis in patient populations with a central venous catheter: a systematic review. *Arch Intern Med* 2003;163(16):1913–1921.

148. Werlin SL, Lausten T, Jessen S, et al. Treatment of central venous catheter occlusions with ethanol and hydrochloric acid. *J Parenter Enteral Nutr* 1995;19(5):416–418.

149. Dwolatzky T, Berezovski S, Friedmann R. A prospective comparison of the use of nasogastric and percutaneous endoscopic gastrostomy tubes for long-term enteral feeding in older people. *Clin Nutr* 2001;20(6):535–540.

150. Boulton-Jones J, Lewis J, Jobling J, et al. Experience of post-pyloric feeding in seriously ill patients in clinical practice. *Clin Nutr* 2004;23:35–41.

151. Gauderer ML, Ponsky JL, Izant RJ Jr. Gastrostomy without laparotomy: a percutaneous endoscopic technique. *J. Pediatr Surg* 1980;15:872–875.

152. Ganga UR, Ryan JJ, Schafer LW. Indications, complications, and long-term results of percutaneous endoscopic gastrostomy: a retrospective study. *S D J Med* 1994;47(5):149–152.

153. Metheny NA, Eisenberg P, Spies M. Aspiration pneumonia in patients fed through nasoenteral tubes. *Heart Lung* 1986;15(3): 256–261.

154. Strong R, Condon S, Soling M, et al. Equal aspiration rates from postpylorus and intragastric-placed small bore nasoenteric feeding tubes: a randomized prospective study. *J Paren Enter Nutr* 1992;16:59–63.

155. Spain DA, DeWeese RC, Reynolds MA, et al. Transpyloric passage of feeding tubes in patients with head injuries does not decrease complications. *J Trauma* 1995;39(6):1100–1102.

Complications of Immunosuppression

Niraj M. Desai   Matthew J. Koch

20

■■■ **INTRODUCTION 212**

■■■ **IMMUNOSUPPRESSIVE AGENTS 212**
Corticosteroids 213
Calcineurin Inhibitors 214
Mammalian Target of Rapamycin Inhibitors 215
Antiproliferative Agents 216
Antibodies 217
Medications in Development 217

■■■ **COMMON PROBLEMS ASSOCIATED WITH IMMUNOSUPPRESSION 218**
Infection 218
Malignancy 219
Impaired Wound Healing 220
Cardiovascular Disease 220
Gastrointestinal Disease 220
Chronic Renal Insufficiency and Failure 221
Endocrine Abnormalities 222

■■■ **SUMMARY 222**

■■■ **REFERENCES 222**

INTRODUCTION

Modern advances in medical therapy have resulted in a large number of individuals with a compromised immune system. The cause of immunodeficiency may be intentional (immunosuppression administration to patients with organ transplants or with autoimmune disease), the unintended consequence of a particular therapy (chemotherapy for cancer), or the result of a disease state (large burns or the acquired immunodeficiency syndrome). As a result of the increasing number of patients receiving immunosuppressive agents, the diagnosis, treatment, and prevention of immunosuppression-related complications has become commonplace. This chapter first reviews immunosuppressive medications and their specific side effects. Complications that commonly occur during immunosuppression are then reviewed from the perspective of the consulting surgeon. A thorough understanding of these complications is essential when providing care to these complex patients.

IMMUNOSUPPRESSIVE AGENTS

Over the past five decades, several classes of immunosuppressive agents have been discovered, with many new compounds becoming part of routine clinical use. These medications are primarily used for the prevention and treatment of rejection and have allowed for an impressive improvement in the survival of solid organ transplants. In addition, immunosuppressive medications have been increasingly used for the treatment of autoimmune diseases. Immunosuppressive agents are used for short time periods in intense doses as induction therapy, for the treatment of rejection, or for the treatment of an autoimmune flare. They are also used chronically in lower doses as maintenance therapy. The available medications can be classified into five major categories: corticosteroids, calcineurin

Niraj M. Desai, Matthew J. Koch: Washington University School of Medicine, St. Louis, MO 63110 inhibitors, mammalian target of rapamycin (mTOR) inhibitors, antiproliferative agents, and antibodies. The immunosuppressive medications and their common side effects are summarized in Table 20-1 (1). The activation of T cells and the inhibitory sites of action for commonly used immunosuppressive agents are shown in Figure 20-1 (2).

Corticosteroids

Corticosteroids were first used clinically in 1949 and since that time have been used for a variety of indications, including allergies, autoimmune diseases, arthritis, asthma, cancer therapies, neurosurgery, organ transplantation, and many others. Steroids are the most commonly prescribed immunosuppressive medication due to their efficacy in a variety of diseases, long experience with their use, and low cost. They are usually used in high doses when therapy is initiated or for the rapid treatment of immune activation (asthma exacerbation, organ rejection). Dosing is often then tapered to a maintenance dose or completely discontinued. Dexamethasone, prednisone,

prednisolone, and methylprednisolone are examples of commonly used steroids.

Corticosteroids have a variety of effects on the immune system. Most importantly, they inhibit the production of several cytokines by T cells and antigen presenting cells (APCs), including IL-1, IL-2, IL-3, IL-6, tumor necrosis factor-α, and γ interferon. Steroids initially enter the cell and bind to intracellular receptors. The steroid-receptor complex then enters the nucleus and binds to sequences of DNA on the promoter region of cytokine genes called glucocorticoid response elements, blocking the transcription of those cytokines. In addition, steroids inhibit the action of nuclear factor-κB, another key element in the cytokine response (3,4). Given the effect on multiple cytokines, steroids inhibit T-cell activation at several stages. Additional immunosuppressive effects of steroids include inhibition of monocyte migration and suppression of chemokine production.

Given the ubiquitous nature of glucocorticoid receptors in most human cells, corticosteroids are associated with adverse effects on a variety of tissues. Transient side effects,

TABLE 20-1

SUMMARY OF IMMUNOSUPPRESSIVE MEDICATION SIDE EFFECTS

Medication	Side Effects
Corticosteroids	Hypertension, glucose intolerance, hyperlipidemia, fluid retention, protein wasting, adipose weight gain, cataracts, glaucoma, peptic ulcers, pancreatitis, osteoporosis, osteonecrosis, mood disturbances, psychosis, acne, delayed wound healing
Cyclosporine	Hypertension, glucose intolerance, hyperlipidemia, nephrotoxicity, electrolyte disturbances, neurotoxicity, gingival hyperplasia, hirsutism
Tacrolimus	Hypertension, glucose intolerance, hyperlipidemia, nephrotoxicity, electrolyte disturbances, neurotoxicity, alopecia
Sirolimus	Hyperlipidemia, anemia, leukopenia, thrombocytopenia, mouth sores, gastrointestinal disturbances, lymphedema, impaired wound healing, pneumonitis
Azathioprine	Leukopenia, thrombocytopenia, gastrointestinal disturbances, pancreatitis
Mycophenolate mofetil/ mycophenolic acid	Leukopenia, thrombocytopenia, gastrointestinal disturbances
Antithymocyte globulin	Fever, chills, rash, leukopenia, thrombocytopenia, allergic reactions
Intravenous immune globulin	Fever, chills, rash, aseptic meningitis, acute renal dysfunction, hypersensitivity reaction
Muromonab-CD3 (OKT3)	Fever, chills, rigors, headache, myalgia, hypertension, flash pulmonary edema, aseptic meningitis, hypersensitivity reaction
Basiliximab/daclizumab	Hypersensitivity reaction (rare)
Alemtuzumab	Fever, rash, nausea, shortness of breath, chest discomfort, hypersensitivity reaction
Rituximab	Fever, rash, nausea, shortness of breath, chest discomfort, hypersensitivity reaction

From Hardinger KL, Koch MJ, Brennan DC. Current and future immunosuppressive strategies in renal transplantation. *Pharmacotherapy* 2004; 24:1159–1176, with permission.

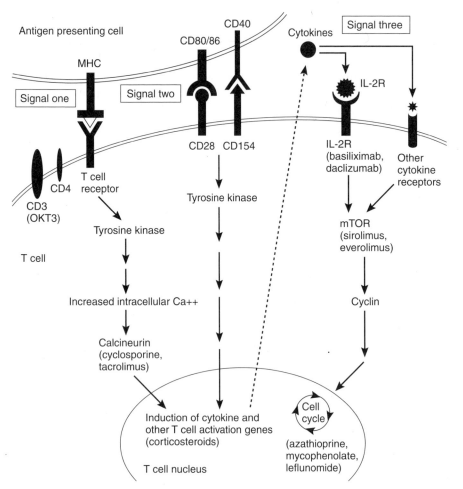

Figure 20-1 Signaling pathways involved in T cell activation. Sites of inhibition by commonly used immunosuppressive medications are indicated in parentheses. (From Helderman JH, Goral S. Transplantation immunobiology. In: Danovitch GM, ed. *Handbook of kidney transplantation*, 3rd ed. Philadelphia, PA: Lippincott Williams & Wilkins;2001: 17–38, with permission.)

such as hypertension and diabetes mellitus, can occur with short-term use of steroids. However, severe complications occur with long-term use, even when steroids are taken at low maintenance doses. The metabolic side effects of steroids are hypertension, diabetes, hyperlipidemia, sodium and fluid retention, protein wasting, and adipose weight gain. Gastrointestinal (GI) side effects include gastritis, duodenal ulcers, and pancreatitis. The ocular complications are glaucoma and cataracts. Osteoporosis often affects vertebral bodies of the spine, while osteonecrosis often affects the femoral head. Psychiatric effects such as mood disturbances and psychosis, cosmetic side effects including acne and the development of Cushingoid features, and delayed wound healing are all observed with steroids (1,3–5). This broad range of side effects associated with chronic steroid use, along with the development of more specific immunosuppressive medications, has led efforts to minimize or completely avoid the use of steroids. For example, clinical trials of kidney transplantation have been performed with only short courses of steroids with promising results so far (6,7). However, for the majority of patients with organ transplants and with autoimmune disease, steroids remain a cornerstone of immunosuppressive therapy.

Calcineurin Inhibitors

The currently available calcineurin inhibitors are cyclosporine and tacrolimus (formerly known as FK-506). Both agents inhibit the activation and proliferation of T lymphocytes by suppressing the production of the cytokines interleukin-2 (IL-2), IL-4, interferon-γ, and tumor necrosis factor-α by T lymphocytes. The agents are biochemically distinct—cyclosporine is an 11 amino acid cyclic polypeptide produced by the fungal species *Tolypocladium inflatum* Gams, and tacrolimus is a macrolide antibiotic produced by the fungus *Streptomyces tsukubaenis*. Both agents have distinct cytoplasmic binding proteins (immunophilins), with cyclosporine binding to cyclophilin and tacrolimus binding to FKBP-12. However, in both cases the drug-immunophilin complex binds calcineurin and thus inhibits its ability to upregulate the activity of certain nuclear regulatory proteins (1,4). Both agents have a relatively narrow therapeutic window and close monitoring of drug levels is necessary to achieve a balance between efficacy and toxicity.

The original oil-based oral cyclosporine formulation depends on bile for absorption and has erratic absorption patterns. In contrast, cyclosporine modified (formerly known as cyclosporine microemulsion) depends less on bile for absorption and exhibits increased bioavailability and more consistent absorption. The two formulas are not considered interchangeable. Appropriate drug levels can sometimes be maintained with a lower relative dose of cyclosporine modified, and monitoring of levels is mandatory if the patient is changed to an alternate formulation. Intravenous cyclosporine is also used in some settings; however, it is usually administered as a 24-hour continuous infusion using approximately one-third of the total oral dose. Tacrolimus does not depend upon bile for absorption and has an excellent oral bioavailability. Owing to its ready absorption, tacrolimus very rarely needs to be given intravenously, with therapeutic levels achievable in almost any patient, even after major abdominal surgery (1). Rather than administering intravenous cyclosporine, it is preferable to convert a patient from cyclosporine to oral tacrolimus if absorption of drug is a concern in the postoperative setting. In contrast to cyclosporine, where administration with food tends to increase bioavailability, administration of tacrolimus with food can decrease the rate and extent of absorption.

Oral cyclosporine and tacrolimus both have approximately an 8-hour half-life and are usually given twice daily. Both agents are metabolized in the liver by the cytochrome P450 IIIA (CYP3A) pathway and are excreted in the bile. Potential drug interactions are important to recognize, and vigilance in monitoring drug levels is required when any agent is added or adjusted that induces or inhibits CYP3A levels (Table 20-2) (1). There is only minimal renal excretion of either drug, and neither is significantly affected by dialysis. Cyclosporine and tacrolimus levels have traditionally been measured as morning trough levels; however, an increasing trend has been to measure the cyclosporine level 2 hours after oral dosing (C_2 level). The appropriate therapeutic levels depend on the type of organ transplant, the length of time since transplantation, and other factors (8).

Calcineurin inhibitors (CNIs) are associated with numerous toxicities. Nephrotoxicity is a critical side effect that is dose dependent and the result of vasoconstriction of the afferent arteriole, resulting in a "prerenal" type of renal dysfunction (4,9,10). Concomitant administration of CNIs with other nephrotoxic medications, such as aminoglycosides, amphotericin B deoxycholate, and nonsteroidal anti-inflammatory drugs, should be avoided. Intravenous contrast should be used cautiously, taking specific measures to protect the kidneys such as hydration, administration of N-acetylcysteine or sodium bicarbonate, and possible adjustment of the CNI dose. Another major side effect of CNIs is glucose intolerance that often results in the development of frank diabetes. The incidence of post-transplant diabetes is higher in those receiving tacrolimus compared to those on cyclosporine (11). The development of diabetes may be mild and require only diet control, or it may be more severe and require insulin or an oral agent to treat.

TABLE 20-2

MEDICATION INTERACTIONS FOR CYTOCHROME P450 IIIA SUBSTRATES— CYCLOSPORINE, TACROLIMUS, AND SIROLIMUS

Increased Immunosuppressant Levels	Decreased Immunosuppressant Levels
Ketoconazole	Rifampin
Fluconazole	Rifabutin
Itraconazole	Phenytoin
Voriconazole	Phenobarbital
Erythromycin	Carbamazepine
Clarithromycin	St. John's wort
Diltiazem	Isoniazid
Verapamil	
Cimetidine	
Danazol	
Grapefruit juice	
Nefazodone	
Fluvoxamine	
Amiodarone	

From Hardinger KL, Koch MJ, Brennan DC. Current and future immunosuppressive strategies in renal transplantation. *Pharmacotherapy* 2004; 24:1159–1176, with permission.

Other common side effects of both agents include hypertension, electrolyte abnormalities, hyperlipidemia, and neurotoxicity. Hypertension, although seen with both CNIs, is often more severe with cyclosporine. This side effect is due to both renal and peripheral vasoconstriction. Electrolyte abnormalities on CNIs include hyperkalemia due to impaired renal excretion of potassium and hypomagnesemia due to wasting of magnesium in the urine (4). Hyperlipidemia is more often seen with cyclosporine than with tacrolimus. Neurologic side effects are more often associated with tacrolimus and may be mild, such as tremor or headache, or may be severe, such as seizures and leukoencephalopathy. Two common cosmetic side effects that are specific to cyclosporine are gingival hyperplasia and hirsutism, while alopecia is sometimes seen with tacrolimus (1). Although the cosmetic side effects of cyclosporine may seem minor compared to the pathophysiologic ones mentioned above, they are important to the patient and can result in medication noncompliance and graft loss. This problem is especially problematic in adolescent patients, and for that reason tacrolimus is the preferred CNI in children and adolescents.

Mammalian Target of Rapamycin Inhibitors

Sirolimus and everolimus are mTOR inhibitors. Both agents are approved for use in Europe but only sirolimus is currently approved for use in the United States. Sirolimus is a macrocyclic antibiotic produced by the bacteria *Streptomyces hygroscopius*. The mTOR inhibitors also bind to FKBP-12 in the cytoplasm of cells (same as tacrolimus); however, the mechanism of action is quite different. The drug/FKBP-12 complex inhibits mTOR, a key regulatory protein kinase that controls cytokine-dependant cell proliferation (1). Similar to the calcineurin inhibitors, the mTOR inhibitors require monitoring of drug levels to achieve proper therapeutic efficacy.

Both sirolimus and everolimus are available in oral form only and are readily absorbed. The half-life of sirolimus is 60 hours, allowing for once daily dosing, while the half-life of everolimus is 24 hours and typical dosing is twice daily. Both drugs are metabolized in the liver and counter transported to the gut lumen leading to elimination in the feces. The CYP3A pathway is involved in drug metabolism; thus potential drug interactions are important to recognize (Table 20-2) (1).

A major distinction between mTOR inhibitors and the CNIs is the lack of renal toxicity from vasoconstriction. However, proteinuria has been associated with the use of mTOR inhibitors, thus they may also be nephrotoxic. When combined with a CNI, mTOR inhibitors appear to actually increase the renal toxicity associated with the CNI (4). This effect is probably most pronounced with cyclosporine, but it is seen with both agents, especially when the CNI is used at regular dosing levels. At lower CNI dosing levels, the renal toxicity may be less pronounced. Given this potential renal toxicity, the combined use of a CNI and an mTOR inhibitor on a chronic basis is often avoided.

Another important toxicity of mTOR inhibitors is hyperlipidemia (hypercholesterolemia and hypertriglyceridemia), affecting upward of 50% of patients (4). In most instances the lipid abnormalities can be managed by placing the patient on either an HMG-CoA reductase inhibitor ("statin") or a fibrate, depending on the specific lipid abnormality. A unique and interesting side effect of mTOR inhibitors is the development of painful mouth sores that are associated with high drug levels and generally resolve with dose reduction. The mTOR inhibitors can also cause hematologic abnormalities such as leukopenia, thrombocytopenia, and anemia that may require dose reduction or changing immunosuppression. Lymphedema is an increasingly recognized complication of mTOR inhibitors and can present any time after initiation (1). Impaired wound healing is an important side effect from the surgeon's perspective that is discussed later in this chapter.

Antiproliferative Agents

A variety of antiproliferative agents is used for immunosuppression. These agents work by inhibiting DNA synthesis and therefore cell proliferation. Azathioprine, mycophenolate mofetil (MMF), and mycophenolate sodium are used in transplant recipients as part of maintenance immunosuppression. Other commonly used antiproliferative agents

include cyclophosphamide (cancer and immune-mediated diseases) and leflunomide (rheumatoid arthritis).

Azathioprine is a purine analog that inhibits lymphocyte and myelocyte proliferation. It is typically administered orally as part of a maintenance immunosuppression regimen, although intravenous dosing at one-half the oral dose is occasionally necessary. Azathioprine should be avoided or the dosing reduced significantly if administered with allopurinol, since xanthine oxidase is necessary for the conversion of azathioprine to inactive metabolites. The major side effect observed is hematologic, with a reversible, dose-dependent leukopenia and anemia most commonly observed. In addition, hepatotoxicity and acute pancreatitis are rarely seen in patients on azathioprine, with both conditions being reversible with timely cessation of therapy (1,4).

MMF and mycophenolate sodium both become mycophenolic acid (MPA) *in vivo*. A product of several *Penicillium* species, MPA affects DNA replication by noncompetitive reversible inhibition of inosine monophosphate dehydrogenase, an important enzyme for *de novo* guanosine synthesis. Because lymphocytes depend upon *de novo* guanosine synthesis, MPA has a more selective cytostatic effect on lymphocytes compared to other cell types that have a salvage pathway. Both drugs are primarily administered orally in two divided doses, although an intravenous form of MMF can be given at the same dosing regimen. The major side effects of both MMF and mycophenolate sodium are related to the GI tract and are generally dose-dependent. Nausea, diarrhea, and bloating are often seen, while esophagitis and gastritis are uncommon and may be related to invasive cytomegalovirus (CMV) disease. Hematologic side effects, including anemia, leukopenia, and thrombocytopenia, are also fairly common and usually improve by temporary medication discontinuation and resumption at lower doses once counts recover (1,4).

Leflunomide is a synthetic isoxazole derivative with anti-inflammatory and immunosuppressive properties used primarily for the treatment of rheumatoid arthritis. The agent disrupts *de novo* pyrimidine synthesis and thus inhibits lymphocyte proliferation. Also of interest is this agent's antiviral property against several DNA viruses. The major side effects are anemia and GI symptoms, such as diarrhea. In addition, leflunomide can cause severe hepatotoxicity in a small percentage of patients, requiring monitoring of liver function tests during therapy and discontinuation of the drug if a significant elevation occurs (1). A few transplant centers have used leflunomide in select recipients; however, concerns over its long half-life (5 to 15 days) and difficulty in obtaining adequate therapeutic levels has limited its use in this population (12, 13). FK778, a leflunomide analog with a much shorter half-life, is under development for use in organ transplant patients (14). This medication is of great interest to transplant physicians given the possibility that it may possess both immunosuppressive and antiviral properties.

Antibodies

Antibodies are often administered for induction therapy in the critical early period after transplantation to decrease the risk of acute rejection and to allow for lower overall intensity of maintenance immunosuppression. They are also used for the treatment of steroid resistant acute rejection. Antibody therapies can be divided into the polyclonal preparations that have a broad range of antibody specificities and the monoclonal preparations that target a single specific molecule to evoke their mechanism of action.

Rabbit-derived and horse-derived polyclonal antithymocyte globulin preparations are currently available. They both contain a variety of antibodies against many lymphocyte surface antigens—these antibodies bind to the surface of the lymphocyte, cause depletion, and thus interfere with cell-mediated and humoral immune responses (1,15). This depletion occurs by both complement-dependent cell lysis and by macrophage phagocytosis. The side effects of this medication include infusion-related ones, such as fever, chills, headache, and, rarely, anaphylaxis. In addition, severe lymphocyte depletion and thrombocytopenia may occur, which can limit the ability to safely administer successive doses (4). Lymphocyte counts remain abnormally low for several months in most patients and may persist for several years in some (16). Thus, it is important to remember that recipients of antithymocyte globulin may develop complications related to persistent lymphopenia weeks, months, or even years after treatment.

Intravenous immune globulins (IVIGs) are also polyclonal antibody preparations that are commonly used to treat autoimmune and inflammatory diseases, and they are increasingly being used in organ transplant recipients. IVIG is prepared by pooling IgG antibody from thousands of normal volunteers. It has complex immunoregulatory properties but is not immunosuppressive and therefore does not lead to the associated complications (17). Similar to antithymocyte globulin, infusion-related side effects are observed. When IVIG is used in high doses, aseptic meningitis can develop that is self-resolving. The medication's high osmotic load can cause tubular injury that may lead to acute renal dysfunction (4). Renal dysfunction associated with IVIG administration has most commonly been reported in the setting of rapid administration and the use of products stabilized with sucrose.

Currently several monoclonal antibodies are available that target the T lymphocyte. In contrast to polyclonal antibodies, each of these agents has a specific target on the T lymphocyte that the antibody binds to and on which it exerts its mechanism of action. The oldest of these agents is muromonab-CD3 (OKT3), a mouse monoclonal antibody against the human T cell surface molecule CD3. OKT3 leads to the rapid depletion of T cells and blocks the action of activated cytotoxic T cells. Severe side effects with initial administration are fairly common due to a cytokine release syndrome that occurs. Fever, chills, rigors, headache, and muscle pain are commonly observed in patients receiving OKT3, especially with the first few doses. In patients that are fluid overloaded, "flash" pulmonary edema can occur and should be monitored for closely. Volume status should be optimized prior to administering this agent. An aseptic meningitis picture has also been observed in patients receiving OKT3 (4).

Two monoclonal antibodies against the IL-2 receptor are basiliximab and daclizumab, both of which are intravenous preparations used for induction therapy only. These antibodies block the IL-2 receptor on T cells, preventing activation and proliferation, but do not lead to depletion and an associated cytokine storm. Both antibodies are of murine origin; however, major portions of each antibody have been replaced by human IgG using molecular biology techniques. Thus they are not perceived as xenogeneic protein by the recipient and are extremely well tolerated with minimal side effects (1).

Antibody preparations from the oncology field are being used "off-label" as immunosuppressive therapy. Alemtuzumab is an anti-CD52 antibody that depletes T and B lymphocytes and monocytes. It has been used for both induction therapy and for the treatment of rejection (1). A prolonged depletion in the white blood cell count can occur, with many patients still having abnormally low counts 6 to 12 months after receiving alemtuzumab (18). Rituximab is directed against the CD20 marker on B cells and is used for prophylaxis and treatment against antibody-mediated immunity (1). Its use in kidney transplantation has increased due to the growing number of transplants performed in sensitized and ABO-incompatible recipients. Both medications are generally well tolerated; however, they can have infusion-related side effects such as fever, rash, nausea, shortness of breath, chest discomfort, and allergic reactions.

Medications in Development

The greater understanding of immune activation at the cellular level has allowed for the development of several monoclonal antibodies that are either approved for limited indications or in development for future clinical use. These agents target the "immune synapse" between the APC and the T lymphocyte (Fig. 20-1). Efalizumab is an antibody that binds the CD11a chain of lymphocyte function-associated antigen (LFA-1) on T cells and is approved for use in patients with psoriasis. Its use in transplant recipients is under investigation. Monoclonal antibodies to CD80 (B7.1) and CD86 (B7.2) on the APC have been developed and tested in a phase I setting (1). Better studied has been LEA29Y, a protein analog to cytotoxic T lymphocyte antigen 4 immunoglobulin (CTLA4Ig) that strongly binds to CD80 and CD86 and interrupts T-cell activation. Clinical trials with LEA29Y in organ transplant recipients are underway and appear promising. Similar to the IL-2 receptor antibodies, these antibodies are all humanized and thus presumably well tolerated by patients (1,19). However, early clinical experience with a monoclonal antibody against CD154 demonstrated major thromboembolic events; thus any new agent will be carefully scrutinized for safety and its efficacy will be compared to current therapy (19).

Small molecule immunosuppressive drug development also continues, with numerous agents being studied. T cell migration between the lymphoid organs, such as lymph nodes and spleen, and the periphery is critical to lymphocyte activation. FTY720 is a structural homolog to sphingosine-1-phosphate, a T cell surface molecule. Administration of FTY720 causes sequestration of lymphocytes in the lymphoid organs and disrupts normal T cell migration. Several clinical studies with this agent have been completed and asymptomatic bradycardia has been the major side effect observed (1,20,21). Janus kinase 3 (JAK3) is an important intracellular signaling protein involved in cytokine mediated T cell proliferation (22). In primates CP-690,550, a JAK3 inhibitor, has demonstrated effective immunosuppressive properties and lacks the side effects associated with currently used drugs such as hypertension, hyperglycemia, and renal dysfunction. This agent is thought to be quite promising and early clinical studies with CP-690,550 have begun (1).

COMMON PROBLEMS ASSOCIATED WITH IMMUNOSUPPRESSION

The complications that occur due to immunosuppression can affect any part of the body and are wide-ranging. Many of them are related to the above-mentioned side effects of a particular immunosuppressive agent; however, additional complications occur that are the result of combination therapy with multiple agents or a consequence of the patient's global immunosuppressed state. This section will cover whole body and organ system based problems associated with immunosuppression, especially as they pertain to the consulting surgeon involved in the care of these patients.

Infection

The majority of the morbidity and mortality from immunosuppression was once primarily due to infection. These infectious complications not only resulted from common pathogens seen in nonimmunosuppressed patients but also were often caused by opportunistic agents that attacked primarily the immune deficient host. With experience, clinicians developed effective prophylactic strategies against the more commonly seen infections. This experience, coupled with the development of newer, more T-cell specific agents, decreased the overall incidence of infectious complications. Despite these advances, infectious complications remain a major concern when caring for immunosuppressed individuals.

The variety of pathogens that has been observed in immunosuppressed patients far exceeds what is seen in the "normal" host, with many of these opportunistic pathogens being observed only in these individuals. Bacterial infections are often resistant to routinely used antibiotics because of previous patient exposure to these agents or colonization of the patient with resistant bacteria during prolonged hospital stays. Vancomycin resistant *Enterococcus* (VRE), methicillin-resistant *Staphylococcus aureus* (MRSA), and extended-spectrum β-lactamase-producing *Escherichia coli* and *Klebsiella* species are such examples. Cystic fibrosis patients awaiting lung transplantation can become colonized with *Pseudomonas aeruginosa*, *Stenotrophomonas maltophilia*, or *Burkholderia cepacia* that are resistant to β lactams, aminoglycosides, and fluoroquinolones, leading to high morbidity and mortality after transplantation (23). Mycobacterial infection with either *Mycobacterium tuberculosis* or atypical mycobacteria occur far more frequently in immunosuppressed patients, but it is still rare in developed countries (23).

Viral infections are often the consequence of reactivation of latent infections once the patient has become immunosuppressed. CMV was an extremely problematic viral infection in organ transplant recipients until prophylaxis with antiviral therapy became routine. CMV disease can occur as a viral syndrome with fever, malaise, leukopenia, and thrombocytopenia, and it can also present as tissue invasive disease causing pneumonitis, hepatitis, retinitis, or GI tract disease (23). Other viral diseases due to Epstein–Barr, herpes simplex, human herpesvirus 6 and 7, varicella zoster, respiratory syncytial, influenza, and adenovirus are all described (23).

Invasive fungal infections are considered the most difficult to treat infections in immunosuppressed patients. *Pneumocystis jiroveci* (formerly known as *Pneumocystis carinii*) causes a pneumonia that is characterized by hypoxemia and dyspnea that is disproportional to physical exam and radiographic findings. This disease was the initial defining illness in 63% of AIDS patients in 1987 and affected up to 15% of transplant recipients (23,24). Fortunately, effective prophylaxis strategies have reduced these rates considerably. *Candida* species can cause mucocutaneous infection, esophagitis, pyelonephritis, candidemia, endocarditis, brain abscess, sinusitis, empyema, peritonitis, and wound infection. *Aspergillus* species most commonly cause lung and upper respiratory tract infections, including sinusitis, tracheobronchitis, necrotizing pneumonia, and empyema. Disseminated disease with brain abscess formation can occur, as can fungal ball formation in preexisting cavities. This organism is especially problematic for lung transplant recipients (23,25). *Cryptococcus neoformans* most commonly causes central nervous system disease and pulmonary disease. In organ transplant recipients, there is a typical timeline of when the more common fungal infections occur—*Candida* in the first few weeks after transplantation, *Aspergillus* and

Pneumocystis in the first 1 to 6 months after transplantation, and *Cryptococcus* after 6 months (23). Of course these times can vary depending on environmental factors and the overall degree of immunosuppression in the individual patient.

Malignancy

Malignancy appears to be a greater problem in those receiving immunosuppression compared to the general population, with the absolute increase in risk depending on the amount of immunosuppression used and the type of malignancy (26–28). The majority of the studies regarding malignancy and immunosuppression are based on transplant recipients, although the findings should be applicable to all immunosuppressed patients. In kidney transplant recipients the risk of developing cancers of the colon, lung, prostate, stomach, esophagus, pancreas, ovary, and breast are approximately twofold greater than the general population for the first 3 years following transplantation. Testicular and bladder cancers are increased threefold, and leukemia, hepatobiliary cancers, and cervical and vulvovaginal cancers are increased approximately fivefold (29). Thus prevention strategies and screening methods for these common cancers are likely to be even more relevant for immunosuppressed individuals.

Skin cancer is the most common malignancy in patients on immunosuppressive therapy, causing serious morbidity and potential mortality. Several studies have shown that the incidence of skin cancers in transplant patients is between 40% to 80% after 20 years of immunosuppressive therapy. Compared to the general population, melanoma occurs 2 to 4 times more often, squamous-cell carcinoma occurs 65 to 250 times more frequently, and basal-cell carcinoma occurs 10 times more often (30). As a result, the number of squamous-cell skin cancers exceeds the number of basal-cell skin cancers in transplant recipients—the opposite of the general population. The key risk factor for development is ultraviolet light exposure, and patients on immunosuppression should be counseled on prevention strategies and careful skin exams to aid early detection.

Treatment of solid organ and skin cancers in patients on immunosuppressive therapy should follow established guidelines for that particular cancer. When possible, surgical resection with adequate margins should be performed to control the primary site of disease. Additional chemotherapy should be administered when indicated. Even with an aggressive approach to cancer treatment, the development of recurrences and distant metastases is common on immunosuppressive therapy. If possible, consideration should be given to immunosuppression reduction or withdrawal. Regardless of whether immunosuppressive therapy can be reduced, frequent monitoring for the development of recurrence and metastases should be performed since the propensity for rapid tumor spread in these patients is well-documented (Fig. 20-2).

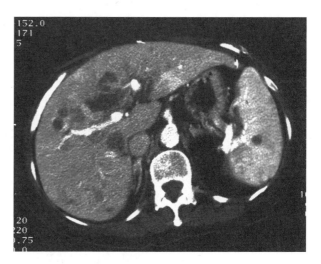

Figure 20-2 Abdominal CT scan demonstrating cancer metastases to the liver and spleen of unknown primary origin in a recipient 4 months after kidney transplantation. A CT scan 3 months earlier was normal.

Two cancers occur in the general population but are observed at much higher rates in immunosuppressed individuals. Post-transplant lymphoproliferative disease (PTLD) represents a variety of B lymphocyte disorders ranging from mild polyclonal hyperplasia to malignant monoclonal lymphoma. In most instances the disease appears to be related to Epstein–Barr virus (EBV)-mediated transformation of B cells. The incidence is estimated to be between 1% and 10% of transplant recipients (31). In one series of 500 liver transplant recipients, 2.4% developed PTLD at a mean of 19.5 months after transplantation (32). Patients may present with fever, fatigue, weight loss, a high EBV viral load, and lymphadenopathy—either by physical exam or by imaging study. Patients can also present with solid organ masses, skin lesions, central nervous system symptoms, and tonsil enlargement, especially in children. Biopsy is sometimes required to confirm the diagnosis, help determine the severity of the disease, and determine therapy. Treatment for milder forms is usually by immunosuppression reduction and antiviral therapy, while more malignant variants require chemotherapy and immunotherapy with anti-CD20 monoclonal antibody (33). Surgical resection or radiation for disease localized to a single lesion has also been reported.

Kaposi sarcoma is characterized by multiple angiomatous lesions. There is an 80- to 500-fold increased incidence in immunosuppressed patients, and human herpes virus 8 (HHV-8) has a causal role. Most patients with Kaposi sarcoma have mucosal or skin lesions, with most skin lesions occurring on the legs. Patients with visceral disease usually present with lesions in the lungs, GI tract, or lymph nodes (30). Immunosuppresion reduction is first-line therapy for Kaposi sarcoma, often resulting in disease regression, with chemotherapy being reserved for persistent disease.

Impaired Wound Healing

Impaired wound healing has been recognized as a consequence of corticosteroid therapy since its introduction. Several studies have documented that steroids administered before or at the time of surgery impair wound healing as measured by tensile strength. Histologic studies have shown that steroids interfere with the migration of monocytes and macrophages into the wound, thus reducing the inflammatory phase of wound healing and reducing the number of fibroblasts in the wound. Studies with corticosteroids have demonstrated a twofold to fivefold increase in wound healing complications compared to control subjects not receiving steroids (5).

More recently, sirolimus and everolimus also have been documented to lead to impaired wound healing. This impairment is related to the antiproliferative effects of the drug on many different cell types. From the transplantation literature, it has been demonstrated that sirolimus causes a fivefold increased incidence of wound infections, lymphoceles, and hernias in kidney recipients and an increased incidence of bronchial anastomosis dehiscence in lung recipients (34,35). Other anecdotal reports describe decreased wound healing in transplant patients on sirolimus undergoing other procedures. Consideration should be given to temporarily substituting an mTOR inhibitor with a CNI at the time of an operative procedure or much earlier in the setting of elective surgery. The use of additional closure methods such as retention sutures should be considered when operating on patients receiving an mTOR inhibitor. Outside of steroids and mTOR inhibitors, the other immunosuppressive medications do not significantly inhibit wound healing. The consequences of wound infections, however, can be severe, and thus vigilant observation for the development of wound complications is recommended.

Cardiovascular Disease

Cardiovascular disease in patients on immunosuppression is frequently observed, but the exact contribution of immunosuppressive agents to cardiovascular complications is difficult to assess since preexisting disease often carries its own risk of cardiovascular complications (36). For example, renal failure patients have a 10 to 20 times higher mortality from cardiovascular events than the general population (37). However, several studies have demonstrated that kidney transplantation reduces this mortality risk when compared to ongoing dialysis; thus the benefit of transplantation overshadows the potential harm caused by immunosuppressive therapy (38,39). Within the population of immunosuppressed patients, differences in cardiovascular mortality have been observed between groups of patients on different immunosuppressive medications, implying a contributory role of these medications to cardiovascular complications. Perhaps the best way to assess the influence of immunosuppressive agents on cardiovascular complications is by examining their impact on the risk factors of cardiovascular disease (37).

Many of the immunosuppressive agents adversely affect cardiovascular risk factors, such as diabetes, hypertension, and hyperlipidemia. As mentioned previously, corticosteroids, tacrolimus, and cyclosporine all cause diabetes, hypertension, and hyperlipidemia to varying degrees. In addition, sirolimus also causes hyperlipidemia to a greater extent than any of the other immunosuppressive agents (1,4,37). Modification of risk factors through diet and exercise is encouraged in patients on immunosuppressive medications. In addition, the aggressive treatment of these risk factors with pharmacologic agents is widely practiced. It is important to remember that patients on long-standing immunosuppression will often have cardiac disease, either as a result of native disease or as a result of these medications. Thus noninvasive stress testing is recommended prior to major elective procedures in this patient population.

Gastrointestinal Disease

Serious and often life-threatening complications involving the entire GI tract have been reported in association with immunosuppressive therapy. Mucosal ulceration leading to bleeding or perforation has been reported with the esophagus, stomach, small intestine, and colon. In addition, biliary tract disease and pancreatitis have also been frequently observed. The most commonly observed problems are gastroduodenal ulcers and colon perforations. Historically, the initial culprit was corticosteroids, with numerous reports documenting GI complications in 10% to 30% of patients on steroids and a high associated mortality (5,40). As additional immunosuppressive agents have been introduced, reduced doses of corticosteroids have been used and the incidence of GI complications has decreased. In addition, the availability of histamine receptor antagonists and proton pump inhibitors has allowed for routine prophylaxis against gastroduodenal ulcer disease and has reduced the incidence of upper GI complications dramatically (41).

The highest rate of GI complications appears to occur in recipients of heart and lung transplants. In one report a 20% rate of GI complications, including perforated duodenal ulcer, pancreatitis, colonic pneumatosis, cholecystitis, appendicitis, and colonic necrosis, was observed within 30 days following cardiac transplantation. Most of these patients underwent successful surgical intervention, with over 90% surviving with normal GI function (42). Another report documented a 40% rate of major GI complications following lung transplantation, with 18% requiring an operative procedure and the remainder being managed with endoscopic intervention or medications. Most of these GI complications occurred within the first month after lung transplantation (43). A more recent analysis of renal transplant recipients documented a 10% rate of severe GI complications following transplantation, with the most common problems being gastroduodenal ulcers, colonic diverticulitis, and pancreatitis (44).

Diagnosis of GI complications in immunosuppressed individuals is often difficult because systemic signs such as abdominal pain, fever, and leukocytosis are often minimal or absent despite significant disease. Abdominal distension and hypoactive bowel sounds may be the only signs of an abdominal catastrophe. A high index of suspicion is required to diagnose these GI complications, with frequent abdominal exams and the liberal use of diagnostic studies being helpful. Plain radiographs, computed tomography scans, contrast studies, selective arteriography, and upper and lower endoscopy have all been reported to be helpful in making the diagnosis in these patients. Once the diagnosis of a major GI complication is made, immediate and aggressive intervention is required to optimize patient outcomes. When operative therapy is necessary, most experienced surgeons advocate a conservative approach in terms of performing the simplest procedure that controls the problem at hand. When small bowel resection is necessary, intestinal continuity can usually be restored safely. However, when large bowel resection is necessary, diversion is preferred over an anastomosis due to the risk of breakdown and the development of further complications. Meticulous surgical care can lead to successful outcomes in patients with major immunosuppression related GI complications.

CMV is a common human pathogen that can lead to significant disease in immunosuppressed individuals as described elsewhere in this chapter. The systemic signs and symptoms of CMV disease include fever, malaise, lethargy, and leukopenia. CMV disease of the GI tract is characterized by mucosal ulcerations, erosions, and hemorrhage that can affect the esophagus, stomach, small bowel, and colon. Lesions in these sites can lead to intestinal tract bleeding or perforation. The diagnosis of CMV disease in the intestinal tract is often made by the presence of GI symptoms in the setting of a high viral load detected by polymerase chain reaction (45). However, significant GI tract CMV disease may be present in the absence of symptoms or a detectable viral load, and investigation with endoscopy and biopsy is recommended when CMV disease is clinically suspected (46). Treatment of GI tract CMV disease is with systemic antiviral therapy. In some situations patients may present with perforation and require surgical intervention, albeit with a high morbidity and mortality.

Chronic Renal Insufficiency and Failure

Renal insufficiency and renal failure are relatively common problems that develop in patients who receive long-term immunosuppressive therapy (10). Although this is primarily a consequence of CNI therapy, other complications of immunosuppression, such as hypertension, diabetes, and dyslipidemia, all contribute to the development of chronic kidney disease. The prolonged use of cyclosporine or tacrolimus leads to tubular atrophy, interstitial fibrosis, and arteriolar hyalinosis in the kidney (47). This development of renal failure is most pronounced in recipients of nonrenal solid organ transplants, primarily due to the dependence on cyclosporine or tacrolimus to prevent rejection and thereby prolong graft and patient survival. Preexisting renal disease from chronic hypoperfusion often contributes as well, particularly in heart and liver recipients. The cumulative incidence of chronic renal failure in the United States at 5 years following transplantation is 10.9% for heart, 21.3% for intestine, 18.1% for liver, and 15.8% for lung recipients (Fig. 20-3) (48).

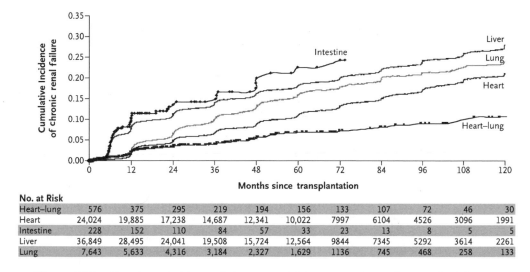

No. at Risk											
Heart–lung	576	375	295	219	194	156	133	107	72	46	30
Heart	24,024	19,885	17,238	14,687	12,341	10,022	7997	6104	4526	3096	1991
Intestine	228	152	110	84	57	33	23	13	8	5	5
Liver	36,849	28,495	24,041	19,508	15,724	12,564	9844	7345	5292	3614	2261
Lung	7,643	5,633	4,316	3,184	2,327	1,629	1136	745	468	258	133

Figure 20-3 Cumulative incidence of chronic renal failure in recipients of nonrenal solid organ transplants in the United States. (From Ojo AO, Held PJ, Port FK, et al. Chronic renal failure after transplantation of a nonrenal organ. *N Engl J Med* 2003;349:931–940, with permission.)

Although the majority of patients on CNI therapy do not develop chronic renal failure, most have some degree of impaired renal function (49). Patients on CNIs have a mean glomerular filtration rate that is approximately 40% less than comparable patients not on CNIs, with this difference being a result of reduced renal blood flow and therefore reduced ultrafiltration (9,47,50). Impaired renal function may or may not be reflected in the plasma creatinine, and it may require calculation or measurement of the creatinine clearance to appreciate the degree of renal dysfunction present. When caring for these patients, it is important to prevent intravascular volume depletion because hypovolemia further exacerbates the chronic effects of CNIs on the kidney. It is also recommended to avoid the use of nephrotoxic medications and to minimize interventions that can further disturb renal function (i.e., intravenous contrast) in patients receiving CNIs.

The management of dialysis access in immunosuppressed patients is often quite complicated. The preferred long-term access is an arterial-venous fistula because infectious complications are often severe in these patients and are much more likely to occur with artificial grafts, peritoneal dialysis catheters, and hemodialysis catheters. The ideal therapy for the recipient of a nonrenal solid organ transplant with renal failure is renal transplantation since the patient is already receiving immunosuppressive therapy. This is an increasingly common scenario, with reports indicating good outcomes (51).

Endocrine Abnormalities

Diabetes mellitus is the most common endocrine abnormality in patients on immunosuppression and is largely due to the use of steroids and CNIs. The diabetes is primarily due to insulin resistance, although it may also result from diminished insulin release. Risk factors for diabetes include African American race, a family history of diabetes, obesity, hepatitis C, and older age. The contribution of steroids to diabetes is dose-related—the majority of individuals receiving high doses of steroids in the immediate period following transplantation demonstrate impairment in glucose tolerance; however, as the dose is reduced most patients return to near normal glucose levels. Since CNIs are most commonly used in conjunction with corticosteroids, their contribution to inducing diabetes is difficult to assess. It is generally accepted that both cyclosporine and tacrolimus can cause diabetes and that the risk is greater with tacrolimus. A recent analysis of renal transplant recipients demonstrated that 18% of patients receiving tacrolimus had developed diabetes by 2 years after transplantation compared to 8% of those receiving cyclosporine (11). Targeting lower, though still therapeutic, CNI levels as well as minimization of steroid dosing will often improve glycemic control (52). Management of patients with immunosuppression-induced diabetes is similar to

others and includes diet and exercise, oral agents, or insulin. The general goal is to maintain a hemoglobin A1c below 7% and to monitor and prevent diabetes-related complications.

Adrenal insufficiency has been a major concern in patients receiving chronic glucocorticoid therapy since an early report of death due to adrenal atrophy in a patient receiving steroids undergoing an operation (53). Thus, for many years these patients received additional large doses of steroids at the time of stress. However, more recent studies have documented the safety of avoiding "stress steroids" in patients receiving maintenance prednisone therapy of 5 to 10 mg per day (54,55). "Stress steroids" should not routinely be given in the perioperative setting to patients on chronic steroid therapy since their administration increases the risk of infection, delays wound healing, and often significantly increases blood glucose levels. When minor or moderate stress is expected, steroids should be continued at maintenance doses and the patient should be observed for signs of adrenal insufficiency, such as hypotension, myalgia, arthralgia, ileus, fever, hyponatremia, and eosinophilia. If signs of adrenal insufficiency develop, a 24- to 48-hour course of "stress steroids" should be given. When a major stressor occurs in a patient on chronic steroid therapy, such as major multiorgan trauma or a ruptured aortic aneurysm, most clinicians agree that adrenal insufficiency should be investigated and administration of "stress steroids" should be considered.

SUMMARY

The complications of immunosuppression remain a challenging problem for patients and their health care providers. Although many people have suffered due to immunodeficiency disease states, there is little doubt that the lives of others have been extended and enhanced by the availability of various medications that allow for the control of autoimmunity, transplant rejection, and cancer. The hope for both groups of patients is based on the growing number of therapeutic agents combined with the increased understanding of the human immune system. Hopefully there will soon be a day when the negative consequences of immunodeficiency can be prevented. Until then, a thorough understanding of the complications associated with immunosuppression, combined with an aggressive approach to diagnosis and treatment, will generally lead to optimal outcomes.

REFERENCES

1. Hardinger KL, Koch MJ, Brennan DC. Current and future immunosuppressive strategies in renal transplantation. *Pharmacotherapy* 2004;24:1159–1176.
2. Helderman JH, Goral S. Transplantation immunobiology. In: Danovitch GM, ed. *Handbook of kidney transplantation*, 3rd ed. Philadelphia, PA: Lippincott Williams & Wilkins; 2001:17–38.

3. Hricik DE, Almawi WY, Strom TB. Trends in the use of glucocorticoids in renal transplantation. *Transplantation* 1994;57:979–989.

4. Danovitch GM. Immunosuppressive medications and protocols for kidney transplantation. In: Danovitch GM, ed. *Handbook of kidney transplantation*, 4th ed. Philadelphia, PA: Lippincott Williams & Wilkins; 2005:72–134.

5. Diethelm AG. Surgical management of complications of steroid therapy. *Ann Surg* 1977;185:251–263.

6. Matas AJ, Kandaswamy R, Humar A, et al. Long-term immunosuppression without maintenance prednisone after kidney transplantation. *Ann Surg* 2004;240:510–516.

7. Khwaja K, Asolati M, Harmon JV, et al. Rapid discontinuation of prednisone in higher-risk kidney transplant recipients. *Transplantation* 2004;78:1397–1399.

8. Nashan B, Cole E, Levy G, et al. Clinical validation studies of Neoral C2 monitoring: a review. *Transplantation* 2002;73:S3–S11.

9. Myers BD, Ross J, Newton L, et al. Cyclosporine-associated chronic nephropathy. *N Engl J Med* 1984;311:699–705.

10. Bennett WM, DeMattos A, Meyer MM, et al. Chronic cyclosporine nephropathy: the Achilles' heel of immunosuppressive therapy. *Kidney Int* 1996;50:1089–1100.

11. Woodward RS, Schnitzler MA, Baty J, et al. Incidence and cost of new onset diabetes mellitus among U.S. wait-listed and transplanted renal allograft recipients. *Am J Transplant* 2003;3:590–598.

12. Williams JW, Mital D, Chong A, et al. Experiences with leflunomide in solid organ transplantation. *Transplantation* 2002;73(3):358–366.

13. Hardinger KL, Wang CD, Schnitzler MA, et al. Prospective, pilot, open-label, short-term study of conversion to leflunomide reverses chronic renal allograft dysfunction. *Am J Transplant* 2002;2:867–871.

14. Jin MB, Nakayama M, Ogata T, et al. A novel leflunomide derivative, FK778, for immunosuppression after kidney transplantation in dogs. *Surgery* 2002;132:72–79.

15. Gaber AO, First MR, Tesi RJ, et al. Results of the double-blind, randomized, multicenter, phase III clinical trial of Thymoglobulin versus Atgam in the treatment of acute graft rejection episodes after renal transplantation. *Transplantation* 1998;66:29–37.

16. Brennan DC, Flavin K, Lowell JA, et al. A randomized, double-blinded comparison of Thymoglobulin versus Atgam for induction immunosuppressive therapy in adult renal transplant recipients. *Transplantation* 1999;67:1011–1018.

17. Kazatchkine MD, Kaveri SV. Immunomodulation of autoimmune and inflammatory diseases with intravenous immune globulin. *N Engl J Med* 2001;345:747–755.

18. Calne R, Moffatt SD, Friend PJ, et al. Campath 1H allows low-dose cyclosporine monotherapy in 31 cadaveric renal allograft recipients. *Transplantation* 1999;68:1613–1616.

19. Vincenti F. What's in the pipeline? New immunosuppressive drugs in transplantation. *Am J Transplant* 2002;2:898–903.

20. Budde K, Schmouder RL, Brunkhorst R, et al. First human trial of FTY720, a novel immunomodulator, in stable renal transplant patients. *J Am Soc Nephrol* 2002;13:1073–1083.

21. Bohler T, Waiser J, Schultz M, et al. FTY720 mediates apoptosis-independent lymphopenia in human renal allograft recipients: different effects on CD62L+ and CCR5+ T lymphocytes. *Transplantation* 2004;15:1424–1432.

22. Nashan B. Review of T-cell activation: impact of Janus kinase 3 inhibition. *Transplantation* 2003;75:1783–1785.

23. Green M, Avery RK, Preiksaitis J. Guidelines for the prevention and management of infectious complications of solid organ transplantation. *Am J Transplant* 2004;10S:6–166.

24. Morris A, Lundgren JD, Masur H, et al. Current epidemiology of Pneumocystis pneumonia. *Emerg Infect Dis* 2004;10:1713–1720.

25. Patterson TF, Kirkpatrick WR, White M, et al. Invasive aspergillosis. Disease spectrum, treatment practices, and outcomes. I3 Aspergillus study group. *Medicine* 2000;79:250–260.

26. Trofe J, Beebe TM, Buell JF, et al. Posttransplant malignancy. *Prog Transplant* 2004;14:193–200.

27. Penn I. The effect of immunosuppression on pre-existing cancers. *Transplantation* 1993;55:742–747.

28. Feng S, Buell JF, Chari RS, et al. Tumors and transplantation: the 2003 third annual ASTS state-of-the-art winter symposium. *Am J Transplant* 2003;3:1481–1487.

29. Kasiske BL, Snyder JJ, Gilbertson DT, et al. Cancer after kidney transplantation in the United States. *Am J Transplant* 2004;4:905–913.

30. Euvrard S, Kanitakis J, Claudy A. Skin cancers after organ transplantation. *N Engl J Med* 2003;348:1681–1691.

31. Green M. Management of Epstein-Barr virus-induced posttransplant lymphoproliferative disease in recipients of solid organ transplantation. *Am J Transplant* 2001;1:103–108.

32. Norin S, Kimby E, Ericzon BG, et al. Posttransplant lymphoma—a single-center experience of 500 liver transplantations. *Med Oncol* 2004;21:273–284.

33. Verschuuren EA, Stevens SJ, van Imhoff GW, et al. Treatment of posttransplant lymphoproliferative disease with rituximab: the remission, the relapse, and the complication. *Transplantation* 2002;73:100–104.

34. Dean PG, Lund WJ, Larson TS, et al. Wound-healing complications after kidney transplantation: a prospective, randomized comparison of sirolimus and tacrolimus. *Transplantation* 2004;77:1555–1561.

35. Groetzner J, Kur F, Spelsberg F, et al. Airway anastomosis complications in de novo lung transplantation with sirolimus-based immunosuppression. *J Heart Lung Transplant* 2004;23:632–638.

36. Kasiske BL, Chakkera HA, Roel J. Explained and unexplained ischemic heart disease risk after renal transplantation. *J Am Soc Nephrol* 2000;11:1735–1743.

37. Boots JMM, Christiaans MHL, van Hoof JP. Effect of immunosuppressive agents on long-term survival of renal transplant recipients: focus on the cardiovascular risk. *Drugs* 2004;64:2047–2073.

38. Wolfe RA, Ashby VB, Milford EL, et al. Comparison of mortality in all patients on dialysis, patients on dialysis awaiting transplantation, and recipients of a first cadaveric transplant. *N Engl J Med* 1999;341:1725–1730.

39. Ojo AO, Hanson JA, Meier-Kriesche H, et al. Survival in recipients of marginal cadaveric donor kidneys compared with other recipients and wait-listed transplant candidates. *J Am Soc Nephrol* 2001;12:589–597.

40. Penn I, Groth CG, Brettschneider L, et al. Surgically correctable intra-abdominal complications before and after renal homotransplantations. *Ann Surg* 1968;168:865–870.

41. Troppmann C, Papalois BE, Chiou A, et al. Incidence, complications, treatment, and outcome of ulcers of the upper gastrointestinal tract after renal transplantation during the cyclosporine era. *J Am Coll Surg* 1995;180:433–443.

42. DiSesa VJ, Kirkman RL, Tilney NL, et al. Management of general surgical complications following cardiac transplantation. *Arch Surg* 1989;124:539–541.

43. Lubetkin EI, Lipson DA, Palevsky HI, et al. GI complications after orthotopic lung transplantation. *Am J Gastroenterol* 1996;91:2382–2390.

44. Sarkio S, Halme L, Kyllonen L, et al. Severe gastrointestinal complications after 1,515 adult kidney transplantations. *Transpl Int* 2004;17:505–510.

45. Goodgame RW. Gastrointestinal cytomegalovirus disease. *Ann Intern Med* 1993;119:924–935.

46. Mayoral JL, Loeffler CM, Fasola CG, et al. Diagnosis and treatment of cytomegalovirus disease in transplant patients based on gastrointestinal tract manifestations. *Arch Surg* 1991;126:202–206.

47. Young EW, Ellis CN, Messana JM, et al. A prospective study of renal structure and function in psoriasis patients treated with cyclosporin. *Kidney Int* 1994;46:1216–1622.

48. Ojo AO, Held PJ, Port FK, et al. Chronic renal failure after transplantation of a nonrenal organ. *N Engl J Med* 2003;349:931–940.

49. Avitzur Y, De Luca E, Cantos M, et al. Health status ten years after pediatric liver transplantation—looking beyond the graft. *Transplantation* 2004;78:566–573.

50. Hollander AA, van Saase JL, Kootte AM, et al. Beneficial effects of conversion from cyclosporine to azathioprine after kidney transplantation. *Lancet* 1995;345:610–614.

51. Coopersmith CM, Brennan DC, Miller B, et al. Renal transplantation following previous heart, liver, and lung transplantation: an 8-year single-center experience. *Surgery* 2001;130:457–462.

52. Gaston RS, Chandrakantan A. Diabetes mellitus after kidney transplantation. *Am J Transplant* 2003;3:512–513.

53. Fraser CG, Preuss FS, Bigford WD. Adrenal atrophy and irreversible shock associated with cortisone therapy. *JAMA* 1952; 149:1542–1543.

54. Bromberg JS, Alfrey EJ, Barker CF, et al. Adrenal suppression and steroid supplementation in renal transplant recipients. *Transplantation* 1991;51:385–390.

55. Bromberg JS, Baliga P, Cofer JB, et al. Stress steroids are not required for patients receiving a renal allograft and undergoing operation. *J Am Coll Surg* 1995;180:532–536.

Complications
of Thoracic Surgery

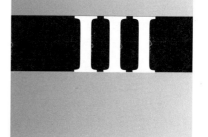

Complications of Intubation, Tracheotomy, and Tracheal Surgery

21

Kevin Fung   Norman D. Hogikyan

■■■ **INTRODUCTION 227**
Terminology 228

■■■ **INTUBATION 228**
Nasal Complications 228
Oral Cavity and Oropharyngeal Complications 229
Acute Laryngeal Complications 229
Chronic Laryngeal Complications 230
Tracheal Complications 233
Tube Complications 233
Cervical Spine Injury 234
Intubation of Incorrect Structure 234
Special Considerations 234

■■■ **TRACHEOTOMY 234**
Intraoperative Complications 234
Early Postoperative Complications 235
Late Postoperative Complications 236

■■■ **SPECIAL CONSIDERATIONS 238**

■■■ **TRACHEAL SURGERY 240**
Intraoperative Complications 240
Postoperative Complications 242

■■■ **REFERENCES 243**

Kevin Fung: University of Western Ontario, London, Ontario, Canada
Norman D. Hogikyan: University of Michigan, Ann Arbor, MI 48109

INTRODUCTION

The development of orotracheal intubation for the administration of anesthesia by William Macewen in 1878 was one of the most important advances in the history of surgery. With the passage of time, however, acute and chronic complications of intubation have become evident. Tracheotomy is currently indicated in patients for prolonged ventilation in order to avoid long-term complications of intubation. Benefits attributed to tracheotomy include enhanced patient comfort, improved pulmonary toilet, decreased ventilator-associated pneumonia, and accelerated ventilator weaning, although strong supportive evidence is lacking (1). Although some view tracheotomy as a routine procedure, the potential complications are significant and can be devastating. As a consequence of prolonged intubation, acquired laryngotracheal stenosis can occur and is the most common indication for tracheal resection. An understanding of the complications of procedures involving the airway, including intubation, tracheotomy, and tracheal surgery, is important for all surgeons.

Terminology

The terms "vocal cord" and "vocal fold" are used in various ways in the literature. Although both terms refer to the same anatomical structures, vocal fold is the more correct contemporary term and will be used throughout the chapter.

INTUBATION

The surgeon should appreciate current techniques to achieve airway control during administration of general anesthesia and their associated complications. Injury can occur to any part of the upper aerodigestive tract as a consequence of the intubation event itself or as a consequence of the endotracheal tube residing in the airway. Injuries are classified according to anatomic location as well as timing—acute (i.e., complications during the intubation event) versus chronic (i.e., complications while the patient is intubated) (2,3). Pertinent risk factors for these injuries are summarized in Table 21-1.

Nasal Complications

Nasotracheal intubation is indicated for surgical procedures involving the oral cavity when endotracheal intubation is expected to be prolonged and when there is a contraindication to orotracheal intubation.

TABLE 21-1

RISK FACTORS FOR INTUBATION COMPLICATIONS

Patient factors
    Unfavorable anatomy—short, thick neck
    Abnormal anatomy—facial skeletal abnormality, trismus
    Preexisting anatomic conditions—loose dentition, nasal septal
       deviation, cervical spine abnormalities
    Preexisting medical conditions—gastroesophageal reflux
       disease (GERD), diabetes, coagulopathy

Tube factors
    Tube too large
    Cuff pressure too high
    Coexisting nasogastric (NG) tube

Technical factors
    Forceful intubation
    Poor visualization of larynx
    Numerous intubation attempts

Acute

Epistaxis

Epistaxis can occur as a result of injury to nasal mucosa during nasotracheal intubation. Injury can occur at the level of the septum (Kiesselbach plexus), lateral nasal wall (branches of internal maxillary artery), nasal turbinates, or nasopharyngeal mucosa. Treatment consists of direct pressure, anterior nasal pack, topical decongestion, or otolaryngologic consultation for cauterization or posterior nasal pack if persistent and profuse. The following preventive measures are suggested.

1. Preoperative recognition and correction of bleeding disorders
2. Preoperative recognition of abnormal anatomy (i.e., deviated nasal septum, septal spur, nasal polyps, enlarged adenoids)
3. Adequate topical decongestion (i.e., pseudoephedrine, oxymetazoline, cocaine)
4. Use of an appropriate size tube (i.e., internal diameter 6.5 mm for men and 6.0 mm for women) (4)
5. Judicious use of lubrication and heat to prepare the tube
6. Proper technique (i.e., angulation of the tube in an inferior and posterior direction along the nasal floor)

Traditionally, it has been believed that in the presence of a midline nasal septum, the right nostril should be used for nasotracheal intubation because endotracheal tubes have a bevel on the tip such that the flat side faces to the left. A recent prospective study randomized nostril side in 128 patients undergoing nasotracheal intubation and found no difference in the incidence of epistaxis or the difficulty of intubation (4).

Chronic

Sinusitis

The osteomeatal complex represents the final common pathway of paranasal sinus drainage. Its patency ensures proper ventilation, aeration, mucociliary clearance, and prevention of effusion and infection. In response to the presence of an endotracheal tube in the nasal cavity, edema and inflammation of the lateral nasal wall mucosa can lead to obstruction of the osteomeatal complex, thereby resulting in effusion and infection within the paranasal sinuses. Obstruction is less common than previously thought. A study of nasotracheally intubated patients demonstrated sinus effusion on ultrasound within 3 days of intubation in 31% of patients (5). No patients developed sinusitis and all effusions resolved with removal of the tube. Longer-term intubation is associated with a higher incidence of sinusitis. At risk are immunocompromised patients and head injury patients with blood in the sinuses. Clinical manifestations of sinusitis include purulent rhinorrhea, fever, facial pain, and unilateral facial swelling. Pus obtained from the osteomeatal complex with endoscopic guidance should be sent for culture and sensitivity. Computed tomography (CT) can demonstrate effusion, but not all effusions represent true bacterial sinusitis. Sinusitis is not an important source of sepsis unless purulent sinusitis exists (2). Treatment involves removal of the tube if possible, a 3-day course of topical decongestant (i.e., pseudoephedrine, oxymetazoline, cocaine), and culture-directed antibiotics, including coverage for anaerobes and *Staphylococcus aureus*. Occasionally, antral lavage is necessary in refractory cases.

Nasal Alar Necrosis

Within hours, pressure necrosis can occur from the nasotracheal tube or its securing ties. This rare complication has been reported in isolated case reports in the literature (6,7). Surgical correction of this devastating cosmetic problem is extremely difficult. Prevention consists of proper cushioning between the nose, the tube, and securing ties.

Oral Cavity and Oropharyngeal Complications

Acute

Dental Injury

Injury to dentition is a relatively common complication of intubation, with a reported incidence of 1 in 150 to 1 in 1,500 intubations (8). This is an avoidable complication. Preventive measures include preoperative recognition of poor dentition or loose teeth and the use of a tooth guard during intubation. Injuries may include dental fracture, avulsion, and partial root avulsion. It is important to ensure that an avulsed tooth is recovered in order to prevent aspiration. Once the tooth is recovered, it should be placed in saline and a dental consultation should be obtained to consider reimplantation (3). In the case of a partial fracture, dental restoration can be considered. In the case of a partial avulsion, the tooth can be splinted or wired to an adjacent tooth.

Lip Injury

The upper lip can be lacerated if it is caught between the laryngoscope blade and the upper teeth. Likewise, the lower lip can be injured as the laryngoscope or the endotracheal tube drags the lip down across the lower teeth. Superficial injuries can be treated conservatively with topical antibiotic ointment, and deeper lacerations can be primarily closed with attention to accurate approximation of the vermillion border.

Temporomandibular Joint Injury

The temporomandibular joint can be dislocated as a consequence of forceful intubation or difficult intubation. At risk are patients with facial skeletal abnormalities. Clinically, the mandible is found to be locked in open position. The mechanism involves disruption of the ligamentous attachment of the temporomandibular disc to the condyle and subsequent displacement of the disc in the anteromedial direction due to the pull of the lateral pterygoid muscle. Immediate manual reduction under anesthesia with muscle relaxation is recommended. Postoperatively, the patient should be on a soft diet for 2 weeks.

Mucosal Injury

Injury to the mucosa of the oral cavity or oropharynx can be superficial, deep, or full-thickness. Risk factors include unfavorable anatomy (i.e., short, thick neck), limited neck extension, and trismus. Injury can manifest as laceration, hematoma, infection, or perforation. Superficial lacerations are treated conservatively while full-thickness lacerations are closed primarily. In the event of hematoma, antibiotics should be administered to prevent infection. Infection outside the pharynx can lead to abscess formation in the retropharyngeal or parapharyngeal spaces and can spread via tissue planes to the mediastinum. Neck abscess should be drained surgically. Perforation can be treated conservatively with nothing by mouth (NPO) and antibiotics if isolated but should be repaired via an external cervical approach with closed suction drainage if large. Definitive airway management with prolonged intubation or tracheotomy may be necessary. It is important to note that positive pressure ventilation in the presence of pharyngeal injury can lead to subcutaneous emphysema, pneumomediastinum, or pneumothorax. These complications are discussed in the section on complications of tracheotomy.

Acute Laryngeal Complications

Mucosal Injury

Mucosal injury to the larynx can be superficial, deep, or transmural. Superficial mucosal injury heals spontaneously within days. Minor mucosal injury can result in troublesome bleeding into the airway (3), and attempts at suctioning can precipitate laryngeal edema. Superficial mucosal injury can also lead to vocal fold hematoma, which resolves spontaneously and does not require intervention except for voice rest. Vocal fold hematoma is more commonly left-sided because of right-handed intubators. Deep mucosal injury can result in cartilage exposure with subsequent chondritis. Symptoms include pain, dysphonia, and odynophagia. Patients with severe edema are treated with steroids and antibiotics (9). Airway obstruction requires definitive airway management. Transmural laryngeal injuries should undergo surgical repair via an open, laryngofissure approach. Laryngotracheal separation can occur from intubation in the setting of acute laryngeal trauma. Awake tracheotomy is the preferred method of airway control in this scenario.

Laryngospasm

Inadequate anesthesia on induction can lead to laryngospasm as a response to noxious stimuli anywhere in the body or stimulation of the airway. Aspiration of gastric contents may be an inciting event. Laryngospasm can also occur following *extubation*. The mechanism of airway obstruction is adduction of the true and false vocal folds, foreshortening of the larynx, pressing the preepiglottic soft tissues against the upper surface of the vocal folds, and complete closure of the larynx (10). Because there is no air movement through the larynx, there is no stridor despite obvious respiratory effort. Management consists of immediate removal of the noxious stimulus, proper positioning (i.e., head extended on a flexed neck) and positive pressure bag and mask ventilation. Lightening the anesthetic may restore tone to vocal fold abductors, thus enabling easier ventilation. If ventilation is not possible, a short-acting muscle relaxant such as succinylcholine should be administered, followed by maintenance of ventilation via a mask or endotracheal intubation if necessary. Prevention consists of adequate anesthesia on induction, avoidance of unnecessary stimuli while the patient is lightly anesthetized, and application of topical lidocaine on the vocal folds following endoscopic laryngeal surgery.

Arytenoid Dislocation/Subluxation

The paired arytenoids are irregular pyramidal-shaped cartilages situated on the cricoid cartilage. The base of the arytenoid cartilage is concave and articulates with the cricoid via the cricoarytenoid joint. This synovial joint allows rotation and translation, which are fundamental movements for proper vocal fold function. Inappropriately forceful or blind intubation can result in arytenoid dislocation or subluxation. Overall, however, this is a very uncommon complication. Clinical features include hoarseness after extubation, odynophagia, weak cough, and dysphagia. Diagnosis is made by bedside awake flexible laryngoscopy, revealing an immobile vocal fold, and the injured arytenoid cartilage is tipped anteriorly and medially (i.e., intubation injury) or posteriorly and laterally (i.e., extubation injury). One would also expect to see contractile activity in vocal fold musculature with phonation on stroboscopic evaluation (11). Definitive diagnosis is made by direct laryngoscopy with palpation of the joint. Laryngeal electromyography (EMG) and CT scan may also be helpful (11). The most important differential diagnosis to rule out is vocal fold paralysis from recurrent laryngeal nerve (RLN) injury. In this case the joint would be freely mobile, and treatment is discussed in the section on complications of tracheal surgery. Voice therapy for dysphonia associated with suspected arytenoid dislocation or subluxation may be helpful in some patients (11), although manual endoscopic reduction is indicated as definitive treatment (12).

Recurrent Laryngeal Nerve Injury

The RLN typically enters the larynx between the cricoid and thyroid cartilages near their articulation and travels a short distance submucosally. A cuffed endotracheal tube might compress the nerve in this region. Patients may develop vocal fold paralysis. Vocal fold paralysis can be an acute injury or can occur as a consequence of long-term intubation and inappropriately high cuff pressure. Patients complain of hoarseness and dysphagia postextubation. Principles of diagnosis and management of RLN injury are discussed in the section on tracheal surgery.

Chronic Laryngeal Complications

Laryngeal injury is common following prolonged intubation. After 10 days of intubation, the incidence of erythema and vocal fold ulceration is 94% and 67%, respectively, and most resolve within 8 weeks (13). The mechanism is straightforward: The posterior position of the endotracheal tube in the airway leads to compression of the mucosa overlying the cricoid cartilage, medial aspect of the arytenoid cartilages, interarytenoid region, and subglottis, leading to ischemic necrosis when the force of compression exceeds mucosal capillary perfusion pressure [i.e., >25 mm Hg (14)]. Following prolonged periods of intubation, granulation and fibrosis can result. Contributing factors include presence of a nasogastric (NG) tube, gastroesophageal reflux disease (GERD), diabetes, systemic vascular disease, and multiple intubation attempts (3).

Laryngotracheal Stenosis

Acquired postintubation stenosis is traditionally classified as glottic, subglottic, and tracheal. The incidence following prolonged intubation has been found to be 4% after 5 to 10 days and 14% beyond 10 days (15). Patients are initially asymptomatic but will develop symptoms weeks to months later. Symptoms may include decreased exercise tolerance, dysphonia, stridor, or dyspnea.

Accurate awake flexible endoscopic examination is important to determine laryngeal function and extent of glottic involvement. If there is combined laryngeal and tracheal damage, the larynx should be addressed first (16). Stenosis at the level of glottic larynx is typically posterior, at the level of the posterior vocal folds, vocal processes of the arytenoid cartilages, and interarytenoid region. A classification system for posterior glottic stenosis has been defined that ranges from a relatively simple interarytenoid scar band (Figs. 21-1A and B) to dense posterior commissure scarring involving both cricoarytenoid joints (Fig. 21-1C) (17). Subglottic stenosis occurs at the level of the cricoid cartilage, the narrowest portion of the airway (Fig. 21-2). Because stenoses can occur simultaneously from the larynx to the trachea, it is imperative to endoscopically assess the entire upper respiratory tract prior to surgical intervention. Awake endoscopy in the outpatient clinic is the optimum way to assess vocal fold mobility, while operative laryngoscopy and bronchoscopy under general anesthesia is often employed to determine the level

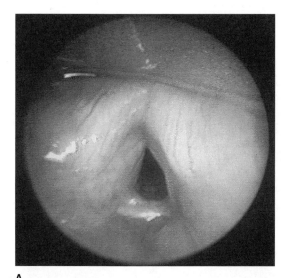

A

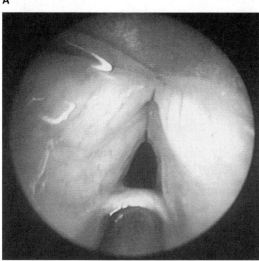

B

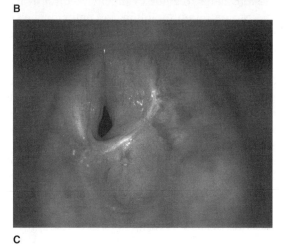

C

Figure 21-1 Two different extremes of posterior glottic stenosis. A relatively simple interarytenoid scar band **(A)** with demonstration of mucosalized tract posterior to scar band by passage of suction tip **(B)**. Severe stenosis with dense posterior commissure scarring **(C)**.

and degree of injury, staging, and to confirm the diagnosis. Endoscopy of the subglottic larynx and trachea using topical anesthesia in the outpatient clinic has also been described as an alternative to operative endoscopy (18). CT scan with fine (2 mm) cuts through the larynx and upper trachea is useful to further delineate the extent of stenosis for diagnosis and surgical planning. Imaging studies, including chest x-ray and lateral neck x-ray, as well as pulmonary function studies, such as flow-volume loops, are imprecise.

Patients without a critical degree of airway compromise can be managed in the elective setting. Initial airway management in the setting of acute respiratory distress includes temporizing measures such as elevation of the head of the bed, cool humidified air, nebulized racemic epinephrine, corticosteroids, and heliox (i.e., a mixture of oxygen and helium that is low in density and flows more efficiently through a constricted airway). Critical airway stenosis that precludes the possibility of intubation is managed with immediate tracheotomy. If critical stenosis is not immediately present, the patient should be transferred to the operating room with an experienced anesthesiologist, otolaryngologist, and operating room staff. Available equipment should include a tracheotomy set, laryngoscope, dilators, rigid bronchoscopes, and endotracheal tubes of various sizes. The bronchoscope can be used to establish an airway rapidly and to dilate the stenotic segment if necessary. If a tracheotomy is performed, it should be done through the area of maximal tracheal damage in order to preserve length for subsequent reconstruction (19). A T-tube can be used to stent the stenotic segment while awaiting surgery.

Definitive surgical management depends on the location and extent of disease.

Glottic stenosis: Posterior glottic stenosis is often a challenging clinical problem. Options for posterior glottic stenosis include directed treatment at the area of stenosis itself, such as simple excision of a scar band, scar excision with endoscopic postcricoid advancement flap (20), open placement of a posterior cartilage graft, or open scar excision via laryngofissure with mucosal graft and postoperative stenting with either a Montgomery T-tube or a solid laryngeal stent for 6 to 8 weeks. Alternatively, enhancement of the airway can be accomplished by reduction or release of glottic tissue that may or may not be directly involved with scar. This includes procedures such as arytenoidectomy or posterior cordotomy.

Subglottic stenosis: If the stenotic segment is <10 mm long, treatment can include endoscopic approaches, such as CO_2 laser excision with a micro-trap door mucosal flap or radial incisions followed by dilation. Additionally, topical mitomycin-C is believed to be a useful adjunct for limiting restenosis (21). When an endoscopic approach is unfavorable, external approaches are warranted, such as cricoid division with cartilage graft or cricotracheal resection and primary thyrotracheal anastomosis.

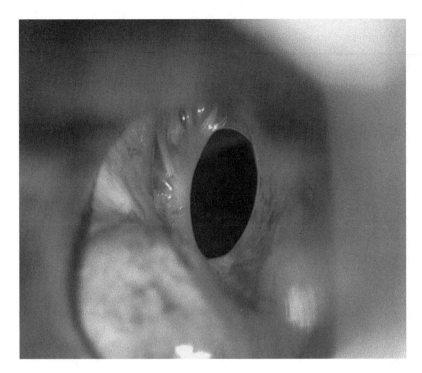

Figure 21-2 Mild short-segment subglottic stenosis.

Tracheal stenosis: Treatment depends on the length of the stenotic segment, whether the stenosis is circumferential or not, and whether it is thin (membranous) or thick (fibrotic). Thin, short-segment stenosis can be managed with endoscopic dilation and CO_2 laser excision. Long-segment stenosis is best managed externally with segmental resection and primary end-to-end anastomosis. The details of tracheal resection for postintubation tracheal stenosis are discussed elsewhere (22). Basic principles include:

1. Accurate preoperative endoscopic evaluation of the anatomy of the stenotic segment
2. Preservation of tracheal blood supply
3. Tension-free anastomosis, which may require one or a combination of various described tracheal mobilization techniques (23)—finger dissection in the pretracheal plane, suprahyoid release, infrahyoid release, hilar release, reimplantation of left mainstem bronchus, and neck flexion
4. Careful patient selection (i.e., no mechanical ventilation, optimization of medical conditions)

Vocal Process Granuloma

Postintubation laryngeal granulomas arise at the medial aspect of the arytenoids, where there is greatest mechanical compression from the endotracheal tube. Terms in the literature used to describe this disease entity include contact ulcer, contact granuloma, and vocal process granuloma.

Patients present with hoarseness after extubation, globus sensation (i.e., sensation of a lump in the throat), or laryngeal pain. Awake laryngoscopy is diagnostic (Figs. 21-3A and B). Typical endoscopic findings include proliferative tissue appearing pale gray to red in color, polypoid, nodular, or ulcerated in shape, and a posterior location. Biopsy should be considered if the appearance is not typical or there is no history of recent intubation.

Thinking of these lesions as wounds rather than as mass lesions helps to guide treatment. Medical treatment includes proton pump inhibitors and antireflux behavior, based on the premise that subclinical reflux can irritate the posterior glottis and delay healing of the granuloma (24). Voice therapy may be useful if voice abuse is felt to be an important contributing factor impeding the healing process (25). These conservative measures usually result in successful resolution. The current otolaryngologic literature supports this nonsurgical approach because of the high rate of recurrence following granuloma excision (25).

Several other treatments are described in the current literature. There is weak evidence supporting the use of antibiotics, systemic steroids, and inhalational steroids (25). Botulinum toxin type A (Botox®; Allergan Inc., Irvine, CA) injection into the thyroarytenoid muscle has demonstrated some efficacy (26). Rationale for this treatment is to reduce the force of vocal fold contact and therefore the trauma to the granuloma. Injection of a large dose, 10 to 15 U, puts the vocal fold at rest and allows the granuloma to heal. Others advocate an additional, smaller dose, 3 to 5 U, injected into the contralateral thyroarytenoid muscle to prevent overcompensation during the healing phase (27). A temporarily weak breathy voice is an expected side effect.

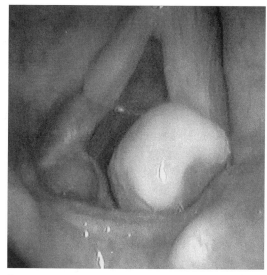

A

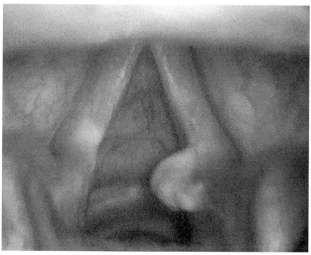

B

Figure 21-3   Bilateral postintubation laryngeal granulomas with large right-sided lesion and smaller left-sided one **(A)**. Unilateral small granuloma **(B)**.

Tracheal Complications

Tracheal Rupture

Intubation can be complicated by penetration of the posterior membranous wall or proximal bronchus, leading to false passage. Penetration can be caused by a long stylet protruding beyond the tip of the endotracheal tube, forceful intubation, or multiple intubation attempts. Clinical manifestations include gastric distension, pneumomediastinum, and pneumothorax. This uncommon complication requires prompt airway control and surgical repair.

Long-term intubation can result in damage to the trachea in a fashion similar to the larynx. Pressure necrosis of the tracheal mucosa leads to ulceration, inflammation, cartilage exposure, granulation, and fibrosis. Pressure injury can manifest as cicatrical scarring of the airway (tracheal stenosis), full-thickness erosion into the esophagus (tracheoesophageal fistula), tracheitis, or loss of cartilaginous support (tracheomalacia). Tracheal stenosis is discussed in the section on laryngeal complications of intubation. Tracheoesophageal fistula (TEF) is discussed in the section on late complications of tracheotomy.

Tracheitis

Mucosal ulceration that becomes full-thickness results in exposed cartilage that can become secondarily infected. Risk factors for tracheitis include patient factors (i.e., advanced age, immunosuppression, diabetes, reflux) and tube factors (i.e., tube too large, cuff pressure too high). Treatment includes broad spectrum antibiotics and pulmonary toilet.

Tracheomalacia

This entity is characterized by abnormal dynamic tracheal collapse secondary to inadequate structural integrity of the tracheal cartilage. Destruction of tracheal cartilage can result from ischemic injury from a cuffed endotracheal tube and from tracheotomy (28). There is distention of the airway with inspiration and collapse with expiration. If severe, tracheomalacia can manifest as airway obstruction. The airway can be stented with positive pressure ventilation or a long endotracheal tube and can be bypassed with a tracheotomy if the affected area is located high in the trachea. Definitive repair consists of tracheal resection with primary anastomosis or tracheoplasty with cartilage graft.

Tube Complications

Cuff Laceration

During the intubation event, the cuff of the endotracheal tube can be lacerated. This manifests as a cuff leak during ventilation. Once recognized, the tube should be changed promptly.

Cuff Leak

A cuff leak can also result from a tube that is too small for the patient's airway. In this scenario the tube should be changed promptly.

Tube Obstruction

Once the patient is successfully intubated, the tube itself could obstruct externally (i.e., patient biting on the tube), internally (i.e., secretions, blood, foreign body), or as a result of the tube twisted on itself. Obstruction manifests as difficulty with ventilation, increased ventilation pressure, decreased breath sounds, hypoxia, and hypercapnia. If the patient is biting on the tube, a bite block should be placed and the level of anesthesia should be increased.

Material within the tube, if present, should be suctioned. Any twists in the tube should be straightened, and the tube should be secured. Intubation of a false passage can manifest in a similar fashion.

Tube Displacement

Either the surgeon or the patient rousing to noxious stimuli could inadvertently extubate the patient. Surgery of the head and neck is prone to this problem because of the need to manipulate these structures during surgery. The following preventive measures are recommended:

1. Arrange the tube and the ventilation circuit so that they are secured in a cephalad direction when the operative field includes both sides of the neck (e.g., thyroid surgery, bilateral neck dissection).
2. Employ nasotracheal intubation for transoral procedures.
3. Secure the tube to the patient's dentition using a circumdental stitch during transoral procedures when nasotracheal intubation is not possible.

Cervical Spine Injury

It is important to recognize patients at risk for developing a cervical spine injury as a consequence of intubation. These include patients with acute head trauma and preexisting conditions (e.g., osteogenesis imperfecta, Down syndrome, Morquio syndrome, lytic bone lesions). If the cervical spine is not cleared by radiology, the neck should be immobilized in a hard collar and in-line manual traction should be applied during intubation. Also useful in such cases are blind nasotracheal intubation, fiberoptic bronchoscopic intubation, or tracheotomy.

Intubation of Incorrect Structure

Incorrect placement of the endotracheal tube into the esophagus, mainstem bronchus, or false passage can result in disastrous consequences. If unrecognized, this complication will lead to hypoxia, brain damage, and death. The anesthesiologist must be able to recognize correct intratracheal tube placement by detection of equal breath sounds, chest rise, tube position at incisors [23 cm for men, 21 cm for women (29)], pulse oximetry, end-tidal CO_2 monitoring, and fiberoptic bronchoscopy.

Special Considerations

Laryngeal Mask Ventilation

This mode of ventilation is commonly used in short elective cases. The main advantage is ease of use. The laryngeal mask is placed at the laryngeal inlet and the cuff is inflated to ensure a seal. If the cuff is overinflated or the mask is placed in a poor position, mucosal injury can occur in the form of abrasions, lacerations, edema, or ulcerations (30). Injury can manifest as hoarseness or airway obstruction.

Jet Ventilation

In endoscopic surgery involving the larynx or trachea, ventilation can be achieved by jet ventilation through a rigid laryngoscope or bronchoscope and obviates the need for translaryngeal intubation. If the vocal folds are not adequately exposed prior to jet ventilation, the jet of air could injure the laryngeal or pharyngeal mucosa, causing edema, hematoma, or laryngospasm. An adequate expiratory pathway must be maintained. If complete expiration does not occur between breaths or if excessive pressure is used, barotrauma can result, manifesting as pneumomediastinum or pneumothorax.

TRACHEOTOMY

The word tracheotomy comes from the Greek and means "cutting the trachea." Asclepiades of Bithynia is credited with performing the first tracheotomy in 100 B.C. The indications for tracheotomy today include upper airway obstruction, long-term ventilation, and need for pulmonary toilet. This procedure can be performed emergently, as in laryngeal trauma, acute airway edema, or obstructing laryngeal neoplasm, or electively, as in critically ill patients who require long-term ventilation.

A retrospective review of 1,130 consecutive open tracheotomies performed over a 10-year period revealed 49 major complications and eight deaths directly attributable to the procedure. The most common complications were tracheal stenosis (21) and hemorrhage (9,31). Although some view tracheotomy as a routine procedure, the significance of the potential complications warrants a detailed understanding. Complications are classified into intraoperative, early postoperative, and late postoperative.

Intraoperative Complications

Damage to Adjacent Structures

As with any surgical procedure, an intimate knowledge of pertinent anatomy is mandatory. During tracheotomy, one must be aware of adjacent structures, including the RLN in the tracheoesophageal groove, the common carotid artery and internal jugular vein laterally, the thyroid isthmus and anterior jugular veins anteriorly, the innominate artery inferiorly, the lung apices inferolaterally, and the esophagus posteriorly.

Recurrent Laryngeal Nerve Injury

The RLN is in the tracheoesophageal groove and therefore should never be injured if dissection is precisely midline. This complication is usually identified when there is dysphonia after plugging the tracheostomy tube or decanulation and is verified with indirect laryngoscopy. Management of RLN injury is discussed in the section on complications of tracheal surgery.

Esophageal Injury

Transmural injury to the posterior wall of the trachea can extend into the esophagus. Management consists of prompt airway stabilization followed by surgical repair. TEF can also be a long-term complication of tracheotomy and is discussed later in this section.

Hemorrhage

Minor hemorrhage can be life-threatening if it interferes with the airway. Bleeding usually originates from the edges of the thyroid isthmus if this structure is divided during the procedure. Depending on surgeon preference, the thyroid isthmus can be divided sharply and suture ligated, carefully divided with monopolar cautery, or left intact. Whatever technique is chosen, it is advisable to check hemostasis at this site prior to incision of the trachea in order to avoid bleeding into the airway and to decrease risk of airway fire associated with the use of cautery in proximity to an open airway (32).

Major hemorrhage from great vessels is life-threatening. Bleeding from the innominate artery is discussed in the section on tracheoinnominate artery fistula. Bleeding from the internal jugular vein or common carotid artery is managed with recognition of the injury, proximal and distal vascular control, and repair or ligation by a surgeon with appropriate expertise.

Airway Fire

Supplemental oxygen may be present in the airway, originating from the ventilator through the endotracheal tube or from mask ventilation if an awake tracheotomy is performed under local anesthesia. In either scenario the surgeon should be aware that an electrical arc from electrocautery, in the presence of supplemental oxygen, can result in airway fire. Airway fire is a devastating but rare complication that has been reported in the literature (32,33). Combustion is easily avoidable with proper precautions. There should be open communication between the anesthesiologist and the surgeon, particularly at the time of surgical entry into the airway. Electrocautery should not be used in the presence of an oxygen-enriched environment and potentially combustible material. In the event of airway fire, supplemental oxygen should be immediately discontinued. All potentially flammable material should be removed from the patient, including the endotracheal tube and surgical drapes. Direct laryngoscopy and rigid bronchoscopy with saline lavage should be performed to extinguish the fire, to reestablish airway control, and to assess damage.

Early Postoperative Complications

The early postoperative period, beginning in the recovery room, is the setting for several important treatable complications. These can be thought of as problems with the tracheotomy tube, problems associated with air outside the tracheobronchial tree, and other problems.

Tube Problems

Cannula Obstruction

The tracheotomy tube itself can be obstructed by blood, secretions, or mucus. This problem is manifested clinically by decreased bilateral breath sounds and hypoxia. Cannula obstruction is easily managed with suction or removal and cleaning of the inner cannula. Prevention of obstruction is achieved by meticulous tracheostomy care, including humidified air and frequent suctioning after instillation of 1–2 cc of sterile saline (3).

Accidental Decannulation

When accidental decannulation occurs, it is important for the surgical staff to replace the tube using the proper introducer and to confirm placement by verifying good ventilation or with flexible endoscopy through the tube. A tube that is blindly placed by well-meaning paramedical personnel can result in false passage. Prevention of decannulation is achieved by securing the tracheostomy tube to the patient with suture and tracheostomy ties. Anticipation is paramount in cases in which recannulation may be difficult, such as in obese patients with abundant cervical subcutaneous tissue, in difficult tracheotomies, and in pediatric cases. In such cases the surgeon can consider placement of guide sutures to assist with recannulation. Nonabsorbable sutures can be placed around adjacent tracheal rings, brought out of the wound on either side of the tracheostomy tube, and taped to the skin. In the event of decannulation, manual tension of these sutures would bring the airway to the skin to permit easy recannulation. The Björk flap is an inferiorly based flap of anterior tracheal wall at the tracheostoma that is sutured to the overlying subcutaneous tissue, and it is another useful technique in cases with the potential for difficult recannulation (34).

False Passage

If the tracheotomy tube is in the subcutaneous tissue between the skin and the trachea, consequences include subcutaneous emphysema, pneumomediastinum, pneumothorax, and hypoventilation (i.e., loss of airway). This problem may occur with initial tube placement or by retraction of the distal end of the tube with patient movement or tube manipulation. Management consists of prompt recognition, reestablishment of the airway, and treatment of the complication. In the early postoperative period, the tracheotomy tract is not well formed, and therefore, recannulation should be performed with appropriate lighting, patient positioning, and equipment.

Air Outside the Tracheobronchial Tree

As a consequence of the surgery itself, positive pressure ventilation into a false passage, or injury to pleura, air can dissect into various tissue planes, resulting in subcutaneous emphysema, pneumomediastinum, or pneumothorax. These complications are uncommon (0.34%) (31). They share similar mechanisms—excessive dissection of tissue planes, cannula blockage, assisted ventilation with excessive pressure (35), excessive coughing against a mechanical ventilator, rupture of subpleural bleb, and discrepancy between size of tracheal opening and size of cannula. Prevention consists of avoiding unnecessary paratracheal dissection, creating an opening into the trachea that is similar in size to that of the cannula, and avoiding tight closure of the tracheotomy site. We do not close the surgical wound around the cannula.

Subcutaneous Emphysema

This complication is heralded by the presence of neck swelling and crepitus. One must first exclude pneumomediastinum and pneumothorax. Management includes removal of skin sutures, replacement of cannula with larger size, insertion of a cuffed tube, adequate sedation, and ventilation of the patient.

Pneumomediastinum and Pneumothorax

Management includes observation, chest tube placement, adequate sedation, or reduction in positive end-expiratory pressure (PEEP).

Other Problems

In patients with chronic upper airway obstruction, tracheotomy results in immediate relief of obstruction but can also result in postobstructive pulmonary edema. This is treated by mechanical ventilation with PEEP and appropriate diuresis.

Late Postoperative Complications

Long-term complications of tracheotomy include stenosis and fistulae. These problems are typically related to direct pressure necrosis at the cuff site (36). Initial mucosal ulceration leads to cartilage exposure, infection, and necrosis. A fibrotic stricture or full-thickness posterior perforation into the esophagus or anterior perforation into the innominate artery can occur (19). Tracheostomy tube cuffs should be kept between 20 and 25 mm Hg because pressures above 25 mm Hg have been shown to occlude submucosal tracheal capillaries (14). Since the advent of high volume, low pressure cuffs, and specially designed tracheotomy tubes for unusual neck anatomy, these complications have decreased.

Tracheal Stenosis

This section will focus on tracheal stenosis as it relates to tracheotomy. The diagnosis and management of tracheal stenosis following intubation are discussed in the section on complications of intubation.

Fortunately, tracheal stenosis following tracheotomy is a rare complication. One study of 2,000 tracheotomies demonstrated the incidence of tracheal stenosis to be 0.5% (37). Technical factors in tracheotomy contributing to development of tracheal stenosis include excessively large opening into the trachea, neglected infection or chondritis, and excessive traction or movement of the tracheotomy tube. Some authors also cite specific tracheostoma techniques (i.e., inferiorly based Björk flap, excision of window, and H-shaped window) as risk factors for development of tracheal stenosis (38). Tracheal stenosis following tracheotomy can be classified anatomically into suprastomal (subglottic), stomal, and infrastomal. Some patients present early, with granulation tissue at the tip of the cannula. Granulation occurs as a result of friction of the tip against the tracheal mucosa. Most patients present following decannulation. Complaints include shortness of breath, exertional dyspnea, cough, or biphasic stridor and respiratory distress if severe. Symptoms may be exacerbated with a viral respiratory illness and may mimic bronchitis, asthma, or pneumonia.

Fistulae

Erosion of the tracheotomy tube into an adjacent structure is a dreaded, potentially life-threatening, and preventable complication. The tube can erode anteriorly into the innominate artery (tracheoinnominate artery fistula) and posteriorly into the esophagus (TEF), and decannulation can result in persistent tracheocutaneous fistula if the wound does not heal completely. Mechanisms include a tracheotomy that is too low (i.e., below the third tracheal ring), a cuff that is inflated too high, and local wound healing problems (i.e., infection, irradiation, and tube movement during mechanical ventilation).

Tracheoesophageal Fistula

The incidence of this uncommon but highly morbid complication is 0.5% (39). TEF is life-threatening because of contamination of the airway and interference with nutrition. TEF is commonly associated with tracheal stenosis since it shares a common pathophysiology. Patients present with a dramatic increase in tracheal secretions, resembling enteral feedings. Coughing may follow oral swallowing. Gastric distension may occur secondary to ventilated air into the stomach. Initial diagnosis is made with endoscopy through the stoma and can be confirmed with methylene blue dye swallow and observation of dye in the trachea. Barium swallow is diagnostic. If the patient is ventilated, one should advance a low-pressure cuffed endotracheal tube below the fistula site and perform gastrostomy for gastric drainage and jejunostomy for enteral nutrition (39). There is evidence that TEFs do not close spontaneously (19). Therefore, management is surgical. Principles of surgical management include multilayered repair with interposition of muscle between the esophagus and trachea.

Tracheoinnominate Artery Fistula

Tracheoinnominate artery fistula (TIF) is a rare, often fatal complication that occurs when a tracheostomy tube erodes anteriorly into the posterior wall of the innominate artery. TIF can also occur as a consequence of tracheal resection and tracheal stenting. Incidence is reported to be 0.3% following tracheotomy and most occur between 1 and 2 weeks postoperatively (40). The mortality rate is 75% (41). Survival depends on prompt recognition and management. Prevention, through the use of the following procedures, is vital:

1. Avoid placing the tracheostoma too low, ideally between the second and third tracheal rings.
2. Be aware of a high innominate artery. One should advocate routine palpation for this possibility intraoperatively.
3. Use a proper sized pliable nonreactive tracheostomy tube whose cuff pressure will not exceed 25 mm Hg (14).
4. Avoid tight closure of the tracheostomy wound to prevent local contamination. Tracheotomy should be performed through a small cutaneous incision without subsequent wound closure.
5. Use flexible connection tubing to the ventilator supported by an adjustable arm to prevent extraneous movement and angulation.
6. Use a flexible endoscope (i.e., nasopharyngoscope or pediatric bronchoscope) to ensure proper position of the tube if position is equivocal.

About 50% of patients with TIF develop a sentinel bleed—that is, a history of minor self-limited bleeding prior to presentation (42). Therefore, the surgeon must be mindful of the possibility of TIF in the setting of delayed posttracheotomy bleeding. In the case of a sentinel bleed, we recommend endoscopy through the tracheostomy tube to examine the distal airway and then endoscopy through the stoma during gradual withdrawal of the tracheostomy tube over the scope to more carefully assess the anterior tracheal wall for erosion. Angiography is not helpful because of time constraints and limited accuracy (43). If imminent TIF is suspected, preparations should be made to go to the operating room promptly by obtaining large bore intravenous access, cross matching blood, and consulting surgical colleagues capable of performing median sternotomy with major vascular repair. Once in the operating room, more detailed endoscopy under general anesthesia can be performed to confirm the diagnosis.

Bleeding from a TIF can occur without a recognized sentinel bleed. In this case immediate bedside management is crucial because of the risk of imminent exsanguination. Tamponade with hyperinflation of the tracheostomy tube cuff is a useful temporizing maneuver. If this fails, the airway should be controlled with an orotracheal tube from above and advanced distal to the bleeding site while the tracheostomy tube is removed. Digital pressure through the stoma against the manubrium of the sternum will tamponade the bleeding source 90% of the time (42). This maneuver can be performed either through the lumen of the trachea or in the pretracheal fascial plane (44). Once the airway has been stabilized in this fashion, the patient should be brought rapidly to the OR for definitive management.

Definitive surgical management of TIF is obtained via a median sternotomy to achieve proximal and distal control of the innominate artery. An upper partial sternotomy that is carried laterally into the right third intercostal space has been described to prevent sternal wound contamination by tracheal secretions (43). The innominate artery is exposed proximal and distal to the TIF. If an aberrant left carotid artery is found, proximal control is obtained distal to its takeoff. Review of the literature reveals that primary repair of the damaged artery is not recommended because of the high failure rate (43). Definitive management should be individualized and may include revascularization or resection of the fistulous segment and coverage with vascularized omentum. The reader is directed to a recent review for a discussion of management options and controversies (45).

Tracheocutaneous Fistula

This is an uncommon complication that results from epithelialization between tracheal mucosa and skin (Fig. 21-4). Normally upon decannulation, the tracheostomy wound closes secondarily within days. Failure of closure results in tracheocutaneous fistula and is seen in patients with prolonged tracheostomy tube placement, poor nutrition, immunosuppression, radiation therapy, and local infection. Clinical manifestations include poor cosmesis, difficult phonation, and local skin irritation from secretions. Single-stage surgical closure has been described whereby a peristomal circular incision is made, creating an epidermal flap that is inverted in order to line the tracheal surface, and the external skin is closed primarily (46). Other authors emphasize the importance of interposing vascularized tissue, such as strap muscles, between the tracheal closure and the overlying skin (47).

Granuloma

Granulation tissue can occur anywhere along the tracheostomy tract, commonly on the anterior tracheal wall near the superior aspect of the stoma. If granulation is broad-based and is not causing airway obstruction, observation is acceptable. Medical management with meticulous stoma care and silver nitrate cautery is also useful. If granulation tissue is pedunculated and causing airway

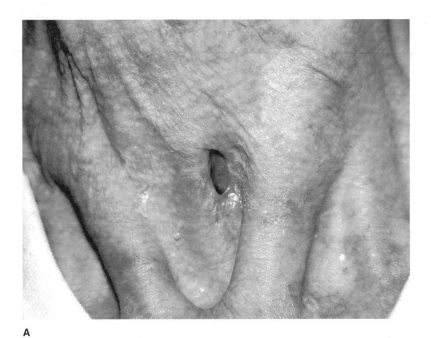

A

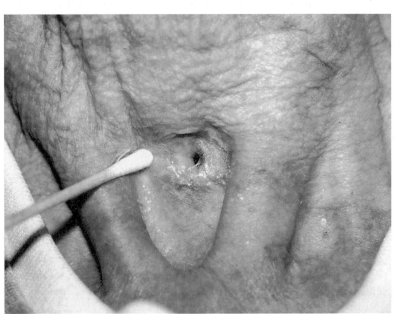

B

Figure 21-4 Tracheocutaneous fistula demonstrating epithelialized tract between tracheal mucosa and skin.

compromise, immediate removal with cupped forceps and cauterization with silver nitrate is warranted.

SPECIAL CONSIDERATIONS

Pediatric Tracheotomy

The incidence of complications following tracheotomy in the pediatric population is higher than in adults. The complication rate in the literature varies considerably, ranging from 7.8% to 77% (31). A recent report by Carr et al. presents a

detailed analysis. The authors found a complication rate of 11% in the early postoperative period (i.e., before the first tube change) and 63% in the late postoperative period (i.e., after the first tube change) (48). In this study the most common complications were stomal granuloma (26%), tracheitis (18%), and aspiration pneumonia (9%), and serious complications were tube obstruction (9%) and accidental decannulation (6%). The reported incidence of tracheal stenosis ranges from 1% to 12% in the literature (49). The incidence of pneumothorax and pneumomediastinum is also quite varied in the literature, ranging from 0% to 60% (49). The tracheotomy-related mortality rate varies from

0.7% (48) to 6% (50). The reason for the high reported rates of complications in children is intuitive—children have more pliable soft tissues of the neck, smaller anatomy, and a tendency to move against a ventilator. Review of the pertinent literature identified the following considerations with pediatric tracheotomy (48,50,51):

1. Vertical skin incision—to permit easier dissection and visualization
2. Guide sutures on the trachea—to permit safer recannulation in case of accidental decannulation
3. Postoperative chest x-ray—to rule out pneumothorax and pneumomediastinum
4. Well-trained paramedical personnel, family, and appropriate use of equipment and monitors
5. Postoperative surveillance bronchoscopies at regular intervals (i.e., every 6 months) or whenever indicated with a change in clinical status (51)

Percutaneous Tracheotomy

The concept of percutaneous tracheotomy originated in 1969 (52) and has been recently popularized (53). Percutaneous tracheotomy has gained popularity because it is a bedside procedure that is relatively brief and inexpensive and requires no operating room time. There are numerous techniques of percutaneous tracheotomy, including progressive dilational technique, nonprogressive dilational technique, and translaryngeal tracheotomy (54). These techniques have been described with or without endoscopic guidance. The problem of accidental decannulation can be troublesome to deal with because there is no formal opening in the trachea; therefore recannulation can be difficult and reintubation may be necessary. A complication unique to this procedure is misguided wire placement, which can be paratracheal, mediastinal, or submucosal.

A recent meta-analysis compared open tracheotomy with percutaneous tracheotomy (55). We have concluded that percutaneous tracheotomy is associated with a higher prevalence of perioperative complications (10% vs. 3%) and open tracheotomy is associated with a higher prevalence of postoperative complications (10% vs. 7%). The rate of major complications was more prevalent in percutaneous tracheotomy, including perioperative death (0.44% vs. 0.03%) and serious cardiorespiratory events (0.33% vs. 0.06%). This trend remained even when comparing endoscopically guided progressive dilational percutaneous tracheotomy to open tracheotomy. All studies were retrospective in design, and a prospective randomized trial is needed to validate these findings. On the basis of this literature and direct clinical experience, the following considerations with percutaneous tracheotomy are recommended:

1. The procedure should be performed by surgeons capable of doing open tracheotomy.
2. Endoscopic guidance is obligatory.
3. Absolute contraindication—emergency airway.

4. Relative contraindications—obesity, enlarged thyroid, coagulopathy, although some authors suggest that this is safe in coagulopathic or heparinized patients because small vessels are compressed rather than transected or cauterized (56).

Cricothyroidotomy

In 1921, Chevalier Jackson published a landmark paper condemning cricothyroidotomy (57). He stated that "high tracheotomy should never be done" because of the high observed rate of laryngeal stenosis (57). This doctrine remained unchallenged until 1976, when Brantigan and Grow published a large series of cardiothoracic surgery patients who underwent cricothyroidotomy for elective airway management (58). Cricothyroidotomy is appropriate in the emergency airway situation because it is rapid and can be life-saving. The controversies are (i) whether cricothyroidotomy should be converted to formal tracheostomy for long-term airway management and (ii) whether elective cricothyroidotomy should be performed.

Jackson reviewed 200 cases of chronic laryngeal stenosis and found that 158 cases were due to "high tracheotomy" (57). Not all cases were true cricothyroidotomies, as most involved division of the cricoid cartilage and 32 cases were performed through the cricothyroid membrane *and* thyroid cartilage. Many patients had an underlying inflammatory disorder of the larynx that may have predisposed to the development of stenosis. Jackson reasoned that the subglottis is the narrowest segment of the airway and that the subglottic mucosa is intolerant to trauma. He therefore advocated "low tracheotomy" below the second tracheal ring in order to prevent laryngeal stenosis. Brantigan and Grow challenged this doctrine in their review of 655 thoracic surgery patients who underwent elective cricothyroidotomy. They observed no cases of chronic subglottic stenosis but found five cases of chronic tracheal stenosis at the cuff site, all requiring tracheal resection. They cite absence of cross-contamination of median sternotomy wounds, simplicity, and safety as the basis of their recommendation that routine elective cricothyroidotomy is appropriate. However, follow-up was limited (i.e., obtained in many cases with telephone calls to patients or referring physicians) and data on vocal quality was lacking. Subsequently, several studies demonstrated variable rates of subglottic stenosis, ranging from 1% to 48%. A meta-analysis of 875 patients who underwent cricothyroidotomy revealed a 4% overall incidence of subglottic stenosis. The authors demonstrated that if patients with contraindications to cricothyroidotomy are excluded, this incidence drops to 1% (59). Contraindications include prolonged endotracheal intubation at 7 days or greater (59), coexisting laryngeal infection (57,60), and upper airway difficulties after endotracheal intubation. Other risk factors for subglottic stenosis following elective cricothyroidotomy include prolonged cannulation beyond 30 days (61) and patients under the age of 18 (59,62). This seemingly low incidence of subglottic stenosis contrasts with a 0.5% incidence of tracheal stenosis following tracheotomy (37). Subglottic stenosis is significantly more difficult to manage than tracheal stenosis and should therefore be prevented whenever possible.

The effect of cricothyroidotomy on voice has been neglected in much of the early, nonotolaryngologic literature on cricothyroidotomy complications. Several studies have documented a high incidence of voice disturbance following cricothyroidotomy, ranging from 40% to 75% (60,63,64). The mechanism involves (i) scarring of the cricothyroid membrane, which limits the pivoting of the thyroid cartilage on the cricoid cartilage that is necessary to increase length and tension of the vocal folds, and (ii) glottic scarring, as a consequence of the close proximity (10 mm) of the true vocal folds with the upper limit of the cricothyroid membrane (59).

In summary, subglottic stenosis can occur following cricothyroidotomy, even in carefully selected patients, and vocal dysfunction is a common complication that is difficult to manage. We recommend that (i) cricothyroidotomy is indicated in the emergency airway setting, (ii) emergency cricothyroidotomy should be expeditiously converted to a formal tracheotomy in an elective setting in order to limit vocal dysfunction and prevent subglottic stenosis, and (iii) elective cricothyroidotomy for long-term airway management *may* be indicated in cases in which it is crucial to maintain separation between the cervical wound and the median sternotomy wound and is contraindicated in patients who have been intubated for 7 days or longer, patients with coexisting laryngeal pathology, occupational and professional voice users, and patients under the age of 18 (59).

TRACHEAL SURGERY

Indications for tracheal resection include primary tracheal tumors, tumors invading the trachea, and stenosis. The most common indication for tracheal resection and reconstruction is postintubation tracheal stenosis (45); therefore, most complications of tracheal surgery can be avoided by prevention of tracheal stenosis. Prevention is achieved by atraumatic intubation technique, proper selection of endotracheal tube, proper inflation of a low-pressure cuff, and avoidance of long-term endotracheal intubation. However, when tracheal resection is indicated, the surgeon must be aware of potential adverse outcomes, their management, and their prevention. Tracheal resection and primary anastomosis is highly successful. A recent series of 23 cases of acquired upper airway stenosis treated with segmental resection and primary reanastomosis had a decannulation rate of 96% (65). The complication rate of tracheal surgery has been found to increase as the anastomotic level rises (45).

Intraoperative Complications

Recurrent Laryngeal Nerve Injury

Given its proximity to the trachea, the RLN is prone to injury during tracheal surgery. This is particularly true in the upper cervical trachea and near the laryngotracheal junction. Meticulous surgical technique and knowledge of pertinent anatomy are the most important safeguards to lessen the likelihood of injury.

The primary clinical manifestations of unilateral RLN injury are a paralyzed vocal fold and dysphonia (66). Some patients will also have dysphagia and signs of aspiration. Airway compromise, usually with stridor due to bilateral vocal fold paralysis, is the hallmark of bilateral RLN injury.

Treatment options for unilateral RLN injury include the nonsurgical alternatives of observation or voice therapy. Surgical treatment options include vocal fold medialization with injection laryngoplasty or laryngeal framework surgery, or laryngeal reinnervation (67). The ideal treatment option, able to restore physiologic movements, is not yet in hand.

Expectant management is appropriate in circumstances where the paralysis may be temporary, such as a neuropraxia due to traction injury or when the symptom severity does not mandate treatment. When observing for possible spontaneous recovery, a period of 6 months to 1 year is generally advocated.

Voice therapy by a speech pathologist should be considered to help ameliorate symptoms during a period when spontaneous recovery is possible, in poor surgical candidates, or for patients whose symptoms are toward the less severe side of the spectrum. Vocal therapy may also be employed as an adjunctive treatment either preoperatively or postoperatively in surgically treated patients.

Although surgical medialization of a paralyzed vocal fold does not restore normal dynamic laryngeal physiology, it is typically a very effective geometrical solution for incomplete glottic closure (Fig. 21-5). Medialization allows the contralateral, normal vocal fold to make better contact with the paralyzed vocal fold during phonation and deglutition.

Injection laryngoplasty is an endoscopic technique in which a substance is injected into the paralyzed vocal fold in order to add bulk and medialize the free edge. A temporary substance, such as a Gelfoam (Upjohn, Kalamazoo, MI), can be used to relieve symptoms when spontaneous recovery of mobility is still possible. A wide variety of other injectable substances of longer duration are also employed, with the search for an ideal permanent injectable substance continuing.

Open laryngeal framework surgery is frequently used to treat patients with unilateral vocal fold paralysis, and the medialization thyroplasty or type-I thyroplasty is the most commonly employed framework procedure. This operation involves precise opening of the thyroid cartilage lateral to the paralyzed vocal fold and placement of an

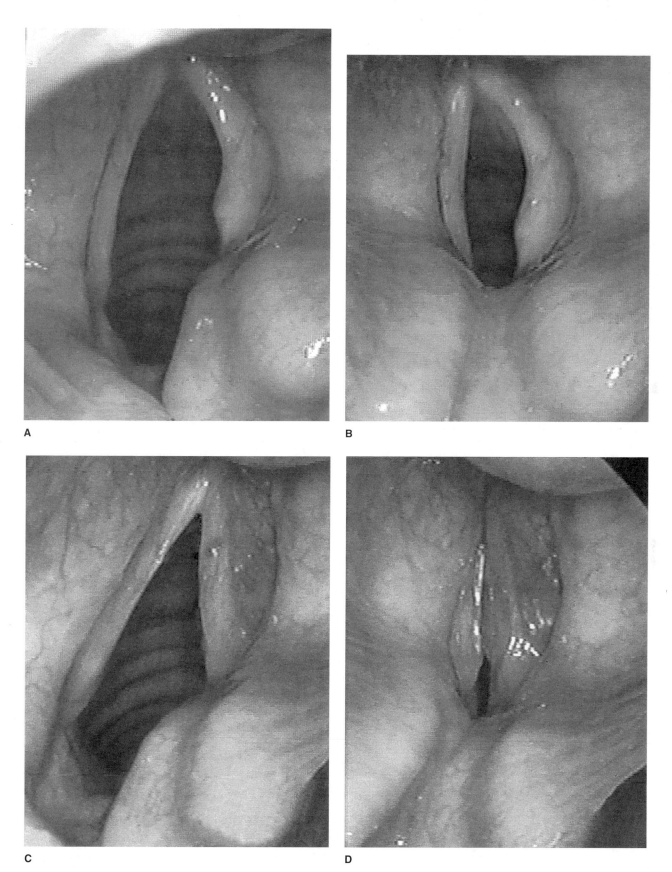

Figure 21-5   Patient with unilateral vocal fold paralysis due to right recurrent laryngeal nerve (RLN) injury during inspiration **(A)** and phonation **(B)** prior to laryngeal framework surgery with type-I thyroplasty. Same patient during inspiration **(C)** and phonation **(D)** post-surgical medialization of the paralyzed vocal fold.

appropriate implant into the paraglottic space (68). The procedure is typically performed under local anesthesia in order to assess voice with varying degrees of medialization to determine the optimum geometry. Options for graft material include Silastic, Gore-Tex (W. L. Gore & Associates, Inc. Flagstaff, AZ), and various prefabricated kits. Efficacy of type-I thyroplasty has been demonstrated using a variety of outcome measures (69,70).

Currently employed laryngeal reinnervation techniques, particularly the ansa cervicalis to RLN nerve transfer (71), can improve voice by restoring bulk and tone to vocal fold musculature (72). They do not, however, restore physiologic movement. Current research in laryngeal reinnervation includes exploring the potential for gene therapy in the treatment of laryngeal paralysis (73,74).

Management of bilateral RLN injury usually requires surgical intervention to establish an adequate airway. Assurance of airway patency is done acutely by intubation followed by tracheotomy or by tracheotomy alone. Once a stable surgical airway has been established, decisions about long-term management can be made. In the setting of possible temporary paralysis, observation is appropriate. If permanent bilateral paralysis exists, tracheotomy can be used as the long-term airway management strategy. Alternatively, procedures to enhance the glottic airway, such as posterior cordotomy or arytenoidectomy, can be performed (75). Informed consent for these procedures must include the knowledge that a degree of voice compromise is an expected trade-off for airway improvement.

Superior Laryngeal Nerve Injury

Injury to the sensory internal branches of this nerve, particularly a bilateral injury, may result in dysphagia and aspiration. The internal branches of the superior laryngeal nerve (SLN) enter the larynx via the thyrohyoid membrane and are in the surgical field when hyoid releasing maneuvers are employed to enhance tracheal reanastomosis. Injury to the external motor branches of the SLN, which innervate the cricothyroid muscles, results in loss of upper vocal range. Voice and swallowing therapy are the primary treatment strategies.

Major Hemorrhage

Major hemorrhage during tracheal surgery is usually from injury to the innominate artery. It is important to secure the airway emergently by placement of a cuffed endotracheal tube at or distal to the bleeding site. Details of management of innominate artery bleeding are discussed in the section on complications of tracheotomy.

Postoperative Complications

Complications following tracheal surgery can be thought of as problems at the site of the anastomosis (i.e., dehiscence, granulation, tracheal stenosis, tracheoinnominate artery fistula) and problems that coexist with the acquired tracheal stenosis (i.e., tracheomalacia, laryngeal dysfunction). In general, prevention of these complications is possible with the following considerations:

1. Accurate preoperative assessment of laryngeal function
2. Accurate endoscopic and radiographic assessment of the extent of stenosis, tracheal anatomy, and presence of associated tracheomalacia
3. Minimizing tension on the anastomosis; appropriate use of releasing maneuvers
4. Avoidance of circumferential tracheal dissection in order to preserve blood supply
5. Awareness of predisposing conditions such as mechanical ventilation, prior radiation therapy, immunosuppression, Wegener granulomatosis, and relapsing polychondritis
6. Multidisciplinary approach, including otolaryngology, thoracic surgery, and anesthesiology
7. Prevention of acquired postintubation stenosis by atraumatic intubation technique, proper selection of endotracheal tube, proper inflation of low-pressure cuff, and avoidance of long-term intubation

Dehiscence

Excessive tension on the anastomosis can result in dehiscence. This results from improper mobilization of the trachea or excessive resection. Clinically, acute dehiscence is manifested by subcutaneous emphysema. Treatment is emergent, consisting of rigid bronchoscopy, reexploration and repair. The repair can be reinforced with a local muscle flap.

Accurate identification of extent of disease and proper preoperative planning prevents this complication. If a long segment of trachea needs to be resected, the surgeon must be aware of techniques to increase mobilization of the larynx and trachea. These include finger dissection in the pretracheal plane, suprahyoid release, infrahyoid release, hilar release, reimplantation of left mainstem bronchus, and neck flexion (23). In the pediatric population, a novel technique termed slide tracheoplasty has been described to manage long-segment congenital tracheal stenosis (76).

Granulation

This is an uncommon complication of tracheal surgery. In a large series of tracheal resections, five out of 317 cases (1.6%) developed granulation tissue at the site of the anastomosis when an absorbable suture material was used (45). When significant granulation occurs, treatment may consist of antibiotics, local injection of corticosteroids such as triamcinolone, and endoscopic removal.

Tracheal Stenosis

Prevention consists of ensuring a tension-free anastomosis and complete removal of all inflamed tissue adjacent to the stenotic segment. Methods of tracheal release are discussed in the section on dehiscence. Management of tracheal stenosis is discussed in the section on complications of intubation.

Tracheoinnominate Artery Fistula

This rare, dreaded complication is discussed in the section on complications of tracheotomy. Predisposing factors following tracheal surgery include the presence of a dehiscent anastomotic suture line adjacent to the innominate artery, presence of a low tracheotomy, or local infection. Interposition of viable tissue (i.e., strap muscle, thymus, pericardium, or omentum) between the anastomotic suture line and the innominate artery is recommended (43).

Tracheomalacia

Tracheomalacia that exists preoperatively should be identified at the time of endoscopy and should be included in the resected tracheal segment. If tracheomalacia develops following tracheal surgery, treatment options include reresection of the diseased trachea or exteriorization of the airway and stenting with a tracheostomy tube or a T-tube (45).

Chronic Aspiration

This may occur as a result of unrecognized coexisting laryngeal dysfunction, RLN injury, or laryngeal releasing maneuvers. Coexisting laryngeal dysfunction must be corrected initially, if possible, before tracheal surgery is attempted.

REFERENCES

1. Heffner JE. The role of tracheotomy in weaning. *Chest* 2001; 120(6):477S–481S.
2. McCulloch TM, Bishop MJ. Complications of translaryngeal intubation. *Clin Chest Med* 1991;12(3):507–521.
3. Loh KS, Irish JC. Traumatic complications of intubation and other airway management procedures. *Anesthesiol Clin North Am* 2002;20(4):953–969.
4. Coe TR, Human M. The peri-operative complications of nasal intubation: a comparison of nostril side. *Anaesthesia* 2001;56(5): 447–484.
5. Weymuller EA, Bishop MJ. Problems associated with prolonged intubation in the geriatric patient. *Otolaryngol Clin North Am* 1990;23:1057–1074.
6. Schultz-Coulon HJ. Repair of postintubational lesions of the cartilaginous nose in infants—sometimes a surgical problem. *Int J Pediatr Otorhinolaryngol* 1984;7(2):119–131.
7. Pettett G, Merenstein GB. Nasal erosion with nasotracheal intubation [Letter]. *J Pediatr* 1975;87(1):149–150.
8. Lockhart P, Feldbau EV, Gabel RA. Dental complications during and after tracheal intubation. *J Am Dent Assoc* 1986;112: 480–483.
9. Weymuller EA. Prevention and management of intubation injury of the larynx and trachea. *Am J Otolaryngol* 1992;13:139–144.
10. Tyler EP. Complications of anesthesia for otolaryngology—head and neck surgery. In: Weissler MC, Pillsbury HC, eds. *Complications of head and neck surgery*. New York: Thieme Medical Publishers; 1995:371 388.
11. Sataloff RT, Bough IB, Spiegel JR. Arytenoid dislocation: diagnosis and treatment. *Laryngoscope* 1994;104:1353–1361.
12. Hoffman HT, Brunberg JA, Winter P, et al. Arytenoid subluxation: diagnosis and treatment. *Ann Otol Rhinol Laryngol* 1991; 100:1–9.
13. Santos P, Afrassiabi A, Weymuller EA. Prospective studies evaluating the standard endotracheal tube and a prototype endotracheal tube. *Ann Otol Rhinol Laryngol* 1989;98:935–940.
14. Heffner JE, Hess D. Tracheotomy management in the chronically ventilated patient. *Clin Chest Med* 2001;22(1):55–69.
15. Stauffer JL, Olson DE, Petty TL. Complications and consequences of endotracheal intubation and tracheotomy: a prospective study of 150 critically ill adult patients. *Am J Med* 1981; 70:65–76.
16. Grillo HC. Treatment of airway complications. *Appl Cardiopulm Pathophysiol* 1989(3):147–159.
17. Bogdasarian RS, Olson NR. Posterior glottic laryngeal stenosis. *Otolaryngol Head Neck Surg* 1980;88:765–772.
18. Hogikyan ND. Transnasal endoscopic examination of the subglottis and trachea using topical anesthesia in the otolaryngology clinic. *Laryngoscope* 1999;109:1170–1173.
19. Wood DE, Mathisen DJ. Late complications of tracheotomy. *Clin Chest Med* 1991;12(3):597–609.
20. Goldenberg AN. Endoscopic postcricoid advancement flap for posterior glottic stenosis. *Laryngoscope* 2000;110:482–485.
21. Rahbar R, Shapshay SM, Healy GB. Mitomycin: effects on laryngeal and tracheal stenosis, benefits, and complications. *Ann Otol Rhinol Laryngol* 2001;110:1–6.
22. Wain JC. Postintubation tracheal stenosis. *Chest Surg Clin N Orth Am* 2003;13:231–246.
23. Heitmiller RF. Tracheal release maneuvers. *Chest Surg Clin N Orth Am* 2003;13:201–210.
24. Koufman JA. The otolaryngologic manifestations of gastroesophageal reflux disease (GERD): a clinical investigation of 225 patients using ambulatory 24-hour pH monitoring and an experimental investigation of the role of acid and pepsin in the development of laryngeal injury. *Laryngoscope* 1991;101:1–64.
25. Hoffman HT, Overholt E, Karnell M, et al. Vocal process granulomas. *Head Neck* 2001;23:1061–1074.
26. Nasri S, Sercarz JA, McAlpin T, et al. Treatment of vocal fold granuloma using botulinum toxin type A. *Laryngoscope* 1995;105(6): 585–588.
27. Berke GS. Voice disorder and phonosurgery. In: Bailey BJ, Calhoun KH, eds. *Head and neck surgery—otolaryngology*, 2nd ed. Philadelphia, PA: Lippincott–Raven Publishers; 1998.
28. Le BT, Eyre JM, Holmgren EP, et al. A tracheostomy complication resulting from acquired tracheomalacia: case report. *J Trauma* 2001;50:120–123.
29. Owen RL, Cheney FW. Endobronchial intubation: a preventable complication. *Anesthesiology* 1987;67:255–257.
30. Briacombe J, Holyoake L, Keller C, et al. Pharyngolaryngeal, neck, and jaw discomfort after anesthesia with the face mask and laryngeal mask airway at high and low cuff volumes in males and females. *Anesthesiology* 2000;93(1):23–31.
31. Goldenberg D, Ari EG, Golz A, et al. Tracheotomy complications: a retrospective study of 1130 cases. *Otolaryngol Head Neck Surg* 2000;123:495–500.
32. Rogers ML, Nickalls RWD, Brackenbury ET, et al. Airway fire during tracheostomy: prevention strategies for surgeons and anaesthetists. *Ann R Coll Surg Engl* 2001;83:376–380.
33. Ng J, Hartigan PM. Airway fire during tracheostomy: should we extubate? *Anesthesiology* 2003;98(5):1303.
34. Malata CM, Foo IT, Simpson KH, et al. An audit of Bjork flap tracheostomies in head and neck plastic surgery. *Br J Oral Maxillofac Surg* 1996;34(1):42–46.
35. Berg LF, Mafee MF, Campos M. Mechanisms of pneumothorax following tracheal intubation. *Ann Otol Rhinol Laryngol* 1988;97: 500–505.
36. Andrews MJ, Pearson FG. The incidence and pathogenesis of tracheal injury following cuffed tube tracheostomy with assisted ventilation: analysis of a two-year prospective study. *Ann Surg* 1971;173:249–263.
37. Chew JY, Cantrell RW. Tracheostomy. *Arch Otolaryngol Head Neck Surg* 1972;96:538–545.
38. Fry TL, Jones RO, Fischer ND, et al. Comparisons of tracheostomy incisions in a pediatric model. *Ann Otol Rhinol Laryngol* 1985;94: 450–453.
39. Reed MF, Mathisen DJ. Tracheoesophageal fistula. *Chest Surg Clin N Orth Am* 2003;13:271–289.
40. Grillo HC, Donahue DM, Mathisen DJ, et al. Postintubation tracheal stenosis: treatment and results. *J Thorac Cardiovasc Surg* 1995;109:486–493.
41. Grillo HC, Mathisen DJ. Cervical exenteration. *Ann Thorac Surg* 1990;49:401–408.

42. Jones JW, Reynolds M, Hewitt RL, et al. Tracheo-innominate artery erosion: successful surgical management of a devastating complication. *Ann Surg* 1976;184:194–204.

43. Allan JS, Wright C. Tracheoinnominate fistula: diagnosis and management. *Chest Surg Clin N Orth Am* 2003;13:331–341.

44. Utley JR, Singer MM, Roe BB, et al. Definitive management of innominate artery hemorrhage complicating tracheostomy. *JAMA* 1972;220:577–579.

45. Lanuti M, Mathisen DJ. Management of complications of tracheal surgery. *Chest Surg Clin N Orth Am* 2003;13:385–397.

46. Lawson DW, Grillo HC. Closure of persistent tracheal stomas. *Surg Gynecol Obstet* 1970;130:995–996.

47. Bishop JB, Bostwick J, Nahai F. Persistent tracheostomy stoma. *Am J Surg* 1980;140:709–710.

48. Carr MM, Poje CP, Kingston L, et al. Complications in pediatric tracheostomies. *Laryngoscope* 2001;111:1925–1928.

49. Kremer B, Botos-Kremer A, Eckel HE, et al. Indications, complications and surgical techniques for pediatric tracheostomies—an update. *J Pediatr Surg* 2002;37:1556–1562.

50. Rodgers BM, Rooks JJ, Talbert JL. Pediatric tracheostomy: long-term evaluation. *J Pediatr Surg* 1979;14(14):258–263.

51. Carron JD, Derkay CS, Strope GL, et al. Pediatric tracheotomies: changing indications and outcomes. *Laryngoscope* 2000;110:1099–1104.

52. Toye FJ, Weinstein JD. A percutaneous tracheotomy device. *Surgery* 1969;65:384–389.

53. Ciaglia P, Firsching R, Syniec C. Elective percutaneous dilatational tracheostomy: a new simple bedside procedure: preliminary report. *Chest* 1985;87:715–719.

54. Sharpe MD, Parnes LS, Drover JW. Translaryngeal tracheostomy: experience of 340 cases. *Laryngoscope* 2003;113(3):530–536.

55. Dulguerov P, Gysin C, Perneger TV, et al. Percutaneous or surgical tracheostomy: a meta-analysis. *Crit Care Med* 1999;27(8):1617–1625.

56. Anderson HL, Bartlett RH. Elective tracheotomy for mechanical ventilation by the percutaneous technique. *Clin Chest Med* 1991;12(3):555–560.

57. Jackson C. High tracheotomy and other errors the chief cases of chronic laryngeal stenosis. *Surg Gynecol Obstet* 1921;32:392–398.

58. Brantigan CO, Grow JB. Cricothyroidotomy: elective use in respiratory problems requiring tracheotomy. *J Thorac Cardiovasc Surg* 1976;71:72–80.

59. Burkey B, Esclamado R, Morganroth M. The role of cricothyroidotomy in airway management. *Clin Chest Med* 1991;12(3):561–571.

60. Cole RR, Aguilar EA. Cricothyroidotomy versus tracheotomy: an otolaryngologist's perspective. *Laryngoscope* 1988;98:131–135.

61. Kuriloff DB, Setzen M, Portnoy W, et al. Laryngotracheal injury following cricothyroidotomy. *Laryngoscope* 1989;99:125–130.

62. Sise MJ, Shackford SR, Cruickshank JC, et al. Cricothyroidotomy for long-term tracheal access: a prospective analysis of morbidity and mortality in 76 patients. *Ann Surg* 1984;200(1):13–17.

63. Gleeson MJ, Pearson FG, Armistead S, et al. Voice changes following cricothyroidotomy. *J Laryngol Otol* 1984;98:1015–1019.

64. Holst M, Hertegard S, Persson A. Vocal dysfunction following cricothyroidotomy: a prospective study. *Laryngoscope* 1990;100:749–755.

65. Wolf M, Shapira Y, Talmi YP, et al. Laryngotracheal anastomosis: primary and revised procedures. *Laryngoscope* 2001;111:622–627.

66. Hoff PT, Hogikyan ND. Unilateral vocal fold paralysis. *Curr Opin Otolaryngol Head Neck Surg* 1996;4:176–181.

67. Zeitels SM, Casiano RR, Gardner GM, et al. Management of common voice problems: committee report. *Otolaryngol Head Neck Surg* 2002;126:333–348.

68. Isshiki N, Morita H, Okamura H, et al. Thyroplasty as a new phonosurgical technique. *Acta Otolaryngol (Stockh)* 1974;78:451–457.

69. Lundy D, Casiano RR, Xue JW, et al. Thyroplasty type I: short versus long-term results. *Otolaryngol Head Neck Surg* 2000;122:533–536.

70. Hogikyan ND, Wodchis WP, Terrell JE, et al. Voice-related quality of life (V-RQOL) following type I thyroplasty for unilateral vocal fold paralysis. *J Voice* 2000;14:378–386.

71. Crumley RL. Update: ansa cervicalis to recurrent laryngeal nerve anastomoses for unilateral laryngeal paralysis. *Laryngoscope* 1991;101:384–387.

72. Olson D, Goding GS, Michael DD. Acoustic and perceptual evaluation of laryngeal reinnervation by ansa cervicalis. *Laryngoscope* 1998;108:1767–1772.

73. Flint PW, Shiotani A, O'Malley BW. IGF-I gene transfer into denervated rat laryngeal muscle. *Arch Otolaryngol Head Neck Surg* 1999;125:274–279.

74. Rubin AD, Mobley B, Hogikyan ND, et al. Delivery of an adenoviral vector to the crushed recurrent laryngeal nerve. *Laryngoscope* 2003;113:985–989.

75. Hillel AD, Benninger M, Blitzer A, et al. Evaluation and management of bilateral vocal cord immobility. *Otolaryngol Head Neck Surg* 1999;121:760–765.

76. Cunningham M, Eavey RD, Vlahakes GJ, et al. Slide tracheoplasty for long-segment tracheal stenosis. *Arch Otolaryngol Head Neck Surg* 1998;124(1):98–103.

Complications

of Esophageal Surgery

22

Andrew C. Chang   Mark D. Iannettoni

▰▰ **ANATOMIC AND PHYSIOLOGIC CONSIDERATIONS 245**

▰▰ **ESOPHAGEAL PERFORATION 247**
Diagnosis 247
Treatment 248

▰▰ **PROCEDURAL COMPLICATIONS 251**
Esophagoscopy 251
Hiatal Hernia Repair 252

▰▰ **LAPAROSCOPIC ANTIREFLUX SURGERY 255**

▰▰ **ESOPHAGEAL RESECTION AND VISCERAL ESOPHAGEAL SUBSTITUTION 255**
Anastomotic Leak 256
Anastomotic Stricture 256
Pulmonary Complications 257
Gastric Outlet Obstruction 258
Diaphragmatic Hiatus Obstruction
    or Herniation 258
Chylothorax 259
Pancreatitis 259
Splenic Injury 259
Peripheral Atheroembolism 259

▰▰ **COMPLICATIONS OF SUBSTERNAL ESOPHAGEAL REPLACEMENT 259**
Complications of Bypassing or Excluding
    the Native Esophagus 260

▰▰ **ESOPHAGEAL DIVERTICULECTOMY 260**

▰▰ **ESOPHAGOMYOTOMY FOR ACHALASIA OR ESOPHAGEAL SPASM 261**

▰▰ **REFERENCES 262**

ANATOMIC AND PHYSIOLOGIC CONSIDERATIONS

Many of the complications of esophageal surgery are related directly to the unique features of esophageal anatomy and physiology. Detailed knowledge of these characteristics is essential for the surgeon to identify potential pitfalls of esophageal surgery and to avert complications. A unique feature of esophageal anatomy is the unusually fatty submucosa, which allows greater mobility of the overlying squamous mucosa. In performing a manual esophageal anastomosis, meticulous technique is necessary so that every suture transfixes the mucosal edge, which at times may retract >1 cm from the cut esophageal margin (Fig. 22-1). The esophagus is also unique in the gastrointestinal (GI) tract because it lacks a serosal layer. The soft and often tenuous muscularis holds sutures poorly and cannot be relied upon to maintain a fixation unless the esophageal stitch transfixes the associated submucosa.

The esophagus is nourished by four to six paired aortic esophageal arteries and by collateral circulation from the inferior thyroid, intercostal and bronchial, inferior phrenic, and left gastric arteries. The segmental blood supply of the esophagus has frequently been incriminated as the cause of anastomotic disruption. However, the submucosal collateral

Andrew C. Chang: University of Michigan, Ann Arbor, MI 48109
Mark D. Iannettoni: University of Iowa, Iowa City, IA 52242

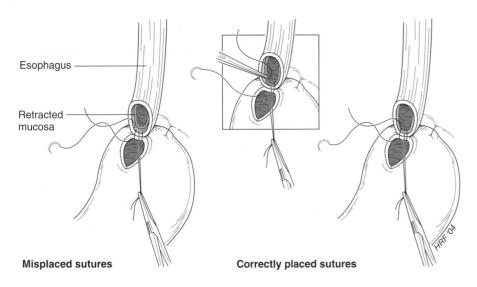

Esophagus

Retracted
mucosa

Misplaced sutures   **Correctly placed sutures**

Figure 22-1 Misplacement of the esophagogastric anastomotic suture. The relatively great mobility of the esophageal mucosa over the fatty submucosa permits the cut mucosal edge to retract proximally. Unless care is taken to identify the mucosa and properly transfix it with each suture, mucosal apposition will not occur and an anastomotic disruption will follow.

circulation of the esophagus is extensive, and even after the cardia has been divided and the intrathoracic esophagus mobilized completely out of the chest, the distal end of the esophagus maintains good arterial bleeding as long as the inferior thyroid arteries remain intact. Poor technique, not poor blood supply, is the likelier explanation for the complication of esophageal anastomotic disruption.

Parasympathetic innervation of the esophagus is supplied by the vagus nerves, and the recurrent laryngeal nerve supplies the upper portion of the esophagus. Recurrent laryngeal nerve injury during esophageal surgery may result in one of the most devastating complications, cricopharyngeal muscle dysfunction, with subsequent incapacitating cervical dysphagia and aspiration pneumonia (1). Injury to the vagal nerve trunks in operations on the distal esophagus may produce neurogenic dysphagia or gastric atony and pylorospasm, which are very troublesome complications after esophageal surgery.

Physiologic considerations influence other complications of surgery on the esophagus. The pathophysiology of gastroesophageal reflux and secondary reflux esophaghitis influences the results of antireflux surgery and the complication of recurrent reflux. The incidence of recurrent reflux in patients undergoing the standard Belsey Mark IV transthoracic hiatal hernia repair in the presence of esophagitis or a stricture is between 25% and 75% (2,3). In the presence of intramural inflammation and esophageal shortening that may accompany reflux esophagitis, the esophageal sutures of the Belsey repair may not be reliable, and tension on the repair sets the stage for recurrence of the hernia (Fig. 22-2). These considerations apply to the Nissen fundoplication and the Hill posterior gastropexy, which also aim to restore an intra-abdominal segment of distal esophagus and require esophageal or periesophageal sutures. To avert the complication of disruption of the repair due to tension on the repair, the esophagus-lengthening Collis gastroplasty can be combined with a fundoplication (4–6). The gastroplasty tube

functions as a new distal esophagus and provides healthy, resilient tissue, the gastric wall, around which to perform the fundoplication. The additional "esophageal length" provided by the gastroplasty tube reduces tension on the repair (Fig. 22-3). The presence of reflux esophagitis and a peptic stricture also complicates an antireflux procedure if the stricture is perforated during attempted dilation.

An intrathoracic esophagogastric anastomotic leak, the most dreaded complication of esophageal surgery, in part owes its morbidity to associated gastroesophageal reflux. An intrathoracic esophagogastric anastomosis is associated almost invariably with the development of reflux esophagitis, compared to a cervical esophagogastric anastomosis, which is rarely associated with clinically significant reflux. Although it has been argued that an intrathoracic esophagogastric anastomosis can be performed reliably and with an exceedingly low morbidity rate (7), the potential for an anastomotic leak and secondary mediastinitis cannot be eliminated totally. For a cervical anastomosis, the consequence of a leak is a salivary fistula and is not life-threatening.

Gastroesophageal reflux after esophageal resection and esophagogastric anastomosis may be responsible for life-threatening aspiration of gastric contents into the tracheobronchial tree in the early postoperative period. For this reason, initial decompression of the intrathoracic stomach with a nasogastric tube and placement of the patient in a 45 degree head-up position are important. Similarly, because of the potential for regurgitation and aspiration after eating, patients who have a fresh esophagogastric anastomosis should not undergo postural drainage as part of their postoperative pulmonary physiotherapy within 1 to 2 hours of mealtime.

Aspiration pneumonia resulting from esophageal obstruction cannot be overestimated. In the patient with a megaesophagus of advanced achalasia, the risk of massive regurgitation and aspiration on induction of general anesthesia is enormous. Awareness of this possibility dictates the

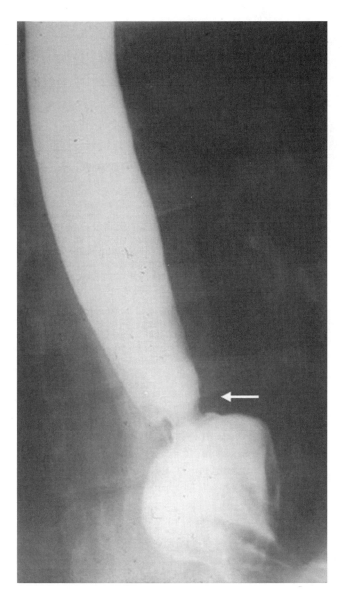

Figure 22-2 A sliding hiatus hernia with a peptic stricture at the esophagogastric junction (*arrow*). Standard antireflux operation (Hill, Belsey, or Nissen) requires reduction below the diaphragm not only of the esophagogastric junction but also of the distal 3 to 5 cm of esophagus. The relative shortening associated with the distal esophagitis in this patient prevented a tension-free standard repair. (Courtesy of M. B. Orringer, MD.)

need for nasogastric tube esophageal decompression and emptying in these patients before rapid-sequence induction of general anesthesia and endotracheal intubation.

ESOPHAGEAL PERFORATION

Perforation of the thoracic esophagus, with resultant mediastinitis, is a devastating complication. Regardless of the cause of perforation (Table 22-1), delay in recognition and definitive management increases mortality and morbidity. Repair of an acute esophageal tear in an otherwise normal esophagus within 6 to 8 hours has a morbidity rate that is

essentially the same as that imposed by elective esophagotomy and primary esophageal closure. If operative intervention is delayed beyond this early period, local inflammation greatly jeopardizes primary healing of the esophageal tear and mortality rises dramatically (8–10).

Esophageal instrumentation accounts for the large majority of iatrogenic perforations, with the cricopharyngeal area most commonly injured (Fig. 22-4). Perforation of the mid- and distal esophagus is most likely to occur following biopsy or dilatation (Fig. 22-5). Spontaneous perforation usually occurs following straining (Boerhaave syndrome) with rupture involving the left posterior aspect of the distal esophagus (11).

Diagnosis

Patients with esophageal perforation typically present with pain directly referring to the site of perforation. The presence of mediastinal air or hydropneumothorax on chest radiograph is confirmatory. However, a normal chest radiograph does not exclude the possibility of esophageal perforation because not every esophageal tear is a full-thickness disruption. For example, pneumatic dilatation of the esophagus for achalasia may result in a tear of the distal esophageal mucosa and submucosa. Air insufflation through a flexible esophagoscope may result in mediastinal, cervical, or subcutaneous air, exaggerating the extent of injury. Following esophagoscopy or esophageal operation, postoperative pain or fever should be considered a result of esophageal perforation until proven otherwise. Contrast esophagogram

TABLE 22-1

CAUSES OF ESOPHAGEAL PERFORATION

Instrumental
Endoscopy
  Direct injury
  Injury occurring during removal of a foreign body
Dilatation
Intubation (esophageal, endotracheal)

Noninstrumental
Barogenic trauma
  Postemetic
  Blunt chest or abdominal trauma
  Other (e.g., labor, convulsion, defecation)
Penetrating neck, chest, or abdominal trauma
Postoperative
Anastomotic disruption
Devascularization following pulmonary resection, vagotomy,
    or repair of hiatal hernia
Injury following ingestion of caustic agent
Erosion by adjacent infection with resultant fistula involving the
    tracheobronchial tree, pericardium, pleural cavity, or aorta
Pathologic
Severe reflux esophagitis
Candidal, herpetic, and opportunistic infection

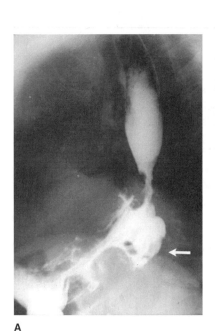

A

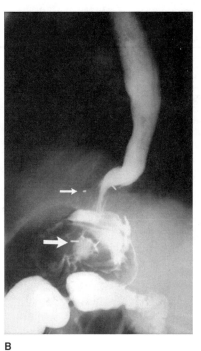

B

Figure 22-3   A: This lateral view from a preoperative esophagogram show a large, sliding hiatus hernia with half of the stomach above the left hemidiaphragm (*arrow*), a proximal stricture, and esophageal dilatation from the obstruction. **B:** Postoperative appearance of the reconstructed distal esophagus following intraoperative dilatation of the stricture and a Collis gastroplasty-Nissen fundoplication. The horizontal gastric folds in the fundoplication around the distal 5 to 7 cm of the functional esophagus can be seen. Also visible are the titanium clips (*small arrow*) marking the diaphragmatic hiatus and those at the new esophagogastric junction (*large arrow*). There is no evidence of esophageal stenosis, and the dilation proximal to the obstruction has resolved. (Courtesy of M. B. Orringer, MD.)

should be performed immediately in order to eliminate delay in establishing proper drainage or definitive repair, or both. Water-soluble contrast esophagogram, followed by dilute barium, best identifies the site of perforation (Fig. 22-6) whether the perforation communicates with either the pleural or peritoneal cavities or is confined to the mediastinum.

Treatment

Once the diagnosis of esophageal perforation is established, oral intake should cease. Aggressive intravenous fluid resuscitation, facilitated by using either a central venous pressure catheter or a pulmonary artery catheter,

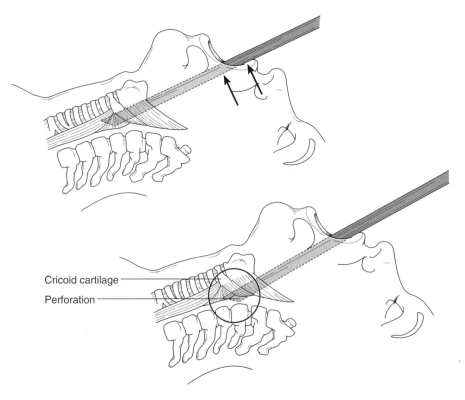

Cricoid cartilage
Perforation

Figure 22-4 The mechanism of rigid endoscopic cervical esophageal perforation. In performing rigid esophagoscopy, it is essential that a gentle, steady, lifting force (*arrows*) be exerted to displace forward the larynx and cricoid cartilage. Failure to overcome the natural pull of the upper esophageal sphincter against the cricoid cartilage results in a typical posterior perforation.

cannot be neglected in the patient with an esophageal perforation.

There is controversy about the best treatment of patients with esophageal perforation. Nonoperative "conservative" therapy is successful in some patients with esophageal perforation, primarily those with preexisting periesophageal and mediastinal fibrosis that contains the injury. For esophageal disruption in which contrast material extends only a few millimeters from the esophageal lumen and the patient is clinically well, antibiotic therapy, chest tube drainage, and observation may suffice (12–14). More frequently, successful outcome following esophageal perforation requires operative intervention (Fig. 22-7).

Perforation of the cervical and upper thoracic esophagus is approached through an oblique cervical incision that parallels the anterior border of the left sternocleidomastoid muscle. The sternocleidomastoid muscle and carotid sheath are retracted laterally and the trachea and thyroid gland medially. If the perforation can be identified, it is closed with absorbable polyglycolic acid sutures. If the injury cannot be visualized adequately for repair, the retroesophageal prevertebral space is dissected bluntly with a finger and the superior mediastinum is drained with two 1-inch Penrose drains brought out through the neck wound. Esophageal perforations to the level of the tracheal bifurcation can generally be treated successfully with a cervical approach. Midthoracic esophageal perforations must be approached through a right thoracotomy and those of the distal third of the esophagus are approached through a left thoracotomy.

Traditional surgical dogma states that esophageal perforations beyond 6 to 12 hours in duration are impossible to repair primarily, the pouting inflamed mucosa at the edge of the tear holding sutures poorly. Recent reports, however, have emphasized that even with delay in repair, successful closure of the esophageal injury may be possible (8,15). Several groups have reported that the majority of esophageal tears can be repaired successfully using

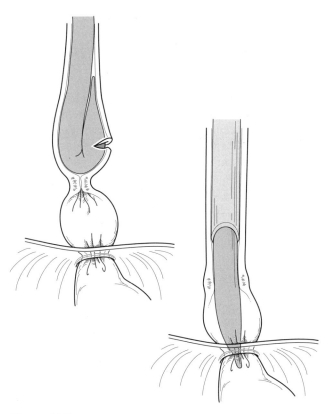

Figure 22-5 Esophageal perforation during an attempt at blind passage of a dilator through a tight stricture. **A:** The dilator has curled proximal to the stenosis, and, as the bougie is advanced, disruption of the esophagus may occur. **B:** When a large esophagoscope that will accommodate up to a 50-French dilator is used, the stricture can be visualized directly for dilatation.

is indicated if there is hypovolemia associated with intrathoracic perforation. Broad-spectrum antibiotic coverage is initiated. The presence of carious teeth increases the morbidity risk of esophageal injury owing to the virulence of swallowed oral bacteria. Oral hygiene

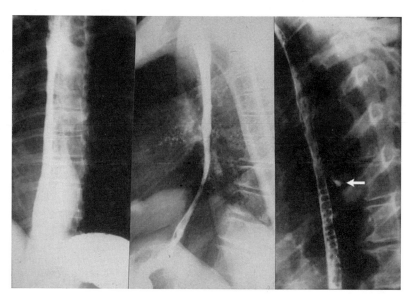

Figure 22-6 Posteroanterior (*left*) and lateral (*center*) views from Gastrografin (meglumine diatrizoate) esophagogram in a patient with acute caustic injury that was incorrectly dilated prematurely within 10 days of caustic ingestion. There was still acute inflammation in this esophagus, and the patient had fever and chest pain following dilation. Despite the negative Gastrografin swallow, dilute barium was administered (*right*), and a perforation (*arrow*) of the midesophagus was demonstrated. (Courtesy of M. B. Orringer, MD.)

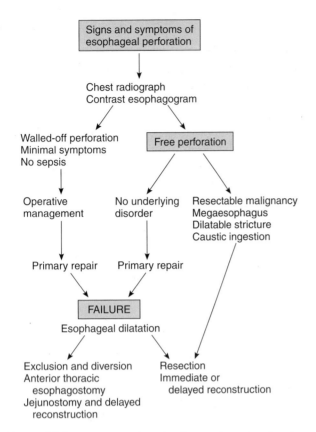

Figure 22-7   Treatment algorithm for esophageal perforation.

meticulous surgical technique that includes identification of adjacent submucosa by dissecting away the overlying muscle, defining the limits of the mucosal tear (Fig. 22-8), reapproximation of the disrupted mucosa and submucosa with a surgical stapler (Auto Suture Endo-GIA II Stapler, U.S. Surgical Corporation, Auto Suture Company Division, Norwalk, CT) (16), and reapproximation of the

muscle over the staple suture line (Fig. 22-9). Limited esophagomyotomy performed 180 degrees opposite the site of injury may permit enough advancement of adjacent esophageal wall for adequate repair of the perforation (17).

In patients with chronic mediastinitis and pleural reaction, the adjacent mediastinal pleura is thickened and provides an excellent flap with which to reinforce the esophageal suture line. Alternatively, if there is not sufficient parietal pleural thickening to provide adequate support for the suture line, reinforcement with either a pedicled intercostal muscle flap, omentum, pericardium, visceral pleura, or diaphragm can be performed (18,19). The mediastinal pleura must be opened from the apex of the chest to the diaphragm to permit wide drainage of the mediastinum. After copious irrigation of the mediastinum and pleural cavity and decortication of acute fibrinous exudate that may have formed over the lung, a large-bore chest tube is left near the esophageal suture line. If disruption occurs, the result will be an esophagopleural cutaneous fistula.

In treating an esophageal perforation, associated esophageal pathology cannot be ignored. Perforation proximal to a carcinoma or a caustic or reflux stricture may necessitate an emergent esophagectomy with either primary or delayed esophageal reconstruction. Patients who present with esophageal perforation and chronic reflux stricture are more likely to develop postoperative dysphagia requiring repeated esophageal dilatation. In this subset of patients consideration should be given to primary esophagectomy if their physiologic status at time of operation permits (20). Alternatively, if it is possible to dilate a benign stricture intraoperatively to relieve the distal obstruction, closure of a proximal esophageal perforation may be successful. A subsequent disruption of the esophageal closure may still eventually heal if dilation of the associated stricture is continued. A perforated pulsion diverticulum of the esophagus may be resected within several hours of the injury; the

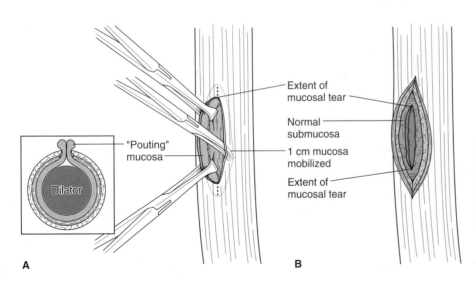

Figure 22-8 Technique of primary repair of esophageal perforation. Mucosa at the site of the tear (*inset*) is grasped with Allis clamps **(A)**, and the adjacent esophageal muscle is mobilized around the entire tear until 1 cm of normal submucosa is exposed around the defect **(B)**. (From Whyte, RI, Iannettoni, MD, Orringer, MB. Intrathoracic perforation: The merit of primary repair. *J Thorac Cardiovasc Surg* 1995;109:140–146, with permission.)

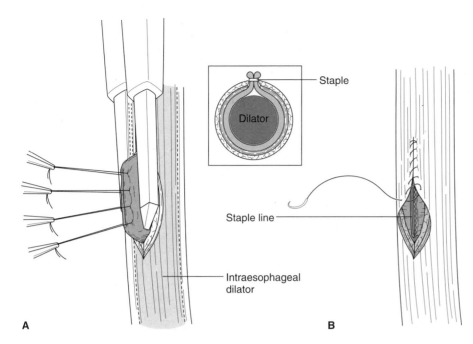

A   B

Figure 22-9 Technique of primary repair of esophageal perforation (continuation of Figure 22-8). Traction sutures placed along the inflamed mucosal edge of the tear elevate the submucosa so that an Endo-GIA II cartridge can be applied and deployed. The esophageal lumen is maintained by passage of an intraesophageal dilator **(A)** (*and inset*). The staple line is covered by approximating the adjacent muscle with a running absorbable suture **(B)**. (From Whyte, RI, Iannettoni, MD, Orringer, MB. Intrathoracic perforation: The merit of primary repair. *J Thorac Cardiovasc Surg* 1995;109:140–146, with permission.)

associated neuromotor esophageal dysfunction responsible for formation of the pouch must be relieved by performing a concomitant esophagomyotomy.

PROCEDURAL COMPLICATIONS

Esophagoscopy

Technologic advances in flexible fiberoptic instruments have facilitated the performance of esophagogastroscopy. There has been a concomitant increase in the number of these studies performed on an outpatient basis. Perforation occurs in as many as 0.8% of all patients during flexible upper endoscopy, with rates as high as 4% for patients undergoing esophageal dilatation (21). Perforation following rigid esophagoscopy occurs in approximately 5% of patients following therapeutic procedures (e.g., biopsy, dilation, or removal of foreign body) and in 1.5% of patients following diagnostic rigid esophagoscopy (22).

For rigid esophagoscopy the following caveats apply:

1. Adequate preoperative and intraoperative sedation and anesthesia are mandatory. In some patients general anesthesia is the only means of creating acceptable conditions for performance of esophagoscopy for both the patient and the surgeon.
2. If a prior barium esophagogram has been performed, the endoscopist should review it. The barium swallow provides information about preexisting pathology and its expected location. For example, a Zenker diverticulum identified with contrast esophagogram should be expected to be encountered at the level of the upper

esophageal sphincter, approximately 15 cm from the upper incisors. A midesophageal carcinoma at the level of the tracheal bifurcation is encountered approximately 25 cm from the upper incisors. An epiphrenic diverticulum located proximal to the esophagogastric junction is encountered before the esophagoscope reaches a point 40 cm from the upper incisors.

3. Failure to introduce the rigid esophagoscope properly through the upper esophageal sphincter may result in a perforation. The cricopharyngeus muscle originates from the cricoid cartilage, and the natural "pull" of this muscle against the cartilage will result in a posterior perforation unless the larynx is "lifted" anteriorly as the esophagoscope is advanced.
4. The esophagoscope should not be advanced unless the lumen is visible.
5. As the esophagoscope is advanced, adjustment must be made for the natural course of the esophagus. Because the distal esophagus courses anteriorly and to the left as it joins the stomach, particularly when performing rigid endoscopy, the instrument must be angled toward the right side of the patient's mouth and the occiput of the head lowered as the esophagoscope is advanced into the distal esophagus.
6. The initial dilatation of a tight esophageal stricture is frequently painful, and patients must be adequately sedated or anesthetized, minimizing patient discomfort and allowing the surgeon to concentrate on the visual field. When a rigid esophagoscope is used for this initial evaluation, flexible gum-tipped Jackson bougies are inserted through the stricture under direct vision, and the pliability and extent of the stenosis are assessed (Fig. 22-10). With a mild "soft"

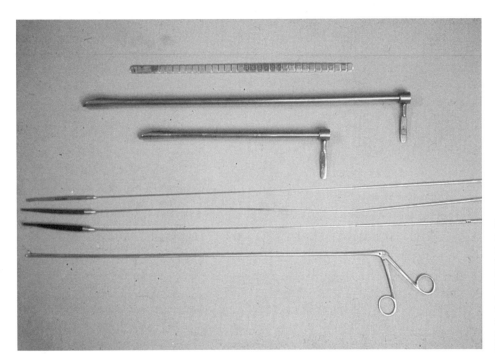

Figure 22-10 The instruments required for evaluating an esophageal stricture. Precisely measured localization of the stricture (in centimeters from the incisor teeth) and adequate biopsies and brushings from the stricture must be obtained. The gum-tipped Jackson dilators, gently manipulated through the stenosis, permit evaluation of the extent and pliability of the obstruction.

stenosis, dilation by advancing the esophagoscope through the stenosis may be possible. With more firm, high-grade strictures, it is safer to pass progressively larger dilators through the narrowing. This can be accomplished using the Savary-Gilliard guidewire and dilating system, with fluoroscopic guidance, or with the Maloney tapered esophageal dilators (Fig. 22-11).

Hiatal Hernia Repair

Hiatal herniorrhaphy, although conceptually quite simple, can result in a number of serious complications (Table 22-2). Acute esophageal perforation can occur when concomitant esophagoscopy is performed during an antireflux operation or when a distal esophageal

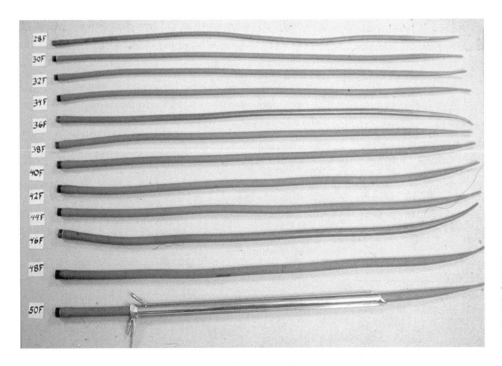

Figure 22-11 Tapered Hurst-Maloney esophageal dilators and a 45-cm Pilling esophagoscope, which accommodates up to a 50-French bougie, thus permitting progressive dilatation of severe peptic strictures under direct vision. (Courtesy of M. B. Orringer, MD.)

TABLE 22-2

COMPLICATIONS OF HIATAL HERNIORRHAPHY

Intraoperative Complications
Perforation
Vagus nerve injury
Hemorrhage
    Splenic laceration
    Short gastric vessel

Postoperative Complications
Perforation
    Stricture
    Suture placement
Dysphagia
    Mechanical
        Tight hiatal closure
        Excessive fundoplication
    Edema
    Gastric atony, pylorospasm
Early anatomic recurrence
    Crural repair disruption
Functional
    Postvagotomy diarrhea
    Ileus
Cardiac tamponade
Chylothorax
Pleural effusion
Incisional pain

From Patel HJ, Tan BT, Yee J, et al. A twenty-five year experience with open primary transthoracic repair of paraesophageal hiatal hernia. *J Thorac Cardiovasc Surg* 2004;127(3):843–849, with permission.

stricture is disrupted during intraoperative dilatation. A delayed perforation, usually within 1 week of surgery, may occur when esophageal sutures placed too deeply during the repair result in local mural necrosis.

Acute esophageal tears recognized before the incision should be approached transthoracically and repaired. The esophageal suture line should be reinforced with either the fundoplication if the tear is in the distal esophagus or with pedicled anterior mediastinal fat or a pedicled intercostal muscle flap if the tear is higher. When an intercostal muscle pedicle is used to reinforce an esophageal suture line, it should be sutured to the esophagus as an onlay patch, not placed circumferentially around the esophagus; regeneration of bone or cartilage from the perichondrium or periosteum mobilized with the flap may result in a late obstructing ring around the esophagus.

When a reflux stricture is perforated during attempted dilation during an antireflux operation, unless the involved tissues are relatively healthy and amenable to repair, resectional therapy is generally a better option. Although most reflux strictures can be dilated, and many regress after an antireflux procedure, disruption of a stricture during attempted dilation is one of the definitions of an "undilatable" stricture that justifies esophageal resection. An option in this situation is to proceed with transthoracic esophagectomy and then to reposition the patient supine and carry out a cervical esophagogastric anastomosis.

Several additional options for the treatment of a disrupted distal stricture are available. Unfortunately, none is without associated morbidity. The Thal fundic patch esophagoplasty uses adjacent gastric fundus to "patch" the narrowed esophagus. This procedure not only relies on the healing of the opened, inflamed distal esophagus to which the stomach is sutured but also requires the addition of an intrathoracic fundoplication (Thal-Woodward procedure) to control gastroesophageal reflux. The incidence of suture line disruption and mechanical complications associated with this operation are very high. The same high complication rate attends the use of an intrathoracic fundoplication (without a Thal procedure) to control reflux.

Gastric ulceration may complicate 3% to 10% of fundoplications and may occur both in supradiaphragmatic fundic wraps and in intra-abdominal fundoplications. In the former, one is dealing with a complication of an iatrogenic paraesophageal hiatal hernia, and operative repair is generally indicated. In the latter, ulceration may be due to relative ischemia in the wrap, and treatment with H_2-receptor blockers, proton pump inhibitors, or cytoprotective agents may suffice.

The development of fever, chest pain, or respiratory distress during the first week after hiatal hernia operation mandates a contrast study, and if a distal esophageal perforation is diagnosed, treatment usually involves reoperation. The site of the perforation is identified intraoperatively, at times by insufflating air through a nasogastric tube. A leak from an intra-abdominal fundoplication suture may be closed and reinforced with adjacent omentum. If the leak is in the chest, pedicled anterior mediastinal fat, intercostal muscle, or pleura is used to reinforce the closure using a transthoracic approach. A jejunostomy feeding tube should be placed to allow nutritional support in case the repair is unsuccessful and an esophageal fistula ensues. A large-bore chest tube should be left near a thoracic esophageal repair or a drain should be placed near a transabdominally repaired fundoplication to ensure external drainage of a recurrent fistula.

Retrosternal dysphagia after an antireflux operation may have one of several causes: (a) distal esophageal edema after intraoperative manipulation, (b) distal esophageal motor dysfunction due to manipulation of the vagus nerves, (c) obstruction due to too tight a fundoplication, or (d) obstruction from excessive closure of the hiatus. Performance of the fundoplication over at least a No. 54 French intraesophageal dilator minimizes the likelihood of the latter complication.

Dysphagia after truncal vagotomy has been recognized for more than 40 years, and it is apparent that neuromotor esophageal dysfunction may follow manipulation of the vagus nerves at the level of the distal esophagus. This complication after antireflux surgery is more likely with a transthoracic than with a transabdominal repair because displacement of the main vagal trunks is more likely with the former approach. Such patients have dysphagia immediately after the antireflux procedure. On barium swallow examination, the distal esophagus is tapered and empties poorly, resembling achalasia or esophageal spasm. Reassurance and maintenance of a soft diet for several days usually constitute adequate therapy, although passage of an esophageal dilator is occasionally required for relief. This problem typically subsides spontaneously, but occasionally reoperation, takedown of the repair, and, at times, even esophageal resection may be needed.

Another complication of intraoperative vagus nerve injury occurring during hiatal hernia repair is impaired gastric motility or pylorospasm resulting in delayed gastric emptying and secondary gastric dilation. This complication has direct implications for the long-term success of the hiatal hernia repair. Sustained gastric dilation may eventually result in disruption of the esophageal sutures used to construct the fundoplication and thus cause failure of the repair. When the patient who has undergone an antireflux operation develops gastric dilation immediately after operation, a 7- to 10-day trial of gastric decompression with a nasogastric tube is indicated. An anticholinergic agent may relieve associated pylorospasm. However, this problem should not be permitted to persist indefinitely, and it is best to perform an early gastric drainage procedure (pyloromyotomy or pyloroplasty) rather than to risk recurrent gastroesophageal reflux.

Vagal nerve injury may result in varying degrees of the "dumping syndrome" (e.g., postprandial diarrhea, cramping, abdominal pain, nausea, diaphoresis, palpitations). This problem generally subsides within a few months, but long-term management with antidiarrheal medication and dietary restriction may be required.

Chylothorax following an antireflux procedure results from injury to the thoracic duct, which passes from the abdomen through the aortic hiatus and then courses in the lower chest anterior to the spine between the esophagus and the aorta. Injury may occur during mobilization of the cardia or during placement of crural sutures. This complication is heralded by prolonged chest tube drainage after a transthoracic repair. The cause of this serosanguinous drainage becomes apparent when the patient's diet is liberalized and fat content increases. If chylothorax is present, the oral administration of 60 to 90 mL of cream for 4 to 6 hours will cause the chest tube drainage to become opalescent and milky. The diagnosis can also be established by staining the fluid with Sudan R, which colorizes globules of fat. Determination of cholesterol and triglyceride levels in the fluid is diagnostic. A cholesterol/triglyceride ratio of <1 is characteristic of a chylous effusion, whereas nonchylous effusions have a ratio of >1. In most cases chylothorax following a hiatal hernia repair can be managed nonoperatively by administering a low-residue elemental diet and maintaining prolonged chest tube suction. If the output of chyle remains significant (>400 to 600 mL per consecutive 8-hour periods) after 7 to 10 days

of this treatment, reoperation with identification and ligation of the injured thoracic duct is indicated.

Acute postoperative hemorrhage after an antireflux operation is most often the result of bleeding from an unsecured divided short gastric vessel high along the greater curvature of the stomach. This possibility should always be borne in mind as the short gastric vessels are divided and ligated before performing a fundoplication. Hemorrhage from these vessels may be a particularly treacherous complication following a transthoracic hiatal hernia repair because the resulting hypovolemic shock may be attributed to other causes [e.g., myocardial infarction (MI)] when there is minimal chest tube drainage and the chest roentgenogram shows no hemothorax. Abdominal exploration, evacuation of blood, and ligation of the bleeding vessel is the proper therapy. Splenic injury also occurs in a small percentage of patients undergoing antireflux surgery, particularly reoperations. The incidence of splenic injury is slightly higher with transabdominal than with transthoracic antireflux operations, particularly in obese patients. Rarely, postoperative hemorrhage manifests as a pericardial effusion causing tamponade and cardiopulmonary collapse. Avulsion of an epicardial vessel occurring during esophageal mobilization for repair of a large hiatal hernia may cause this development. Rapid diagnosis by surface echocardiogram followed by sternotomy, relief of tamponade, and repair of the bleeding vessel is indicated (23).

A barium contrast study may reveal a "silent" localized extravasation of contrast material at the site of fundoplication sutures that were placed too deeply. If the patient is asymptomatic and the "leak" is very small, no therapy may be required; the supporting fundoplication has prevented a more major disruption. A more disconcerting radiographic finding on "routine" postoperative barium swallow is the asymptomatic migration of the fundoplication or gastric fundus into the chest as a result of disruption of the posterior crural repair. This iatrogenic paraesophageal hiatal hernia is subject to the same mechanical complications of paraesophageal herniation as in the patient who has had no surgery. Reoperation is necessary to reduce the fundoplication back into the abdomen and to replace the posterior crural sutures before postoperative adhesions form between the herniated stomach and adjacent tissues. Conservative management of this problem is ill-advised.

Controversy remains regarding the role of surgical therapy for patients with Barrett esophagus. Both symptoms and requirements for antisecretory medications decrease significantly following antireflux operation (24). However, no long-term data are available proving postoperative regression of Barrett esophagus, regarded as a precursor lesion to esophageal adenocarcinoma. Currently, patients with Barrett esophagus undergoing hiatal herniorrhaphy should continue surveillance esophagoscopy with biopsies to screen for the progression from metaplasia to dysplasia and esophageal adenocarcinoma (25).

LAPAROSCOPIC ANTIREFLUX SURGERY

Since 1991, when the first reports of laparoscopic antireflux surgery were published, minimally invasive surgical approaches to the diaphragmatic esophageal hiatus have been used with increasing frequency. Mortality rates for laparoscopic fundoplication have been low (0% to 1.4%), morbidity rates are acceptable, and conversion rates to the open procedure are from 0% to 14% (26).

In obese patients, in those with intra-abdominal adhesions from prior surgery, and in patients with an unusually large left hepatic lobe, visualization of the operative field may be difficult. Persistence with a "closed" operation may be dangerous. These factors are indications for open hiatal hernia repair. Perforations of the distal esophagus or gastric fundus have been reported during laparoscopic fundoplication. Blind dissection posterior to the esophagus should be avoided to prevent this complication. When recognized at the time of, or soon after, operation, laparoscopic repair is feasible, but repair may also warrant conversion to an open procedure.

Early postoperative dysphagia may result from an overly tight fundoplication. Performance of the fundoplication over at least a size 54 French Maloney dilator minimizes the likelihood of this complication. Postoperative dysphagia due to fibrotic stenosis of the muscular esophageal hiatus, attributed to diathermy injury during the esophageal dissection, has been treated with laparoscopic hiatal division. Persistent dysphagia after a laparoscopic fundoplication, refractory to dilatation therapy, may necessitate reoperation, takedown of the wrap, and construction of a looser fundoplication. Our approach to such reoperative procedures is a transthoracic one, generally with a combined esophageal lengthening Collis gastroplasty and Nissen fundoplication. Additional complications of laparoscopic fundoplication include pneumothorax or pneumomediastinum from CO_2 tracking into the chest during the operation, incisional hernias at port sites, and herniation of the fundoplication through the diaphragmatic hiatus.

As experience with laparoscopic fundoplication has grown, this approach has been used to repair paraesophageal hiatal hernias, which are often associated with an attenuated, abnormally wide esophageal hiatus. In 1983, Pearson et al. reported that esophageal shortening was common in these patients, most of whom had combined sliding and paraesophageal hiatus hernias. They used a combined Collis gastroplasty-fundoplication operation in this group (27,28). With the laparoscopic approach, one cannot assess the degree of tension on the distal esophagus that results from reduction of the esophagogastric junction below the diaphragm, and manual palpation of the esophagus is not possible. With the diaphragms pushed upward by CO_2 instillation into the abdomen, a false ease of reduction of the esophagogastric junction into the abdomen may occur. Several groups have developed minimally invasive techniques for combined Collis gastroplasty and fundoplication, with acceptable short-term results (29,30). Fundoplications that have "slipped" through the hiatus into the chest after laparoscopic repair may reflect, at least in part, a lack of recognition by the original surgeon that there was unacceptable tension on the repair. Recurrent herniation of an intact or a partially disrupted fundoplication is the most common reason for failure of laparoscopic fundoplication. Body habitus is an important but often overlooked factor in recurrence after laparoscopic antireflux operation; a significant number of patients who experience disruption of repairs are obese.

Another laparoscopic technique for the repair of paraesophageal hiatal hernias involves the use of mesh to repair the diaphragmatic defect. This is an ill-conceived operation because the constant diaphragmatic motion against the adjacent esophagus at the hiatus may result in esophageal or gastric erosion and perforation.

ESOPHAGEAL RESECTION AND VISCERAL ESOPHAGEAL SUBSTITUTION

For patients undergoing esophageal resection and substitution with either stomach or intestine, the leading causes of death are (1) respiratory insufficiency associated with the physiologic insult of a combined thoracic and abdominal operation and (2) sepsis from mediastinitis resulting from disruption of an intrathoracic anastomosis. As a result, some groups have adopted a policy of performing no intrathoracic esophageal anastomoses and prefer a cervical esophagogastric anastomosis. A cervical esophagogastric anastomotic leak generally represents little more morbidity than a salivary fistula, and spontaneous closure with local wound care is the rule. Investigators have reported a dramatic reduction in the incidence of postoperative cervical esophagogastric anastomotic leak to less than 3% with a side-to-side stapled cervical esophagogastric anastomosis (31) constructed with the Auto Suture Endo-GIA II Stapler (U.S. Surgical Corporation, Auto Suture Company Division, Norwalk, CT). We have also reported that a transhiatal esophagectomy without thoracotomy and cervical esophagogastric anastomosis is applicable in most patients requiring esophageal resection and reconstruction for both benign and malignant disease. This procedure minimizes the operative insult by avoiding thoracotomy. The incidence of postoperative pulmonary complications is thereby reduced, and the possibility of mediastinitis resulting from an intrathoracic leak is virtually eliminated.

We recommend a No. 14 French rubber catheter feeding jejunostomy tube secured with a Witzel maneuver in every patient undergoing esophagectomy and esophageal reconstruction. The jejunostomy tube is considered an "insurance policy" if anastomotic disruption necessitates an alternate means of nourishment. If use of the tube is not required postoperatively, it is removed after several weeks. Alternatively, if an anastomotic leak occurs, a feeding jejunostomy tube is safer and more effective in providing calories than intravenous hyperalimentation.

Anastomotic Leak

After completion of a cervical esophageal anastomosis, the neck wound is loosely closed with only four or five 4-0 sutures over a 1/4-in Penrose drain placed adjacent to the anastomosis. If an anastomotic leak does occur, the neck wound is opened at the bedside in its entirety and gentle wound packing with gauze is initiated. The leak's size can be estimated by having the patient drink water and evaluating the amount that escapes from the neck wound with a disposable bedside suction catheter. Generally, within several days of opening the wound, the drainage diminishes considerably, and the patient may resume oral intake while maintaining steady gentle pressure over the wound to occlude the fistula. Passage of tapered Maloney dilators (generally, 40 and 46 French) at the bedside during the first week after drainage of the cervical fistula ensures that no element of obstruction from either local edema or spasm contributes to continued drainage (32).

More than 98% of cervical esophagogastric anastomotic leaks are small and respond to the open drainage and packing as described. A small proportion, however, are associated with catastrophic complications: major gastric tip necrosis necessitating takedown of the anastomosis, construction of cervical esophagostomy and resection of nonviable stomach; vertebral body osteomyelitis; epidural abscess with resultant paraplegia; pulmonary microabscesses from an internal jugular vein abscess; and tracheoesophagogastric anastomotic fistula (33).

Early disruption of an intrathoracic esophageal anastomosis occurring within the first 10 days after operation is characterized by mediastinitis. Symptoms include fever, chest pain, tachycardia, tachypnea, respiratory distress, peripheral cyanosis, vasoconstriction, hypotension, and shock. A chest roentgenogram that demonstrates hydrothorax or pneumothorax leaves little question about the diagnosis. The complication should be documented with a contrast study.

In an asymptomatic patient found to have a small (>1 cm) contained anastomotic leak on a routine postoperative barium swallow, observation alone may be sufficient. In most cases, however, anastomotic disruption warrants immediate reexploration, irrigation of the chest and mediastinum, repair of the fistula, if possible, and chest tube drainage. A localized anastomotic leak with viable adjacent tissue may be amenable to direct suture repair. A pedicled flap of anterior mediastinal fat, intercostal muscle flap, pleura, or omentum should be mobilized to reinforce the repair. Decompression of the esophageal substitute with a nasogastric tube, placement of a jejunostomy tube for nutritional support, and appropriate antibiotics complete therapy.

Following removal of chest tubes, a barium swallow examination should be performed to be certain that healing has occurred. If disruption of the anastomosis recurs, a controlled esophagopleural cutaneous fistula should be established. Rib resection with placement of a large-bore drainage tube adjacent to the fistula may be required to ensure that all drainage from the esophageal leak can flow freely out of the chest. Gastric contents that are aspirated through the nasogastric tube can be returned to the alimentary tract through the jejunostomy tube to minimize electrolyte imbalance and to simplify fluid and electrolyte replacement.

During reexploration of the chest for a disrupted esophageal anastomosis, extensive local necrosis with major anastomotic dehiscence mandates reversal of the anastomosis, resection of nonviable stomach, and replacement of the remaining stomach into the abdomen. Only nonviable distal esophagus should be resected. A diverting lateral cervical esophagostomy with oversewing of the divided proximal intrathoracic esophagus should not be attempted. Disruption of the intrathoracic esophageal suture line is likely, and if subsequent reconstruction is possible, management of the remaining segment of intrathoracic esophagus presents a considerable technical problem. The best alternative is to mobilize the esophagus circumferentially into the neck through the thoracic incision. After the thoracotomy is closed, end esophagostomy, with the patient returned to the supine position, should be performed. The submucosal collateral circulation of the esophagus is excellent, and most of the length of the thoracic esophagus will remain viable as long as at least one inferior thyroid artery remains intact. After delivering the divided thoracic esophagus out of the neck incision, the maximum length of remaining esophagus should be preserved to facilitate later reconstruction. This is done by developing a subcutaneous tunnel anteriorly to the left clavicle onto the chest wall in order to construct an anterior thoracic esophagostomy. The patient can much more easily care for an esophagostomy stoma placed on the relatively flat upper anterior chest wall because a stomal appliance is more readily adapted to this location than to the usual site of a cervical esophagostomy (Fig. 22-12). A feeding jejunostomy is required until later esophageal reconstruction can be performed.

When colon or jejunum has been used to replace the esophagus and necrosis of the graft is documented at reexploration for an anastomotic leak, there is little recourse but to remove the nonviable graft and insert a feeding tube. If the patient survives the sequelae of the mediastinal sepsis, later reconstruction can be considered.

Anastomotic Stricture

Although the management of a cervical anastomotic leak is generally straightforward and seldom associated with death, the long-term sequelae of a cervical leak are not

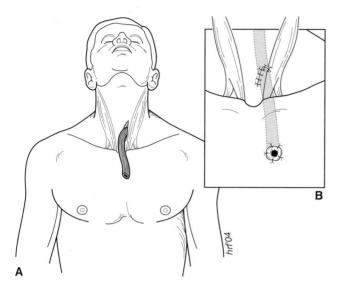

A

B

Figure 22-12 Construction of an anterior thoracic esophagostomy instead of a traditional end-cervical esophagostomy. **A:** The mobilized thoracic esophagus is placed on the anterior chest wall so that the location of the stoma can be determined. **B:** All viable remaining esophagus is preserved and tunneled subcutaneously, and an end anterior thoracic esophagostomy is constructed. Stomal appliances are readily applied to the flat surface of the anterior chest, and, when performing a later colon interposition, 7 to 12 cm of esophagus is available for the reconstruction.

inconsequential. As many as 50% of cervical esophagogastric anastomotic leaks result in an anastomotic stricture as healing occurs, and this represents an unsatisfactory outcome of an operation that was intended to provide comfortable swallowing. The implications are similar in patients who survive an intrathoracic esophageal anastomotic leak. One group has reported an anastomotic leak rate averaging 13% in nearly 1,100 transhiatal esophagectomy patients with nearly half of these patients developing subsequent anastomotic strictures (34). The observation is consistent with reports in the literature, with an incidence of anastomotic leak from 5% to 26% and stenosis from 10% to 31% (35–37). Without question, the prevention of anastomotic leak is key to a successful functional outcome in these patients. In an initial experience with side-to-side stapled cervical esophagogastric anastomosis, which has been associated with an anastomotic leak rate of <3%, a dramatic reduction in the need for late postoperative anastomotic dilatations was noted (31).

In the patient who has experienced an esophageal anastomotic leak, early passage of a 46 French or larger dilator within 1 week of drainage is performed to maintain a satisfactory lumen and to prevent late high-grade stenosis. A cervical fistula generally heals within 7 to 10 days of external drainage. When the patient returns for follow-up, a 46 French or larger Maloney dilator is passed through the anastomosis. If the patient has no dysphagia and there is no resistance to passage of the dilator, the return of cervical dysphagia dictates the need for subsequent dilatations. In

patients with anastomotic narrowing that prevents the free passage of a 46 French or larger Maloney dilator, a more aggressive program of esophageal dilatation is undertaken. With an early program of weekly dilatations, anastomotic healing in a patent configuration is often achieved. Patients whose anastomotic stricture produces resistance as the dilator is passed may need more frequent dilatations. In this situation the patient is taught over several weeks to pass a 46 or 48 French dilator with the assistance of a family member or friend. Once facility with passage of the dilator is achieved, the patient is issued a dilator with instructions to pass it daily for 1 week, then every other day for 1 week, and then at increasingly longer intervals until the longest duration between dilatations without the recurrence of dysphagia can be established. With this aggressive initial program of dilatation, long-term comfortable swallowing with little or no need for subsequent dilatations is generally achieved. Few patients require anastomotic revision. Occasionally, endoscopic injection of steroids into a refractory anastomotic scar facilitates the management of this problem (38,39).

Pulmonary Complications

Respiratory insufficiency after esophageal resection and reconstruction is exceedingly common and is associated with a mortality rate of up to 40% (40,41). Patients with esophageal squamous cell cancer, particularly those treated with preoperative chemoradiation, may have a greater risk for postoperative pulmonary morbidity, including pleural effusion, pneumonia, and respiratory insufficiency following esophagectomy (42). A vital part of minimizing postoperative pulmonary complications is rigorous preoperative pulmonary physiotherapy. We insist on total abstinence from cigarette smoking for a minimum of 2 weeks before esophagectomy. Home use of an incentive inspirometer and instruction in deep-breathing exercises are also begun 2 weeks preoperatively. This investment of time and energy in improving the patient's preoperative respiratory status is rewarded by a lower incidence of postoperative pulmonary complications. Patients are extubated immediately after operation and resume pulmonary physiotherapy as early as possible. Adequate postoperative analgesia, particularly epidural anesthesia, is of great value in minimizing postoperative pulmonary problems.

One of the most disastrous complications after esophageal resection is the development of a fistula between the tracheobronchial tree and either the esophagus or esophageal substitute. Fistulae generally occur at the anastomotic site. Among 207 patients with malignant esophagorespiratory fistulas treated at the Memorial Sloan-Kettering Cancer Center in New York City, Burt et al. reported 13 patients who developed their fistulae after resections for esophageal carcinoma (43). Once a fistula between the airway and adjacent alimentary tract develops, there is little option to prevent continued contamination of the respiratory tree other than to identify and to divide the fistula and to repair the airway, generally a major undertaking in a desperately ill patient.

Gastric Outlet Obstruction

The need for a routine gastric drainage procedure following the vagotomy that inevitably accompanies esophagectomy has been debated. Most patients who undergo an esophagectomy and esophagogastric anastomosis without concomitant drainage procedure do not develop difficulty with gastric outlet obstruction (44,45). However, in a prospective trial in which 200 patients undergoing esophageal resection were randomized to receive either a pyloroplasty or no gastric drainage procedure, gastric emptying was found to be four times longer in those who did not have pyloroplasty (46). Adverse postprandial symptoms were fewer in those who had a drainage procedure, and there was no morbidity from the pyloroplasty. For the occasional patient who does develop significant gastric outlet obstruction after esophageal resection (Fig. 22-13), the outcome may be aspiration pneumonia and impaired nutrition due to inability to eat. Reoperation to perform a drainage procedure may be very difficult after the stomach has been mobilized into the chest. For these reasons, we advocate performance of a gastric drainage procedure in every patient undergoing esophagectomy and esophageal reconstruction, preferring a Ramstedt-type extramucosal pyloromyotomy, which avoids the intra-abdominal suture line of a pyloroplasty. After performing the pyloromyotomy, metallic clips placed at the level of the pylorus aid in interpreting subsequent radiologic studies used to evaluate gastric emptying. In more than 1,500 such pyloromyotomies performed during esophageal bypass or replacement with stomach, our group has experienced one leak postoperatively. This leak resulted in fatal peritonitis.

Intrathoracic gastric outlet obstruction may also result from failure to enlarge the diaphragmatic hiatus adequately before mobilizing the stomach into the chest. The diaphragmatic hiatus should accommodate at least three fingers comfortably alongside the mobilized stomach to prevent this complication.

Diaphragmatic Hiatus Obstruction or Herniation

The hiatus must be enlarged sufficiently to prevent the esophageal substitute from becoming obstructed at the level of the diaphragm, and the esophageal replacement, whether stomach or intestine, should be carefully sutured to the edge of the diaphragmatic hiatus to prevent subsequent herniation of abdominal viscera through the hiatus into the chest (Fig. 22-14). This complication may occur acutely within the first several days of operation or years after esophagectomy (47,48). Such a hernia may be an asymptomatic finding on a postoperative chest roentgenogram on which

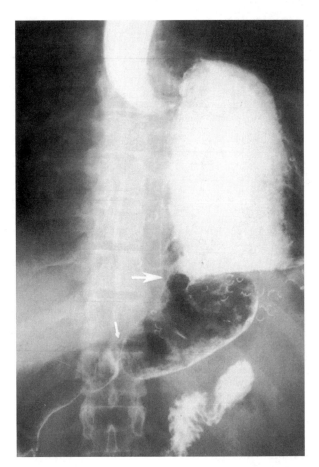

Figure 22-13 A barium study of a patient with regurgitation and dilatation of the intrathoracic stomach following esophagectomy for distal-third carcinoma. This complication was the result of two technical errors: failure to enlarge the diaphragmatic hiatus sufficiently, with resultant relative obstruction at the diaphragmatic hiatus (*large arrow*), and failure to perform a gastric drainage procedure, with resultant pyloric obstruction (*small arrow*). (Courtesy of M. B. Orringer, MD.)

intestinal gas is seen above the level of the hiatus, or the patient may present with vague left upper quadrant abdominal or lower thoracic discomfort, nausea, and vomiting.

Because the risk of incarceration and strangulation of the herniated viscera is substantial, reduction of the hernia is advised. Most herniations of intestine alongside the intrathoracic stomach occur through a relatively patulous hiatus. Reduction of the hernia and narrowing of the hiatus are readily achieved through the abdomen. This situation can generally be prevented. When the esophageal substitute has been brought through the diaphragmatic hiatus and the anastomosis has been completed, several heavy diaphragmatic crural sutures should be used to narrow the hiatus so that it admits three fingers alongside the stomach or colon. Then a few interrupted sutures between the edge of the diaphragmatic hiatus and the visceral esophageal substitute should be used to limit the migration of other intra-abdominal viscera through the hiatus into the chest. Finally, the divided triangular ligament of the mobilized liver should be sutured to

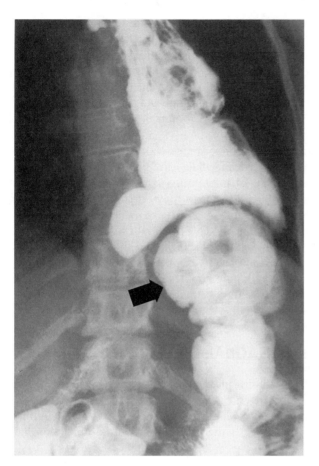

Figure 22-14 Herniation of the splenic flexure of the colon (*arrow*) through the diaphragmatic hiatus following esophageal replacement with stomach for a caustic stricture. No sutures had been placed between the intrathoracic stomach and the edge of the diaphragmatic hiatus to prevent this complication. (Courtesy of M. B. Orringer, MD.)

the edge of the hiatus to provide an additional barrier to herniation at this site.

Chylothorax

Owing to the proximity of the thoracic duct and the esophagus, chylothorax following esophagectomy is a recognized complication. Ligation of the divided periesophageal tissues at the time of esophagectomy minimizes this complication. This complication occurring in the debilitated patient with esophageal obstruction is not well tolerated, with reported mortality as high as 50% (49,50). Patients with chronic esophageal obstruction are often nutritionally depleted. Further loss of protein-rich chyle is not well tolerated. Only a few days should be expended trying to treat this complication nonoperatively. With aggressive operative intervention and direct ligation of the point of duct injury, patient salvage is the rule (51). Thoracic duct ligation at the point where the thoracic duct emerges through the diaphragmatic hiatus can be accomplished either by right posterolateral thoracotomy or minimally invasive techniques.

Pancreatitis

Postoperative pancreatitis may occur following esophagectomy due to pancreatic injury during performance of a Kocher maneuver or gastric mobilization. This possibility should be suspected in patients who develop unexplained fever, respiratory distress, or prolonged ileus after esophagectomy. The diagnosis is confirmed by elevated serum amylase and lipase levels. Standard treatment of pancreatitis with nasogastric tube decompression of the GI tract and intravenous fluids is usually sufficient, although progression to fatal hemorrhagic pancreatitis may occur.

Splenic Injury

Injury to the spleen may occur during esophagectomy, particularly during mobilization of the stomach for esophageal replacement. Careful avoidance of traction on the short gastric vessels during gastric mobilization and early division of adhesions between the stomach and the spleen on opening the abdomen minimize this complication. Routine splenectomy as part of the oncologic treatment for esophageal carcinoma is not advocated.

Peripheral Atheroembolism

Thromboembolic sequelae after transhiatal esophagectomy have been reported in two patients and attributed to inadvertent dislodgement of debris from the diseased aorta in the process of mobilizing the esophagus through the diaphragmatic hiatus (52).

COMPLICATIONS OF SUBSTERNAL ESOPHAGEAL REPLACEMENT

Several unique complications of esophageal replacement are related to retrosternal positioning of the esophageal substitute. Obstruction at the level of the retrosternal neohiatus may be due to failure to create an adequate opening. When creating a retrosternal tunnel, one must dilate this space until the entire hand and forearm can be inserted retrosternally, ensuring sufficient room for either the stomach or the colon. Compression and obstruction of the retrosternal esophageal substitute at the superior opening into the anterior mediastinum is a function of the posterior prominence of the clavicular head, which narrows the anterior thoracic inlet. When performing a retrosternal interposition of stomach or colon, which requires relocation of the cervical esophagus anteriorly from its usual position to the left and posterior to the trachea, the medial third of the clavicle, the adjacent manubrium, and usually the medial first rib should be resected to ensure an adequate opening into the anterior mediastinum.

Complications of Bypassing or Excluding the Native Esophagus

Management of the diseased native esophagus is controversial when performing retrosternal replacement of the esophagus. An esophagus that is severely strictured from a caustic injury may be left in the posterior mediastinum and bypassed with retrosternal colon. The potential complications arising from the residual diseased esophagus, however, usually mandate that it is removed whenever possible. There is a small but increased risk of late development of carcinoma in the strictured esophagus. Caustic injury may destroy the lower esophageal sphincter mechanism, and such a patient may develop reflux symptoms and severe esophagitis in the native esophagus.

Although substernal bypass of the excluded esophagus with either stomach or colon has been used for treatment of both benign and malignant disease, the complications from such an approach are appreciable. When esophageal replacement is necessary for benign disease, most authors advocate resection of the esophagus. The excluded esophagus may become a posterior mediastinal mucocele that causes respiratory distress due to tracheobronchial compression. Disruption of the distal end of the excluded esophagus will result in left subphrenic abscess.

It is always preferable to place the esophageal substitute in the posterior mediastinum in the original esophageal bed because (i) this is the shortest distance between the neck and the abdominal cavity; (ii) if subsequent anastomotic dilation is required, it is safer and more direct to perform it when one does not have to negotiate the anterior angulation of the cervical esophagus that has been anastomosed to a retrosternal graft; and (iii) the incidence of postoperative cervical anastomotic leak is lower. In the original esophageal bed in the neck, adjacent tissues buttress the anastomosis: the spine posteriorly, the carotid sheath laterally, the trachea medially, and the strap muscles anteriorly. An esophageal anastomosis to a retrosternal colon or stomach is subcutaneous in the neck and is relatively unsupported. Coughing or a Valsalva maneuver against a closed upper esophageal sphincter results in distention of the retrosternal esophageal substitute with increased pressure on the anastomosis. If esophageal bypass is performed in patients with unresectable esophageal carcinoma, the distal esophagus should be decompressed into a Roux-en-Y limb or jejunum rather than excluded (53,54).

ESOPHAGEAL DIVERTICULECTOMY

Pulsion diverticula of the esophagus, whether oropharyngeal (Zenker diverticulum) or intrathoracic, result from associated distal esophageal obstruction, most often neuromotor dysfunction. If the underlying neuromotor abnormality

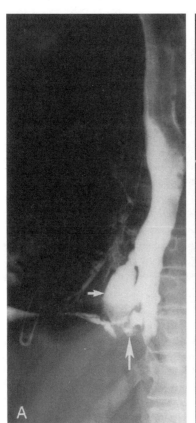 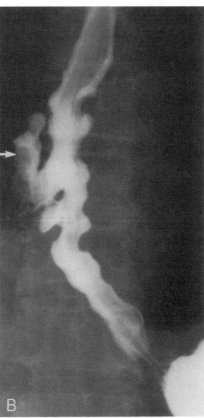

Figure 22-15 A: Esophagogram showing an esophagopleural cutaneous fistula (*large arrow*) and a recurrent esophageal diverticulum (*small arrow*) in a patient who had undergone prior resection of the diverticulum *without* an esophagomyotomy. **B:** The patient's underlying esophageal neuromotor problem is evident in this view from the same study, showing a typical corkscrew esophagus. The relative obstruction secondary to intermittent spasm distal to the esophageal suture line had not been relieved when the diverticulum was resected; hence disruption of the suture line with fistula formation and recurrence of the diverticulum (*arrow*) followed. (Courtesy of M. B. Orringer, MD.)

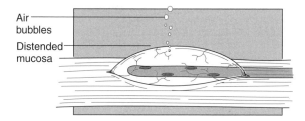

Figure 22-16 Testing for inadvertent esophageal perforation following esophagomyotomy. The esophageal mucosa is distended by insufflating air down an intraesophageal nasogastric tube. Air bubbles escaping from the esophagus submerged under saline indicate a perforation.

responsible for the formation of the diverticulum is not addressed at the time of diverticulectomy, failure to relieve the distal obstruction may result in disruption of the suture line (Fig. 22-15). With an adequate esophagomyotomy that relieves distal obstruction, the incidence of leak from a diverticulectomy suture line is exceedingly low. Following resection of a diverticulum, the esophagus should be insufflated with air through an indwelling nasogastric tube positioned within the esophagus, and an air leak should be sought by immersing the pouting esophageal submucosa in saline solution (Fig. 22-16). The most opportune time to treat a pinhole leak is at the time of operation, and a single 5-0 monofilament stitch may avert a great deal of postoperative morbidity. Alternatively, if a cervical esophageal leak occurs after diverticulectomy and esophagomyotomy, the neck wound must be opened, irrigated, and drained, as described earlier for the treatment of cervical anastomotic disruption. Nutrition may be maintained with either nasogastric feedings or total parenteral support. Broad-spectrum antibiotics are administered. If a cervical salivary fistula does occur, spontaneous closure within 7 to 10 days should be expected. If an intrathoracic esophageal suture line leak occurs within several days of diverticulectomy, immediate reexploration of the chest with closure of the fistula and reinforcement with anterior mediastinal fat, adjacent pleura, intercostal muscle, or omentum is indicated.

ESOPHAGOMYOTOMY FOR ACHALASIA OR ESOPHAGEAL SPASM

The megaesophagus of achalasia may contain 1 to 2 L of stagnant intraesophageal contents. Induction of general anesthesia in such a patient represents the most dangerous part of the operation. Because a nasogastric tube interferes with deep breathing and adequate clearing of pulmonary secretions, one should not use an intraesophageal nasogastric tube preoperatively to decompress the dilated esophagus. Rather, the patient is restricted to a clear liquid diet for 2 days before the operation, and immediately before induction of general anesthesia, with the patient in a sitting position, a nasogastric tube is passed and the esophagus is

aspirated and evacuated. Rapid-sequence induction of anesthesia is then carried out while constant pressure is maintained on the cricoid cartilage to prevent regurgitation of esophageal contents into the pharynx until the endotracheal tube balloon is inflated. Once the airway is protected, rigid esophagoscopy is carried out, and the esophagus is further evacuated and irrigated.

After completion of esophagomyotomy for either achalasia or esophageal spasm, integrity of the esophageal mucosa is documented by insufflating air into the esophagus through an indwelling intraesophageal nasogastric tube. As described earlier, identification and closure of an inadvertent esophageal injury at this point is far simpler than when the perforation is detected hours to days after operation. Patients with achalasia are frequently referred for operation following failed pneumatic dilatation or, more recently, unsuccessful intrasphincteric injection of botulinum toxin. Patients who have previously undergone botulinum toxin injection are more likely to have periesophageal fibrosis and increased risk of esophageal perforation during esophagomyotomy. Periesophageal fibrosis is less prevalent among patients previously treated by pneumatic dilatation and does not affect surgical outcomes following esophagomyotomy (55,56).

Regardless of the approach used, potential complications exist and require reoperation in 10% to 15% of patients following esophagomyotomy. If a complete distal esophagomyotomy is not performed, dysphagia and regurgitation will continue in the immediate postoperative period (57). Alternatively, if the esophagomyotomy is carried onto the stomach to ensure adequate relief of the esophageal obstruction, the uncoordinated lower esophageal sphincter may be converted to an incompetent one, with ensuing long-term complications of reflux esophagitis. A "long" esophagomyotomy, over 5 cm with extension onto the stomach, has been associated with "diverticularization" of the mucosa in long-term follow-up (58,59).

Controversy exists about the need for a concomitant antireflux procedure with the distal esophagomyotomy (60–62). Most esophageal surgeons advocate partial fundoplication to prevent the subsequent development of gastroesophageal reflux following esophagomyotomy for achalasia (63). A Belsey-type partial fundoplication has been recommended when esophagomyotomy is approached transthoracically, whereas Toupet (posterior) or Dor (anterior) fundoplication is recommended following transabdominal esophagomyotomy. When performing a fundoplication to ensure lower esophageal sphincter competence in an atonic esophagus, care must be exercised to avoid subsequent obstruction due to an overly aggressive fundoplication.

Among the more difficult problems of surgery for achalasia is the development of recurrent dysphagia and regurgitation due to esophageal obstruction after esophagomyotomy. In patients with a tortuous megaesophagus and a supradiaphragmatic pouch of esophagus, delayed esophageal emptying may occur even after a satisfactory esophagomyotomy.

Patients who have undergone previous esophagomyotomy and have recurrent symptoms have only a 40% to 70% chance of experiencing a good result from a repeated esophagomyotomy (64,65). Patients with achalasia are at risk for the development of esophageal squamous cell carcinoma and should undergo routine surveillance upper endoscopy following esophagomyotomy. In patients with either recurrent or persistent symptoms of achalasia with or without associated reflux esophagitis, esophagectomy may provide the best option, eliminating the esophageal obstruction as well as the potential for late development of carcinoma (66).

REFERENCES

1. Henderson RD, Boszko A, VanNostrand AW, et al. Pharyngoesophageal dysphagia and recurrent laryngeal nerve palsy. *J Thorac Cardiovasc Surg* 1974;68:507–512.
2. Salama FD, Lamont G. Long-term results of the Belsey Mark IV antireflux operation in relation to the severity of esophagitis. *J Thorac Cardiovasc Surg* 1990;100:517–519.
3. Orringer MB, Skinner DB, Belsey RH. Long-term results of the Mark IV operation for hiatal hernia and analyses of recurrences and their treatment. *J Thorac Cardiovasc Surg* 1972;63:25–33.
4. Pearson FG, Langer B, Henderson RD. Gastroplasty and Belsey hiatus hernia repair. An operation for the management of peptic stricture with acquired short esophagus. *J Thorac Cardiovasc Surg* 1971;61:50–63.
5. Orringer MB, Orringer JS, Dabich L, et al. Combined Collis gastroplasty—fundoplication operations for scleroderma reflux esophagitis. *Surgery* 1981;90:624–630.
6. Pearson FG. Hiatus hernia and gastroesophageal reflux: indications for surgery and selection of operation. *Semin Thorac Cardiovasc Surg* 1997;9:163–168.
7. Lam TC, Fok M, Cheng SW, et al. Anastomotic complications after esophagectomy for cancer. A comparison of neck and chest anastomoses. *J Thorac Cardiovasc Surg* 1992;104:395–400.
8. Michel L, Grillo HC, Malt RA. Esophageal perforation. *Ann Thorac Surg* 1982;33:203–210.
9. White RK, Morris DM. Diagnosis and management of esophageal perforations. *Am Surg* 1992;58:112–119.
10. Bufkin BL Jr, Miller JI, Mansour KA. Esophageal perforation: emphasis on management. *Ann Thorac Surg* 1996;61:1447–1451.
11. Zwischenberger JB, Savage C, Bidani A. Surgical aspects of esophageal disease: perforation and caustic injury. *Am J Respir Crit Care Med* 2002;165:1037–1040.
12. Cameron JL, Kieffer RF, Hendrix TR, et al. Selective nonoperative management of contained intrathoracic esophageal disruptions. *Ann Thorac Surg* 1979;27:404–408.
13. Andersen OS, Giustra PE. Nonoperative management of contained esophageal perforation. *Arch Surg* 1981;116:1214–1217.
14. Michel L, Grillo HC, Malt RA. Operative and nonoperative management of esophageal perforations. *Ann Surg* 1981;194:57–63.
15. Flynn AE, Verrier ED, Way LW, et al. Esophageal perforation. *Arch Surg* 1989;124:1211–1214.
16. Whyte RI, Iannettoni MD, Orringer MB. Intrathoracic esophageal perforation: the merit of primary repair. *J Thorac Cardiovasc Surg* 1995;109:140–146.
17. Orringer MB. Complications of esophageal surgery and trauma. In: Greenfield LJ, ed. *Complications in surgery and trauma*, 2nd ed. Philadelphia, PA: JB Lippincott Co; 1990:313.
18. Gouge TH, Depan HJ, Spencer FC. Experience with the Grillo pleural wrap procedure in 18 patients with perforation of the thoracic esophagus. *Ann Surg* 1989;209:612–617.
19. Wright CD, Mathisen DJ, Wain JC, et al. Reinforced primary repair of thoracic esophageal perforation. *Ann Thorac Surg* 1995;60:245–248.
20. Iannettoni MD, Vlessis AA, Whyte RI, et al. Functional outcome after surgical treatment of esophageal perforation. *Ann Thorac Surg* 1997;64:1606–1609.

21. Hernandez L, Jacobson J, Harris M. Comparison among the perforation rates of Maloney, balloon, and Savary dilation of esophageal strictures. *Gastrointest Endosc* 2000;51:460–462.
22. Kubba H, Spinou E, Brown D. Is same-day discharge suitable following rigid esophagoscopy? Findings in a series of 655 cases. *Ear Nose Throat J* 2003;82:33–36.
23. Patel HJ, Tan BB, Yee J, et al. A 25-year experience with open primary transthoracic repair of paraesophageal hiatal hernia. *J Thorac Cardiovasc Surg* 2004;127(3):843–849.
24. Khaitan L, Ray WA, Holzman MD, et al. Health care utilization after medical and surgical therapy for gastroesophageal reflux disease: a population-based study, 1996 to 2000. *Arch Surg* 2003;138:1356–1361.
25. Bowers SP, Mattar SG, Smith CD, et al. Clinical and histologic follow-up after antireflux surgery for Barrett's esophagus. *J Gastrointest Surg* 2002;6:532–539.
26. Watson DI, Baigrie RJ, Jamieson GG. A learning curve for laparoscopic fundoplication. Definable, avoidable, or a waste of time? *Ann Surg* 1996;224:198–203.
27. Pearson FG, Cooper JD, Ilves R, et al. Massive hiatal hernia with incarceration: a report of 53 cases. *Ann Thorac Surg* 1983;35:45–51.
28. Maziak DE, Todd TR, Pearson FG. Massive hiatus hernia: evaluation and surgical management. *J Thorac Cardiovasc Surg* 1998;115:53–60.
29. Johnson AB, Oddsdottir M, Hunter JG. Laparoscopic Collis gastroplasty and Nissen fundoplication. A new technique for the management of esophageal foreshortening. *Surg Endosc* 1998;12:1055–1060.
30. Luketich JD, Grondin SC, Pearson FG. Minimally invasive approaches to acquired shortening of the esophagus: laparoscopic Collis-Nissen gastroplasty. *Semin Thorac Cardiovasc Surg* 2000;12:173–178.
31. Orringer MB, Marshall B, Iannettoni MD. Eliminating the cervical esophagogastric anastomotic leak with a side-to-side stapled anastomosis. *J Thorac Cardiovasc Surg* 2000;119:277–288.
32. Orringer M, Lemmer J. Early dilation in the treatment of esophageal disruption. *Ann Thorac Surg* 1986;42:536–539.
33. Iannettoni MD, Whyte RI, Orringer MB. Catastrophic complications of the cervical esophagogastric anastomosis. *J Thorac Cardiovasc Surg* 1995;110:1493–1500.
34. Orringer MB, Marshall B, Iannettoni MD. Transhiatal esophagectomy: clinical experience and refinements. *Ann Surg* 1999;230:392–400.
35. Dewar L, Gelfand G, Finley RJ, et al. Factors affecting cervical anastomotic leak and stricture formation following esophagogastrectomy and gastric tube interposition. *Am J Surg* 1992;163:484–489.
36. Vigneswaran WT, Trastek VF, Pairolero PC, et al. Transhiatal esophagectomy for carcinoma of the esophagus. *Ann Thorac Surg* 1993;56:838–844.
37. Gandhi SK, Naunheim KS. Complications of transhiatal esophagectomy. *Chest Surg Clin N Orth Am* 1997;7:601–610.
38. Kirsch M, Blue M, Desai RK, et al. Intralesional steroid injections for peptic esophageal strictures. *Gastrointest Endosc* 1991;37:180–182.
39. Lee M, Kubik C, Polhamus C, et al. Preliminary experience with endoscopic intralesional steroid injection therapy for refractory upper gastrointestinal strictures. *Gastrointest Endosc* 1995;41:598–601.
40. Law SY, Fok M, Cheng SW, et al. A comparison of outcome after resection for squamous cell carcinomas and adenocarcinomas of the esophagus and cardia. *Surg Gynecol Obstet* 1992;175:107–112.
41. Gillinov AM, Heitmiller RF. Strategies to reduce pulmonary complications after transhiatal esophagectomy. *Dis Esophagus* 1998;11:43–47.
42. Doty JR, Salazar JD, Forastiere AA, et al. Postesophagectomy morbidity, mortality, and length of hospital stay after preoperative chemoradiation therapy. *Ann Thorac Surg* 2002;74:227–231.
43. Burt M, Diehl W, Martini N, et al. Malignant esophagorespiratory fistula: management options and survival. *Ann Thorac Surg* 1991;52:1222–1228.
44. Urschel JD, Blewett CJ, Young JE, et al. Pyloric drainage (pyloroplasty) or no drainage in gastric reconstruction after

esophagectomy: a meta-analysis of randomized controlled trials. *Dig Surg* 2002;19:160–164.

45. Ludwig DJ, Thirlby RC, Low DE. A prospective evaluation of dietary status and symptoms after near-total esophagectomy without gastric emptying procedure. *Am J Surg* 2001;181: 454–458.

46. Fok M, Cheng SW, Wong J. Pyloroplasty versus no drainage in gastric replacement of the esophagus. *Am J Surg* 1991;162: 447–452.

47. Katariya K, Harvey JC, Pina E, et al. Complications of transhiatal esophagectomy. *J Surg Oncol* 1994;57:157–163.

48. Heitmiller RF, Gillinov AM, Jones B. Transhiatal herniation of colon after esophagectomy and gastric pull-up. *Ann Thorac Surg* 1997;63:554–556.

49. Merigliano S, Molena D, Ruol A, et al. Chylothorax complicating esophagectomy for cancer: a plea for early thoracic duct ligation. *J Thorac Cardiovasc Surg* 2000;119:453–457.

50. Wemyss-Holden SA, Launois B, Maddern GJ. Management of thoracic duct injuries after oesophagectomy. *Br J Surg* 2001;88: 1442–1448.

51. Orringer MB, Bluett M, Deeb GM. Aggressive treatment of chylothorax complicating transhiatal esophagectomy without thoracotomy. *Surgery* 1988;104:720–726.

52. Magee MJ, Landreneau RJ, Keenan RJ, et al. Peripheral atheroembolism from the aorta complicating transhiatal esophagectomy. *Am Surg* 1994;60:634–637.

53. Kirschner M. Ein neues verfahren der oesophagus plastik. *Arch Klin Chir* 1920;114:606–663.

54. Meunier B, Stasik C, Raoul J-L, et al. Gastric bypass for malignant esophagotracheal fistula: a series of 21 cases. *Eur J Cardiothorac Surg* 1998;13:184–189.

55. Patti MG, Feo CV, Arcerito M, et al. Effects of previous treatment on results of laparoscopic Heller myotomy for achalasia. *Dig Dis Sci* 1999;44:2270–2276.

56. Wiechmann RJ, Ferguson MK, Naunheim KS, et al. Video-assisted surgical management of achalasia of the esophagus. *J Thorac Cardiovasc Surg* 1999;118:916–923.

57. Patti MG, Molena D, Fisichella PM, et al. Laparoscopic Heller myotomy and Dor fundoplication for achalasia: analysis of successes and failures. *Arch Surg* 2001;136:870–877.

58. Chen L-Q, Chughtai T, Sideris L, et al. Long-term effects of myotomy and partial fundoplication for esophageal achalasia. *Dis Esophagus* 2002;15:171–179.

59. Ellis FH Jr. Failure after esophagomyotomy for esophageal motor disorders. Causes, prevention, and management. *Chest Surg Clin N Orth Am* 1997;7:477–487.

60. Richards WO, Sharp KW, Holzman MD. An antireflux procedure should not routinely be added to a Heller myotomy. *J Gastrointest Surg* 2001;5:13–16.

61. Peters JH. An antireflux procedure is critical to the long-term outcome of esophageal myotomy for achalasia. *J Gastrointest Surg* 2001;5:17–20.

62. Lyass S, Thoman D, Steiner JP, et al. Current status of an antireflux procedure in laparoscopic Heller myotomy: outcomes of laparoscopic fundoplication for gastroesophageal reflux disease and paraesophageal hernia. *Surg Endosc* 2003;17:554–558.

63. Ellis FH Jr, Watkins E Jr, Gibb SP, et al. Ten to 20-year clinical results after short esophagomyotomy without an antireflux procedure (modified Heller operation) for esophageal achalasia. *Eur J Cardiothorac Surg* 1992;6:86–89.

64. Gorecki PJ, Hinder RA, Libbey JS, et al. Redo laparoscopic surgery for achalasia. *Surg Endosc* 2002;16:772–776.

65. Ellis FH Jr, Crozier RE, Gibb SP. Reoperative achalasia surgery. *J Thorac Cardiovasc Surg* 1986;92:859–865.

66. Devaney EJ, Lannettoni MD, Orringer MB, et al. Esophagectomy for achalasia: patient selection and clinical experience. *Ann Thorac Surg* 2001;72:854–858.

Complications of Pulmonary and Chest Wall Surgery

23

Harvey I. Pass   Shane Yamane

■■■ PREOPERATIVE ASSESSMENT 264

■■■ ARRHYTHMIAS 265

■■■ POSTRESECTION PULMONARY EDEMA 266
Pathogenesis 266
Preventative Maneuvers 267
Treatment 267

■■■ CARDIAC HERNIATION 267

■■■ LOBAR TORSION 267

■■■ ATELECTASIS 267

■■■ BRONCHOPLEURAL FISTULA 268

■■■ SPACES AND AIR LEAKS 270

■■■ INTRAOPERATIVE HEMORRHAGE 272
Right Hilum 272
Left Hilum 272

■■■ POSTOPERATIVE HEMORRHAGE 272

■■■ CHYLOTHORAX 273

■■■ ESOPHAGOPLEURAL FISTULA 273

■■■ COMPLICATIONS OF CHEST WALL
RESECTION 274

■■■ FLAIL CHEST 274

■■■ SEROMA 274

■■■ WOUND INFECTION 274

■■■ SCAPULA ENTRAPMENT 274

■■■ REFERENCES 275

Harvey I. Pass and Shane Yamane: Wayne State University, Detroit, MI 48201

Lung resection remains the only curative treatment option for patients with lung carcinoma. Despite greater surveillance and enhanced imaging modalities, the locally advanced lung cancer with involvement of the chest wall remains a surgical challenge. Complications after resectional therapy can never be totally eliminated (1), but the effects can be minimized with careful attention to preoperative assessment, meticulous surgical technique, and surgical maneuvers to minimize potential problems.

PREOPERATIVE ASSESSMENT

The initial evaluation of a patient's risk of lung resection has been clinical assessment and pulmonary function tests. Nagasaki et al. studied 961 patients undergoing resection for lung carcinoma and found three high risk factors: age >70 who require major resection, positive cardiac history, and any patient with severely restricted pulmonary reserve (2). Gender, stage, and cell type were found to have little influence on morbidity. In a study of 476 patients undergoing thoracotomy, Kohman et al. evaluated 37 preop risk factors (3). Only age >60, need for pneumonectomy, and premature ventricular contractions on preop EKG were associated with increased mortality, accounting for only 12% of observed mortality. Accurate preoperative assessment requires more physiologic measurements.

Ferguson et al. evaluated the preoperative risk factors of 165 patients undergoing pulmonary resection and found the single greatest predictor of postoperative morbidity and mortality to be the preoperative diffusing capacity of the lung for carbon dioxide ($DLCO_2$) (4). The $DLCO_2$ estimates pulmonary capillary surface area and can reveal diffusion defects and emphysematous changes even with acceptable spirometric values. This increased sensitivity justifies the addition of $DLCO_2$ to preoperative assessment. In a retrospective review, Ferguson et al. found that the most reliable predictor of postoperative complication was percent-predicted postoperative $DLCO_2$ (5). They concluded that a preoperative diffusing capacity <60% of predicted was an increased risk for complications after pneumonectomy (6).

Maximum oxygen consumption during exercise (VO_{2max}) has been evaluated to predict postoperative complication. Bechard and Wetstein (7) evaluated minimal risk when VO_{2max} was >20 mL/kg/min. Patients with VO_{2max} <50 mL/kg/min. accounted for 75% of all postoperative complications. Bolliger and Perruchoud (8) concluded that VO_{2max} <10 mL/kg/min. is predictive of high postoperative complications and may be considered prohibitive. A value >20 mL/kg/min or >75% predicted normal is safe for major pulmonary resection, including pneumonectomy.

Exercise oximetry has been shown to predict prolonged hospitalization, intensive care stay, and major morbidity (9,10), but randomized trials are needed to determine this test's reliability.

Vigorous preoperative respiratory therapy, smoking cessation, bronchodilator therapy, and even short course steroid use has shown improvement in operability of lung cancer patients with marginal pulmonary reserve (11). More conservative operations for the marginal patient may still allow for a curative resection.

ARRHYTHMIAS

Both atrial and ventricular arrhythmias can occur following pulmonary resection. As early as the 1940s investigators noted an increased incidence of arrhythmias after lung resections (12,13). Postoperative arrhythmias have been reported at an incidence of 3.4% to 30%. Atrial arrhythmias, fibrillation, flutter, and supraventricular tachycardia are the most common (14–16). Arrhythmias most often occur on the second or third postoperative day. Shields and Ujiki (15) studied 125 consecutive patients and reported a 22% mortality rate for patients with an arrhythmia postoperatively versus 7% for those in sinus rhythm. The Mayo Clinic retrospectively reviewed 236 pneumonectomy patients and found a 25% 30-day mortality in patients developing a tachyarrhythmia.

Age as a risk factor for postoperative arrhythmia, although intuitive, has conflicting support within the literature. Some authors (14) report a near linear relationship between age and arrhythmia, but Krowka et al. (17) studied 236 pneumonectomy patients and failed to show a correlation between age and arrhythmia. Advanced age increases the likelihood of coexistent risk factors for arrhythmias, which supports the findings of Wheat and Burford, who reported a 50% incidence of postoperative arrhythmias in patients 70 years and older undergoing pulmonary resection (16).

A direct relationship exists between extent of resection and postoperative arrhythmias. In a series of 301 patients, Mowry and Reynolds (14) reported a 19.4% rate of arrhythmias after pneumonectomy versus a 3.1% rate following lobectomy. Other series (15,16) have shown a less dramatic difference between extent of resection and arrhythmia. Likewise, Krowka et al. (17) failed to demonstrate a firm relationship between preoperative pulmonary function and arrhythmia. Volume overload on chest x-ray after pneumonectomy has been correlated to an increased incidence of arrhythmia.

Accurate preoperative identification of patients at risk for postoperative arrhythmia remains elusive. Digoxin and β-blockers preoperatively have often been used for prevention. Although digoxin has been the drug of choice to prevent postoperative arrhythmias, potential side effects and newer agents have reduced its popularity. Digoxin is thought to reduce conduction through the AV node via enhanced vagal tone. Digoxin is known to slow ventricular response rate in supraventricular tachycardias, but it is relatively ineffective at converting the heart to sinus rhythm. In the immediate postoperative period, digoxin has reduced efficacy due to more pronounced andrologic influences. Underlying lung disease and ventricular dysfunction have reduced the use of low-dose β blockade for arrhythmia prophylaxis preoperatively.

A prophylactic calcium channel blocker (verapamil) significantly reduces post-thoracotomy arrhythmias (18). In addition, verapamil has been shown to reduce right ventricular systolic and diastolic pressures, which, when elevated, are thought to predispose to atrial arrhythmias. Van Mieghem et al. (19) showed that a 10-mg bolus of verapamil reduced the incidence of atrial arrhythmias by 50%. Associated bradycardia and hypotension have led to the discontinuation of this drug in many patients. Diltiazem, also a calcium channel blocker, has shown similar efficacy in reducing atrial arrhythmias, with a lower side effect profile than verapamil, leading to greater use of this agent post-thoracotomy (20,21). Amar (22) compared digoxin to diltiazem and found diltiazem to be safer and more effective at preventing atrial arrhythmias in pneumonectomy patients. The incidence of arrhythmias in the digoxin-treated patients was similar to the untreated arm. Amiodarone has been used to treat postoperative atrial arrhythmias; however, an association with pulmonary toxicity and adult respiratory distress syndrome (ARDS) has prevented its widespread acceptance in the postpulmonary resection patients.

Once postoperative arrhythmias such as atrial fibrillation occur, treatment follows several steps. First, the heart function (rate and contractility) should be acutely controlled. Atrial fibrillation with rapid ventricular response results in poor cardiac filling and decreased cardiac output. Digoxin is administered intravenously in divided doses to a loading dose of 1 mg in adults. Digoxin does not slow ventricular rate acutely, and, as mentioned previously, does not reliably convert patients to sinus rhythm. Acute rate control is obtained with diltiazem given as a bolus followed by a continuous infusion. Underlying causes such as electrolyte abnormalities—particularly potassium and magnesium—are evaluated, as are hypoxia, anemia, and volume overload. For unstable patients with atrial fibrillation, immediate electrocardioversion is required. Refractory atrial fibrillation is rare, and electrocardioversion for stable atrial fibrillation is not usually needed unless a long preoperative history of atrial fibrillation exists. Patients requiring pharmacologic conversion should be kept on these medications for at least 3 months after surgery.

Prophylaxis against atrial arrhythmias is usually administered only for pneumonectomy patients. Although no data indicates that this prevents atrial fibrillation, it should prevent rapid ventricular response if atrial fibrillation occurs. If a pneumonectomy is performed unexpectedly, the patient is loaded with digoxin postoperatively and maintained on daily doses. All pulmonary resection patients require cardiac monitoring for the first 24 hours. We generally extend this period for pneumonectomy patients, older patients, and patients with comorbidities predisposing to cardiac events.

POSTRESECTION PULMONARY EDEMA

Noncardiogenic pulmonary edema after lung resection was first described by Gibbon and Gibbon in 1942 (23,24). Zeldin et al. (25) reviewed ten cases of postresection pulmonary edema (PPE) and identified three risk factors: right pneumonectomy, high perioperative fluid administration, and high urine output (UOP) as a sign of volume overload. Verheijen-Breemhaar (26) et al. reviewed 243 pneumonectomy patients and found that PPE occurred in 4.5%, a mortality rate of 27%, increased in right versus left

pneumonectomy, a more positive fluid balance, and in patients who required reoperation for bleeding. Patel et al. (27) retrospectively studied 197 pneumonectomy patients in England and found a 15% incidence of postoperative pulmonary edema and a mortality rate of 43%.

Waller et al. reported a larger series involving 402 lung resection patients from Leeds, England (28). In this series, PPE occurred in 5.1% of right pneumonectomies, 4% of left pneumonectomies, and 1% of all lobectomies. The mortality rate was 55%. Interestingly, these authors did not observe a correlation between perioperative fluid administration and PPE. Turnage and Lunn (29) retrospectively reviewed charts on 806 pneumonectomy patients at the Mayo Clinic and found 21 cases (2.6%) who experienced PPE. Affected patients had a 100% mortality rate and histologic evidence of ARDS at autopsy. Patients who had a right-sided resection had a threefold higher incidence of PPE as compared to left pneumonectomy patients. No significant difference was found between the affected patients and age-matched and sex-matched control groups with regard to administration of perioperative fluids. The authors concluded that although PPE is more common following right pneumonectomy, the etiology was still uncertain. Shapira and Shahian (30) reviewed the literature in their report and confirmed that pulmonary edema developed in approximately 4% of patients following a major lung resection.

Pathogenesis

Fluid overload has been implicated in the pathogenesis of PPE since the early work of Gibbon and Gibbon (23,24) and almost certainly plays a major role. Zeldin et al. (25) confirmed the role of overhydration in the canine model. The authors concluded that following pneumonectomy the entire cardiac output is directed to the remaining lung with resultant increase in the intracapillary pressure, which predisposes to edema formation. Increased cardiac output from catecholamine release secondary to pain or from excessive fluid administration exacerbates this situation.

Interruption of mediastinal lymphatics probably plays a role in the formation of PPE. In normal lungs it has been estimated that lymph flow can increase sevenfold to tenfold without leading to pulmonary edema. Following pneumonectomy, a proportional amount of lymphatic channels is removed with the specimen. In addition, mediastinal and subcarinal dissection can effectively compromise the lymphatic drainage from the remaining lung. Little et al. (31) studied the effect of pneumonectomy and mediastinal lymphatic interruption in a canine model. Following pneumonectomy, the contralateral lung was more prone to extravascular fluid development due to the loss of parenchymal and hilar lymphatics. Nohl-Oser (32) has further described the lymphatic drainage of the lung and mediastinum and reported that the lymphatics from the right and left lungs are notably different. The majority of lymphatic channels from the left lung cross the midline.

Therefore a right pneumonectomy is more likely to disrupt lymphatic drainage from the remaining left lung, possibly contributing to edema formation.

Preventative Maneuvers

Following pneumonectomy, the entire cardiac output is directed to the remaining lung, with resultant elevation in pulmonary capillary pressure. Efforts should be made to restrict fluid administration during the intraoperative and early postoperative periods. Total positive fluid balance in the first 24 hours perioperatively should not exceed 20 mL per kg—typically, <2 L intraoperatively followed by <50 mL per hour postoperatively for an average adult. UOP >0.5 mL per kg is unnecessary in the early postoperative period unless renal insufficiency exists. Placement of a central venous pressure monitoring line is often useful in assessing intravascular volume and will aid in the decision to administer diuretic or inotropic therapy.

Avoidance of mediastinal shift and overdistention of the remaining lung is also essential. Experimental work by Raffensperger et al. (33) in dogs confirmed that overdistention of the contralateral lung following pneumonectomy led to deterioration in lung function. These changes were reflected by an increase in the alveolar-arterial gradient. It is now believed that acute hyperinflation of the remaining lung is probably a significant factor in the development of PPE.

Adequate pain control is essential to minimize catecholamine release with resultant increase in cardiac output. Lumbar or thoracic epidural anesthesia has proved extremely useful in this situation by providing adequate pain control without oversedation of the patient.

Treatment

Development of PPE is associated with a mortality rate in excess of 50%. Current therapy is supportive and essentially the same as for ARDS. This generally consists of fluid restriction, diuretic therapy, and maintenance of adequate oxygenation and nutritional support. Most patients require intubation and mechanical ventilation. Prolonged ventilation may increase barotrauma and bronchial stump dehiscence. Inspired oxygen concentrations of 80% to 100%, as well as high positive end-expiratory pressures, may be required to maintain adequate arterial saturation. Peak inspiratory pressures >30 mm Hg should be avoided if possible. Empiric antibiotic use is probably of little benefit because the underlying process is not infectious in nature.

Mathison et al. (34) reported the use of inhaled nitric oxide in ten patients with PPE. In addition to standard supportive therapy, inhaled nitric oxide at 10 to 20 parts per million was administered. Overall mortality was 30%. In refractory cases extracorporeal membrane oxygenation (ECMO) may improve survival, but the role for this last stand therapy has not been fully defined.

CARDIAC HERNIATION

Cardiac herniation following lung resection requiring pericardial resection is a rare but lethal complication. Herniation of the heart through the pericardial defect with entrapment and both venous and arterial obstruction decreases cardiac output and increases central venous pressure. Cardiac herniation is reported to occur following both left and right pneumonectomies, and symptoms include tachycardia, hypotension, and jugular venous distension. The event usually occurs early in the postoperative period before intracardiac adhesions have occurred. Precipitating events can include coughing, position changes, positive pressure ventilation, or excessive negative pressure applied to the pneumonectomy space. Posteroanterior chest radiograph may diagnose right sided herniation, but lateral film may be required to show the posterior displacement of a left sided herniation.

When suspected, patients require prompt reexploration and closure of the pericardial defect. To prevent herniation at resection, most recommend closure of the pericardiotomy. Materials include pleura, vicryl mesh, and Gore-Tex.

All right sided pericardial defects must be closed because of the severe consequences of herniation into the right chest. Large left sided defects do not require routine closure.

LOBAR TORSION

Lobar torsion is most commonly associated with the mobilized right middle lobe after right upper lobectomy (35). Torsion on the left following either upper or lower lobectomies has been reported. Right middle lobe torsion can be prevented by tacking the lobe to the remaining upper or lower lobe either with suturing or application of stapling devices. Schuler (36) reported a 16% mortality rate in 31 patients with torsion. Rotation of the pulmonary lobe around its bronchovascular pedicle results in occlusion of pulmonary veins, infarction, and eventual gangrene of the involved parenchyma. Angulation of the bronchus also compromises bronchial circulation, endangering lung parenchyma. Postoperative pulmonary infarct in the absence of torsion has been described from venous thrombosis, pulmonary artery (PA) occlusion, and intraoperative bronchial circulation damage (37).

Early recognition is essential to prevent irreversible damage. Chest radiographs may demonstrate hilar displacement, bronchial cutoff, and lobar consolidation. Nuclear perfusion scans and pulmonary angiography can also support the diagnosis.

ATELECTASIS

Atelectasis following thoracotomy is the most common postoperative complication. The absolute incidence of atelectasis is difficult to determine because of varying definitions in the literature. Although atelectasis is generally accepted to occur in 20% to 30% of thoracotomies, the actual incidence may be as high as 70% (2,38,39).

Physiological significant atelectasis results in decreased lung compliance, functional residual capacity, and vital capacity. This results clinically in increased work of breathing and impaired gas exchange (40,41). Patients present with varying degrees of fever, tachycardia, tachypnea, and impaired gas exchange. Atelectasis also makes the lung more susceptible to infection (42). Physical exam findings include crackles and tubular breath sounds, indicating the involvement of entire segments or lobes. Sudden cessation of an air leak may occur with atelectasis. The radiologic appearance of atelectasis varies with the extent of involvement. Linear horizontal densities in the basilar segments are typical of small areas of atelectasis and usually occur near the diaphragm. Progression may lead to involvement of entire segments and eventually lobar collapse.

At least two mechanisms prevent alveolar collapse. The first is a sigh breath, usually two times the normal resting tidal volume (V_T). The sigh recruits collapsed alveoli. Inadequate pain control with resultant shallow breathing and inadequate V_Ts in the intubated patient result in progressive alveolar collapse and atelectasis. The second mechanism is surfactant. Produced by type II pneumocytes, surfactant reduces the surface tension within the alveoli, preventing preferential collapse of smaller alveoli. Malnutrition, sepsis, parenchymal injury, and prolonged collapse all reduce surfactant production and predispose to alveolar collapse.

A condition known as absorption atelectasis occurs with proximal airway occlusion. Gases in the distal alveoli are absorbed, resulting in alveolar collapse. In addition, a higher concentration of oxygen in the trapped or anesthetic gases is more readily absorbed, thereby hastening the process.

Several maneuvers can be extremely valuable in the prevention of postoperative atelectasis. Patients must refrain from smoking for as long as possible before thoracotomy. Any bronchospasm detected either clinically or on preoperative pulmonary function testing should be minimized with medical therapy. Patient training and use of incentive spirometry should be initiated in the preoperative period and continued postoperatively. Adequate analgesia is essential to prevent splinting and to allow adequate pulmonary toilet. We use epidural analgesics routinely for 3 to 5 days postoperatively because they provide excellent pain relief with minimal adverse effects (43). Patient positioning in the early postoperative period is also important. Functional residual capacity declines by about 40% in the supine position as compared to upright. Routine elevation of the head of the bed to 45 degrees and early ambulation promote effective inspiration.

Treatment of postoperative atelectasis involves many of the principles used in its prevention. Airways must remain free of retained secretions, and collapsed lung tissue must be reexpanded. Adequate postoperative analgesia is essential to allow for deep breathing, effective cough, and therapeutic physiotherapy. Epidural analgesia is an effective means of obtaining adequate analgesia without significant sedation. Contraindications to placement of an epidural catheter include bleeding diathesis, spinal deformity, neurologic deficit, or local infection in the area of catheter placement. Side effects and symptoms of overdosing include respiratory depression, nausea, pruritus, urinary retention, and hypotension secondary to peripheral vasodilatation.

Patients with thick or copious secretions require a more aggressive approach. Nasotracheal suctioning is effective when performed by personnel experienced in passing the catheter into the trachea. A nasal trumpet may facilitate the process while decreasing patient discomfort. Caution should be exercised when passing the catheter blindly after pneumonectomy or a bronchoplastic procedure. Prolonged suctioning can precipitate hypoxia and should be performed only intermittently for short periods following administration of supplemental oxygen. Routine use of flexible bronchoscopy for the prevention of postoperative atelectasis has been studied prospectively and found to offer no advantage over other less invasive techniques (44,45). However, in the setting of significant pulmonary collapse or after bronchoplastic procedures, fiberoptic bronchoscopy is a safe and effective method to aspirate secretions under direct vision. Bronchoscopy can be easily performed at the bedside using local analgesia and, if necessary, can be repeated often (46). Finally, percutaneous cricothyroidotomy, or "minitracheostomy," has been found to be effective for preventing atelectasis from retained secretions (47–50). Treatment of postoperative atelectasis should be graded according to the patient's clinical status and risk factors, as described by Massard and Wihlm (51).

BRONCHOPLEURAL FISTULA

The incidence of bronchopleural fistula after pulmonary resection is <5% (52–54). Predisposing factors include the patient's nutritional status and the presence of sepsis. Lung cancer patients are frequently malnourished, and the ability of tissues to heal is decreased. Sepsis also retards bronchial healing, and many patients with an obstructive endobronchial neoplasm have distal pneumonitis producing chronic low-grade infection. Neoadjuvant treatment of clinically advanced lung cancer includes chemotherapy and radiation. Chemotherapy can be debilitating to the patient and a significant factor in the development of a bronchial fistula. Radiation destroys small blood vessels, creates fibrous tissue, and is associated with an increased incidence of bronchial fistula (55). Vester et al. (52) reported that of the 33 patients who developed a bronchopleural fistula after resection for bronchogenic carcinoma, 20 had received radiation or chemoradiation. It is mandatory that special care be given to the bronchial stump in all patients who have received neoadjuvant therapy.

Numerous studies indicate that the causes of bronchopleural fistula include devitalization and devascularization by excessive dissection, parabronchial infection related to nonabsorbable suture, residual bronchial disease, poor approximation of the mucosa, the length of the stump, and the surgeon's lack of experience (56). The avoidance of the complication of a bronchopleural fistula implies prevention, and several technical factors can minimize this complication.

Preoperative bronchoscopy is an important step in evaluating the status of the bronchial mucosa at the site of the planned resection. If inflammation is present, specific attention is made to the stump closure along with coverage by flaps of tissue for reinforcement and added blood supply. If surgery for the cancer is semielective, it can be delayed for nutritional optimization and antibiotics.

It is important for the surgeon to know the anatomic location of the bronchial arteries and to preserve as many as possible. This is particularly true when carrying out mediastinal lymphadenectomy. Feeding bronchial arteries traverse the subcarinal area, and dissection must be done carefully to preserve these nutrient vessels. The right mainstem bronchus receives its blood supply from vessels posterior to the trachea and bronchus, and it is appropriate not to dissect this area if possible. The lymphadenectomy between the vena cava and trachea is done carefully to minimize damage to the blood supply to the lateral walls of the trachea. On the left side, a large bronchial artery has its origin from the distal transverse aorta and, on occasion, can be preserved despite removal of lymph nodes in the aorticopulmonary window. An excessively long bronchial stump accumulates excessive secretions, and its distal margin has a limited blood supply. The bronchus should always be divided as proximally as possible, but closure must not compromise the adjacent trachea or bronchial lumen.

The method of bronchial stump closure is generally the surgeon's preference. Stapled bronchial closure is associated with a fistula rate of 1.7% to 2.6% (52,57). Al-Kattan et al. reviewed 530 consecutive pneumonectomies and found a hand-sewn bronchial closure fistula rate of 1.3% (58). In 1982, Lawrence et al. (53) studied 378 patients undergoing pulmonary resection and found no significant difference between the hand-sewn and stapled bronchial closure. If the cancer is close to the bronchial orifice, by bronchoscopy or during hilar dissection the stapling techniques should not be used. Whenever the proximal extent of tumor is uncertain, the bronchus is transected by knife and suture closure is performed. After neoadjuvant therapy, the bronchial tissues can be thick and fibrotic. A thickened bronchus does not hold the staples, and excessive tension permits edges of the bronchus to separate. In this instance it is recommended that the hand-suture technique be performed with absorbable or nonabsorbable monofilament suture.

The same principles used in dissecting and closing the bronchus for a pneumonectomy apply to the bronchus after lobectomy. If the tissues are too thick or the cancer is too close to the margin of resection, stapling is not used. Special attention must be given to the bronchial stump of a bilobectomy. Vester et al. (52) reported ten bronchial fistulas in 965 patients receiving either bilobectomy or lobectomy, with nine fistulas after bilobectomy. The increased incidence of fistula after a bilobectomy undoubtedly relates to the extensive dissection of the bronchus and devitalization. It is important to consider tissue coverage of the bronchial stump after bilobectomy to minimize this complication. This is particularly true if the patient has received neoadjuvant therapy.

All right pneumonectomy stumps should be covered with some form of tissue. The left pneumonectomy stump, if done correctly, retracts deeply into the mediastinum, and the decision for tissue coverage requires careful judgment. All pneumonectomy patients who have received neoadjuvant therapy should have both the right and left pneumonectomy stumps covered with tissue.

Al-Kattan et al. (58) recommend burying the bronchial stump beneath the mediastinal tissues. Azygos vein, adjacent pleura, pericardium, and esophageal wall can all be used for this. A broad-based pleural flap can also be used to cover the bronchial stump. The pleura contains few blood vessels and does not enhance the healing process with additional blood supply. For this reason, other tissue coverage is generally recommended. Pedicled muscle flaps include the intercostal muscle and the serratus anterior (59,60). We use a broad-based mediastinal fat pad for coverage of both the right and left pneumonectomy stumps. Its blood supply is not as generous as a muscle flap, but secure tissue coverage is obtained. Use of the omentum is not recommended for routine coverage of a pneumonectomy stump. It requires the placement of an additional incision in the abdomen and a longer operating time than the flaps described above.

Patients who develop a bronchial fistula 3 to 4 weeks after pneumonectomy expectorate serosanguineous fluid, may become dyspneic, and frequently develop subcutaneous emphysema. Chest radiograph illustrates a decreasing amount of fluid in the pneumonectomy space and the presence of subcutaneous air. In the hospital the patient should be positioned with the operated side down to prevent spillage of the pleural fluid into the contralateral lung. A chest tube is inserted to remove all the fluid without delay. Balanced pleural drainage is preferable, but a standard underwater-seal drainage system is adequate. The drainage system is not connected to suction to prevent mediastinal shift and hemodynamic compromise. Flexible fiberoptic bronchoscopy should be done to evaluate the pneumonectomy stump and clear the airway of secretions and fluid. With the development of vascular tissue flaps for stump coverage, new antibiotics, and the success of antibiotic irrigation in combating empyema, reoperation and bronchial stump reclosure can be considered up to 14 days after the initial operation.

The management of a bronchopleural fistula that occurs several weeks or months after pneumonectomy is best accomplished with the open-window thoracostomy or Eloesser flap (61). The presence of a chronic bronchopleural fistula requires direct closure because it will not heal on its own, and the pneumonectomy space cannot be closed or sterilized until the fistula has healed. Puskas et al. (62) described successful closure of chronic bronchopleural fistulas in 40 of 47 patients (85%) using direct suture closure of the bronchial stump in 37 patients. All these closures were buttressed with vascularized pedicle flaps of omentum, muscle, or pleura. At the time of fistula closure the empyema cavity can be obliterated using myoplasty and thoracoplasty techniques. Any residual cavity that remains can be successfully sterilized using the Claggett (63) technique. These techniques have significantly decreased the need for a disfiguring thoracoplasty, which is the alternative method of treating postpneumonectomy empyema and fistula.

If a pneumonectomy fistula occurs in a long bronchial stump, consideration can be given to the transsternal approach for reamputation of the stump. Fibrin glue can successfully close a small fistula up to 4 mm in size, and its use should be considered when a small fistula has been identified. Closure of small fistulas in both pneumonectomy and lobar stumps has been achieved. Fibrin glue is instilled through catheters passed through the channel of a fiberoptic bronchoscope. This technique is associated with low morbidity and can be the initial therapeutic maneuver if the fistula is small (64,65).

Bronchial fistula after lobectomy is rare, and it is more common for a lobar bronchial fistula to occur after a bilobectomy than a standard lobectomy. Early dehiscence of a bronchial stump after lobectomy is evidenced by a persistent and moderate air leak, a sudden increase in the size of an air leak, or the development of a space after chest tubes have been removed. Other symptoms include fever and a cough productive of serosanguineous fluid or purulent material from a developing empyema. If a fistula is suspected, bronchoscopy should be carried out. Complete separation of a bronchial closure is obvious, but small defects in a lobar bronchus may be difficult to identify. A to-and-fro motion of secretions at the stump, necrotic tissue, and granulations are all indicators of a fistula. If the chest tubes have been removed, a new chest tube must be inserted into the developing space as soon as the diagnosis of a lobar stump fistula is made. A decision is then made about appropriate therapy.

In general, it is better to treat lobar bronchial fistula in a long-term conservative manner, for several reasons. First, acute debridement of a dehisced lobar stump may result in little remaining bronchus to reapproximate, and closure would compromise a mainstem bronchus. Second, to achieve closure of viable bronchial tissue, a completion pneumonectomy may be required, with increased morbidity and mortality. Third, the probable infected space may predispose the fistula closure to failure, resulting in an increase in morbidity and mortality.

Reoperation for a lobar fistula consists of several options. The bronchus can be resected to obtain more healthy tissue, and the stump is reapproximated with a fine, nonabsorbable, monofilament suture. If the bronchial tissues are necrotic, amputation of the bronchus at a higher level must be considered. Sleeve lobectomy can be considered after an upper-lobe bronchial fistula, but the possibility of anastomotic failure and difficulty in reexpansion of the residual lung tissue must be considered. All reoperative bronchial closures must be covered by a viable tissue flap.

Despite the fact that adequate tube drainage after lobar bronchial fistula may result in a more protracted course, a successful long-term result can usually be achieved. Myoplasty or thoracoplasty, or both, may be necessary to close the fistula and obliterate the associated space, but they are accomplished at less risk when the patient's condition is able to withstand a second operation. Tube drainage is maintained until the residual lung tissue is adherent to the parietal pleura, and the fistula is then treated as a chronic problem. A small fistula may eventually close with fibrotic resolution of the space, but most remain open. Basic criteria to be carried out include control of the underlying disease process and a clean, dependently drained space (65).

SPACES AND AIR LEAKS

Normal adaptive mechanisms to compensate for lung volume reduction are (a) expansion of the residual lung, (b) mediastinal shift, (c) narrowing of the intercostal space, and (d) elevation of the diaphragm. Reduction of the postoperative air space directly correlates to duration of air leak and postoperative complications. Induction chemoradiation therapy for lung cancer can result in mediastinal fibrosis limiting its movement. Fibrotic lung does not fully expand, and air leaks do not seal. The elderly lung cancer patient with emphysematous lungs is prone to prolonged air leak.

Most air leaks close within 7 days. Persistent air leaks from small bronchi or disrupted alveoli can be termed alveolo-pleural fistulas. These small leaks result from denuded visceral pleura, incomplete lung fissures, raw surface of a segmentectomy, and nonanatomic resections. Use of stapling devices to complete fissures or for wedge resections minimizes air leaks. If the lung is emphysematous, the staple lines should be reinforced with bovine pericardium or Gore-Tex. At the conclusion of the resection the lung should be expanded to 20 to 25 cm H_2O pressure under saline immersion to evaluate all surfaces for air leaks. Small air leaks are closed with fine sutures. Leakage from a bronchial stump is repaired. A pedicled pleural flap can be used to cover both bronchial stumps and tissue leaks, secured to the lung parenchyma with absorbable suture.

Air leaks lasting longer than 7 days may be managed in several ways. Suction can be discontinued because it is possible that the increased negative intrapleural pressure is maintaining the air leak. A chest radiograph is obtained in 24 hours, and if a space is developing, the suction is restarted. Chest-tube suction is maintained for the initial postoperative 7 days because it has been our experience that if the lung collapses in the early postoperative period, reexpansion can be difficult, with a resultant residual space. A second maneuver is to withdraw the anterior chest tube by 1 or 2 inches. A chest-tube hole may be directly adjacent to a small air leak; repositioning the tube allows the lung to expand, and the leaking lung surface adheres to the parietal pleura.

If the lung remains expanded after discontinuation of suction, consideration can be given to removing the chest tubes, despite the presence of a small air leak. This technique can be successful, but if a space does develop, a chest tube must be reinserted. Suction is maintained until the air leak stops or the patient is discharged with a Heimlich valve attached to the leaking chest tube. The patient is seen at weekly intervals in the office. The leak usually stops by the time of the first office visit, and the tube is then removed. It may be necessary to leave the tube in place for an additional 2 to 3 weeks until the air leak stops. If the air leak persists 4 weeks after hospital discharge, the patient is considered to have an empyema, and open drainage is instituted. The tube is then shortened by 1 or 2 inches at weekly intervals until it is removed. This method of tube management is predicated on the fact that the patient does not have an infected space and the lung is expanded.

There are no specific guidelines for the indications of reoperation of a patient with a persistent air leak at 7 to 14 days. Factors in this decision include the patient's general condition, the emphysematous nature of the remaining lung, the speculated cause of the persistent air leak, and the presence and magnitude of an intrapleural space. Reoperation and necessary decortication can create new air leaks, and careful judgment is required to reoperate for a persistent air leak. A large and increasing air leak may make reoperation necessary.

The development of a postoperative space is commonly related to a persistent and large air leak, but other causes include resection of two lobes on the right side, only the basal segments of either lobe remaining, fibrosis in the remaining lung that limits expansion, and incomplete decortication from prior pleural effusion or infection. Postoperative atelectasis and a fixed mediastinum due to irradiation or prior inflammation also contribute to the development of a space. All these factors are seen in patients undergoing resection for lung cancer. Kirsch et al. (66) reported on the natural history of the pleural space and noted that 74% undergo spontaneous resolution, 13% require temporary drainage, 7% are persistently sterile, and only 6% become infected.

Practical steps can be carried out in the management of a postoperative space. The first is to be certain that the residual lung tissue is clear of all secretions and that postoperative atelectasis is aggressively treated. Early postoperative consideration must be given to increasing the amount of chest-tube suction. We routinely start with 20 cm of water suction immediately after the operation and recommend increasing suction to 30 or 40 cm of water pressure if there is a space in association with an air leak. Evacuation of the air permits the raw lung surface to reach the parietal pleura, and small air leaks close. Suction should be increased in increments of only 10 cm of water to evaluate the patient's ability to tolerate it. We do not use suction set at more than 40 cm of water pressure because of patient discomfort.

Intraoperative maneuvers to minimize postoperative airspace include pleural tent. Even if a constructed pleural tent is not airtight, the large pleural flap can cover residual lung tissue and expedite the closure of parenchymal air leaks, which effectively eliminates a space problem. Transplantation of the diaphragm and crushing of the phrenic nerve have been advocated to minimize the postoperative space but have not been used in our experience. Disadvantages include the time involved to transplant the diaphragm and the loss of diaphragmatic motion, which decreases the patient's ability to cough, as well as long-term pulmonary function. The most extensive intraoperative procedure is to bring the chest wall to the lung tissue by either a tailoring or an osteoplastic thoracoplasty. A tailoring thoracoplasty entails subperiosteal resection of the first and second ribs along with a portion of the third rib to decrease the size of the apex. An osteoplastic thoracoplasty is a subperiosteal resection of the posterior portions of ribs 2, 3, 4, and 5, with wire fixation of these ribs to the posterior sixth rib. Thoracoplasty in association with an extended pulmonary resection is not recommended because it will result in inadequate postoperative ventilation due to paradoxical chest wall motion.

If the air leak stops and there is a persistent space, the chest tube is removed and the space is treated as if it were sterile. The patient can be safely discharged without antibiotic therapy and is followed with periodic chest radiographs. The sterile space obliterates with fibrous tissue over time.

If an empyema does develop in a postoperative space, tube drainage is mandatory. If the space is small, it is managed with open-tube drainage, and the tube is slowly backed out as the space obliterates. If closure of an infected space does not occur after several weeks, or if the space is large, there are two surgical options, thoracoplasty and muscle flap obliteration.

The pedicle muscle flap is the most effective method of obliterating almost any infected residual space, and the muscle can be used to close any residual bronchial fistula (67). The pectoralis major is particularly well suited for placement into the apex of the chest and avoids the deformity of a thoracoplasty. Other tissues that can be used include the omentum, serratus anterior muscle, and latissimus dorsi muscle—if the previous thoracotomy has not transected it.

INTRAOPERATIVE HEMORRHAGE

Hilar dissection in patients with central lung cancers can be very difficult. Tissue planes of the PA following neoadjuvant radiation therapy are often obliterated. Meticulous sharp dissection is often required to resect tumors from these structures. Neoadjuvant therapy and prior mediastinoscopy create fibrosis of the paratracheal tissues, making mediastinal lymphadenectomy difficult. Various technical maneuvers can be used to minimize intraoperative hemorrhage.

Right Hilum

With difficult access to the PA in hilar dissection from central tumor or other technical reason, a proximal approach to the PA is to open the pericardium at the level of the superior pulmonary vein and extend the pericardiotomy onto the superior vena cava above the azygos. Ligation and division of the azygos is without consequence and enhances exposure. The main right PA medial to the superior vena cava can be isolated, and, if a difficult lobectomy is expected, a Rumel tourniquet can be applied.

A more medial approach to the right PA requires a wide pericardiotomy and exposure of the artery between the ascending aorta and superior vena cava. This dissection is mostly blunt finger dissection, and care is used not to disrupt the main artery. Tumor involvement at this level is rare, and proximal control can be obtained. The artery may be ligated at this level for pneumonectomy with either heavy permanent suture or stapling device.

Upper lobe tumor blocking the anterior approach to the PA, but not involving the mainstem bronchus, may be approached by first dividing the bronchus. The artery's posterior aspect is then readily visible and ligation and division performed. Despite proximal arterial control, a defect in a large lobar branch may cause significant atrial back bleeding, necessitating clamping of the pulmonary veins.

Involvement of either superior or inferior pulmonary vein requires opening of the pericardium for proximal control. The atrium may be included in the vascular stapling device for adequacy of margin, or a clamp and sew technique with a large vascular clamp and running monofilament suture may be employed.

Tumor may involve the superior vena cava. If minimally involved, a partially occluding vascular clamp may be used to resect part of the vena cava wall. If more extensively involved, the innominate veins are isolated and controlled with provisional ligatures. The pericardium is opened, and a tourniquet is applied at the caval-atrial junction. The vena cava can be bypassed by a catheter technique, as described by Piccione et al. (68), and the defect closed by a pericardial patch graft. Vena cava may also be replaced by Gore-Tex in the technique of Dartevelle et al. (69).

Left Hilum

Left-sided lung cancer frequently involves the aorticopulmonary window. The PA cannot be safely dissected outside the pericardium, which is opened medial or lateral to the phrenic nerve, extending to the aortic arch. The main PA is identified and the left main artery is then dissected free, usually necessitating transection of the ligamentum arteriosum for exposure. The right PA should be identified to prevent injury to the main PA. Control of the left main artery with a Rumel tourniquet may be performed for a difficult lobectomy. The left main PA can be approached posteriorly after division of the left mainstem bronchus.

Involvement of the transverse aortic arch may occur with large hilar tumors that have been treated with neoadjuvant therapy. Meticulous sharp dissection is required to separate these fibrotic tissues. Care must be exercised to avoid dissection between the adventitia of the aorta. Direct tumor involvement with its poor prognosis precludes en bloc resection of the aorta.

POSTOPERATIVE HEMORRHAGE

Postoperative bleeding usually occurs from the primary resection site or from intercostal incisional bleeding. Extrapleural resections may produce persistent chest wall oozing that is difficult to control. Suture slippage may produce sudden massive blood loss in the recovery unit or ICU and necessitates emergent reoperation. Another cause of postoperative bleeding is from coagulopathy related to transfusion of several units of banked blood intraoperatively.

Patients on aspirin for coronary or cerebral vascular disease are common, and such therapy should be stopped 2 weeks prior to the operation. Generalized oozing after an extended dissection in patients still on aspirin prior to surgery may require platelet transfusion.

Symptoms of postoperative hemorrhage are tachycardia, hypotension, and chest tube drainage >200 mL per hour into chest drainage system. Upright chest radiograph is required to evaluate for accumulation in the chest since tube drainage is not a reliable indicator.

Blood replacement is guided by intraoperative loss, patient's physiologic status, and chest tube loss. Bleeding 200 mL per hour for 4 consecutive hours is indication for reoperation. Decision to reoperate is guided by rate and trend of blood loss, patient clinical status, speculative source for bleeding, and coagulation profile.

Prevention is the key to avoiding postoperative bleeding complications. Cautery to the chest wall is used liberally.

The mediastinum is carefully inspected for large bronchial arteries that may have clotted and will rebleed postoperatively. PA and veins are inspected for defects in closure, controlled with fine interrupted suture. Large vessels should be suture ligated to prevent slippage. The anterior and posterior portions of the thoracotomy are inspected for intercostal bleeding.

CHYLOTHORAX

Postoperative chylothorax occurs more frequently after pneumonectomy than after lobectomy. The thoracic duct enters the chest through the aortic hiatus and is on the right side of the vertebral bodies until it crosses to the left at T5 or 6. The duct ascends posterior to the aortic arch before exiting the mediastinum and joining into the left subclavian vein. The duct may have multiple channels and tributaries in the region of the subcarinal space. Damage may occur anywhere along the mediastinum. Subcarinal lymphadenectomy, mobilization of the left mainstem bronchus, or dissection of involved lymph nodes may all result in unrecognized injury to the thoracic duct. Any milky drainage during dissection must be investigated, and any defect in the main duct or its branches must be ligated with interrupted permanent suture. Because the patients have been NPO (nothing by mouth) for several hours prior to surgery, chyle may appear golden-yellow rather than milky.

Chylothorax is most often suspected when chest tube drainage turns a milky opaque character. Persistent drainage of serous fluid 1,000 mL in 24 hours should raise the possibility of thoracic duct leak. With resumption of oral intake the drainage will turn the classic milky character. Chylomicrons and lipoprotein electrophoresis on pleural fluid analysis, as well as triglyceride levels more than 100 mg per dL, indicate chyle.

Rapid filling of the pneumonectomy space with tracheal deviation away from the operative side suggest chylothorax. Initial management is conservative with chest tube drainage and total parenteral nutrition. Miller (70) reports spontaneous closure in about half of patients. Maximum observation time is 2 weeks. Reoperation at 7 days may be required for massive fluid loss and patient deterioration. Further nutritional deficits and clinical deterioration invite complication and possible mortality; therefore, conservative management beyond 2 weeks is not recommended.

At reoperation the chest is opened on the side of the fistula. The patient is administered cream or olive oil 2 to 3 hours prior. The fistula area is often inflamed and does not hold sutures well. Dissection to better define the leak results in bleeding. Supradiaphragmatic ligation of the main duct should be performed. The tissues between the aorta and azygos are bluntly dissected with an angled clamp and mass ligated with heavy silk. Clips may further damage the duct and should be avoided. Although more

accessible through a right lower thoracotomy, this ligation may be performed through either thorax.

Other operations to control chylothorax include pleurectomy, pleural peritoneal shunt, fibrin glue sealant, and thoracoscopic ligation of duct. The gold standard remains operative ligation of the duct.

ESOPHAGOPLEURAL FISTULA

The intrathoracic esophagus runs in close proximity to the lower trachea and right mainstem bronchus. A large hilar cancer may involve the muscular wall by direct invasion. The esophagus is also directly posterior to the subcarinal space and may be injured by subcarinal lymphadenectomy from either chest.

Careful review of preoperative imaging will show proximity of the tumor to the esophagus. Nasogastric tube placement prior to the procedure helps delineate the entire thoracic esophagus. Any full thickness defects should be immediately closed in two layers with fine absorbable monofilament. The repair is easily buttressed with an adjacent flap. Muscularis injuries alone should be repaired using similar suture in a single layer closure.

The subcarinal space may contain large bronchial arteries that have been supplying tumor and lymph nodes. Extensive use of cautery in this area to control bleeding should be avoided and individual ligation performed.

Esophageal fistula may occur both early and late in the postoperative course. Presenting signs and symptoms of empyema include fever, chest pain, loss of appetite, decreased fluid level in pneumonectomy space, or the appearance of an air fluid level in previously opacified hemithorax. Tube thoracostomy may demonstrate food particles. Bronchoscopy is performed to evaluate for bronchopleural fistula; immediate esophogram confirms the leak. Massard et al. (71) recommend routine barium swallow for any postpneumonectomy empyema, especially if it occurs late after operation.

Treatment of early esophageal fistula is direct repair. The pneumonectomy space is opened and careful debridement performed. The esophagus is repaired in two layers and buttressed with vascularized intercostals muscle flap, serratus anterior, or omentum. Gastrostomy for drainage and feeding jejunostomy are recommended. The pneumonectomy space is lavaged with antibiotic solution, and, if sterilized, the chest tube may be removed. Long-term open drainage by the Claggett technique may be required. Esophageal exclusion with later reconstruction is another option; however, one stage repair is recommended (72). Late esophageal fistula requires rib resection and adequate drainage of the pleural space, as well as gastrostomy and jejunostomy for alimentation. When the patient's condition is stabilized, direct repair as previously described is performed. The omentum's vascularity and adhesive properties make an excellent buttress in this case. Thoracoplasty and myoplasty are used to obliterate the pleural space. Esophageal fistula carries a high mortality and morbidity. The fistula requires aggressive therapy because it will not close spontaneously.

COMPLICATIONS OF CHEST WALL RESECTION

Despite advances in preoperative evaluation with high resolution CT scans, discrimination between tumor invasion, adhesion, or simple contact between tumor and parietal pleura cannot always be determined preoperatively. Approximately 5% of lung cancers involve the parietal pleura and chest wall. Completeness of resection is one of the main factors affecting long-term survival in patients with lung cancer and chest wall invasion (73). With aggressive resection to clear margins involving the chest wall, some specific complications should be watched for.

FLAIL CHEST

Chest wall reconstruction for prevention of flail chest needs to be performed only if more than three contiguous ribs in the anterolateral chest wall are resected. Any full thickness defect with the possibility of paradoxical movement with respiration should be reconstructed. Skeletal reconstruction of 5 cm or lesser resections of full thickness chest wall anywhere in the chest is not necessary due to the lack of respiratory compromise. Posterior chest wall resections have skeletal support from the scapula, and defects <10 cm do not require reconstruction.

Reconstructive techniques utilizing flaps and free grafts can be used to provide soft tissue coverage of large chest wall defects. Thoracic cage skeletal fixation has been described using bone grafts from tibia, fibula, iliac crest, and rib transposition. Fascia lata can also be used for reconstruction. Myocutaneous flaps available for chest wall reconstruction include the rectus abdominis, latissimus dorsi, and pectoralis major.

The choice of prosthetic material for chest wall reconstruction depends on surgeon preference. Prosthetic materials used to reconstruct the chest wall include various mesh materials, such as polypropylene, polytetrafluoroethylene, marlex, and Teflon (74). Rigid fixation with prosthetics includes wire fixation and methylmethacrylate.

Mechanical ventilation may be required in the immediate postoperative period for respiratory insufficiency; however, within 6 or 7 days adhesions provide adequate stabilization of the chest wall.

SEROMA

After respiratory complications, wound seroma is the most common complication following chest wall reconstruction

for locally advanced lung cancer. Deschamps et al. (75) reviewed the Mayo clinic experience with prosthetic chest wall reconstruction in 197 patients. In their series they presented progression of prosthetic mesh closure of large chest wall defects from polypropylene mesh (PM) from 1977 to 1986 to polytetrafluoroethylene (PTFE) from 1986 to 1992. Seroma occurred in 7.1% of patients, none of whom went on to develop infection. Twelve seromas were small; six of them resolved spontaneously and six resolved after repeated aspiration. Seromas not resolving with conservative measures require wound exploration and obliteration of the involved space.

WOUND INFECTION

Perhaps the most feared complication of prosthetic closure of chest wall defects is infection of the graft material. From the Mayo Clinic experience (75), wound infection occurred in 4.6% of all patients undergoing chest wall reconstruction. Early management of infections of prosthetic mesh reconstructions involved removal of the mesh. Because the underlying lung was adherent to the pleura and no pneumothorax space developed, no further therapy was required. Later in their series, four patients with infections of PTFE prostheses were managed by wound opening, debridement, and packing. All wounds closed by secondary intention without further complications. Prosthetic mesh placed into known contaminated wounds resulted in wound infection rates of 100%. Skeletal support following prosthetic mesh removal is then provided by autologous tissue transfers, as described above.

Omentum, with its high vascularity, allows for use in coverage of infected spaces and readily accepts skin graft. Omentum can be used to fill residual space left from myocutaneous flaps, and, with production of angiogenic factors, accelerates healing of infected spaces (75,76).

SCAPULA ENTRAPMENT

Because of scapula coverage, posterior defects of the chest wall do not need to be closed unless the scapula tip becomes trapped in the defect. If the chest wall defect is located posteriorly near the tip of the scapula, during movement of the arm the tip can become trapped (75). Closure of the defect in the chest wall, as discussed above, is indicated in this instance.

Lung cancer is the leading cause of cancer-related death in the United States and a continuing challenge to the thoracic surgeon. Lung resection with and without chest wall resection presents surgical and postoperative challenges. Preoperative assessment, meticulous attention to operative technique, and vigilance for postoperative complications will continue to advance the practice and safety of surgical resection of lung cancer.

REFERENCES

1. Ginsberg RJ, Hill LD, Eagan RT, et al. Modern thirty-day operative mortality for surgical resections in lung cancer. *J Thorac Cardiovasc Surg* 1983;86:654.
2. Nagasaki F, Flehinger BJ, Martini N. Complications of surgery in the treatment of carcinoma of the lung. *Chest* 1982;82:25.
3. Kohman LJ, Meyer JA, Ikins PM, et al. Random versus predictable risks of mortality after thoracotomy for lung cancer. *J Thorac Cardiovasc Surg* 1986;91:551.
4. Ferguson MK, Little L, Rizzo L, et al. Diffusing capacity predicts morbidity and mortality after pulmonary resection. *J Thorac Cardiovasc Surg* 1988;96:894.
5. Ferguson MK, Reeder LB, Mich R. Optimizing selection of patients for major lung resection. *J Thorac Cardiovasc Surg* 1995;109:275.
6. Ferguson MK. Assessment of operative risk for pneumonectomy. *Chest Surg Clin Am* 1999;9:339.
7. Bechard D, Wetstein L. Assessment of exercise oxygen consumption as preoperative criterion for lung resection. *Ann Thorac Surg* 1987;44:344.
8. Bollinger CT, Perruchoud AP. Functional evaluation of lung resection candidate. *Eur Respir J* 1998;11:198.
9. Rao V, Todd TRV, Kuus A, et al. Exercise oximetry versus spirometry in the assessment of risk prior to lung resection. *Ann Thorac Surg* 1995;60:603.
10. Ninin M, Somers E, Landreneau RJ. Standardized exercise oximetry predicts post pneumonectomy outcome. *Ann Thorac Surg* 1997;64:328.
11. Peters RM, Clausen JL, Tisi GM. Extending resectability for carcinoma of the lung in patients with impaired pulmonary function. *Ann Thorac Surg* 1978;26:250.
12. Bailey CC, Betts RH. Cardiac arrhythmias following pneumonectomy. *N Engl J Med* 1943;229:356.
13. Currens JH, White PD, Churchill ED. Cardiac arrhythmias following thoracic surgery. *N Engl J Med* 1943;229:360.
14. Mowry FM, Reynolds EW. Cardiac rhythm disturbances complicating resection surgery of the lung. *Ann Intern Med* 1964;61:688.
15. Shields TW, Ujiki GT. Digitalization for prevention of arrhythmias following pulmonary surgery. *Surg Gynecol Obstet* 1968;126:743.
16. Wheat MW, Burford THE. Digitalis in surgery: extension of classical indications. *J Thorac Cardiovasc Surg* 1961;41:162.
17. Krowka MJ, Pairolero PC, Trastek VE, et al. Cardiac dysrhythmia following pneumonectomy. *Chest* 1987;91:490.
18. Lindgren L, Lepantalo M, Von Knorring J, et al. Effect of verapamil on right ventricular pressure and atrial tachyarrhythmia after thoracotomy. *Br J Anaesth* 1991;66:205.
19. Van Mieghem W, Coolen L, Malysse I, et al. Amiodarone and the development of ARDS after lung surgery. *Chest* 1994;105:1642.
20. Salerno DM, Dias VC, Kleiger RE, et al. Efficacy and safety of intravenous diltiazem for treatment of atrial fibrillation and atrial flutter. *Am J Cardiol* 1989;63:1046.
21. Ellenbogen KA, Dias VC, Plumb VJ, et al. A placebo-controlled trial of continuous intravenous diltiazem infusion for 24-hour heart rate control during atrial fibrillation and atrial flutter: a multi center study. *J Am Coll Cardiol* 1991;18:891.
22. Amar D. Cardiac arrhythmias. *Chest Surg Clin N Am* 1998; 8:479.
23. Gibbon JR, Gibbon MH, Kraul CW. Jr. Experimental pulmonary edema following lobectomy and blood transfusion. *J Thorac Surg* 1942;12:60.
24. Gibbon JR, Gibbon MH Jr. Experimental pulmonary edema following lobectomy and plasma infusion. *Surgery* 1942;12:694.
25. Zeldin RA, Normandin D, Landtwing D, et al. Postpneumonectomy pulmonary edema. *J Thorac Cardiovasc Surg* 1984;87:359.
26. Verheijen-Breemhaar L, Bogaard JM, Van Den Berg B, et al. Postpneumonectomy pulmonary edema. *Thorax* 1988;43:323.
27. Patel RL, Townsend ER, Fountain SW. Elective pneumonectomy: factors associated with morbidity and mortality. *Ann Thorac Surg* 1992;54:840.
28. Waller DA, Gebitekin C, Saunders NR, et al. Noncardiogenic pulmonary edema complicating lung resection. *Ann Thorac Surg* 1993;55:140.
29. Turnage WS, Lunn JJ. Postpneumonectomy pulmonary edema: a retrospective analysis of associated variables. *Chest* 1993; 103(6):1646.
30. Shapira OM, Shahian DM. Postpneumonectomy pulmonary edema. *Ann Thorac Surg* 1993;56:190.
31. Little AG, Langmuir VK, Singer AH, et al. Hemodynamic pulmonary edema in dog lungs after contralateral pneumonectomy and mediastinal lymphatic interruption. *Lung* 1984;162:139.
32. Nohl-Oser HC. An investigation of the anatomy of the lymphatic drainage of the lungs as shown by the lymphatic spread of bronchial carcinoma. *Ann R Coll Surg Engl* 1972;51:157.
33. Raffensperger JG, Luck SR, Inwood RJ, et al. The effect of overdistention of the lung on pulmonary function in beagle puppies. *J Pediatr Surg* 1979;14(6):757.
34. Mathisen DJ, Kuo EY, Hahn C, et al. Inhaled nitric oxide for adult respiratory distress syndrome after pulmonary resection. *Ann Thorac Surg* 1998;65:1894.
35. Wong PS, Goldstraw P. Pulmonary torsion: a questionnaire survey and a survey of the literature. *Ann Thorac Surg* 1992; 54:286.
36. Schuler JG. Intraoperative lobar torsion producing pulmonary infarction. *J Thorac Cardiovasc Surg* 1973;65:951.
37. Kim H, Roldan CA, Shively BK. Pulmonary vein thrombosis. *Chest* 1993;104:624.
38. Iverson LIG, Ecker RR, Fox HE, et al. A comparative study of IPPB, the incentive spirometer, and blow bottles: the prevention of atelectasis following cardiac surgery. *Ann Thorac Surg* 1978; 25:197.
39. O'Donohue WJ. National survey of the usage of lung expansion modalities for the prevention and treatment of postoperative atelectasis following abdominal and thoracic surgery. *Chest* 1985;87:76.
40. Ali J, Serrette C, Wood LDH, et al. Effect of post-operative intermittent positive pressure breathing on lung function. *Chest* 1984;85:192.
41. Stock MC, Downs JB, Gauer PK, et al. Prevention of postoperative pulmonary complications with CPAP, incentive spirometry, and conservative therapy. *Chest* 1985;87:151.
42. Nguyem DM, Mulder DS, Shennib H. Altered cellular immune functioning of the atelectatic lung. *Ann Thorac Surg* 1981;51:76.
43. Lubenow TR, Faber LP, McCarthy RJ, et al. Postthoracotomy pain management using continuous epidural analgesia in 1,324 patients. *Ann Thorac Surg* 1994;58:924.
44. Bartlett RH. Pulmonary pathophysiology in surgical patients. *Surg Clin North Am* 1980;60:1323.
45. Jawroski A, Goldberg SK, Walkenstein MD, et al. Utility of immediate postlobectomy fiberoptic bronchoscopy in preventing atelectasis. *Chest* 1988;94:38.
46. Mahajan VK, Catron PW, Huber GL. The value of fiber-optic bronchoscopy in the management of pulmonary collapse. *Chest* 1978;73:817.
47. Au J, Walker WS, Inglis D, et al. Percutaneous cricothyroidostomy (minitracheostomy) for bronchial toilet: results of therapeutic and prophylactic use. *Ann Thorac Surg* 1989;48:850.
48. Wain JC, Wilson DJ, Mathisen DJ. Clinical experience with minitracheostomy. *Ann Thorac Surg* 1990;49:881.
49. Randell TT, Tierala EK, Lepantalo MJ, et al. Prophylactic minitracheostomy after thoracotomy: a prospective, random control, clinical trial. *Eur J Surg* 1991;157:501.
50. Mastboom WJ, Wobbes T, van den Dries A, et al. Bronchial suction by minitracheostomy as an effective measure against sputum retention. *Surg Gynecol Obstet* 1991;173:187.
51. Massard G, Wihlm JM. Postoperative atelectasis. *Chest Surg Clin North Am* 1998;8:503.
52. Vester SR, Faber LP, Kittle CF, et al. Bronchopleural fistula after stapled closure of bronchus. *Ann Thorac Surg* 1991;52:1253.
53. Lawrence GH, Ristroph R, Wood JA, et al. Methods for avoiding dire surgical complications: bronchopleural fistula after pulmonary resection. *Am J Surg* 1982;144:136.
54. Williams NS, Lewis CT. Bronchopleural fistula: a review of 86 cases. *Br J Surg* 1976;63:530.
55. Warram J. A collaborate study. Preoperative irradiation of cancer of the lung: final report of a therapeutic trial. *Cancer* 1975; 36:914.

56. Kaplan DK, Whyte RJ, Donnelly RD. Pulmonary resection using automatic stapling devices. *Eur J Cardiothorac Surg* 1987;1:152.

57. Forrester-Wood CP. Bronchopleural fistula following pneumonectomy for carcinoma of the bronchus. *J Thorac Cardiovasc Surg* 1980;80:406.

58. Al-Kattan K, Cattalani L, Goldstraw T. Bronchopleural fistula after pneumonectomy with a hand suture technique. *Ann Thorac Surg* 1994;58:1433.

59. Pairolero PC, Arnold PG, Piehler JM. Intrathoracic transposition of extrathoracic skeletal muscle. *J Thorac Cardiovasc Surg* 1983; 86:809.

60. Regnard JF, Icard P, Deneuville M, et al. Lung resection after high doses of mediastinal radiotherapy (sixty grays or more). *J Thorac Cardiovasc Surg* 1994;106:607.

61. Puskas JD, Mathisen DJ, Grillo HC, et al. Treatment strategies for bronchopleural fistula. *J Thorac Cardiovasc Surg* 1995;109(5): 989–995.

62. Eloesser L. An operation for tuberculosis empyema. *Surg Gynecol Obstet* 1935;60:1096.

63. Claggett OT, Gerace JE. A procedure for the management of post-pneumonectomy empyema. *J Thorac Cardiovasc Surg* 1963;45:141.

64. Spotnitz WD, Dalton MS, Baker JW, et al. Successful use of fibrin glue during 2 years of surgery at a university medical center. *Am Surg* 1989;55:1660.

65. Torre M, Chiesa G, Ravini M, et al. Endoscopic gluing of bronchopleural fistula. *Ann Thorac Surg* 1994;58:901.

66. Kirsch MM, Rotman H, Behrendt DM, et al. Complications of pulmonary resection. *Ann Thorac Surg* 1975;20:215.

67. Arnold PG, Pairolero PC. Intrathoracic muscle flaps: an account of their use in the management of 100 consecutive patients. *Ann Surg* 1990;211:656.

68. Piccione W, Faber LP, Warren WH. Superior vena caval reconstruction using autologous pericardium. *Ann Thorac Surg* 1990;50:417.

69. Dartevelle F, Chapelier A, Pastorino U, et al. Long-term follow-up after prosthetic replacement of the superior vena cava combined with resection of mediastinal-pulmonary malignant tumors. *J Thorac Cardiovasc Surg* 1991;102:259.

70. Miller JI. Chylothorax. In: Shields TW, ed. *General thoracic surgery*, 4th ed. Baltimore, MD: Williams & Wilkins; 1994:714.

71. Massard G, Ducrocq X, Hentz JG, et al. Esophagopleural fistula: an early and long-term complication after pneumonectomy. *Ann Thorac Surg* 1994;58:1437.

72. Asaoka U, Imaizumi M, Kajita M, et al. One stage repair for an oesophageal fistula after pneumonectomy using an omental pedicle flap. *Thorax* 1988;43:943.

73. Magdeleinat P, Alifano M, Benbrahem C, et al. Surgical treatment of lung cancer invading the chest wall: results and prognostic factors. *Ann Thorac Surg* 2001;71:1094.

74. McCormack PM. Use of prosthetic materials in chest wall reconstruction: assets and liabilities. *Surg Clin North Am* 1989;69:965.

75. Deschamps C, Tirnaksiz BM, Darbandi R, et al. Early and long-term results of prosthetic chest wall reconstruction. *J Thorac Cardiovasc Surg* 1999;117:588.

76. Al-Kattan KM, Breach NM, Kaplan DK, et al. Soft-tissue reconstruction in thoracic surgery. *Ann Thorac Surg* 1995;60:1372.

Complications of Extracorporeal Circulation

24

Jennifer S. Lawton

■ INTRODUCTION 277

■ MECHANISMS 278

■ CARDIOVASCULAR COMPLICATIONS 278
Prevention 278

■ PULMONARY COMPLICATIONS 279
Risk Factors 279
Prevention 279

■ IMMUNE AND ALLERGIC COMPLICATIONS 279

■ PROTAMINE REACTION 279

■ HEPARIN-INDUCED THROMBOCYTOPENIA 279
Risk Factors 280
Prevention 280

■ HEMATOLOGIC COMPLICATIONS 280
Risk Factors 281
Prevention 281

■ ENDOCRINE COMPLICATIONS 281

■ FLUID BALANCE AND RENAL
COMPLICATIONS 281
Risk Factors 282
Prevention 282

■ CENTRAL NERVOUS SYSTEM
COMPLICATIONS 282
Risk Factors 282
Prevention 282

■ GASTROINTESTINAL COMPLICATIONS 283
Risk Factors 284
Prevention 284

■ REFERENCES 284

Jennifer S. Lawton: Washington University School of Medicine, St. Louis, MO 63110

INTRODUCTION

Extracorporeal circulation is a form of temporary circulatory support that is nonphysiologic and usually nonpulsatile. This form of circulatory support may or may not include an in-line oxygenator. Extracorporeal circulation may be used to provide hemodynamic support, gas exchange, or body temperature regulation. Extracorporeal circulation, in the form of cardiopulmonary bypass (CPB), allows for the performance of cardiothoracic surgery in a quiet, bloodless field. This chapter focuses on CPB as it is used for the performance of cardiothoracic surgery.

Extracorporeal circulation was first used to perform the intracardiac repair of an atrial septal defect by John Gibbon on May 6, 1953 (1). Technologic advances since that time have made the use of CPB readily available and technically feasible, with a subsequent decline in the morbidity and mortality of cardiothoracic surgery. Unfortunately, the use of CPB requires systemic anticoagulation and introduces the blood to nonendothelial surfaces that result in detrimental changes evident throughout the body. These detrimental changes result in postoperative complications that increase morbidity, mortality, and the cost and length of hospitalization for patients undergoing cardiothoracic surgery.

In a series of 10,634 patients, investigators reported that 15% of patients having coronary artery bypass grafting had one or more complications, and those patients who had complications experienced an eightfold to tenfold increase in operative mortality (2). Although it is uncertain what portion of postoperative complications can be attributed to CPB alone, it is clear that prolonged CPB time is a significant risk factor for all postoperative complications. The complications of CPB have come under intense interest and critical scrutiny recently due to the more widespread adaptation of off-pump coronary artery bypass grafting and the development of minimally invasive techniques. The use of off-pump techniques to avoid the complications associated with CPB seems intuitively beneficial. However, large, prospective randomized trials have yet to determine the actual benefits of performing surgery without CPB (3).

MECHANISMS

Fortunately, most patients who undergo CPB recover without significant complication. The mechanisms responsible for injury may include any of the following: a generalized low flow state, relative ischemia and reperfusion injury, exposure to anticoagulation and its reversal, hemodilution and the destruction of the blood constituents, the embolization of gas or particulate matter, the placement of intravascular cannulae, mishaps related to pumps and tubing, and the activation of a systemic inflammatory response. Complications directly related to the CPB machine may include power interruption, air introduction via physical jarring of the machine or circuit manipulation, oxygenator failure, dislodgement of a connection, pump head reversal, tubing rupture, improper occlusion, and stopcock dislodgement or turning. Complications secondary to CPB are grouped according to organ system, with emphasis on pathophysiology, risk factors, prevention, and management. This chapter will focus on adult patients only.

CARDIOVASCULAR COMPLICATIONS

Injury to the heart during CPB may be manifested as poor myocardial function at the time of separation from bypass. Myocardial dysfunction attributed to CPB alone is often

difficult to distinguish from dysfunction as a result of preexisting injury or damage due to poor myocardial protection. Myocardial dysfunction following CPB that improves after a limited time is called myocardial stunning. Myocardial stunning is a reversible postischemic contractile dysfunction that persists after reperfusion despite the absence of irreversible damage and despite the return of normal perfusion (4). Stunning occurs in up to 10% of patients and is associated with mortality as high as 17% (1,5). Myocardial stunning attributed to CPB may result from fluid overload and edema, activation of complement and neutrophils, microemboli, damage to the coronary endothelium by cardioplegic arrest and reperfusion, inadequate protection during aortic cross clamping, and global ischemia and reperfusion (1,6).

Injury to the heart structures during CPB may occur. Epicardial vessels can be injured with manipulation of the heart. The coronary sinus may be perforated due to the placement of a retrograde cardioplegia catheter, and the sinus node may be injured secondary to purse-string sutures or retraction.

Cardiopulmonary bypass also contributes to postoperative arrhythmias, including supraventricular tachycardia, atrial fibrillation, ventricular tachycardia, and heart block. The altered electrolyte balance following ischemia, cardioplegia administration, and reperfusion may play a role in this complication. The etiology of arrhythmias is multifactorial and may include inflammation secondary to surgical trauma and manipulation, air embolism, elevated catecholamine levels, and ischemic injury (7,8).

Vascular complications of CPB include direct injury to the vessel wall secondary to cannula placement, aortic dissection or posterior wall perforation secondary to cannula placement, or embolization of particulate matter. The placement of intravascular cannulae can also result in retroperitoneal hematoma, vessel transection, and ischemia or malperfusion of the lower extremity.

Risk factors associated with cardiovascular complications following CPB include peripheral vascular disease, emergency surgery, presence of unstable angina, length of CPB, and poor preoperative ventricular function.

Prevention

Strategies to prevent cardiovascular complications include frequent delivery of cardioplegia, complete coronary revascularization when possible, minimization of bypass time, and confirmation of cannulae placement using transesophageal echocardiography, pressure waveforms, or pulsatility. Myocardial dysfunction following CPB may be multifactorial and challenging to treat. A pulmonary artery catheter is often helpful in decision making. Cardiac output should be optimized by the manipulation of preload, heart rate, contractility, and afterload. Technical problems related to the surgery should be excluded using echocardiography or cardiac catheterization. Stunned myocardium that does not respond to maximum inotrope doses may be supported by using an intra-aortic balloon pump (IABP) and, ultimately, a ventricular assist device.

Postoperative arrhythmias are typically treated by temporary pacing or by pharmacologic means. Blood vessel injury or transection requires operative repair, and an iatrogenic aortic dissection requires replacement of the ascending aorta to reestablish the normal aortic lumen.

PULMONARY COMPLICATIONS

Lung injury is the most common serious injury following CPB (9). Lung injury may range from minor subclinical functional changes to adult respiratory distress syndrome (10). Lung injury is due to many factors, including leukoembolization secondary to complement activation, increased interstitial edema and atelectasis, increased vascular permeability, decreased colloid osmotic pressure due to hemodilution, bronchospasm, and decreased surfactant production (1,9,11).

During CPB the lungs remain in an altered state of deflation, which contributes to atelectasis. The diaphragm becomes passively displaced cephalad by the abdominal contents in the paralyzed patient. Deflation, combined with preferential ventilation to the nondependent regions of the lung, leads to ventilation-perfusion mismatch (11). The lungs receive blood largely from the bronchial arteries, as pulmonary artery blood flow may be minimal, contributing to pulmonary ischemia during CPB (10,12). The sequestration of neutrophils in the lung microvasculature results in the release of oxygen free radicals and proteolytic enzymes with resultant edema and increased capillary permeability (1). A cycle of poor gas exchange, increased pulmonary vascular resistance, increased capillary permeability, and more edema ensues.

Risk Factors

Risk factors associated with pulmonary dysfunction following CPB include duration of CPB, advanced age, elevated pulmonary artery pressure, poor preoperative pulmonary function, tobacco use, chronic bronchitis, obesity, preoperative pulmonary edema, poor ventricular function, history of cerebrovascular disease, and emergency surgery (9,13).

Prevention

Strategies that minimize lung injury following CPB include limiting the duration of CPB, use of leukocyte filters, continuous hemofiltration while on CPB, preventing low colloid osmotic pressure with albumin priming, and venting the left heart if pulmonary artery pressures are elevated (9,10).

The administration of a series of sighs or slow, sustained breaths prior to reinflation of the lungs and separation from CPB improves ventilation to atelectatic segments (11). Support of the patient with significant lung injury following CPB includes positive pressure ventilation, diuresis, hemodynamic support, and, occasionally, extracorporeal membrane oxygenation. Pharmacologic manipulations have not proven useful in limiting postoperative lung injury (10). In the future, large, randomized trials of off-pump bypass surgery compared to on-pump surgery may elucidate the role of CPB on lung injury. An isolated role may be difficult to elicit due to the deleterious pulmonary effects related to general anesthesia and sternotomy.

IMMUNE AND ALLERGIC COMPLICATIONS

Mechanical shear stress, contact with the nonendothelial surfaces of the CPB circuit and the wound, and the formation of heparin-protamine complexes lead to the activation of the plasma enzyme systems and formed elements of blood (1). This reaction is called the whole body inflammatory response or cascade. The magnitude of the inflammatory response has been demonstrated to adversely influence clinical outcome following CPB (14). Reduced levels of reactive mediators have been demonstrated with off-pump bypass surgery, but it is unclear how this reduction translates to clinical benefit (15–17). Activation of multiple mediators by CPB ultimately leads to tissue damage and organ injury. These mediators, their sites of origin, and the mechanisms of injury are summarized in Table 24-1 (1,9,18).

PROTAMINE REACTION

During protamine administration patients may experience hypotension or a severe catastrophic reaction, which leads to massive pulmonary vasoconstriction, systemic hypotension, and right heart failure. Hypotension may be avoided by the slow administration of protamine and by the administration of vasopressors. The often-fatal idiosyncratic reaction that includes hypotension, bronchospasm, pulmonary vasoconstriction, and right heart failure is typically refractory to medical therapy and often requires reheparinization and reinstitution of CPB for hemodynamic support. Therapy may then include pulmonary vasodilators, systemic vasoconstriction, steroids, antihistamines, and aminophylline (19).

HEPARIN-INDUCED THROMBOCYTOPENIA

Heparin-induced thrombocytopenia results from the production of immunoglobulin G antibodies that recognize platelet factor 4 when bound to heparin (20). This reaction leads to platelet activation and to activation of the coagulation cascade. Unfractionated heparin from porcine intestinal mucosa is preferred over heparin obtained from

TABLE 24-1

INFLAMMATORY MEDIATORS AND MECHANISMS OF INJURY DURING CARDIOPULMONARY BYPASS

Mediator	Effects
Complement: anaphylatoxins C3a, C4a, C5a	Increased vascular permeability Histamine release from mast cells and basophils Smooth muscle contraction Leukocyte migration Cytokine release Neutrophils and mast cell enzyme release C3a-caused platelet aggregation C5a-caused neutrophil aggregation and adherence to endothelium
Cytokines: TNF-α, IL-6, IL-8, IL-10	Altered myocardial contractility Chemoattraction of neutrophils IL-10 may be protective
Arachidonic acid metabolites	Thromboxane A_2-caused vasoconstriction, platelet aggregation Prostaglandins (E_1, E_2, I_2)-caused vasodilatation, platelet antiaggregant Leukotriene-caused chemoattractant, increased vascular permeability
Clotting and fibrinolytic systems/ kallikrein–bradykinin system	Bradykinin leads to vasodilatation, smooth muscle contraction, Increased vascular permeability Kallikrein activates plasminogen to plasmin Endothelial cells facilitate plasminogen activation
Endotoxin (intestinal mucosa)	Activation of complement Increased release of cytokines

TNF, tumor necrosis factor.

bovine lung due to its reduced risk of antibody formation (20). The diagnosis of heparin-induced thrombocytopenia must be considered when thrombocytopenia occurs following CPB. If the diagnosis is suspected, heparin should be immediately discontinued. Administration of thrombin inhibitors is essential in the prevention of thrombotic complications related to heparin-induced thrombocytopenia. Direct thrombin inhibitors lepirudin, bivalirudin, or argatroban are recommended, with the choice depending on renal and hepatic function (20).

Risk Factors

Length of CPB is key in the degree of inflammatory reaction invoked and is correlated with mediator and cytokine levels. Heparin exposure is essential for the development of heparin-induced thrombocytopenia. Previous exposure to protamine, fish allergy, diabetes mellitus, and exposure to protamine-containing insulin have been implicated as risk factors for protamine reaction. Previous exposure is the most important predictor (21–24).

Prevention

Strategies to limit the inflammatory response to CPB include leukocyte filtration, ultrafiltration, heparin-bonded circuits, aprotinin use, anticytokine antibodies, and steroids (1,25–28). These methods have typically targeted only one specific portion of this complicated process and therefore have not consistently benefited patient outcome. Large, prospective randomized clinical trials are needed to establish the clinical benefit of many of these strategies (18,29).

HEMATOLOGIC COMPLICATIONS

The interaction of blood with air and with the nonendothelial surface of the CPB circuit results in a myriad of effects on the hematologic system. Postoperative bleeding requiring return to the operating room occurs in up to 5% of patients (9). The most dreaded complication is clotting of the oxygenator or the CPB circuit. The most common complication pertaining to hemostasis is due to qualitative and quantitative platelet defects. Platelets are diluted and destroyed during CPB and are often defective due to preoperative medications such as aspirin and dipyridamole. A variety of events contribute to the hematologic complications following CPB. Coagulation factors are hemodiluted by the pump prime. The fibrinolytic system is activated following contact of factor XII with the circuit and by stimulation of endothelial cells. Thrombin is generated by the coagulation cascade. Cardiotomy and vent suctions result in turbulence and shear stress of the blood elements, while platelet aggregation leads to impaired function. Platelet function is further inhibited by hypothermia (1,9,30). Heparin resistance is due to antithrombin III depletion preoperatively by heparin therapy, resulting in increased doses of heparin and the need for antithrombin III repletion. Heparin rebound is defined as persistence of active, unmetabolized heparin following the administration and complete metabolism of protamine. Both may contribute to postoperative bleeding (1,31).

Risk Factors

Factors that result in an increased risk of bleeding following CPB include repeat surgery, surgery requiring hypothermia below 27°C, preoperative use of aspirin or anticoagulants, significant liver disease or congestion, end stage renal disease, and congenital or acquired coagulation protein deficiency (1,9,32,33). Prolonged CPB time is also a risk factor for postoperative hematologic complications (34).

Prevention

Multiple strategies may be employed to prevent hematologic complications following CPB. The antifibrinolytics epsilon-aminocaproic acid and aprotinin may be used to

---

TABLE 24-2
TREATMENT OF BLEEDING FOLLOWING CPB

Correct abnormal laboratory values:
 Platelet transfusion
 Cryoprecipitate administration
 Fresh frozen plasma administration
 Additional protamine
Correct hypothermia:
 Use a blood product warmer for massive transfusions
 Warm the patient with a topical warming device
Avoid systemic hypertension that places tension on suture lines
Administer supplemental protamine dose to treat heparin
 rebound
Avoid hemodilution and support blood volume and
 hemodynamics with packed red blood cell transfusion
Increase positive end-expiratory pressure on ventilator
Maintain a high suspicion of tamponade if cardiac output
 decreases, chest tube output decreases, and CVP increases
Surgical exploration if bleeding remains excessive

CVP, central venous pressure.

---

reduce mediastinal blood loss and transfusion requirements (32). Maintenance of a hematocrit level >22% during CPB will significantly reduce the incidence of postoperative bleeding and morbidity and may improve long-term survival (35). Controlled, gentle cardiotomy suction decreases shear forces and preserves platelets (33). Repletion of antithrombin III by the administration of fresh frozen plasma corrects heparin resistance. The treatment of bleeding following CPB begins with the investigation of causative factors. A management strategy is summarized in Table 24-2 (36).

ENDOCRINE COMPLICATIONS

Pain, stress, hypothermia, hemodilution, and the contact of blood with a nonendothelial surface lead to physiologic responses during CPB. Multiple changes are noted in endogenous hormone levels despite their relative lack of physiologic control during CPB. Hemodilution results in a decrease in total and ionized calcium, parathyroid hormone, T_3, and T_4 (9,37). Hyperglycemia is noted during CPB secondary to decreased insulin secretion, decreased peripheral glucose utilization secondary to hypothermia, and elevated levels of circulating cortisol and epinephrine (9,30,38). Increased levels of norepinephrine, aldosterone, renin, angiotensin, and vasopressin are noted. There is an increase in free fatty acids and lipid metabolism. Decreased levels of atrial natriuretic factor and adrenocorticotropin hormone are noted during CPB (30,38).

Many of the hormonal changes noted are inevitable during CPB and are limited only by the length of CPB. Increasing the depth of anesthesia during CPB or providing pulsatile perfusion may blunt some hormonal responses. The significance of hormonal responses on ultimate outcome is unknown (38).

FLUID BALANCE AND RENAL COMPLICATIONS

During CPB the intravascular volume of the body is removed, hemodiluted, and then returned. The normal physiologic responses to intravascular volume change are eliminated during CPB as central venous pressure is artificially controlled. The adult patient may gain 1 to 15 lb following CPB; the amount of weight gained increases with the length of CPB (30). Fluid accumulation occurs mainly in the extracellular, extravascular interstitial space (39). Renal impairment is observed in 12% of patients following CPB, and the incidence of renal failure requiring hemodialysis is approximately 1% to 5% (9,40). Renal failure following CPB results in an eightfold increase in morbidity and mortality. Mortality rates increase by 20-fold in patients who require hemodialysis (40,41).

Renal insufficiency may be attributed to a combination of hemodilution, low perfusion pressure and decreased renal blood flow on CPB, hypothermia, microembolization, circulating hormones (renin, aldosterone, vasopressin, and angiotensin II) that cause renal vasoconstriction, injury secondary to inflammatory mediators, and hemolysis (1,9). Despite the beneficial effects of increased blood flow secondary to decreased viscosity, the hemodilution of CPB results in fluid retention as a decrease in plasma colloid osmotic pressure leads to increased capillary permeability (30,39). Hypothermia reduces glomerular filtration, renal blood flow, and osmolar clearance (39). Aldosterone and vasopressin promote conservation of sodium and water and renal vasoconstriction (39). Hemolysis results in hemoglobin cast formation in renal tubules (30,39).

Risk Factors

Factors that are predictive of postoperative fluid accumulation include obesity, female sex, diabetes mellitus, emergency surgery, advanced age, congestive heart failure, and preoperative anemia (30,39). Risk factors associated with renal dysfunction following CPB include preoperative renal dysfunction, age >70 years, diabetes mellitus, blood transfusion, previous cardiac surgery, congestive heart failure, use of IABP, unstable angina, low cardiac output, emergency surgery, and duration of CPB (9,42–44).

Prevention

Strategies to prevent renal failure focus upon the prevention of oliguria by maximizing cardiac output and utilizing diuretic therapy, the limitation of CPB time, maintenance of an alkaline urine if hemolysis is ongoing, and the avoidance of nephrotoxic drugs or dyes.

Strategies to manage renal injury are based on the maintenance of fluid and electrolyte balance and the use of hemodialysis when indicated. Hemodilution with a crystalloid prime solution and hyperglycemia provide modest diuresis in most patients following CPB. Fluid losses should be repleted and preload maximized. Often the most important strategy in the postoperative period is the improvement of cardiac output with resulting improved renal perfusion.

CENTRAL NERVOUS SYSTEM COMPLICATIONS

Significant neurologic injury is the most disabling of all complications relating to CPB. CNS injury ranges from minor cognitive deficit to overt stroke. Injury may include delirium, encephalopathy, confusion, agitation, disorientation, drowsiness, decreased alertness, memory deficit, seizure, or other neuropsychiatric disturbances (45).

Neurologic deficits are often difficult to quantify and categorize. Many studies have underestimated the number of patients with deficits because findings may be subtle and difficult to document (46,47). The incidence of stroke following CPB ranges from 1% to 7% (48,49). The incidence of encephalopathy is as high as 7% (50), and up to 53% of patients undergoing cardiac surgery experience postoperative cognitive deficits (51,52). Neurologic injury is particularly devastating because it significantly increases mortality, length of hospital stay, and cost of hospitalization and requires inpatient and outpatient rehabilitation (46,50).

Neurologic injury is attributed to global or regional hypoperfusion, hemorrhage, or embolic phenomenon. Global hypoperfusion is particularly important in patients with hypertension who require a higher mean arterial pressure during CPB to provide adequate blood flow to the brain. The presence of significant carotid artery disease increases this risk, particularly in the cerebrum.

The number of cerebral emboli detected during CPB has been correlated with the degree of neurologic deficit postoperatively (53). Embolic phenomena may occur as a result of cannulation of the aorta, clamping the aorta, intracardiac debris or clot, or gaseous or particulate matter from the cardiotomy suction and the CPB machine (30,54). Air emboli may result from the reversal or kinking of pump or vent lines, the vortexing of air entering an empty venous reservoir, air entry around vent lines, an intravenous infusion line in a patient with a patent foramen ovale, the clotting or detachment of the oxygenator, inadequate deairing of open cardiac chambers, a break in the integrity of the arterial line, and the introduction of air bubbles in solution into the internal mammary artery graft lumen (55).

Microembolization may include gas, lipid particles, atheroma, calcific debris, bone marrow, glove powder, aggregates of blood cells or fibrin, or particles of silicone or polyvinyl chloride tubing (9,56). Using transcranial Doppler ultrasonography, CPB has been demonstrated to significantly increase the number of microemboli compared to the use of off-pump coronary artery bypass techniques (57–59). The number of microemboli has been demonstrated to increase significantly with perfusionist manipulations such as injection of drugs into the CPB circuit or the acquisition of blood samples from the circuit (60).

Risk Factors

Risk factors for stroke in patients undergoing CPB are summarized in Table 24-3 (46,61,62). Technical strategies may be employed to reduce neurologic injury during CPB (Table 24-4). Prior to cannulation, care should be given to the site of cannulation and the placement of the aortic cross clamp in the patient with the calcified aorta.

Prevention

Alternatives include femoral artery cannulation, axillary artery cannulation, cold fibrillatory arrest for the placement of proximal coronary artery anastomoses or for the replacement of a mitral valve, the use of off-pump coronary artery bypass techniques with placement of proximal anastomoses

TABLE 24-3
RISK FACTORS FOR STROKE FOLLOWING CARDIOPULMONARY BYPASS

Preoperative	Intraoperative
Age	Atherosclerosis of the ascending aorta
Peripheral vascular disease (especially carotid artery disease)	Duration of cardiopulmonary bypass
Renal insufficiency or failure	Return to cardiopulmonary bypass after separation
Diabetes mellitus	Use of IABP
Previous stroke	Presence of left ventricular thrombus
Urgent or emergency surgery	Severe valvular calcification
Ejection fraction <40%	
Recent myocardial infarction	
Hypertension	

IABP, intra-aortic balloon pump.

on internal mammary artery grafts, replacement of the entire ascending aorta, and the placement of proximal anastomoses on the descending aorta. Other strategies include the use of a higher perfusion pressure during CPB (63) and the use of aprotinin in patients undergoing repeat surgery (64). A management strategy for the treatment of air embolism during CPB is summarized in Table 24-5 (65).

Two different blood gas management techniques may be used during CPB. Hypothermia results in an elevation of the pH. Using the pH stat method, carbon dioxide is added to the CPB circuit to correct the alkalotic pH to 7.4. Using the α stat method, the numerical pH result is corrected to account for hypothermia and no carbon dioxide is added. Carbon dioxide added when using the pH stat method results in arteriolar dilatation in the brain. Despite increased blood flow to the brain with the pH stat method, cerebral autoregulation of blood flow is lost (66). The use of α stat blood gas management during hypothermia maintains cerebral blood flow autoregulation and improves myocardial functional recovery when compared to pH stat management (1,66).

The use of off-pump coronary artery bypass technique provides fewer microemboli to the brain and allows for a "no touch" aorta technique (57). Large, randomized prospective trials will be necessary to determine whether this approach significantly reduces the incidence of neurologic injury. Treatment following CPB and central nervous system injury includes neurologic consultation, supportive care, aggressive physical and occupational therapy, the limitation of cerebral edema when appropriate, and the correction of any contributing metabolic derangements.

GASTROINTESTINAL COMPLICATIONS

The incidence of gastrointestinal complications following CPB is approximately 1% (67). Gastrointestinal complications of CPB are often subtle and difficult to detect because patients are sedated. Diagnosis often requires transportation of the critically ill patient to various radiology departments.

TABLE 24-4
STRATEGIES TO MINIMIZE NEUROLOGIC INJURY DURING CARDIOPULMONARY BYPASS

Address symptomatic carotid artery stenosis preoperatively
Image ascending aorta using epiaortic ultrasound probe to guide cannulation site
Plan "no touch" technique for calcified aorta
Minimize frequency of aortic cross clamping
Careful deairing maneuvers: vent aorta and use Trendelenburg position when removing cross clamp
Maintain adequate mean arterial pressure
Minimize cardiotomy suction
Consider use of aprotinin
Perform careful and thorough debridement and irrigation of intracardiac debris
Minimize cardiopulmonary bypass and deep hypothermic circulatory arrest time
Consider retrograde cerebral perfusion during circulatory arrest
Adhere to cooling and warming guidelines to prevent air precipitation

TABLE 24-5
MANAGEMENT OF MASSIVE AIR EMBOLUS DURING CARDIOPULMONARY BYPASS

Stop the pump immediately
Clamp both arterial and venous lines
Place the patient into deep Trendelenburg position
Ventilate with 100% oxygen
Remove the aortic cannula to deair the aorta
Place the arterial cannula in the SVC for retrograde cerebral perfusion, clamp the SVC proximally, and cool the patient
Compress the heart manually
Compress the carotid arteries manually
Once the aorta is deaired, replace the aortic cannula and resume CPB at a high pressure
Turn off any nitrous gas
Consider the administration of steroids and mannitol

CPB, cardiopulmonary bypass; SVC, superior vena cava.

Intraoperative monitoring of splanchnic perfusion is not routinely performed. Injury to the small and large bowel, gallbladder, liver, and pancreas during CPB results from regional malperfusion secondary to hypoperfusion, vasoactive substances, cytotoxins, and microemboli. Angiotensin II release results in splanchnic vasoconstriction that may be harmful in patients with arteriosclerosis of the splanchnic vessels (68,69). Reduced gastrointestinal blood flow combined with systemic anticoagulation may cause gastrointestinal bleeding, gastritis, cholecystitis, ischemic colitis, hepatic damage, and pancreatitis. Relative hypoperfusion is particularly detrimental to the liver and pancreas due to the lack of intrinsic autoregulation mechanisms during CPB (70).

Approximately 10% to 20% of patients will manifest mild jaundice secondary to blood transfusion, hemolysis, and liver injury (1). Hepatic injury can also occur during manual compression of the liver to augment venous return or to fill venous cannulas with blood prior to initiation of CPB. Acute pancreatitis occurs in <1% of patients, but 30% of patients will have temporary asymptomatic elevation of serum amylase or lipase (12,71). Mortality is greatly increased when severe gastrointestinal complications occur following CPB, likely the reflection of a generalized low cardiac output state.

Risk Factors

Risk factors for gastrointestinal injury following CPB include advanced age, emergency surgery, prolonged duration of CPB, low cardiac output, prolonged use of vasopressors, peripheral vascular disease, and congestive heart failure (12,68). Risks of pancreatitis include previous history of recurrent pancreatitis, renal insufficiency, and high-dose calcium administration (12,71).

Prevention

Strategies to decrease gastrointestinal complications include the use of an increased perfusion flow rate rather than peripheral vasoconstrictors for maintaining perfusion pressure on CPB and limitation of bypass time (72). Optimization of cardiac output improves splanchnic perfusion. Manual compression of the liver should not be used to augment venous return. The management of gastrointestinal complication focuses on prompt recognition and treatment, which often requires further surgery.

REFERENCES

1. Edmunds LH, ed. *Cardiac surgery in the adult.* New York: McGraw-Hill; 1997.
2. Hammermeister KE, Burchfiel C, Johnson R, et al. Identification of patients at greatest risk for developing major complications at cardiac surgery. *Circulation* 1990;82(Suppl 5):IV380–IV389.
3. Parolari A, Alamanni F, Cannata A, et al. Off-pump vs. on-pump coronary artery bypass: meta-analysis of currently available randomized trials. *Ann Thorac Surg* 2003;76:37–40.
4. Braunwald E, Kloner RA. The stunned myocardium: prolonged, post-ischemic ventricular dysfunction. *Circulation* 1982;66:1146–1149.
5. Menasche P. Strategies to improve myocardial protection during extracorporeal circulation. *Shock* 2001;16(Suppl 1):20–23.
6. Jain U. Myocardial ischemia after cardiopulmonary bypass. *J Card Surg* 1995;10(Suppl 4):520–526.
7. Kalman J. Arrhythmias and pacing. In: Buxton B, Frazier OH, Westaby S, eds. *Ischemic heart disease surgical management.* London: Mosby; 1999:87–89.
8. Jayam VKS, Flaker GC, Jones JW. Atrial fibrillation after coronary bypass: etiology and pharmacologic prevention. *Cardiovasc Surg* 2002;10(4):351–358.
9. Brodie JE, Johnson RB. *The manual of clinical perfusion,* 2nd ed. Augusta, GA: Glendale Medical Corp; 1997.
10. Ng CSH, Wan S, Yim APC, et al. Pulmonary dysfunction after cardiac surgery. *Chest* 2002;121:1269–1277.
11. Sladen RN, Berkowitz DE. Cardiopulmonary bypass and the lung. In: Gravlee GP, Davis RF, Utley JR, eds. *Cardiopulmonary bypass principles and practice.* Baltimore, MD: Williams & Wilkins; 1993:467–487.
12. Cohn LH, Edmunds LH, eds. *Cardiac surgery in the adult,* 2nd ed. New York: McGraw-Hill; 2003.
13. Rady MY, Ryan T, Starr NJ. Early onset of acute pulmonary dysfunction after cardiovascular surgery: risk factors and clinical outcome. *Crit Care Med* 1997;25(11):1831–1839.
14. Holmes JH, Connolly NC, Paull DL, et al. Magnitude of the inflammatory response to cardiopulmonary bypass and its relation to adverse clinical outcomes. *Inflamm Res* 2002;51(12):579–586.
15. Okubo N, Hatori N, Ochi M, et al. Comparison of m-RNA expression for inflammatory mediators in leukocytes between pump and off-pump coronary artery bypass grafting. *Ann Thorac Cardiovasc Surg* 2003;9(1):43–49.
16. Wildhirt SM, Schulze C, Schulz C, et al. Reduction of systemic and cardiac adhesion molecule expression after off-pump versus conventional coronary artery bypass grafting. *Shock* 2001;16(Suppl 1):55–59.
17. Schulze C, Conrad N, Schutz A, et al. Reduced expression of systemic proinflammatory cytokines after off-pump versus conventional coronary artery bypass grafting. *Thorac Cardiovasc Surg* 2000;48(6):364–369.
18. Wan S, LeClerc JL, Vincent JL. Inflammatory response to cardiopulmonary bypass: mechanisms involved and possible therapeutic strategies. *Chest* 1997;112:676–692.
19. Hensley FA, Larach DR, Martin DE. Intraoperative anesthetic complications and their management. In: Waldhausen JA, Orringer MB, eds. *Complications in cardiothoracic surgery.* St. Louis, MO: Mosby–Year Book; 1991:12–14.
20. Warkentin TE, Greinacher A. Heparin-induced thrombocytopenia and cardiac surgery. *Ann Thorac Surg* 2003;76: 638–648.
21. Weiler JM, Gellhaus MA, Carter JG, et al. A prospective study of the risk of an immediate adverse reaction to protamine sulfate during cardiopulmonary bypass surgery. *J Allergy Clin Immunol* 1990;85(4):713–719.
22. Brooks JC. Noncardiogenic pulmonary edema immediately following rapid protamine administration. *Ann Pharmacother* 1999; 33(9):927–930.
23. Levy JH, Schwieger IM, Zaidan JR, et al. Evaluation of patients at risk for protamine reaction. *J Thorac Cardiovasc Surg* 1989;98(2):200–204.
24. Comunale ME, Maslow A, Robertson LK, et al. Effect of site of venous protamine administration, previously alleged risk factors, and preoperative use of aspirin on acute protamine-induced pulmonary vasoconstriction. *J Cardiothor Vasc Anes* 2003;17(3):309–313.
25. Kaul TK, Fields BL. Leukocyte activation during cardiopulmonary bypass: limitations of the inhibitory mechanisms and strategies. *J Cardiovasc Surg (Torino)* 2000;41(6):849–862.
26. Lei Y, Haider HK, Chusnsheng W, et al. Dose-dependent effect of aprotinin on aggravated pro-inflammatory cytokines in patients with pulmonary hypertension following cardiopulmonary bypass. *Cardiovasc Drugs Ther* 2003;17(4):343–348.

27. Gott JP, Cooper WA, Schmidt FE, et al. Modifying risk for extracorporeal circulation: trial of four anti-inflammatory strategies. *Ann Thor Surg* 1998; 66(3):747–753.
28. Schmartz D, Tabardel Y, Preiser JC, et al. Does aprotinin influence the inflammatory response to cardiopulmonary bypass in patients? *J Thorac Cardiovasc Surg* 2003;125(1):184–190.
29. Paparella D, Yau TM, Young E. Cardiopulmonary bypass induced inflammation: pathophysiology and treatment. An update. *Eur J Cardiothor Surg* 2002;21:232–244.
30. Buxton B, Frazier OH, Westaby S, eds. *Ischemic heart disease surgical management.* London: Mosby; 1999.
31. Ranucci M. Antithrombin III. A key factor in extracorporeal circulation. *Minerva Anestesiol* 2002;68(5):454–457.
32. Barrons RW, Jahr JS. A review of post-cardiopulmonary bypass bleeding, aminocaproic acid, tranexamic acid, and aprotinin. *Am J Ther* 1996;3(12):821–838.
33. Weerasinghe A, Taylor KM. The platelet in cardiopulmonary bypass. *Ann Thorac Surg* 1998;66:2145–2152.
34. Woodman RC, Harker LA. Bleeding complications associated with cardiopulmonary bypass. *Blood* 1990;76(9):1680–1697.
35. Habib RH, Zacharias A, Schwann TA, et al. Adverse effects of low hematocrit during cardiopulmonary bypass in the adult: should current practice be changed? *J Thorac Cardiovasc Surg* 2003; 125(6):1438–1450.
36. Horrow JC. Management of coagulopathy associated with cardiopulmonary bypass. In: Gravlee GP, Davis RF, Utley JR, eds. *Cardiopulmonary bypass principles and practice.* Baltimore, MD: Williams & Wilkins; 1993:436–466.
37. Klemperer JD. Thyroid hormone and cardiac surgery. *Thyroid* 2002;12(6):517–521.
38. Kennedy DT, Butterworth JF. Endocrine function during and after cardiopulmonary bypass: recent observations. *J Clin Endo Metab* 1994;78(5):997–1002.
39. Utley JR. Renal function and fluid balance with cardiopulmonary bypass. In: Gravlee GP, Davis RF, Utley JR, eds. *Cardiopulmonary bypass principles and practice.* Baltimore, MD: Williams & Wilkins; 1993:488–508.
40. Conlon PJ, Stafford-Smith M, White WD, et al. Acute renal failure following cardiac surgery. *Nephrol Dial Transplant* 1999;14: 1158–1162.
41. Rinder CS, Fontes M, Matthew JP, et al. Neutrophil CD11b upregulation during cardiopulmonary bypass is associated with postoperative renal injury. *Ann Thorac Surg* 2003;75(3): 899–905.
42. Suen WS, Mok CK, Chiu SW, et al. Risk factors for development of acute renal failure (ARF) requiring dialysis in patients undergoing cardiac surgery. *Angiology* 1998;49(10):789–800.
43. Ranucci M, Pavesi M, Mazza E, et al. Risk factors for renal dysfunction after coronary surgery: the role of cardiopulmonary bypass technique. *Perfusion* 1994;9(5):319–326.
44. Boldt J, Brenner T, Lehmann A. Is kidney function altered by the duration of cardiopulmonary bypass? *Ann Thorac Surg* 2003; 73(3):906–912.
45. Taggart DP, Westaby S. Neurological and cognitive disorders after coronary artery bypass grafting. *Curr Opin Cardiol* 2001;16: 271–276.
46. Stamou SS, Hill PC, Dangas G. Stroke after coronary artery bypass: incidence, predictors, and clinical outcome. *Stroke* 2001; 32:1508–1513.
47. Sotaniemi KA. Long-term neurologic outcome after cardiac operation. *Ann Thorac Surg* 1995;59:1336–1339.
48. John R, Choudhri AF, Weinberg AD, et al. Multicenter review of preoperative risk factors for stroke after coronary artery bypass grafting. *Ann Thorac Surg* 2000;69:30–36.
49. Trehan N, Mishra M, Sharma OP, et al. Further reduction in stroke after off-pump coronary artery bypass grafting: a 10-year experience. *Ann Thorac Surg* 2001;72(3):S1026–S1032.
50. McKhann GM, Grega MA, Borowicz LM, et al. Encephalopathy and stroke after coronary artery bypass grafting. *Arch Neurol* 2002;59:1422–1428.
51. Newman MF, Kirchner JL, Phillips-Bute B, et al. Longitudinal assessment of neurocognitive function after coronary-artery bypass surgery. *N Engl J Med* 2001;344(6):395–402.
52. Baker RA, Andrew MJ, Knight JL. Evaluation of neurological assessment and outcomes in cardiac surgical patients. *Semin Thorac Cardiovasc Surg* 2001;13(2):149–157.
53. Mark DB, Newman MF. Protecting the brain in coronary artery bypass graft surgery. *JAMA* 2002;287(11):1448–1450.
54. Appelblad M, Engstrom G. Fat contamination of pericardial suction blood and its influence on in vitro capillary-pore flow properties in patients undergoing routine coronary artery bypass grafting. *J Thorac Cardiovasc Surg* 2002;124(2): 377–386.
55. Pae WE, Williams DR, Troncelliti EK, et al. Prevention of complications during cardiopulmonary bypass. In: Waldhausen JA, Orringer MB, eds. *Complications in cardiothoracic surgery.* St. Louis, MO: Mosby–Year Book; 1991:39–44.
56. Mills SA. Cerebral injury and cardiac operations. *Ann Thorac Surg* 1993;56(5 Suppl):S86–S91.
57. Bowles J, Lee JD, Dang CR, et al. Coronary artery bypass performed without the use of cardiopulmonary bypass is associated with reduced cerebral microemboli and improved clinical results. *Chest* 2001;119:25–30.
58. Malheiros SM, Massaro AR, Gabbai AA, et al. Is the number of microemboli signals related to neurologic outcome in coronary bypass surgery? *Arg Neuropsiguiatr* 2001;59(1):1–5.
59. Lee JD, Lee SJ, Tsushima WT, et al. Benefits of off-pump bypass on neurologic and clinical morbidity: a prospective randomized trail. *Ann Thorac Surg* 2003;76(1):18–25.
60. Borger MA, Feindel CM. Cerebral emboli during cardiopulmonary bypass: effect of perfusionist interventions and aortic cannulas. *J Extra Corpor Technol* 2002;34(1):29–33.
61. Likosky DS, Leavitt BJ, Marin CAS, et al. Intra- and postoperative predictors of stroke after coronary artery bypass grafting. *Ann Thorac Surg* 2003;76:428–435.
62. Tuman KJ, McCarthy RJ, Rajafi H, et al. Differential effects of advanced age on neurologic and cardiac risks of coronary artery operations. *J Thorac Cardiovasc Surg* 1992;104(6): 1510–1517.
63. Gold JP, Charlson ME, Williams-Russo P, et al. Improvement of outcomes after coronary artery bypass. A randomized trial comparing intraoperative high versus low mean arterial pressure. *J Thorac Cardiovasc Surg* 1995;110(5):1302–1311.
64. Levy JH, Pifarre R, Schaff HV, et al. A multi-center, double-blind, placebo-controlled trial of aprotinin for reducing blood loss and the requirement for donor-blood transfusion in patients undergoing repeat coronary artery bypass grafting. *Circulation* 1995; 92:2236–2244.
65. Mills NL, Morris JM. Air embolism associated with cardiopulmonary bypass. In: Waldhausen JA, Orringer MB, eds. *Complications in cardiothoracic surgery.* St. Louis, MO: Mosby–Year Book; 1991: 60–67.
66. Rogers AT, Newman SP, Stump DA, et al. Neurologic effects of cardiopulmonary bypass. In: Gravlee GP, Davis RF, Utley JR, eds. *Cardiopulmonary bypass principles and practice.* Baltimore, MD: Williams & Wilkins; 1993:542–576.
67. Halm MA. Acute gastrointestinal complications after cardiac surgery. *Am J Crit Care* 1996;5(2):109–118.
68. Zacharias A, Schwann TA, Parenteau GL, et al. Predictors of gastrointestinal complications in cardiac surgery. *Tex Heart Inst J* 2000;27:93–99.
69. Reilly PM, Bulkley GB. Vasoactive mediators and splanchnic perfusion. *Crit Care Med* 1993;21(Suppl 2):S55–S68.
70. Shangraw RE. Metabolic and splanchnic visceral effects of cardiopulmonary bypass. In: Gravke GP, Davis RF, Utley JR, eds. *Cardiopulmonary bypass principles and practice.* Baltimore, MD: Williams & Wilkins; 1993:509–541.
71. Fernandez-del Castillo C, Harringer W, Warshaw Al, et al. Risk factors for pancreatic cellular injury after cardiopulmonary bypass. *N Engl J Med* 1991;325(6):382–387.
72. Plestis KA, Gold JP. Importance of blood pressure regulation in maintaining adequate tissue perfusion during cardiopulmonary bypass. *Semin Thorac Cardiovasc Surg* 2001;13(2): 170–175.

Complications of Surgical Coronary Revascularization

25

Traves D. Crabtree   Marc R. Moon

■ INTRODUCTION 286

■ OVERALL MORBIDITY AND MORTALITY 287

■ NEUROLOGIC COMPLICATIONS 287

■ POSTOPERATIVE ARRHYTHMIAS 288

■ STERNAL WOUND COMPLICATIONS 290

■ POSTOPERATIVE MYOCARDIAL ISCHEMIA 291

■ COMPLICATIONS OF CONDUIT HARVEST SITES 291

■ COMPLICATIONS RELATED TO HEMOSTASIS 292

■ RENAL COMPLICATIONS 292

■ POSTOPERATIVE PULMONARY COMPLICATIONS 292

■ GI COMPLICATIONS 292

■ ON-PUMP VERSUS OFF-PUMP CORONARY ARTERY BYPASS SURGERY 293

■ SUMMARY 293

■ REFERENCES 294

Traves D. Crabtree, Marc R. Moon: Washington University School of Medicine, St. Louis, MO 63110

INTRODUCTION

Despite advances in percutaneous techniques for coronary revascularization, coronary artery bypass surgery remains an integral component of the treatment regimen for patients with coronary artery disease. Critical analysis of clinical outcomes, in addition to improvements in critical care management and myocardial protection techniques, has significantly improved outcomes related to surgical revascularization. Based on previous comparisons with nonsurgical techniques, current guidelines for coronary artery bypass grafting (CABG) include left main coronary artery stenosis, triple-vessel disease, single- or double-vessel disease that includes left anterior descending stenosis in patients with poor left ventricular (LV) function, and disease refractory to nonsurgical management (1). CABG is recommended for diabetic patients with significant coronary disease, particularly for those with LV dysfunction (2,3).

Continued efforts to decrease morbidity and mortality associated with surgical revascularization have resulted in persistent survival advantage and decreased need for reinterventions relative to nonsurgical revascularization techniques. Based upon many randomized controlled trials of patients with stable angina, CABG has been shown to provide a significant survival advantage in moderate to high-risk patients at 5, 7, and 9 years follow-up compared to medical management (4–8). A recent meta-analysis of randomized trials also demonstrates a significant long-term survival advantage of CABG over percutaneous transluminal coronary angioplasty (PTCA) and a substantial decrease in the number of repeat interventions required following CABG relative to PTCA (9). These differences were most notable in patients with multivessel disease or diabetes. These studies, however, fail to completely capture the purported benefit of newer coronary stents and drug-eluting devices that may decrease the need for reintervention. Long-term investigations comparing contemporary coronary stent technology to CABG are currently unavailable but may have an impact on clinical practice in the future.

OVERALL MORBIDITY AND MORTALITY

With regard to monitored outcome variables, coronary revascularization is one of the most scrutinized procedures performed. With the development of the Society of Thoracic Surgeons (STS) database, surveillance of perioperative morbidity and mortality and identification of significant comorbid conditions have allowed for an unprecedented model of quality control on a local, regional, and national basis. The STS database has also permitted the development of risk stratification models that can estimate perioperative mortality and morbidity based on multiple potential risk factors and comorbid conditions. A recent report from the STS database of over 500,000 isolated coronary revascularization procedures performed between 1997 and 2000 demonstrated an overall 30-day operative mortality of 2.61% (10). Risk factors for perioperative death included increasing age, renal dysfunction, emergency surgery, cardiogenic shock, and repeat operations. Perioperative mortality is closely linked to postoperative morbidity, and many of the risk factors identified for mortality correlate with the development of surgery-related complications.

Table 25-1 summarizes the incidence of several major complications associated with CABG based on review of the STS database (10). The characteristics of the population undergoing coronary revascularization have changed considerably over the past decade, increasing the complexity of the surgery as well as postoperative care. Review of the STS database demonstrates that from 1990 to 1999 patients have become significantly older and are more likely to have a history of smoking, diabetes, renal failure, hypertension, stroke, chronic lung disease, worsening heart failure, and multivessel disease. Risk stratification models have also shown that predicted operative risk has risen from 2.6% in 1990 to 3.4% in 1999 while the observed operative mortality has decreased

TABLE 25-1

INCIDENCE OF MAJOR COMPLICATIONS FOLLOWING ISOLATED CORONARY REVASCULARIZATION (STS DATABASE, 1997-2000)

Complication	Incidence (%)
30-day mortality	2.61
Permanent stroke	1.67
Renal failure requiring dialysis	3.53
Prolonged mechanical ventilation (>48 hrs)	5.79
Deep sternal wound infection	0.60
Reoperation for bleeding	5.06

From Prabhakar G, Haan CK, Peterson ED, et al. The risks of moderate and extreme obesity for coronary artery bypass grafting outcomes: a study from the Society of Thoracic Surgeons' database. *Ann Thorac Surg* 2002;74:1125–1130; discussion 1130–1131, with permission.

from 3.9% to 3.0% (11). Although advances in surgical and perioperative care have resulted in improvement in clinical outcomes, the increasing complexity of the patients will require continuing efforts to understand and improve outcomes related to CABG.

NEUROLOGIC COMPLICATIONS

One of the most devastating complications following coronary revascularization is the development of stroke. The reported incidence of stroke following CABG is 1.1% to 2.9% with an associated in-hospital mortality of 22% to 24.8% and a 5-year mortality of 56% (12–16). Risk factors for the development of stroke by multivariate analysis include the presence of a calcified aorta, prior stroke, increasing age, carotid artery disease, increasing duration of cardiopulmonary bypass, unstable angina, renal failure, peripheral vascular disease, smoking history, and diabetes mellitus (12,13,16,17). The most significant risk factor among these is the presence of an atherosclerotic ascending aorta, with atheroemboli accounting for the majority of severe ischemic strokes. The presence of mobile plaques in the ascending aorta has been associated with a stroke rate as high as 33.3% following coronary bypass surgery (18,19). Manipulation of the aorta with or without the institution of cardiopulmonary bypass is a significant risk factor for stroke following coronary revascularization (20). Emboli account for >80% of strokes after cardiac surgery with watershed infarcts contributing to the other sources of ischemic events (21).

Preoperative identification of risk factors allows for risk stratification and patient education but may also help to plan the operation in order to decrease the rate of stroke. Patients with symptomatic carotid artery stenosis or critical asymptomatic stenosis diagnosed preoperatively may undergo endarterectomy prior to bypass surgery or at the time of the bypass operation. Preoperative carotid duplex scanning is performed in patients with a history of a transient ischemic attack (TIA), stroke, amaurosis fugax, or in patients with a carotid bruit. Patients with <80% stenosis, corresponding to an internal carotid artery to common carotid artery (IC:CC) velocity ratio <4.0, typically undergo CABG alone. For patients with high-grade carotid stenosis (IC:CC velocity ratio >4.0) carotid endarterectomy is necessary before cardiopulmonary bypass to minimize the risk of stroke. The approach differs depending on the degree of cardiac disease. Timing of endarterectomy for patients with significant but asymptomatic carotid stenosis remains a subject of debate. For patients with unstable angina and preserved left ventricular function, simultaneous carotid endarterectomy and CABG are performed. For patients with stable angina and severe left ventricular dysfunction, carotid endarterectomy is performed 1 to 2 days prior to coronary revascularization. Patients who undergo combined CABG and carotid endarterectomy often have significant hemodynamic fluctuation in the immediate postoperative period due to carotid body manipulation. Although these fluctuations do not affect patients with normal left ventricular function, the occurrence makes patients with poor left ventricular function difficult to manage perioperatively.

The application of transesophageal echocardiography and sensitive epiaortic echocardiography has improved the ability to diagnose and characterize a severely atherosclerotic aorta (22). This diagnosis poses a formidable challenge to the surgeon. The advancement of "no-touch" techniques that avoid manipulation or clamping of the diseased ascending aorta may be used with or without cardiopulmonary bypass (23,24). Application of such techniques has been shown to significantly decrease the incidence of stroke in high-risk patients undergoing coronary revascularization (25). Another option for patients with a severely atherosclerotic aorta involves institution of circulatory arrest and replacement of the ascending aorta to limit the incidence of stroke in this population (26). Recently developed intra-aortic filters may be used in conjunction with the aortic cannula to decrease the embolic load during cardiopulmonary bypass and may play a future role in reducing the rate of stroke (27,28).

Areas of controversy regarding the conduct of the operation and its effect upon neurologic outcome include the use of a single or sequential clamp technique, temperature management strategies during and after bypass, and perioperative management of hyperglycemia.

Unfortunately, there are few treatment options for patients who develop an intraoperative or perioperative stroke. A small number of patients with a thromboembolic etiology may benefit from early (<6 to 8 hours) thrombolytic therapy.

Neurocognitive changes or encephalopathy may occur following bypass surgery. Encephalopathy is present in 3.0% to 6.9% of patients undergoing CABG and is associated with an increased length of stay and mortality relative to patients without encephalopathy (15,29). Significant

risk factors for postoperative encephalopathy or neurocognitive changes include increasing age, the presence of a carotid bruit, hypertension, diabetes mellitus, pulmonary disease, excessive alcohol consumption, and history of a previous stroke (15,29). More stringent neuropsychometric tests have estimated that 19% to 26% of patients have persistent cognitive deficits for >2 months following coronary revascularization surgery (30). The etiology of these subtle deficits is incompletely understood, although microembolization may play a role. Although the use of cardiopulmonary bypass has been implicated, recent studies have failed to identify long-term differences in neurocognitive testing 3 to 12 months postbypass between patients undergoing on-pump revascularization versus off-pump revascularization (31,32).

POSTOPERATIVE ARRHYTHMIAS

Postoperative arrhythmias are a common problem following coronary bypass surgery, with atrial fibrillation accounting for the majority of occurrences. The incidence of postoperative atrial fibrillation following coronary revascularization is 23% to 40%, with even higher rates reported among patients undergoing combined bypass and valve surgery (33–38). The pathophysiology of atrial fibrillation is related to the development of reentrant circuits within the atrium or pulmonary veins. Potential risk factors for atrial fibrillation include advanced age, male gender, chronic obstructive pulmonary disease (COPD), left atrial enlargement, a preoperative history of paroxysmal atrial fibrillation, increasing severity of coronary artery disease, and preoperative digoxin use (34,37,38). Among these, advanced age is the most consistent predictor of postoperative atrial fibrillation. Following coronary revascularization, the incidence of atrial fibrillation is 26% in patients younger than 70 and 45% in patients older than 70 (33).

Atrial fibrillation typically develops between postoperative day 1 and day 5 and is often asymptomatic. Some patients develop hypotension or experience shortness of breath, chest pain, palpitations, or confusion with acute onset of atrial fibrillation. Acute hypotension or a low cardiac output state account for most symptoms and are often related to a rapid ventricular response to the atrial rhythm. In these circumstances urgent treatment to control the ventricular rate is required. In addition to acute symptoms, the development of postoperative atrial fibrillation significantly increases the risk of stroke following coronary revascularization (38,39). The loss of normal atrial contraction results in the development of thrombus within the atrium that serves as a source for emboli. Such thrombus may develop within 48 hours from the onset of fibrillation. The morbidity associated with postoperative atrial fibrillation results in prolonged hospital stay, prolonged ICU stay, increased hospital costs, and need for hospital readmission after discharge (33,35,38–40).

Many trials have examined the prevention of postoperative atrial fibrillation by perioperative pharmacotherapy. Prophylactic administration of β-blockers has consistently been shown to decrease postoperative atrial fibrillation in randomized controlled trials, especially in patients who received preoperative β-blockade. Other trials have demonstrated that preoperative administration of amiodarone decreases the rate of postoperative atrial fibrillation after bypass surgery (41,42). Criticisms of amiodarone prophylaxis have included an inability to reproduce these results in subsequent trials using similar regimens of amiodarone and failure of trials to demonstrate a benefit over β-blockers (43,44). A recent meta-analysis of randomized trials suggests that preoperative administration of β-blockers, sotalol, and amiodarone are all effective at preventing postoperative atrial fibrillation in cardiac patients (45). Despite the ability of these agents to decrease the rate of postoperative atrial fibrillation, their prophylactic administration has not resulted in a significant decrease in the length of stay or in overall hospital costs (43,45–47).

A practical limitation of preoperative prophylaxis with β-blockers or amiodarone in patients requiring coronary revascularization is the inability to provide an adequate therapeutic regimen prior to surgery. In most patients current surgical practice involves CABG within 1 to 2 days of catheterization, making preoperative treatment impractical. Recent randomized trials have demonstrated that immediate postoperative administration of metoprolol or amiodarone significantly decreases the incidence of postoperative atrial fibrillation (46,48). Prophylactic administration of other agents such as digoxin, calcium channel blockers, and magnesium sulfate have shown mixed results (39,49–55).

A novel technique for the prevention of postoperative atrial fibrillation involves biatrial overdrive pacing in the early postoperative period. Pacing wires are placed in both atria intraoperatively and the patient undergoes overdrive pacing for 4 to 5 days postoperatively. Randomized studies have demonstrated a significant reduction in postoperative atrial fibrillation with biatrial pacing (56–59). Although this technique decreases the incidence of atrial fibrillation, these studies have not demonstrated a consistent decrease in hospital length of stay (56–59).

Initial treatment of atrial fibrillation is based on the severity of symptoms. Immediate electrical cardioversion is indicated in the presence of hemodynamic instability, worsening left ventricular dysfunction, or ischemia. Among patients who are relatively asymptomatic, initial management strategies include identification and treatment of underlying abnormalities such as hypoxia, hypovolemia or hypervolemia, hypokalemia, hypomagnesemia, and elimination of chronotropic drugs. Agents used for rate control include metoprolol and diltiazem, which can be given intravenously initially and subsequently as an oral maintenance dose. Although used less frequently, digoxin can be given when other agents are contraindicated. These agents are titrated to a resting ventricular heart rate of 80 to 110 beats per minute, provided that there is an absence of symptoms or hemodynamic compromise.

Rate control with β-blockers or calcium channel blockers may also result in conversion to sinus rhythm. Other antiarrhythmic agents may also be given specifically to convert patients to sinus rhythm. Administration of intravenous amiodarone has been shown to restore sinus rhythm within 24 hours in 77% to 83% of cardiac surgical patients (60–62). Other agents such as propafenone and sotalol have not been as effective as amiodarone for conversion to sinus rhythm (63,64). Side effects of long-term amiodarone administration include pulmonary fibrosis, hepatic toxicity, and hypothyroidism, although these side effects occur infrequently with short-term (≤ 6 weeks) treatment (65).

Table 25-2 outlines an approach to the management of postoperative atrial fibrillation. In patients who are hemodynamically stable, amiodarone 150 mg is administered intravenously, followed by initiation of oral amiodarone, 400 mg three times a day. If the patient has a controlled

TABLE 25-2

TREATMENT OPTIONS FOR ACUTE MANAGEMENT OF POSTOPERATIVE ATRIAL FIBRILLATION

Drug	Initial IV Dose	Maintenance Dose
Amiodarone	150 mg bolus $\pm$ 0.5 mg/min drip	400 mg po tid $\times$ 5 days (load) followed by 200–400 mg po qd for 4–6 weeks
Metoprolol	2.5–5 mg bolus q 5–10 min (max. 3 doses)	12.5–100 mg po bid
Atenolol	5–10 mg q 5–10 min	25–100 mg po qd or bid[a]
Diltiazem	2.5–5 mg bolus q 10 min $\pm$ initiation of IV drip at 5–15 mg/hour	30–90 mg po qid

[a]Extended release form may be dosed once daily.

heart rate at the onset of atrial fibrillation ($\leq$100 bpm), the intravenous loading dose can be eliminated. If the heart rate remains >120 beats per minute, intravenous amiodarone bolus is repeated or metoprolol or diltiazem is administered for rate control. A diltiazem drip may also be used for rate control in this setting. Fortunately, among patients without a preoperative history of atrial arrhythmias, over 98% will return to sinus rhythm within 8 weeks after cardiac surgery (66).

A new technique involving temporary atrial cardioversion electrodes, placed intraoperatively similar to standard pacing electrodes, may provide for early low energy cardioversion in patients who develop atrial fibrillation prior to discharge (67,68). Low energy cardioversion has been shown to decrease the total time a patient remains in atrial fibrillation but has not been shown to decrease the length of hospitalization relative to pharmacologically treated controls (69). Further studies are needed to thoroughly examine the efficacy and safety of these devices before they are used routinely.

Many patients will convert to sinus rhythm immediately after initiation of treatment. Patients who do not convert within the first 24 to 48 hours are at risk for mural thrombus within the atrium that may serve as a source of emboli. Patients who remain in atrial fibrillation for >24 hours may be started on a low-dose heparin drip at 500 to 800 units per hour. Anticoagulation with heparin followed by coumadin has been shown to decrease the risk of thromboembolic events in patients with persistent postoperative atrial fibrillation (70,71). In the absence of anticoagulation, attempts at pharmacologic cardioversion with agents such as amiodarone or electrical cardioversion have been associated with a 1% to 7% risk of thromboembolism (72,73). Patients with persistent or recurrent atrial fibrillation are maintained on coumadin for 4 to 6 weeks postoperatively to minimize the risk of thromboembolic events.

STERNAL WOUND COMPLICATIONS

According to the STS database, the incidence of sternal wound infections in 2002 was 0.4% among isolated coronary artery bypass procedures (74). A previous surveillance of over 2,400 patients demonstrated an overall chest infection rate of 3% among coronary artery bypass patients, with 1.6% superficial infections and 1.4% deep sternal wound infections (75,76). It is expected that this rate will increase due to a trend toward increasing comorbidities and decreasing left ventricular function among patients undergoing bypass surgery. The most common organisms isolated from sternal wound infections are staphylococcal species. The average time from operation to diagnosis of sternal wound infection is 15 to 19 days, with most diagnosed after discharge (77).

Risk factors for the development of sternal wound infections include steroid use, diabetes mellitus, reoperation for

bleeding, increasing operative duration, heart failure, increased number of grafts performed, and prolonged mechanical ventilation (75,78). Previous reports have identified the use of bilateral internal mammary arteries as a significant risk factor for the development of deep sternal wound infections (79,80). Most recent studies have demonstrated a similar infection rate with use of bilateral internal mammary arteries versus use of a single internal mammary artery in nondiabetics (81,82). A purported advantage of use of both internal mammary arteries is a decrease in recurrent angina post-CABG and a decrease in overall cardiac morbidity (81,82). Skeletonization of the internal mammary artery during mobilization rather than creation of a large pedicle may decrease the rate of sternal wound infections (83). Use of bilateral internal mammary arteries with or without skeletonization may still increase the risk of sternal wound complications in high-risk patients such as obese diabetic women, patients with COPD, and in patients undergoing a repeat sternotomy (84,85).

Because diabetes is a significant risk factor for sternal wound infections and because hyperglycemia has a determined effect upon wound healing, investigations of the impact of improved glucose control perioperatively have been performed. Continuous perioperative intravenous infusion of insulin decreased the rate of deep sternal wound infections to 0.8% from 2.0% among patients receiving standard subcutaneous insulin injections ($p = 0.01$) (86). Continuous infusion of insulin has been shown to decrease overall hospital mortality among diabetics undergoing CABG relative to controls (2.5% vs. 5.3%, $p <0.0001$) (87). One protocol for insulin infusion consists of three regimens—a conservative regimen, a moderate regimen, and an aggressive regimen. The choice of regimen is based on the patient's preoperative insulin dose or oral hypoglycemic agent, recent hemoglobin A1-C level, and most recent preoperative blood glucose level. Depending on the regimen and the blood glucose level, which is monitored every 1 to 2 hours, insulin infusion may range between 0.5 units per hour to 10 units per hour.

Signs and symptoms of chest wound infections include purulent drainage, erythema, sternal instability, fever, and pain. Clinical history and physical examination are frequently diagnostic, although a CT scan may help delineate the deep extent of the infectious process. Wound cultures should be performed to direct antibiotic therapy. Surgical debridement is invariably necessary. Care must be taken to debride all necrotic sternal tissue or bone and avoid injury to underlying structures, such as the thinwalled right ventricle, which can be adherent to the posterior sternum. Historical management strategies for deep sternal wound infections included sternal wound debridement followed by sternal rewiring using a closed drainage system. However, early coverage of the wound with pectoralis myocutaneous advancement flaps and greater omental transposition into the wound have been associated with a decreased length of stay, mortality, and recurrent infection rate versus the standard approach (88). Coverage of the wound can be performed after adequate debridement of all necrotic or infected tissue, usually within 3 to 5 days. Most patients can be extubated shortly after sternal debridement. After 3 to 5 days of dressing changes, definitive closure of the wound is performed. Patients who present late or have significant sepsis can expect a prolonged ICU and hospital stay and an increased mortality rate.

POSTOPERATIVE MYOCARDIAL ISCHEMIA

Although uncommon after coronary revascularization, myocardial ischemia or infarction can occur and is frequently difficult to diagnose in the early postoperative period. Postoperative myocardial infarction (MI) is estimated to occur in 1% to 2% of patients undergoing CABG (89). Risk factors for postoperative ischemia include the presence of preoperative unstable angina and increasing bypass time, with a bypass time of >100 minutes associated with a MI rate of 7.7% (89). Off-pump coronary revascularization may be associated with a hypercoagulable state in the early postoperative period requiring aggressive antiplatelet therapy (90,91). Complicated revascularizations, such as those requiring coronary endarterectomy or grafting of small diffusely diseased vessels, may also require aggressive antiplatelet therapy to avoid early graft failure.

The diagnosis of myocardial ischemia in the early postoperative period can be challenging. The presence of Q waves is not associated with significant myocardial tissue damage and is not predictive of early mortality following coronary revascularization (92). Prospective studies have demonstrated that conventional biochemical markers for postoperative infarction, such as CK-MB, troponin T, and troponin I, are unreliable in determining graft occlusion postbypass because there is significant overlap in these values among patients with and without graft occlusion (93). If postoperative infarction or severe ischemia is identified, efforts should be made to evaluate graft function with reexploration or urgent catheterization to identify and correct the cause of ischemia.

COMPLICATIONS OF CONDUIT HARVEST SITES

One of the most frequent sources of complaints following bypass surgery is related to the saphenous vein harvest site. The incidence of leg wound complications following saphenous vein harvesting is 1% to 28%, with variability related to differences in the definition of leg wound complications as well as variations in harvesting techniques (75,77,94–97). Common minor complications include dermatitis, cellulitis, greater saphenous nerve paresthesias, persistent leg swelling, seromas, and lymphoceles. Major leg wound complications requiring additional surgical procedures occur in less than 0.7% of patients, with nonhealing wounds and wound necrosis accounting for the majority (95,98). Risk factors for the development of major leg wound complications include female gender, peripheral vascular disease, and use of an intra-aortic balloon pump (95). These risk factors emphasize the contribution of vasculopathy and peripheral ischemia to the development of complications.

Several techniques are used to harvest the saphenous vein, including a single incision extending over the entire length of the vein, several smaller intermittent incisions with skin bridges, and endoscopic techniques that further limit the extent of incisions. Endoscopic techniques have recently been developed to decrease wound complications associated with standard open techniques. Prospective studies have provided varying results regarding the ability of endoscopic vein harvest techniques to decrease the local wound complication rate compared to standard open techniques (97,99,100). The learning curve, the cost of additional equipment, and the time required for endoscopic harvesting have been limiting factors. The technique does not appear to affect vein quality (101–103). The most important caveats to limiting leg wound complications include identification of at-risk patients and careful handling of tissue with minimization of the dissection necessary to procure the vein.

With improvements in prevention of radial artery spasm and reports of good long-term patency in radial artery grafts, this conduit has been used with increasing frequency for coronary revascularization (104,105). Complications associated with radial artery harvesting have been uncommon, with hand ischemia occurring rarely (106,107). Neurologic complications, including sensation abnormalities of the hand or forearm or decreased thumb strength, have been reported to be as high as 30% among patients in the early postoperative period (108). Longer follow-up has demonstrated that most of these symptoms resolve over time, with donor arm weakness in 0.7% and cutaneous paresthesias in 3.7% of patients 8 weeks postoperatively (108,109). Risk factors for the development of these complications include diabetes, peripheral vascular disease, smoking history, and elevated serum creatinine levels. Preoperative demonstration of adequate collateral blood supply from the ulnar distribution using an Allen test is adequate for preventing significant ischemic injury with radial artery harvesting. Careful surgical technique with avoidance of injury or traction on the superficial radial nerve may help limit the degree of neurologic injury associated with radial artery harvesting. Newer techniques of endoscopic radial artery harvesting are currently under investigation (110).

COMPLICATIONS RELATED TO HEMOSTASIS

Postoperative bleeding is a significant early complication following CABG. The incidence of reexploration for bleeding is 2% to 4% for isolated coronary revascularization and accounts for the majority of patients requiring reoperation (74,111,112). The most common etiology of bleeding at the time of reoperation is a surgical cause (67%); diffuse bleeding related to coagulopathy accounts for the remainder (33%) (111). Reoperation for bleeding is associated with an in-hospital mortality three times higher than for patients not requiring reoperation (112). Reexploration is also associated with a higher rate of postoperative renal failure, prolonged mechanical ventilation, adult respiratory distress syndrome (ARDS), sepsis, atrial arrhythmias, sternal wound infection, and increased length of stay (112,113). Risk factors for reexploration for bleeding include prolonged CPB time (>150 min), older age, smaller body surface area, and increasing number of distal anastamoses (112). Emergent reexploration, occasionally at the bedside, may be necessary in patients who develop postoperative cardiac tamponade. Tamponade occurs in 0.3% to 0.5% of postoperative cardiac patients and should be suspected in all patients who develop hypotension or decreased cardiac output (74).

A thorough preoperative history should identify most patients with a bleeding diathesis and allow for diagnostic evaluation and planning. Although aspirin administration has been shown to improve graft patency postoperatively, it is also associated with an increase in postoperative blood loss and transfusion requirements (114–116). Very little can be done to combat this problem preoperatively as almost all patients are on aspirin prior to surgery. Administration of clopidogrel in the preoperative period has also been shown to increase the number of patients requiring reoperation for bleeding, increased red blood cell transfusion, and transfusion of other blood products (117). Perioperative administration of aprotinin, a protease inhibitor that works to inhibit fibrinolysis, has been shown to decrease the rate of reoperation for bleeding, postoperative chest tube drainage, and requirement for blood transfusions (118–120). Aprotinin may be used in patients at high risk for postoperative bleeding complications. Limiting postoperative transfusion requirements is crucial not only because of the need to decrease the morbidity and cost associated with transfusion therapy but also because transfusion of blood products may be an independent predictor of mortality following bypass surgery (121). Other agents that have been shown to decrease bleeding and the requirement for blood transfusions include tranexamic acid and aminocaproic acid (119,122,123). Despite its procoagulant effects, aprotinin does not affect the occurrence of postoperative MI or overall cardiac-related mortality (124). Although these agents may facilitate hemostasis following coronary revascularization, the most important factor is meticulous surgical technique and control of surgical bleeding at the time of operation.

RENAL COMPLICATIONS

There is wide variation in the literature regarding the incidence of postoperative acute renal failure following coronary revascularization. This inconsistency is related to variability in the definition of renal failure, ranging from an isolated increase in serum creatinine to the requirement for dialysis. Acute renal failure defined as a rise in serum creatinine of at least 1 mg per dL above baseline has been reported as 7.9% to 14.9% following revascularization, with an associated mortality of 14% to 21.5% (125,126). According to the STS database (1999–2002), the incidence of acute renal failure requiring dialysis following revascularization is 3.4% (74). Mortality associated with the need for dialysis after coronary bypass surgery has been reported to be as high as 28% (125). Risk factors for the development of renal failure requiring dialysis include elevated preoperative creatinine, increasing duration of cardiopulmonary bypass, cerebrovascular disease, diabetes, advanced age, postoperative hypotension (systolic blood pressure <90 mm Hg for >1 hour), left ventricular dysfunction, and atherosclerosis of the ascending aorta (125–127). Maintenance of adequate systemic perfusion during and after bypass is the only way to minimize the risk of renal failure following cardiac surgery.

POSTOPERATIVE PULMONARY COMPLICATIONS

Respiratory failure and pulmonary complications are a significant cause of morbidity and mortality among post-CABG patients. Respiratory failure defined as the requirement for mechanical ventilatory support for more than 72 hours occurs in 5.6% of patients undergoing isolated coronary revascularization, with an associated 30-day mortality of 24.3% (128). Preoperative risk factors for prolonged ventilation include unstable angina, COPD, preoperative renal failure, female gender, and age >70 (129). Intraoperative risk factors for respiratory failure include increasing cardiopulmonary bypass time, while postoperative risk factors for respiratory failure include the presence of sepsis, gastrointestinal bleeding, renal failure, sternal wound infection, postoperative stroke, and reoperation for bleeding (128). The most important intervention to prevent respiratory complications postoperatively is aggressive pulmonary toilet with early ambulation, especially in the elderly.

GI COMPLICATIONS

Although rare, gastrointestinal complications following coronary revascularization are associated with high morbidity and mortality. Gastrointestinal complications have been reported to occur in 0.7% to 2.1% of patients undergoing coronary revascularization (130–132). The most common complications include GI bleeding, bowel ischemia, and pancreatitis. Other less frequent complications include perforated duodenal ulcer, pseudomembranous colitis, hepatic failure, and cholecystitis. Overall mortality in patients with postoperative GI complications is 34% to 87% (131–133). A significant cause of the poor outcomes associated with these complications is that they are often associated with a delay in diagnosis.

One of the most challenging diagnoses to make in the postoperative CABG patient is intestinal ischemia. Mortality for patients developing intestinal ischemia postoperatively is 64% to 80% (131–133), and 50% to 90% of cases of postoperative intestinal ischemia are secondary to nonocclusive mesenteric ischemia, with embolic and thrombotic causes accounting for the remainder (133,134). Early recognition of signs and symptoms is the most essential component in the prevention of the excessive mortality associated with ischemia. The presence of postoperative abdominal pain, bloating, persistent ileus, sepsis, or lower GI bleeding should prompt an early evaluation for ischemia. Unfortunately, many of these patients remain intubated or sedated in the postoperative period, which makes it more difficult to follow the physical examination, thus contributing to a delay in diagnosis. Serum lactate levels may be used as an adjunct to physical exam findings in identifying patients with ischemia; however, it should be noted that serum lactate may be unreliable in identifying patients with early intestinal ischemia and more likely reflects very advanced disease in the setting of high lactate levels. Flexible sigmoidoscopy should be instituted early to identify signs of mucosal ischemia. Similar to the prevention of renal failure, maintenance of adequate systemic perfusion and cardiac output both intraoperatively and postoperatively allows for better prevention of GI complications.

The cornerstone of treatment involves optimizing perfusion based on the mechanism of ischemia. Vasopressor agents should be discontinued if possible with optimization of the patient's volume status and cardiac function. If necrotic bowel is suspected, prompt surgical intervention is essential, with thromboembolectomy and resection of residual nonviable bowel. Early surgical intervention—defined as performance of laparotomy within 6 hours of the onset of symptoms—has been shown to decrease mortality in patients with postoperative intestinal ischemia (133).

ON-PUMP VERSUS OFF-PUMP CORONARY ARTERY BYPASS SURGERY

A current area of controversy is the impact of off-pump coronary bypass grafting on outcomes in patients requiring revascularization. Although beating-heart coronary revascularization is not a novel concept, newer technology has improved the ability to manipulate the heart while maintaining hemodynamic stability and has improved the ability to stabilize the isolated coronary vessel for performance of distal anastamoses. A central objective of off-pump surgery is to decrease neurologic and neurocognitive complications and to decrease morbidity related to cardiopulmonary bypass. Review of the STS database shows a decrease in the risk-adjusted operative mortality from 2.9% with conventional CABG to 2.3% with off-pump CABG and a decrease in the risk-adjusted major complication rate from 14.15% to 10.62% in 118,140 CABG procedures performed from 1998 to 2000 (135).

Questions remain about the potential selection bias of patients undergoing off-pump CABG. Previous randomized trials comparing outcomes between on-pump and off-pump surgery failed to demonstrate significant differences in postoperative neurologic injury, neurocognitive dysfunction, or overall mortality (31,136–138). In addition, randomized trials have failed to demonstrate significant improvements in quality of life following revascularization (31,139). Studies have suggested that off-pump surgery may be associated with decreased incidence of postoperative atrial fibrillation, decreased length of hospital stay, and decreased hospital costs versus the use of cardiopulmonary bypass (136–138,140). Other studies have failed to reproduce such benefits (136,138,139,141,142).

One of the purported advantages of off-pump coronary revascularization is the limitation of blood transfusion requirements (137). Off-pump techniques prove to be very beneficial in patients with a difficult, severely atherosclerotic aorta by allowing for limited or complete avoidance of aortic manipulation. Improvements in technology and in individual comfort level with this technique may provide an additional tool for dealing with challenging patients and may have an advantage over on-pump coronary revascularization in selected patients.

SUMMARY

As the use of percutaneous techniques for coronary artery disease becomes more prevalent, the population of patients undergoing CABG has become more complex. Surgical patients are now significantly older and have more comorbidities than historical cohorts. In spite of these factors, improvements in intraoperative and postoperative management and concerted efforts to improve on quality control practices have allowed for improvements in outcomes for patients undergoing coronary revascularization. As acuity continues to rise, it will be even more challenging to deal with the complications associated with surgical coronary revascularization. To meet this challenge, a multidisciplinary approach among medicine, cardiology, and cardiac surgery will be necessary to improve clinical management and to foster research directed at the treatment of patients with coronary artery disease.

REFERENCES

1. Eagle KA, Guyton RA, Davidoff R, et al. ACC/AHA guidelines for coronary artery bypass graft surgery: executive summary and recommendations: a report of the American College of Cardiology/American Heart Association Task Force on Practice Guidelines (committee to revise the 1991 guidelines for coronary artery bypass graft surgery). *Circulation* 1999;100:1464–1480.
2. Seven-year outcome in the Bypass Angioplasty Revascularization Investigation (BARI) by treatment and diabetic status. *J Am Coll Cardiol* 2000;35:1122–1129.
3. Niles NW, McGrath PD, Malenka D, et al. Northern New England Cardiovascular Disease Study Group. Survival of patients with diabetes and multivessel coronary artery disease after surgical or percutaneous coronary revascularization: results of a large regional prospective study. *J Am Coll Cardiol* 2001;37:1008–1015.
4. Coronary Artery Surgery Study (CASS): a randomized trial of coronary artery bypass surgery. Survival data. *Circulation* 1983;68:939–950.
5. Murphy ML, Hultgren HN, Detre K, et al. Treatment of chronic stable angina. A preliminary report of survival data of the randomized Veterans Administration cooperative study. *N Engl J Med* 1977;297:621–627.
6. Varnauskas E. Twelve-year follow-up of survival in the randomized European coronary surgery study. *N Engl J Med* 1988;319:332–337.
7. Yusuf S, Zucker D, Peduzzi P, et al. Effect of coronary artery bypass graft surgery on survival: overview of 10-year results from randomised trials by the coronary artery bypass graft surgery trialists collaboration. *Lancet* 1994;344:563–570.
8. Second interim report by the European Coronary Surgery Study Group. Prospective randomised study of coronary artery bypass surgery in stable angina pectoris. *Lancet* 1980;2:491–495.
9. Hoffman SN, TenBrook JA, Wolf MP, et al. A meta-analysis of randomized controlled trials comparing coronary artery bypass graft with percutaneous transluminal coronary angioplasty: one-to eight-year outcomes. *J Am Coll Cardiol* 2003;41:1293–1304.
10. Prabhakar G, Haan CK, Peterson ED, et al. The risks of moderate and extreme obesity for coronary artery bypass grafting outcomes: a study from the Society of Thoracic Surgeons' database. *Ann Thorac Surg* 2002;74:1125–1130; discussion 1130–1131.
11. Ferguson TB Jr, Hammill BG, Peterson ED, et al. A decade of change-risk profiles and outcomes for isolated coronary artery bypass grafting procedures, 1990–1999: a report from the STS National Database Committee and the Duke Clinical Research Institute. Society of Thoracic Surgeons. *Ann Thorac Surg* 2002;73:480–489; discussion 489–490.
12. Ascione R, Reeves BC, Chamberlain MH, et al. Predictors of stroke in the modern era of coronary artery bypass grafting: a case control study. *Ann Thorac Surg* 2002;74:474–480.
13. John R, Choudhri AF, Weinberg AD, et al. Multicenter review of preoperative risk factors for stroke after coronary artery bypass grafting. *Ann Thorac Surg* 2000;69:30–35; discussion 35–36.
14. Puskas JD, Winston AD, Wright CE, et al. Stroke after coronary artery operation: incidence, correlates, outcome, and cost. *Ann Thorac Surg* 2000;69:1053–1056.
15. McKhann GM, Grega MA, Borowicz LM Jr, et al. Encephalopathy and stroke after coronary artery bypass grafting: incidence, consequences, and prediction. *Arch Neurol* 2002;59:1422–1428.
16. Almassi GH, Sommers T, Moritz TE, et al. Stroke in cardiac surgical patients: determinants and outcome. *Ann Thorac Surg* 1999;68:391–397; discussion 397–398.
17. Gardner TJ, Horneffer PJ, Manolio TA, et al. Stroke following coronary artery bypass grafting: a ten-year study. *Ann Thorac Surg* 1985;40:574–581.
18. Barbut D, Lo YW, Hartman GS, et al. Aortic atheroma is related to outcome but not numbers of emboli during coronary bypass. *Ann Thorac Surg* 1997;64:454–459.
19. Barbut D, Lo YW, Gold JP, et al. Impact of embolization during coronary artery bypass grafting on outcome and length of stay. *Ann Thorac Surg* 1997;63:998–1002.
20. Calafiore AM, Di Mauro M, Teodori G, et al. Impact of aortic manipulation on incidence of cerebrovascular accidents after surgical myocardial revascularization. *Ann Thorac Surg* 2002;73:1387–1393.
21. Salazar JD, Wityk RJ, Grega MA, et al. Stroke after cardiac surgery: short-and long-term outcomes. *Ann Thorac Surg* 2001;72:1195–1201; discussion 1201–1202.
22. Davila-Roman VG, Barzilai B, Wareing TH, et al. Intraoperative ultrasonographic evaluation of the ascending aorta in 100 consecutive patients undergoing cardiac surgery. *Circulation* 1991;84:III47–III53.
23. Mills NL, Everson CT. Atherosclerosis of the ascending aorta and coronary artery bypass. Pathology, clinical correlates, and operative management. *J Thorac Cardiovasc Surg* 1991;102:546–553.
24. Royse AG, Royse CF, Ajani AE, et al. Reduced neuropsychological dysfunction using epiaortic echocardiography and the exclusive Y graft. *Ann Thorac Surg* 2000;69:1431–1438.
25. Gaudino M, Glieca F, Alessandrini F, et al. Individualized surgical strategy for the reduction of stroke risk in patients undergoing coronary artery bypass grafting. *Ann Thorac Surg* 1999;67:1246–1253.
26. Wareing TH, Davila-Roman VG, Daily BB, et al. Strategy for the reduction of stroke incidence in cardiac surgical patients. *Ann Thorac Surg* 1993;55:1400–1407; discussion 1407–1408.
27. Banbury MK, Kouchoukos NT, Allen KB, et al. Emboli capture using the Embol-X intraaortic filter in cardiac surgery: a multi-centered randomized trial of 1,289 patients. *Ann Thorac Surg* 2003;76:508–515; discussion 515.
28. Harringer W, International Council of Emboli Management Study Group. Capture of particulate emboli during cardiac procedures in which aortic cross-clamp is used. *Ann Thorac Surg* 2000;70:1119–1123.
29. Roach GW, Kanchuger M, Mangano CM, et al. Adverse cerebral outcomes after coronary bypass surgery. Multicenter Study of Perioperative Ischemia Research Group and the Ischemia Research and Education Foundation investigators. *N Engl J Med* 1996;335:1857–1863.
30. van Dijk D, Keizer AM, Diephuis JC, et al. Neurocognitive dysfunction after coronary artery bypass surgery: a systematic review. *J Thorac Cardiovasc Surg* 2000;120:632–639.
31. Van Dijk D, Jansen EW, Hijman R, et al. Cognitive outcome after off-pump and on-pump coronary artery bypass graft surgery: a randomized trial. *Jama* 2002;287:1405–1412.
32. Kilo J, Czerny M, Gorlitzer M, et al. Cardiopulmonary bypass affects cognitive brain function after coronary artery bypass grafting. *Ann Thorac Surg* 2001;72:1926–1932.
33. Aranki SF, Shaw DP, Adams DH, et al. Predictors of atrial fibrillation after coronary artery surgery. Current trends and impact on hospital resources. *Circulation* 1996;94:390–397.
34. Borzak S, Tisdale JE, Amin NB, et al. Atrial fibrillation after bypass surgery: does the arrhythmia or the characteristics of the patients prolong hospital stay? *Chest* 1998;113:1489–1491.
35. Mathew JP, Parks R, Savino JS, et al. MultiCenter Study of Perioperative Ischemia Research Group. Atrial fibrillation following coronary artery bypass graft surgery: predictors, outcomes, and resource utilization. *JAMA* 1996;276:300–306.
36. Shore-Lesserson L, Moskowitz D, Hametz C, et al. Use of intraoperative transesophageal echocardiography to predict atrial fibrillation after coronary artery bypass grafting. *Anesthesiology* 2001;95:652–658.
37. Ducceschi V, D'Andrea A, Liccardo B, et al. Perioperative clinical predictors of atrial fibrillation occurrence following coronary artery surgery. *Eur J Cardiothorac Surg* 1999;16:435–439.
38. Almassi GH, Schowalter T, Nicolosi AC, et al. Atrial fibrillation after cardiac surgery: a major morbid event? *Ann Surg* 1997;226:501–511; discussion 511–513.
39. Creswell LL, Schuessler RB, Rosenbloom M, et al. Hazards of postoperative atrial arrhythmias. *Ann Thorac Surg* 1993;56:539–549.
40. Lahey SJ, Campos CT, Jennings B, et al. Hospital readmission after cardiac surgery. Does "fast track" cardiac surgery result in cost saving or cost shifting? *Circulation* 1998;98:II35–II40.
41. Daoud EG, Strickberger SA, Man KC, et al. Preoperative amiodarone as prophylaxis against atrial fibrillation after heart surgery. *N Engl J Med* 1997;337:1785–1791.
42. Guarnieri T, Nolan S, Gottlieb SO, et al. Intravenous amiodarone for the prevention of atrial fibrillation after open heart

surgery: the Amiodarone Reduction in Coronary Heart (ARCH) trial. *J Am Coll Cardiol* 1999;34:343–347.

43. Dorge H, Schoendube FA, Schoberer M, et al. Intraoperative amiodarone as prophylaxis against atrial fibrillation after coronary operations. *Ann Thorac Surg* 2000;69:1358–1362.

44. Redle JD, Khurana S, Marzan R, et al. Prophylactic oral amiodarone compared with placebo for prevention of atrial fibrillation after coronary artery bypass surgery. *Am Heart J* 1999;138: 144–150.

45. Crystal E, Connolly SJ, Sleik K, et al. Interventions on prevention of postoperative atrial fibrillation in patients undergoing heart surgery: a meta-analysis. *Circulation* 2002;106:75–80.

46. Connolly SJ, Cybulsky I, Lamy A, et al. Double-blind, placebo-controlled, randomized trial of prophylactic metoprolol for reduction of hospital length of stay after heart surgery: the beta-Blocker Length Of Stay (BLOS) study. *Am Heart J* 2003;145: 226–232.

47. Lee SH, Chang CM, Lu MJ, et al. Intravenous amiodarone for prevention of atrial fibrillation after coronary artery bypass grafting. *Ann Thorac Surg* 2000;70:157–161.

48. Yagdi T, Nalbantgil S, Ayik F, et al. Amiodarone reduces the incidence of atrial fibrillation after coronary artery bypass grafting. *J Thorac Cardiovasc Surg* 2003;125:1420–1425.

49. Seitelberger R, Hannes W, Gleichauf M, et al. Effects of diltiazem on perioperative ischemia, arrhythmias, and myocardial function in patients undergoing elective coronary bypass grafting. *J Thorac Cardiovasc Surg* 1994;107:811–821.

50. Kowey PR, Taylor JE, Rials SJ, et al. Meta-analysis of the effectiveness of prophylactic drug therapy in preventing supraventricular arrhythmia early after coronary artery bypass grafting. *Am J Cardiol* 1992;69:963–965.

51. Podesser B, Schwarzacher S, Zwolfer W, et al. Combined perioperative infusion of nifedipine and metoprolol provides antiischemic and antiarrhythmic protection in patients undergoing elective aortocoronary bypass surgery. *Thorac Cardiovasc Surg* 1993;41:173–179.

52. Toraman F, Karabulut EH, Alhan HC, et al. Magnesium infusion dramatically decreases the incidence of atrial fibrillation after coronary artery bypass grafting. *Ann Thorac Surg* 2001;72: 1256–1261; discussion 1261–1262.

53. Speziale G, Ruvolo G, Fattouch K, et al. Arrhythmia prophylaxis after coronary artery bypass grafting: regimens of magnesium sulfate administration. *Thorac Cardiovasc Surg* 2000;48:22–26.

54. Parikka H, Toivonen L, Pellinen T, et al. The influence of intravenous magnesium sulphate on the occurrence of atrial fibrillation after coronary artery by-pass operation. *Eur Heart J* 1993; 14:251–258.

55. Kaplan M, Kut MS, Icer UA, et al. Intravenous magnesium sulfate prophylaxis for atrial fibrillation after coronary artery bypass surgery. *J Thorac Cardiovasc Surg* 2003;125:344–352.

56. Daoud EG, Dabir R, Archambeau M, et al. Randomized, double-blind trial of simultaneous right and left atrial epicardial pacing for prevention of post-open heart surgery atrial fibrillation. *Circulation* 2000;102:761–765.

57. Fan K, Lee KL, Chiu CS, et al. Effects of biatrial pacing in prevention of postoperative atrial fibrillation after coronary artery bypass surgery. *Circulation* 2000;102:755–760.

58. Greenberg MD, Katz NM, Iuliano S, et al. Atrial pacing for the prevention of atrial fibrillation after cardiovascular surgery. *J Am Coll Cardiol* 2000;35:1416–1422.

59. Levy T, Fotopoulos G, Walker S, et al. Randomized controlled study investigating the effect of biatrial pacing in prevention of atrial fibrillation after coronary artery bypass grafting. *Circulation* 2000;102:1382–1387.

60. Cochrane AD, Siddins M, Rosenfeldt FL, et al. A comparison of amiodarone and digoxin for treatment of supraventricular arrhythmias after cardiac surgery. *Eur J Cardiothorac Surg* 1994;8: 194–198.

61. Di Biasi P, Scrofani R, Paje A, et al. Intravenous amiodarone vs propafenone for atrial fibrillation and flutter after cardiac operation. *Eur J Cardiothorac Surg* 1995;9:587–591.

62. Galve E, Rius T, Ballester R, et al. Intravenous amiodarone in treatment of recent-onset atrial fibrillation: results of a randomized, controlled study. *J Am Coll Cardiol* 1996;27:1079–1082.

63. Campbell TJ, Gavaghan TP, Morgan JJ. Intravenous sotalol for the treatment of atrial fibrillation and flutter after cardiopulmonary bypass. Comparison with disopyramide and digoxin in a randomised trial. *Br Heart J* 1985;54:86–90.

64. Costeas C, Kassotis J, Blitzer M, et al. Rhythm management in atrial fibrillation—with a primary emphasis on pharmacological therapy: Part 2. *Pacing Clin Electrophysiol* 1998;21:742–752.

65. Dimopoulou I, Marathias K, Daganou M, et al. Low-dose amiodarone-related complications after cardiac operations. *J Thorac Cardiovasc Surg* 1997;114:31–37.

66. Kowey PR, Stebbins D, Igidbashian L, et al. Clinical outcome of patients who develop PAF after CABG surgery. *Pacing Clin Electrophysiol* 2001;24:191–193.

67. Liebold A, Haisch G, Rosada B, et al. Internal atrial defibrillation—a new treatment of postoperative atrial fibrillation. *Thorac Cardiovasc Surg* 1998;46:323–326.

68. Liebold A, Wahba A, Birnbaum DE. Low-energy cardioversion with epicardial wire electrodes: new treatment of atrial fibrillation after open heart surgery. *Circulation* 1998;98:883–886.

69. Bechtel JF, Christiansen JF, Sievers HH, et al. Low-energy cardioversion versus medical treatment for the termination of atrial fibrillation after CABG. *Ann Thorac Surg* 2003;75:1185–1188.

70. Petersen P, Boysen G, Godtfredsen J, et al. Placebo-controlled, randomised trial of warfarin and aspirin for prevention of thromboembolic complications in chronic atrial fibrillation. The Copenhagen AFASAK study. *Lancet* 1989;1:175–179.

71. The effect of low-dose warfarin on the risk of stroke in patients with nonrheumatic atrial fibrillation. The Boston area anticoagulation trial for atrial fibrillation investigators. *N Engl J Med* 1990;323:1505–1511.

72. Arnold AZ, Mick MJ, Mazurek RP, et al. Role of prophylactic anticoagulation for direct current cardioversion in patients with atrial fibrillation or atrial flutter. *J Am Coll Cardiol* 1992;19: 851–855.

73. Bjerkelund CJ, Orning OM. The efficacy of anticoagulant therapy in preventing embolism related to D.C. electrical conversion of atrial fibrillation. *Am J Cardiol* 1969;23:208–216.

74. Society of Thoracic Surgeons. STS NCD Executive Summary Spring 2003.

75. Slaughter MS, Olson MM, Lee JT Jr, et al. A fifteen-year wound surveillance study after coronary artery bypass. *Ann Thorac Surg* 1993;56:1063–1068.

76. Olsen MA, Lock-Buckley P, Hopkins D, et al. The risk factors for deep and superficial chest surgical-site infections after coronary artery bypass graft surgery are different. *J Thorac Cardiovasc Surg* 2002;124:136–145.

77. L'Ecuyer PB, Murphy D, Little JR, et al. The epidemiology of chest and leg wound infections following cardiothoracic surgery. *Clin Infect Dis* 1996;22:424–429.

78. Lu JC, Grayson AD, Jha P, et al. Risk factors for sternal wound infection and mid-term survival following coronary artery bypass surgery. *Eur J Cardiothorac Surg* 2003;23:943–949.

79. Borger MA, Rao V, Weisel RD, et al. Deep sternal wound infection: risk factors and outcomes. *Ann Thorac Surg* 1998;65:1050–1056.

80. Risk factors for deep sternal wound infection after sternotomy: a prospective, multicenter study. *J Thorac Cardiovasc Surg* 1996;111: 1200–1207.

81. Buxton BF, Komeda M, Fuller JA, et al. Bilateral internal thoracic artery grafting may improve outcome of coronary artery surgery. Risk-adjusted survival. *Circulation* 1998;98:II1–II6.

82. Lev-Ran O, Mohr R, Amir K, et al. Bilateral internal thoracic artery grafting in insulin-treated diabetics: should it be avoided? *Ann Thorac Surg* 2003;75:1872–1877.

83. Sofer D, Gurevitch J, Shapira I, et al. Sternal wound infections in patients after coronary artery bypass grafting using bilateral skeletonized internal mammary arteries. *Ann Surg* 1999;229: 585–590.

84. Pevni D, Mohr R, Lev-Run O, et al. Influence of bilateral skeletonized harvesting on occurrence of deep sternal wound infection in 1,000 consecutive patients undergoing bilateral internal thoracic artery grafting. *Ann Surg* 2003;237:277–280.

85. Matsa M, Paz Y, Gurevitch J, et al. Bilateral skeletonized internal thoracic artery grafts in patients with diabetes mellitus. *J Thorac Cardiovasc Surg* 2001;121:668–674.

86. Furnary AP, Zerr KJ, Grunkemeier GL, et al. Continuous intravenous insulin infusion reduces the incidence of deep sternal wound infection in diabetic patients after cardiac surgical procedures. *Ann Thorac Surg* 1999;67:352–360; discussion 360–362.

87. Furnary AP, Gao G, Grunkemeier GL, et al. Continuous insulin infusion reduces mortality in patients with diabetes undergoing coronary artery bypass grafting. *J Thorac Cardiovasc Surg* 2003;125:1007–1021.

88. Brandt C, Alvarez JM. First-line treatment of deep sternal infection by a plastic surgical approach: superior results compared with conventional cardiac surgical orthodoxy. *Plast Reconstr Surg* 2002;109:2231–2237.

89. Iyer VS, Russell WJ, Leppard P, et al. Mortality and myocardial infarction after coronary artery surgery. A review of 12,003 patients. *Med J Aust* 1993;159:166–170.

90. Cartier R, Robitaille D. Thrombotic complications in beating heart operations. *J Thorac Cardiovasc Surg* 2001;121:920–922.

91. Mariani MA, Gu YJ, Boonstra PW, et al. Procoagulant activity after off-pump coronary operation: is the current anticoagulation adequate? *Ann Thorac Surg* 1999;67:1370–1375.

92. Svedjeholm R, Dahlin LG, Lundberg C, et al. Are electrocardiographic Q-wave criteria reliable for diagnosis of perioperative myocardial infarction after coronary surgery? *Eur J Cardiothorac Surg* 1998;13:655–661.

93. Holmvang L, Jurlander B, Rasmussen C, et al. Use of biochemical markers of infarction for diagnosing perioperative myocardial infarction and early graft occlusion after coronary artery bypass surgery. *Chest* 2002;121:103–111.

94. Utley JR, Thomason ME, Wallace DJ, et al. Preoperative correlates of impaired wound healing after saphenous vein excision. *J Thorac Cardiovasc Surg* 1989;98:147–149.

95. Paletta CE, Huang DB, Fiore AC, et al. Major leg wound complications after saphenous vein harvest for coronary revascularization. *Ann Thorac Surg* 2000;70:492–497.

96. Garland R, Frizelle FA, Dobbs BR, et al. A retrospective audit of long-term lower limb complications following leg vein harvesting for coronary artery bypass grafting. *Eur J Cardiothorac Surg* 2003;23:950–955.

97. Bitondo JM, Daggett WM, Torchiana DF, et al. Endoscopic versus open saphenous vein harvest: a comparison of postoperative wound complications. *Ann Thorac Surg* 2002;73:523–528.

98. DeLaria GA, Hunter JA, Goldin MD, et al. Leg wound complications associated with coronary revascularization. *J Thorac Cardiovasc Surg* 1981;81:403–407.

99. Puskas JD, Wright CE, Miller PK, et al. A randomized trial of endoscopic versus open saphenous vein harvest in coronary bypass surgery. *Ann Thorac Surg* 1999;68:1509–1512.

100. Schurr UP, Lachat ML, Reuthebuch O, et al. Endoscopic saphenous vein harvesting for CABG—a randomized, prospective trial. *Thorac Cardiovasc Surg* 2002;50:160–163.

101. Crouch JD, O'Hair DP, Keuler JP, et al. Open versus endoscopic saphenous vein harvesting: wound complications and vein quality. *Ann Thorac Surg* 1999;68:1513–1516.

102. Griffith GL, Allen KB, Waller BF, et al. Endoscopic and traditional saphenous vein harvest: a histologic comparison. *Ann Thorac Surg* 2000;69:520–523.

103. Meyer DM, Rogers TE, Jessen ME, et al. Histologic evidence of the safety of endoscopic saphenous vein graft preparation. *Ann Thorac Surg* 2000;70:487–491.

104. Acar C, Ramsheyi A, Pagny JY, et al. The radial artery for coronary artery bypass grafting: clinical and angiographic results at five years. *J Thorac Cardiovasc Surg* 1998;116:981–989.

105. Maniar HS, Barner HB, Bailey MS, et al. Radial artery patency: are aortocoronary conduits superior to composite grafting? *Ann Thorac Surg* 2003;76:1498–1503; discussion 1503–1504.

106. Dumanian GA, Segalman K, Mispireta LA, et al. Radial artery use in bypass grafting does not change digital blood flow or hand function. *Ann Thorac Surg* 1998;65:1284–1287.

107. Serricchio M, Gaudino M, Tondi P, et al. Hemodynamic and functional consequences of radial artery removal for coronary artery bypass grafting. *Am J Cardiol* 1999;84:1353–1356, A8.

108. Denton TA, Trento L, Cohen M, et al. Radial artery harvesting for coronary bypass operations: neurologic complications and

109. Budillon AM, Nicolini F, Agostinelli A, et al. Complications after radial artery harvesting for coronary artery bypass grafting: our experience. *Surgery* 2003;133:283–287.

110. Connolly MW, Torrillo LD, Stauder MJ, et al. Endoscopic radial artery harvesting: results of first 300 patients. *Ann Thorac Surg* 2002;74:502–505; discussion 506.

111. Hall TS, Brevetti GR, Skoultchi AJ, et al. Re-exploration for hemorrhage following open heart surgery: differentiation of the causes of bleeding and the impact on patient outcomes. *Ann Thorac Cardiovasc Surg* 2001;7:352–357.

112. Dacey LJ, Munoz JJ, Baribeau YR et al, Northern New England Cardiovascular Disease Study Group. Reexploration for hemorrhage following coronary artery bypass grafting: incidence and risk factors. *Arch Surg* 1998;133:442–447.

113. Moulton MJ, Creswell LL, Mackey ME, et al. Reexploration for bleeding is a risk factor for adverse outcomes after cardiac operations. *J Thorac Cardiovasc Surg* 1996;111:1037–1046.

114. Verstraete M, Brown BG, Chesebro JH, et al. Evaluation of antiplatelet agents in the prevention of aorto-coronary bypass occlusion. *Eur Heart J* 1986;7:4–13.

115. Kallis P, Tooze JA, Talbot S, et al. Pre-operative aspirin decreases platelet aggregation and increases post-operative blood loss—a prospective, randomised, placebo controlled, double-blind clinical trial in 100 patients with chronic stable angina. *Eur J Cardiothorac Surg* 1994;8:404–409.

116. Ferraris VA, Ferraris SP, Joseph O, et al. Aspirin and postoperative bleeding after coronary artery bypass grafting. *Ann Surg* 2002;235:820–827.

117. Yende S, Wunderink RG. Effect of clopidogrel on bleeding after coronary artery bypass surgery. *Crit Care Med* 2001;29:2271–2275.

118. Murkin JM, Lux J, Shannon NA, et al. Aprotinin significantly decreases bleeding and transfusion requirements in patients receiving aspirin and undergoing cardiac operations. *J Thorac Cardiovasc Surg* 1994;107:554–561.

119. Laupacis A, Fergusson D. Drugs to minimize perioperative blood loss in cardiac surgery: meta-analyses using perioperative blood transfusion as the outcome. The International Study of Peri-operative Transfusion (ISPOT) investigators. *Anesth Analg* 1997;85:1258–1267.

120. Alvarez JM, Jackson LR, Chatwin C, et al. Low-dose postoperative aprotinin reduces mediastinal drainage and blood product use in patients undergoing primary coronary artery bypass grafting who are taking aspirin: a prospective, randomized, double-blind, placebo-controlled trial. *J Thorac Cardiovasc Surg* 2001;122: 457–463.

121. Engoren MC, Habib RH, Zacharias A, et al. Effect of blood transfusion on long-term survival after cardiac operation. *Ann Thorac Surg* 2002;74:1180–1186.

122. Mongan PD, Brown RS, Thwaites BK. Tranexamic acid and aprotinin reduce postoperative bleeding and transfusions during primary coronary revascularization. *Anesth Analg* 1998;87:258–265.

123. Bernet F, Carrel T, Marbet G, et al. Reduction of blood loss and transfusion requirements after coronary artery bypass grafting: similar efficacy of tranexamic acid and aprotinin in aspirin-treated patients. *J Card Surg* 1999;14:92–97.

124. Alderman EL, Levy JH, Rich JB, et al. Analyses of coronary graft patency after aprotinin use: results from the International Multicenter Aprotinin Graft Patency Experience (IMAGE) trial. *J Thorac Cardiovasc Surg* 1998;116:716–730.

125. Conlon PJ, Stafford-Smith M, White WD, et al. Acute renal failure following cardiac surgery. *Nephrol Dial Transplant* 1999;14:1158–1162.

126. Suen WS, Mok CK, Chiu SW, et al. Risk factors for development of acute renal failure (ARF) requiring dialysis in patients undergoing cardiac surgery. *Angiology* 1998;49:789–800.

127. Davila-Roman VG, Kouchoukos NT, Schechtman KB, et al. Atherosclerosis of the ascending aorta is a predictor of renal dysfunction after cardiac operations. *J Thorac Cardiovasc Surg* 1999;117:111–116.

128. Canver CC, Chanda J. Intraoperative and postoperative risk factors for respiratory failure after coronary bypass. *Ann Thorac Surg* 2003;75:853–857; discussion 857–858.

129. Legare JF, Hirsch GM, Buth KJ, et al. Preoperative prediction of prolonged mechanical ventilation following coronary artery bypass grafting. *Eur J Cardiothorac Surg* 2001;20:930–936.

130. Perugini RA, Orr RK, Porter D, et al. Gastrointestinal complications following cardiac surgery. An analysis of 1477 cardiac surgery patients. *Arch Surg* 1997;132:352–357.

131. Huddy SP, Joyce WP, Pepper JR. Gastrointestinal complications in 4473 patients who underwent cardiopulmonary bypass surgery. *Br J Surg* 1991;78:293–296.

132. Byhahn C, Strouhal U, Martens S, et al. Incidence of gastrointestinal complications in cardiopulmonary bypass patients. *World J Surg* 2001;25:1140–1144.

133. Ghosh S, Roberts N, Firmin RK, et al. Risk factors for intestinal ischaemia in cardiac surgical patients. *Eur J Cardiothorac Surg* 2002;21:411–416.

134. Pinson CW, Alberty RE. General surgical complications after cardiopulmonary bypass surgery. *Am J Surg* 1983;146:133–137.

135. Cleveland JC Jr, Shroyer AL, Chen AY, et al. Off-pump coronary artery bypass grafting decreases risk-adjusted mortality and morbidity. *Ann Thorac Surg* 2001;72:1282–1288; discussion 1288–1289.

136. Angelini GD, Taylor FC, Reeves BC, et al. Early and midterm outcome after off-pump and on-pump surgery in Beating Heart Against Cardioplegic Arrest Studies (BHACAS 1 and 2): a pooled analysis of two randomised controlled trials. *Lancet* 2002;359:1194–1199.

137. Puskas JD, Williams WH, Duke PG, et al. Off-pump coronary artery bypass grafting provides complete revascularization with reduced myocardial injury, transfusion requirements, and length of stay: a prospective randomized comparison of two hundred unselected patients undergoing off-pump versus conventional coronary artery bypass grafting. *J Thorac Cardiovasc Surg* 2003;125:797–808.

138. Nathoe HM, van Dijk D, Jansen EW, et al. A comparison of on-pump and off-pump coronary bypass surgery in low-risk patients. *N Engl J Med* 2003;348:394–402.

139. van Dijk D, Nierich AP, Jansen EW, et al. Early outcome after off-pump versus on-pump coronary bypass surgery: results from a randomized study. *Circulation* 2001;104:1761–1766.

140. Ascione R, Caputo M, Calori G, et al. Predictors of atrial fibrillation after conventional and beating heart coronary surgery: a prospective, randomized study. *Circulation* 2000;102:1530–1535.

141. Bull DA, Neumayer LA, Stringham JC, et al. Coronary artery bypass grafting with cardiopulmonary bypass versus off-pump cardiopulmonary bypass grafting: does eliminating the pump reduce morbidity and cost? *Ann Thorac Surg* 2001;71:170–173; discussion 173–175.

142. Shennib H, Endo M, Benhamed O, et al. Surgical revascularization in patients with poor left ventricular function: on- or off-pump? *Ann Thorac Surg* 2002;74:S1344–S1347.

Complications

of Valvular Cardiac

Surgery

Steven F. Bolling

■ **PROSTHETIC HEART VALVES 299**
Mechanical Valves 299
Tissue Valves 299
Prosthetic Valve Endocarditis 299
Perivalvular Leak 300
Supraventricular Arrythmias 300

■ **COMPLICATIONS OF MITRAL VALVE SURGERY 300**
Atrioventricular Groove Rupture 300
Injury to the Circumflex Artery 300
Posterior Myocardial Perforation 301
Embolus 301
Entrapment of the Noncoronary Cusp of the Aortic Valve 301
Leaflet Entrapment by Retained Valvular Tissue 302
Acute Valve Dysfunction Due to Suture Looping 302
Low Cardiac Output 302
Perivalvular Leak 302
Prosthetic Valve Thrombosis 302
Late Tamponade 303

■ **COMPLICATIONS OF MITRAL VALVE REPAIR 303**
Residual Mitral Stenosis or Regurgitation 303
Persistent Mitral Regurgitation 303

Left Ventricular Outflow Tract Obstruction or Abnormal Systolic Anterior Motion (SAM) of the Anterior Leaflet 303
Hemolysis 303

■ **COMPLICATIONS OF AORTIC VALVE SURGERY 304**
Complications Related to the Aortic Valve Annulus 304
Complications Related to Myocardial Preservation 304
Complications Related to the Aorta and the Aortotomy 304
AV Node Block 304

■ **COMPLICATIONS OF TRICUSPID VALVE SURGERY 304**
Persistent Right Ventricular Failure 304
Rhythm Disturbances 304
Recurrent/Residual Tricuspid Regurgitation 305

■ **REFERENCES 305**

More than 100,000 operations for cardiac valve repair or replacement are performed in the United States each year. Over the past 20 years, surgeons and their teams have achieved marked improvements in the outcome of patients with valvular heart disease. Intraoperative echocardiographic assessment of valvular function, improvements in

Steven F. Bolling: University of Michigan, Ann Arbor, MI 48109

prosthetic valves, advances in reconstructive techniques, and guidelines for timing of surgical intervention are all contributing factors in the improved prognosis (1,2). However, one of the most important advances has been the recognition and avoidance of the complications of valvular surgery (Table 26-1).

PROSTHETIC HEART VALVES

The prosthetic valves available today are of two primary categories: mechanical and tissue (biologic) valves. The mechanical prostheses include the caged-ball, tilting disc, and bileaflet valves. Tissue valves include porcine (stented and stentless) and pericardial valves. In addition, allografts (human tissue homografts) are available for use in both the aortic and mitral positions, and autografts (pulmonic valve) are available for use in the aortic position (3).

TABLE 26-1

COMPLICATIONS OF VALVE SURGERY

General complications
- Mechanical valve thromboembolism
- Anticoagulation-related bleeding
- Structural valve degeneration
- Prosthetic valve endocarditis
- Perivalvular leak
- Supraventricular arrhythmias

Procedure-specific complications
Mitral valve replacement complications
- Atrioventricular groove rupture
- Circumflex artery injury
- Posterior myocardial perforation
- Debris, fat, or air embolism
- Aortic valve cusp entrapment
- Mitral valve prosthesis leaflet entrapment/suture looping
- Ventricular output failure
- Prosthetic valve thrombosis
- Late cardiac tamponade

Mitral valve repair complications
- Residual mitral stenosis or regurgitation
- Persistent mitral regurgitation
- LV outflow obstruction
- Hemolysis

Aortic valve complications
- Mitral leaflet detachment
- Inadequate myocardial preservation
- Aortic wall dissection or embolization
- Atrioventricular node block

Tricuspid valve complications
- Persistent right ventricular failure
- Complete heart block
- Recurrent or residual tricuspid regurgitation

Mechanical Valves

All the mechanical valves share the advantage of long-term durability but have increased risk of thromboembolism and the risk of bleeding secondary to the need for anticoagulation to prevent thromboembolism (4). Rates of thrombotic complications are low (1% to 3%) when the patients are adequately anticoagulated. However, anticoagulation-related bleeding remains one of the most common causes of valve-related morbidity (1% to 3% per patient-year) and mortality (0.1% to 0.5% per patient-year), as safe, stable, and effective anticoagulation is difficult to achieve (5).

Tissue Valves

A significant advantage of tissue valves is the avoidance of need for anticoagulation. These valves have a very low thromboembolic complication rate; however, risk does exist in patients with atrial fibrillation or with an enlarged left atrium, a history of previous emboli, an atrial clot, or significantly reduced left ventricular (LV) function. These patients should be considered for anticoagulation therapy in spite of having a tissue prosthesis. Structural valve degeneration is the most important complication of the bioprosthetic valve. The risk of valve failure increases over time, and this rate is accelerated in younger patients. The probability of structural failure with currently available porcine valves (Hancock or Carpentier-Edwards) increases beginning at about 8 years after operation and reaches over 60% at 15 years. This finite durability is a major impediment to long-term success of biologic prostheses. The failure rate in the elderly patient ($\geq$70) is significantly less than in younger age groups. Some of these durability issues may be improved with the new anticalcification fixation techniques now being used (6–10).

Prosthetic Valve Endocarditis

Prosthetic heart valves carry an increased risk for the development of endocarditis that can be precipitated by any cause of transient bacteremia. Prosthetic valve endocarditis (PVE) encompasses 15% to 30% of all cases of endocarditis, is reported in 1% to 2% of all valve implants, and is associated with an overall higher mortality rate than native valve endocarditis (11,12). PVE that occurs in the early postoperative period is frequently due to *Staphylococcus epidermidis*, either due to a break in technique in the operating room or from skin contamination. Late onset PVE is related to bacteremic seeding of the valve. Common portals of entry include dental procedures, operations, gastrointestinal endoscopy, intravenous catheter contamination, intravenous drug abuse, and infections of the skin, lungs, bowel, and urinary tract.

Physical examination, microbiological results, laboratory testing, and imaging procedures are all useful to diagnose

PVE. The most common presenting symptoms for PVE are fever, fatigue, malaise, and dyspnea. Pyrexia, newly noted heart murmur, and microscopic hematuria are frequent clinical signs. Thirty percent of patients present with septic emboli, which can involve the spleen, kidneys, cerebral vasculature, and coronary system. Septic pulmonary emboli from tricuspid valve endocarditis can produce patchy infiltrates on chest radiograph. Echocardiograms may show a rocking motion of the prosthesis and the presence of vegetations. Blood cultures are the mainstay of diagnosis and are positive in over 90% of cases.

Although carefully selected antimicrobial therapy, specific for the infecting organisms, is important in the care of PVE, it is rare that antimicrobial therapy alone will cure PVE. Most patients require operative removal of the valve and reconstruction of its function. Indications for acute surgical intervention in PVE include the presence of new onset unmanageable congestive heart failure or cardiogenic shock. Surgical intervention should not be delayed in the presence of acute infective PVE when congestive heart failure ensues. However, surgical intervention is futile if complications of the infection (such as severe embolic cerebral damage) or other comorbid conditions make the prospect of recovery remote.

Anesthesia, intraoperative monitoring, cardioplegia, and exposure of the valve are similar to other valvular procedures. Excision of the valve and debridement of the annulus and abscesses must be meticulous and extensive. All necrotic and infected tissue must be removed. After local antibiotic irrigation, the annulus and areas of tissue loss can often be reconstructed using autologous pericardium (13).

Abscess formation is the most commonly reported PVE manifestation; it occurs in 20% of cases and is most often caused by *Staphylococcus aureus*. *Enterococcus* species have been reported in 5% to 17%, and gram-negative rod infections are rare (1% to 9%). Other secondary manifestations of endocarditis include aortic mycotic infections, cardiac conduction defects, sinus of Valsalva aneurysms, and valve thrombosis. Fungal infections occur more frequently in patients with prosthetic valves who are immunocompromised or intravenous drug users. Fungal vegetations, due to their bulky size, can produce valvular stenosis (14–16).

Postoperative care should include at least 6 weeks of selected intravenous antibiotics. Hospital mortality is related primarily to ongoing sepsis, multisystem organ failure, or failure to eradicate the local infection followed by recurrent perivalvular leak. Valve replacement in hemodynamically stable patients with PVE has a favorable outcome in 80% to 95% of cases (17). The reinfection rate ranges from 1% to 13%.

Perivalvular Leak

Perivalvular leak is an uncommon complication with current surgical techniques using Teflon pledgets. The incidence of perivalvular leak for both mechanical and biologic valves is about 0% to 1.5% per patient-year of valve life. Perivalvular leak is slightly more common with the bileaflet valve than with the porcine valve because of the use of the everting suture technique and less bulky sewing ring (18).

Supraventricular Arrythmias

Atrial arrhythmias, primarily atrial fibrillation or, less commonly, atrial flutter, occur in 10% to 40% of patients after valve surgery and can contribute to neurologic morbidity. The usual onset is 1 to 3 days after operation, with a peak incidence at 48 hours; however, arrythymias may occur at any time, including shortly after discharge. Increasing age is the most consistent predisposing factor; other conditions include a history of rheumatic fever, the durations of aortic cross-clamp time and cardiopulmonary bypass, the method of cardioplegia, and abrupt stoppage of β-blocking agents. Acidosis, hypokalemia, or hypoxemia may contribute to the onset of the arrhythmia and should be corrected prior to initiating definitive therapy. Amiodarone is the first-line agent for both rate control and conversion to sinus rhythm in these patients (19,20).

COMPLICATIONS OF MITRAL VALVE SURGERY

Atrioventricular Groove Rupture

In many patients, particularly the elderly, there is extensive calcification in the posterior mitral annulus and leaflet. Rupture of the AV groove is usually related to vigorous traction on the posterior leaflet of the valve or to calcium excision in a calcified posterior leaflet. This can cause separation of the AV groove, leading to massive hemorrhage. This complication is prevented by understanding the pathologic process of calcification of the mitral annulus and avoiding rupture by either placing traction sutures on the edge of the posterior leaflet or by only very careful calcium debridement in isolated spots. A safer procedure may be to attach the prosthesis to the atrial wall, leaving the entire calcified mass intact. This approach may result in a smaller valve area but a successful operation (21).

Injury to the Circumflex Artery

The circumflex coronary artery in the AV groove can be injured or occluded by placement of the mitral valve sutures too far radially beyond the annulus during valve replacement, particularly on the left lateral edge of the annulus (Fig. 26-1). This complication presents as decreased cardiac output, poor LV lateral wall motion on intraoperative echocardiogram, or bleeding posteriorly from the heart. Correction requires the reinstitution of cardiopulmonary bypass, removal of the stitch, and, occasionally, a saphenous

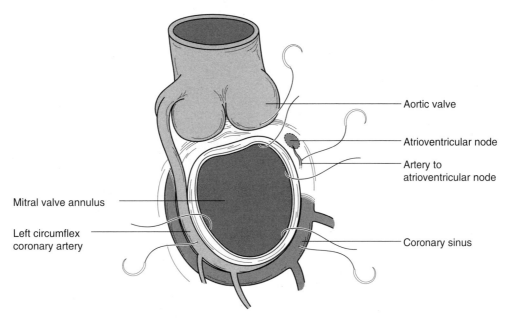

Figure 26-1   Suture injuries to structures surrounding the mitral valve annulus. Improper placement of sutures in the annulus can damage the left circumflex artery, aortic valve, atrioventricular node, or coronary sinus.

vein bypass graft to the circumflex coronary. Placing the sutures at the junction of the mitral valve annulus and the valve leaflet prevents this complication. Circumflex artery injury is rare during mitral valve repair as the sutures are placed parallel to the valve rather than across the annulus.

Posterior Myocardial Perforation

Myocardial rupture is a catastrophic complication of mitral valve surgery. The incidence is 0.5% to 2% in mitral valve replacement. This complication is caused by perforation or stretching of the LV by the prosthesis or by a strut. It should be recognized in the operating room, and treatment requires reinstitution of cardiopulmonary bypass. The perforation is located, and repair may be done with the use of Teflon strips, both externally and internally. The valve prosthesis must be removed to accomplish the repair. With preservation of the posterior mitral leaflet and papillary muscles, this complication is rare.

Embolus

Emboli from the heart can be debris from valve debridement, fat particles, or air. This complication results when there is failure to remove all debris, often from an extensively calcified valve, or through technical errors that allow air to remain in the LV outflow tract. Embolism typically occurs upon removal of the cross-clamp and resumption of normal cardiac ejection. Prevention is critical and involves copious irrigation of the LV to remove all debris. In addition, a sponge placed in the ventricle to catch debris may be helpful (Fig. 26-2). Air embolism may be prevented by an LV vent, by

an aortic root aspirating vent, or by needle-venting the LV apex. Removal of all air can be confirmed by the intraoperative transesophageal echocardiogram (TEE) (22,23).

Entrapment of the Noncoronary Cusp of the Aortic Valve

Though rare, this can occur in the area of 10 o'clock to 12 o'clock of the mitral valve, near the anterolateral commissure

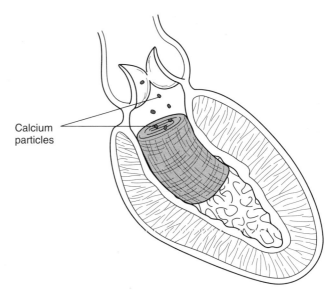

Figure 26-2 A sponge placed in the left ventricle during debridement of the aortic or mitral valve annulus can catch the debris. This may prevent small pieces from becoming lodged in the spaces along the wall of the ventricle, only to embolize once contractile cardiac function resumes.

of the mitral valve. At this point the commissure is very close to the aortic valve's noncoronary cusp, and this cusp may be entrapped if the mitral valve suture is placed too deeply (Fig. 26-1). This complication may be diagnosed only after removal of the aortic cross clamp, when the heart dilates due to severe aortic regurgitation and when aortic insufficiency is observed on TEE. Avoiding excessively deep bites can prevent entrapment. Treatment of entrapment requires reinstitution of cardiopulmonary bypass, recross clamping, removal of the mitral prosthesis, and resuturing the area at this point. In some cases, the aortic root may need to be opened and the aortic valve inspected.

Leaflet Entrapment by Retained Valvular Tissue

Many prosthetic valves involve the opening and closing of either single or double leaflets. With these valves care must be taken that retained native valve structures, chords, or tips of papillary muscles do not interfere with the leaflet action (Fig. 26-3). Tissue retention can produce significant obstruction or regurgitation. Echocardiography is the best way to demonstrate valve malfunction. This complication is prevented by using proper supra, sub, or annular suturing technique. To ensure that the leaflets open and close without interference at implantation, a rubber-shod instrument can be used to test the valve. To fix this problem, the mitral valve is removed and the tissue that prevents opening and

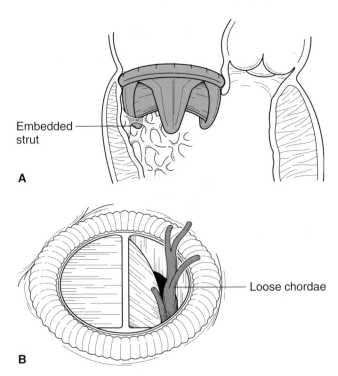

Figure 26-3 Dysfunction of prosthetic valves due to interference from periannular structures. **A:** Mitral valve struts can become entrapped along the wall of the ventricle and in the valve remnant, chordae, or papillary muscles. **B:** Remnants of the papillary muscles preventing full closure of the valve.

closing below the valve should be removed. The valve is then replaced.

Acute Valve Dysfunction Due to Suture Looping

This complication causes early bioprosthetic valve dysfunction and severe mitral regurgitation (MR) from immobility of a leaflet. Leaflet looping is preventable by carefully pushing the valve down during insertion or by use of a dental mirror to inspect the valve struts and ensure that no suture is looped over them before the valve sutures are tied down. Management of this done is by removing and reimplanting the valve.

Low Cardiac Output

Low cardiac output following mitral valve replacement is a frequent complication that has been documented since this procedure's inception. It has also been one of the most difficult problems to treat because it has many causes. In patients with MR, depression of cardiac performance is common after initial valve replacement. The normally cone-shaped ventricle assumes a spherical shape if there is removal of the papillary muscle-annular continuity. This concept was first promulgated in 1964, and laboratory and clinical studies have substantiated that papillary muscle-annular continuity is important for the maintenance of normal cardiac output. The normal LV geometric relationship can be best maintained by mitral valve repair or, if that is not possible, by preserving the posterior leaflet and papillary muscles with the insertion of a totally intact valve into the mitral apparatus. The prognosis for the patient with low cardiac output from loss of LV geometry is grave and accounts for substantial early and late mortality following mitral valve replacement (MVR) (24).

Perivalvular Leak

Perivalvular leak, early or late, producing severe regurgitation may occur in patients whose tissue is friable, in patients with endocarditis, or in patients who have extensive calcification. Patients have a loud holosystolic murmur. The diagnosis is made by echocardiogram and a rise in left atrial pressure with a prominent V wave. Using pledgeted sutures can prevent this complication, particularly when fragile or minimal annular tissue is found. If there is an abscess, a pericardial or Teflon bolster may be necessary to improve the fixation of the valve.

Prosthetic Valve Thrombosis

Thrombosis of a mechanical mitral valve can be noted by low cardiac output refractory to all forms of support. This rare complication can occur early in patients with low cardiac output and less than full anticoagulation. The thrombosed mechanical prosthesis has restricted leaflet motion on echocardiography. Definitive diagnosis is made by fluoroscopy. Although immediate operation may be required, thrombolytic therapy is an option if the patient is not moribund. At operation the prosthesis is inspected and can be reimplanted, or a thrombectomy may be sufficient. If there is an obvious cause for the thrombosis that can be fixed, such as an impinging suture, the clot can be removed and the LV irrigated copiously to ensure complete thrombus removal. If not, the valve should be re-replaced (25).

Late Tamponade

Patients who have undergone recent mitral valve replacement requiring anticoagulation may have late cardiac tamponade. This is due to accumulation of blood in the pericardial space. The diagnosis should be considered in any patient on anticoagulants who has low cardiac output days to weeks after placement of a mitral valve. It is frequent in patients who have become excessively anticoagulated. Echocardiography is diagnostic for this with great accuracy. The treatment is to reopen the incision and evacuate the fluid collection, which should result in immediate improvement of the patient's hemodynamic stability. Directed needle aspiration is also possible.

COMPLICATIONS OF MITRAL VALVE REPAIR

Residual Mitral Stenosis or Regurgitation

Residual stenosis is diagnosed by TEE, high left atrial pressure, and low cardiac output in the immediate postrepair period while still in the operating room (25–27). It usually results from inadequate relief of the stenosis; mitral valve replacement should be considered. Postrepair MR after operation for mitral stenosis is usually the result of an excessive commissurotomy. Significant MR is detected by TEE. Usually, the incisions in the leaflet have missed the fused commissures or a chorda supporting a section of the valve has been inadvertently cut. The aorta must be clamped, cardioplegia reinstituted, and the left atrium reopened. If the MR originates at the commissures, a pledgeted stitch can correct this complication. If regurgitation persists, valve replacement is mandated.

Persistent Mitral Regurgitation

Residual MR after operation for MR is probably the most vexing of all problems for the mitral repair surgeon. Residual MR almost always results from a lack of understanding of the exact geometry of the underlying pathology and an inability to recreate a functional intraventricular zone of leaflet coaptation. Correction of this residual deficit requires a reconsideration of the valve structure and either re-repair or replacement.

Left Ventricular Outflow Tract Obstruction or Abnormal Systolic Anterior Motion (SAM) of the Anterior Leaflet

A ring placement for mitral repair can be complicated by LV outflow obstruction due to the posterior leaflet being too "tall." This geometry pushes the anterior leaflet into the LV outflow tract during systole. This problem can be diagnosed by an increased left atrial pressure and reduced cardiac output; TEE can confirm the diagnosis. Often this is a dynamic finding and is associated with hypovolemia and hypercontractility. Discontinuation of pressors and correction of intravascular volume deficit solve this in many cases. Some authors advocate the use of β-blockers. If these maneuvers do not alleviate the obstruction, a second pump run can be initiated to reduce the height of the posterior leaflet, perhaps with a sliding valvuloplasty. As a last resort, mitral valve replacement is possible. Similarly, a "tilted" placement of a prosthetic mitral valve can obstruct the LV outflow tract (Fig. 26-4). This generally requires repositioning or replacement of the valve.

Hemolysis

Insertion of an annuloplasty mitral valve ring requires sutures placed around the annulus. If there is dehiscence of a suture, the result is a moving nonsupported ring that can hemolyze red blood cells. Hemolysis may also occur in the absence of dehiscence when a small jet of insignificant MR hits a stitch or the ring itself. Either one may produce only a very minor derangement or severe hemolysis with resulting anemia. β-blockade, to reduce the force of the blood shear, and pentoxyfyline, to make the red cells more "pliable," may be satisfactory therapy. For some patients requiring intermittent transfusion, reoperation is the only choice.

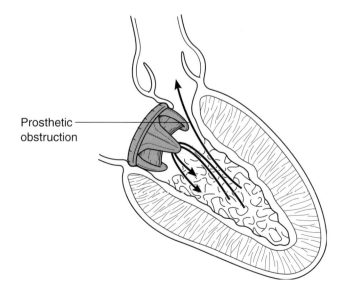

Prosthetic obstruction

Figure 26-4 Obstruction of the left ventricular outflow tract by a prosthetic mitral valve.

COMPLICATIONS OF AORTIC VALVE SURGERY

Complications Related to the Aortic Valve Annulus

Calcific degeneration is the most common cause of aortic valve dysfunction, and calcium is nearly always present in the aortic valve annulus at the time of operation, particularly in the elderly patient. The native valve is excised using scissors, knife, or a rongeur to remove all calcium. To avoid embolism of debris down the coronaries or into the LV cavity, copious rinsing is critical; a sponge placed in the ventricle can be helpful (Fig. 26-2). Vigorous debridement can result in detachment of the anterior mitral leaflet, which is in continuity with the aortic valve annulus. This results in an opening from the aortic root into the left atrium. This defect should be repaired with pledgeted sutures through the anterior leaflet of the mitral valve and the aortic valve annulus. These sutures are then used to secure the prosthesis.

Complications Related to Myocardial Preservation

Inadequate myocardial preservation during the aortic valve replacement procedure is the most common cause of postoperative ventricular dysfunction. Most surgeons employ hypothermic cardioplegic preservation during aortic valve replacement. Concomitant coronary artery occlusive disease can result in uneven distribution of the cardioplegia solution. For this reason most surgeons use retrograde cardioplegia as an adjunct to protection or as the sole method to distribute the cardioplegia. The use of topical cooling solutions around the heart during aortic valve replacement also helps to ensure adequate myocardial preservation. One effective routine is to measure the septal temperature continuously during operation and maintain it at 10°C to monitor the adequacy of myocardial preservation (28).

Complications Related to the Aorta and the Aortotomy

Either a transverse or an oblique aortotomy is used to provide access to the valve. Some forms of degenerative disease that affect the aortic valve also can affect the aorta itself, resulting in a thin and friable structure. Calcification of the ascending aorta frequently accompanies calcific degeneration of the aortic valve. Calcification can severely limit the area available for cannulation of the ascending aorta and may force the surgeon to cannulate the femoral artery to provide adequate cardiopulmonary bypass. In addition, calcified plaques can fracture when the aortic cross clamp is applied, causing arterial embolization or later dissection of the aorta. With a severely diseased aorta that is too calcified for the safe application of a cross clamp, the technique of deep hypothermia and circulatory

arrest may be a preferable option. Segmental endarterectomy and decalcification are occasionally required to successfully close the aorta. Aortas that are friable or calcified should be closed using strips of felt to buttress the suture line.

AV Node Block

The atrioventricular node is very close to the junction of the right coronary cusps and the noncoronary cusps of the aortic valve and may be damaged by placement of deep stitches, overly aggressive debridement, or annular abscess (similar to Fig. 26-1). In most circumstances atrioventricular conduction disturbances at the conclusion of the procedure do not require the placement of permanent pacing electrodes. Edema from the procedure itself can cause temporary A-V conduction block, which resolves within the first postoperative week (29,30).

COMPLICATIONS OF TRICUSPID VALVE SURGERY

Persistent Right Ventricular Failure

The prognosis and complications after tricuspid valve operation depend less on the valve surgery itself than on the duration of tricuspid disease, particularly tricuspid regurgitation and right ventricular (RV) hemodynamic abnormalities. In one series only 13% of patients with chronic tricuspid regurgitation and severe RV failure had a good outcome, while 78% of the patients who had no history of congestive heart failure and less RV dysfunction had a good outcome (31). The difficult preoperative decision is whether a patient's tricuspid regurgitation is the result of tricuspid valve disease or is due to primary RV failure. Tricuspid valve surgery is likely to be curative in the former case but possibly lethal in the latter. Unfortunately, there are no completely reliable preoperative methods to predict recovery of RV systolic function postoperatively. Sound clinical judgment based on a careful examination of the patient over time, along with the response to optimal fluid and electrolyte management, remains the best preoperative indicator. Right ventricular failure has become more easily manageable with the use of vasodilators and phosphodiesterase inhibitors, such as milirinone, and inhaled nitric oxide (32).

Rhythm Disturbances

The most common heart rhythm problem following tricuspid valve surgery is complete heart block (CHB). The risk of CHB is time-related; the incidence at 5 weeks has been reported to be 5%, but it is 25% by 10 years. The early risk is largely iatrogenic, having to do with suture placement near the location of the AV node, which is at the junction of the anterior and septal leaflets of the tricuspid valve (33). This can be minimized by judicious placement of valve sutures, particularly near the triangle of Koch. Placing the sutures at the base of the valve leaflet rather than deeper in the annulus ensures the greatest distance from the conduction system. The risk of CHB is greater when TV replacement or annuloplasty is combined with mitral valve procedures than after tricuspid valve procedures alone, due to swelling on both sides of the AV node or His bundle. Heart block appears to occur less frequently after annuloplasty than after replacement of the tricuspid valve—a difference of 6% versus 24% in one series involving 47 patients. Late CHB is due to scar formation around the prosthetic valve annulus, particularly when a mitral or aortic prosthesis nearly abuts it. CHB usually necessitates a permanent epicardial pacemaker system for the patient.

Recurrent/Residual Tricuspid Regurgitation

Comparative studies of recurrent/residual tricuspid regurgitation after tricuspid annuloplasty are few. One prospective, randomized study compared ring to stitch annuloplasty. At 64 months' follow-up, there was a significantly greater incidence of moderate or severe postoperative tricuspid regurgitation in the DeVega stitch group (34). However, in both groups control of tricuspid regurgitation was poor, particularly with elevated pulmonary vascular resistance or organic tricuspid disease. Although long-term survival was termed excellent, recurrence of at least moderate tricuspid regurgitation occurs in many patients; most do not require reoperation. A very recent study advocated an aggressive approach of TV annuloplasty, even with minor tricuspid regurgitation, if the annulus was dilated. This study showed infrequent recurrent tricuspid regurgitation in the group treated with annuloplasty for less severe dilation (35).

REFERENCES

1. Bonow RO, Carabello B, de Leon AC, et al. ACC/AHA guidelines for the management of patients with valvular heart disease. Executive summary. *J Heart Valve Dis* 1998;7:672.
2. Carabello BA, Crawford FA. Medical progress: valvular heart disease. *N Engl J Med* 1997;337:32.
3. Rahimtoola SH. Choice of prosthetic heart valve for adult patients—review article. *J Am Coll Cardiol* 2003;41(6):893–904.
4. Akins CW. Results with mechanical cardiac valvular prostheses. *Ann Thorac Surg* 1995;60:1836.
5. Hammermeister KE, Henderson WG, Burchfiel CM, et al. Comparison of outcome after valve replacement with a bioprosthesis versus a mechanical prosthesis: initial 5 year results of a randomized trial. *J Am Coll Cardiol* 1987;10:719.
6. Chaitman BR, Bonan R, Lepage G, et al. Hemodynamic evaluation of the Carpentier-Edwards porcine xenograft. *Circulation* 1979;60:1170.
7. Wernly JA, Crawford MH. Choosing a prosthetic heart valve. *Cardiol Clin* 1998;16:491.
8. Edwards TJ, Livesey SA, Simpson IA, et al. Biological valves beyond fifteen years: the Wessex experience. *Ann Thorac Surg* 1995;60:S211.
9. Bernal JM, Rabasa JM, Lopez R, et al. Durability of the Carpentier-Edwards porcine bioprosthesis: role of age and valve position. *Ann Thorac Surg* 1995;60:S248.
10. Doty JR, Flores JH, Millar RC, et al. Aortic valve replacement with Medtronic freestyle bioprosthesis: operative technique and results. *J Card Surg* 1998;13:208.
11. Steusse DC, Vlessis AA. Epidemiology of native valve endocarditis. In: Vlessis AA, Bolling SF, eds. *Endocarditis: a multidisciplinary approach.* Armonk, NY: Futura Publishing, 1999:77.
12. Vlessis AA, Hovaguimian H, Jaggers J, et al. Infective endocarditis: ten-year review of medical and surgical therapy. *Ann Thorac Surg* 1996;61:1217.
13. Schwartz CF, Bolling SF. Mitral valve endocarditis. In: Vlessis AA, Bolling SF, eds. *Endocarditis: a multidisciplinary approach.* Armonk, NY: Futura Publishing, 1999:263.
14. Husebye DG, Pluth JR, Piehler JM, et al. Reoperation on prosthetic heart valves. An analysis of risk factors in 552 patients. *J Thorac Cardiovasc Surg* 1983;86:543–552.
15. Lytle BW, Cosgrove DM, Taylor PC, et al. Reoperation for valve surgery: perioperative mortality and determinants of risk for 1,000 patients. *Ann Thorac Surg* 1986;42:632–643.
16. Teoh KH, Ivanov J, Weisel RD, et al. Survival and bioprosthetic valve failure. *Circulation* 1989;80(Suppl. 1):8–15.
17. David TE, Bos J, Christakis GT, et al. Heart valve operations in patients with active infective endocarditis. *Ann Thorac Surg* 1990;49:701.
18. Lindblom D. Long-term clinical results after aortic valve replacement with the Bjork-Shiley prosthesis. *J Thorac Cardiovasc Surg* 1988;95:658–667.
19. Kalus JS, White CM, Caron MF, et al. Indicators of atrial fibrillation risk in cardiac surgery patients on prophylactic amiodarone. *Ann Thorac Surg* 2004;77(issue 4):1288–1292.
20. Kobayashi J, Kosakai Y, Isobe F, et al. Rationale of the Cox maze procedure for atrial fibrillation during redo mitral valve operations. *J Thorac Cardiovasc Surg* 1996;112:1216.
21. Najafi H, Dye WS, Javid H, et al. Mitral valve replacement: review of seven years' experience—review article. *Am J Cardiol* 1969;24(3):386–392.
22. Bucerius J, Gummert JF, Borger MA, et al. Stroke after cardiac surgery: a risk factor analysis of 16,184 consecutive adult patients. *Ann Thorac Surg* 2003;75(2):472–478.
23. Jennifer C, O'Brien B, Schneck M. Risk of stroke following valve replacement surgery. *Semin Cerebrovasc Dis Stroke* 2003;3(4): 214–218.
24. Fenster MS, Feldman MD. Mitral regurgitation: an overview. *Curr Prob Cardiol* 1995;20:193.
25. David TE, Uden DE, Strauss HD. The importance of the mitral apparatus in left ventricular function after correction of mitral regurgitation. *Circulation* 1983;68:II76.
26. Akins CW, Hilgenberg AD, Buckley MJ, et al. Mitral valve reconstruction versus replacement for degenerative or ischemic mitral regurgitation. *Ann Thorac Surg* 1994;58:668.
27. Roberts WC, McIntosh CL, Wallace RB. Mechanisms of severe mitral regurgitation in mitral valve prolapse determined from analysis of operatively excised valves. *Am Heart J* 1987; 113:1316.
28. Carr JA, Savage EB. Aortic valve repair for aortic insufficiency in adults: a contemporary review and comparison with replacement techniques—review article. *Eur J Cardiothorac Surg* 2004; 25(1):6–15.
29. David TE, Komeda M, Brofman PR. Surgical treatment of aortic root abscess. *Circulation* 1989;80(Suppl. 1):269–274.
30. Magovern JA, Pennock JL, Campbell DB, et al. Aortic valve replacement and combined aortic valve replacement and coronary artery bypass grafting: predicting high risk groups. *J Am Coll Cardiol* 1987;9:38–43.
31. Bernal JM, Gutiérrez-Morlote J, Llorca J, et al. Tricuspid valve repair: an old disease, a modern experience. *Ann Thorac Surg* 2004;78(6):2069–2074.
32. Thorburn CW, Morgan JJ, Shanahan MX, et al. Long-term results of tricuspid valve replacement and the problem of prosthetic valve thrombosis. *Am J Cardiol* 1983;51:1128–1132.
33. Breyer RH, McClenathan JH, Michaelis LL, et al. Tricuspid regurgitation. A comparison of nonoperative management, tricuspid annuloplasty and tricuspid valve replacement. *J Thorac Cardiovasc Surg* 1976;72:867–874.
34. Peterffy A, Jonasson R, Henze A. Haemodynamic changes after tricuspid valve surgery. A recatheterization study in forty-five patients. *Scand J Thorac Cardiovasc Surg* 1981;15:161–170.
35. Dreyfus GD, Corbi PJ, John Chan KM, et al. Secondary tricuspid regurgitation or dilatation: which should be the criteria for surgical repair? *Ann Thorac Surg* 2005;79(1):127–132.

Complications

of Thoracoscopy

Michael A. Smith   Richard J. Battafarano

■■■ BACKGROUND 306

■■■ RISK ASSESSMENT 307

■■■ GENERAL COMPLICATIONS 308

■■■ INTRAOPERATIVE COMPLICATIONS 308
Hemorrhage 308
Intraoperative Cardiogenic Disturbances 308
Ventilatory Complications 309

■■■ POSTOPERATIVE COMPLICATIONS 309
General Considerations 309
Residual Air Space and Prolonged Air Leaks 309
Empyema 310
Sputum Retention and Pneumonia 311
Completion of Cancer Resection 311

■■■ SUMMARY 312

■■■ REFERENCES 312

BACKGROUND

The use of endoscopy for diagnostic and therapeutic procedures of the chest was introduced in 1910 by the Swedish physician Hans Christian Jacobeus (1). Over the

Michael A. Smith: Keck School of Medicine, University of Southern California, Los Angeles, CA 90033
Richard J. Battafarano: Barnes-Jewish Hospital, St. Louis, MO 63110

following decades thoracoscopy developed into a routine procedure for the diagnosis and management of pleural space complications of tuberculosis. As antimicrobial therapy for tuberculosis developed, the use of thoracoscopy waned. However, during the past decade many technological advances have laid the foundation for the rebirth of thoracoscopy. Currently, video-assisted thoracic surgery (VATS) is an increasingly popular approach for diagnostic and therapeutic procedures of the lung, pleura, esophagus, and mediastinum (Table 27-1). In some ways the minimally invasive nature of this approach has changed the way patients are managed. This is especially true for biopsy of peripheral pulmonary nodules and densities, which historically have been followed with serial imaging studies.

When considering whether to proceed with a VATS approach for a given diagnostic or therapeutic procedure, it is important to consider the advantages and disadvantages as well as contraindications for each individual patient. VATS is often preferable to open procedures because it reduces surgical trauma, decreases pain and postoperative narcotic use, and preserves pulmonary function (2). These factors may allow older or sicker patients who are poor candidates for thoracotomy to undergo diagnostic or therapeutic interventions (3). The appeal of the VATS approach for diagnostic procedures is relatively well recognized in the thoracic community. Because of significant disadvantages, many are less enthusiastic about the use of VATS for major anatomic resections.

The disadvantages of VATS include a steep learning curve, the loss of tactile sensation, concern about adequacy of therapy for cancer resections, poor access to and ability to control vital structures in the event of emergent blood loss, and the high cost of specialized equipment. In addition, there

TABLE 27-1

MINIMALLY INVASIVE PROCEDURES OF THE CHEST

Pulmonary
    Wedge resection
    Lobectomy
    Pneumonectomy

Esophageal
    Fundoplication
    Myotomy
    Leiomyoma resection
    Esophagectomy

Cardiac
    Pericardial window

Nervous system
    Sympathectomy

Other
    Thymectomy
    Mediastinal mass excision

are contraindications to thoracoscopy (Table 27-2) that also diminish the prospect of using this approach in certain patients. The technical accomplishment of VATS procedures requires certain conditions to be safe and effective. The most important requirement is that the surgeon be able to see the operative field. Therefore, two absolute contraindications to VATS are a fused pleural space from prior surgery

TABLE 27-2

CONTRAINDICATIONS TO THORACOSCOPY

Absolute
    Fused pleural space
        Prior thoracotomy
        Severe inflammatory process
        Prior pleurodesis
    Inability to tolerate single lung ventilation
        Prior pneumonectomy
        Severe respiratory failure
    Hemodynamically unstable patient
        Cardiac arrest
        Severe trauma

Relative
    High risk of incomplete resection or dissemination
        Tumor >4 cm
        Central pulmonary lesions
        Endobronchial tumor
        Hilar lymphadenopathy
    Fused fissures
    Prior hilar radiation
    Chest wall involvement
    Coagulopathy
    Obesity

or inflammation and an inability to tolerate single lung ventilation secondary to preexisting lung disease or cardiopulmonary instability. In general, resection of tumors >4 cm in diameter is also a contraindication for a VATS approach. Relative contraindications include endobronchial tumor seen on bronchoscopy, obesity, coagulopathy, hilar lymphadenopathy, fused fissures, prior hilar radiation, and chest wall involvement for pulmonary resections for technical difficulty of safe operative dissection. It is important for surgeons to understand the potential complications associated with the thoracoscopic approach in order to identify the patients most likely to benefit from this minimally invasive technique. If there are no absolute contraindications, many surgeons will begin with the VATS technique and will convert to open thoracotomy if they are unable to proceed safely.

RISK ASSESSMENT

In an effort to avoid complications in the intraoperative and postoperative period, a preoperative risk assessment must be performed. Many algorithms have been developed to systematically stratify the risk of candidates for chest surgery based upon preoperative data such as age, exercise capacity, spirometric values, and measures of gas exchange and diffusing capacity. No single factor has been proven predictive for the development of complications. In an effort to improve predictive ability, various factors have been combined into scoring systems. The Cardiopulmonary Risk Index (CPRI) and the Physiological and Operative Severity Score for the Enumeration of Mortality and Morbidity (POSSUM) are general scoring systems that have been used for lung resection with variable predictive ability (4–6). Additional scoring systems specifically developed for lung resection, such as the Predictive Respiratory Quotient (PRQ) (7) and the Predicted Postoperative Product (8), have not gained widespread use.

Most surgeons do not rely completely on a particular scoring system to determine a patient's surgical fitness. However, many of the factors that make up these scoring systems, along with surgical judgment, are used to make the ultimate decision. Some of these factors include patient age, pulmonary function, clinical stage of disease, and presence of comorbid illnesses. Patients who would normally be considered high risk because of advanced age, poor pulmonary function, and low functional status may actually experience better outcomes with fewer complications using a VATS approach (9,10). However, their risks are still substantial when compared to the general population and should not be underestimated. Another consideration specific to VATS is the clinical stage and location of disease. More central lung lesions are more difficult to deal with from both a diagnostic and therapeutic standpoint. The close proximity of central lung lesions to major pulmonary vessels can increase the risk of approaching these using a VATS approach (11). For this reason it is important to set size and location criteria for VATS approaches to lung lesions. Disregarding these criteria will make the patient vulnerable to complications.

GENERAL COMPLICATIONS

VATS is simply a minimally invasive approach to perform essentially the same operation that is done with the open approach. Although the VATS approach may be less traumatic, the anatomic and physiologic consequences of the operation remain the same. Therefore, all potential complications that may be associated with the open procedure may also be encountered in the same operation performed by VATS. However, there are intraoperative complications that are specific to VATS. The overall mortality rate for VATS approaches ranges from 0.5% to 2.5%, while morbidity rates vary from 4% to 14% (9,12–14).

INTRAOPERATIVE COMPLICATIONS

The initial reservation with minimally invasive surgery in the chest was concern for safety. However, over the years it has been shown that minimally invasive chest surgery can be performed for a variety of procedures with safety comparable to open thoracotomy. To a great degree, safety depends on good surgical judgment for conversion to open thoracotomy for technical reasons or when an open operation is more appropriate. The most common, immediately life-threatening intraoperative complications of chest surgery are massive hemorrhage, cardiogenic disturbances, and ventilatory problems.

Hemorrhage

Massive intraoperative hemorrhage is the most worrisome complication for surgeons when considering minimally invasive procedures in the chest because of the difficulty in obtaining central control of the pulmonary artery and veins using the VATS technique. Massive hemorrhage in the chest can result from great vessel injury or, more commonly, injury to a pulmonary artery or vein branch sustained during pulmonary dissection. The pulmonary artery and its branches are especially thin-walled and easily injured during manipulation or traction employed to increase exposure. In contrast, the walls of the pulmonary vein are more resilient and withstand surgical manipulation much better. The risk of a difficult dissection and pulmonary artery injury can be anticipated in patients who have had induction chemotherapy or prior irradiation. In addition, patients with mediastinal granulomatosis or prior silica exposure will have regional bronchopulmonary lymph nodes densely adherent to branch pulmonary arteries. In such cases it is prudent to begin the surgical dissection by

encircling the ipsilateral main pulmonary artery and both pulmonary veins, so as to have proximal and distal control in the event of vessel injury. Another reported cause of major intraoperative bleeding is mechanical failure of vascular staplers (15,16). Some authors recommend placement of vascular clamps centrally prior to vessel division to minimize the sequelae of misfiring staplers.

Because the pulmonary circulation is a low-pressure, high-flow system, arterial and venous injury can almost always be immediately controlled with local pressure at the injury site. After local control of the bleeding is obtained, the surgeon, knowing the injury's site and magnitude, must make an immediate decision on what will be required to control the bleeding. In the setting of VATS the operative view can be lost very quickly. Therefore, attempts to place a vascular clamp to control bleeding should be avoided. In case of a pulmonary artery injury, this may, in fact, exacerbate the injury. A better alternative to controlling bleeding during VATS or open thoracotomy is to gain immediate control with gentle application of pressure using a sponge-stick through the utility incision or a port site. This will give ample time to gain better exposure with an open incision and repair the injury if needed. Rarely, injury to the main pulmonary artery, the left atrium medial to the pulmonary vein, or the superior or inferior vena cava will require cardiopulmonary bypass to control the situation for adequate repair.

In addition, injuries to bronchial arteries, parenchymal surfaces, and pleural adhesions, as well as intercostal and internal mammary vessels, can also lead to significant intraoperative blood loss if they go unnoticed. It is important to use careful dissection techniques at all times during the operation to avoid injuries to these structures and to control them quickly when they occur.

Intraoperative Cardiogenic Disturbances

As mentioned previously, adequate exposure is extremely important when using a VATS approach. The insufflation of CO_2 aids in the compression of lung parenchyma and the effacement of subpleural lesions and acts as a retractor when combined with changes in patient position. Initially, there was reluctance to use CO_2 insufflation because of concern about hemodynamic compromise. Intrapleural CO_2 insufflation has been shown to have adverse hemodynamic consequences in laboratory animal studies (17). However, in the clinical setting low-pressure (<10 mm Hg) insufflation of CO_2 during thoracoscopy is safe and without significant hemodynamic consequences except for elevation of central venous pressure. The pressures and flow rates should be kept <10 mm Hg and 2 L per minute, respectively, to avoid significant central venous pressures or rapid mediastinal movement. In addition, intrapleural CO_2 insufflation should be initiated only if there are no significant adhesions present to prevent pleural and parenchymal injury.

Patients with preexisting heart disease are at risk for more typical intraoperative cardiogenic disturbances, such as ischemia and arrhythmias. It is important to identify these patients based upon history, physical exam, and preoperative testing to determine the need for preoperative prophylactic measures to avoid cardiac ischemia and to select those who need intraoperative Swan-Ganz catheter monitoring. Patients without preexisting cardiac dysfunction can also develop intraoperative arrhythmias due to hypothermia, hypoxemia, hypokalemia, hyperkalemia, hypovolemia, or acidosis. When they occur, these problems must be corrected as soon as possible. Electrical cardioversion may be necessary in the case of hemodynamically significant arrhythmias. However, the arrhythmia may be recalcitrant to electrical cardioversion if the underlying disturbance is not corrected (i.e., hypothermia, hyperkalemia). In addition, manipulation and compression of the heart for exposure can also lead to arrhythmias and ischemia. Often, these maneuvers cannot be completely avoided, but they must be limited in duration and frequency, using close communication between the surgeon and anesthesiologist to help identify the effects on blood pressure and rhythm.

Ventilatory Complications

A host of ventilatory problems can put the patient's gas exchange and hemodynamic stability at risk. If ventilation is established through a double lumen endobronchial tube or a single lumen tube with a bronchial blocking balloon, it is essential for the surgeon, as well as the anesthesiologist, to be confident that proper positioning has been established prior to starting the resection. The surgeon must also be aware of the presentation of tube displacement. High airway pressure and absent CO_2 in the ventilator circuit indicates that the bronchial cuff or bronchial blocking balloon has herniated into the trachea, causing tracheal obstruction. Deflation of the cuff or balloon solves the problem and advancement of the tube or balloon prevents the problem from reoccurring. While conducting a right-sided resection with ventilation only on the left, persistent hypoxemia suggests that the balloon on the left limb of the double lumen tube has advanced too far and has occluded the left upper lobe orifice. This problem is sometimes first detected by the attentive surgeon, who recognizes that the mediastinum's usual ventilatory movement is absent because of progressive atelectasis of the left upper lobe. Repositioning the tube solves the problem.

In general, patients undergoing lung surgery are more susceptible to pneumothorax secondary to barotrauma because of preexisting emphysema from smoking. Pneumothorax can occur at the time of induction and onset of positive pressure ventilation or at any point during the actual operation on the contralateral side. The surgeon should be aware of this development since airway pressures will increase and the rhythmic movement of the mediastinum will be absent. Indeed, the mediastinum will sometimes balloon out toward the operative side, causing obstruction of venous return and hemodynamic compromise. Opening the mediastinal pleura easily remedies the problem.

POSTOPERATIVE COMPLICATIONS

General Considerations

Several complications can arise after chest surgery. Many can be fatal if not recognized and managed early and aggressively. Attention to details of patient symptoms, clinical exam, and routine chest x-rays, in addition to having a high index of suspicion during the postoperative period, will help the clinician identify complications and manage them effectively.

Residual Air Space and Prolonged Air Leaks

During the normal conduct of partial lung resection or any VATS procedure, there can be small injuries to the visceral pleura resulting in air leaks. These small visceral pleural injuries can be minimized with meticulous technique. Normally these small air leaks resolve with apposition of pleural surfaces once the lung is reexpanded. A residual air space exists when there is failure to fill the chest cavity after reexpansion of the lung. Greater amounts of parenchymal resection increase the risk of residual air space. Thus, bilobectomies and lobectomies have a higher rate of residual air space than segmentectomies and wedge resections. Usually the space is noted at the apex after upper lobectomy, but it can also be found at the base near the diaphragm after other types of resections. In many patients residual air space in the absence of a persistent air leak will not be associated with any significant morbidity. The space gradually disappears over several weeks secondary to reabsorption of gases within the space, further reexpansion of the lung, shift of the mediastinum to the operative side, and elevation of the ipsilateral hemidiaphragm. When a residual air space is associated with symptoms such as pain, dyspnea, hemoptysis, or fever, a bronchopleural fistula should be suspected and requires appropriate intervention with thoracostomy tube placement.

As with open lung resection, prolonged air leak is the most common cause of morbidity and prolonged hospital stay after minimally invasive partial lung resection. It also increases patient discomfort, cost of care, and utilization of resources. Prolonged air leak is responsible for approximately 25% of all morbidity after lung resection. An air leak that persists more than 5 to 7 days after surgery is generally considered a prolonged air leak. It occurs in 4% to 15% of cases after partial lung resection with open thoracotomy (18,19). VATS series report rates of prolonged air leak between 1.4% and 16% (9,13,14,20). The data is a bit more difficult to evaluate for the thoracoscopic approach.

Many series combine anatomic resections with wedge resections when recording data on air leak rates after thoracoscopy, giving a lower reported rate of prolonged air leak because of the larger denominator. In addition, some series differ in their criteria for prolonged air leak (i.e., 5 days vs. 7 days vs. 10 days). In general, the air leak rate after VATS anatomic resection is likely higher than after open anatomic resection because of the more difficult management of incomplete fissures. As with open lung resection, the most consistent risk factor for prolonged air leak after VATS is severe obstructive pulmonary disease. Other potential risk factors for prolonged air leak include advanced age, pleural adhesions, preoperative steroid use, and induction chemo/radiation therapy.

Preoperative awareness of increased risk for prolonged air leaks should engender extra measures in addition to meticulous technique during the operation to help prevent them. The use of bovine pericardial strips as a buttress along the lung staple line to decrease air leaks was first described for lung volume reduction surgery (21). However, their efficacy for completing fissures during lobectomy and segmentectomy is unclear. Previously, Venuta et al. (22) found that the use of pericardial strips to complete interlobar fissures for pulmonary lobectomy significantly reduced the duration of postoperative air leaks and hospital stay. The use of pericardial buttressing strips has been described in conjunction with the VATS approach (23) and has been shown to lower the prolonged air leak rate after VATS lung volume reduction surgery (24,25).

Other measures to reduce the incidence of prolonged air leak in the high-risk patient are maneuvers that displace the potential residual space to an extrapleural position, thereby making apposition of pleural surfaces more likely. One common practice is the creation of a pleural tent. In a prospective randomized study of 200 patients undergoing upper lobectomy (26), it was found that pleural tenting reduced the duration of air leaks and hospital costs. Similarly, other randomized and retrospective studies (27,28) showed that pleural tenting following lobectomy shortens the duration of chest tube drainage and hospital costs. The use of pleural tents has also been described with the VATS approach (22). A second way to limit the potential residual pleural air space is to elevate the diaphragm by insufflating air into the peritoneal cavity. Pneumoperitoneum has been described to treat air leaks and residual spaces after lung volume reduction surgery (29). Subsequently, De Giacomo et al. (30) described its use after pulmonary resection. In a prospective randomized study of 16 patients undergoing bilobectomy, Cerfolio et al. showed that intraoperative creation of pneumoperitoneum decreased the incidence of air leaks and shortened hospital stay without increasing morbidity (31).

A third measure that has been used for prolonged air leak is the use of biologic sealants. Prior reports have shown (32,33) that fibrin glue is not effective in reducing the duration of air leaks after lobectomy. However, Fabian et al. (34) showed in a randomized study that fibrin glue reduced the rate of postoperative air leak from 15% to 2% after lung resection. Similarly, Wain et al. (35) found that fibrin glue-treated patients had a mean air leak time of 31 hours while untreated patients had a mean air leak time of 52 hours. Although this difference was significant, there was no reduced time to chest tube removal and earlier hospital discharge. Because thoracoscopic procedures were excluded from both of these sealant trials, further study is needed to determine efficacy, patient selection, and cost effectiveness of fibrin sealants for preventing prolonged air leak for VATS pulmonary resection.

Despite preventive measures, many patients go on to develop prolonged air leak. Although this is the most common problem thoracic surgeons deal with in the postoperative period, there is no consensus on its management. Most surgeons believe that conversion from suction to water seal is an effective way of encouraging an air leak to seal. Development of a pneumothorax in the setting of an expiratory air leak is uncommon. This is supported by a study by Cerfolio et al. (36), in which 33 patients with postoperative air leak were randomized to continued suction versus water seal on postoperative day 2. They found that 67% of the patients treated with water seal had air leak resolution by postoperative day 3 versus 7% of the patients who remained on suction. Air leaks that do not resolve on water seal should be placed on a Heimlich valve once the fluid drainage is minimal. The patient can be discharged with the chest tube and Heimlich valve in place as long as there is no new or enlarging pneumothorax on chest x-ray (CXR). Outpatient chest tube management is well tolerated and desirable for the patient as it avoids prolonged hospitalization. Most air leaks stop after several days and the chest tube can be removed at that time.

Empyema

Empyema occurs in approximately 2% of patients after VATS procedures (12,13). This complication is often associated with a bronchopleural fistula after pulmonary resection. In addition to the presence of bronchopleural fistula, other factors, such as poor pulmonary function, lower preoperative serum hemoglobin, right pneumonectomy, and lack of bronchial stump reinforcement, have been shown to be associated with the development of postresection empyema (37). Some believe that the use of neoadjuvant and adjuvant therapy protocols also contributes to the development of postresection empyema.

The diagnosis of empyema is suspected in any patient with signs and symptoms of infection after lung resection. Development of serosanguinous sputum, purulent chest tube, or wound drainage are also highly suspicious findings. Imaging studies consistent with empyema are pleural opacity with or without an air-fluid level after partial lung resection or a new or falling air-fluid level after pneumonectomy.

Once the diagnosis of postoperative empyema is made or strongly suspected, immediate management includes closed chest tube thoracostomy as well as appropriate antibiotic therapy. Once adequate drainage has been established and the patient is stabilized, the appropriate definitive management can be decided. Factors determining definitive management include presence or absence of bronchopleural fistula, partial lung resection versus pneumonectomy, stability of the patient, and the need for positive pressure ventilation. The traditional management approach involves three separate procedures: open drainage, closure of the fistula (if present), and closure of the cavity as described above. Several weeks of dressing changes are usually required to get the pleural cavity clean and covered with healthy granulation tissue. Patients deemed unsuitable for definitive closure can be managed with open window thoracostomy and dressing changes indefinitely.

Sputum Retention and Pneumonia

Poor airway hygiene is a significant life-threatening problem after chest surgery. Acutely, it can cause hypoxia, tachycardia, and hemodynamic embarrassment. Postoperative pain and compromised mental status leading to an inability to deep breathe and cough are the main factors contributing to retention of airway secretions. In many cases postoperative pain leads to more narcotic use with subsequent compromised mental status and sputum retention. These airway secretions can go on to plug the airways, causing atelectasis, lobar collapse, pneumonia, and respiratory failure. Specific patients at risk for postoperative sputum retention are current smokers, patients with a history of chronic obstructive pulmonary disease, cerebrovascular accident, or ischemic heart disease, and those without regional analgesia (38). In case-controlled studies, the VATS approach has been shown to be associated with less immediate postoperative pain compared to the thoracotomy approach by objective assessment of analgesic requirements (39,40) and by subjective scales (2). However, one prospective randomized trial comparing VATS lobectomy with thoracotomy showed only a trend toward less narcotic use that was not statistically significant (41). The lack of statistical significance in this study may have been related to small sample sizes and low statistical power. In general, it is believed that the VATS approach indeed lowers postoperative pain and the need for analgesia. Diminished pain and need for narcotic analgesia should lower the risk of sputum retention and poor postoperative airway hygiene.

In addition to a surgical approach, there are other measures to reduce the incidence of sputum retention. The most important tactic is smoking cessation prior to surgery. Vaporciyan et al. (42) found in a retrospective analysis of 237 patients undergoing pneumonectomy that patients who continued to smoke within 1 month of operation were at increased risk for developing pneumonia and adult respiratory distress syndrome (ARDS). Chest physiotherapy, including coughing, early ambulation, incentive spirometry, and percussion with postural drainage, is the standard approach for postoperative prophylaxis and therapy for sputum retention. However, patients with recalcitrant sputum retention may require more invasive measures, such as transcricoid saline injection, to stimulate coughing. Bronchoscopy may ultimately be required to aspirate secretions and stimulate a more vigorous cough. Many recommend liberal use of minitracheostomies in high-risk patients as a form of prophylaxis and treatment. The minitracheostomy tube allows immediate and repeated aspiration of the tracheobronchial tree. It is placed percutaneously through the cricothyroid membrane either at the time of surgery or at the bedside postoperatively. In a prospective randomized trial of 102 high-risk patients, Bonde et al. (43) found that prophylactic use of minitracheostomy significantly lowered the incidence of sputum retention. Similarly, Au et al. (44) reported decreased need for suction bronchoscopy in patients who had undergone minitracheostomy placement. More studies are needed to determine how much these benefits carry over to the VATS approach.

Completion of Cancer Resection

As stated previously, some surgeons have been less enthusiastic about the application of the VATS approach to the management of primary lung malignancy as well as metastasectomy with curative intent. Inability to adequately palpate lesions and loss of spatial relationships make completeness of resection the major concern. Completeness of resection can be problematic from the standpoint of achieving negative margins as well as the ability to avoid intrapleural and port site tumor seeding when using a VATS approach. The ability to achieve negative margins can be directly correlated to size and location of pulmonary lesions. Therefore, lesions that are >4 cm in size and centrally located are generally not amenable to a VATS approach. Although microscopic spillage of tumor cells during thoracotomy for esophageal and lung cancer resection has been described (45–47), reports of actual esophageal and lung cancer tumor dissemination are rare. However, there have been several case reports of tumor dissemination after VATS resections (48–53). These are anecdotal case reports without a denominator, and it is unknown whether the recurrences are related to the VATS approach or to the cancer's aggressive nature. Therefore, this complication's true incidence is unknown. It is thought that disruption of the tumor during dissection or forced extraction of unprotected specimens through small exit sites with extensive direct contact with the chest wall make VATS resection of a malignancy more susceptible to pleural dissemination and port site recurrence. Measures to prevent these potential mechanisms of tumor cell dissemination are meticulous use of oncologic surgical technique with conversion to open thoracotomy if necessary to prevent compromise of these principles. Further important measures include the use of a protective impermeable bag for specimen retrieval, an adequate exit port during the tumor removal, and sterile water lavage of all port sites and the pleural cavity before the conclusion of the surgery (53). When these oncologic principles are followed, the development of port site tumor recurrences is low.

SUMMARY

The revival of thoracoscopy for the management of diseases of the chest is one of the most important recent advancements in thoracic surgery. With proper judgment and skill, the surgeon can safely apply this approach to a wide variety of cardiothoracic procedures. Although the approach is minimally invasive, the risks for complications must not be overlooked. Anticipation and attention to the details of patient selection, intraoperative technique, and postoperative patient management will help with prevention, early identification, and successful management of complications after thoracoscopy.

REFERENCES

1. Jacobeus HC. Ueber die möglichkeit die zytoskopie bei untersuchung seroser hohlungen anzuwenden. *Munch Med Wochenschr* 1910;57:2090–2092.
2. Demmy TL, Curtis JJ. Minimally invasive lobectomy directed toward frail and high-risk patients: a case-control study. *Ann Thorac Surg* 1999;68:194–200.
3. Lewis RJ, Caccavale RJ, Sisler GE, et al. One hundred consecutive patients undergoing video-assisted thoracic operations. *Ann Thorac Surg* 1992;54:421–426.
4. Epstein SK, Faling LJ, Daly BD, et al. Predicting complications after pulmonary resection. Preoperative exercise testing vs a multifactorial cardiopulmonary risk index. *Chest* 1993;104:694–700.
5. Melendez JA, Carlon VA. Cardiopulmonary risk index does not predict complications after thoracic surgery. *Chest* 1998;114:69–75.
6. Brunelli A, Fianchini A, Gesuita R, et al. POSSUM scoring system as an instrument of audit in lung resection surgery. Physiological and operative severity score for the enumeration of mortality and morbidity. *Ann Thorac Surg* 1999;67:329–331.
7. Melendez JA, Barrera R. Predictive respiratory complication quotient predicts pulmonary complications in thoracic surgical patients. *Ann Thorac Surg* 1998;66:220–224.
8. Pierce RJ, Copland JM, Sharpe K, et al. Preoperative risk evaluation for lung cancer resection: predicted postoperative product as a predictor of surgical mortality. *Am J Respir Crit Care Med* 1994;150:947–955.
9. DeCamp MM Jr, Jaklitsch MT, Mentzer SJ, et al. The safety and versatility of video-thoracoscopy: a prospective analysis of 895 consecutive cases. *J Am Coll Surg* 1995;181:113–120.
10. Jaklitsch MT, DeCamp MM Jr, Liptay MJ, et al. Video-assisted thoracic surgery in the elderly. A review of 307 cases. *Chest* 1996;110:751–758.
11. Demmy TL, Wagner-Mann CC, James MA, et al. Feasibility of mathematical models to predict success in video-assisted thoracic surgery lung nodule excision. *Am J Surg* 1997;174:20–23.
12. Jancovici R, Lang-Lazdunski L, Pons F, et al. Complications of video-assisted thoracic surgery: a five-year experience. *Ann Thorac Surg* 1996;61:533–537.
13. Yim AP, Liu HP. Complications and failures of video-assisted thoracic surgery: experience from two centers in Asia. *Ann Thorac Surg* 1996;61:538–541.
14. Krasna MJ, Deshmukh S, McLaughlin JS. Complications of thoracoscopy. *Ann Thorac Surg* 1996;61(4):1066–1069.
15. Yim AP, Ho JK. Malfunctioning of vascular staple cutter during thoracoscopic lobectomy. *J Thorac Cardiovasc Surg* 1995;109:1252.
16. Watanabe A, Abe T, Yamauchi A, et al. Reinforcement of a bronchial stump in VATS lobectomy. *Thorac Cardiovasc Surg* 2000;48:242–243.
17. Jones DR, Graeber GM, Tanguilig GG, et al. Effects of insufflation on hemodynamics during thoracoscopy. *Ann Thorac Surg* 1993;55:1379–1382.
18. Deslauriers J, Ginsberg RJ, Dubois P, et al. Current operative morbidity associated with elective surgical resection for lung cancer. *Can J Surg* 1989;32:335–339.
19. Rice TW, Okereke IC, Blackstone EH. Persistent air-leak following pulmonary resection. *Chest Surg Clin N Am* 2002;12: 529–539.
20. Gharagozloo F, Tempesta B, Margolis M, et al. Video-assisted thoracic surgery lobectomy for stage I lung cancer. *Ann Thorac Surg* 2003;76:1009–1014; discussion 1014–1015.
21. Cooper JD. Technique to reduce air leaks after resection of emphysematous lung. *Ann Thorac Surg* 1994;57:1038–1039.
22. Venuta F, Rendina EA, De Giacomo T, et al. Technique to reduce air leaks after pulmonary lobectomy. *Eur J Cardiothorac Surg* 1998;13:361–364.
23. Eugene J, Dajee A, Kayaleh R, et al. Reduction pneumonoplasty for patients with a forced expiratory volume in 1 second of 500 milliliters or less. *Ann Thorac Surg* 1997;63:186–190; discussion 190–192.
24. Hazelrigg SR, Boley TM, Naunheim KS, et al. Effect of bovine pericardial strips on air leak after stapled pulmonary resection. *Ann Thorac Surg* 1997;63:1573–1575.
25. Stammberger U, Klepetko W, Stamatis G, et al. Buttressing the staple line in lung volume reduction surgery: a randomized three-center study. *Ann Thorac Surg* 2000;70:1820–1825.
26. Brunelli A, Al Refai M, Monteverde M, et al. Pleural tent after upper lobectomy: a randomized study of efficacy and duration of effect. *Ann Thorac Surg* 2002;74:1958–1962.
27. Okur E, Kir A, Halezeroglu S, et al. Pleural tenting following upper lobectomies or bilobectomies of the lung to prevent residual air space and prolonged air leak. *Eur J Cardiothorac Surg* 2001;20:1012–1015.
28. Robinson LA, Preksto D. Pleural tenting during upper lobectomy decreases chest tube time and total hospitalization days. *J Thorac Cardiovasc Surg* 1998;115:319–326; discussion 326–327.
29. Handy JR Jr, Judson MA, Zellner JL. Pneumoperitoneum to treat air leaks and spaces after a lung volume reduction operation. *Ann Thorac Surg* 1997;64:1803–1805.
30. De Giacomo T, Rendina EA, Venuta F, et al. Pneumoperitoneum for the management of pleural air space problems associated with major pulmonary resections. *Ann Thorac Surg* 2001;72: 1716–1719.
31. Cerfolio RJ, Holman WL, Katholi CR. Pneumoperitoneum after concomitant resection of the right middle and lower lobes (bilobectomy). *Ann Thorac Surg* 2000;70:942–946; discussion 946–947.
32. Fleisher AG, Evans KG, Nelems B, et al. Effect of routine fibrin glue use on the duration of air leaks after lobectomy. *Ann Thorac Surg* 1990;49:133–134.
33. Wong K, Goldstraw P. Effect of fibrin glue in the reduction of post-thoracotomy alveolar air leak. *Ann Thorac Surg* 1997;64:979–981.
34. Fabian T, Federico JA, Ponn RB. Fibrin glue in pulmonary resection: a prospective, randomized, blinded study. *Ann Thorac Surg* 2003;75:1587–1592.
35. Wain JC, Kaiser LR, Johnstone DW, et al. Trial of a novel synthetic sealant in preventing air leaks after lung resection. *Ann Thorac Surg* 2001;71:1623–1628; discussion 1628–1629.
36. Cerfolio RJ, Bass C, Katholi CR. Prospective randomized trial compares suction versus water seal for air leaks. *Ann Thorac Surg* 2001;71:1613–1617.
37. Deschamps C, Bernard A, Nichols FC III, et al. Empyema and bronchopleural fistula after pneumonectomy: factors affecting incidence. *Ann Thorac Surg* 2001;72:243–247; discussion 248.

38. Bonde P, McManus K, McAnespie M, et al. Lung surgery: identifying the subgroup at risk for sputum retention. *Eur J Cardiothorac Surg* 2002;22:18–22.
39. Yim AP, Ko KM, Chau WS, et al. Video-assisted thoracoscopic anatomic lung resections. The initial Hong Kong experience. *Chest* 1996;109:13–17.
40. Walker WS, Pugh GC, Craig SR, et al. Continued experience with thoracoscopic major pulmonary resection. *Int Surg* 1996;81: 255–258.
41. Kirby TJ, Mack MJ, Landreneau RJ, et al. Lobectomy—video-assisted thoracic surgery versus muscle-sparing thoracotomy. A randomized trial. *J Thorac Cardiovasc Surg* 1995;109(5):997–1001.
42. Vaporciyan AA, Merriman KW, Ece F, et al. Incidence of major pulmonary morbidity after pneumonectomy: association with timing of smoking cessation. *Ann Thorac Surg* 2002;73:420–425; discussion 425–426.
43. Bonde P, Papachristos I, McCraith A, et al. Sputum retention after lung operation: prospective, randomized trial shows superiority of prophylactic minitracheostomy in high-risk patients. *Ann Thorac Surg* 2002;74:196–202; discussion 202–203.
44. Au J, Walker WS, Inglis D, et al. Percutaneous cricothyroidostomy (minitracheostomy) for bronchial toilet: results of therapeutic and prophylactic use. *Ann Thorac Surg* 1989;48:850–852.
45. Natsugoe S, Tokuda K, Matsumoto M, et al. Molecular detection of free cancer cells in pleural lavage fluid from esophageal cancer patients. *Int J Mol Med* 2003;12:771–775.
46. Okumura M, Ohshima S, Kotake Y, et al. Intraoperative pleural lavage cytology in lung cancer patients. *Ann Thorac Surg* 1991;51:599–604.
47. Buhr J, Berghauser KH, Gonner S, et al. The prognostic significance of tumor cell detection in intraoperative pleural lavage and lung tissue cultures for patients with lung cancer. *J Thorac Cardiovasc Surg* 1997;113:683–690.
48. Downey RJ, McCormack P, LoCicero JIII, The Video-Assisted Thoracic Surgery Study Group. Dissemination of malignant tumors after video-assisted thoracic surgery: a report of twenty-one cases. *J Thorac Cardiovasc Surg* 1996;111:954–960.
49. Walsh GL, Nesbitt JC. Tumor implants after thoracoscopic resection of a metastatic sarcoma. *Ann Thorac Surg* 1995;59: 215–216.
50. Buhr J, Hurtgen M, Kelm C, et al. Tumor dissemination after thoracoscopic resection for lung cancer. *J Thorac Cardiovasc Surg* 1995;110:855–856.
51. Dixit AS, Martin CJ, Flynn P. Port-site recurrence after thoracoscopic resection of oesophageal cancer. *Aust N Z J Surg* 1997; 67:148–149.
52. Sartorelli KH, Partrick D, Meagher DP Jr. Port-site recurrence after thoracoscopic resection of pulmonary metastasis owing to osteogenic sarcoma. *J Pediatr Surg* 1996;31:1443–1444.
53. Ang KL, Tan C, Hsin M, et al. Intrapleural tumor dissemination after video-assisted thoracoscopic surgery metastasectomy. *Ann Thorac Surg* 2003;75:1643–1645.

Complications of
Vascular Surgery

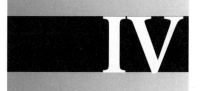

IV

Complications

of Arterial Surgery

28

Gilbert R. Upchurch, Jr.   *Jonathan L. Eliason*
James C. Stanley

■ INTRODUCTION 317

■ EXTRACRANIAL CAROTID ARTERIES 317
Early Complications 317
Late Complications 320

■ AORTA 321
Early Complications 322
Late Complications 324

■ LOWER EXTREMITY REVASCULARIZATION 329
Early Complications 330
Late Complications 331

■ REFERENCES 334

INTRODUCTION

Life-threatening and organ-threatening complications may accompany the most carefully performed arterial surgery. Although vascular surgery has undergone significant changes over the last 20 years, many of the complications that occur during open arterial surgery remain the same (1). Ultimately, successful operative outcome depends on avoiding complications, as well as recognizing and

Gilbert R. Upchurch, Jr., James C. Stanley: University of Michigan, Ann Arbor, MI 48109
Jonathan L. Eliason: Wilford Hall Medical Center, Lackland AFB, TX 78236

promptly managing complications when they occur. Individual discussions of specific complications affecting operations on the extracranial carotid arteries, the aorta, and the lower extremity arteries are highlighted in this chapter as these three regions of the vasculature account for most arterial reconstructions. A general working knowledge of the complications that occur in each of these vascular beds is essential to the contemporary practice of surgery.

EXTRACRANIAL CAROTID ARTERIES

Carotid endarterectomy (CEA) is the most commonly performed peripheral vascular operation in the United States (2). To achieve its primary goal, stroke prevention, CEA must be performed with a low complication rate. The incidence of stroke after CEA varies widely. Experienced surgeons report established morbidity and mortality standards to be between 3% and 7% (3,4). This variation in postoperative morbidity and mortality may be secondary to the presenting symptoms, ranging from asymptomatic to that of a frank stroke. Surgeon volume of carotid procedures may also influence variability (5). Specific complications and complication rates (Tables 28-1 and 28-2) deserve individual comment.

Early Complications

Myocardial Infarction

Cardiac complications remain the most common source of nonstroke-related mortality after CEA. In an important

TABLE 28-1

COMMON EARLY AND LATE COMPLICATIONS FOLLOWING CAROTID ENDARTERECTOMY

EARLY
Stroke
Myocardial infarction
Cranial nerve injury:
   Vagus nerve (recurrent laryngeal, superior laryngeal)
   Hypoglossal nerve
   Facial nerve (marginal mandibular branch)
Hemodynamic instability:
   Hypotension and bradycardia
   Hypertension
Neck hematoma
Acute internal carotid artery thrombosis

LATE
Recurrent carotid artery stenosis (neointimal hyperplasia 0 to 24
   months, recurrent atherosclerosis >24 months)
Pseudoaneurysm (patch infection, suture line failure, arterial wall
   disruption)

early study, DeBakey et al. (6) noted that the risk of perioperative myocardial infarction was three times higher in patients who had hypertension or symptomatic coronary artery disease than in those who did not. Myocardial infarction is also the most common cause of late deaths in patients who have undergone prior CEA. The 10-year survival after CEA when patients with coronary artery disease underwent coronary artery bypass grafting (CABG) prior to CEA was 55%, compared to 32% among those whose coronary artery disease remained uncorrected (7).

Given this increased risk of myocardial infarction following CEA, many authors have advocated combined CEA and CABG (8,9). Although single institutional experiences have reported acceptable results, current recommendations are that combined CEA/CABG be performed only in the setting of symptomatic internal carotid artery (ICA) disease. This subject is controversial and prospective evidence-based

data does not exist to establish rigid guidelines (10). A recent study by Brown et al. suggested that the stroke and death rate nationally following CEA/CABG may be higher than reported from isolated centers of excellence (11). In this study the combined CEA/CABG stroke and death rate was 17.7%. Perhaps somewhat surprisingly, the diagnosis of stroke was often delayed and most strokes were not limited to the same hemisphere as the CEA.

Cerebral Ischemia or Infarction

This complication may occur during endarterectomy as a result of internal carotid occlusion and inadequate collateral flow to the brain. The risk of cerebral ischemia is greater among patients with contralateral carotid occlusion or prior stroke affecting the ipsilateral hemisphere (12). A variety of techniques have been used to lessen cerebral ischemia during CEA. One approach is to place an indwelling carotid shunt in all patients. However, many surgeons find the operation more difficult when a shunt is in place and believe that added complications might be associated with its use, including intimal tears, embolization of proximal atherosclerotic debris, and air emboli. The most appropriate use of a shunt requires development of criteria to determine the adequacy of cerebral flow during carotid artery occlusion. Some surgeons perform CEA under local or regional anesthesia, and if carotid cross-clamping initiates neurologic dysfunction, then a shunt is placed (13,14). Use of selective shunting under regional anesthesia appears to offer a reasonable means of recognizing intraoperative cerebral ischemia during carotid clamping. In addition, it may reduce cardiovascular complications, such as perioperative blood pressure instability accompanying general anesthesia.

One of the original techniques used for assessing the adequacy of cerebral blood flow in anesthetized patients was measurement of the carotid artery "stump pressure" or "back pressure." Pressure measurements are made after the common and external carotid arteries are clamped. A 20-gauge needle, connected to a pressure transducer, is inserted into the carotid artery distal to the common carotid artery

TABLE 28-2

EARLY COMPLICATIONS FOLLOWING CAROTID ENDARTERECTOMY FROM CONTEMPORARY, LARGE, SINGLE INSTITUTIONAL SERIES

Primary Author	Year of Report	Study Period	Carotid Endarterectomies Performed	Mortality (%)	Stroke (%)	Cranial Nerve Injury (%)	Postoperative Bleeding (%)
Ballotta (101)	2004	1990–2002	1,150	3 (0.3)	11 (0.9)	48 (4.5)	Not stated
Conrad (102)	2003	1990–1999	1,045	9 (0.9)	32 (3.0)	26 (2.5)	18 (1.7)
Darling (103)	2003	1994–1999	3,429	20 (1.1)	30 (1.7)	10 (0.6)	40 (2.3)
Ecker (104)	2003	1988–2000	1,000	9 (0.9)	10 (1.0)	7 (0.7)	Not stated
Illig (105)	2003	1993–2000	1,168	(0.6)	(2.7)	(0.8)	(2.7)

clamp. A mean stump pressure below 25 mm Hg (15) or 50 mm Hg (16) has often been used as an indication for the placement of a shunt. However, neurologic deficits are known to occur in patients operated on under regional anesthesia with stump pressures above these levels (17).

Continuous electroencephalographic (EEG) monitoring during carotid artery occlusion has been proposed to provide a sensitive technique for monitoring the efficacy of cerebral blood flow. Approximately 15% of patients evaluated in this fashion will require shunting during CEA (18). Some patients with stump pressures above 75 mm Hg will develop EEG evidence of cerebral ischemia. For example, the EEG remained normal in of 39 of 1,009 patients subjected to endarterectomy under local anesthesia who showed obvious cerebral ischemia. In 52 other patients of this series, the EEG became abnormal but the clinical status did not suggest cerebral ischemia. Thus, although the EEG may provide a means of monitoring cerebral perfusion during CEA, it is not completely reliable.

A second cause of perioperative stroke is embolization of thrombus or atheromatous debris from within the diseased carotid artery. This complication may occur during dissection of the carotid artery, placement or release of a clamp, or from platelet aggregates accumulating at the endarterectomy site during the operation or in the immediate postoperative period. Carotid artery dissection should always be performed with minimal manipulation of the vessel using the so-called "no touch technique." Similarly, at the completion of the endarterectomy the vessel lumen should be carefully irrigated with heparinized saline and all pieces of loose intima or media removed. Perioperative use of aspirin or other antiplatelet grafts will reduce deposition of platelets on the surface of the endarterectomized vessel.

A third cause of stroke following CEA is acute thrombosis of the ICA. This complication almost always results from subintimal hemorrhage under a loose flap or inadequate proximal or distal endarterectomy end points. Completion duplex of the carotid artery has altered the traditional algorithm for treatment of acute ICA thrombosis, and it has been suggested that a normal completion duplex eliminates the need to return the patient immediately to the operating room (19). Intraoperative use of carotid duplex has recently gained favor over cerebral angiography. One could not be faulted for an aggressive approach and for re-exploring the closed artery if a significant abnormality is recognized by duplex ultrasonography.

A final cause of postendarterectomy stroke is intracerebral hemorrhage. This problem typically occurs on the second or third day after CEA, often during a period of severe hypertension (20). Neurologic deficits occurring on the second or third postoperative day should lead to duplex scanning or angiography to ensure the patency of the carotid artery. If a significant carotid artery defect is identified, the patient should be returned to the operating room and the vessel repaired. Computed tomography (CT) or magnetic resonance imaging (MRI) of the brain should be obtained if the carotid artery is normal. The presence of intracerebral hemorrhage carries a poor prognosis, and some have recommended craniotomy and evacuation of the hematoma in selected patients (13).

Cranial Nerve Injury

Cranial nerve injury is not an uncommon complication following CEA, accompanying as many as 39% of these procedures (21). Certain cranial nerve injuries are not detectable on casual examination, in that one-third of these injuries produce no clinical symptoms like hoarseness, difficulty in swallowing, or changes in speech (22,23). The most common injuries involve the recurrent laryngeal nerve with subsequent hoarseness and the hypoglossal nerve with resultant tongue deviation toward the side of the injury and difficulty in mastication. Recurrent laryngeal nerve injury is usually a manifestation of injury to the ipsilateral vagus nerve, most often by a retractor. Other injuries involve the superior laryngeal nerve with resultant fatigability of the voice and the marginal mandibular nerve with subsequent drooping of the lower lip. Less commonly injured nerves are the greater auricular nerve, which results in numbness over the lower earlobe, the spinal accessory nerve, and the glossopharyngeal nerve.

Many cranial nerve traction injuries resolve within 6 months. However, bilateral injuries may be severely disabling or even life-threatening. This is especially true in the case of bilateral recurrent laryngeal nerve injury. All patients who undergo CEA should be subjected to careful cranial nerve examination before and after operation. In addition, bilateral carotid endarterectomies should not be performed simultaneously but should be staged with an appropriate neurologic examination between operations.

Hemorrhage

Hemorrhage after CEA may in part reflect the fact that many patients receive antiplatelet agents such as aspirin preoperatively and anticoagulation with heparin intraoperatively. However, reoperation for evacuation of a hematoma or control of bleeding occurs in only 1% of experienced practices (24). Acute airway compromise may occur, and opening of the neck at the bedside on rare occasions may obviate the need for creation of an emergent surgical airway, allowing for an orderly return to the operating room.

Hypertension and Hypotension

Hypertension and hypotension associated with CEA have been attributed to a number of factors. Hypotension and bradycardia are thought to be secondary to increased baroreceptor activity during dissection of the carotid artery or stimulation of the sinus nerve following removal of a rigid atherosclerotic plaque. Hypertension may be caused by interruption of carotid sinus nerve activity due to its transection or changes in the arterial wall compliance. In an early study (25) severe hypertension complicated 19% of carotid endarterectomies and hypotension affected an additional 28% of cases. Such alterations in blood pressure were associated with a 9% incidence of postoperative neurologic deficits, in contrast to no neurologic complications among normotensive patients.

Postoperative hypertension is much more common in chronically hypertensive patients. Patients who have undergone bilateral CEA are particularly prone to develop hypertension, and, in addition, they appear to lose their normal compensatory respiratory and circulatory responses to hypoxia (26). Because of the potential severity of these complications, hypertension should be controlled and volume deficits corrected in all patients prior to elective CEA (25).

Late Complications

Recurrent Carotid Stenosis

Symptomatic recurrence of carotid stenosis occurs in <3% of patients, whereas careful follow-up using noninvasive tests has documented the asymptomatic recurrence rate to be between 9% and 12% (27). Two forms of recurrent carotid disease have been identified (28). One type occurs within the first 2 years as neointimal hyperplasia and is characterized by proliferation of mesenchymal cells, perhaps of smooth-muscle origin (Fig. 28-1). The second type usually develops after 2 years and represents recurrent atherosclerosis. The mechanisms by which these two forms of recurrent carotid stenosis evolve are unknown, but there is evidence that they represent a continuum and are a consequence of vascular wall injury (29). In this regard, extensive platelet aggregation within the endarterectomized vessel may be associated with release of platelet-derived growth factor that acts as a stimulus to cellular proliferation. Aspirin and other antiplatelet agents may

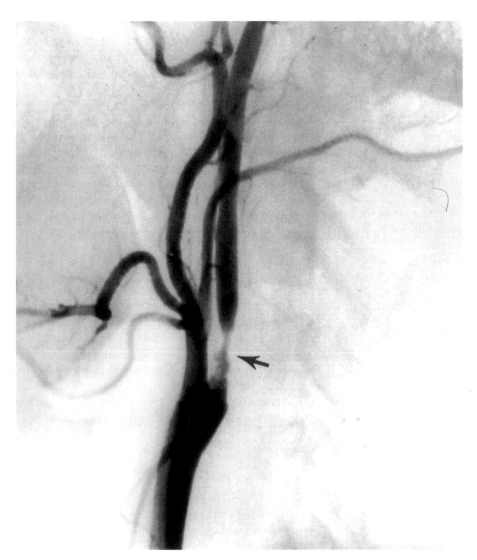

Figure 28-1 Recurrent carotid stenosis secondary to neointimal hyperplasia following carotid endarterectomy.

prevent platelet aggregation with adherence to the vessel wall, and heparin may inhibit arterial smooth-muscle proliferation after endothelial cell injury. Unfortunately, there is little clinical evidence that antiplatelet drugs prevent recurrent carotid stenosis (27). Other factors have been identified with hypercellular responses after endarterectomy, including hypercholesterolemia and female gender (30). The incidence of recurrent carotid stenosis is three times higher in women than it is in men. Recurrent carotid stenosis also occurs more often in patients with diffuse vascular disease and has been most striking in those with a history of heavy cigarette smoking (27).

High-grade stenoses or symptomatic recurrent carotid artery stenoses should be assessed by arteriography and treated. Operations for recurrent carotid artery stenosis can be demanding, especially those that occur within the first 2 years. In these cases there is usually extensive scarring around the artery, making the dissection difficult. Special attention should be paid to the identification and preservation of the cranial nerves. Patch-graft angioplasty is recommended in closing the carotid arteriotomy in these instances. Replacement of the affected carotid artery with an expanded polytetrafluoroethylene (ePTFE) or saphenous vein graft has also been described (31). Carotid stenting (discussed elsewhere in this book) as a means to lessen the risks of those reoperations has gained favor in the treatment of recurrent carotid artery disease.

False Aneurysm

False aneurysm formation after CEA is an especially rare complication, occurring in <0.05% of cases (32). Causes of aneurysm formation include suture line failure, arterial wall degeneration, and infection, especially of a patch used in the arteriotomy closure (Fig. 28-2). Management of carotid artery false aneurysms usually entails arterial closure with a saphenous vein patch or carotid artery replacement with an interposition vein graft.

TABLE 28-3

COMMON EARLY AND LATE COMPLICATIONS FOLLOWING INFRARENAL ABDOMINAL AORTIC ANEURYSM REPAIR

EARLY
Myocardial infarction
Hemorrhage
Respiratory failure
Renal failure
Embolization
Mesenteric ischemia
Spinal cord ischemia
Ureteral injuries
Chylous ascites

LATE
Graft infection (aortoduodenal fistula, anastomotic pseudo-aneurysm)
Graft thrombosis
Structural graft failure
Aneurysm proximal/distal to repair
Abdominal wall hernia
Impotence/retrograde ejaculation

AORTA

Aortic reconstruction is one of the most common vascular surgery procedures with significant variation in mortality and morbidity based on both patient and provider variables (33,34). Both the aging of society and the introduction of endovascular aortic aneurysm repair has affected the number of aortic procedures. The importance of comorbid diseases on mortality associated with elective and emergent abdominal aortic aneurysm repair has been well documented in two large population-based studies (35,36). Specific complications and complication rates (Table 28-3 and 28-4) are discussed individually.

TABLE 28-4

EARLY COMPLICATIONS FOLLOWING INTACT ABDOMINAL AORTIC ANEURYSM REPAIR FROM CONTEMPORARY SERIES

Primary Author	Year of Report	Study Period	Patients Undergoing Elective Open AAA Repair (n)	Mortality (%)	Myocardial Infarction (%)	Acute Renal Failure (%)	Respiratory Failure (%)	Ischemic Colitis (%)
Bertges (44)	2000	1994–1999	314	6 (1.9)	7 (2.9)	11 (4.5)	23 (7.3)	4 (1.6)
Elkouri (106)	2004	1999–2001	261	3 (1.2)	14 (5.4)	11 (4.2)	20 (7.7)	Not stated
Hertzer (39)	2002	1989–1998	1,135	14 (1.2)	16 (1)	19 (1.7)	48 (4)	11 (1)
Menard (107)	2003	1990–2000	572	6 (1.0)	7 (1.2)	13 (2.3)	30 (5.2)[a]	1 (0.2)

[a]Number reflects clinically significant pneumonia only, not additional sources of respiratory failure.

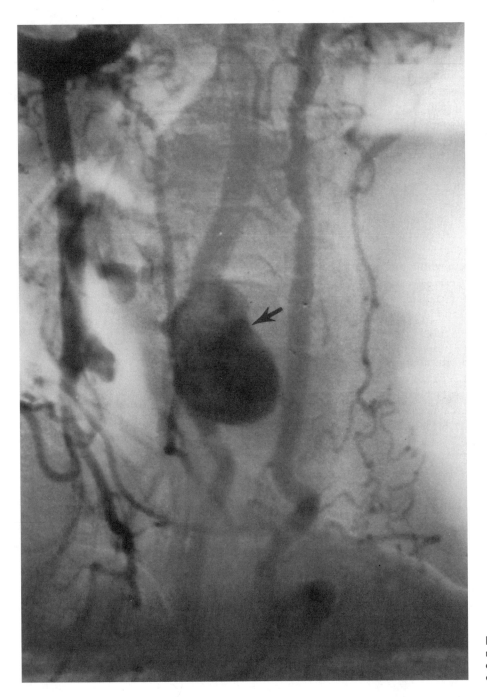

Figure 28-2 False aneurysm of right carotid artery following carotid endarterectomy with patch graft closure.

Early Complications

Myocardial Ischemia and Infarction

Cardiac complications are the most relevant causes of perioperative mortality and late postoperative death following aortic surgery (37). In one report fatal myocardial infarction accounted for 37% of early postoperative deaths among 343 consecutive patients with abdominal aortic aneurysms (38). In this regard, severe coronary artery disease was present in 36% of 1,000 patients with abdominal aortic aneurysms subjected to mandatory coronary arteriography before routine aortic surgery.

Recent results suggest that the rate of this dreaded complication has markedly decreased, with only 1% of 1,135 patients sustaining a perioperative myocardial infarction following abdominal aortic aneurysm repair (39).

Aggressive preoperative cardiac management of patients who are to undergo aortic operations includes selective exercise or chemical stress thallium testing, as well as coronary arteriography (40) and preoperative coronary artery angioplasty or bypass. Eagle et al. and Froehlich et al. have established the criteria for pursuing extensive cardiac studies (41,42). The combined performance of CABG and abdominal aortic aneurysm repair has been reported (43) but can be advocated only in patients with both symptomatic coronary and aneurysmal disease. Modern intraoperative and postoperative care (44) includes hemodynamic monitoring with Swan-Ganz pulmonary artery catheters and transesophageal echocardiography. Such a program has been reported to result in less than a 2% perioperative mortality rate and, more important, a 75% 5-year survival rate with only a 5% late cardiac mortality (45). These data contrast with a 25% to 35% cardiac mortality at 5 years following major aortic surgery in older series.

Hemorrhage

Hemorrhage contributes to early morbidity and mortality following elective aortic surgery (46). Certain factors may be associated with excessive operative blood loss during aortic surgery. Venous anomalies such as duplication of the inferior vena cava, circumferential renal vein, left-sided inferior vena cava, and retroaortic left renal vein, which occur in approximately 5% of cases, may be easily injured and lead to considerable hemorrhage. Absence of an anterior left renal vein is indicative of a retroaortic left renal vein, which may be torn during posterior dissection of the proximal infrarenal aorta. The small lumbar vein originating from the midportion of the posterior left renal vein is particularly disposed to injury. Careful ligation of all vessels transected during the aortic dissection not only reduces operative blood loss but also lessens the incidence of troublesome postoperative hemorrhage. Similarly, careful temperature control and blood component replacement therapy will lessen the incidence of coagulopathies associated with excessive blood loss and administration of large quantities of banked blood. The benefits of using autotransfusion devices during aortic surgery repair has been supported by some (47) but contested by others (48).

Accurate blood and fluid replacement is important in preventing operative hypotension associated with unclamping of the aorta (37). Vasodilators used to decrease peripheral resistance and afterload during aortic cross-clamping should be discontinued prior to declamping so that further decreases in peripheral resistance with declamping will not result in hypotension. Reperfusion of ischemic extremities releases substances into the systemic circulation that have an adverse effect on blood pressure, including lactic acid, potassium, cytokines, and other vasoactive metabolic products (49). An expeditious operation, slow aortic declamping, and good communication with the anesthesiologist should lessen hazardous reperfusion events.

Renal Insufficiency

Renal insufficiency accompanying aortic surgery is more likely to occur with hemorrhage, shock, and inadequate blood replacement (50). Acute renal failure is associated with >30% mortality in the setting of an elective aneursymectomy (35). Renal failure affects >70% of patients with ruptured abdominal aortic aneurysms. In this setting acute renal failure is associated with a 53% mortality rate, being directly related to total aortic clamp time, the time delay from rupture to aneurysm resection, and blood loss (51). Renal atheroembolism with aortic clamping is another recognized cause of renal failure accompanying aortic surgery. Renal failure is also a relatively common complication following resection of thoracoabdominal aneurysms (52). Postoperative dialysis is required in 5% of these patients having normal preoperative renal function and in 17% of those with preoperative serum creatinine levels >2 mg per dL (53). Intraoperative renal artery perfusion with cold balanced salt solutions may have a protective effect in those with impaired preoperative renal function.

Embolization

Lower extremity embolization, often from dislodgement of mural debris during operative dissection, is a serious complication of aortic surgery. Embolization may also occur from accumulated thrombus in the static column of blood above the aortic clamp. Although larger emboli can often be retrieved with a balloon catheter, smaller artheroembolic particles cannot be removed and will lead to microvascular occlusions, producing cutaneous ischemia, including so-called trash foot, if the digital arteries are affected (54). The frequency of such complications ranges from 2% to 5%.

Technical maneuvers to lessen the complication of embolization during aortic surgery include careful dissection of iliac vessels prior to clamp application, distal iliac clamp application prior to proximal aortic clamp application, effective systemic heparin anticoagulation, thorough aspiration of the lumen of the aortic prosthesis prior to implantation to remove any adherent debris, prevention of blood accumulation in the graft while the anastomoses are being performed, and vigorous flushing of the proximal and distal vessels prior to reestablishment of extremity arterial blood flow. Patients with arteroembolism experience extreme pain in the foot and toes associated with the inflammatory response to cholesterol emboli. Epidural anesthesia may help to blunt the sympathetic response associated with this type of ischemic pain.

Colon Ischemia

Colon ischemia has been reported to accompany 0.2% to 10% of abdominal aortic aneurysm resections (55,56). Intestinal ischemia is less common following aortofemoral bypass or aortoiliac endarterectomy for occlusive disease. A prospective study (57) using routine colonoscopy documented colon ischemia in 4.3% of elective aortic procedures for occlusive disease, 7.4% for aneurysmal disease, and 60% when treating ruptured abdominal aortic aneurysms. Overall mortality for colon ischemia in this setting is approximately 50% and approaches 90% with transmural infarction. Colonic ischemia is more likely to accompany aortic resection with improper inferior mesenteric artery ligation, ruptured aneurysms with arterial and venous compression by hematoma within the mesocolon, operative trauma to vessels within the mesocolon, hypotension with diminished perfusion of colon blood vessels, inadequate collaterals to the inferior mesenteric arterial circulation, and damage to collateral vessels when they do exist. Presence of a large meandering mesenteric artery carrying blood from the left colic branch of the inferior mesenteric to the left branch of the middle colic artery just beyond its origin from the superior mesenteric artery indicates superior mesenteric artery occlusive disease. In such cases reconstruction of the superior mesenteric artery or inferior mesenteric artery reimplantation into the vascular graft may be necessary to avoid colon ischemia. Inferior mesenteric artery back pressure <40 mm Hg in patients undergoing abdominal aortic aneurysm resection also suggests a need to restore antegrade flow in this vessel (58). Some have advocated routine reimplantation of the inferior mesenteric artery into the aortic graft, but it does not ensure prevention of significant mesenteric ischemia (59). Intraoperative Doppler confirmation of blood flow at both the mesenteric and antimesenteric borders of the sigmoid colon is a useful means of confirming the adequacy of collateral blood flow to the colon during aortic reconstructive surgery.

Patients with severe colon ischemia often present 1 to 2 days postoperatively with liquid brown or bloody diarrhea, left-sided abdominal pain, abdominal distension, acidosis, oliguria, and fever. Less severe ischemia may not become apparent until 5 to 7 days after surgery. Any patient who undergoes aortic surgery and develops these signs and symptoms requires urgent colonoscopy. If transmural infarction is suspected, laparotomy and resection of the affected colon should be undertaken with creation of a proximal colostomy and a Hartmann pouch or mucous fistula distally. Mucosal ischemia, if not severe, may be managed by hydration, hemodynamic stabilization, and intravenous administration of antibiotics. Mucosal ischemia may resolve within 7 to 10 days. If deeper structures are affected and perforation does not occur, stricture formation may occur in 6 to 10 weeks. In one study of 472 cases of abdominal aortic aneurysm resection, 33% of the elective mortality was associated with acute gastrointestinal complications, of which ischemic colitis was the most common (55).

Spinal Cord Ischemia

Spinal cord ischemia accompanies 0.2% of elective abdominal aortic aneurysm resections and 2% of emergent resections for ruptured aneurysms. Spinal cord ischemia is not predictable from preoperative arteriograms (60). Among 51 reported cases of postoperative spinal cord ischemia following abdominal aortic surgery, 45% occurred with ruptured aneurysms, 33% with elective aneurysmectomy, and 20% with treatment for aortoiliac occlusive disease (61). Spinal cord ischemia is more common with resection of thoracoabdominal aneurysms, occurring in approximately 10% of these procedures, and >40% of patients with aneurysms caused by dissections (53). The primary cause of spinal ischemia has been attributed to interruption of the cord's blood supply. Clamping of the suprarenal aorta and concomitant hypotension appear to contribute to this complication. The former relates to the aortic origin of the spinal artery of Adamkiewicz, which has been found as high as T8 and as low as L4. Impaired hypogastric artery perfusion, embolization, and postoperative hypotension may also cause lower spinal cord ischemia during abdominal aortic surgery (62).

No universal intervention has been found to protect against spinal cord ischemia. Recent research has centered on the gradient between spinal fluid pressure and systemic arterial blood pressure below the aortic cross-clamp. In order to maintain at least a 10-mm gradient, withdrawal of spinal fluid to decrease intraspinal canal pressure has been advocated (63). Spinal cord monitoring using somatosensory evoked potentials, as well as various drug interventions, has also been proposed to lessen the risk of this complication (64,65).

Ureteral Injuries

Ureteral injuries may occur during dissection and repair of large aortic or iliac aneurysms, especially with treatment of inflammatory lesions (66) (Fig. 28-3). Most ureteric injuries are associated with devascularization due to excessive or injudicious skeletonization of the ureter. Inadvertent inclusion of a portion of the ureteral wall in a suture is an infrequent cause of ureteral injury. Aortofemoral graft limbs should be tunneled posterior to the ureters so as to prevent compression of the ureters.

Late Complications
Prosthetic Aortic Graft Infection

This complication affects between 1% and 6% of implanted aortic grafts, with an average incidence of 0.7% for aortoiliac grafts and 1.6% for aortofemoral grafts (67). Mortality from infected grafts in the aortoiliac or aortofemoral positions is over 50%. In a series of 92 patients with 84 infected aortoiliac or aortofemoral grafts, >70% had salutory outcomes, with follow-up ranging from 10 months to 12 years (68). However, 25% of the patients required amputation, most at a level above the knee. Thus, amputation morbidity remains high, even with relatively successful management of the vascular graft infection.

Factors contributing to graft infection include intraoperative contact of the graft with skin, contaminated lymph,

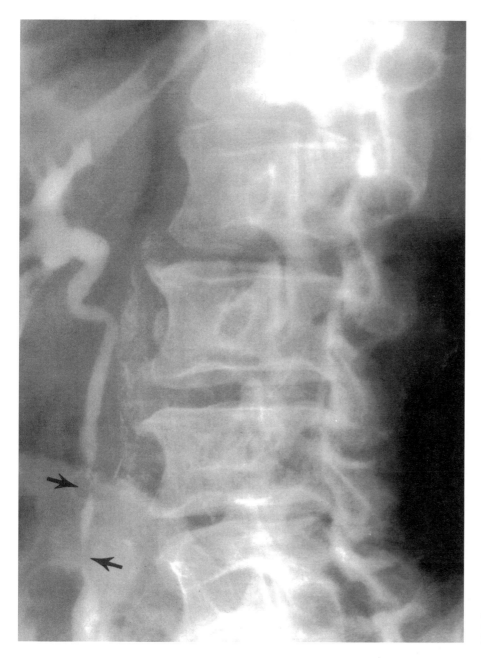

Figure 28-3 Ureteral injury due to excessive dissection and devascularization during aortic reconstruction leading to an ischemic stenosis.

intraoperative breaks in sterile technique, extension from wound sepsis or contamination, arterial wall infection, and transient bacteremias. Bacteria have been found in aneurysm contents, with up to 43% of arterial walls cultured during routine vascular procedures harboring bacteria, the most common organism being *Staphylococcus epidermidis* (69). A significant increase in graft infection occurs in patients with positive arterial wall cultures undergoing secondary operations. The bacteriology of graft sepsis has changed. In 1977, *Staphylococcus aureus* was the leading pathogen (70), with a recent shift to *S. epidermidis* as the most likely cause of infection. *S. epidermidis* organisms are sometimes difficult to culture from infected grafts. Segments of grafts should be

cultured not only on plates, but also in broth following sonication (71).

A number of tests may be performed if a diagnosis of graft infection is suspected, including indium labeled white blood cell imaging, MRI, and CT (Fig. 28-4). Direct operative inspection of the graft suspected to be infected is usually required to establish the presence or absence of infection when other studies are equivocal. Failure of graft incorporation, accumulation of perigraft fluid or debris, and a Gram stain providing evidence of bacteria or leukocytes all support the existence of a graft infection.

The traditional means of treating an infected graft is its removal first, followed by secondary revascularization. In

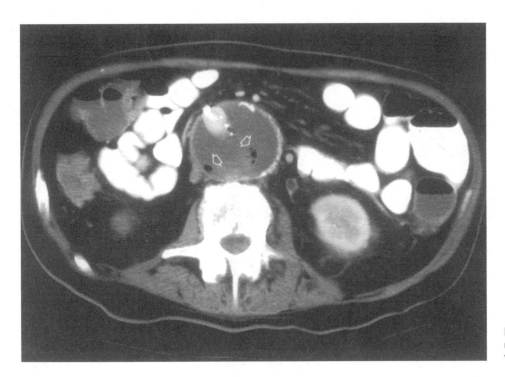

Figure 28-4 Infected graft in a redundant aortic aneurysm sac with visible gas bubbles.

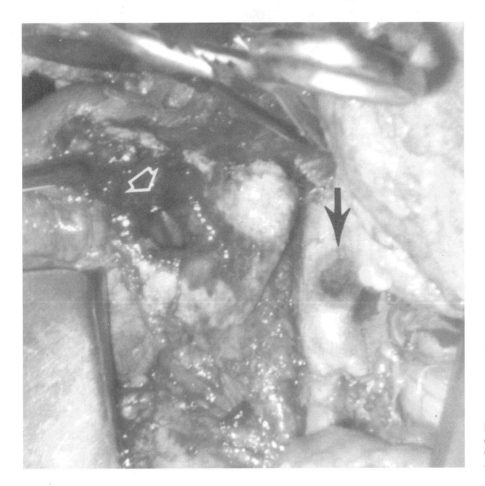

Figure 28-5 Bile staining (*solid arrow*) of an infected aortic graft as consequence of a duodenal erosion (*open arrow*).

most series this method has been supplanted by revascularization first, either during the same operation as the graft removal or 2 to 5 days before graft removal (72). Significant differences in mortality or new graft infections do not occur using this latter technique; however, there is a significantly lower rate of extremity amputation. The use of the superficial femoral vein to replace the infected graft has recently been advocated (73). Others have suggested use of antibiotic-soaked grafts or cryopreserved grafts (74,75).

Aortoenteric graft intestinal erosion is a distinct subcategory of graft infection (Fig. 28-5). This complication often follows a lack of retroperitoneal tissue coverage of the implanted graft during the primary aortic reconstruction. Graft sepsis and intestinal bleeding are usually the first manifestations of this complication. Spread of graft infection to involve the entire conduit occurs in many cases (Fig. 28-6). In general, the entire prosthetic graft in this setting must be excised.

In the case of an isolated aortobifemoral graft limb infection, after demonstration of good incorporation of the proximal graft limb at the graft bifurcation, the limb only may be removed, leaving the remainder of the graft in place. In this setting the proximal limb may be divided, soft tissue interposed between the limb and the main body of the graft, and the distal limb removed from the groin after closure of the abdominal incision. If the body of an aortic graft requires removal, the aortic stump must be securely closed with a double layer of monofilament cardiovascular suture and covered with omentum or presacral fascia.

Structural Graft Failure

Serious structural graft failure is rare. Most large prostheses placed in the aortoiliofemoral area function well, exhibiting 85% to 95% long-term patencies. However, fabric prostheses may exhibit friability, inability to hold sutures, rents in the wall, aneurysm formation, and both early and late dilation (76). Defective grafts have been described for all types of prosthetic material, including expanded Teflon and Dacron of knitted, woven, and velour construction. Structural failures in grafts usually reflect mechanical failures in their construction. Fabricated Dacron grafts, because of their design, have been noted to increase in

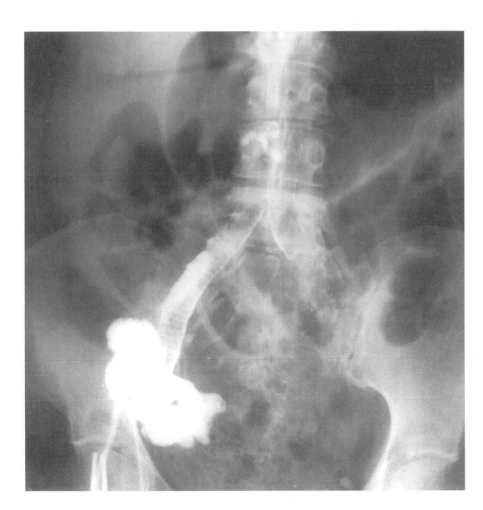

Figure 28-6 Infected aortic graft limb with opaque contrast injected through an open sinus tract in the groin. Primary infection was an aortoduodenal erosion.

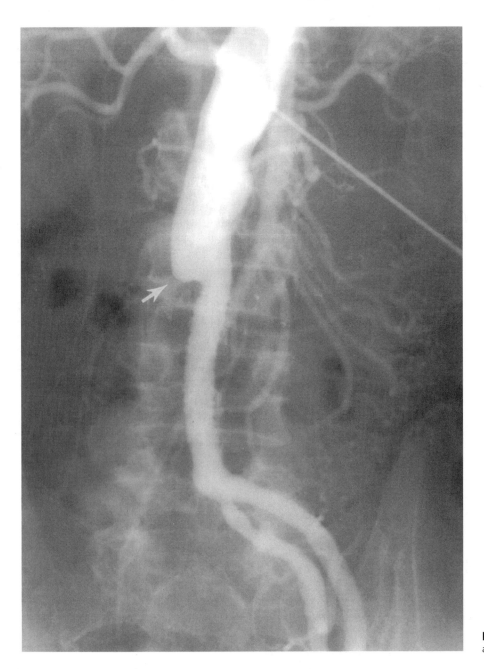

Figure 28-7   Late limb occlusion of an aortoiliac bypass graft.

diameter approximately 15% to 20% following insertion. Graft dilation such as this must be taken into consideration when choosing the proper prosthetic graft size for implantation.

Graft Thromboses

Early aortoiliofemoral graft thromboses are usually technical in nature, including intimal flaps, anastomotic narrowing, graft twisting or kinking, compression of the graft limb by the inguinal ligament, unrecognized inflow disease, inadequate runoff because of unappreciated distal disease, and undiagnosed hypercoagulability (77). Late graft thromboses are usually secondary to progressive downstream atherosclerosis or anastomotic intimal fibrodysplasia (Figs. 28-7 and 28-8).

The most important factor contributing to long-term aortoiliofemoral graft occlusion is inadequate outflow. In the case of an aortofemoral bypass for occlusive disease, as opposed to aneurysm disease, this relates to patency of the deep femoral artery. Progressive atherosclerosis of the superficial femoral or infrapopliteal arteries may contribute to graft thrombosis, especially in patients who continue to smoke (77). Impaired inflow is a much less common cause of late graft thrombosis (78), and when it

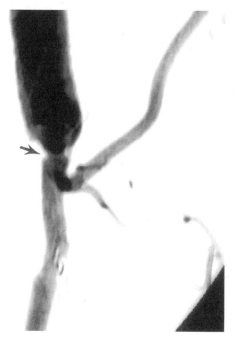

Figure 28-8 Intimal hyperplasia resulting in an anastomotic stenosis of an aortobifemoral bypass graft (*arrow*).

does occur it is most often associated with low placement of grafts originating on the terminal aorta. Less frequent causes of late graft thromboses include kinking or excessive angulation of graft limbs, accumulation of mural thrombus, and pseudoaneurysm formation.

A comprehensive study (79) reported 1,748 aortic reconstructions in 1,647 patients with aortoiliac occlusive disease. This series included 1,186 aortofemoral bypasses, 76 aortoiliac bypasses, 176 combined aortoiliac and aortofemoral bypasses, 181 cases of aortoiliac endarterectomy, and 129 remote bypasses. Early perioperative or postoperative graft occlusion decreased from 8.3% from 1954 to 1963 to 3.2% from 1974 to 1983. Late anastomotic thromboses affected 13.1% of aortofemoral bypasses, 10.5% of aortoiliac bypasses, 10.8% of bypasses combining aortoiliac and aortofemoral limbs, and 13.8% of aortoiliac endarterectomies. Anastomotic stenoses, defined as a reduction in lumen size to the degree of threatened thrombosis, occurred in 4.5% of aortofemoral bypasses, 3.9% of aortoiliac bypasses, and 2.2% of aortoiliac endarterectomies. Secondary repair of complications affecting aortofemoral bypass procedures resulted in 77% 5 year patency, 77% 10-year patency, 73% 15-year patency, and 68% 20-year patency.

Anastomotic Aneurysms

Anastomotic aneurysms affect up to 6% of all aortoiliofemoral grafts (Fig. 28-9). In a large experience with 4,214 vascular reconstructions between 1957 and 1974,

there was a 1.7% incidence of anastomotic aneurysms, occurring with a 3% incidence in the femoral region, 1.2% in the iliac region, and 0.2% in the aortic region (80). The most common cause of false aneurysm formation was structural deficiency of the host vessel, followed by hypertension, mechanical stress, graft or suture defects, and infection. Elective repair of anastomotic aneurysms is successful in >80% of cases, whereas emergency repair is successful in 60% of cases. Late recurrences range from 11% to 14%.

Femoral false aneurysms are usually obvious on physical examination. If rupture occurs it can usually be compressed prior to emergency operative intervention. However, aortic false aneurysms may remain silent until they become very large and rupture with life-threatening hemorrhage. Overall mortality for treating anastomotic aneurysms in the femoral region is 3.5%, with an amputation rate of 2.8% (21). Repair of false aortic aneurysms carries a greater risk and usually involves insertion of a new segment of graft after debridement or excision of the involved native vessel. Endovascular graft placement in this setting may prove less hazardous (81).

Impotence

Iatrogenic impotence has been reported to range from 21% to 88% in men undergoing conventional aortic reconstruction. In a unique experience employing a nerve-sparing approach with minimal aortic dissection and reperfusion of at least one hypogastric vessel, impotence was eliminated and retrograde ejaculation was reduced from 43% to 3% (82). Inasmuch as 70% to 80% of patients with aortoiliofemoral arterial occlusive disease may already be impotent, it is important to document the presence or absence of impotence prior to surgery (83).

Vasculogenic impotence involves an inability to sustain an erection (84). Neurogenic impotence refers to the inability to achieve any erection at all. A penile systolic-brachial index below 0.6 supports the presence of vasculogenic impotence. When vasculogenic impotence exists, consideration should be given to restoring internal iliac artery blood flow or occasionally performing a more direct revascularization of the penis. In the presence of neurogenic impotence, a penile implant is acceptable treatment. Most patients developing vasculogenic impotence from aortic surgery will not benefit from further revascularization unless clear evidence of impaired pelvic perfusion exists. The use of newer drugs for erectile dysfunction benefits many of these patients.

LOWER EXTREMITY REVASCULARIZATION

All patients who undergo lower extremity revascularization should be subjected to rigorous postoperative follow-up

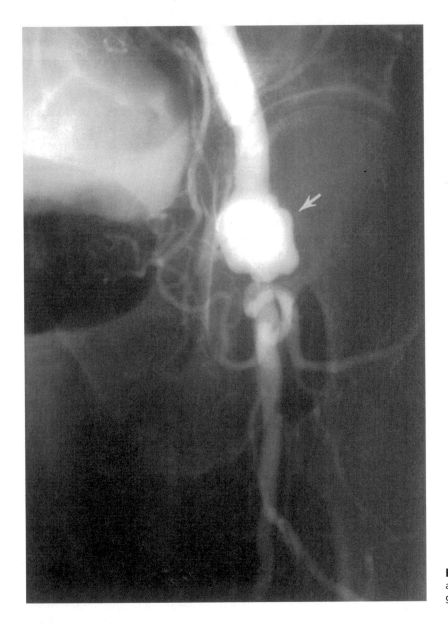

Figure 28-9 Femoral artery anastomotic aneurysm affecting an aortobifemoral bypass graft limb.

TABLE 28-5

COMMON EARLY AND LATE COMPLICATIONS FOLLOWING LOWER EXTREMITY BYPASS

EARLY
Myocardial infarction
Hemorrhage
Bypass graft thrombosis
Lower extremity swelling (lymphocele, venous insufficiency)

LATE
Graft thrombosis (neointimal hyperplasia 1 to 24 months, recurrent atherosclerosis >24 months)
Graft infection
Retained arteriovenous fistula

---

(85), as surveillance is considered mandatory to detect impending graft failure, which may occur in many patients. Specific complications and complication rates deserve note (Tables 28-5 and 28-6).

Early Complications

Myocardial Ischemia and Infarction

The major cause of early and late death after lower extremity revascularization is myocardial infarction (86). Operative mortality rates between 3% and 5% accompany these procedures and are almost entirely due to perioperative cardiac events. Patients treated for tibial or peroneal occlusive disease have a particularly high incidence of

TABLE 28-6

COMPLICATION RATES FOLLOWING LOWER EXTREMITY BYPASS FROM CONTEMPORARY, LARGE, SINGLE INSTITUTIONAL SERIES

Primary Author	Year of Report	Study Period	Extremity Bypass Procedures	Mortality (%)	Myocardial Infarction (%)	Stroke (%)	Perioperative Graft Failure (%)	Postoperative Bleeding (%)
Chew (108)	2001	1983–1999	165[a]	3 (1.8)	(9)[b]	Not stated	18 (11)	(5.4)
Goshima (109)	2004	1990–2002	318	3 (1.3)	9 (3.9)	3 (1.3)	8 (3.5)	3 (1.3)
Pomposelli (110)	2003	1990–2000	1032[c]	10 (1.0)	31 (3)[b]	3 (0.3)	43 (4.2)	Not stated
Raffetto (111)	2002	Not stated	352	(1.1)	9 (2.6)	1 (0.3)	24 (6.8)	3 (0.8)
Roddy (93)	2003	1968–1999	5880	183 (3.1)	(2.9)[b]	Not stated	108 (1.8)[d]	126 (2.1)

[a]Surgical technique using composite vein grafts only.
[b]Percentage also reflects patients with other severe cardiac morbidity such as congestive heart failure and arrhythmia.
[c]Surgical technique using only the dorsalis pedis artery as the target vessel.
[d]Perioperative graft failure defined as immediate limb loss.

underlying coronary artery disease that contributes to myocardial complications.

Hemorrhage

Hemorrhage occurs after lower extremity revascularization in 1% to 3% of cases (87). Serious hemorrhage is usually secondary to anastomotic bleeding or unligated branches of implanted vein grafts. Less often, bleeding is due to coagulation defects, often related to excessive administration of heparin, and use of dextran, or antiplatelet agents such as aspirin and Plavix.

Bypass Graft Thrombosis

Acute bypass graft thrombosis occurring within 24 hours of surgery affects approximately 5% of lower extremity revascularizations. The most common causes of early graft thromboses are technical, including injury to vein grafts during harvest, intimal flaps from an incomplete endarterectomy or a clamp injury, improper graft tunneling causing twisted or kinked conduits, and grafts placed under excessive tension. Early graft failure is twice as high in bypass grafts placed for limb salvage compared to those used in treating claudication (88). Poor arterial inflow and outflow have also been associated with early graft thromboses, as are infrapopliteal bypasses compared to above-the-knee bypass grafts. Hypovolemia or diminished cardiac output can also contribute to graft thrombosis. A hypercoagulable state may affect approximately 5% of patients undergoing infrainguinal bypass (89), and unexplained acute graft thromboses deserve an evaluation for such. The use of statins may lessen these graft failures (90,91).

Most complications affecting lower extremity revascularizations are correctable if recognized early. In this regard, an objective assessment of the reconstruction in the operating room is critical. Completion angiography has been replaced by intraoperative duplex examination as the most common means of assessing the adequacy of graft placement (92), with standard criteria predictive of early bypass graft failure (93). Immediate postoperative ankle-brachial indices (ABIs) should also be performed to establish a baseline against which to compare future ABIs.

Lymphoceles and Lymph Drainage

These complications occur most commonly following groin dissection and usually result from lymphatic channel interruption or a transected lymph node. Lymphatic drainage through a surgical incision is usually treated initially with strict bed rest and leg elevation. Frequent applications of sterile dressings or povidine-iodine soaked gauze to the wound lessen the incidence of wound infection. Patients with small-volume intermittent drainage may be safely managed nonoperatively for short periods by this means, especially in the setting of an autogenous vein graft. The need for operative intervention depends on the leak's magnitude, as well as the type of vascular graft. Large quantities of lymph drainage or the presence of a prosthetic graft that would be at risk for infection necessitate prompt surgical exploration, with identification and ligature control of the leaking lymphatic.

Late Complications

Late Graft Occlusion

This complication of lower extremity revascularization appears as a result of two distinct pathological entities (94). Those occurring within 12 to 24 months after graft insertion

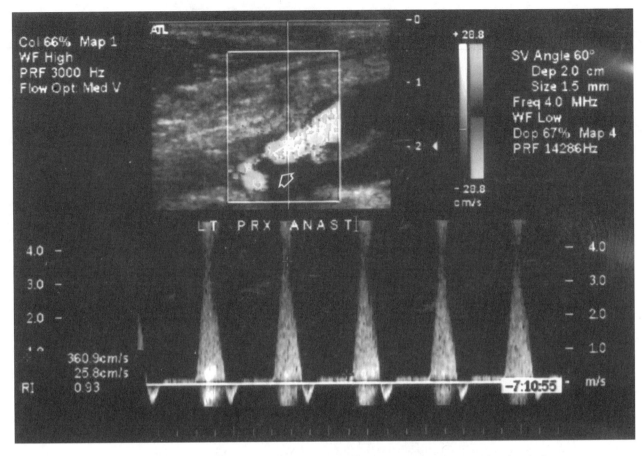

Figure 28-10   Femoral popliteal bypass stenosis due to intimal hyperplasia evident by duplex scan on direct image (*arrow*) and elevated blood flow velocities.

are most often due to neointimal hyperplasia and are usually found at the site of the distal anastomosis (Figs. 28-10 and 28-11). Graft occlusions that occur beyond 24 months are most often due to progression of atherosclerosis (95). In one study, 87% of graft occlusions secondary to progression of atherosclerosis occurred beyond the first year of implantation (96).

Graft Infection

Graft infection is a serious complication of lower extremity revascularization. Mortality after lower extremity graft infection averages 9% (97), and >50% of patients with this complication require amputation. The incidence of graft infection is three times higher when using synthetic grafts compared to saphenous vein grafts. The overall incidence of infection in expanded polytetrafluoroethylene (PTFE) or Dacron grafts is approximately 3% (97). If only one anastomosis is involved, local treatment with antibiotics, wound debridement, and muscle coverage have been attempted in selected cases. However, in most cases total graft excision and revascularization by an alternate route is required.

Lower Extremity Edema

Edema is a common and troublesome complication affecting as many as two-thirds of patients after lower extremity revascularization (98,99). Three mechanisms contribute to development of edema. First, loss of arteriolar smooth muscle function due to chronic ischemia can lead to uncontrolled hyperemia and increased pressures within the microcirculation, especially when the leg is dependent. Second, interruption of lymphatic drainage occurs during the vascular dissection. Third, harvesting of the ipsilateral greater saphenous vein as the conduit for a bypass may cause some patients to have worsened venous insufficiency. Postoperative edema, although often very obvious, is usually self-limited and resolves in 3 to 4 months. Compression therapy in the form of support stockings or elastic wraps may alleviate symptoms in these patients.

Complications of *in situ* Saphenous Vein Bypass Reconstructions

These complications include persistence of large arteriovenous fistulas (Fig. 28-12), obstruction by residual

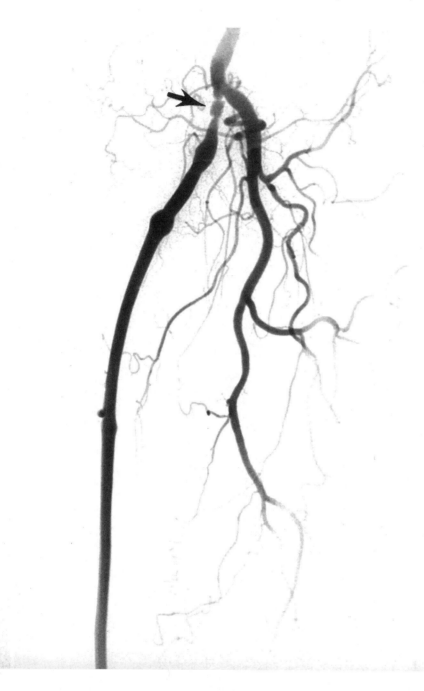

Figure 28-11 Femoral artery to popliteal artery vein bypass stenosis (*arrow*).

valve leaflets, vasospasm, and luminal platelet aggregation (100). Although small arteriovenous fistulas are usually of little consequence, large fistulas communicating with the deep system require interruption. These fistulas may be identified by intraoperative Doppler examination or intraoperative arteriography. Their late persistence often causes areas of cutaneous erythema and painful induration. Residual competent valve leaflets are another cause of early graft thrombosis when retrograde passing of a valvulotome or valve cutter temporarily coapts the valve leaflet against the vein wall in the open position. Identification of these collapsed leaflets on intraoperative angiography is difficult. Sometimes direct mechanical manipulation of the vein will cause the leaflet to go into the closed position, allowing for identification and eventual incision. Platelet aggregates invariably attach to damaged endothelium from mechanical or ischemic injury and may on occasion require a longitudinal venotomy for removal, followed by vein patch angioplasty to close the defect. Attempts at platelet removal by balloon catheter in this setting may only cause more platelet aggregation (100).

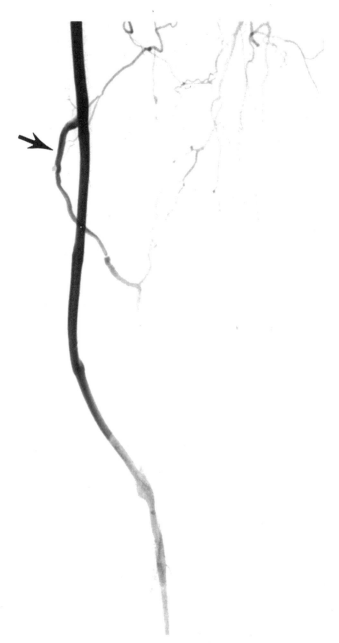

Figure 28-12 Retained vein graft fistula (*arrow*) following *in situ* vein bypass.

REFERENCES

1. Stanley JC, Messina LM, Wakefield TW. Complications of vascular surgery and trauma. In: Greenfield LJ, ed. *Complications in surgery and trauma*, 2nd ed. Philadelphia, PA: JB Lippincott Co; 1989:359–387.
2. Stanley JC, Barnes RW, Ernst CB, et al. Vascular surgery in the United States: workforce issues. Report of the society for vascular surgery and the international society for cardiovascular surgery, North American chapter, committee on workforce issues. *J Vasc Surg* 1996;23:172–181.
3. Biller J, Feinberg WM, Castaldo JE, et al. Guidelines for carotid endarterectomy: a statement for healthcare professionals from a Special Writing Group of the Stroke Council, American Heart Association. *Circulation* 1998;97:501–509.
4. Moore WS, Barnett HJM, Beebe HG, et al. Guidelines for carotid endarterectomy: a multidisciplinary consensus statement from the Ad Hoc Committee, American Heart Association. *Circulation* 1995;91:566–579.
5. Cowan JA Jr, Dimick JB, Thompson BG, et al. Surgeon volume as an indicator of outcomes after carotid endarterectomy: an effect independent of specialty practice and hospital volume. *J Am Coll Surg* 2002;195:814–821.
6. DeBakey ME, Crawford ES, Cooley DA, et al. Cerebral arterial insufficiency: one to 11-year results following arterial reconstructive operation. *Ann Surg* 1965;161:921–945.
7. Hertzer NR, Arison R. Cumulative stroke and survival ten years after carotid endarterectomy. *J Vasc Surg* 1985;2:661–668.
8. Hertzer NR, Loop FD, Beven EG, et al. Surgical staging for simultaneous coronary and carotid disease: a study including prospective randomization. *J Vasc Surg* 1989;9:455–463.
9. Perler BA, Burdick JF, Williams GM. The safety of carotid endarterectomy at the time of coronary artery bypass surgery: analysis of results in a high-risk patient population. *J Vasc Surg* 1985;2:558–562.
10. Ricotta JJ, Peterson MJ, Char DJ. Management of concomitant carotid and coronary arterial disease. In: Ernst CB, Stanley JC, eds. *Current therapy in vascular surgery*, 4th ed. St Louis: Mosby; 2001:101–104.
11. Brown KR, Kresowik TF, Chin MH, et al. Multistate population-based outcomes of combined carotid endarterectomy and coronary artery bypass. *J Vasc Surg* 2003;37:32–39.
12. Graham AM, Gewertz BL, Zarins CK. Predicting cerebral ischemia during carotid endarterectomy. *Arch Surg* 1986;121:595–598.
13. Imparato AM, Riles TS, Lamparello PJ, et al. The management of TIA and acute strokes after carotid endarterectomy. In: Bernhard VM, Towne JB, eds. *Complications in vascular surgery*. New York: Grune & Stratton; 1985:725.
14. Till JS, Toole JF, Howard VJ, et al. Declining morbidity and mortality of carotid endarterectomy. The Wake Forest University Medical Center experience. *Stroke* 1987;18:823–829.
15. Moore WS, Hall AD. Carotid artery back pressure. A test of cerebral tolerance to temporary carotid occlusion. *Arch Surg* 1969;99:702–710.
16. Hays RJ, Levinson SA, Wylie EJ. Intraoperative measurement of carotid back pressure as a guide to operative management for carotid endarterectomy. *Surgery* 1972;72:953–960.
17. Kwaan JHM, Peterson GJ, Connolly JE. Stump pressure. An unreliable guide for shunting during carotid endarterectomy. *Arch Surg* 1980;115:1083–1085.
18. Baker JD, Glucklich B, Watson CW, et al. An evaluation of electroencephalographic monitoring for carotid study. *Surgery* 1975;78:787–794.
19. Ascher E, Markevich N, Kallakuri S, et al. Intraoperative carotid artery duplex scanning in a modern series of 650 consecutive primary endarterectomy procedures. *J Vasc Surg* 2004;39:416–420.
20. Caplan LR, Skillman J, Ojemann R, et al. Intracerebral hemorrhage following carotid endarterectomy. A hypertensive complication? *Stroke* 1978;9:457–460.
21. Evans WE, Hayes JP, Vermilion B. Anastomotic femoral false aneurysms. In: Bernhard VM, Towne JP, eds. *Complications in vascular surgery*. New York: Grune & Stratton; 1985:205.
22. Evans WE, Mendelowitz DS, Liapis C, et al. Motor speech deficit following carotid endarterectomy. *Ann Surg* 1982;196:461–464.
23. Hertzer NR. Postoperative management and complications of extracranial carotid reconstruction. In: Rutherford RB, ed. *Vascular surgery*. Philadelphia, PA: WB Saunders; 1984:1300.
24. Thompson JE. Complications of carotid endarterectomy and their prevention. *World J Surg* 1979;3:155–165.
25. Bove EL, Fry WJ, Gross WS, et al. Hypotension and hypertension as consequences of baroreceptor dysfunction following carotid endarterectomy. *Surgery* 1979;85:633–637.
26. Wade JG, Larson CP, Hickey RF, et al. Effect of carotid endarterectomy on carotid chemoreceptor and baroreceptor function in man. *N Engl J Med* 1970;282:823–829.
27. Clagett GP, Rich NM, McDonald PT, et al. Etiologic factors for recurrent carotid artery stenosis. *Surgery* 1983;93:313–318.

28. Stoney RJ, String ST. Recurrent carotid stenosis. *Surgery* 1976; 80:705–710.

29. Imparato AM, Bracco A, Kim GE. Intimal and neointimal fibrous proliferation causing failure of arterial reconstructions. *Surgery* 1972;72:1007–1017.

30. Rapp J, Stoney RJ. Recurrent carotid stenosis. In: Bernhard VM, Towne JB, eds. *Complications in vascular surgery.* New York: Grune & Stratton; 1986:767.

31. Roddy SP, Darling RC III, Ozsvath KJ, et al. Choice of material for internal carotid artery bypass grafting: vein or prosthetic? Analysis of 44 procedures. *Cardiovasc Surg* 2002;10:540–544.

32. Reul GJ, Cooley DA. False aneurysm of the carotid artery. In: Bergan JJ, Yao JST, eds. *Reoperative arterial surgery.* New York: Grune & Stratton; 1986:538.

33. Dimick JB, Upchurch GR. Jr. The quality of care for patients with abdominal aortic aneurysms. *Cardiovasc Surg* 2003;11:331–336.

34. Dimick JB, Stanley JC, Axelrod DA, et al. Variation in death rate after abdominal aortic aneurysmectomy in the United States: impact of hospital volume, gender, and age. *Ann Surg* 2002; 235:579–585.

35. Katz DJ, Stanley JC, Zelenock GB. Operative mortality rates for intact and ruptured abdominal aortic aneurysms in Michigan: an eleven-year statewide experience. *J Vasc Surg* 1994;19: 804–817.

36. Katz DJ, Stanley JC, Zelenock GB. Gender differences in abdominal aortic aneurysm prevalence, treatment, and outcome. *J Vasc Surg* 1997;25:561–568.

37. Dauchot PJ, DePalma P, Grum D, et al. Detection and prevention of cardiac dysfunction during aortic surgery. *J Surg Res* 1979;26:574–580.

38. Hertzer NR. Fatal myocardial infarction following abdominal aortic aneurysm resection. Three hundred forty-three patients followed 6-11 years postoperatively. *Ann Surg* 1980;192: 667–673.

39. Hertzer NR, Mascha EJ, Karafa MT, et al. Open infrarenal abdominal aortic aneurysm repair: the Cleveland clinic experience from 1989–1998. *J Vasc Surg* 2002;35:1145–1154.

40. Beven EC. Routine coronary angiography in patients undergoing surgery for abdominal aortic aneurysm and lower extremity occlusive disease. *J Vasc Surg* 1986;3:682–684.

41. Eagle KA, Brundage BH, Chaitman BR, et al. Guidelines for perioperative cardiovascular evaluation for noncardiac surgery. Report of the American College of Cardiology/American Heart Association Task Force on Practice Guidelines (Committee on Perioperative Cardiovascular Evaluation for Noncardiac Surgery). *J Am Coll Cardiol* 1996;27:910–948.

42. Froehlich JB, Karavite D, Russman PL, et al. American College of Cardiology/American Heart Association preoperative assessment guidelines reduce resource utilization before aortic surgery. *J Vasc Surg* 2002;36:758–763.

43. Ohuchi H, Gojo S, Sato H, et al. Simultaneous abdominal aortic aneurysm repair during the on-pump coronary artery bypass grafting. *Ann Thorac Cardiovasc Surg* 2003;9:409–411.

44. Bertges DJ, Rhee RY, Muluk SC, et al. Is routine use of the intensive care unit after elective infrarenal abdominal aortic aneurysm repair necessary? *J Vasc Surg* 2000;32:634–642.

45. Hertzer NR, Young JR, Beven EG, et al. Late results of coronary bypass in patients with infrarenal aortic aneurysms. The Cleveland Clinic Study. *Ann Surg* 1987;205:360–367.

46. Diehl JT, Call RP, Hertzer NR, et al. Complication of abdominal aortic reconstruction. An analysis of peri-operative risk factors in 557 patients. *Ann Surg* 1983;197:49–56.

47. O'Hara PJ, Hertzer NR, Santilli PH, et al. Intraoperative autotransfusion during abdominal aortic reconstruction. *Am J Surg* 1983;145:215–220.

48. Clagett GP, Valentine RJ, Jackson MR, et al. A randomized trial of intraoperative autotransfusion during aortic surgery. *J Vasc Surg* 1999;29:22–31.

49. Haimovici H. Metabolic syndrome secondary to acute arterial occlusions. In: Haimovici H, ed. *Vascular emergencies.* East Norwalk, CT: Appleton & Lange; 1982:267.

50. Bush HL. Renal failure following abdominal aortic reconstruction. *Surgery* 1983;93:107–109.

51. Wakefield TW, Whitehouse WM Jr, Wu SC, et al. Abdominal aortic aneurysm rupture: statistical analysis of factors affecting outcome of surgical treatment. *Surgery* 1982;91:586–596.

52. Hassoun HT, Miller CC III, Huynh TT, et al. Cold visceral perfusion improves early survival in patients with acute renal failure after thoracoabdominal aortic aneurysm repair. *J Vasc Surg* 2004;39:506–512.

53. Crawford ES, Crawford JL, Safi HJ, et al. Thoracoabdominal aortic aneurysms: preoperative and intraoperative factors determining immediate and long-term results of operations in 605 patients. *J Vasc Surg* 1986;3:389–404.

54. Starr DS, Lawrie GM, Morris GC. Prevention of distal embolism during arterial reconstruction. *Am J Surg* 1979;138:764–769.

55. Crowson M, Fielding JWL, Black J, et al. Acute gastrointestinal complications of infrarenal aortic aneurysm repair. *Br J Surg* 1984;71:825–828.

56. Zelenock GB, Strodel WE, Knol JA, et al. A prospective study of clinically and endoscopically documented colonic ischemia in 100 patients undergoing aortic reconstructive surgery with aggressive colonic and direct pelvic revascularization, compared with historic controls. *Surgery* 1989;106:771–780.

57. Hagihara PF, Ernst CB, Griffin WO Jr. Incidence of ischemic colitis following abdominal aortic reconstruction. *Surg Gynecol Obstet* 1979;149:571–573.

58. Ernst CB, Hagihara PF, Daugherty ME, et al. Inferior mesenteric artery stump pressure: a reliable index for safe IMA ligation during abdominal aortic aneurysmectomy. *Ann Surg* 1978;197:641–646.

59. Mitchell KM, Valentine RJ. Inferior mesenteric artery reimplantation does not guarantee colon viability in aortic surgery. *J Am Coll Surg* 2002;194:151–155.

60. Szilagyi DE, Hageman JH, Smith RF, et al. Spinal cord damage in surgery of the abdominal aorta. *Surgery* 1978;83:38–56.

61. Elliott JP, Szilagyi DL, Hageman JH, et al. Spinal cord ischemia: secondary to surgery of the abdominal aorta. In: Bernhard VM, Towne JB, eds. *Complications in vascular surgery.* New York: Grune & Stratton; 1985:291.

62. Picone AL, Green RM, Ricotta JR, et al. Spinal cord ischemia following operations on the abdominal aorta. *J Vasc Surg* 1986; 3:94–103.

63. McCullough JL, Hollier LH, Nugent M. Paraplegia after thoracic aortic occlusion: influence of cerebrospinal fluid drainage. Experimental and early clinical results. *J Vasc Surg* 1988; 7:153–160.

64. Joob AW, Dunn C, Miller E, et al. Effect of left atrial to left femoral artery bypass and renin-angiotensin system blockade on renal blood flow and function during and after thoracic aortic occlusion. *J Vasc Surg* 1987;5:329–335.

65. Laschinger JC, Cunningham JN Jr, Catinella FP, et al. Detection and prevention of intraoperative spinal cord ischemia after crossclamping of the thoracic aorta: use of somatosensory evoked potentials. *Surgery* 1982;92:1109–1117.

66. Lambardini MM, Ratliff RK. The abdominal aortic aneurysm and the ureter. *J Urol* 1967;98:590–596.

67. Szilagyi DE, Smith RF, Elliott JP, et al. Infection in arterial reconstruction with synthetic grafts. *Ann Surg* 1972;176:321–333.

68. Reilly LM, Altman H, Lusby RJ, et al. Late results following surgical management of vascular graft infection. *J Vasc Surg* 1984; 1:36–44.

69. MacBeth GA, Rubin JR, McIntyre KE, et al. The relevance of arterial wall microbiology to the treatment of prosthetic graft infections: graft infection vs. arterial infection. *J Vasc Surg* 1984;1: 750–756.

70. Liekweg WG, Greenfield LJ. Vascular prosthetic infections: collected experience and results of treatment. *Surgery* 1977;81: 335–342.

71. Tollefson DF, Bandyk DF, Kaebnick HW, et al. Surface biofilm disruption: enhanced recovery of microorganisms from vascular prostheses. *Arch Surg* 1987;122:38–43.

72. Reilly LM, Stoney RJ, Goldstone J, et al. Improved management of aortic graft infection: the influence of operation sequence and staging. *J Vasc Surg* 1987;5:421–431.

73. Clagett GP, Valentine RJ, Hagino RT. Autogenous aortoiliac/femoral reconstruction from superficial femoral-popliteal veins: feasibility and durability. *J Vasc Surg* 1997; 25: 255–270.

74. Bandyk DF, Novotney ML, Johnson BL, et al. Use of rifampin-soaked gelatin-sealed polyester grafts for in situ treatment of primary aortic and vascular prosthetic infections. *J Surg Res* 2001;95:44–49.

75. Kieffer E, Gomes D, Chiche L, et al. Allograft replacement for infrarenal aortic graft infection: early and late results in 179 patients. *J Vasc Surg* 2004;39:1009–1017.

76. Stanley JC, Lindenauer SM, Graham LM, et al. Vascular grafts. In: Moore W, ed. *Vascular surgery. A comprehensive review.* New York: Grune & Stratton; 1986:365–390.

77. Lalka SG, Bernhard VM. Noninfectious complications in vascular surgery. In: Moore W, ed. *Vascular surgery. A comprehensive review.* New York: Grune & Stratton; 1986:959.

78. Brewster DC, Darling RC. Optimal methods of aortoiliac reconstruction. *Surgery* 1978;84:739–748.

79. Szilagyi DE, Elliott JP, Smith RF, et al. A 30-year survey of the reconstructive surgical treatment of aortoiliac occlusive disease. *J Vasc Surg* 1986;3:421–436.

80. Szilagyi DE, Smith FR, Elliott JP, et al. Anastomotic aneurysms after vascular reconstruction: problems of incidence, etiology and treatment. *Surgery* 1975;78:800–816.

81. Berchtold C, Eibl C, Seelig MH, et al. Endovascular treatment and complete regression of an infected abdominal aortic aneurysm. *J Endovasc Ther* 2002;9:543–548.

82. Flanigan DP, Schuler JJ, Keifer T, et al. Elimination of iatrogenic impotence and improvement of sexual function after aortoiliac revascularization. *Arch Surg* 1982;117:544–550.

83. Nath RL, Menzoian JO, Kaplan KH, et al. The multidisciplinary approach to vasculogenic impotence. *Surgery* 1981;89:124–133.

84. DePalma RG, Emsellem HA, Edwards CM, et al. A screening sequence for vasculogenic impotence. *J Vasc Surg* 1987;5:228–236.

85. Ferris BL, Mills JL Sr, Hughes JD, et al. Is early postoperative duplex scan surveillance of leg bypass grafts clinically important? *J Vasc Surg* 2003;37:495–500.

86. Hertzer NR. Fatal myocardial infarction following lower extremity revascularization: 273 patients followed 6 to 11 postoperative years. *Ann Surg* 1981;193:492–498.

87. Brewster DC. Early complications of vascular repair below the inguinal ligament. In: Bernhard VM, Towne JB, eds. *Complications in vascular surgery.* New York: Grune & Stratton; 1985:37.

88. Brewster DC, LaSalle AJ, Robison JG, et al. Femoropopliteal graft failures. Clinical consequences and success of secondary reconstructions. *Arch Surg* 1983;118:1043–1047.

89. Donaldson MC, Mannick JA, Whittemore AD. Causes of primary graft failure after in situ saphenous vein bypass grafting. *J Vasc Surg* 1992;15:113–120.

90. Abbruzzese TA, Havens J, Belkin M, et al. Statin therapy is associated with improved patency of autogenous infrainguinal bypass grafts. *J Vasc Surg* 2004;39:1178–1185.

91. Henke PK, Blackburn S, Proctor MC, et al. Patients undergoing infrainguinal bypass to treat atherosclerotic vascular disease are underprescribed cardioprotective medications: effect on graft patency, limb salvage, and mortality. *J Vasc Surg* 2004;39:357–365.

92. Bandyk DF. Postoperative surveillance of femorodistal grafts: the application of echo-Doppler (duplex) ultrasonic scanning. In: Bergan JJ, Yao JST, eds. *Reoperative arterial surgery.* New York: Grune & Stratton; 1986:59.

93. Roddy SP, Darling RCIII, Maharaj D, et al. Gender-related differences in outcome: an analysis of 5880 infrainguinal arterial reconstructions. *J Vasc Surg* 2003;37:399–402.

94. LoGerfo FW, Quist WC, Cantlemo NL, et al. Integrity of vein grafts as a function of initial intimal and medial preservation. *Circulation* 1983;68(Suppl. 2):117–124.

95. Veith FJ, Gupta S, Daly V. Management of early and late thrombosis of expanded polytetrafluoroethylene (PTFE) femoropopliteal bypass grafts: favorable prognosis with appropriate reoperation. *Surgery* 1980;87:581–587.

96. Whittemore AD, Clowes AW, Couch NP, et al. Secondary femoropopliteal reconstruction. *Ann Surg* 1981;193:35–42.

97. Durham JR, Rubin JR, Malone JM. Management of infected infrainguinal bypass grafts. In: Bergan JJ, Yao JST, eds. *Reoperative arterial surgery.* New York: Grune & Stratton; 1986:359.

98. Eickhoff JH, Engell HG. Local regulation of blood flow and the occurrence of edema after arterial reconstruction of the lower limbs. *Ann Surg* 1982;195:474–478.

99. Schubart PJ, Porter JM. Leg edema following femorodistal bypass. In: Bergan JJ, Yao JST, eds. *Reoperative arterial surgery.* New York: Grune & Stratton; 1986:331.

100. Leather RP, Karmody AM, Shah DM, et al. The in situ saphenous vein arterial bypass. In: Bergan JJ, Yao JST, eds. *Reoperative arterial surgery.* New York: Grune & Stratton; 1986:299.

101. Ballotta E, Da Giau G, Piccoli A, et al. Durability of carotid endarterectomy for treatment of symptomatic and asymptomatic stenosis. *J Vasc Surg* 2004;40(2):270–278.

102. Conrad MF, Shepard AD, Pandurangi K, et al. Outcome of carotid endarterectomy in African Americans: is race a factor? *J Vasc Surg* 2003;38:129–137.

103. Darling RC III, Mehta M, Roddy SP, et al. Eversion carotid endarterectomy: a technical alternative that may obviate patch closure in women. *Cardiovasc Surg* 2003;11:347–352.

104. Ecker RD, Pichelmann MA, Meissner I, et al. Durability of carotid endarterectomy. *Stroke* 2003;34:2941–2944.

105. Illig KA, Shortell CK, Zhang R, et al. Carotid endarterectomy then and now: outcome and cost-effectiveness of modern practice. *Surg* 2003;134:705–712.

106. Elkouri S, Gloviczki P, McKusick MA, et al. Perioperative complications and early outcomes after endovascular and open surgical repair of abdominal aortic aneurysms. *J Vasc Surg* 2004;39:497–505.

107. Menard MT, Chew DKW, Chan RK, et al. Outcome in patients at high risk after open surgical repair of abdominal aortic aneurysm. *J Vasc Surg* 2003;37:285–292.

108. Chew DKW, Conte MS, Donaldson MC, et al. Autogenous composite vein bypass graft for infrainguinal arterial reconstruction. *J Vasc Surg* 2001;33:259–265.

109. Goshima KR, Mills JL Sr, Huches JD. A new look at outcomes after infrainguinal bypass surgery: traditional reporting standards systematically underestimate the expenditure of effort required to attain limb salvage. *J Vasc Surg* 2004;39:330–335.

110. Pomposelli FB, Kansal N, Hamdan AD, et al. A decade of experience with dorsalis pedis artery bypass: analysis of outcome in more than 1000 cases. *J Vasc Surg* 2003;37:307–315.

111. Raffetto JD, Chen MN, LaMorte WW, et al. Factors that predict site of outflow target artery anastomosis in infrainguinal revascularization. *J Vasc Surg* 2002;35:1093–1099.

Complications of Venous Disease and Therapy

29

Thomas W. Wakefield   Peter K. Henke

▬▬ INCIDENCE, RISK FACTORS, AND
CATEGORIES 337
Phlegmasia Alba Dolens/Phlegmasia Cerulea
   Dolens 338
Axillary/Subclavian Vein Thrombosis 338
Superficial Thrombophlebitis 339

▬▬ VENOUS DISEASE DIAGNOSIS 339

▬▬ VENOUS THROMBOEMBOLISM
PROPHYLAXIS 342

▬▬ STANDARD THERAPY FOR VENOUS
THROMBOEMBOLISM 344

▬▬ ALTERNATIVE AND FUTURE TREATMENTS 346

▬▬ VENA CAVA FILTERS 348

▬▬ THROMBOLYTIC AND SURGICAL PROCEDURES
FOR DEEP VENOUS THROMBOSIS AND
PULMONARY EMBOLISM 350

▬▬ VENOUS VARICOSITIES 351

▬▬ CHRONIC VENOUS INSUFFICIENCY 352

▬▬ REFERENCES 354

Thomas W. Wakefield, Peter K. Henke: University of Michigan,
Ann Arbor, MI 48109

INCIDENCE, RISK FACTORS, AND CATEGORIES

Deep venous thrombosis involves >250,000 patients per year, affecting approximately 50 to 200 per 100,000 population, and pulmonary embolism involves >200,000 patients per year, affecting approximately 20 to 200 per 100,000 population. The incidence of deep venous thrombosis has remained constant since 1980 (1) and increases with age, such that the incidence is approximately 300 per 100,000 in those older than 85. Deep venous thrombosis and pulmonary embolism (together termed venous thromboembolism) are noted in approximately 1% of Medicare inpatient discharges. The cost of treatment has been estimated to be in the billions of dollars per year.

Virchow triad of stasis, vessel wall injury, and hypercoagulability underlies the clinical events that predispose to the development of deep venous thrombosis. Today a more sophisticated understanding of events that occur at the level of the vein wall include the influence of the inflammatory response on thrombus amplification, organization, and recanalization. Varicosities of the limb likely have an etiology separate from, and not usually related to, venous

TABLE 29-1

VENOUS DISEASE AND LEVELS OF MEDICAL EVIDENCE FOR SPECIFIC THERAPIES

Venous Disease Therapies	Highest Supporting Level of Evidence
VTE prophylaxis & treatment	I
Vena cava filters	I (mostly III)
Thrombolysis, PE, DVT	I, II (mostly III, IV)
Thrombectomy	III
Varicosity excision	III
Perforator ligation	II
Deep reconstruction	IV
Angioplasty	III

VTE, venous thromboembolism; PE, pulmonary embolism; DVT, deep venous thrombosis.

TABLE 29-2

HYPERCOAGULABLE TESTING

Standard coagulation tests
Mixing studies (if APTT is elevated)
Antithrombin antigen and activity
Protein C antigen and activity
Protein S antigen
APC resistance test
Factor V genetic analysis
Prothrombin 20210A genetic analysis
Homocysteine level
Antiphospholipid/anticardiolipin antibody screen
Factor VIII levels
Platelet count/platelet aggregation testing
Functional plasminogen
Heparin antibodies

APTT, activated partial thromboplastin time.

thrombophlebitis. When making treatment decisions for venous disease, it is important to keep in mind the supporting levels of medical evidence for each therapy (Table 29-1).

Acquired risk factors for venous thromboembolism include age (1,000-fold thrombosis difference in the very young vs. the very old), malignancy (3% to 20% among those with venous thrombosis), surgery and trauma (up to 50% to 60% incidence without prophylaxis), immobilization (airflight incidence between 1/10 and 1/10,000), oral contraceptive use (fourfold to eightfold increase), hormone replacement therapy (twofold to fourfold increase), pregnancy (10-fold increase) and the puerperium, obesity, neurologic disease, cardiac disease, and antiphospholipid antibodies (10-fold increase) (2).

Genetic causes include deficiencies of natural coagulation inhibitors (antithrombin, protein C, and protein S; 10-fold increase), Factor V Leiden (incidence up to 20% in an unselected and 50% in a selected population of patients with venous thromboembolism; threefold to eightfold increase in thrombosis with heterozygous and 80-fold with homozygous state), prothrombin 20210A (incidence up to 6% in a selected population of patients with venous thrombosis; threefold increase in thrombosis), blood group non-O (twofold to fourfold increase), hyperhomocystinemia (5% to 10% of population: twofold increase in thrombosis), dysfibrinogenemia (incidence 3%), dysplasminogenemia (incidence <1%), reduced heparin cofactor II activity, elevated levels of clotting factors such as factors XI, IX, VII, VIII, X, and II, and plasminogen activator inhibitor-1 (twofold to threefold increase) (3).

When a patient presents with an idiopathic venous thromboembolism or there is a family history of venous thromboembolism, a work-up for a hypercoagulable state is suggested (2,3). Common etiologies include deficiency of natural anticoagulants, production of altered procoagulants, and elevated prothrombic factors. Appropriate tests are available in most hospital laboratories (Table 29-2).

Hematologic diseases associated with an increased incidence of venous thromboembolism include disseminated intravascular coagulation, heparin-induced thrombocytopenia, antiphospholipid antibody syndrome, thrombotic thrombocytopenic purpura, hemolytic uremic syndrome, and myeloproliferative disorders such as polycythemia vera and essential thrombocythemia.

Most cases of deep venous thrombosis affect the lower limb and include the popliteal, femoral, or iliac veins. Presenting symptoms include unilateral limb pain and swelling, but deep venous thrombosis is sometimes silent, with pulmonary embolism as the first manifestation.

Phlegmasia Alba Dolens/Phlegmasia Cerulea Dolens

Massive iliofemoral deep venous thrombosis may cause phlegmasia alba dolens (the white swollen leg) and phlegmasia cerulean dolens (the blue swollen leg). When capillaries occlude, venous gangrene may result. Occlusion occurs as arterial inflow becomes obstructed due to extreme venous hypertension. Alternatively, arterial emboli or spasm may occur. The toes on the involved limb turn blue and black, and the skin blisters. Venous gangrene can be differentiated from arterial ischemia by generalized swelling and limb blueness as opposed to the pale, cold limb of acute arterial ischemia. Venous gangrene is often associated with an underlying malignancy, and phlegmasia cerulea dolens virtually always precedes it. Amputation rates of 20% to 50% are noted, with pulmonary embolism rates of 12% to 40% and mortality of 20% to 40% (4).

Axillary/Subclavian Vein Thrombosis

Thrombosis of the axillary/subclavian vein is an uncommon event accounting for <5% of all cases of acute deep venous thrombosis. Nevertheless, axillary and subclavian venous thrombosis has been associated with pulmonary embolism in up to 10% to 15% of cases and can be the source of significant disability (5). Primary axillary or subclavian vein thrombosis results from intermittent obstruction of the vein in the thoracic outlet (Paget-von Schrötter syndrome) in relatively healthy muscular individuals, with strenuous exercise often precipitating the thrombosis. Thrombosis may also occur in patients with hypercoagulable states. Secondary axillary and subclavian vein thrombosis most commonly results from indwelling catheters or pacemaker wires. Less common secondary causes include congestive heart failure, nephrotic syndrome, mediastinal tumors, and malignancy. Most patients present with pain, edema, and cyanosis of the arm. Superficial venous distension may be apparent in the arm, forearm, shoulder, and anterior chest wall, and this finding can aid in the diagnosis.

Superficial Thrombophlebitis

Superficial thrombophlebitis occurs in over 125,000 patients per year and is associated with varicose veins, pregnancy, thromboangiitis obliterans (Behçet disease), and indwelling catheters. Complications of superficial thrombophlebitis have been associated with male gender and a history of venous thromboembolism (6). Clinically, a painful, firm, palpable cord with inflammation and tenderness along the affected vein, and occasionally edema, are noted. There may be a history of venous puncture or intravenous canalization, trauma, physical inactivity, oral contraceptives, malignancy, or infection. The presence of migratory superficial thrombophlebitis suggests the presence of cancer [e.g., carcinoma of the pancreas (Trousseau sign)]. The incidence of deep venous thrombosis associated with superficial thrombophlebitis is estimated to be between 0.75% and 40%. The association of a noncontiguous deep venous thrombosis with superficial thrombophlebitis is as high as 25% to 75% in patients who present with involvement of both systems (7). Pulmonary embolism, the most lethal and under-recognized complication associated with this entity, occurs from 0% to 17% (1).

Suppurative superficial thrombophlebitis is associated with intravenous catheter use or multiple puncture sites secondary to intravenous drug abuse, most often in the upper extremity. The clinical presentation is similar to that of nonsuppurative superficial thrombophlebitis, although there is often also pyrexia, leukocytosis, and bacteremia. Local intravenous catheter site infections occur in up to 8% of cases and bacteremia is detected in approximately 1 of every 400 intravenous catheterizations (7). Immunocompromised and burn patients are particularly susceptible to superficial thrombophlebitis.

Hypercoagulability in the setting of superficial thrombophlebitis is not uncommon. The risk of superficial thrombophlebitis in the absence of varicose veins, malignancy, or autoimmune disorders is approximately 13-fold higher for deficiencies of inhibitors of coagulation (antithrombin, protein C, or protein S), sixfold higher for Factor V Leiden mutation, and fourfold higher for the prothrombin gene mutation (8). The same indications for hypercoagulable work-up in patients with deep venous thrombosis should be applied to patients with superficial thrombophlebitis (6). This category includes patients *without* an associated history of trauma or inactivity, venipuncture, malignancy, or varicose veins and *with* severe superficial thrombophlebitis, recurrence, family history, early age at presentation, and resistance to therapy.

VENOUS DISEASE DIAGNOSIS

The diagnosis of deep venous thrombosis *cannot* be made solely on the basis of presenting symptoms and signs, as up to 50% of patients with acute deep venous thrombosis are asymptomatic. When symptoms are present, patients often complain of a dull ache or pain in the calf or leg. The most common physical finding is edema of the involved calf or ankle (9). When there is extensive proximal deep venous thrombosis, there may be massive edema, cyanosis, and dilated superficial collateral veins.

Objective tests must be used in making the diagnosis of deep venous thrombosis. Tests of historical interest include hand-held Doppler examination, impedance plethysmography, radiolabeled fibrinogen scanning, and phlebography. Because of its high sensitivity, specificity, and reproducibility, duplex ultrasound imaging has replaced contrast phlebography. Duplex ultrasound imaging includes both a B-mode image and Doppler flow analysis and carries sensitivity and specificity rates of >95% (10) (Figs. 29-1 and 29-2). Magnetic resonance imaging (MRI) may be helpful to diagnose pelvic vein and caval thrombosis, but MRI and spiral computed tomography (CT) scanning are unlikely to replace duplex ultrasound as the primary diagnostic test. Even at the calf level, duplex imaging is an accurate technique in symptomatic patients. In addition to its accuracy, duplex ultrasound is painless, requires no contrast, can be serially repeated, and is performed safely during pregnancy. The test is also able to image other potential causes of the patient's symptoms. Combining clinical characteristics with the D-dimer assay may decrease the number of negative duplex scans (11). Importantly, a single complete and technically adequate negative compression duplex scan is accurate enough to base the withholding of anticoagulation with minimal long-term adverse thromboembolic complications (12).

Other conditions may be confused with deep venous thrombosis. For example, muscle strain or contusion may mimic deep venous thrombosis, while cellulitis may cause edema, localized pain, and erythema. Iliac vein obstruction in the retroperitoneum by a tumor or mass may lead to unilateral massive leg edema. The presence of a Baker

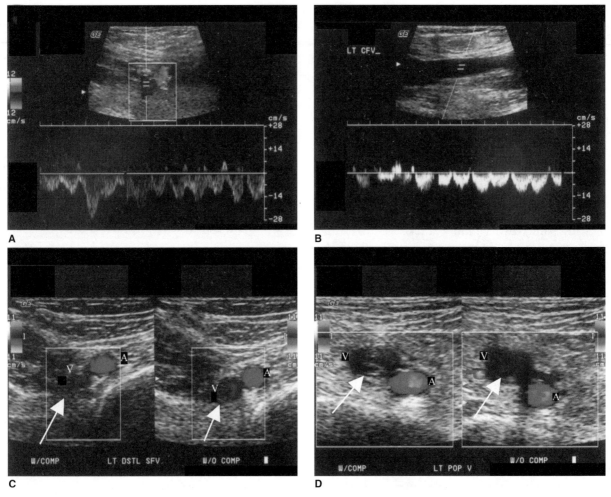

Figure 29-1 By duplex ultrasound, normal venous flow is demonstrated in the left external iliac vein (**A**) and the left common femoral vein (**B**). There is partial thrombus in the left distal superficial femoral vein (**C**) and left popliteal vein (**D**). Arrows point to thrombus. A, artery; V, vein.

cyst may also produce unilateral leg pain and edema. Other causes of leg swelling (usually bilateral) include cardiac, renal, or hepatic abnormalities.

Diagnosis of incompetent venous perforators, in planning for venous stasis ulceration treatment, can be done by duplex. Although sensitivity is >80% and reproducible, it is recommended that a full subfascial exploration be performed at the time of surgery, as preoperative duplex marking may miss up to 20% of perforators (13). Ascending venography may also be of benefit in this regard. The duplex scan can also be used to diagnose femoropopliteal venous reflux reliably, which contributes to primary venous varicosities in 50% (14). Saphenopopliteal reflux should also be documented, as this may contribute to persistent and recurrent venous varicosities.

A definitive diagnosis of chronic venous insufficiency is essential for selecting patients who will benefit most from any given intervention. A standard severity classification scoring system, which includes a Venous Severity Score as well as the more traditional CEAP (Clinical Etiology Anatomic Pathophysiologic) system, has been developed (15). The latter is a standard way to categorize venous insufficiency, and it includes etiology and anatomical information. The classification allows cross-communication between physicians, as well as documentation of therapeutic outcome for any given procedure. It differentiates between reflux and obstructive components that may aid with therapy.

If further interventions are planned, venous insufficiency is diagnosed with both duplex ultrasound imaging assessing valvular reflux and air plethysmography. Air plethysmography is a moderately complex noninvasive venous assessment that assesses for calf muscle pump function, as well as reflux and obstructive components of venous insufficiency. A recent report suggests this is most sensitive for reflux assessment, both in the deep and superficial perforator systems (16). However, there is no correlation with the parameters of air plethysmography and severity of clinical disease. Similarly, foot venous pressures or ambulatory venous pressure measurements are invasive methods to quantify venous hypertension. A needle is placed in the medial vein of the great toe and pressures are taken both at rest and after calf ejection with compression. Unlike the air

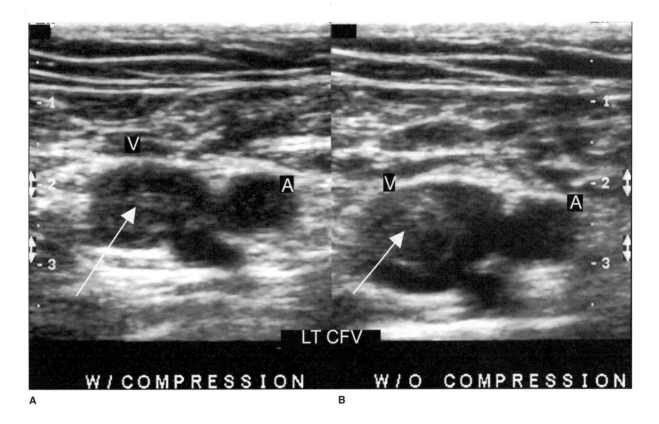

Figure 29-2   By duplex ultrasound, note that with compression **(A)** and without compression **(B)**, the thrombosed left common femoral vein is dilated with intraluminal partially echogenic thrombus *(arrows)*. A, artery; V, vein.

plethsymography, foot venous pressure does correlate with venous clinical severity symptomatology (17). This test may be used for preprocedural and postprocedural quantification of therapy, although it has not gained widespread popularity because of its invasive nature and procedural pain for the patient.

Almost any pulmonary symptom can mimic a pulmonary embolism. Chest x-ray changes are infrequently present, and hemoptysis represents pulmonary infarction and suggests a far advanced state of abnormality. The diagnostic modalities for pulmonary embolism are in flux. In the most recent past the tests used included ventilation/perfusion scanning (V/Q) and pulmonary arteriography. Unfortunately, V/Q scanning is diagnostic in only approximately one-third of cases, and

pulmonary arteriography has morbidity and occasional mortality. Spiral CT scanning has shown significant promise and in many institutions has become the test of choice (Fig. 29-3). A national multicenter study evaluating its role in the diagnosis of pulmonary embolism is currently being conducted (PIOPED II), and its results should allow for an accurate determination when to use this test and how it compares with V/Q imaging and pulmonary arteriography. Certain biomarkers of cardiac injury, including troponin and brain natruretic peptide, have now been recognized to be useful in acute pulmonary embolism (18). For example, if the biomarkers are positive, further testing with echocardiography is indicated to determine right ventricular strain and to direct thrombolytic therapy.

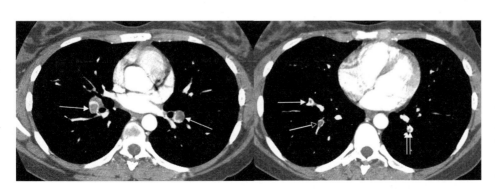

Figure 29-3   Spiral CT scan revealing evidence of pulmonary embolism. **A:** Note the thrombi in the descending pulmonary arteries; **B:** Note the thrombi in the right anterior segmental pulmonary artery *(closed arrow)*, lateral segmental pulmonary artery *(open arrow)*, and posterior segmental pulmonary artery *(double arrow)*.

VENOUS THROMBOEMBOLISM PROPHYLAXIS

Methods for venous thromboembolism prophylaxis include pharmacologic, mechanical, and combinations of them (19,20). The following discussion is based on the current recommendations from the Sixth ACCP Consensus Conference on Antithrombotic Therapy (20). Pharmacologic agents include unfractionated heparin, low-molecular-weight heparin (LMWH), warfarin, dextran, and aspirin. Enoxaparin and dalteparin are the low-molecular-weight heparins approved by the U.S. Food and Drug Administration (FDA). Prophylactic dosages for enoxaparin are either 30 mg subcutaneously every 12 hours or 40 mg once daily, whereas dalteparin dosage is either 2,500 or 5,000 anti-Xa units subcutaneously once daily.

Mechanical methods include pneumatic compression devices and elastic stockings. Mechanical prophylaxis with pneumatic compression devices reduces the incidence of deep venous thrombosis, although this has not been proven with the same rigor as with heparin agents. It is commonly believed that the effectiveness of pneumatic compression devices is based on overcoming venous stasis and increasing lower extremity blood flow and, possibly, by increasing native fibrinolytic activators, although the latter is still controversial. These devices use three patterns of compression: rapid graduated sequential compression, graduated sequential compression, and intermittent compression. The rapid graduated compression is available only in calf length, but the remaining techniques are available as calf or thigh devices.

Concerning general surgical patients (Fig. 29-4), the incidence of deep venous thrombosis is as high as 25% overall without prophylaxis. The risk of pulmonary embolism is 1.6%, with 0.9% fatal. Patients have been categorized into levels of risk (Table 29-3). In low-risk patients no specific venous thromboembolism prophylaxis is indicated other than early ambulation. In moderate-risk patients, prophylaxis includes low-dose heparin (LDH), low-molecular-weight heparin, pneumatic compression devices (PCD), or elastic stockings. For higher-risk patients, low-dose heparin, low-molecular-weight heparin, or pneumatic compression devices should be used, whereas for very-high-risk patients, low-dose heparin or low-molecular-weight heparin plus pneumatic compression devices are recommended. Full-dose warfarin may also be used, but few general surgeons use full-dose oral anticoagulation during surgery because of bleeding. Importantly, aspirin alone is not recommended for general surgery patients.

In reviewing individual regiments for general surgical procedures, low-dose heparin has been found to reduce the total incidence of deep venous thrombosis from 25% to 8% and to reduce the risk of fatal pulmonary embolism by approximately 50%. Low-molecular-weight heparin reduces deep venous thrombosis incidence for general surgical patients to 6% with a lower risk of bleeding. Physical

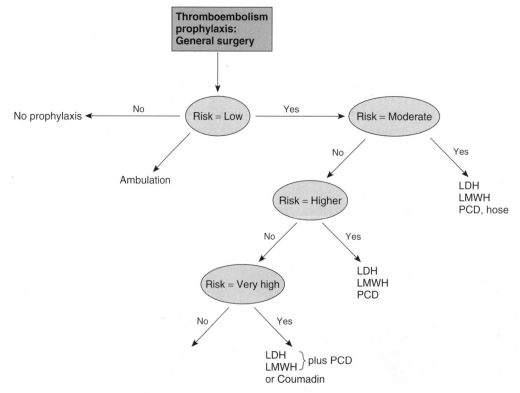

Figure 29-4 VTE prophylaxis for general surgery patients. LHD, low-dose heparin; LMWH, low-molecular-weight heparin; PCD, pneumatic compression device.

TABLE 29-3

RISK FACTOR STRATIFICATION FOR VENOUS THROMBOEMBOLISM PROPHYLAXIS

Low risk	Minor surgery in patients <40 years with no additional risk factors
Moderate risk	Minor surgery in patients with additional risk factors; nonmajor surgery in patients 40–60 years with no additional risk factors; major surgery in patients <40 years with no additional risk factors
High risk	Nonmajor surgery in patients >60 years or with additional risk factors; major surgery in patients >40 years or with additional risk factors
Highest risk	Major surgery in patients >40 years plus prior venous thromboembolism, cancer, or hypercoagulable states; hip or knee replacement, hip fracture surgery; major trauma; spinal cord injury

Adapted from Geerts WH, Heit JA, Clagett GP, et al. Prevention of venous thromboembolism. *Chest* 2001;119:132S–175S.

measures, such as pneumatic compression devices, reduce deep venous thrombosis, but their ability to reduce the incidence of pulmonary embolism is unknown. Likewise, the use of graded elastic support stockings in prevention of pulmonary embolism and proximal deep venous thrombosis is controversial. Dextran, although not as effective in preventing deep venous thrombosis (decreasing the incidence only to 18%), lowers the incidence of fatal pulmonary embolism and is equal to low-dose heparin in preventing pulmonary embolism. Finally, warfarin, although effective in the prevention of leg deep venous thrombosis and thus pulmonary embolism, is difficult to use, is difficult to monitor, and is associated with bleeding.

For orthopedic surgery patients, the incidence of deep venous thrombosis is as high as 45% to 57% for total hip replacement, 40% to 84% for total knee replacement, and 36% to 60% for hip fracture surgery patients without prophylaxis. For these groups total pulmonary embolism incidence is 0.7% to 30%, 1.8% to 7%, and 4.3% to 24%, respectively. For total hip replacement, low-molecular-weight heparin, adjusted-dose warfarin, or adjusted-dose unfractioned heparin is recommended. When to begin the prophylaxis (preoperative or postoperative) is a point of controversy, as both approaches have been used successfully. Comparing with adjusted-dose warfarin prophylaxis, the rate of in-hospital symptomatic venous thromboembolism was 0.3% for low-molecular-weight heparin and 1.1% for warfarin, with major bleeding at 1.2% for low-molecular-weight heparin and 0.5% for warfarin.

Adjuvant physical modalities may provide additional benefit. For total knee replacement, low-molecular-weight heparin, adjusted-dose warfarin, or pneumatic compression devices should be used. For both total hip and knee surgery, mechanical measures are indicated when there are contraindications to anticoagulation. For hip fracture surgery, preoperative or postoperative low-molecular-weight heparin or adjusted-dose warfarin is suggested. Prolonged post-hospital prophylaxis may improve both total deep venous thrombosis and pulmonary embolism rates, as

some studies suggest that up to one-third of episodes of venous thromboembolism occur after discharge.

Solid evidence is lacking for venous thromboembolism prophylaxis of trauma patients (Fig. 29-5). Duplex ultrasound screening is appropriate when dictated by clinical indications, and inferior vena cava filters are routinely used in patients with proximal deep venous thrombosis when anticoagulation is contraindicated (21,22). Without venous thromboembolism prophylaxis, deep venous thrombosis may occur in up to 50% of high-risk cases. Pulmonary embolism is the third most common cause of death in trauma patients surviving beyond the first day. Trauma risk factors include spinal cord injury; lower extremity or pelvic fractures; surgical procedures; advanced age; femoral venous lines or major venous repairs; prolonged immobility; and prolonged duration of hospital stay. Acceptable prophylaxis includes low-molecular-weight heparin and pneumatic compression devices when bleeding risk is high. The benefits of

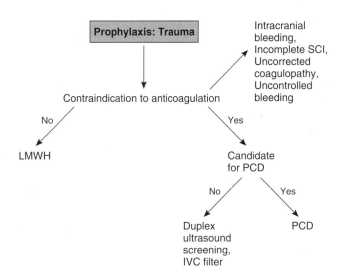

Figure 29-5 VTE prophylaxis for trauma patients. SCI, spinal cord injury; LMWH, low-molecular-weight heparin; PCD, pneumatic compression device; IVC, inferior vena cava.

combined therapy are unknown. Contraindications to early initiation of low-molecular-weight heparin include intracranial bleeding, incomplete spinal cord injury with paraspinal hematoma, severe uncorrected coagulopathy, and uncontrolled bleeding.

In neurosurgery deep venous thrombosis and pulmonary embolism occur frequently, generally equivalent to general surgery patient risk. Risk factors include intracranial surgery, malignant tumors, leg weakness, increased age, and lengthy surgery. Pneumatic compression devices with or without elastic stockings are recommended when anticoagulation cannot be used. Combining low-dose heparin or postoperative low-molecular-weight heparin with pneumatic compression devices with or without elastic stockings may be more effective than either technique alone. Overall rates of deep venous thrombosis and proximal deep venous thrombosis were reduced by approximately 50% with combined treatment. Pulmonary embolism is a frequent cause of death in patients with spinal cord injury. Low-molecular-weight heparin with or without mechanical measures is recommended for 3 months or until the completion of the rehabilitation phase of recovery. Although adjusted-dose warfarin or low-molecular-weight heparin has been suggested in the rehabilitation phase, low-dose heparin, pneumatic compression devices, and elastic stockings are inadequate alone.

Less evidence exists on venous thromboembolism prophylaxis for medically ill patients. Low-dose heparin appears to be effective for those with myocardial infarction in whom deep venous thrombosis is a risk. Pneumatic compression devices and possibly elastic stockings should be used if heparin is contraindicated. For patients with stroke and lower extremity paralysis, low-dose heparin and low-molecular-weight heparin have been recommended. Pneumatic compression devices and elastic stockings are likely to be ineffective in this situation. Low-dose heparin and low-molecular-weight heparin have been recommended in those patients with congestive heart failure or pulmonary infections. In a study of medical intensive care unit patients who underwent routine upper and lower extremity duplex scan surveillance, the incidence of venous thrombosis was as high as 39%, despite deep venous thrombosis prophylaxis in 80% of cases. Fixed low-dose warfarin (1 mg per dL) or low-molecular-weight heparin is recommended in patients with long-term upper body indwelling venous catheters to prevent axillary-subclavian vein thrombosis. This therapy is especially important in patients with malignancy.

A recent warning from the FDA concerning heparin prophylaxis (especially enoxaparin low-molecular-weight heparin) in the presence of spinal and epidural catheters warns of epidural and spinal hematoma formation. Factors that may contribute to this problem include coagulopathy, traumatic catheter or needle insertion, repeated insertion attempts, use of continuous epidural catheters, anticoagulant dosage, concurrent administration of medications that increase bleeding, vertebral column abnormalities, older age, and female gender (23).

STANDARD THERAPY FOR VENOUS THROMBOEMBOLISM

The primary treatment of venous thromboembolism is systemic anticoagulation, which reduces the risk of pulmonary embolism and the extension and recurrence of venous thrombosis (Fig. 29-6). Immediate systemic anticoagulation should be undertaken with heparin, as it has been shown that the recurrence rate for venous thromboembolism is approximately fourfold to sixfold higher if anticoagulation is not therapeutic in the first 24 hours (24). After adequate treatment of acute deep venous thrombosis, recurrent deep venous thrombosis may occur in one-third of patients over an 8-year period (25). Thus, these patients should always be considered at higher risk for thrombosis during environmental stresses that increase risk of venous thromboembolism (e.g., transcontinental flight, surgery), and aggressive venous thromboembolism prophylaxis should be in place at these times.

Traditionally, systemic intravenous unfractionated heparin has been undertaken for 5 days, during which time oral anticoagulation with warfarin is instituted. Because of dosing inconvenience as well as bleeding risks of unfractionated heparin, low-molecular-weight heparin has recently been advanced as primary therapy for venous thromboembolism. In summaries of multiple studies and meta-analyses, low-molecular-weight heparin is equivalent or superior to unfractionated heparin regarding thrombus recurrence, with a lower risk for major hemorrhage (26). Low-molecular-weight heparin is derived from the lower molecular weight range of standard heparin with less direct thrombin inhibition and more antifactor Xa activity. The advantages of low-molecular-weight heparin include a lower risk of bleeding, less antiplatelet activity (which also decreases the risk for bleeding), a lower incidence of heparin-induced thrombocytopenia, less interference with protein C and complement activation, and a lower risk of osteoporosis. Because low-molecular-weight heparins can be administered subcutaneously and are weight-based, they may be given in the outpatient setting and do not require frequent monitoring except in certain circumstances, such as renal failure and morbid obesity (27).

Warfarin should be started only after heparinization is therapeutic to prevent the rare complication of warfarin-induced skin necrosis. The goal for warfarin dosing is an international normalized ratio (INR) between 2.0 to 3.0. The recommended duration of anticoagulation after a first episode of venous thromboembolism is 3 to 6 months (28). After a second episode of venous thromboembolism, the usual recommendation is lifelong warfarin unless the patient is very young at the time of presentation or there are other mitigating factors.

Recurrent venous thromboembolism is increased significantly in the presence of homozygous Factor V Leiden and prothrombin 20210A mutation, protein C/S deficiency, antithrombin deficiency, antiphospholipid antibodies,

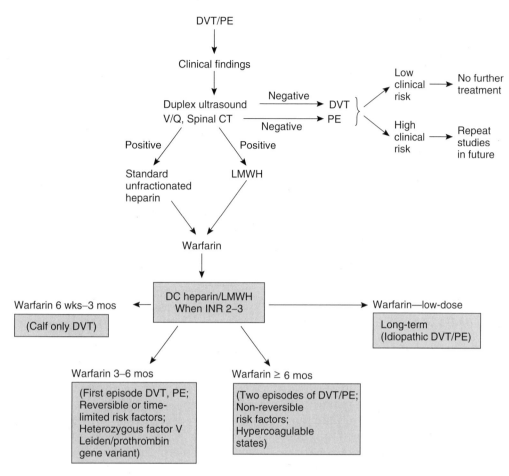

Figure 29-6 Treatment algorithm for VTE. LMWH, low-molecular-weight heparins; VTE, venous thromboembolism; PE, pulmonary embolism; DVT, deep venous thrombosis.

and cancer (3). The heterozygous Factor V Leiden/prothrombin 20210A state does not carry the same high risk of recurrence as the homozygous condition, and the period of oral anticoagulation may be shortened. Combined heterozygous deficiency states likely are additive.

Calf thrombi may be treated with 6 weeks of warfarin, while idiopathic deep venous thrombosis requires >6 months of warfarin. A recent multicenter trial has suggested that for idiopathic deep venous thrombosis, low-dose warfarin (INR 1.5 to 2.0) is superior to placebo over a 4-year follow-up period, with a 64% risk reduction for recurrent deep venous thrombosis after the completion of an initial 6 months of standard warfarin therapy (29). A second study has suggested that full-dose warfarin (INR 2.0 to 3.0) is superior to low-dose warfarin in similar patients without a difference in bleeding morbidity (30).

The most common and potentially life-threatening complication of anticoagulation is bleeding. With unfractioned heparin, the bleeding risk is approximately 10% over the first 5 days. With the addition of warfarin, and keeping the INR at 2 to 3, the incidence of major bleeding is approximately 6% per year. Specifically for deep venous thrombosis and pulmonary embolism, major bleeding has been reported in 0% to 7% of patients, with fatal bleeding in 0% to 2% of patients (23). A recent meta-analysis showed a significant rate of hemorrhagic complications, estimated at 9.1% for anticoagulation continued beyond 3 months (31). Careful dose adjustments and use of a specialized anticoagulation clinic can minimize bleeding complications.

Another major complication is heparin-induced thrombocytopenia, which occurs in 0.6% to 30% of patients in whom heparin is administered. Although historical morbidity and mortality have been high, early diagnosis and appropriate treatment have decreased these to 6% and 0%, respectively (32). Heparin-induced thrombocytopenia usually begins 3 to 14 days after heparin administration and is caused by a heparin-dependent antibody immunoglobulin G, which binds to platelets and induces them to aggregate when exposed to heparin (33). Both bovine and porcine unfractioned heparin, as well as low-molecular-weight heparin, have been associated with heparin-induced thrombocytopenia. Both arterial and venous thromboses have been reported, and even small exposures to heparin, as with the heparin coating on indwelling catheters or tubing, have been known to cause the syndrome (34). The diagnosis should be suspected in a patient who experiences a 50%

drop in platelet count or when there is a fall in platelet count below 100,000/μL during heparin therapy or in any patient who experiences thrombosis during heparin administration (2,35).

An enzyme-linked immunosorbent assay detects anti-heparin antibody in plasma and is now the test of choice. Cessation of heparin is the most important step. Warfarin is contraindicated in this condition until an adequate alternative anticoagulant has been established. Low-molecular-weight heparins (enoxaparin and dalteparin) have high cross-reactivity with standard heparin antibodies on the serotonin release assay and, therefore, should not be substituted for standard heparin in patients with heparin-induced thrombocytopenia. The direct thrombin inhibitors hirudin (Lepirudin/Refludan) and argatroban are the alternatives of choice (36). These agents show no cross-reactivity to heparin antibodies.

ALTERNATIVE AND FUTURE TREATMENTS

Two new therapeutic agents have demonstrated significant promise of greater efficacy with less bleeding risk in both venous thromboembolism prophylaxis and treatment. These include a direct thrombin inhibitor and a specific factor Xa inhibitor (Fig. 29-7). The direct thrombin inhibitor, ximelagatran/melagatran, has shown considerable efficacy for both prophylaxis and treatment of deep

venous thrombosis. This drug can be taken orally and may become an alternative to warfarin without the need for the same monitoring as warfarin and with no increase in bleeding potential. In a large prospective study comparing oral ximelagatran, which is metabolized to the active melagatran, to placebo, the recurrent deep venous thrombosis and pulmonary embolism rate was reduced from approximately 12% to 2% (37). However, this drug causes liver function elevations in approximately 6% of cases.

The specific factor Xa inhibitor pentasaccharide (Fondaparinux) has also shown significant promise for both the prophylaxis and treatment of deep venous thrombosis. This drug potentiates by approximately 300 times the neutralization of factor Xa by antithrombin without inactivating thrombin. In orthopedic surgical patients this agent has shown superiority to low-molecular-weight heparin with both acute and more chronic usage.

Large prospective randomized studies for both deep venous thrombosis and pulmonary embolism treatment have been conducted (38). For deep venous thrombosis, in a study with 2,205 patients (>30% outpatients) the rate of recurrent deep venous thrombosis or major hemorrhage was 3.9% and 1.1% for pentasaccharide compared to low-molecular-weight-heparin (4.1% and 1.2%, respectively). For pulmonary embolism, a study with 2,213 patients (with >15% outpatients) showed that the rate of recurrent pulmonary embolism or major hemorrhage was 3.8% and 1.3% for pentasaccharide compared to 5% and 1.1%, respectively, for unfractioned heparin. Mortality rates were equal.

TABLE 29-4

ALTERNATIVE AGENTS FOR ANTICOAGULATION

Drug	Mechanism of Action
Oral heparins SNAC-UFH SNAD-LMWH	Heparin is bound noncovalently to carrier proteins enabling passage through GI mucosa
Direct thrombin inhibitors Recombinant hirudin and analogues Desirudin Lepirudin Bivalirudin Argatroban H376/95 (melagatran)	Binds to thrombin and inhibits its activity directly without need for cofactors (e.g., antithrombin III); melagatran administered orally, while other agents are given intravenously
Ancrod (defibrination agent)	Serine protease that cleaves fibrinopeptide A from fibrinogen, resulting in less stable fibrin clot more easily degraded by plasmin
P-selectin inhibitors (rPSGL-Ig)	Decreases amplification of thrombosis by reducing leukocyte-platelet interactions
Factor VIIa inhibitors	Competes with factor VIIa-TF complex
Tissue-factor pathway inhibitor	Inhibits the factor VIIa-TF complex
Activated Protein C tPA	Inactivates factors Va and VIIIa, as well as inhibitors of
Fondaparinux (synthetic pentasaccharide)	Inhibits factor Xa without inhibiting thrombin

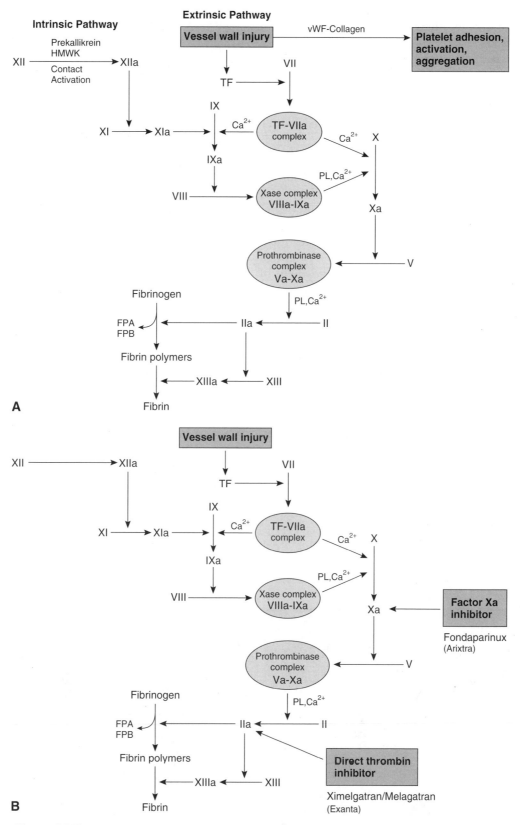

Figure 29-7 Coagulation pathway **(A)** and location of action of direct thrombin inhibitor and specific factor Xa inhibitor **(B)**.

Other novel agents are in various stages of development, such as oral heparin and oral low-molecular-weight heparin, ancrod, P-selectin inhibitors, Factor VIIa inhibitors, tissue-factor pathway inhibitors, and activated protein C (Table 29-4). Pharmacologic reversal once a patient is therapeutic on these agents will need to be defined before their widespread use in surgical and critically ill patients.

VENA CAVA FILTERS

Vena cava filters are used to prevent pulmonary embolism, with an average efficacy of >95% (20,22,39–41). Well accepted indications for filter placement include contraindication to anticoagulation, complications of anticoagulation, failure of anticoagulation, and as treatment after pulmonary embolectomy (Table 29-5). Although clinical evidence is limited, prophylactic placement of inferior vena cava (IVC) filters is commonly performed for high-risk trauma patients, for patients with poorly adherent free-floating thrombi (Fig. 29-8), for patients with malignancy at risk of hemorrhage if anticoagulated, and for elderly patients with isolated long bone fractures. Filter designs currently approved for permanent insertion include the Greenfield filter, the Simon-Nitinol filter, the Vena Tech filter, the Trap-Ease filter, and the bird's nest and Günther Tulip filters. The filter design with the longest and widest patient follow-up is the Greenfield filter (22,39). It is recommended that prospective registries be used to track any mechanical device for patient safety, efficacy, and complications, since randomized prospective studies comparing different filter designs are unlikely to be conducted.

Filter complications are categorized as periprocedural, early device-related, and long-term device-related (41,42) (Table 29-5). Periprocedural complications include bleeding, pulmonary embolism at the time of filter deployment (43), device-specific misplacement, or inability to insert the

TABLE 29-5

VENA CAVA FILTER PLACEMENT INDICATIONS AND COMPLICATIONS

Indications	Complications
Contraindication to anticoagulation Complication of anticoagulation Failure of anticoagulation	Placement —Site bleed/thrombosis —Malposition —Pulmonary embolism —Guidewire entrapment
	Device —Migration —Occlusion —1° failure
	Late —Strut fracture —Penetration —Wire ensnarement (other procedure) —1° failure

device. The most common complication is bleeding, but cessation of heparin around the time of insertion can lessen this risk. As the venous system is generally low pressure, the risk of bleeding is not high relative to arterial puncture. The use of gentle firm pressure with sheath removal is important. Periprocedural pulmonary embolism may occur if the filter is deployed through a thrombus (44). Duplex assessment of distal iliac vein thrombus involvement and cavography to assess iliac vein patency can minimize this complication. Conversely, many filters can be placed through jugular or upper arm veins as the delivery systems are now lower profile, with 6 to 12 French outer diameters.

Early device-related complications usually involve filter deployment. As user experience has increased, failure to

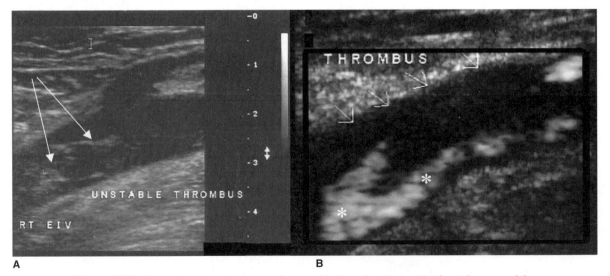

Figure 29-8 By duplex ultrasound, note the unstable thrombus (*arrows*) in the right external iliac vein in which the thrombus is loosely adherent. The thrombus is noted using gray scale **(A)** and using duplex sonography **(B)**. The flow channel is indicated by the stars.

deploy the filter has become very uncommon. Vena cava filters are generally placed at the level of L2/L3 for inferior vena cava placement and T12-L1 for suprarenal filter placement. Misplacement of the filter may occur if cavography or ultrasound imaging is not used. For example, there is a >20-fold increased risk of misplacement if only external bony landmarks are employed (22). Alternative imaging with intravascular and transabdominal ultrasound may be used in the critically ill or massively obese. If misplacement is evident and the filter's efficacy is thought to be compromised, the decision whether or not to place a more proximal filter needs to be made on an individual basis. No increase in direct thrombotic complications has been observed in patients with two filters (45).

Long-term device-related complications, including filter migration, are less common than previously thought, as respiratory variation may account for as much as 20 mm of movement as depicted on plain abdominal x-rays taken at different time points. Current rates of migration of >20 mm rates are 9% to 11% (41). A large vena cava (>28 mm diameter) needs to be imaged before the filter is placed, and either bilateral iliac venous filters or a bird's nest IVC filter should be used. Excessive filter tilt is another potential complication. This may occur with strut deployment into a vessel orifice or misplacement of the sheath device at the time of placement. Some reports have suggested that increased filter tilt may decrease the effectiveness of the filter for trapping pulmonary embolism, but little objective data support this contention unless the tilt is >15% off axial midline (21).

Device failure, defined as recurrent pulmonary embolism despite a technically good placement, may occur in 2% to 5% of patients (22,40,45). One way to decrease this risk is to have the patient concurrently anticoagulated if the patient has a particularly malignant form of hypercoagulability and if there are no contraindications to anticoagulation. For example, if the patient has a limited contraindication to anticoagulation for which the filter is placed but a persistent risk of venous thromboembolism, anticoagulation in the setting of a filter may be indicated. If this is not an option, the patient may have a suprarenal Greenfield filter placed. Suprarenal filter placement indications include a failed infrarenal filter, a patient who is pregnant and requires filter placement but cannot be anticoagulated, and a patient with an extensive IVC thrombus for whom the thrombus tail obstructs where the infrarenal filter would normally be placed. Generally, this location carries no greater complication rate than the infrarenal location. In a series of 124 consecutive patients with suprarenal Greenfield filters, no renal failure secondary to renal vein thrombosis was documented (46). In patients with malignancy the risk of thrombotic renal vein occlusion may be higher (47).

Inferior vena cava occlusion after filter placement is a dreaded complication that may occur in the early or late setting and may lead to phlegmasia cerulea dolens in up to 24% of patients who are unable to be anticoagulated (48). Various rates of IVC occlusion have been documented with all filter types and may be highest with the bird's nest filter or the Trap-Ease-type filter (49–51). The lack of prospective randomized trials with regard to specific filter type, particularly in the long term, limits data about IVC occlusion rates. The best information comes from the Greenfield database, with approximately 3,200 patients over 27 years, showing an overall IVC occlusion rate of approximately 2% to 4% (39,45). Filter occlusion may be caused by the filter performing its function by trapping a massive pulmonary embolism or as a complication of the filter causing a new inferior vena cava thrombosis.

When an inferior vena cava occludes acutely, the patient may become hypotensive. It is important to differentiate an acute massive pulmonary embolism (filter failure) in a patient with a patent inferior vena cava from an occluded inferior vena cava and normal pulmonary artery. This distinction can be made by bedside detection of jugular venous distention. If distension is evident, it is likely the patient has right heart failure and thrombolytics and vasopressor agents may be appropriate (41). However, if the patient has intravascular volume depletion due to an occluded IVC, large volume resuscitation is mandatory. Any patient with an inferior vena cava filter who develops sudden lower extremity edema needs an urgent caval duplex examination, and, if technically unsatisfactory, a cavogram.

Several strategies are available to treat inferior vena cava occlusion. For an acute thrombus, full anticoagulation with heparin followed by catheter-directed thrombolysis may alleviate the problem. If the thrombus is older, catheter suction embolectomy and dissolution by a mechanical thrombus fragmentation device may be performed (52,53). If occlusion is recent, one may place a protective suprarenal filter and then navigate in the peri-filter plane to recanalize the inferior vena cava, using a Gianturco stent to push the filter against the IVC wall (54). If the symptoms are recent, thrombolytic therapy can be performed.

Chronic occlusions with minimal symptoms should be managed expectantly. If the filter becomes full of thrombus, its effectiveness for trapping pulmonary embolism is markedly reduced and a suprarenal filter needs to be placed, as pulmonary embolism may occur in up to 33% of patients (55).

Temporary and retrievable filters have been used with some success in countries outside the United States. The concept that a filter can be placed for a defined period of time and then retrieved percutaneously to avoid potential long-term complications is appealing for young, temporarily high venous thromboembolism risk patients. Two retrievable types of filters have been reported—the Günther Tulip and the Recovery Nitinol filter. Evidence of their efficacy is promising, but so far only small patient numbers and short follow-ups have been reported (56,57). Retrieval complications have so far been few. However, the need for a permanent filter later is common (56).

Prophylactic inferior vena cava filters that are placed for patients at high risk for venous thromboembolism, such as those with major trauma, have low immediate complication rates, and long-term deep venous thrombosis has been documented in up to 44% (58,59). Whether this high deep venous thrombosis rate would have occurred without filter placement is unknown. Long-term morbidity after prophylactic IVC filter placement is usually due to development of deep venous thrombosis and subsequent chronic venous insufficiency (60). In one series of pediatric patients who had filters placed for prophylaxis from 19 months to 14 years (61), pulmonary embolism, inferior vena caval thrombosis, or migration was documented.

Less common filter complications include ensnared guide wires, either at the time of placement (more common with a jugular approach) or at a remote time, with a wire for another procedure or device (e.g., central venous access) (42,62). The J-wire can become caught by the strut apex fixation. Standard endovascular techniques using snares and catheters to straighten the J-wire allow disengagement. If a wire is placed for venous access and the operator is unaware that a filter is present, significant problems may occur if the wire cannot be pulled out. It is incumbent on the operator to remove the wire carefully, and if retrieval is not easy, fluoroscopy is used to identify where the wire is ensnared. If guidewires are removed forcefully, the filter may fracture and end up in the heart.

Filter strut fracture may be demonstrated at late follow-up by duplex ultrasonography or by CT scan. Fracture rarely causes a complication, as the struts and the device are well incorporated via attachment sites. Strut fracture is more common in the suprarenal location as greater vena cava motion occurs in this area. Penetration of hooks into the aorta or small bowel has been documented but rarely has clinical consequences. Retroperitoneal hemorrhage has been documented (63). Renal penetration with resultant hydronephrosis and small bowel obstruction have been documented by case reports only (64–66). Intracardiac migration of a filter is rare (<0.1%) and usually necessitates either an open surgical procedure or a catheter-based procedure with a snare to remove the filter (67).

THROMBOLYTIC AND SURGICAL PROCEDURES FOR DEEP VENOUS THROMBOSIS AND PULMONARY EMBOLISM

Systemic thrombolytic therapy was initially investigated for use in acute deep venous thrombosis in the late 1970s and 1980s, with little data to support its use over standard heparinization, despite more complete thrombus resolution (68). The lack of benefit was primarily because of significantly increased risks of bleeding. Recently, better patient selection with catheter-directed venous thrombolysis shows promise for extensive lower extremity deep venous thrombosis allowing faster thrombus resolution with decreased bleeding risks and a decreased incidence of late post-thrombotic syndrome (69,70). Early thrombolysis

in massive iliofemoral deep venous thrombosis is effective, especially if thrombi are <7 days old (71–73). Postlytic venous patency over 2-year follow-up approximates 60% to 85% (73).

The use of thrombolytic therapy for pulmonary embolism is effective in selected patients. Thrombolysis has been shown to decrease right ventricular injury and strain and, in longer-term follow-up, to decrease the pulmonary hypertension and perfusion deficits that may persist after standard heparin anticoagulation for massive pulmonary embolism (74,75). Intravascular catheter-directed thrombolysis may be safer than systemic bolus administration for pulmonary embolism, although data are limited (76).

Numerous trials of thrombolysis for venous thromboembolism have confirmed that the primary complication is bleeding. The most important consideration of thrombolytic therapy for patients with venous thromboembolism is to balance the significant bleeding risk against the benefit of hastened thrombus resolution. Rates of bleeding have ranged up to 30% with fatalities in 1% to 2%. Bleeding risk is increased threefold with thrombolysis as compared to heparin alone. Both tissue plasminogen activator and urokinase plasminogen activator have been used with similar efficacy and risk. Analysis of pulmonary embolism trials with various dosing and delivery strategies of thrombolytic agents demonstrates significant bleeding complications in the range of 25%. This figure is lessened if one considers only fatal hemorrhage or bleeding necessitating surgery or transfusion and is in the range of approximately 8% to 10% (74). Intracranial hemorrhage is the most feared complication of thrombolysis, with a rate of ~1.2%, and approximately 50% of these patients do not leave the hospital after hemorrhagic stroke (77). Risk factors for intracranial hemorrhage include older age, female gender, history of neurological trauma, and elevated diastolic blood pressure.

Strategies to reduce bleeding complications include minimizing secondary invasive catheter procedures, minimizing the thrombolytic dose for effect, and careful monitoring of heparin and fibrinogen levels. Ultrasound-guided needle cannulation of the femoral or jugular vein may also decrease postlytic vessel bleeding. Adjuncts such as GpIIb/IIIa antagonists (e.g., aciximab) have been successful in decreasing the overall dose of lytic therapy in the arterial system, as well as in hastening arterial thrombosis dissolution, but they have not been tested in the venous circulation. Standard therapies for excessive bleeding include protamine to reverse heparin effect. In patients with a hemodynamically significant pulmonary embolism, it is recommended that intravenous heparin be used, as this can be readily stopped and protamine can be administered if significant bleeding occurs. Low-molecular-weight heparin has a longer half-life, and full reversal may not be possible. Cryoprecipitate or fresh frozen plasma may be required to provide clotting factors and fibrinogen in cases of severe hemorrhage. Prevention is also key. Standard contraindications to lytic therapy include recent surgery, trauma, and ongoing bleeding.

Secondary pulmonary embolism is very rare with thrombolysis of iliofemoral deep venous thrombosis, occurring in <1% of cases (72,74). Rethrombosis of the iliocaval segment may occur if the patient is not adequately anticoagulated or has poor venous inflow. After iliac vein thrombolysis, construction of an arterio-venous fistula may be useful, though no comparative trials exist.

Pulmonary embolectomy for massive pulmonary embolism has fallen into disfavor over the last decade, although a recent series has shown an 80% survival with carefully selected patients undergoing prompt treatment (78). The authors emphasize that patients who have had a prehospital arrest and those older than 80 should not be considered for this surgery. Placement of an IVC filter is advocated for everyone at the time of embolectomy to reduce the risk of early recurrent fatal pulmonary embolism (Table 29-5). Fatal postembolectomy pulmonary hemorrhage accounts for most deaths. A transvenous percutaneous suction catheter technique is also useful for large pulmonary embolism if attempted acutely (79), but with the advent of mechanical thrombolysis devices it is not commonly used.

Open catheter iliofemoral venous embolectomy is not widely performed, given perceived morbidity and no well-confirmed benefit over anticoagulation. One randomized prospective study suggested less long-term morbidity from venous hypertension and post-thrombotic syndrome (80,81). There are no data comparing the efficacy of catheter-directed thrombolysis against open thrombectomy, but in the authors' opinion the fewer invasive catheter-based technique is as efficacious with less procedural risks. Ways to decrease postembolectomy rethrombosis include use of a groin arterio-venous fistula, decompressive fasciotomy, and only performing this procedure for deep venous thrombosis <7 days old (80,82,83). This procedure has a high venous rethrombosis rate, which is likely due to endothelial damage at the time of surgery. Wound hematomas are common and necessitate removal to decrease local compression and infectious potential. Other risks include those associated with groin exposure, including nerve injury and lymph leaks. Another caveat for open thromboembolectomy is that when the catheter is advanced proximally into the iliac vein, the anesthesiologist should add 20 to 30 mm Hg positive ventilator pressure to maintain venous pressure to decrease the risk of air embolism. The use of a rotational thrombectomy device may also be useful in this setting, comparable to open embolectomy, although patient numbers are small (84).

Catheter-directed thrombolysis is well accepted for axillary and subclavian venous thrombosis, particularly effort thrombosis in young patients (70). More rapid thrombolysis decreases long-term risk of swelling and dependence of venous collateralization for outflow (85). Subclavian vein angioplasty and stenting for exertional axillary-subclavian venous thrombosis have been reported (86). However, the stents may crimp, migrate, or erode through the vein, given

upper shoulder outlet motion. A thoracic outlet decompression procedure is efficacious, as thoracic outlet compression most often causes the underlying venous stenosis. It is important that the patient undergoes positional phlebography if the axillary/subclavian axis is patent to confirm extrinsic compression of the axillary and subclavian veins at the thoracic outlet. Generally, thoracic outlet decompression follows thrombolysis. Operative timing, whether immediate or after a delay to allow for the vein wall inflammatory response to subside, is controversial. In cases of secondary axillary/subclavian deep venous thrombosis due to indwelling catheters, anticoagulation along with removal of the catheter is indicated. The duration of anticoagulation should be individualized, reflecting the patient's thrombotic risk—usually <3 months.

Patch venoplasty is also recommended if persistent venous narrowing is present after thoracic outlet decompression. The main complications of thoracic outlet decompression are bleeding, lymphatic leak, infection, recurrent thrombosis, and brachial plexus nerve injury (87).

VENOUS VARICOSITIES

Most venous varicosities are tributaries of the greater or lesser saphenous venous systems. The overall incidence ranges from 18% to 52% of selected populations and close to 7% in the general population, with women more commonly affected than men (88,89). The pathophysiology of venous varicosities is a combination of superficial venous insufficiency at either the popliteal/lesser saphenous junction or the femoral/greater saphenous junction (90). Medial venous perforator incompetence also plays a role. Although venous hypertension was once thought to be the primary etiology of venous varicosities, it is now believed that development of varicositis is due to congenitally weak venous valves that dilate over time. In patients with venous varicosities, <25% have documented duplex reflux or other evidence of deep venous insufficiency. Primary thrombotic complications of varicose veins are quite unusual. A known complication of venous varicosities is ulceration, although this is fairly unusual in the setting solely of superficial venous incompetence. Most patients with ulcers related to varicose veins have had varicosities for >10 years with incompetent perforators (91). Standard nonoperative therapy includes stocking compression, elevation, and good skin care.

Phlebectomy has been performed for more than a millennium. Standard indications include pain, swelling, ulceration, bleeding, and cosmetic purposes (92,93). The technique is very safe and can be done under regional anesthesia, and cosmesis is very good (92,94). Sclerotherapy with hypertonic saline or detergent for spider angiomata and small varicosities (<2 mm) is also standard therapy that achieves very good results (95). Sclerotherapy causes an intraluminal fibrotic response but does not cause thrombophlebitis (96). Contraindications to phlebectomy include active cellulitis, acute deep venous thrombosis, and severe comorbid disease.

The primary complication of sclerotherapy is extravasation of the sclerosant, which can be minimized by careful technique under loupe magnification using a 30-gauge microsurgical needle. If extravasation occurs in the dermis, rapid dilution with a 10-fold volume of sterile normal saline is indicated (97). Skin breakdown and pain may result, but severe cosmetic problems are rare. Most commonly, transient pigmentation and neovascularity in the area of the varicosity occurs in approximately 3% to 4% of cases (98). Blisters and cellulitis may also occur with an incidence of approximately 1% (99). Deep perforator sclerotherapy can result in intra-arterial injection, leading to arterial thrombosis and cutaneous tissue neurosis. If this complication does occur, full heparinization and vasodilation may decrease tissue damage (97). Deep venous thrombosis after sclerotherapy occurs with a <0.01% incidence (not significantly increased over the general population) and compares to 0.2% to 0.4% deep venous thrombosis rate after open phlebectomy (97,98). Both phlebectomy and sclerotherapy have similar return to full activity (~72 hours) and postprocedure impairment.

The complications of open phlebectomy are mostly minor and non-life-threatening. Infection is very rare. An antiseptic leg and groin wash twice the night before surgery is recommended. There is no need for systemic antibiotic prophyaxis. Hematoma and lymphocele occur in <0.5% of cases. Avoiding dissection of the anterior tibial dorsal veins decreases lymphocele formation (98). To decrease the risk of perioperative hematoma, it is important to obtain a careful history of the patient's medications, including herbal supplements, high-dose vitamin E, aspirin, or other anticoagulants, as these may potentiate a hematoma due to venous oozing. Generally, venous hematomas resolve spontaneously and do not require additional surgical therapy or transfusion. Use of a tourniquet may decrease bleeding associated with varicosity excision (100).

As an office procedure, venous varicosity excision has been performed using tumescent anesthesia where a dilute amount of low-concentration lidocaine (0.5%) with very dilute epinephrine (1:1,000,000) allows for a large area to be anesthetized. Earlier return to usual activities may be an additional benefit (101).

Peripheral nerve injury is the most common complication of open phlebectomy, with approximately 40% to 50% of patients having some hypesthesia in the area of the incisions, usually within the greater saphenous nerve distribution (97,102). Permanent nerve injury occurs approximately 1% of the time. With calf vein excision in the lesser saphenous distribution, the sural nerve is at greatest risk.

Recurrence of venous varicosities is also a known complication, and some surgeons consider this part of the natural history. Recurrence of venous varicosities is thought to occur by recruitment of collaterals or recanalization of the obliterated vein. To avoid this complication, it is important preoperatively to have the patient stand and to mark all the veins to avoid missing any varicosities that disappear once the patient is recumbent. Duplex-directed varicose excision may also decrease incision number and decrease varicosity recurrence by directing excision and ligation of incompetent perforators (94).

Treatment for primary superficial thrombophlebitis begins with a venous duplex ultrasound scan to evaluate for deep venous thrombosis (7) (Table 29-6). The most important factor to decrease secondary suppurative superficial thrombophlebitis is to limit intravenous peripheral catheters to 48 to 72 hours per site. Treatment consists of catheter removal, warm compresses, elevation, and antibiotics if cellulitis exists. If purulent discharge, bacteremia, or sepsis occur, complete excision of the affected venous segment with open packing is necessary.

Superficial vein thrombophlebitis may also occur after varicosity excision or sclerotherapy (96,97). A short course of low-molecular-weight heparin for 10 to 14 days, in addition to local warm compresses, may be beneficial in decreasing pain and hastening thrombosis resolution. Long-term anticoagulation is not indicated, as the risks of warfarin outweigh the benefits. Other rare complications include pulmonary embolism with a high ligation and sclerotherapy (103) and tibial arterial injury due to the stripping device.

A controversial area in varicosity management is whether or not to strip the entire greater saphenous vein versus performing a limited saphenofemoral disconnection (104). It is the authors' practice to preserve the greater saphenous vein if it is not dilated and to perform saphenofemoral or saphenopopliteal disconnection on a case-by-case basis, directed by duplex-detected reflux. This strategy allows salvage of the greater saphenous vein if needed for other purposes, and spares the patient some risk of greater saphenous nerve injury. However, with significant saphenous vein insufficiency, stripping improves results as compared to high ligation (105).

Newer devices such as powered catheter phlebectomy, as well as laser and radio frequency ablation devices, are now on the market, but long-term follow-up is not yet available (101,105–107). Though early, there is evidence that there is less pain and perhaps earlier return to work than with a standard saphenous stripping. There is a learning curve, and cutaneous thermal injury is a potential complication that is not present with other surgical techniques.

CHRONIC VENOUS INSUFFICIENCY

Chronic venous insufficiency affects women much more commonly than men, with a ratio of ten to one (108). The progression of disease related to venous hypertension is, on average, 13 years, and leg varicosities are the most common presentation, followed by edema and heaviness.

TABLE 29-6

TREATMENT OPTIONS FOR SUPERFICIAL THROMBOPHLEBITIS

Suppurative SVT
Secondary to intravenous catheter placement;
The best treatment is prevention—removing intravenous catheters within 48 to 72 h;
Treat with catheter removal, warm compresses, elevation; if cellulitis, add antibiotics;
If purulent discharge is noted with bacteremia or sepsis, excise the entire segment.

Unexpected SVT
Complete duplex scanning of the deep and superficial venous systems to rule out concomitant DVT should be obtained;
Hypercoagulable work-up should be considered in patients;
  without a history of: associated trauma or inactivity, venipuncture, malignancy, varicose veins; and
  with severe thrombophlebitis, recurrence, family history, early age at presentation and resistance to therapy;
Treatment as discussed below.

Above-knee superficial venous thrombosis associated with or without varicose veins
Obtain bilateral duplex examination;
If the superficial venous thrombosis is located above the knee but is not approaching the saphenofemoral junction, then medical therapy
  with heat, elevation, elastic compression stockings, and NSAIDs can be employed, although close follow-up and repeat duplex
  scanning within 1 wk is recommended;
If a superimposed cellulitis develops, antibiotics should be added;
If bleeding occurs secondary to erosion through the skin, direct pressure to stop bleeding and surgical excision at a later time should be
  performed;
If the superficial venous thrombosis approaches the saphenofemoral junction, anticoagulant therapy should be considered for 6 wk
  to 3 mo;
If the saphenofemoral junction is involved or there is evidence of DVT, anticoagulation for 3–6 mo is recommended;
If there is a contraindication to anticoagulation or in the presence of severe pain, flush ligation at the saphenofemoral junction and stripping
  of the phlebitic vein should be performed;
If PE is documented, anticoagulation for 6 mo is recommended.

SVT, superficial venous thrombosis; DVT, deep venous thrombosis; NSAIDs, nonsteroidal anti-inflammatory drugs; PE, pulmonary embolism.
From Sullivan V, Wakefield TW. Superficial venous thrombosis. In: Pearce WH, Matsumara JS, Yao JST, eds. *Trends in vascular surgery*, 2003.

However, ulceration affects up to 30% of patients and causes most of the associated morbidity (25). The pathophysiology of venous ulceration may be a chronic deep vein obstruction, related to deep venous thrombosis with failure of full resolution, or it may be related to valvular dysfunction without proximal obstruction, associated with incompetent perforators. To generalize, the results with venous reconstructive surgery for severe manifestations such as pain or persistent ulceration, or both, are better if the etiology is primary valvular dysfunction rather than for postphlebitic disease (109,110).

Standard therapy for venous stasis ulceration includes elevation, compression, and local wound care. Patient compliance is a must (111). The main complications with local venous ulcer therapy are allergic reaction to the agent used and failure of therapy due to intractable venous stasis ulceration.

A recent article using decision analysis suggested that compression stockings are cost-effective and are better than routine care for ulcer healing (112). It is important to decrease local bacterial colonization, promote a granulating wound bed, and provide an environment that allows healing. It is the authors' opinion that the Unna boot is most effective in this regard for a *noninfected* venous stasis ulcer. The wound is protected, and the constant compression of the dressing decreases venous hypertension that impairs healing. Care must be taken to place compression

dressings so that the Unna boot is firmly applied but is not so tight as to create skin breakdown. If the patient has evidence of cellulitis, systemic antibiotics are recommended. However, no evidence supports routine antibiotic use for prolonged periods, as this may increase bacterial resistance. Various wound care measures such as saline, colloid, or vacuum are also appropriate, given the individual patient. A recent prowound healing agent, Sulodexide, appears to be promising in healing ulcers relative to saline and compression (113), but whether this agent is more effective than other topical growth factor agents, such as platelet-derived growth factor, remains to be proven.

Multimodality therapy for venous stasis ulceration addresses the contribution of the perforating and superficial venous system to this problem (114). For many years the Linton procedure was the standard therapy for obliteration of venous perforators that contribute to nonhealing or recurrent venous ulcers. The technique involves an open subfascial approach with ligation of the perforating venous branches. However, wound complications are very common.

More recently, subfascial perforator surgery has been advanced (109). This technique involves remote endoscopic access to visualize and ligate the subfascial perforators. This technique allows the ulcer and surrounding skin to be free from any incisions and removes the nidus of venous hypertension communicating to the skin ulcer. A recent retrospective study showed approximately 86%

improved ulcer healing with a mean follow-up of 3 months to 1 year with a combination of subfascial perforator surgery and saphenofemoral disconnection (115). Complications were rare, with transient neurologic symptoms and an overall deep venous thrombosis incidence of <0.1%. Recurrent ulceration secondary to missed perforators can be treated with a repeat subfascial perforator surgery procedure. A review of the subfascial perforator surgery national registry showed a 2-year recurrence of ulcers in 28% (116). Failure of this procedure was significantly higher in patients who had postphlebitic etiology for venous insufficiency relative to patients with primary valvular insufficiency (117). A recent randomized prospective study failed to show any benefit over nonoperative management, except in patients with very large ulcers (118).

Less common techniques, including primary valvuloplasty and axillary vein to popliteal vein valve transplant, are selectively performed. The efficacy of these techniques is less clear, as medical evidence outside of case series is unavailable and long-term patient follow-up is scant. Primary complications are bleeding and thrombosis. Adjuncts to decrease these problems include meticulous hemostasis and periprocedural use of sequential compression devices, as well as judicious perioperative anticoagulation. Some investigators advocate the use of intravenous Dextran followed by coumadinization (119)—a safer approach than full heparin anticoagulation. Nerve injury and other injuries are quite rare. Long-term arm swelling related to axillary vein segmental removal is minimal as long as the patient has a competent cephalic vein that enters distal to the area where the vein segment with valve is removed. Preoperative arm ascending venography is essential in selecting the axillary venous segment to use and in confirming that a usable valve is present.

Surgical reconstruction of the iliofemoral veins and inferior vena cava in the setting of malignancy is accepted therapy, though not common. The risks are bleeding and thrombosis. Anticoagulants, perioperative sequential compression devices to maintain brisk venous flow, and arteriovenous fistulae are adjuncts that can be used to improve patency rates. Evidence outside of small retrospective series is lacking, and referral to a center that has expertise and experience with these cases is probably the most practical measure to ensure fewer complications. In a series of 18 patients there were no deaths and no major complications, except prolonged ileus related to the surgery itself. No anticoagulation was used, and overall clinical patency was approximately 80% (120).

Reconstruction of the IVC and iliofemoral veins for venoocclusive disease may be done in limited settings. The expectations for venous reconstruction surgery need to be realistic, as venous physiology makes these repairs much less durable than arterial reconstructions. Early graft occlusion has been reported in 20% of patients, with bleeding and infection in 12% and 7%, respectively (110). Thrombectomy was required in approximately 7% of

patients. Overall secondary patency was 54% at 3 years, and thus the procedure can be recommended in properly selected patients (121). By far the most effective procedure is a saphenous vein femorofemoral crossover bypass for chronic iliac venous obstruction. Deep vein angioplasty and stenting have promise as less invasive techniques for obstructive venous hypertension. Case series have suggested early patency rates >70% with little need for secondary procedures for occlusive complications (122). Endovascular therapies seem as efficacious as open, although combined series are small. Endovascular venoplasty and stenting appears to work much better in the iliac vein than in other locations, and it is currently the definitive approach for the patient with iliac vein compression syndrome (May-Thurner syndrome) (123).

REFERENCES

1. Heit JA, Silverstein MD, Mohr DN, et al. The epidemiology of venous thromboembolism in the community. *Thromb Haemost* 2001;86:452–463.
2. Bauer KA, Rosendaal FR, Heit JA. Hypercoaguability: too many tests, too much conflicting data. *Hematolgy* 2002;1:353–368.
3. Henke PK, Schmaier A, Wakefield TW. Thrombosis due to hypercoagulable states. In: Rutherford RB, ed. *Rutherford's textbook of vascular surgery*, 6th ed. Philadelphia, PA: Elsevier; 2004.
4. Perkins JM, Magee TR, Galland RB. Phlegmasia caerulea dolens and venous gangrene. *Br J Surg* 1996;83:19–23.
5. Prandoni P, Bernardi E. Upper extremity deep vein thrombosis. *Cur Op Pulm Med* 1999;5:222–226.
6. Quenet S, Laport S, Decousus H. et al. Factors predictive of venous thrombotic complications in patients with isolated superficial vein thrombosis. *J Vasc Surg* 2003;38:944–949.
7. Sullivan V, Wakefield TW. Superficial venous thrombosis. In: Pearce WH, Matsumara JS, Yao JST, eds. *Trends in vascular surgery*, 2003.
8. Martinelli I, Cattaneo M, Taioli E, et al. Genetic risk factors for superficial vein thrombosis. *Thromb Haemost* 1999;82:1215–1217.
9. Fowl RJ, Strothman GB, Bleabea J, et al. Inappropriate use of venous duplex scans: an analysis of indications and results. *J Vasc Surg* 1996;23:881–886.
10. Douglas MG, Sumner DS. Duplex scanning for deep vein thrombosis: has it replaced both phlebography and noninvasive testing? *Sem Vasc Surg* 1996;9:3–12.
11. Wells PS, Anderson DR, Rodger M, et.al. Evaluation of D-dimer in the diagnosis of suspected deep vein thrombosis. *N Engl J Med* 2003;349:1227–1235.
12. Schellong SM, Schwarz T, Halbritten K, et al. Complete compression ultrasonography of the leg veins as a single test for the diagnosis of DVT. *Thromb Haemost* 2003;89:228–234.
13. Pierik EGJM, Toonder IM, van Urk H, et al. Validation of duplex ultrasonography in detecting competent and incompetent perforating veins in patients with venous ulceration of the lower leg. *J Vasc Surg* 1997;26:49–52.
14. Sakurai T, Matsushita M, Nishikimi N, et al. Hemodynamic assessment of femoropopliteal venous reflux in patients with primary varicose veins. *J Vasc Surg* 1997;26:260–264.
15. Rutherford RB, Padberg FT Jr, Comerota AJ, et al. Venous severity scoring: an adjunct to venous outcome assessment. *J Vasc Surg* 2000;31:1307–1312.
16. Criado E, Farber MA, Marston WA, et al. The role of air plethysmography in the diagnosis of chronic venous insufficiency. *J Vasc Surg* 1998;27:660–670.
17. Fukuoka M, Okada M, Sugimoto T. Foot venous pressure measurement for evaluation of lower limb venous insufficiency. *J Vasc Surg* 1998;27:671–676.
18. Kucher N, Goldhaber SZ. Cardiac biomarkers for risk stratification of patients with acute pulmonary embolism. *Circulation* 2003;108:2191–2194.

19. Wakefield TW, Proctor MC. Current status of pulmonary embolism and venous thrombosis prophylaxis. *Sem Vasc Surg* 2000;13:171–181.

20. Geerts WH, Heit JA, Clagett GP, et al. Prevention of venous thromboembolism. *Chest* 2001;119:132S–175S.

21. Rogers FB, Strindberg G, Shackford SR, et al. Five-year follow-up of prophylactic venal caval filters in high risk trauma patients. *Arch Surg* 1998;133:406–411.

22. Streiff MB. Venal caval filters: a comprehensive review. *Blood* 2000;95:3669–3677.

23. Levine MN, Raskob G, Landefeld S, et al. Hemorrhagic complications of anticoagulant treatment. *Chest* 1998;114(5):511S–523S.

24. Hull RD, Raskob GE, Brant RF, et al. Relation between the time to achieve the lower limit of the APTT therapeutic range and recurrent venous thromboembolism during heparin treatment for deep vein thrombosis. *Arch Intern Med* 1997;157:2562–2568.

25. Prandoni P, Lensing AW, Cogo A, et al. The long-term clinical course of acute deep venous thrombosis. *Ann Intern Med* 1996;125:1–7.

26. van den Belt AGM, Prins MH, Lensing AWA, et al. Fixed dose subcutaneous low molecular weight heparins versus adjusted dose unfractionated heparin for venous thromboembolism. *Cochrane Peripheral Vascular Diseases Group Cochrane Database of Systematic Reviews* 1, 2003.

27. Ageno W, Turpie AG. Low-molecular-weight heparin in the treatment of pulmonary embolism. *Sem Vasc Surg* 2000;13: 189–193.

28. Hyers TM, Agnelli G, Hull RD, et al. Antithrombotic therapy for venous thromboembolic disease. *Chest* 2001;119(1):176S–193S.

29. Ridker PM, Goldhaber SZ, Danielson E, et al. Long-term, low-intensity warfarin therapy for the prevention of recurrent venous thromboembolism. *N Engl J Med* 2003;348:1425–1434.

30. Kearon C, Ginsberg JS, Kovacs MJ, et al. Comparison of low-intensity warfarin therapy with conventional-intensity warfarin therapy for long-term prevention of recurrent venous thromboembolism. *N Engl J Med* 2003;349:631–639.

31. Linkins LA, Choi PT, Douketis JD. Clinical impact of bleeding in patients taking oral anticoagulant therapy for venous thromboembolism. *Ann Intern Med* 2003;139:893–900.

32. Almeida J, Coats R, Liem TK, et al. Reduced morbidity and mortality rates of the heparin-induced thrombocytopenia syndrome. *J Vasc Surg* 1998;27:309–316.

33. Greinacher A, Michels I, Mueller-Eckhardt C. Heparin-associated thrombocytopenia: the antibody is not heparin specific. *Thromb Haemost* 1992;67:545–549.

34. Laster J, Silver D. Heparin costs: catheters and heparin-induced thrombocytopenia. *J Vasc Surg* 1988;7:667–672.

35. Alving B. How I treat heparin-induced thrombocytopenia and thrombosis. *Blood* 2001;101:1–14.

36. Greinacher A, Volpel H, Janssens U, et al. Recombinant hirudin (Lepirudin) provides safe and effective anticoagulation in patients with heparin-induced thrombocytopenia. *Circulation* 1999;99:73–80.

37. Schulman S, Wahlander K, Lundstrom T, et al. Secondary prevention of venous thromboembolism with the oral direct thrombin inhibitor ximelagatran. *N Eng J Med* 2003;349:1713–1721.

38. Matisse investigators. The Matisse-DVT and PE trials. *Thromb Haemost* 2003;1(Suppl 1) July: abstracts OC331, OC332.

39. Greenfield LJ, Proctor MC. Vena caval filters for the prevention of pulmonary embolism. *N Engl J Med* 1998;339:47–48.

40. Ferris EJ, McCowan TC, Carver DK, et al. Percutaneous inferior vena caval filters: follow-up of seven designs in 320 patients. *Radiology* 1993;188:851–856.

41. Greenfield LJ, Proctor MC. Filter complications and their management. *Sem Vasc Surg* 2000;13:213–216.

42. Joels CS, Sing RF, Heniford BT. Complications of inferior vena caval filters. *Am Surg* 2003;69:654–659.

43. Promisloff RA. Pulmonary embolism after insertion of a Greenfield filter. *JAOA* 2002;102:558–560.

44. Kinney TB, Rose SC, Lim GW, et al. Fatal paradoxic embolism occurring during IVC filter insertion in a patient with chronic pulmonary embolism. *JVIR* 2001;12:770–772.

45. Greenfield LJ, Proctor MC. Recurrent thromboembolism in patients with venal caval filters. *J Vasc Surg* 2001;33:510–514.

46. Henke PK, Varma MH, Procter MC, et al. Suprarenal Greenfield filter placement: the Ann Arbor experience. In: Yao JT, Pearce WH, eds. *Modern trends in vascular surgery*, 2000.

47. Marcy PY, Magne N, Frenay M, et al. Renal failure secondary to thrombotic complications of suprarenal inferior vena cava filter in cancer patients. *Cardiovasc Interv Radiol* 2001;24:257–259.

48. Harris EJ Jr, Kinney EV, Harris EJ Sr, et al. Phlegmasia complicating percutaneous inferior vena caval interruption: a word of caution. *J Vasc Surg* 1995;22:606–611.

49. Thomas JH, Cornell KM, Siegel EL, et al. Vena caval occlusion after bird's nest filter placement. *Am J Surg* 1998;176:598–600.

50. The FDA Website, Center for Devices and Radiological Health. MAUDE database. *www.fda.gov* 2003.

51. Schutzer R, Ascher E, Hingorani A, et al. Preliminary results of the new 6F TrapEase inferior vena cava filter. *Ann Vasc Surg* 2003;17:103–106.

52. Reekers JA. Current practice of temporary venal caval filter insertion: a multicenter registry. *JVIR* 2000;13:1363–1364.

53. Poon W, Luk SH, Yam KY, et al. Mechanical thrombectomy in inferior vena cava thrombosis after caval filter placement: a report of three cases. *Cardiovasc Inter Radiol* 2002;25:440–443.

54. Joshi A, Carr J, Chrisman H, et al. Filter-related, thrombotic occlusion of the inferior vena cava treated with a Gianturco stent. *JVIR* 2003;14:381–385.

55. Tardy B, Mismetti P, Page Y, et al. Inferior vena caval thrombosis: clinical study of 30 consecutive cases. *Eur Resp J* 1996;9: 2012–2016.

56. Wicky S, Doenz F, Meuwly JY, et al. Clinical experience with retrievable Gunther Tulip vena cava filters. *J Endovasc Ther* 2003;10:994–1000.

57. Asch MR. Initial experience in humans with a new retrievable inferior vena cava filter. *Radiology* 2002;225:835–844.

58. Wojcik R, Cipolle MD, Fearen I, et al. Long-term follow-up of trauma patients with a venal caval filter. *J Trauma* 2000;49: 839–843.

59. Greenfield LJ, Proctor MC, Michaels AJ, et al. Prophylactic vena caval filters in trauma: the rest of the story. *J Vasc Surg* 2000; 32:490–497.

60. Patton JH Jr, Fabian TC, Croce MA, et al. Prophylactic Greenfield filters: acute complications and long-term follow-up. *J Trauma* 1996;41:231–237.

61. Cahn MD, Rohrer MJ, Martella MB, et al. Long-term follow-up of a Greenfield inferior vena caval filter placement in children. *J Vasc Surg* 2001;34:820–825.

62. Dardik A, Campbell KA, Yeo CJ, et al. Vena caval filter ensnarement and delayed migration: an unusual series of cases. *J Vasc Surg* 1997;26:869–874.

63. Woodward EB, Farber A, Wagner WH, et al. Delayed retroperitoneal arterial hemorrhage after inferior vena caval filter insertion: case report and literature review of caval perforations by IVC filters. *Ann Vasc Surg* 2002;16:193–196.

64. Raghavan S, Akhtar A, Bastani B. Migration of inferior vena cava filter into renal hilum. *Nephron* 2002;91:333–335.

65. Porcellini M, Stassano P, Musumeci A, et al. Intracardiac migration of nitinol TrapEase venal caval filter and paradoxical embolism. *Eur J Card Surg* 2002;22:460–461.

66. Slappy ALJ, Kennedy RJ, Hakaim Parra RO, et al. Delayed transcaval renal penetration of a Greenfield filter presenting as symptomatic hydronephrosis. *J Urol* 2002;167:1778–1779.

67. Loehr SP, Hamilton C, Dyer R. Retrieval of entrapped guide wire in an IVC filter facilitated with use of a myocardial biopsy forceps and snare device. *JVIR* 2001;12:1116–1118.

68. Arcasoy SM, Vachani A. Local and systemic thrombolytic therapy for acute venous thromboembolism. *Clin Chest Med* 2003;24: 73–91.

69. Comerota AJ. Quality-of-life improvement using thrombolytic therapy for iliofemoral deep vein thrombosis. *Rev Cardiovasc Med* 2002;3:S61–S67.

70. Meissner MH. Thrombolytic therapy for acute deep vein thrombosis and the venous registry. *Rev Cardiovasc Med* 2002;3: S53–S60.

71. Semba CP, Dake MD. Iliofemoral deep vein thrombosis: aggressive therapy with catheter-directed thrombolysis. *Radiology* 1994;191:487–494.

72. Mewissen MW. Catheter-directed thrombolysis for lower extremity deep vein thrombosis. *Tech Vasc Intvent Radiol* 2001;4:111–114.

73. Bjarnason H, Kruse JR, Asinger DA, et al. Iliofemoral deep vein thrombosis: safety and efficacy outcome during 5 years of catheter-directed thrombolytic therapy. *JVIR* 1997;8:405–418.

74. Goldhaber SZ. Thrombolytic therapy in venous thromboembolism. *Clin Chest Med* 1995;16:307–320.

75. Konstantinides S, Geibel A, Heusel G, et al. Heparin plus alteplase compared with heparin alone in patients with submassive pulmonary embolism. *N Engl J Med* 2002;347:1143–1150.

76. Comerota AJ, Aldridge SC, Cohen G, et al. A strategy of aggressive regional therapy for acute iliofemoral venous thrombosis with contemporary venous thrombectomy or catheter-directed thrombolysis. *J Vasc Surg* 1994;20:244–254.

77. Levine MN, Goldhaber SZ, Califf RM, et al. Hemorrhagic complications of thrombolytic therapy in the treatment of myocardial infarction and venous thromboembolism. *Chest* 1992;102: 365S–373S.

78. Aklog L, Williams CS, Byrne JG, et al. Acute pulmonary embolectomy: a contemporary approach. *Circulation* 2002;105:1416–1419.

79. Greenfield LJ, Peyton R, Brown PP, et al. Transvenous management of pulmonary embolic disease. *Am Surg* 1974;180:461–468.

80. Plate G, Eklof B, Norgren L, et al. Venous thrombectomy for iliofemoral venous thrombosis—10-year results of a prospective randomized study. *Eur J Vasc Endo Surg* 1997;14:367–374.

81. Juhan CM, Alimi YS, Barthelemy PJ, et al. Late results of iliofemoral venous thrombectomy. *J Vasc Surg* 1997;25:417–422.

82. Plate G, Akesson H, Einarsson E, et al. Thrombectomy with temporary A-V fistula: the treatment of choice in iliofemoral thrombosis. *J Vasc Surg* 1984;1:867–876.

83. Eklof B, Arfvidsson B, Kistner RL, et al. Indications for surgical treatment of iliofemoral venous thrombosis. *Hem-Onc Clin N A* 2000;14:471–482.

84. Gandini R, Maspes F, Sodani G, et al. Percutaneous ilio-caval thrombectomy with the Amplatz device: preliminary results. *Eur Radiol* 1999;9:951–958.

85. Sharafuddin MJ, Sun S, Hoballah JJ. Endovascular management of venous thrombotic diseases of the upper torso and extremities. *JVIR* 2002;13:975–990.

86. Meier GH, Pollak JS, Rosenblatt M, et al. Initial experience with venous stents in exertional axillary-subclavian vein thrombosis. *J Vasc Surg* 1996;24:974–983.

87. Axelrod DA, Proctor MC, Geisser ME, et al. Outcomes after surgery for thoracic outlet syndrome. *J Vasc Surg* 2001;33:1220–1225.

88. Cesarone MR, Belcaro G, Nicolaides AN, et al. "Real" epidemiology of varicose veins and chronic venous diseases: the San Valentino Vascular Screening Project. *Angiology* 2002;53: 119–130.

89. London NJM, Nash R. ABC's of arterial and venous disease: varicose veins. *BMJ* 2000;320:1391–1394.

90. vanRij AM, Jiang P, Soloman C, et al. Recurrence after varicose veins surgery: a prospective long-term clinical study with duplex ultrasound scanning and air plethysmography. *J Vasc Surg* 2003;38:935–943.

91. Hoare MC, Nicolaides AN, Miles CR, et al. The role of primary varicose veins in venous ulceration. *Surgery* 1982;92:450–453.

92. Ramelet AA. Phlebectomy. *Int Angiol* 2002;21:46–51.

93. Keith LM Jr, Smead WILL. Saphenous vein stripping and its complications. *Surg Clin N A* 1983;63:1303–1312.

94. Criado E, Lujan S, Izquierdo L, et al. Conservative hemodynamic surgery for varicose veins. *Sem Vasc Surg* 2002;15:27–33.

95. Weiss RA, Weiss MA. Ambulatory phlebectomy compared to sclerotherapy for varicose and telangiectatic veins: indications and complications. *Adv Derm* 1996;11:3–17.

96. Green D. Sclerotherapy for the permanent eradication of varicose veins: theoretical and practical considerations. *J Am Acad Dermatol* 1998;38:461–475.

97. Goldman MP. Complications of sclerotherapy in venous surgery. In: Gloviczki P, Yao JST, eds. *Handbook of venous disorders*, 2nd ed. London: Hoddard & Stoughton; 2001.

98. French LE, Braun F, Masouye I, et al. Post-stripping sclerodermiform dermatitis. *Arch Dermatol* 1999;135:1387–1391.

99. Ramelet AA. Complications of ambulatory phlebectomy. *Dermatol Surg* 1997;23:947–954.

100. Rigby KA, Palfreyman SJ, Beverley C, et al. Surgery for varicose veins: use of tourniquet. *The Cochrane Database of Systematic Reviews* 2003;3:1–19.

101. Bergan JJ. Varicose veins: hooks, clamps, and suction. Application of new techniques to enhance varicose vein surgery. *Sem Vasc Surg* 2002;15:21–26.

102. Morrison C, Dalsing MC. Signs and symptoms of saphenous nerve injury after greater saphenous vein stripping: prevalence, severity, and relevance for modern practice. *J Vasc Surg* 2003;38: 886–890.

103. Yamaki T, Nozaki M, Sasaki K. Acute massive pulmonary embolism following high ligation combined with compression sclerotherapy for varicose veins. *Dermatol Surg* 1999;25:321–325.

104. Rutgers PH, Kitslaar PJ. Randomized trial of stripping versus high ligation combined with sclerotherapy in the treatment of the incompetent greater saphenous vein. *Am J Surg* 1994;168: 311–315.

105. Zotto LM. Treating varicose veins with transilluminated powered phlebectomy. *AORN Journal* 2002;76:981–990.

106. Rautio T, Ohinmaa A, Perala J, et al. Endovenous obliteration versus conventional stripping operation in the treatment of primary varicose veins: a randomized controlled trial with comparison of the costs. *J Vasc Surg* 2002;35:958–965.

107. Fischer R, Chandler JG, De Maeseneer MG, et al. The unresolved problem of recurrent saphenofemoral reflux. *J Am Coll Surg* 2002;195:80–94.

108. Boccalon H, Janbon C, Saumet JL, et al. Characteristics of chronic venous insufficiency in 895 patients followed in general practice. *Int Angiol* 1997;16:226–234.

109. Gloviczki P. Subfascial endoscopic perforator vein surgery: indications and results. *Vasc Med* 1999;4:173–180.

110. Jost CJ, Gloviczki P, Cherry KJ Jr, et al. Surgical reconstruction of iliofemoral veins and the inferior vena cava for nonmalignant occlusion disease. *J Vasc Surg* 2001;33:320–328.

111. Kunimoto BT. Management and prevention of venous leg ulcers: a literature-guided approach. *Ostomy/Wound Management* 2001; 47(6):36–49.

112. Korn P, Patel ST, Heller JA, et al. Why insurers should reimburse for compression stockings in patients with chronic venous stasis. *J Vasc Surg* 2002;34:1–8.

113. Coccheri S, Scondotto G, Agnelli G, et al. Randomized, double blind, multicentre, placebo controlled study of sulodexide in the treatment of venous leg ulcers. *Thromb Haemost* 2002;87:947–952.

114. Padberg FT Jr. Surgical intervention in venous ulceration. *Cardiovasc Surg* 1999;7:83–90.

115. Tawes RL, Barron ML, Coello AA, et al. Optimal therapy for advanced chronic venous insufficiency. *J Vasc Surg* 2003;37: 545–551.

116. Gloviczki P, Bergan JJ, Rhodes JM, et al. North American Study Group. Mid-term results of endoscopic perforator vein interruption for chronic venous insufficiency: lessons learned from the North American Subfascial Endoscopic Perforator Surgery registry. *J Vasc Surg* 1999;29:489–502.

117. Kalra M, Gloviczki P. Surgical treatment of venous ulcers: role of subfascial endoscopic perforator vein ligation. *Surg Clin N Am* 2003;83:671–705.

118. Wittens CH, van Gent BW, Hop WC, et al. The Dutch subfascial endoscopic perforating vein surgery (SEPS) trial: a multicenter trial comparing ambulatory compression therapy versus surgery in patients with venous leg ulcers. *Abstract: Annual Vascular Meeting*, 2003.

119. Bergan JJ MD, Kumins NH, Owens EL, et al. Surgical and endovascular treatment of lower extremity venous insufficiency. *JVIR* 2002;13:563–568.

120. Sarkar R, Eilber FR, Gelabert HA, et al. Prosthetic replacement of the inferior vena cava for malignancy. *J Vasc Surg* 1998;28:75–83.

121. Alimi YS, DiMauro P, Fabre D, et al. Iliac vein reconstruction to treat acute and chronic venous occlusive disease. *J Vasc Surg* 1997;25:673–681.

122. Juhan C, Hartung O, Alimi Y, et al. Treatment of nonmalignant obstructive iliocaval lesions by stent placement: mid-term results. *Ann Vasc Surg* 2001;15:227–232.

123. Thorpe PE, Osse FS, Dang HP. Endovascular reconstruction for chronic iliac vein and inferior vena cava obstruction. In: Gloviczki P, Yao JST, eds. *Handbook of venous disorders*, 2nd ed. London: Hoddard & Stoughton; 2001.

Complications of Endovascular Therapy

30

Matthew J. Eagleton   Sunita D. Srivastava

■ INTRODUCTION 357

■ ARTERIAL INTERVENTIONS 357
Diagnostic Angiography 357
Contrast Nephropathy 357
Puncture Site Complications 359
Catheter and Guidewire Related Complications 360

■ SUPRA-AORTIC INTERVENTIONS 360
Cerebral Angiography 360
Carotid Artery Angioplasty and Stenting 361
Brachiocephalic Angioplasty and Stenting 361

■ AORTOILIAC INTERVENTIONS 362
Aortoiliac Angioplasty and Stenting 362
Aortic Endografts for Aneurysmal Disease 364
Mesenteric Artery Angioplasty and Stenting 370
Renal Artery Angioplasty and Stenting 370

■ LOWER EXTREMITY INTERVENTIONS 371
Femoropopliteal Angioplasty and Stenting 371
Tibial Angioplasty and Stenting 373
Thrombolysis 373

■ VENOUS INTERVENTIONS 375
Vena Cava Filters 375
Venous Angioplasty and Stenting 376
Endovascular Therapy for Pulmonary Embolism 376

■ CONCLUSIONS 377

■ REFERENCES 377

INTRODUCTION

The number of patients undergoing endovascular interventions is increasing. At some point most surgeons will manage patients who require an endovascular procedure, or they will be called on to manage one of the complications of an intervention. Outlined in this chapter are the main complications encountered with several of the most common endovascular therapies.

ARTERIAL INTERVENTIONS

Diagnostic Angiography

A number of complications can occur during the performance of routine angiography. Most of these complications are not specific to diagnostic angiography but can occur during the performance of any number of vascular interventions. More common complications include those associated with the administration of radiologic contrast agents and injury to the artery used for access.

Contrast Nephropathy

Contrast nephropathy is the development of acute renal failure or insufficiency secondary to the parenteral administration of radiologic contrast agents. Contrast nephropathy

Matthew J. Eagleton, Sunita D. Srivastava: University of Michigan, Ann Arbor, MI 48109 is the third leading cause of acute renal failure in hospitalized patients (1). The incidence of contrast nephropathy varies widely and depends on the definition of renal insufficiency used by the varying studies (2,3). Contrast nephropathy generally presents as an elevation in serum creatinine 1 to 2 days after dye administration. Creatinine values peak after 3 to 5 days and return to baseline by 7 to 10 days (2,4). The acute renal failure is usually nonoliguric in nature. Urinalysis reveals a range of findings from normal to granular casts, tubular epithelial cells, and protein. The diagnosis of contrast nephropathy is typically easy to make, given the temporal relationship of the onset of renal failure to the contrast load. Other causes of acute renal failure, such as hypovolemia and atheroembolization of the renal arteries, should be excluded.

The pathogenesis of contrast nephropathy is complex and involves a synergistic effect of direct renal tubular epithelial cell toxicity and renal medullary ischemia. Three main factors contribute to its development, including osmotic effects, renal hemodynamic effects, and renal tubular effects (3,5). Contrast media are small molecules that become concentrated in urine up to 100-fold within the first 4 hours after administration. The increase in osmolarity causes an increase in intratubular hydrostatic pressure and decreases filtration pressure in glomeruli, leading to osmotic diuresis and increased sodium and water excretion. The increased sodium load to the macula densa in the distal tubule causes a decrease in the glomerular filtration rate (6). This response is more pronounced with contrast agents that have a high osmolarity compared to those that are iso-osmolar or hypo-osmolar. The osmotic diuresis also places an increased metabolic demand on the distal nephron and may aggravate medullary hypoxia (7).

Contrast agents can cause direct cytotoxicity leading to contrast nephropathy. Cytotoxicity is suggested by evidence of cell injury on histologic evaluation and by the presence of enzymuria, particularly N-acetyl-β-glucosaminidase and alkaline phosphatase (8,9).

Contrast agents affect renal blood flow in a biphasic pattern. Initially there is a brief increase in renal blood flow, followed by a steady decline. Decreased blood flow is due to the induction of renal vasoconstriction caused by rheologic changes, erythrocyte deformability, and the release of a variety of endothelial factors, including endothelin, adenosine, calcium, and oxygen free-radicals (6,10–12).

Alterations in renal function are seen in almost every patient who receives a contrast load, but not every patient develops contrast nephropathy (13). There are a variety of risk factors for development of acute renal failure following contrast dye administration (Table 30-1). Alone, chronic renal insufficiency is the most important risk factor; combined with diabetes mellitus negative effects are synergistic. In one series of 1,800 patients undergoing cardiac catheterization, the rate of contrast nephropathy was

TABLE 30-1

RISK FACTORS FOR CONTRAST NEPHROPATHY

Chronic renal insufficiency
Diabetes mellitus
Congestive heart failure
High dose contrast agent
Nephrotoxic drugs (i.e., antibiotics)
Agents that decrease renal perfusion (i.e., NSAIDs)

14.5% for all patients. When adjusted for the presence of risk factors, the development of contrast nephropathy increases from 1.2% in patients with no risk factors to 100% in patients with four or more risk factors (14).

Contrast nephropathy, despite generally resolving over the course of 7 to 10 days, is not a benign complication. Few patients go on to require dialysis, but up to 30% will have residual renal impairment and there is some suggestion that patients affected by contrast nephropathy have increased mortality rates (15,16). Management of these patients is similar to other patients who develop acute renal failure. A thorough investigation should be made to identify contributing factors, such as hypovolemia or nephrotoxic medications, with correction. Monitoring of serum chemistries and assessment of fluid status should be performed.

Although there is no antidote for the nephrotoxic effects of radiologic contrast media, several strategies have been devised with the hope of decreasing morbidity. Nonionic and low-osmolality contrast agents were developed to lower the complications of radiologic dye. These agents are associated with a lower incidence of contrast nephropathy compared to high-osmolarity agents (17). Preprocedural administration of intravenous fluid is a simple, inexpensive measure that treats hypovolemia and should theoretically offer protection to patients who are going to receive radiologic contrast agents. Protective effects, however, have never been proven. Dopamine was thought to be protective, given its renal vasodilatory effects, but several studies reveal it to have no effect on the development of contrast nephropathy in patients with underlying risk factors, and in one study dopamine increased the risk in diabetic patients (18,19). Acetylcysteine is an antioxidant that has been evaluated in several studies for reducing the incidence of contrast nephropathy. A meta-analysis of seven randomized prospective trials comparing orally administered acetylcysteine with hydration alone have shown it to significantly reduce the risk of developing contrast nephropathy in patients with underlying chronic renal insufficiency (20). Fenoldopam mesylate is a potent vasodilator that increases renal plasma flow. Periprocedural intravenous administration of fenoldopam mesylate has been shown to significantly reduce the development of contrast nephropathy when compared to saline alone (21,22).

Puncture Site Complications

The incidence of puncture site complications ranges from 0.3% to 35% (23–29). Lower rates are associated with diagnostic procedures, while higher rates follow interventional procedures due to the use of larger sheaths (30). Factors that increase the risk of puncture site complications are significant atherosclerotic disease in the artery that is being accessed, obesity, and the use of antithrombotic or fibrinolytic pharmacotherapies (27). The more complex the procedure, the higher the rate of puncture site complications (24). In only 9% of all cases is surgical therapy necessary (23).

Hemorrhage

Hemorrhage is the most common puncture site complication, occurring in 8% of diagnostic procedures and 18% of arterial interventions (23,25–28). Patients present with a painful, pulseless mass at the puncture site. Assessment with duplex ultrasound is necessary to exclude pseudoaneurysm. Hemorrhage may not be obvious on physical exam if the bleeding tracks into the retroperitoneum. In these situations computed tomography will verify the diagnosis. Management entails application of pressure over the puncture site followed by continued close observation. If hemorrhage persists, surgical intervention is required. Other indications for surgical intervention include significant overlying skin changes and hematoma causing symptomatic compression of adjacent nervous or venous structures.

Pseudoaneurysm

Diagnostic procedures are associated with the development of pseudoaneurysms at the puncture site in <1% of patients having diagnostic procedures and in up to 5% of those undergoing interventions (23,26,27,29,31). Pseudoaneurysms can be detected by the palpation of a pulsatile mass on physical exam and confirmed by duplex ultrasound. The most common anatomic factor associated with femoral pseudoaneurysm formation is aberrant puncture, entering the vessel in either the external iliac artery or superficial femoral artery (32–35). Both these locations make compression following sheath and catheter removal more difficult and less successful. The use of periprocedural anticoagulation also increases the risk of pseudoaneurysm formation (29). Small pseudoaneurysms <3 cm can resolve spontaneously, provided patients are not anticoagulated (29,36).

Persistent pseudoaneurysms and those that cause symptoms require intervention. Untreated lesions may cause pain, neuropathy, arteriovenous fistulas with steal syndrome, or rupture. Treatment was classically performed with surgical repair, and urgent surgical intervention is recommended when there is an expanding pseudoaneurysm, an expanding hematoma, severe pain, femoral nerve compression, or groin infection (36). When surgical repair is required, management can often be accomplished by lateral suture of the arterial communication. With large pseudoaneurysms, proximal control of the distal external iliac artery through a retroperitoneal incision may be required prior to repair.

Recently, nonsurgical treatment of pseudoaneurysms has proven effective. Initial experience was with ultrasound guided compression of the pseudoaneurysm origin. Compression is applied for 30 minutes or longer. Success rates for compression therapy vary and are significantly affected by the presence of on-going anticoagulation. In anticoagulated patients failure rates are as high as 41% (31). When anticoagulation is not present, success rates approach 90% (37). An alternative is ultrasound guided thrombin injection. This therapy has proven effective in over 90% of patients, including those with ongoing anticoagulation (31,38). The major risk of this procedure is induction of thrombus in the native vessel and subsequent occlusion or distal embolization. Thrombus occurs in up to 3% of patients undergoing thrombin injection and requires surgical intervention (31). The risk is limited if treatment of lesions comprised of short, wide necks >10 mm and small native artery diameters are excluded. The use of covered stents has been described to treat postprocedural pseudoaneurysms, but experience with this modality is not widespread (39,40).

Arteriovenous Fistula

The development of an arteriovenous fistula complicates diagnostic angiography in <1% of cases and interventional procedures in up to 2% of cases (23,27,28). The incidence is higher when the puncture site is more caudal on the femoral artery, due to the juxtaposition of the superficial femoral artery, deep femoral artery, and adjacent veins in this region. On physical examination a bruit will be heard over the puncture site, and duplex ultrasound easily confirms the diagnosis. Most arteriovenous fistulae spontaneously thrombose (29,36). Patients with this complication can be safely monitored with ultrasound until closure. Indications for intervention include the development of congestive heart failure due to the fistula, limb ischemia, venous insufficiency, or distal embolization. In these instances surgical intervention is warranted. Employing covered stents to treat the lesion has been described, but their use is not widespread (39,40)

Neuropathy

Nerve injury due to compression from local bleeding is the most common and debilitating complication after transaxillary arteriography. Due to the close proximity of the axillary artery and brachial plexus, even a small hematoma can produce significant nerve compression. Patients can present with sensory and motor deficits that can affect the median, radial, and ulnar nerve distribution. This complication occurs in <1% of transaxillary procedures (28). The incidence of femoral neuropathy after a femoral artery puncture is about 0.2% (41). Femoral neuropathy occurs more frequently with retroperitoneal hemorrhage. Prompt surgical decompression is necessary in patients who have neurologic symptoms to reduce the incidence of prolonged deficits (28,41,42).

Vascular Closure Device Complications

Several devices have been developed over the past decade to assist in arterial puncture site closure. Approaches include collagen plug mediated devices and suture mediated devices. These devices have shown to significantly decrease the amount of time necessary to obtain hemostasis (43–45), but their effectiveness for reducing access complications has not been proven. Several reports have shown similar complication rates compared to hemostasis obtained by manual compression (46–49). Some investigators have reported increased complications with closure devices (50,51). Complications specific to the use of these percutaneous arterial closure devices include embolization of collagen plugs, arterial occlusion, and infection (52–54). These events occur in <2% of device deployments (54).

Catheter and Guidewire Related Complications

Thrombosis

Arterial thrombosis is rare (<1% of cases) following both diagnostic and interventional procedures (23,26,27). Thrombosis is affected by the size of the catheter in relation to the size of the arterial lumen and the length of the catheter exposed to the blood (55–57). This relationship affects the size of the thrombus that develops on the catheter. Thrombotic complications present with a variety of symptoms. If the region supplied by the occluded artery has a vast collateral blood supply, no significant symptoms may arise and the only finding may be loss of distal palpable pulses. This finding is typical of brachial artery thrombosis following upper extremity arterial access. Most episodes of thrombosis are treated with thrombectomy, but if severe underlying atherosclerotic disease is present, arterial bypass may be required.

Arterial Dissection

Arterial dissection is rare, occurring in <1% of cases (23,26,27). Arterial dissection more frequently occurs after interventional procedures and with antegrade arterial punctures. Occasionally no intervention is required, especially if

a retrograde dissection has occurred. More severe dissections present with complete arterial occlusion and loss of a pulse on physical examination. The surgical procedure required to repair these dissections depends on the defect's extent and location. Short focal lesions can be treated by endarterectomy, but more extensive dissections may require arterial bypass.

Embolization

Embolization complicates diagnostic arteriography and arterial interventions at a rate approaching 6% (23,27). Embolization can result from dislodgement of atheroemboli and the development and embolization of thrombus on the introducer sheath, and it can involve foreign bodies such as sheared-off portions of angiographic catheters. When embolization occurs, the surgeon should consider intervention to prevent sequelae. Options include immediate percutaneous or surgical thrombectomy (or removal of foreign body) and selective thrombolysis (42,58,59). Cholesterol syndrome is due to the dislodgement of cholesterol crystals from atheromatous vessels, particularly the aorta. Cholesterol emboli lodge in small arterioles and most often affect the skin in the form of livedo reticularis, the kidneys resulting in renal failure, and the digits resulting in "blue toe syndrome" (60–62). The incidence and sequelae of embolization during cerebral angiography and carotid artery interventions have been extensively studied and will be discussed in more detail below.

SUPRA-AORTIC INTERVENTIONS

Cerebral Angiography

Many of the complications encountered with cerebral angiography are similar to those of routine peripheral or coronary angiography. The consequence of embolization, however, is more profound, as the outcome may be a cerebral vascular accident. Overall complication rates for cerebral angiography parallel peripheral angiography and coronary angiography, ranging from 0.6% to 10% (63–66). Complications include strokes (occurring at an incidence of approximately 0.5%) and transient ischemic attacks (TIAs) (occurring at an incidence of approximately 0.4%) (66). The incidence of embolization and subsequent cerebral ischemic event increases if the patients have symptomatic carotid artery stenosis (65,67). Embolization during cerebral angiography, however, is not always symptomatic. Sources of embolization include microscopic air embolization or silent thromboembolism (68,69). Bendszus et al. evaluated diffusion-weighted magnetic resonance imaging before and after angiography to assess embolic events in 100 consecutive patients undergoing diagnostic angiography (70). In this study, 23% of patients had evidence of embolization without neurologic symptoms. The appearance of lesions was associated with difficult vessel access, higher contrast loads, increased fluoroscopy time, and the use of multiple catheters.

Carotid Artery Angioplasty and Stenting

Stroke

Stroke is the most feared complication of cerebrovascular interventions. With the growing use of carotid artery stenting, a more thorough evaluation of associated complications is being realized. The incidence of cerebrovascular events following carotid artery stenting varies according to classification schemes. Events are categorized as major strokes, minor strokes, and TIAs.

Technical success in carotid artery stenting approaches 100% (71–75). Thirty-day rates of major stroke range from 1.3% to 3.6%, while rates of minor stroke and TIA range from 0% to 1.3% and 3.4% to 10.7%, respectively. Patients with severely elevated baseline systolic blood pressure are at higher risk for hemodynamic instability and neurologic events during carotid artery stenting (76).

Unfortunately, it is rare that an operation can correct distal cerebral embolization. Distal thrombolysis should be attempted if arterial occlusion is visualized angiographically, although it is impossible to ascertain whether the occlusion is secondary to atheromatous embolization or thromboembolization. Treatment is continued until lysis is achieved, there is systemic evidence of fibrinolysis, a limiting total dose of thrombolytic has been delivered, or there is evidence of intracranial hemorrhage (77).

Most carotid artery stent-related strokes are due to distal atheroemboli or thromboemboli dislodged at the time of the procedure. In order to decrease the incidence of these complications, several cerebral protection devices have been developed. Several series evaluating the efficacy of cerebral protection devices have shown an 80% reduction in acute neurologic events related to embolism compared to unprotected procedures (78–81). Cerebral protection devices are also associated with complications. These complications are infrequent (occurring <1% of the time) and include focal dissection of the internal carotid artery and failure of device deployment. Internal carotid artery vasospasm occurs in up to 15% of patients, half of whom respond to vasodilatory therapy with nitroglycerin (78). In patients in whom occlusive protection devices are used (i.e., balloon occluders), transient alterations in mental function are documented in 15% of patients (82).

Hemodynamic Instability

Carotid artery angioplasty and stenting involves dilation of the carotid bulb. This maneuver can cause immediate cardiovascular hemodynamic alterations, similar to the blood pressure and heart rate changes associated with carotid endarterectomy. In the review by Ohki et al. nearly one-third of patients had an alteration in heart rate. Ten percent of the patients had transient asystole, while 20% developed transient bradycardia (83). Approximately 30% developed concomitant hypotension, half of whom required infusion of phenylephrine. All underwent monitoring in an intensive care unit.

Myocardial Infarction and Death

Most patients who undergo carotid artery stenting are considered to be at high operative risk. In one of the first large series, 77% of patients would have been ineligible for the North American Symptomatic Carotid Endarterectomy Trial (NASCET) due to the presence of medical comorbidities (84). Included in this group of comorbidities is significant coronary artery disease, which is present in 80% of patients in some series (73). Despite this level of risk, rates of perioperative myocardial infarction were only 0% to 0.6% (72,74). The 30-day death rates have been reported to be between 0% and 4.5% (55,75,85–88). The majority of deaths were related to either periprocedural myocardial infarction, fatal stroke, or intracranial hemorrhage.

Restenosis and Late Stroke

The natural history of in-stent restenosis is unknown. A restenosis rate following carotid artery stenting has been reported to be 3% at 1 year (89). Two types of restenosis have been described: narrowing within the stent and stenosis at the end of the stent, often caused by a kink in the artery. Most restenoses are treated with another stent or balloon angioplasty, with one-third developing repeated episodes of recurrent stenosis. Several studies have used life-table analysis to determine long-term restenosis and stroke free rates. Lal et al. report an in-stent restenosis rate (restenosis defined as >80% stenosis) of 6.4% at 60 months (90). Over half of these occurred at 15 months or less, and none were associated with neurologic deficits. Hobson et al. reported a similar time period of recurrent stenosis (75). Investigators have reported an 89% freedom from stroke rate at 48 months with a recurrent stenosis rate of 45% (91). At most institutions asymptomatic patients who develop a restenosis >80%, or those who are symptomatic and have a >50% stenosis, are considered for reintervention. Reintervention can entail angioplasty, angioplasty with a cutting balloon, repeat carotid artery stenting, and carotid artery resection with interposition graft (73,89,92).

Brachiocephalic Angioplasty and Stenting

Embolization and Stroke

The incidence of acute cerebral ischemia following subclavian artery intervention is low. In one series there was only one incidence of TIA in 76 interventions (93). The risk of vertebral artery embolization is almost negligible due to the "delay" phenomenon described by Ringelstein and Zeumer (94). Following proximal subclavian artery angioplasty, the reversal of flow from retrograde to antegrade does not occur immediately but gradually. Distal embolization involving the brachial artery and left internal mammary artery has been reported in 1.1% of patients (95). Brachial artery embolization can be easily managed with a brachial artery cutdown and embolectomy. Embolization to the left internal mammary artery may have a profound effect in patients who have had coronary artery bypass grafting. Patients may experience acute myocardial infarction and corresponding hemodynamic compromise. Treatment is generally catheter directed thrombolytic therapy.

Technical Complications

Technical complications have been described in 11% of patients undergoing treatment of subclavian artery stenosis or occlusion (93,95,96). These complications include stent migration, failure to cross the occlusive lesion, arterial dissection, acute thrombosis, arterial rupture, and inadvertently covering the vertebral artery. Arterial dissection is treated by placement of a stent. Acute thrombosis is treated with locally delivered thrombolysis and subsequent balloon angioplasty. Arterial rupture is one of the most feared complications of endovascular therapies. Rupture is detected by visualization of contrast extravasation on completion angiogram. Prompt recognition is important in order to avoid exsanguinations or limb loss. An angioplasty balloon can be reinserted and inflated at the site of rupture, providing a tamponade effect (97). Prolonged balloon inflation may be sufficient to provide hemostasis and no further intervention may be necessary. If balloon inflation fails, a treatment option is placement of a covered stent to exclude the artery's ruptured area. This maneuver has proven effective in the treatment of a variety of brachiocephalic injuries and is associated with shorter operative times, less blood loss, and equivalent patency rates compared to open surgery (98).

Not all subclavian artery ruptures following percutaneous transluminal angioplasty or stent placement are immediately identified. Disruption may present in a delayed fashion in the form of a pseudoaneurysm. This complication may present with symptoms due to compression on surrounding structures, including the recurrent laryngeal nerve (hoarseness), sympathetic chain (Horner syndrome), and brachial plexus (weakness or paresthesias). Although an endovascular approach may be effective at ameliorating the pseudoaneurysm, symptomatic lesions are best treated with open surgery to accomplish aneurysmal decompression.

Stent Infection

One incidence of subclavian artery stent infection has been described in the literature (99). The patient presented 6 days after stent placement with *Staphylococcus aureus* bacteremia and stigmata of septic emboli to the ipsilateral hand. CT evaluation revealed a phlegmon surrounding the stented portion of the artery; angiography detected a pseudoaneurysm at the site. The patient underwent resection of the affected portion of the artery with autogenous vascular reconstruction. The underlying etiology of the stent infection is unknown, but it was hypothesized that prolonged femoral access and an infected left arm venous access contributed.

Mortality

Mortality rates from brachiocephalic interventions are low, reported at 0% to 4.8% (93,95,96,100). Deaths in the immediate postprocedural period (30 days) have rarely been attributable directly to the endovascular procedure. In a few cases deaths were due to strokes that occurred at the time of angioplasty and stent placement (95). Long-term mortality tends to be unrelated to the brachiocephalic disease but related to coexisting or subsequently developed comorbidities.

Restenosis and Occlusion

Immediate success in the treatment of subclavian artery stenosis is between 95% and 100% (93,96,100,101). Angioplasty alone has a lower success rate (80% to 85%) compared to primary arterial stenting (97% to 100%) (93,96,101,102). Complete occlusion of the vessel and lesions longer than 2 cm correlate with lower success rates. Short-term patency (1 year) is lower in patients who have undergone only angioplasty (76%) compared to patients receiving primary stenting (95%) (101). Longer-term outcomes (4 years) favor primary angioplasty, with a patency rate of 68% compared to a primary patency rate stenting of 59%. This difference was due to the development of in-stent stenosis. The development of restenosis can be due to misplacement of the stent, particularly in ostial lesions. Up to half of patients who develop a restenosis become symptomatic (93). Restenosis can be treated, when necessary, by balloon angioplasty.

AORTOILIAC INTERVENTIONS

Aortoiliac Angioplasty and Stenting

Technical Complications

Iliac artery percutaneous transluminal angioplasty (PTA) and stent placement is technically successful in 95% and 97% of patients, respectively (103). Stenotic segments are more effectively treated than occlusions. Technical complications occur in <6% of interventions and include subintimal dilation, dissection, arterial rupture, inability to cross the lesion, and distal embolization. In one series, 2.8% developed complications requiring surgery and 0.9% required reconstructive bypass (104). Clinically significant distal embolization occurs in 1% of patients undergoing iliac artery PTA and stent placement. Doppler ultrasound has detected silent peripheral embolization in 90% of patients following iliac PTA (105). Symptomatic embolization can be treated by a variety of endovascular methods, including suction thrombectomy and thrombolytic therapy. If these modalities are not successful, surgical thromboembolectomy is necessary.

Iliac artery dissection during PTA is reported in 0.5% to 1% of patients (91,106). Half of these patients developed significant luminal compromise. Dissections can be treated by prolonged balloon inflation to tack down the flap or by placement of an intra-arterial stent. If endovascular therapy is not successful, operative treatments include iliac endarterectomy, iliofemoral bypass, femoral–femoral bypass, and aortobifemoral bypass grafting. Arterial dissection has been reported in 10% of patients undergoing iliac artery stent placement; 70% of the dissections cause hemodynamically significant stenosis requiring an additional stent placement (107).

Vessel injury is related to balloon oversizing and to the degree of arterial calcification. Iliac artery rupture during balloon dilation and stent placement has been reported in 0.9% of cases (108,109). Vessel disruptions can present with uncontained hemorrhage, contained hemorrhage, or pseudoaneurysm formation (Fig. 30-1). The key to initial management is maintenance of endovascular access across the site of disruption with a guidewire. Control of hemorrhage can be obtained with the insertion of an angioplasty balloon to tamponade the site of injury. If prolonged balloon tamponade does not achieve hemostasis, the placement of a covered stent can be used to seal the injury. Uncontrolled hemorrhage warrants emergent surgical intervention, but balloon occlusion proximal to the site of injury can afford some time to prepare for surgery. Risk factors for rupture are similar to those for dissection and include the presence of a high-grade stenosis with heavy calcification. Other risk factors include the use of oversized balloons and manual inflation without manometric control.

Other complications of iliac artery PTA and stent placement include nondeflating angioplasty balloons and stent migration. Modern angioplasty catheters are very reliable, but despite many safeguards deployment failures can occur. The most common cause of failure of angioplasty balloons is kinking or plugging of the deflation lumen (110). Injection of carbon dioxide or saline can clear the deflation lumen. In addition, a fine wire can be inserted through the inflation lumen. If these techniques are not successful, the balloon can be punctured percutaneously with a 21-gauge needle, depending on the balloon's location and its relationship to surrounding structures.

The exact incidence of iliac stent migration is not known, and this is not a frequently reported complication. Migration is probably not an uncommon complication that occurs when a self-expanding stent abruptly jumps cranially upon deployment (111). Movement may not cause significant morbidity, but it may result in the complete dislodgment of the stent. Unfortunately, once these stents have been deployed they are difficult to retrieve. Management options for this complication include emergent vascular surgery, observation, stent retrieval using

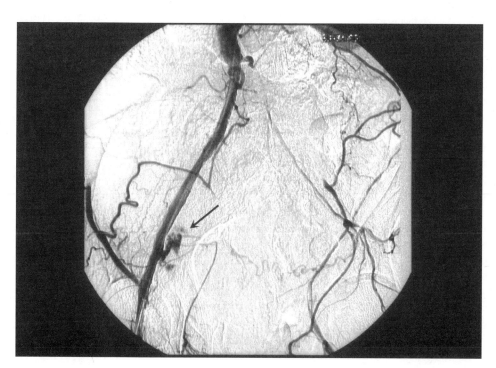

Figure 30-1 Angiogram from a patient undergoing iliac artery angioplasty that resulted in a perforation. This is demonstrated by the arrow. The hemorrhage was controlled by brief occlusion of the perforation site with an angioplasty balloon and subsequent placement of an iliac artery stent.

endovascular snares and large introducer sheaths, and aortoiliac bifurcation reconstruction using balloon-expandable stents.

Infection

Stent infection following iliac artery stent placement is rare but has been reported to occur both acutely and in a delayed fashion after several years (112–114). In one case, after thrombolytic therapy and subsequent iliac artery stent placement the patient developed fever, groin pain, and ipsilateral lower extremity petechiae (113). The patient developed symptoms of systemic inflammatory response with evidence of multisystem organ failure, and *Staphylococcus aureus* grew from blood cultures. Treatment subsequently required excision of the stent and the involved segment of artery, followed by above-the-knee amputation. Another report describes a similar clinical scenario (114). The resected iliac artery revealed severe necrotizing arteritis, and cultures grew *S. aureus* and *S. epidermidis*. Disruption and fracture of the arterial intima and media during angioplasty may predispose this portion of the artery to seeding by bacteria. Bacteria have been shown to colonize a stent surface irreversibly and to prevent tissue incorporation (115). No studies have examined the efficacy of periprocedural antibiotic prophylaxis, but, given the seriousness of stent infection, many authors advocate antibiotic use.

Restenosis

Restenosis following iliac artery PTA occurs in 5% to 11% of patients. The incidence of recurrent stenosis and the development of recurrent symptoms depend on the indication for the primary intervention (103,116). Patients treated for limb salvage have higher restenosis and symptom recurrence rates than those treated for claudication. Outcomes are impaired by young age and the presence of poor distal runoff (116,117). Four-year primary patency rates for iliac PTA are 65% for stenosis and 54% for occlusion in patients with claudication and 53% for stenosis and 44% for occlusion in those with limb threatening ischemia (118). In a meta-analysis evaluating outcomes of iliac artery PTA and stent placement in 1,300 patients, 4-year primary patency rates were 77% for stenotic lesions treated with iliac stenting and 61% for occlusive lesions in patients with claudication and 67% and 53%, respectively, in patients with limb-threatening ischemia (118). The risk of long-term failure was reduced by 39% after stent placement compared to PTA alone. Iliac artery stent patency rates are significantly lower in women and in patients with renal insufficiency and critical ischemia (119).

Late iliac artery thrombosis can develop in 10% of patients (107). Most of these lesions can be treated with thrombolytic therapy followed by repeat angioplasty of in-stent restenosis or endovascular or surgical therapy for more distally occlusive lesions. Patency is reported to be 87% at 1 year (120). Prospective studies reveal that elevated plasma fibrinogen levels are a major risk factor for arterial thrombosis and iliac artery stent restenosis (121).

Mortality

Mortality rates following PTA and stenting of the iliac artery are low and range from 0% to 1.2% (104,108,122). Some mortalities have been directly attributable to the intervention. These include deaths from overwhelming cholesterol embolization, the development of septicemia following reperfusion of ischemic limbs, and contrast reaction.

Aortic Endografts for Aneurysmal Disease

Iliac Artery Rupture

The primary mode of placement of aortic endografts is via a femoral artery cutdown and deployment of grafts through the iliac artery system and into the aorta. Disease, such as atherosclerosis, or tortuosity can lead to complications involving the iliac artery during placement. If the delivery system used to place the endograft is significantly larger than the iliac artery, the vessel can rupture during placement. Iliac artery rupture has been reported in 1% to 2% of cases (123,124). Several maneuvers can be used to traverse complex iliac arteries. Iliac artery stenosis can be predilated with balloon angioplasty to allow safe passage of the delivery system. Preprocedural stenting of the iliac arteries is generally dissuaded as it makes placement prohibitive. If tortuous iliac arteries are present, the use of a stiff guidewire may help reduce the tortuosity and allow easier access (Fig. 30-2). In some instances the use of two stiff guidewires (also known as a "buddy wire") may straighten the tortuosity. If these techniques do not allow adequate placement of the endograft, an iliac artery conduit can be used. This technique involves the suturing of a prosthetic graft to the midcommon iliac artery. The endograft is placed through the prosthetic graft and common iliac artery, and the iliac limb of the graft is seated in the prosthetic graft. The distal limb of the prosthetic graft is then anastomosed to the common femoral artery. The distal end of the common iliac artery is oversewn to allow retrograde flow through the external iliac artery and into the hypogastric artery.

Pelvic Ischemia

Iliac artery aneurysms coexist with abdominal aortic aneurysms (AAAs) in up to 30% of patients undergoing endograft repair (125–129). This circumstance can present a problem with aortic endograft placement, as the iliac arteries may be too large for the iliac limbs to form a seal. In these situations the iliac limb of the aortic endograft may be parked in the external iliac artery, covering the hypogastric artery. If this is a planned event, the hypogastric artery is

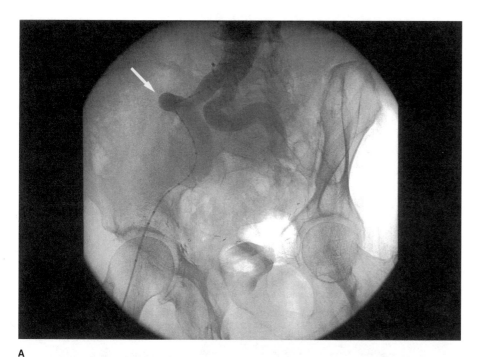

A

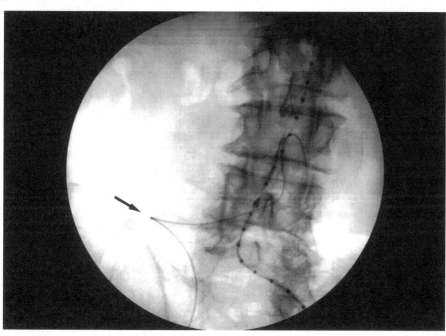

B

Figure 30-2 Angiogram from a patient undergoing endograft repair of an abdominal aortic aneurysm. **A:** The preoperative study revealed tortuous iliac arteries *(arrow)*. **B:** Placement of a "floppy" guidewire allows the iliac artery to retain a tortuous course *(arrow)*.

often embolized preoperatively to cause its occlusion and prevent an endoleak. The presence of an internal iliac artery aneurysm would necessitate the same treatment. Rarely, bilateral hypogastric artery embolization is required, usually performed in a staged fashion.

Complications from hypogastric artery embolization can occur in up to 50% of patients (126). Buttock claudication is the predominant complaint after hypogastric artery occlusion. Buttock claudication occurs in 12% to 50% of patients, but few have symptoms that persist beyond several months (125–129). Up to 25% of men

complain of new onset erectile dysfunction (128,129). Significant pelvic devascularization leading to colonic ischemia requiring bowel resection is of theoretical concern, but this entity has not been described in any of the larger series. Patients requiring embolization of the more distal branches of the hypogastric artery are at a higher risk of developing pelvic symptoms (130). Bilateral hypogastric artery embolization has not been associated with increased symptoms when compared to unilateral embolization (126,127,129). Coil embolization of the hypogastric artery can be avoided altogether if it is not aneurysmal. If as little

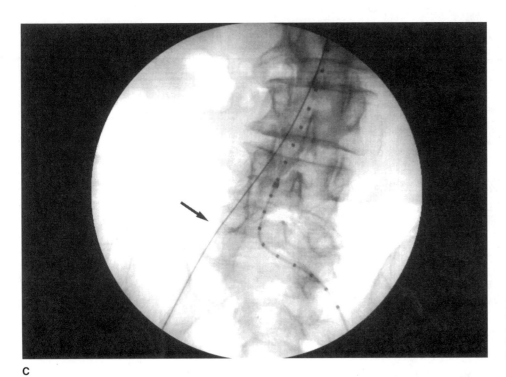

Figure   30-2C   *(continued)*
C: Placement of a stiff guidewire straightens the iliac artery *(arrow)* and allows for subsequent endograft placement.

C

as 5 mm of normal diameter common iliac artery is present prior to its bifurcation and there is 15 mm of acceptable artery distal to the bifurcation, coil embolization of the internal iliac artery is not necessary in order to obtain a distal iliac artery seal (131).

Endoleaks

An endoleak is the persistence of blood flow outside of the endograft within the aneurysm sac (AS) (132). Endoleaks are classified according to their etiology. Five types of endoleaks have been described (Table 30-2) (133,134). A type I endoleak (Fig. 30-3) arises from inadequate sealing at either the proximal aortic (allowing antegrade flow) or distal iliac (allowing retrograde flow) attachment sites. Type II endoleaks (Fig. 30-4) arise from patent aortic branch vessels. Such vessels include patent lumbar arteries or the inferior mesenteric artery. These allow retrograde flow into the AS, continued pressurization, and potential

risk for rupture. Type III endoleaks develop from defects in the fabric of the graft or at the junction zone between modular components (Fig. 30-5). Type IV endoleaks develop secondary to diffuse leaking of blood between the interstices of the fabric or where the graft is sutured to a stent. Type V endoleaks occur when the AS remains pressurized and the aneurysm enlarges, but no flow can be demonstrated within the AS using currently available imaging modalities. A type V endoleak is one in which the defect is large enough to allow blood flow into the sac and to transmit pressure to the sac, but the exit site is not present or too small to be detected by conventional imaging techniques (135).

Type I and type III endoleaks are associated with a significant risk of aneurysm enlargement and possible rupture. These endoleaks should be treated if they are detected (136,137). Treatment may be accomplished by the placement of additional endograft components, including a proximal aortic extension cuff or an additional iliac limb.

TABLE 30-2
TYPES OF ENDOLEAKS

Type I	Inadequate sealing at either the proximal aortic or distal iliac landing zones. Allows antegrade or retrograde flow into the aneurysm sac.
Type II	Patent aortic branch vessel (i.e., lumbar artery) providing retrograde flow into the aneurysm sac.
Type III	Defects in the fabric of the graft or at the junction zone between modular components providing flow into the aneurysm sac.
Type IV	Diffuse leaking of blood between the interstices of the fabric or where the graft is sutured to the stents.
Type V (controversial)	Aneurysm sac pressurized and enlarges despite no identifiable blood flow into the sac.

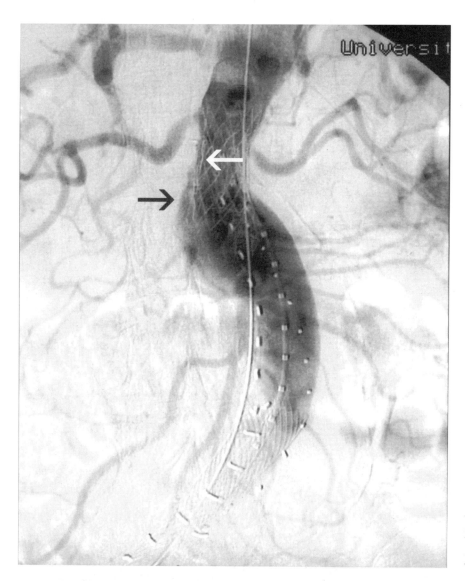

Figure 30-3 Aortogram demonstrating a type I endoleak. The white arrow demonstrates the lateral aspect of the stent graft. The black arrow points to contrast leaking around the proximal seal of the endograft, filling the aneurysm sac.

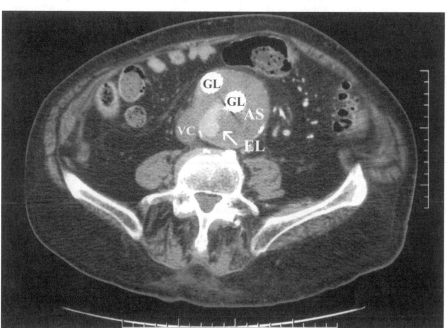

Figure 30-4 CT scan demonstrating a type II endoleak. GL represents the graft limbs, and AS is the aortic sac. There is contrast outside the graft limbs within the aneurysm sac that is characteristic of a type II endoleak (EL). This patient had an expanding aneurysm, and selective angiography revealed a patent inferior mesenteric artery. This artery was embolized and there was subsequent regression of the aneurysm size.

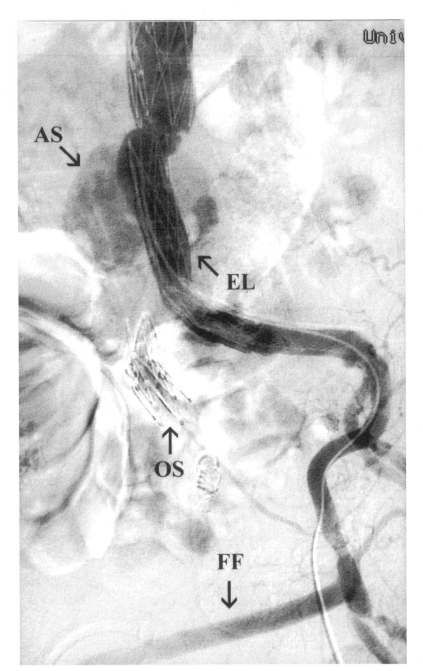

Figure 30-5 Aortogram demonstrating a type III endoleak. This patient had a homemade graft inserted that was of aorto-uni-iliac design. There is an occluding stent in the contralateral iliac artery (OS) with a femoral–femoral bypass graft (FF). The patient presented 5 years after the initial graft insertion with back pain and acute expansion of the aneurysm sac. Aortogram reveal a leak from the body of the graft (EL) filling the aneurysm sac (AS). The endograft was relined with a new graft that sealed the endoleak.

If the leak is a proximal type I endoleak and the graft is juxtaposed to the inferior border of the renal arteries, a large balloon-expandable stent can be placed in the proximal aspect of the endograft to increase radial force, causing better juxtaposition of the graft to the aortic wall. If less invasive interventions are unsuccessful at treating these types of endoleaks, removal of the endograft with conventional surgical repair is indicated. Fabric tears are easily managed if the site of the leak is localized. This complication can be managed by placement of an aortic cuff or an iliac extension to cover the hole. If the leak is more diffuse, the entire endograft can be relined or the device can be explanted.

Type II endoleaks are rarely associated with aneurysm rupture (138). At least 10% to 15% of patients will be identified with a type II endoleak during the endograft's lifespan (139–142). Chronic anticoagulation therapy is not associated with an increased risk of type II endoleak formation, but type II leaks are less likely to spontaneously resolve if the patient requires warfarin (143). No intervention is generally undertaken when a type II endoleak is diagnosed unless it is associated with an increase in aneurysm size or associated with aortic pulsatility on physical examination. In these situations arteriography is required to identify the source of the endoleak. An aortogram is performed, followed by selective injections into each iliac limb, the superior mesenteric artery, and hypogastric arteries. Superselective arterial access is then obtained, which allows embolization of the feeding vessels. Alternatively, direct sac puncture can be performed with embolization of the feeding vessels (144). The sac is then filled with glue, coils, or other embolization material.

Endograft Structural Failure

One of the most worrisome long-term complications associated with aortic endografting is material failure. Structural failure is difficult to identify as patients are often asymptomatic and may not present with acute changes. Three modes of structural failure have been described in aortic endografting, involving fabric erosion, suture disruption, and metal fracture (145). The development of endoleaks secondary to graft erosion has been documented in first-generation grafts (Fig. 30-5) (146,147). Areas of graft erosion are hypothesized to be secondary to the interaction of the stent material with the fabric. Repeated aortic pulsations cause friction between the stent and the fabric, causing eventual graft deterioration and the development of a type III endoleak. In many aortic endografts the graft material is attached to a metal skeleton with sutures. In several series in which patients developed new endoleaks, a graft explantation suture disruption was discovered within the graft (148,149). The mechanism leading to suture disruption is similar to graft erosion. It is not known, however, if suture disruption directly leads to endograft failure or if the resultant destabilization of the graft results in further deterioration.

The most common structural problem identified with aortic endograft systems has been metallic stent fracture (150). Jacobs et al. reported the outcome of 686 patients who underwent endovascular aneurysm repair. Sixty patients had material failure. Three-fourths of these failures were due to metallic stent fracture. Metal failure was caused by two processes: stress fatigue and metal corrosion. Stress fatigue resulted from repeated aortic pulsations. Metal corrosion occurs predominantly in nitinol stents (151). More recent stent-graft designs have improved nitinol processing and do not exhibit the same extent of corrosion (152–154).

Limb Thrombosis

Endograft limb thrombosis after endovascular aortic endografting occurs in 11% of patients (155–160). A variety of factors have been hypothesized to place patients at increased risk for limb thrombosis. The lack of metallic support within the limbs of endografts has been suggested to increase risk for thrombosis. In one series, 5% of supported limbs required a subsequent intervention to maintain patency while 44% of unsupported limbs required this degree of intervention (157). Oversizing of the graft limb also increases the risk of thrombosis. The infolding of the graft material due to the oversizing decreases the inner diameter, which increases the incidence of thrombosis (158). Extension of the iliac limb into the external iliac artery may place the limb at increased risk of thrombosis due to size mismatch between the graft and the smaller external iliac artery. Damage to the external iliac artery or femoral artery at the time of graft placement (i.e., dissection) can subsequently cause an outflow obstruction and graft limb thrombosis (155).

Management of patients with limb thrombosis depends on the severity of the induced ischemia. Nearly one-third of patients present with mild symptoms and require no intervention (156). Most patients, however, present with more severe ischemia and require a femoral–femoral bypass in order to reperfuse the affected limb. Few patients are successfully treated with thrombolysis or graft thrombectomy followed by endovascular repair. Most episodes of graft limb thrombosis present within the first 6 months; no limb occlusions have been described after 30 months (155–157,161).

Graft Migration

Distal stent-graft migration complicates abdominal aortic endografting in 9% to 45% of patients. Migration is a risk for developing a type I endoleak and delayed rupture or late conversion to open repair (162). The pathophysiology of endograft migration is complex, but blood flow is the main displacing force (163). As the tube of the endograft curves, the change in velocity of the blood causes an increase in the displacement force. Resistance to migration is afforded by friction between the graft and the aortic wall and by the graft's columnar strength. Barbs or hooks encompassed in graft design may provide some additional protection (164).

Angulation of the aortic neck may decrease the frictional force and increase the risk of graft migration (162,165). Other hypotheses about the cause of device migration have focused on the morphologic changes in the aneurysm and aortic neck after endovascular AAA repair. Aortic neck dilation, longitudinal sac shrinkage, and graft shortening have been described (166–169). The aortic neck has been documented to significantly dilate during the first 2 years after endograft repair (170). In a review in which the incidence of graft migration was 15%, the two independent risk factors for endograft migration were neck dilation following repair and a baseline AAA size of >55 mm. Others have argued that neck dilation is not a significant event if adequate graft oversizing was performed at initial endograft placement (171).

Technical Complications and Conversion to Open Surgery

Technical complications have been described in up to one-fourth of endograft placements (172). The occurrence of critical events is independent of operator experience, perhaps reflecting the fact that more anatomically difficult cases are attempted with increasing experience (173). Deployment difficulties include graft foreshortening necessitating the placement of additional distal covered extensions, suprarenal graft displacement, infrarenal graft displacement, and device-related issues such as iliac limb kinking or twisting. Conversion to open surgery has been reported in only 1% to 3% of patients during endograft repair (137,142,174,175). According to the Eurostar registry, however, 18% of patients with endograft placement required a secondary intervention (176). Most of these interventions (76%) were through a transfemoral approach, while the rest required a transabdominal (12%) or extra-anatomic (11%) approach. The rates of freedom from intervention at 1, 3, and 4 years were 89%, 67%, and 62%, respectively. Other large series have mirrored these results (159,161).

Aneurysm Rupture

The risk of rupture following aneurysm repair is low. One series reports a freedom from risk of rupture of 98.7% at 2 years (177). In another series the risk of rupture approached 1% per year (142). The presence of an endoleak and the development of graft migration increase the risk of subsequent AAA rupture.

Mortality

Aortic endograft repair of AAA is associated with a low mortality rate in the range of 1% to 3% (137,142,161,175). Most deaths are related to cardiovascular morbidity. Long-term survival is lower, with 1-year survival rates of 90% and 3-year survival rates of 70% (161). The need for a secondary procedure increases the mortality risk, as 8% of patients requiring a transfemoral secondary intervention died. Mortality rose to 18% for those requiring a transabdominal intervention.

Mesenteric Artery Angioplasty and Stenting

Technical Complications

Primary technical success for mesenteric interventions has been reported at 63% to 81% for PTA and 96% to 100% for primary stenting, with overall clinical success (as measured by resolution or significant reduction in symptoms) in up to 88% of patients (178–180). Unsuccessful PTA is managed with subsequent stent placement. In one series, 50% of the immediate clinical failures were due to misdiagnosis of chronic mesenteric ischemia, and in the follow-up period underlying gastrointestinal cancer was identified (178). Clinical success was not attributable to the number of mesenteric vessels that were treated. Complications described at the site of PTA include arterial dissection,

which is managed with placement of a stent in some cases and observation alone in others (179). Episodes of post-procedural bowel ischemia have been described, affecting 7% to 8% of patients undergoing mesenteric artery endovascular therapy (181,182). The etiology of this complication, presumed to be embolization, dissection, or the underlying reason for mesenteric intervention, has not been explained.

Restenosis

Approximately 15% to 20% of patients who have had a successful endovascular mesenteric intervention have recurrent symptoms, generally occurring within the first year (178–181). In most cases recurrent symptoms are due to the development of restenosis, which can be treated with repeat PTA and, if necessary, secondary stent placement. Primary and assisted-primary patency rates for mesenteric stent placement have been reported to be 70% and 90%, respectively, at 18 months (180). If endovascular therapy continues to fail, surgical revascularization should be performed—provided the patient is an acceptable operative candidate.

Mortality

Mortality rates associated with mesenteric PTA and stent placement have been reported to be between 0% and 11% (178,180,181). In all cases of early mortality, death was attributable to bowel ischemia. Five-year survival rates approach 70% and do not depend on whether the patients underwent primary PTA or stenting, the number of mesenteric vessels treated, or whether the superior mesenteric artery, specifically, had an intervention performed upon it (178).

Renal Artery Angioplasty and Stenting

Technical Complications

Renal artery stenting is associated with technical success rates between 91% and 98% (183,184). Complications associated with renal artery PTA and stenting include renal artery rupture (1.7%), aortic dissection at the level of the renal artery (2.2%), flow-limiting renal artery dissection (1.1%), and renal artery thromboembolism (1.1%) (183). Renal artery rupture, if diagnosed at the time of occurrence, can be managed with reversal of anticoagulation and tamponade of the rupture site with inflation of an angioplasty balloon. Rupture is not always identified at the time of the procedure and may present in a delayed fashion with hypotension, drop in hematocrit, and the development of a perinephric hematoma on imaging studies. Depending on the patient's hemodynamic stability, the delayed diagnosis of renal artery rupture may require no further intervention.

In cases of uncontrolled hemorrhage or failure of less invasive therapies, operative repair of the ruptured renal artery is required. Treatment may require a simple arterial repair, arterial reconstruction, or nephrectomy.

Renal artery dissection can be managed by placement of additional stents if dissection involves the main renal artery. When the dissection involves a branch vessel, the problem becomes more difficult to manage and may result in infarction of the portion of the kidney supplied by that branch. Renal artery thrombosis and embolism may be treated with suction thrombectomy or the administration of a thrombolytic agent. Some instances of acute renal artery thrombosis during the procedure require acute surgical revascularization (184). Stent dislodgement has been reported in 2% of patients undergoing renal stent placement (185). Two-thirds of these patients required abortion of the endovascular procedure and conversion to surgical repair. The others had the stents retrieved with the use of an endovascular snare. Failure to use a guiding sheath has been identified as a risk for stent dislodgment during placement.

Renal Function Complications

Approximately 6% to 25% of patients undergoing renal artery PTA and stent placement have an elevation in serum creatinine lasting longer than 30 days (183,184). Over half of these patients required hemodialysis, but not all required long-term dialysis. The etiology of acute renal failure is variable and in some instances is due to distal renal artery embolization or branch vessel thrombosis resulting in renal infarction. Renal infarction has been documented in approximately 3% of patients.

Infection

Stent infections are not common complications. Several incidences of renal artery stent infection have been described (186–188). The common bacteria in all these cases was *S. aureus*, but in two of the case reports at least one additional bacterium was isolated from blood cultures, including *Proteus mirabilis* and *Klebsiella pneumoniae*. Risk factors for the development of renal artery stent infection do not differ from risk factors for all stent infections. These include breaks in sterile technique, repeated puncture of the same vessel for arterial access, reuse of an indwelling catheter, increased procedure time, and puncture site hematoma formation (186). Patients present with fever, local pain, and leukocytosis. If bacteremia is associated with a particularly virulent pathogen, patients may present with a profound systemic inflammatory response manifested by hypotension, tachycardia, and multisystem organ failure. An intrarenal abscess may form due to embolization from the infected stent. CT scans are sensitive for the diagnosis of stent infection and show an intense inflammatory response around the affected stent and renal artery. Renal artery pseudoaneurysm formation is

associated with the renal artery stent infection (187,188). Death secondary to overwhelming infection has been described as a result of renal artery stent infection (188). Treatment involves intravenous antibiotic administration and resuscitation guided by the clinical scenario. Resection of the infected stent is mandatory, including removal of surrounding infected and devitalized tissue. Excision is followed by autogenous renal artery reconstruction. Some interventionalists recommend the routine use of prophylactic antibiotics prior to renal PTA and stenting (187).

Restenosis

Follow-up angiography is not routine after renal artery PTA or stenting. Patients are reevaluated if they develop worsening renal function or hypertension. In one series, 20.5% of patients developed worsening renal function or hypertension after initially having a positive clinical response to endovascular therapy (184). When these cases underwent angiography, 14 of the 15 patients had evidence of significant in-stent restenosis. Half of these lesions were successfully treated with either angioplasty alone, repeat stent placement, or open surgery. The other half had no intervention as the degree of restenosis was <50%. Other series have reported restenosis rates ranging between 11% and 44% at 2 years (189,190). Restenosis is secondary to either intimal hyperplasia or progression of atherosclerosis.

Mortality

Thirty-day mortality rates following renal artery PTA and stent are low, between 0% and 1.4% (183–185). Mortality has not been directly associated with the renal artery intervention, but to complications from comorbidities.

LOWER EXTREMITY INTERVENTIONS

Femoropopliteal Angioplasty and Stenting

Technical Complications

Initial technical success of femoropopliteal PTA is between 76% and 95% (191–195). Failure is mainly attributable to the inability to cross occlusions and tight stenoses, inability to inflate the angioplasty balloon, or inability to enter the patent distal lumen. Early failures <24 hours occur in 23% of patients (192).

Complications occurring during PTA include arterial disruption, thrombosis, distal embolization, and arterial dissection. Complications occur more frequently in femoropopliteal interventions compared to iliac artery interventions (13% of cases), and half of these complications are significant enough to require operation, transfusion, or an extended hospital stay. Arterial disruption can present with the development of hematoma, pseudoaneurysm, or arteriovenous fistula. Management includes reversal of anticoagulation and the use of a balloon catheter to occlude the arterial injury. The use of covered stents has been described to effectively treat this complication (196). Operative intervention may be required if bleeding is not controlled.

Embolization can occur from thrombus or atheromatous debris from disrupted plaque. Treatment involves the administration of catheter-directed thrombolytic therapy or surgical thromboembolectomy (Fig. 30-6). Acute thrombosis at the angioplasty site has been described in 2.5% of patients and generally occurs at sites of plaque ulceration (193). As with embolization, thromboses are generally treated with thrombolytic therapy, and, if not successful, open thrombectomy. Arterial dissection can also occur following PTA. This complication is often treated with the placement of an intraarterial stent (Fig. 30-7). Most of the complications related to PTA are best managed by arterial bypass. Complication rates depend on the indication for intervention and the patient's age. Older patients and those who were treated for limb-threatening ischemia have worse outcomes.

Technical success following femoropopliteal artery stenting is reported to be 92% (197). In one series 27% of cases of femoropopliteal recanalization were complicated by immediate thrombosis requiring thrombolytic therapy (198). One-fifth of these patients could not have patency reestablished. Distal embolization has been reported in 10% of the patients and is treated as outlined above (199).

Patency and Amputation

Primary patency rates for femoropopliteal PTA are 38% to 45% at 5 years (194). Patency rates are improved in patients whose initial lesions were <5 cm in length (200). Failure of the intervention depends on indication, lesion type, and distal runoff. Patients with critical ischemia, occlusive lesions, and poor runoff have worse outcomes (191). The occurrence of a complication at the time of initial PTA also adversely affects long-term results. Limb salvage is 86% to 91% at 5 years.

Primary patency rates for femoropopliteal artery stenting are 29% to 48% at 3 years (198,199,201). Assisted patency and secondary patency rates increase to 59% to 70% in selected series (198,201). Long-term patency is better for shorter lesions (<10 cm in length) and is worse for patients who require the use of thrombolytic therapy as part of initial treatment and for those treated for femoropopliteal artery occlusion. In-stent restenosis, as evaluated by intravascular ultrasound, is caused by neointimal hyperplasia and stent remodeling leading to lumen area reduction (202). The extent of changes is most significant at stent edges. Patency may be improved by the use of expanded polytetrafluoroethylene (ePTFE) stent-graft relative to bare stents (203).

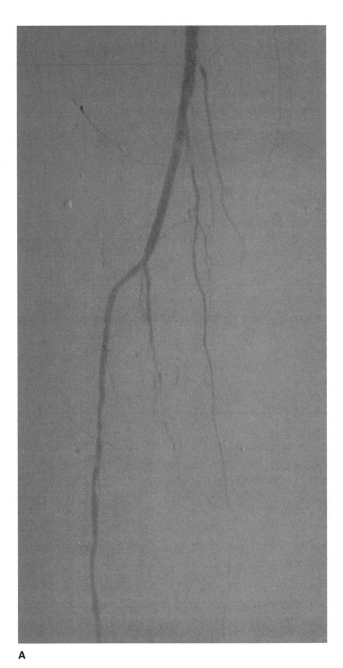

A

Figure 30-6 A: Lower extremity angiogram revealing the outflow tract of a patient with a more proximal popliteal artery stenosis.

Mortality

Mortality rates after femoropopliteal PTA are low, ranging between 0% and 4.3% (191,194,197,200). Deaths are often related to comorbidities, but death from complications directly related to endovascular therapy has been described, including retroperitoneal hemorrhage (201). Survival rates at 5 years are 51% to 73%, with at least a 6% per year mortality.

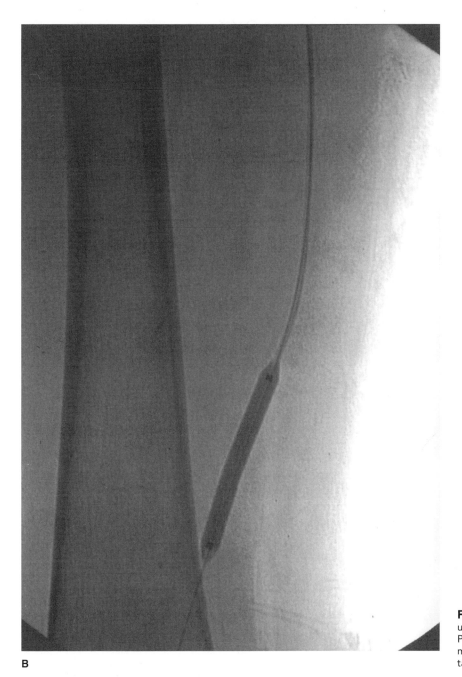

B

Figure 30-6 *(continued)* **B:** This lesion underwent primary balloon angioplasty. Postprocedure ankle-brachial index measurements were significantly lower than those taken before the procedure.

Tibial Angioplasty and Stenting

Few studies provide enough data to adequately evaluate complications following endovascular intervention in the tibial arteries. Technical success has been described in 87% to 92% of patients (204,205). Complications related to tibial PTA include the need for emergency vascular surgery (0.7% of patients), procedurally related deaths (0.4%), amputation (0.4%), and the development of compartment syndrome after tibial recanalization (0.4% of cases) (204). Limb salvage was reported in 91% of these limbs, but 5-year survival was only 31%.

Thrombolysis

Thrombolytic therapy is used to treat acute arterial or venous occlusions. The main risk associated with thrombolytic therapy is bleeding. A variety of agents is used for thrombolytic therapy, including streptokinase derivatives, urokinase compounds (UK), tissue plasminogen activator, and its recombinant forms (rt-PA). An analysis of data collected in a prospective single-institution registry revealed an overall complication rate of 55.9% in patients undergoing thrombolytic therapy for both arterial and venous disease (206). In patients receiving thrombolytic

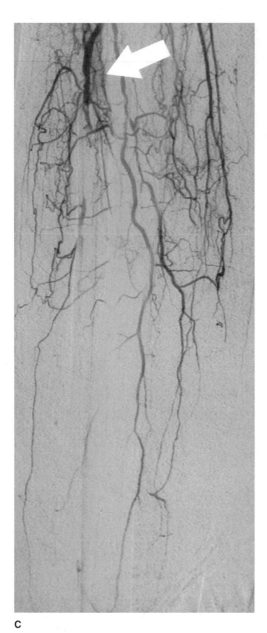

c

Figure 30-6 *(continued)* **C:** Repeat angiography revealed a thromboembolus occluding the outflow tract. Attempts at thrombolysis were unsuccessful and the patient underwent popliteal thromboembolectomy.

therapy for arterial disease, complications included development of hematoma or pseudoaneurysm (30.6% UK vs. 57.7% rt-PA), bleeding requiring transfusion (11.9% UK vs. 18.7% rt-PA), and intracranial bleeding (0.8% UK vs. 3.3% rt-PA). Mortality rates were 2.9% for UK and 1.6% for rt-PA.

In patients being treated for venous disease, the complications reported were hematoma formation (18.4% UK vs. 28.6% rt-PA) and bleeding requiring transfusion (14.3% UK vs. 42.9% rt-PA). There were no episodes of intracranial bleeding in venous patients, but mortality rates were 2% for UK compared to 19% for rt-PA. The causes of mortality were not reported in the venous group, but in the arterial

group some were related to the development of intracranial hemorrhage. There are fewer complications with the use of thrombolytic therapy to treat venous disease, and there appears to be fewer complications with the use of UK compared to rt-PA.

Two major randomized prospective trials have evaluated the use of thrombolytic therapy for lower extremity ischemia: Surgery versus Thrombolysis for Ischemia of the Lower Extremity (STILE) and Thrombolysis or Peripheral Artery Surgery (TOPAS) (207,208). In these trials complications occurred with an incidence of 22% to 41% and included hemorrhage, distal embolization, and catheter-related problems. Life-threatening hemorrhage occurred in 6.2% of patients undergoing thrombolytic therapy in the STILE trial and in 12.5% of patients treated with thrombolytics in the TOPAS trial. The TOPAS trial did show that when aspirin and therapeutic heparin were withheld during thrombolytic therapy the rate of intracranial hemorrhage decreased from 5% to 0.5% (208). Aggressive control of hypertension is also beneficial in decreasing the risk of intracranial hemorrhage (209). Distal embolization occurred in 14% of cases. Embolization is generally self-limiting; as the thrombolysis progresses, the embolization is cleared. Embolization requiring surgery occurs in approximately 2% of cases.

In order to minimize the risks of thrombolytic therapy, several criteria have been accepted as contraindications (Table 30-3). The use of micropuncture needles and small catheters may decrease the risk of bleeding complications. Monitoring of laboratory values, such as fibrinogen level, have been of no value in predicting which patients are at increased risk of bleeding (209). In the presence of hemorrhage, heparin and thrombolytic agent should be discontinued. If necessary, thrombolytic agents can be reversed with cryoprecipitate, fresh frozen plasma, tranexamic acid, aminocaproic acid, or aprotinin. These interventions are rarely necessary, as most thrombolytic agents have short half-lives in the range of minutes.

TABLE 30-3

CONTRAINDICATIONS TO THROMBOLYTIC THERAPY

Absolute Contraindications
Stroke or transient ischemic attack within the past 2 months
Gastrointestinal bleeding within the past 10 days
Neurosurgery or intracranial trauma within the past 3 months

Relatively Major Contraindications
Cardiopulmonary resuscitation within the past 10 days
Major nonvascular surgery or trauma within the past 10 days
Uncontrolled hypertension
Intracranial tumor
Recent eye surgery

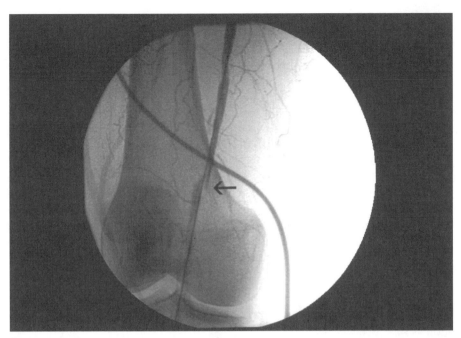

A

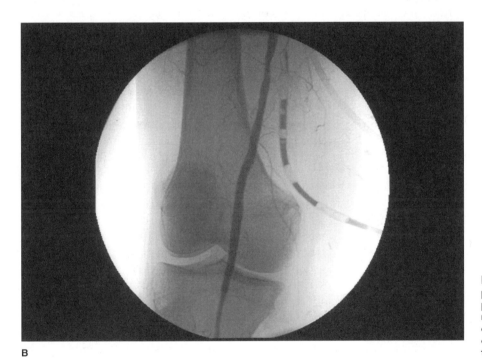

B

Figure 30-7 A: Angiogram of a patient who underwent balloon angioplasty of a popliteal artery stenosis. This resulted in an arterial dissection that occluded flow in the vessel. **B:** Placement of an intra-arterial stent successfully treated the dissection.

VENOUS INTERVENTIONS

Vena Cava Filters

Technical Complications

Complications during placement of an inferior vena cava (IVC) filter are rare. Problems can include bleeding, embolism, inability to insert the device, misplacement, migration, and guidewire entrapment. Embolism is a rare occurrence, but it can occur if the device is inserted through

deep venous thrombosis. If it is suspected that thrombus is lining the IVC or involves both of the iliac veins, an alternative approach places the filter through the internal jugular vein. Occasionally IVC filter placement is hindered by difficulty in passing the filter through the iliac venous system. This problem is particularly difficult for the left iliac venous system. With newer delivery systems that provide a lower profile and increased flexibility, this complication is rare.

Acute migration of IVC filters occurs when there is lack of apposition to the caval wall with cranial displacement.

Possible mechanisms for this complication include the deployment of the filter into thrombus preventing the limb from attaching to the caval wall or placement in an IVC that is larger than the filter (210). Few IVC filters are approved for placement in vena cavas >28 mm, making this an important anatomic characteristic to identify. Filter migration (movement of >10 mm) has been described in 30% to 76% of filter placements (211). Improved stent designs have lowered this risk to between 3% and 10%. In some instances the device fails to open at the time of release. This phenomenon has been described in 2% to 42% of cases, depending on the brand of filter used (210,212). Migrated filters can occasionally be left in place, or they may be snared and removed through a large sheath, often requiring a vein cutdown for complete removal.

Postdeployment Complications

Excessive tilt of a filter is another potential complication. Failure to adequately locate the renal veins prior to placement increases the risk of this complication as filter struts lodged in the orifice of a branching vein will offset the filter's alignment. Excessive filter tilting increases the risk of subsequent pulmonary embolism (213). If a filter is tilted by >14 degrees, a second filter should be placed above the level of the initial filter.

Recurrent pulmonary embolism is one of the most serious complications of filter placement, reported in 2% to 5% of Greenfield filters (210). This complication is most often seen in patients who have a malignancy and remain with a hypercoaguable state. In 1% to 2% of patients, the filter traps a massive thrombus, filling the volume of the filter with clot and leading to IVC occlusion. These patients can present with evidence of acute caval occlusion and subsequent decreased cardiac preload. Affected patients will have hypotension and lower extremity swelling. These cases can be distinguished from recurrent acute PE, as that may present with hypotension but will have increased jugular distension. Cavography can confirm the diagnosis, and thrombolytic therapy may be used to restore patency. If the patient is asymptomatic, no intervention is required, as most clots will lyse spontaneously (210).

Full thickness erosion of filter struts is seen infrequently. This problem may be caused by an inflammatory response of the caval wall to the struts. Rates of strut perforation are surprisingly high and have been reported in 30% to 95% of filters (211). Most cases of perforation remain asymptomatic, but erosion into surrounding structures has been described (214). These structures have included the duodenum and aorta and have resulted in ulceration, hemorrhage, arteriovenous fistula, and heart failure. These serious complications require surgical intervention.

Venous Angioplasty and Stenting

Technical complications during venous PTA and stent placement are rare. In a large series of patients treated for chronic venous insufficiency, no technical complications occurred and all lesions were technically successfully treated (215). Forty-four of 304 limbs treated, however, required reintervention in the follow-up period due to symptomatic restenosis. Primary patency of these stents at 24 months was 71%, with an assisted patency rate of 97%. No deaths were associated with this procedure, nor were any deaths evident in the follow-up period. Patency rates are lower in those venous segments that required recanalization due to complete occlusion (216). Patients treated for the May–Thurner syndrome have similarly negligible complication rates and comparable patency rates (217). Complications associated with stenting of the superior vena cava in the superior vena cava syndrome have been described in case reports and in one instance was associated with cardiac tamponade.

Endovascular Therapy for Pulmonary Embolism

Technical Failure

The most common complication in endovascular treatment of pulmonary embolism is failure to resolve the thromboembolus. Technical failures occur in 5% to 39% of cases. Most reports indicate that the success of endovascular therapy is directly related to the age of the pulmonary embolism. Greenfield noted that embolectomy success was highest for major pulmonary embolism and massive acute pulmonary embolism (100% and 82% success, respectively) and worst for chronic pulmonary embolism (56% success) (218). In most series, failed procedures occurred in patients who had a history of previous pulmonary embolism, who had elevated pulmonary artery pressure suggestive of chronic pulmonary embolism, or who had chronic thrombus found at the time of pulmonary embolectomy (219). Endovascular therapy for pulmonary embolism is less effective in patients who are >72 hours beyond the initial event and should be performed only in patients with a recent pulmonary embolism and a pulmonary artery pressure <50 mm Hg. Most initial treatment failures require operative thromboembolectomy, or the patients succumb to the hemodynamic compromise induced by the pulmonary embolism. Perforation of the pulmonary artery is a rare occurrence and has only been described twice in the Greenfield series (218). In one instance the complication was believed to be secondary to the suction pulmonary embolectomy device, and with subsequent modifications no perforations have been described.

Mortality

Mortality rates mirror treatment failure rates and range from 5% to 28%. Initial problems with cardiac arrest were attributed to large volume contrast bolus injections into the main pulmonary artery (218). Most short-term deaths are secondary to cardiovascular collapse secondary to irreversible right heart failure (218–220). Other causes of death include intracerebral hemorrhage, sepsis, and multisystem organ failure. Survival is directly attributable to the procedure's success. Short-term mortality rates are as high as 73% in patients with failure of thrombus resolution but decrease to 17% with successful treatment (218).

Recurrent Thromboembolism

The incidence of recurrent deep venous thrombosis (4%) and recurrent pulmonary embolism (4%) has been described in only one study (218). These episodes occurred prior to the development of percutaneous placed vena cava filters. The episodes of recurrent pulmonary embolism presented in the interval between pulmonary embolectomy and subsequent vena cava clip placement—which was performed in the operating room as a separate procedure. The placement of a vena cava filter at the time of pulmonary embolectomy, as well as the use of heparin anticoagulation, is beneficial in preventing the risk of recurrent pulmonary embolism.

CONCLUSIONS

Endovascular therapies are becoming more prevalent. Many of the complications that occur are similar among the different interventions. An understanding of the potential adverse events is helpful to the surgeon who is either requesting the intervention or performing it. Most of the complications can be managed in a noninvasive fashion, but when they cannot be, conventional surgery is required.

REFERENCES

1. Hou S, Bushinsky D, Wish J, et al. Hospital-acquired renal insufficiency: a prospective study. *Am J Med* 1983;74:243–248.
2. Murphy S, Barrett B, Parfrey P. Contrast nephropathy. *J Am Soc Nephrol* 2000;11:177–182.
3. Berg K. Nephrotoxicity related to contrast media. *Scand J Urol Nephrol* 2000;34:317–322.
4. Solomon R. Nephrology forum: contrast-medium-induced acute renal failure. *Kidney Int* 1998;53:230–242.
5. Barrett B. Contrast nephropathy. *J Am Soc Nephrol* 1994;5:125–137.
6. Katzberg R. Urography in the 21st century: new contrast media, renal handling, imaging characteristics, and nephrotoxicity. *Radiology* 1997;204:297–312.
7. Liss P, Nygren A, Olsson U, et al. Effect of contrast media and mannitol on renal medullary blood flow and red cell aggregation in the rat kidney. *Kidney Int* 1996;49:1268–1275.
8. Berg K, Jakobsen J. Nephrotoxicity related to x-ray contrast media. *Adv X-ray Cont* 1993;1:10–18.
9. Rudnick M, Berns J, Cohen R, et al. Contrast-media associated nephrotoxicity. *Semin Nephrol* 1997;17:15–26.
10. Cantley L, Spokes K, Clark B, et al. Role of endothelin and prostaglandins in radiocontrast-induced renal artery constriction. *Kidney Int* 1993;44:1217–1223.
11. Bakris G, Burnett J. A role for calcium in radiocontrast-induced reduction in renal hemodynamics. *Kidney Int* 1985;27:465–468.
12. Bakris G, Lass N, Osama Gaber A, et al. Radiocontrast medium-induced decline in renal function: a role for oxygen free radicals. *Am J Physiol* 1990;258:F115–F120.
13. Katholi R, Taylor G, McCann W, et al. Nephrotoxicity from contrast media: attenuation with theophylline. *Radiology* 1995;195:17–22.
14. Rich M, Crecelius C. Incidence, risk factors, and clinical course of acute renal insufficiency after cardiac catheterization in patients 70 years of age or older. *Arch Intern Med* 1995;150:1237–1242.
15. Porter G. Contrast-associated nephropathy. *Am J Cardiol* 1989;64:22E–26E.
16. Levy E, Viscoli C, Horwitz R. The effect of acute renal failure on mortality: a cohort analysis. *J Am Med Assoc* 1996;275:1489–1494.
17. Rudnick M, Goldfarb S, Wexler L, et al. Nephrotoxicity of ionic and nonionic contrast media in 1196 patients: a randomized trial. *Kidney Int* 1995;47:254–261.
18. Weisberg L, Kurnik P, Kurnik B. Dopamine and renal blood flow in radiocontrast-induced nephropathy in humans. *Ren Fail* 1993;15:61–68.
19. Abizaid A, Clark C, Mintz G, et al. Effects of dopamine and aminophylline on contrast-induced acute renal failure after coronary angioplasty in patients with preexisting renal insufficiency. *Am J Cardiol* 1999;83:260–263.
20. Birck R, Krzossok S, Markowetz F, et al. Acetylcysteine for prevention of contrast nephropathy: meta-analysis. *Lancet* 2003;362:598–603.
21. Tumlin J, Wang A, Murray P, et al. Fenoldopam mesylate blocks reductions in renal plasma flow after radiocontrast dye infusion: a pilot trial in the prevention of contrast nephropathy. *Am Heart J* 2002;143:894–903.
22. Kini A, Mitre C, Kim M, et al. A protocol for prevention of radiographic contrast nephropathy during percutaneous coronary intervention: effect of selective dopamine receptor agonist fenoldopam. *Catheter Cardiovasc Interv* 2002;55:169–173.
23. Messina L, Brothers T, Wakefield T, et al. Clinical characteristics and surgical management of vascular complications in patients undergoing cardiac catheterization: interventional versus diagnostic procedures. *J Vasc Surg* 1991;13:593–600.
24. Muller D, Podd J, Shamir K. Vascular access site complications in the era of complex percutaneous coronary interventions. *Circulation* 1990;82:510.
25. Young N, Chi K-K, Ajaka J, et al. Complications with outpatient angiography and interventional procedures. *Cardiovasc Intervent Radiol* 2002;25:123–126.
26. Franco C, Goldsmith J, Veith F, et al. Management of arterial injuries produced by percutaneous femoral procedures. *Surgery* 1993;113:419–425.
27. Cragg A, Nakagawa N, Smith T, et al. Hematoma formation after diagnostic angiography: effect of catheter size. *J Vasc Interv Radiol* 1991;2:231–233.
28. Chitwood R, Shepard A, Shetty P, et al. Surgical complications of transaxillary arteriography: a case-control study. *J Vasc Surg* 1996;23:844–850.
29. Kresowick T, Khoury M, Miller B, et al. A prospective study of the incidence and natural history of femoral vascular complications after percutaneous transluminal coronary angioplasty. *J Vasc Surg* 1991;13:328–336.
30. Dowling K, Todd D, Siskin G, et al. Early ambulation after diagnostic angiography using 4-F catheters and sheaths: a feasibility study. *J Endovasc Ther* 2002;9:618–621.
31. Lonn L, Olmarker A, Geterud K, et al. Treatment of femoral pseudoaneurysms. Percutaneous US-guided thrombin injection versus US-guided compression. *Acta Radiol* 2002;43:396–400.
32. Spies J, Berlin L. Complications of femoral artery puncture. *Am J Roentgen* 1998;170:9–11.
33. Lilly M, Reichman W, Srazen A, et al. Anatomic and clinical factors associated with complications of transfemoral arteriography. *Ann Vasc Surg* 1990;4:264–269.
34. Altin R, Flicker S, Naidech H. Pseudoaneurysm and arteriovenous fistula after femoral catheterization: association with low femoral punctures. *Am J Radiol* 1989;152:629–631.
35. Rapoport S, Sniderman K, Morse S, et al. Pseudoaneurysm: a complication of faulty technique in femoral arterial puncture. *Radiology* 1985;154:529–530.

36. Toursarkissian B, Allen B, Petrinec D, et al. Spontaneous closure of selected iatrogenic pseudoaneurysms and arteriovenous fistulae. *J Vasc Surg* 1997;25:803–809.

37. Cox G, Young J, Gray B, et al. Ultrasound-guided compression of postcatheterization pseudoaneurysms: results of treatment in one hundred cases. *J Vasc Surg* 1994;19:683–686.

38. Elford J, Burrell C, Freeman S, et al. Human thrombin injection for the percutaneous treatment of iatrogenic pseudoaneurysms. *Cardiovasc Intervent Radiol* 2002;25:115–118.

39. Waigand J, Uhlich F, Gross M, et al. Percutaneous treatment of pseudoaneurysms and arteriovenous fistulas after invasive vascular procedures. *Catheter Cardiovasc Interv* 1999;47:157–164.

40. Thalhammer C, Kirchherr A, Uhlich F, et al. Postcatheterization pseudoaneurysms and arteriovenous fistulas: repair with percutaneous implantation of endovascular covered stents. *Radiology* 2000;214:127–131.

41. Kent K, Mosucci M, Gallagher S, et al. Neuropathy after cardiac catheterization: incidence, clinical patterns, and long-term outcome. *J Vasc Surg* 1994;19:1008–1014.

42. Mills J, Wiedeman J, Robison J, et al. Minimizing mortality and morbidity from iatrogenic arterial injuries: the need for early recognition and prompt repair. *J Vasc Surg* 1986;4:22–27.

43. Tron C, Koning R, Eltchaninoff H, et al. A randomized comparison of a percutaneous suture device versus manual compression for femoral artery hemostasis after PTCA. *J Intervent Cardiol* 2003;16:217–221.

44. Sanborn T, Gibbs H, Brinker J, et al. A multicenter randomized trial comparing a percutaneous collagen hemostasis device with conventional manual compression after diagnostic angiography and angioplasty. *J Am Coll Cardiol* 1993;22:1273–1279.

45. Wetter D, Rickli H, von Smekal A, et al. Early sheath removal after coronary artery interventions with use of a suture-mediated closure device: clinical outcome and results of Doppler US evaluation. *J Vasc Interv Radiol* 2000;11:1033–1037.

46. Michalis L, Rees M, Patsouras D, et al. A prospective randomized trial comparing the safety and efficacy of three commercially available closure devices (Angioseal, Vasoseal and Duett). *Cardiovasc Intervent Radiol* 2002;25:423–429.

47. Kornowski R, Brandes S, Teplitsky I, et al. Safety and efficacy of a 6 French Perclose arterial suturing device following percutaneous coronary interventions: a pilot evaluation. *J Invasive Cardiol* 2002;14:741–745.

48. Sesana M, Vaghetti M, Albiero R, et al. Effectiveness and complications of vascular access closure devices after interventional procedures. *J Invasive Cardiol* 2000;12:395–399.

49. Meyerson S, Feldman T, Desai T, et al. Angiographic access site complications in the era of arterial closure devices. *Vasc Endovasc Ther* 2002;36:137–144.

50. Starnes B, O'Donnell S, Gillespie D, et al. Percutaneous arterial closure in peripheral vascular disease: a prospective evaluation of the Perclose device. *J Vasc Surg* 2003;38:263–271.

51. Dangas G, Mehran R, Kokolis S, et al. Vascular complications after percutaneous coronary interventions following hemostasis with manual compression versus arteriotomy closure devices. *J Am Coll Cardiol* 2001;38:638–641.

52. Goyen M, Manz S, Kroger K, et al. Interventional therapy of vascular complications caused by the hemostatic puncture closure device angio-seal. *Catheter Cardiovasc Interv* 2000;49:142–147.

53. Carere R, Webb J, Miyagishima R, et al. Groin complications associated with collagen plug closure of femoral arterial puncture sites in anticoagulated patients. *Catheter Cardiovasc Diag* 1998;43:124–129.

54. Hoffer E, Bloch R. Percutaneous arterial closure devices. *J Vasc Interv Radiol* 2003;14:865–885.

55. Egglin T, O'Moore P, Feinstein A, et al. Complications of peripheral arteriography: a new system to identify patients at increased risk. *J Vasc Surg* 1995;22:787–794.

56. Dawson P, Strickland N. Thromboembolic phenomena in clinical angiography: role of materials and techniques. *J Vasc Interv Radiol* 1991;2:125.

57. Formanek G, Frech R, Amplatz K. Arterial thrombus formation during clinical percutaneous catheterization. *Circulation* 1970;41:833–839.

58. van Andel G. Arterial occlusion following angiography. *Br J Radiol* 1980;53:747–753.

59. Bolasny B, Killen D. Surgical management of arterial injuries secondary to angiography. *Ann Surg* 1971;174:962–964.

60. Fine M, Kapoor W, Falanga V. Cholesterol crystal embolization: a review of 221 cases in the English literature—angiology. *J Vasc Dis* 1987;7:769–784.

61. Deschamps P, Leroy D, Mandard J, et al. Cholesterol embolism in the lower limbs. *Br J Dermatol* 1977;97:93–97.

62. Hendrickx I, Monti M, Manasse E, et al. Severe cutaneous cholesterol emboli syndrome after coronary angiography. *Eur J Cardiothorac Surg* 1999;15:215–217.

63. Dion J, Gates P, Fox A, et al. Clinical events following neuroangiography: a prospective study. *Stroke* 1987;18:997–1004.

64. Hankey G, Warlow C, Sellar R. Cerebral angiographic risk in mild cerebrovascular disease. *Stroke* 1990;21:209–222.

65. Davies K, Humphrey P. Complications of cerebral angiography in patients in patients with symptomatic carotid territory ischeamia screened by carotid ultrasound. *J Neurol Neurosurg Psychiatry* 1993;56:967–972.

66. Johnston D, Chapman K, Goldstein L. Low rate of complications of cerebral angiography in routine clinical practice. *Neurology* 2001;57:2012–2014.

67. Theodotou B, Whaley R, Mahaley M. Complications following tranfemoral cerebral angiography for cerebral ischemia: report of 159 angiograms and correlation with surgical risk. *Surg Neurol* 1987;28:90–92.

68. Markus H, Loh A, Israel D, et al. Microscopic air embolism during cerebral angiography and strategies for its avoidance. *Lancet* 1993;341:784–787.

69. Woolfenden A, O'Brien M, Schwartzberg R, et al. Diffusion weighted MRI in transient global amnesia precipitated by cerebral angiography. *Stroke* 1997;28:2311–2314.

70. Bendszus M, Koltzenburg M, Burger R, et al. Silent embolization in diagnostic cerebral angiography and neurointerventional procedures: a prospective study. *Lancet* 1999;354:1594–1597.

71. Roubin G, Yadav S, Vitek J. Carotid stent-supported angioplasty: a neurovascular intervention to prevent stroke. *Am J Cardiol* 1998;78:8–12.

72. Malek A, Higashida R, Phatouros C, et al. Stent angioplasty for cervical carotid artery stenosis in high-risk symptomatic NASCET-ineligible patients. *Stroke* 2000;31:3029–3033.

73. Ross C, Naslund T, Ranval T. Carotid stent-assisted angioplasty: the newest addition to the surgeons' armamentarium in the management of carotid occlusive disease. *Am Surg* 2002;68:967–975.

74. New G, Iyer S, Diethrich E, et al. Safety, efficacy, and durability of carotid artery stenting for restenosis following carotid endarterectomy: a multicenter study. *J Endovasc Ther* 2000;7:345–352.

75. Hobson R II, Lal B, Chaktoura E, et al. Carotid artery stenting: analysis of data for 105 patients at high risk. *J Vasc Surg* 2003;37:1234–1239.

76. Howell M, Krajcer Z, Dougherty K, et al. Correlation of periprocedural systolic blood pressure changes with neurologic events in high-risk carotid stent patients. *J Endovasc Ther* 2002;9:810–816.

77. Schwarten D. Extracranial brachiocephalic angioplasty. In: Baum S, Pentecost M, eds. *Abram's angiography: interventional radiology*. Boston, MA: Little, Brown and Company; 1997:339–355.

78. Castriota F, Cremonesi A, Manetti R, et al. Impact of cerebral protection devices on early outcome of carotid stenting. *J Endovasc Ther* 2002;9:786–792.

79. Wilentz J, Chati Z, Krafft V, et al. Retinal embolization during carotid angioplasty and stenting: mechanisms and role of cerebral protections systems. *Catheter Cardiovasc Diag* 2002;56:320–327.

80. Macdonald S, McKevitt F, Venables G, et al. Neurologic outcomes after carotid stenting protected with Neuroshield filter compared to unprotected stenting. *J Endovasc Ther* 2002;9:777–785.

81. Martin J-B, Pache J-C, Treggiari-Venzi M, et al. Role of the distal balloon protection technique in the prevention of cerebral embolic event during carotid stent placement. *Stroke* 2001;32:479–484.

82. Cremonesi A, Manetti R, Setacci F, et al. Protected carotid stenting: clinical advantages and complications of embolic protection devices in 442 consecutive patients. *Stroke* 2003;34:1936–1943.

83. Ohki T, Veith F, Grenell S, et al. Initial experience with cerebral protection devices to prevent embolization during carotid artery stenting. *J Vasc Surg* 2002;36:1175–1185.

84. Yadav J, Roubin G, Iyer S, et al. Elective stenting of the extracranial carotid arteries. *Circulation* 1997;95:376–381.

85. Wholey M, Wholey M, Bergeron P, et al. Current global status of carotid stent placement. *Catheter Cardiovasc Diag* 1998;44:1–6.

86. Bergeron P, Becquemin J-P, Jausseran J-M, et al. Percutaneous stenting of the internal carotid artery: the European CAST-1 study. *J Endovasc Surg* 1999;6:155–159.

87. Henry M, Amor M, Masson I, et al. Angioplasty and stenting of the extracranial carotid arteries. *J Endovasc Surg* 1998;5:293–304.

88. Al-Mubarak N, Roubin G, Gomez C, et al. Carotid artery stenting in patients with high neurologic risks. *Am J Cardiol* 1999;83: 1411–1413.

89. Willfort-Ehringer A, Ahmadi R, Gschwandtner M, et al. Single-center experience with carotid stent restenosis. *J Endovasc Ther* 2002;9:299–307.

90. Lal B, Hobson R II, Goldstein J, et al. In-stent recurrent stenosis after carotid artery stenting: life table analysis and clinical relevance. *J Vasc Surg* 2003;38:1162–1169.

91. Becker G, Palmaz J, Rees C, et al. Angioplasty-induced dissections in human iliac arteries: management with Palmaz balloon-expandable intraluminal stents. *Radiology* 1990;176:31–38.

92. Bendok B, Roubin G, Katzen B, et al. Cutting balloon to treat carotid in-stent stenosis: technical note. *J Invasive Cardiol* 2003;15:227–232.

93. Rodriguez-Lopez J, Werner A, Martinez R, et al. Stenting for atherosclerotic occlusive disease of the subclavian artery. *Ann Vasc Surg* 1999;13:254–260.

94. Ringelstein E, Zeumer H. Delayed reversal of vertebral artery blood flow following percutaneous transluminal angioplasty for subclavian steal syndrome. *Neuroradiology* 1984;26:189–198.

95. Sullivan T, Gray B, Bacharach J, et al. Angioplasty and primary stenting of the subclavian, innominate, and common carotid arteries in 83 patients. *J Vasc Surg* 1998;28:1059–1065.

96. Al-Mubarak N, Liu M, Dean L, et al. Immediate and late outcomes of subclavian artery stenting. *Catheter Cardiovasc Interv* 1999;46:169–172.

97. Lin P, Bush R, Weiss V, et al. Subclavian artery disruption resulting from endovascular intervention: treatment options. *J Vasc Surg* 2000;32:607–611.

98. Xenos E, Freeman M, Stevens S, et al. Covered stents for injuries of subclavian and axillary arteries. *J Vasc Surg* 2003;38:451–454.

99. Malek A, Higashida R, Reilly L, et al. Subclavian arteritis and pseudoaneurysm formation secondary to stent infection. *Cardiovasc Intervent Radiol* 2000;23:57–60.

100. Hadjipetrou P, Cox S, Piemonte T, et al. Percutaneous revascularization of atherosclerotic obstruction of aortic arch vessels. *J Am Coll Cardiol* 1999;33:1238–1245.

101. Schillinger M, Haumer M, Schillinger S, et al. Risk stratification for subclavian artery angioplasty: is there an increased rate of restenosis after stent implantation? *J Endovasc Ther* 2001;8: 550–557.

102. Korner M, Baumgartner I, Do D, et al. PTA of the subclavian and innominate arteries: long-term results. *Vasa* 1999;28:117–122.

103. Tegtmeyer C, Hartwell G, Selby J, et al. Results and complications of angioplasty in aortoiliac disease. *Circulation* 1991;83: I53–I60.

104. Belli A, Cumberland D, Knox A, et al. The complication rate of percutaneous peripheral balloon angioplasty. *Clin Radiol* 1990;41:380–383.

105. Al-Hamali S, Baskerville P, Fraser S, et al. Detection of distal emboli in patients with peripheral arterial stenosis before and after iliac angioplasty: a prospective study. *J Vasc Surg* 1999;29:345–351.

106. Gardiner G Jr, Meyerovitz M, Stokes K, et al. Complications of transluminal angioplasty. *Radiology* 1986;159:201–208.

107. Ballard J, Sparks S, Taylor F, et al. Complications of iliac artery stent deployment. *J Vasc Surg* 1996;24:545–555.

108. Palmaz J, Laborde J, Rivera F, et al. Stenting of the iliac arteries with the Palmaz stent: experience from a multicenter trial. *Cardiovasc Intervent Radiol* 1992;15:291–297.

109. Allaire E, Melliere D, Poussier B, et al. Iliac artery rupture during balloon dilatation: what treatment? *Ann Vasc Surg* 2003;17: 306–314.

110. Trost D, Jagust M, Weiss M, et al. Percutaneous puncture of nondeflating angioplasty balloons. *J Vasc Interv Radiol* 1999;10: 924–926.

111. Parham W, Puri S, Bitar S, et al. Management of iliac stent movement complicating peripheral vascular intervention: a rescue technique when stent deployment malfunctions. *J Invasive Cardiol* 2003;15:277–279.

112. Bunt T, Gill H, Smith D, et al. Infection of a chronically implanted iliac artery stent. *Ann Vasc Surg* 1997;11:529–532.

113. Deiparine M, Ballard J, Taylor F, et al. Endovascular stent infection. *J Vasc Surg* 1996;23:529–533.

114. Therasse E, Soulez G, Cartier P, et al. Infection with fatal outcome after endovascular metallic stent. *Radiology* 1994;192:363–365.

115. Palmaz J. Intravascular stents: tissue-stent interaction and design consideration. *Am J Roentgen* 1993;160:613–618.

116. Johnston K, Rae M, Hogg-Johnston S, et al. 5-year results of a prospective study of percutaneous transluminal angioplasty. *Ann Surg* 1987;206:403–413.

117. Yasuhara H, Shigematsu H, Muto T. Risk factors for restenosis after balloon angioplasty in focal iliac stenosis. *Surgery* 1998;123:658–665.

118. Bosch J, Hunink M. Meta-analysis of the results of percutaneous transluminal angioplasty and stent placement for aortoiliac occlusive disease. *Radiology* 1997;204:87–96.

119. Timaran C, Stevens S, Freeman M, et al. Predictors for adverse outcome after iliac angioplasty and stenting for limb-threatening ischemia. *J Vasc Surg* 2002;36:507–513.

120. Vorwerk D, Guenther R, Schurmann K, et al. Late reobstruction in iliac arterial stents: percutaneous treatment. *Radiology* 1995;197:479–483.

121. Schillinger M, Exner M, Mlekusch W, et al. Fibrinogen predicts restenosis after endovascular treatment of the iliac arteries. *Thromb Haemost* 2002;2002:959–965.

122. Murphy K, Encarnacion C, Le V, et al. Iliac artery stent placement with the Palmaz stent: follow-up study. *J Vasc Interv Radiol* 1995;6:321–329.

123. Zarins C, White R, Schwarten D, et al. AneuRx stent graft versus open surgical repair of abdominal aortic aneurysms: multicenter prospective clinical trial. *J Vasc Surg* 1999;29:292–305.

124. May J, White G, Waugh R, et al. Improved survival after endoluminal repair with second-generation prostheses compared with open repair in the treatment of abdominal aortic aneurysms: a 5-year concurrent comparison using life table method. *J Vasc Surg* 2001;33:S21–S26.

125. Lee WA, O'Dorisio J, Wolf YG, et al. Outcome after unilateral hypogastric artery occlusion during endovascular aneurysm repair. *J Vasc Surg* 2001;33:921–926.

126. Wolpert LM, Dittrich KP, Hallisey MJ, et al. Hypogastric artery embolization in endovascular abdominal aortic aneurysm repair. *J Vasc Surg* 2001;33:1193–1198.

127. Criado FJ, Wilson EP, Velazquez OC, et al. Safety of coil embolization of the internal iliac artery in endovascular grafting of abdominal aortic aneurysms. *J Vasc Surg* 2000;32:684–688.

128. Schoder M, Zaunbauer L, Holzenbein T, et al. Internal iliac artery embolization before endovascular repair of abdominal aortic aneurysms: frequency, efficacy, and clinical results. *Am J Radiol* 2001;177:599–605.

129. Mehta M, Veith FJ, Ohki T, et al. Unilateral and bilateral hypogastric artery interruption during aortoiliac aneurysm repair in 154 patients: a relatively innocuous procedure. *J Vasc Surg* 2001;33:S27–S32.

130. Kritpracha B, Pigott JP, Price CI, et al. Distal internal iliac artery embolization: a procedure to avoid. *J Vasc Surg* 2003;37: 943–948.

131. Wyers MC, Shermerhorn ML, Fillinger MF, et al. Internal iliac occlusion without coil embolization during endovascular abdominal aortic aneurysm repair. *J Vasc Surg* 2002;36: 1138–1145.

132. White GH, Yu W, May J. Endoleak: a proposed new terminology to describe incomplete aneurysm exclusion by an endoluminal graft. *J Endovasc Surg* 1996;3:124–125.

133. White GH, May J, Waugh RC, et al. Type I and type II endoleaks: a more useful classification for reporting results of endoluminal AAA repair. *J Endovasc Surg* 1998;5:189–191.

134. White GH, May J, Waugh RC, et al. Type III and type IV endoleaks: toward a complete definition of blood flow in the sac after endoluminal AAA repair. *J Endovasc Surg* 1998;5:305–309.

135. Ouriel K, Greenberg R, Clair D. Endovascular treatment of aortic aneurysm. *Current Problems in Surgery* 2002;39:233.

136. Zarins CK, White RA, Hodgson KJ, et al. Endoleak as a predictor of outcome after endovascular aneurysm repair: AneuRx multi-center clinical trial. *J Vasc Surg* 2000;32:90–107.

137. Holzenbein T, Kretschmer G, Thurnher S, et al. Midterm durability of abdominal aortic aneurysm endograft repair: a word of caution. *J Vasc Surg* 2001;33:S46–S54.

138. Buth J, Harris·PL, van Marrewijk C, et al. The significance and management of different types of endoleaks. *Semin Vasc Surg* 2003;16:95–102.

139. Chuter TAM, Faruqi RM, Sawhney R, et al. Endoleak after endovascular repair of abdominal aortic aneurysm. *J Vasc Surg* 2001;34:98–105.

140. Buth J, Laheji RJF. Early complications and endoleaks after endovascular abdominal aortic aneurysm repair: report of a multicenter study. *J Vasc Surg* 2000;31:134–146.

141. Dattilo JB, Brewster DC, Fan C-M, et al. Clinical failures of endovascular abdominal aortic aneurysm repair: Incidence, causes, and management. *J Vasc Surg* 2002;35:1137–1144.

142. Zarins CK. The US AneuRx clinical trial: 6-year clinical update 2002. *J Vasc Surg* 2003;37:904–908.

143. Fairman RM, Carpenter JP, Baum RA, et al. Potential impact of therapeutic warfarin treatment on type II endoleaks and sac shrinkage rates on midterm follow-up examination. *J Vasc Surg* 2002;35:679–685.

144. Baum RA, Carpenter JP, Cope C, et al. Aneurysm sac pressure measurements after endovascular repair of abdominal aortic aneurysms. *J Vasc Surg* 2001;33:32–41.

145. Jacobs T, Teodorescu V, Morrissey N, et al. The endovascular repair of abdominal aortic aneurysm: an update analysis of structural failure modes of endovascular grafts. *Semin Vasc Surg* 2003;16:103–112.

146. Stelter W, Umscheid T, Ziegler P. Three-year experience with modular stent-graft devices for endovascular AAA treatment. *J Endovasc Surg* 1997;4:362–369.

147. Beebe HG, Cronenwett JL, Katzen BT, et al. Results of an aortic endograft trial: impact of device failure beyond 12 months. *J Vasc Surg* 2001;33:S55–S63.

148. Alimi YS, Chakfe N, Rivoal E, et al. Rupture of an abdominal aortic aneurysm after endovascular graft placement and aneurysm size reduction. *J Vasc Surg* 1998;28:178–183.

149. Riepe G, Heilberger P, Umschield T, et al. Frame dislocation of body middle rings in endovascular stent tube grafts. *J Endovasc Surg* 1999;17:28–34.

150. Jacobs TS, Won J, Graveraux EC, et al. Mechanical failure of prosthetic human implants: a 10-year experience with aortic stent graft devices. *J Vasc Surg* 2003;37:16–26.

151. Heintz C, Riepe G, Birken L. Corroded nitinol wires in explanted aortic endografts: an important mechanism of failure? *J Endovasc Ther* 2001;8:248–253.

152. Trepanier C, Tabrizian M, Yahia L, et al. Effect of modification of oxide layer on NiTi stent corrosion resistance. *J Biomed Mater Res (Appl Biomater)* 1998;43:433–440.

153. Duerig TW, Pelton AR, Stockel D. An overview of nitinol medical applications. *Mater Sci Eng* 1999;A273-275:149–160.

154. Starosvetsky E, Gotman I. Corrosion behavior of titanium nitride coated Ni-Ti shape memory surgical alloy. *Biomaterials* 2001;22:1853–1859.

155. Fairman RM, Baum RA, Carpenter JP, et al. Limb interventions in patients undergoing treatment with an unsupported bifurcated aortic endograft system: a review of the phase II EVT trial. *J Vasc Surg* 2002;36:118–126.

156. Carroccio A, Faries PL, Morrissey NJ, et al. Predicting iliac limb occlusion after bifurcated aortic stent grafting: anatomic and device-related causes. *J Vasc Surg* 2002;36:679–684.

157. Baum RA, Shetty SK, Carpenter JP, et al. Limb kinking in supported and unsupported abdominal aortic stent-grafts. *J Vasc Interv Radiol* 2000;11:1165–1171.

158. Amesur NB, Zajko AB, Orons PD, et al. Endovascular treatment of iliac limb stenoses or occlusion in 31 patients treated with the Ancure endograft. *J Vasc Interv Radiol* 2000;11:421–428.

159. Ohki T, Veith FJ, Shaw P, et al. Increasing incidence of midterm and long-term complications after endovascular graft repair of abdominal aortic aneurysms: a note of caution based on a 9-year experience. *Ann Surg* 2001;234:323–335.

160. Carpenter JP, Neschis DG, Fairman RM, et al. Failure of endovascular abdominal aortic aneurysm graft limbs. *J Vasc Surg* 2001;33:296–303.

161. Sampram ES, Karafa MT, Mascha EJ, et al. Nature, frequency, and predictors of secondary procedures after endovascular repair of abdominal aortic aneurysm. *J Vasc Surg* 2003;37:930–937.

162. Cao P, Verzini F, Zannetti S, et al. Device migration after endoluminal abdominal aortic aneurysm repair: analysis of 113 cases with a minimum follow-up period of 2 years. *J Vasc Surg* 2002;35:229–235.

163. Lawrence-Brown MMD, Semmens JB, Hartley D, et al. How is durability related to patient selection and graft design with endoluminal grafting for abdominal aortic aneurysm? In: Greenlaugh R, ed. *The durability of vascular and endovascular surgery.* London: WB Saunders; 1999:375–385.

164. Resch T, Malina M, Lindblad B, et al. The impact of stent design on proximal stent-graft fixation in the abdominal aorta: an experimental study. *Eur J Vasc Endovasc Surg* 2000;20:190–195.

165. Albertini J-N, Kalliafas S, Travis S, et al. Anatomical risk factors for proximal perigraft endoleak and graft migration following endovascular repair of abdominal aortic aneurysms. *Eur J Vasc Endovasc Surg* 2000;19:308–312.

166. Resch T, Ivancev K, Brunkwall J, et al. Distal migration of stent-grafts after endovascular repair of abdominal aortic aneurysms. *J Vasc Interv Radiol* 1997;10:257–264.

167. Harris P, Brennan J, Martin J, et al. Longitudinal aneurysm shrinkage following endovascular aortic aneurysm repair: a source of intermediate and late complications. *J Endovasc Surg* 1999;6:11–16.

168. White GH, May J, Waugh R, et al. Shortening of endografts during deployment in endovascular AAA repair. *J Endovasc Ther* 1999;6:4–10.

169. Prinssen M, Wever JJ, Mali WPTM, et al. Concerns for the durability of the proximal abdominal aortic aneurysm endograft fixation from a 2-year and 3-year longitudinal computed tomography angiography study. *J Vasc Surg* 2001;33:S64–S69.

170. Badran MF, Gould DA, Raza I, et al. Aneurysm neck diameter after endovascular repair of abdominal aortic aneurysms. *J Vasc Interv Radiol* 2002;13:887–892.

171. Lee JT, Lee J, Aziz I, et al. Stent-graft migration following endovascular repair of aneurysms with large proximal necks: anatomical risk factors and long-term sequelae. *J Endovasc Ther* 2002;9:652–664.

172. Naslund TC, Edwards WH, Neuzil DF, et al. Technical complications of endovascular abdominal aortic aneurysm repair. *J Vasc Surg* 1997;26:502–510.

173. Fairman RM, Velazequez OC, Baum RA, et al. Endovascular repair of aortic aneurysms: critical events and adjunctive procedures. *J Vasc Surg* 2001;33:1226–1232.

174. Moore WS, Matsumura JS, Makaroun MS, et al. Five-year interim comparison of the Guidant bifurcated endograft with open repair of abdominal aortic aneurysm. *J Vasc Surg* 2003;38:46–55.

175. Becker GJ, Kovacs M, Mathison MN, et al. Risk stratification and outcomes of transluminal endografting for abdominal aortic aneurysm: 7-year experience and long-term follow-up. *J Vasc Interv Radiol* 2003;12:1033–1046.

176. Laheji RJF, Buth J, Harris PL, et al. Need for secondary interventions after endovascular repair of abdominal aortic aneurysms. Intermediate-term follow-up results of a European collaborative registry (EUROSTAR). *Br J Surg* 2000;87:1666–1673.

177. Ouriel K, Clair DG, Greenberg RK, et al. Endovascular repair of abdominal aortic aneurysms: device-specific outcome. *J Vasc Surg* 2003;37:991–998.

178. Matsumoto A, Angle J, Spinosa D, et al. Percutaneous transluminal angioplasty and stenting in the treatment of chronic

mesenteric ischemia: results and longterm followup. *J Am Coll Surg* 2002;194(Suppl. 1):S22–S31.

179. Steinmetz E, Tatou E, Favier-Blavoux C, et al. Endovascular treatment as first choice in chronic intestinal ischemia. *Ann Vasc Surg* 2002;16:693–699.

180. Sharafuddin M, Olson C, Sun S, et al. Endovascular treatment of celiac and mesenteric arteries stenoses: application and results. *J Vasc Surg* 2003;38:692–698.

181. Kasirajan K, Dolmatch B, Ouriel K, et al. Delayed onset of ascending paralysis after thoracic aortic stent graft deployment. *J Vasc Surg* 2000;31:196–199.

182. Sheeran S, Murphy T, Khwaja A, et al. Stent placement for treatment of mesenteric artery stenoses or occlusions. *J Vasc Interv Radiol* 1999;10:861–867.

183. Ivanovic V, McKusick M, Johnson C III, et al. Renal artery stent placement: complications at a single tertiary care center. *J Vasc Interv Radiol* 2003;14:217–225.

184. Bush R, Najibi S, MacDonald J, et al. Endovascular revascularization of renal artery stenosis: technical and clinical results. *J Vasc Surg* 2001;33:1041–1049.

185. Bakker J, Goffette P, Henry M, et al. The Erasme study: a multicenter study on the safety and technical results of the Palmaz stent used for the treatment of atherosclerotic ostial renal artery stenosis. *Cardiovasc Intervent Radiol* 1999;22:468–474.

186. DeMaioribus C, Anderson C, Popham S, et al. Mycotic renal artery degeneration and systemic sepsis caused by infected renal artery stent. *J Vasc Surg* 1998;28:547–550.

187. Deitch J, Hansen K, Regan J, et al. Infected renal artery pseudoaneurysm and mycotic aortic aneurysm after percutaneous transluminal renal artery angioplasty and stent placement in a patient with a solitary kidney. *J Vasc Surg* 1998;28:340–344.

188. Bukhari R, Muck P, Schlueter F, et al. Bilateral renal artery stent infection and pseudoaneurysm formation. *J Vasc Interv Radiol* 2000;11:337–341.

189. Henry M, Amor M, Henry I, et al. Stents in the treatment of renal artery stenosis: long-term follow-up. *J Endovasc Surg* 1999;6:42–51.

190. Tullis M, Zierler R, Glickerman D, et al. Results of percutaneous transluminal angioplasty for atherosclerotic renal artery stenosis: a follow-up study with duplex ultrasonography. *J Vasc Surg* 1997;25:46–54.

191. Hunink M, Donaldson M, Meyerovitz M, et al. Risks and benefits of femoropopliteal percutaneous balloon angioplasty. *J Vasc Surg* 1993;17:183–194.

192. Stanley B, Teague B, Raptis S, et al. Efficacy of balloon angioplasty of the superficial femoral artery and popliteal artery in the relief of leg ischemia. *J Vasc Surg* 1996;23:679–685.

193. Golledge J, Ferguson K, Ellis M, et al. Outcomes of femoropopliteal angioplasty. *Ann Surg* 1999;229:146–153.

194. Johnston K. Femoral and popliteal arteries: reanalysis of results of balloon angioplasty. *Radiology* 1992;183:767–771.

195. Bolia A, Miles K, Brennan J, et al. Percutaneous transluminal angioplasty of occlusions of the femoral and popliteal arteries by subintimal dissection. *Cardiovasc Intervent Radiol* 1990;13:357–364.

196. Werner G, Ferrari M, Figulla H. Superficial femoral artery rupture after balloon angioplasty: treatment with implantation of a balloon-expandable graft. *J Vasc Interv Radiol* 1999;10:1115–1117.

197. Cheng S, Ting A, Wong J. Endovascular stenting of superficial femoral artery stenosis and occlusions: results and risk factor analysis. *Cardiovasc Surg* 2001;9:133–140.

198. Gordon I, Conroy R, Arefi M, et al. Three-year outcome of endovascular treatment of superficial femoral artery occlusion. *Arch Surg* 2001;136:221–228.

199. Strecker E, Boos I, Gottman D. Femoropopliteal artery stent placement: evaluation of long-term success. *Radiology* 1997;205:375–383.

200. Lofberg A-M, Karacagil S, Ljungman C, et al. Percutaneous transluminal angioplasty of the femoropopliteal arteries in limbs with chronic critical lower limb ischemia. *J Vasc Surg* 2001;34:114–121.

201. Conroy R, Gordon I, Tobis J, et al. Angioplasty and stent placement in chronic occlusion of the superficial femoral artery: technique and results. *J Vasc Interv Radiol* 2000;11:1009–1020.

202. van Lankeren W, Gussenhoven E, van Kints M, et al. Stent remodeling contributes to femoropopliteal artery restenosis: an intravascular ultrasound study. *J Vasc Surg* 1997;25:753–756.

203. Saxon R, Coffman J, Gooding J, et al. Long-term results of ePTFE stent-graft versus angioplasty in the femoropopliteal artery: single center experience from a prospective, randomized trial. *J Vasc Interv Radiol* 2003;14:303–311.

204. Dorros G, Jaff M, Dorros A, et al. Tibioperoneal (outflow lesion) angioplasty can be used as primary treatment in 235 patients with critical limb ischemia: five-year follow up. *Circulation* 2001;104:2057–2062.

205. Faglia E, Mantero M, Caminiti M, et al. Extensive use of peripheral angioplasty, particularly infrapopliteal, in the treatment of ischaemic diabetic foot ulcers: clinical results of a multicentric study of 221 consecutive diabetic subjects. *J Intern Med* 2002;252:225–232.

206. Ouriel K, Gray B, Clair D, et al. Complications associated with the use of urokinase and recombinant tissue plasminogen activator for catheter-directed peripheral arterial and venous thrombolysis. *J Vasc Interv Radiol* 2000;11:295–298.

207. The STILE Investigators. Results of a prospective randomized trial evaluating surgery versus thrombolysis for ischemia of the lower extremity. *Ann Surg* 1994;220:251–268.

208. Ouriel K, Veith F, Sasahara A. A comparison of recombinant urokinase with vascular surgery as initial treatment for acute arterial occlusion of the legs. *N Engl J Med* 1998;338:1105–1111.

209. McNamara T, Goodwin S, Kandarpa K. Complications of thrombolysis. *Semin Interv Radiol* 1994;11:134–144.

210. Greenfield L, Proctor M. Filter complications and their management. *Semin Interv Radiol* 2000;13:213–216.

211. Joels C, Sing R, Heniford B. Complications of inferior vena cava filters. *Am Surg* 2003;69:654–659.

212. Reed R, Teitelbaum G, Taylor F, et al. Incomplete opening of LGM (VenaTech) filters inserted via transjugular approach. *J Vasc Interv Radiol* 1991;2:441–445.

213. Rogers F, Strindberg G, Shackford S, et al. Five-year follow-up of prophylactic vena cava filters in high-risk trauma patients. *Arch Surg* 1998;133:406–412.

214. Campbell J, Calcagno D. Aortic pseudoanerusym from aortic perforation with a bird's nest vena cava filter. *J Vasc Surg* 2003;38:596–599.

215. Raju S, Owen S, Neglen P. The clinical impact of iliac venous stents in the management of chronic venous insufficiency. *J Vasc Surg* 2002;35:8–15.

216. Raju S, McAllister S, Neglen P. Recanalization of totally occluded iliac and adjacent venous segments. *J Vasc Surg* 2002;36:903–911.

217. Lamont J, Pearl G, Patetsios P, et al. Prospective evaluation of endoluminal venous stents in the treatment of the May-Thurner syndrome. *Ann Vasc Surg* 2002;16:61–64.

218. Greenfield L, Proctor M, Williams D, et al. Long-term experience with transvenous catheter pulmonary embolectomy. *J Vasc Surg* 1993;18:450–458.

219. Timsit F, Reynaud P, Meyer G, et al. Pulmonary embolectomy by catheter device in massive pulmonary embolism. *Chest* 1991;100:655–658.

220. De Gregario M, Gimeno M, Mainar A, et al. Mechanical and enzymatic thrombolysis for massive pulmonary embolism. *J Vasc Interv Radiol* 2002;13:163–169.

Complications
of Gastrointestinal
Surgery

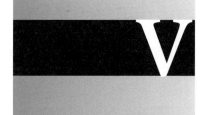

Complications
of Gastric Surgery

31

Michael W. Mulholland

■■■ **PEPTIC ULCERATION 386**
Hemorrhage 386
Perforation 390

■■■ **GASTRIC CANCER 396**

■■■ **MORBID OBESITY 398**

■■■ **REFERENCES 404**

Gastric operations constitute an increasingly large proportion of the general surgical workload. Although the incidences of complicated peptic ulceration and gastric cancer have declined significantly over the past several decades, gastric operations for treatment of morbid obesity have undergone explosive growth. Complications from gastric operations are common and frequently severe.

Nationwide trends for complications of gastric surgery are clearest in how they relate to the treatment of gastric cancer. Epidemiologic studies in the United States demonstrate that gastric cancer has decreased in incidence over the last two decades (1). Despite this reduction in incidence, gastric cancer remains one of the most common causes of cancer-related deaths in the United States, and surgical resection offers the only chance of cure (1–4).

Michael W. Mulholland: University of Michigan, Ann Arbor, MI 48109

In one recent study the overall incidence of gastric cancer and subsequent gastric resection was reported to have declined from 1988 to 2000 (5). Use of a nationwide database has shown that the number of patients with a discharge diagnosis of gastric cancer decreased from 25 cases per 100,000 U.S. adults in 1988 to 20 cases per 100,000 in 2000 (Fig. 31-1). These results were mirrored by declining rates of gastric resection, with a 29% decrease from 5.6 cases per 100,000 adults in 1988 to 4.0 cases per 100,000 in 2000 (Fig. 31-1). The overall proportion of hospitalized gastric cancer patients undergoing gastric resection remained constant at approximately 22%.

Gastric resection for cancer has a relatively high rate of postoperative complication and operative mortality. In-hospital mortality did not significantly change over the 1988–2000 timeframe, with an overall mortality rate of 7.4% for the nationwide group. Rates of adverse outcomes were not uniform but varied in relation to hospital experience with the operation. Low volume centers had an 8.3% mortality rate, medium volume hospitals had a 7.1% mortality rate, and high volume centers had a 6.5% mortality rate (Fig. 31-2). The safety of gastric resection improved from 1988 to 2000 at high volume medical centers, decreasing from 7.1% in 1988 to 1992, to 6.5% in 1993 to 1996, to 5.8% in 1997 to 2000. A decline in mortality was not observed at low or medium volume hospitals.

Despite stagnant overall mortality rates, patients are spending less time in the hospital after gastric resection. The decrease in length of stay suggests improved efficiency and better use of resources over time. Shorter hospital stay

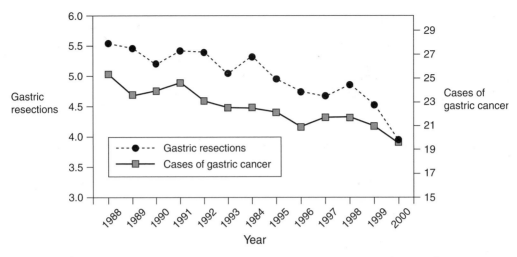

Figure 31-1 Incidence of gastric cancer and gastric cancer resection in the United States, per 100,000 adults, from 1988 through 2000.

may also result from the cost-saving efforts of healthcare payers during the same interval (Fig. 31-3).

PEPTIC ULCERATION

Hemorrhage

Although peptic ulcer disease remains a major worldwide health problem, the United States has experienced a decline in both the incidence of uncomplicated ulceration and the rate of hospitalization for complicated disease (6). Bleeding, perforation, and obstruction are the three major complications of peptic ulcer, with bleeding the most common. Despite appreciation of the role of *Helicobacter pylori* infection in peptic ulcer pathogenesis and improvements in therapeutic endoscopy, mortality from bleeding ulcers

has remained stable (8% to 10%) over the past 30 years (6–8). Contemporary patients are increasingly elderly and have frequent coexisting illnesses. Advanced age and the existence of concurrent illness are the most important prognostic factors in patients with bleeding peptic ulcers. Patients older than 60 have a significantly higher mortality than those younger than 60. The presence and number of comorbidities are closely related to mortality (9–13).

Pathogenesis

Infection with the gram-negative bacterium, *Helicobacter pylori*, is very strongly linked to the development of peptic ulceration. This infectious association has fundamentally changed the treatment of patients with peptic disease. Although *H. pylori* infection rates have wide geographic variability, the organism is present in as much as 30% to 50% of

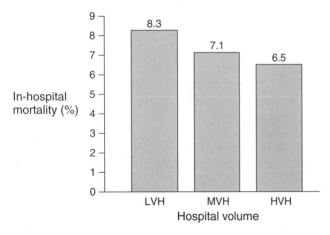

Figure 31-2 In-hospital mortality as a function of varying hospital volume. Low hospital volumes are defined as performing four or fewer resections per year. Medium volume hospitals are defined as performing five to eight resections per year. High volume hospitals are defined as performing nine or more resections per year.

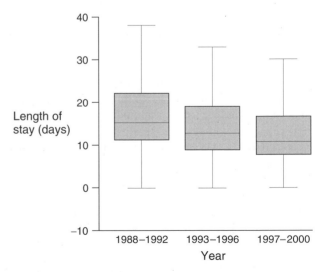

Figure 31-3 Length of stay after gastric resection by time period from 1988 through 2000.

the population. Most infected individuals remain without symptoms; only 6% to 20% of colonized individuals develop peptic ulcer disease (14). Conversely, *H. pylori* is present in >90% of patients with ulcer disease. Surprisingly, the prevalence of *H. pylori* is 15% to 20% lower in patients with ulcer hemorrhage relative to patients with nonbleeding ulcers (6,15). The significance of this negative correlation is unknown.

With mucosal colonization, a variety of bacterial and host responses are elicited. *H. pylori* produces the enzyme urease. Urease hydrolyzes urea to produce ammonia, which, in turn, increases luminal pH, thus providing a favorable microenvironment for *H. pylori* survival. Urease production appears to be crucial to the pathogenicity of *H. pylori*; mutants of *H. pylori* that do not produce urease are unable to establish colonization. The bacterium attaches to the gastric epithelium beneath the mucous layer. Following attachment, *H. pylori* causes direct cellular injury and changes gastric secretory physiology. Vacuolating cytotoxin (*vac*A), the product of the cytotoxin-associated gene (*cag*A), and growth-inhibitory (GI) factor act as *H. pylori* toxins to produce gastric mucosal injury.

H. pylori infection produces abnormalities in gastric acid secretion (Table 31-1). Levels of serum gastrin are elevated in patients infected with *H. pylori*. Hypergastrinemia secondary to *H. pylori* infection occurs in response to the cytokines tumor necrosis factor-α and interleukin-8, which are produced in response to mucosal infection. Local secretion of the inhibitory hormone somatostatin is also diminished. The imbalances in gastrin and somatostatin production are manifested clinically as elevated basal and maximal acid outputs. Abnormalities in gastric secretion return to normal after *H. pylori* eradication, supporting the idea that infection is the cause of increased acid production (16).

Nonsteroidal anti-inflammatory drugs (NSAIDs) are ubiquitous and have been associated with both gastric and duodenal ulcer diseases. The inhibitory effect of NSAIDs upon prostaglandin production in the gastric mucosa is the cause of NSAID ulcerogenic actions. NSAID use is an important risk factor for ulcer hemorrhage, and NSAIDs significantly increase the risk of bleeding in *H. pylori*-infected individuals (17). Ingestion of NSAIDs is associated with a twofold increase in risk of bleeding in patients who are infected with *H. pylori* relative to patients who are *H. pylori*-negative (12). Only 10% of patients with bleeding ulcers are both *H. pylori*-negative and without a history of NSAID exposure (15).

Endoscopic Treatment

Peptic ulcer disease constitutes a significant proportion of upper gastrointestinal hemorrhage. A widely variable proportion of patients (20% to 68%) present with melena, while 14% to 30% develop hematemesis and 18% to 50% present with both hematemesis and melena (6,8,18). Initial management is focused on stabilization and then upon diagnosis. Patients should be aggressively resuscitated with intravenous fluids and blood components. Patients presenting with shock, elderly patients (>60 years), and those with recurrent bleeding are at increased risk of death and should be treated in an intensive care unit (9–13). A nasogastric tube should be inserted and the stomach lavaged with warm saline. Lavage is not effective in stopping bleeding; the measure is performed to allow subsequent endoscopic visualization of the bleeding site. The use of intravenous histamine$_2$-blockers for acute ulcer bleeding has not been shown to be beneficial (6,19,20). Proton pump inhibitors may improve outcome in patients with bleeding ulcers (21–23). However, these drugs should not be considered the crucial aspect of therapy during the acute episode.

Upper gastrointestinal endoscopy, not contrast radiography, is the preferred diagnostic modality for upper GI hemorrhage. Endoscopy can define the nature and site of the bleeding lesion. Endoscopic findings also provide information that predicts the risk of recurrent bleeding (Table 31-2). Endoscopic therapy, performed immediately, defines the nature of the bleeding lesion and is effective in most patients (>80%). When necessary, tissue biopsy can be obtained for histology and for the diagnosis of *H. pylori* infection.

TABLE 31-1

GASTRIC SECRETORY RESPONSES TO *HELICOBACTER PYLORI* INFECTION

Acid secretion
   Increased basal acid output
   Increased maximal acid output
   Increased responsiveness to gastrin-releasing peptide
Hormonal
   Increased basal gastrin levels
   Increased meal induced gastrin release
   Decreased acid inhibition by cholecystokinin
   Decreased antral distension inhibition of gastrin release
Duodenal bicarbonate secretion
   Decreased mucosal bicarbonate secretion

TABLE 31-2

ENDOSCOPIC ULCER APPEARANCE AND RISK OF RECURRENT HEMORRHAGE

Risk	Appearance	Recurrent Bleeding
Low	Clean base	0%–15%
	Flat spot	
High	Adherent clot	40%–90%
	Nonbleeding visible vessel	
	Active hemorrhage	

Endoscopy should not be performed until patients have been hemodynamically stabilized. Following resuscitation, endoscopy should be performed emergently in high-risk patients such as the elderly, those with significant blood loss, and patients experiencing rebleeding episodes. Performance of initial endoscopy within 24 hours of the bleeding episode has been associated with improved outcome (24).

The endoscopic appearance of the ulcer bed and ulcer size provide information that predicts the likelihood of rebleeding. Ulcers are categorized on the basis of endoscopic appearances: clean base, flat spot, adherent clot, nonbleeding visible vessel, or active bleeding. Each of these appearances is associated with a defined risk of rebleeding (Table 31-2). Although patients with clean base ulcers have a very low recurrent bleeding rate, those with visible vessels or active bleeding have recurrent bleeding rates of 43% and 55%, respectively (4,25–27). Because of the risk of recurrent hemorrhage associated with these endoscopic findings, patients who have a nonbleeding visible vessel or active bleeding at the time of endoscopy should undergo immediate endoscopic therapy (27). For patients with low risk visual findings, endoscopic therapy is not recommended, as intervention has not been shown to reduce the already low risk of rebleeding (27).

Endoscopic therapy options include thermal coagulation and injection of vessel sclerosants or vasoconstrictor agents. Thermal coagulation involves direct application of heat or electrocoagulation to the bleeding site. The electrocoagulation device or heat probe is passed through the endoscope and positioned so that it overlies the visible bleeding vessel. Initial hemostasis is accomplished by direct vessel compression with coaptation of vessel walls. Energy is applied in order to produce tissue coagulation.

Endoscopic injection therapy involves injection of solutions into the base of the ulcer, resulting in tamponade, vasoconstriction, and eventual sclerosis of the ulcer bed and surrounding blood vessels. A dilute solution (1:10,000) of epinephrine is most commonly used for this purpose. Other injection agents include polidocanol, ethanol, and thrombin. With either heater probe or injection, the initial success rate is estimated at 75% to 90% (19,27,28). Complications, either immediate bleeding or perforation, have been reported in <1% of cases (6,27).

The major complication of endoscopic therapy is delayed rebleeding, approximately 10% to 30% after initial endoscopic hemostasis (6,18,19,29). Almost all patients who rebleed after endoscopic therapy do so within 96 hours of the initial endoscopic procedure (18). In one report, all fatal rebleeding events occurred within the first 24 hours of the initial bleeding episode (30). High-risk patients include those with hemodynamic instability, comorbid disease, or visible ulcer vessels, and they should be monitored in an intensive care unit. Patients with limited bleeding and low risk findings, such as a clean ulcer base on endoscopy, may be discharged within 24 hours.

Surgery has been the usual treatment for failure of endoscopic therapy. Recent data suggest that endoscopic retreatment is also a safe alternative (29). Endoscopic retreatment has a success rate of 50% to 70% in patients who rebleed after initial endoscopic therapy. Endoscopic retreatment must be employed with caution. The perforation rate during endoscopic retreatment is increased, and a significant delay in definitive therapy must not occur for those patients who fail the second attempt at endoscopic hemostasis.

Surgical treatment of rebleeding should be considered for patients who are at highest risk for continued bleeding, including patients with large ulcers and large bleeding vessels, the elderly (>60), patients with active hemorrhage, and patients who develop hypotension. These factors have been associated with failure of endoscopic therapy (9,30,31).

Operative Treatment

Operative therapy is indicated when endoscopic therapy is either not possible or unsuccessful or when bleeding is so rapid that endoscopy is not feasible. Because the indications for surgical therapy are identical to those for endoscopic therapy, a surgeon should be consulted for the care of every patient with upper gastrointestinal hemorrhage from the outset (Table 31-3). Patient characteristics such as advanced age (>60 years) and the presence of significant comorbid disease predict a superior outcome with early surgery (13,19). Elderly patients or those with cardiovascular compromise cannot sustain repetitive hypotension or the episodic anemia related to delayed surgical therapy.

When surgery is performed for hemorrhage, there are two therapeutic goals. First, the bleeding must be controlled. Second, therapy that minimizes ulcer recurrence should be provided. Direct suture ligature of the ulcer or bleeding site is used to control hemorrhage. When the site of ulcer bleeding is a gastric ulcer, the ulcer should be resected. In addition to hemostasis, ulcer resection provides gastric tissue for histology to evaluate for the presence of gastric cancer. For ulcers located on the lesser curve of the stomach near the gastroesophageal junction, resection may

---

TABLE 31-3

INDICATIONS FOR OPERATION IN BLEEDING PEPTIC ULCERATION

Continuous or recurrent hemorrhage
Ongoing transfusion requirement
Hypotension
Age >60 years with ongoing hemorrhage
Failed endoscopic hemostasis
Ulcer inaccessible to endoscopic therapy

be hazardous and direct suture ligature of the ulcer base is more appropriate, with biopsy to exclude cancer.

For bleeding duodenal ulcers, a Kocher maneuver is first performed to mobilize the duodenum from the retroperitoneum (Fig. 31-4). Through a duodenotomy, the bleeding vessel at the base of the ulcer is visualized and ligated. In placing sutures, care should be taken to avoid the common bile duct as it passes deep to the first and second portions of the duodenum.

After hemostasis is achieved, a decision must be made about the performance of a definitive antiulcer procedure. The surgical literature on this issue predates the current understanding of the pathogenetic role of *H. pylori* in ulcer disease. Currently available but dated literature suggests that the performance of an antiulcer procedure in addition to oversewing the ulcer produces a lower rate of rebleeding compared to oversewing of the ulcer alone. Postoperative morbidity and mortality are reported to be similar (32,33).

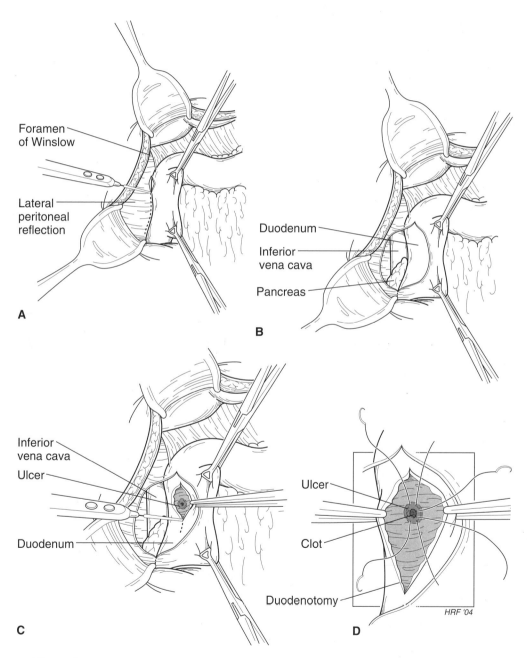

Figure 31-4 Operative maneuvers in management of bleeding duodenal ulcer. **A:** The duodenum is mobilized from the retroperitoneum by a Kocher maneuver. **B:** As the duodenum is reflected anteriorly, the retroperitoneal duodenum, the posterior aspect of the pancreatic head, and the inferior vena cava are visualized. **C:** Direct visualization of the ulcer is obtained by a longitudinal duodenotomy. **D:** Circumferential sutures are used to control vessels entering the ulcer base peripherally. Vessels entering perpendicularly are controlled using a U-stitch.

However, these studies are flawed in that they do not address the effect of *H. pylori* eradication on bleeding recurrence after surgery.

In the past, vagotomy and pyloroplasty had been recommended in hemodynamically unstable patients when the operative goals need to be achieved expeditiously. When performed electively, operative mortality approximates 1% and ulcer recurrence rates average 10% to 12% (Table 31-4). The incidence of dumping, a syndrome of postprandial flushing and vasomotor effects, ranges from 1% to 10% (34,35). Elective highly selective vagotomy is also associated with low mortality but with somewhat higher recurrence rates of 10% to 15%. In most series highly selective vagotomy has fewer postoperative symptoms, with an incidence of dumping of <5%. Elective vagotomy and antrectomy is associated with an ulcer recurrence rate of 1% (34,35).

Not surprisingly, surgical results are less salutary when hemorrhage prompts urgent operation. When performed emergently, vagotomy and pyloroplasty has a recurrent bleeding rate of 17%, with a duodenal leak rate of 3%. Vagotomy and gastrectomy has a lower rebleeding rate of 3%, but a significantly higher frequency of duodenal leak at 13%. Reoperations for bleeding and overall mortality are similar between these two procedures (36).

Prevention of recurrent bleeding requires treatment of underlying *H. pylori* infection and discontinuation of NSAIDs. With anti-*H. pylori* therapy and avoidance of NSAIDs, a 95% ulcer cure rate for uncomplicated peptic ulcers has been reported. The combination of omeprazole, amoxicillin, and clarithromycin has been most widely used and is associated with elimination of *H. pylori* in 90% of patients. An alternative regimen combines omeprazole, metronidazole, and either amoxicillin or clarithromycin. When NSAIDs cannot be discontinued, use of the synthetic prostaglandin analog Misoprostol decreases the incidence of recurrent bleeding, especially in the elderly (37,38).

A number of controlled trials are now available, demonstrating that for patients with bleeding as a complication of *H. pylori*-positive ulcers, eradication of infection prevents recurrent ulceration and bleeding. Two randomized trials have reported the results of treatment of *H. pylori* in patients following duodenal ulcer hemorrhage (39,40). Patients treated with antibiotics had a 0% incidence of recurrent bleeding during the year following treatment, while 33% and 27% rates of repeat bleeding were noted in control groups. Two additional trials have compared recurrent bleeding during maintenance ranitidine therapy (11% to 13%) to bleeding subsequent to *H. pylori* eradication (2% to 5%) (41,42). Although it seems likely that effective antibiotic therapy would eliminate duodenal ulcer disease in postoperative patients and thus permit more limited surgical therapy for control of hemorrhage, this approach has not yet been subjected to clinical trial.

Perforation

Hospitalization rates for duodenal ulcer perforation have not decreased with the introduction of powerful antisecretory drugs or with antibiotic treatment of peptic ulcer. In the majority of affected patients, perforation is the first manifestation of duodenal ulcer disease.

The patient usually experiences sudden, severe epigastric pain, followed shortly by diffuse abdominal pain. Chemical irritation of the parietal peritoneum by acidic gastric contents causes severe pain. If gastric contents contact the diaphragm, the patient will also experience referred pain in the area of the right scapula. Respiration worsens symptoms. Physical examination typically reveals a silent abdomen with muscular rigidity and epigastric tenderness. Moderate fever and tachycardia are often present; hypotension is unusual initially. Laboratory examination reveals leukocytosis. Hyperamylasemia, attributed to absorption of duodenal contents from the peritoneal cavity, is common. Upright abdominal films demonstrate pneumoperitoneum in 80% of cases. If pneumoperitoneum is absent, computed tomography (CT) with oral contrast may be used to demonstrate perforation.

The fasting human stomach contains 10^2 to 10^3 organisms; oral bacteria, including lactobacilli and aerobic streptococci, predominate. Infectious complications associated with duodenal perforation are closely related to the length of time that elapses before definitive treatment. Peritoneal cultures obtained between 6 to 12 hours of perforation are positive in <50% of cases, but culture positivity increases rapidly thereafter. Beyond 24 hours coliforms and fungal species are increasingly frequent.

Nonoperative management of perforated duodenal ulcer is rarely justified in modern medical practice. Reports of nonoperative management are highly biased by exclusion of patients with gastric ulcer, perforations of >24 hours duration, clinical deterioration, associated shock, diagnostic uncertainty, or comorbid medical illnesses (43). In one report, initial treatment with intravenous fluids, nasogastric suction, and antibiotics was coupled with contrast radiography to evaluate for intraperitoneal leakage of gastric contents. Lack of clinical improvement was an indication for emergent operation. In this series, 28% of patients initially

TABLE 31-4

RESULTS OF ELECTIVE OPERATION FOR PEPTIC ULCER

Procedure	Mortality	Recurrent Ulcer	Dumping
Truncal vagotomy	1%	10%–12%	1%–10%
Proximal gastric vagotomy	0.5%	8%–20%	2%–3%
Truncal vagotomy and antrectomy	1%	1%	10%–20%

managed nonoperatively had clinical deterioration within 24 hours, and perforated neoplasms were discovered in 27% of patients initially treated as perforated ulcer. Older patients were less likely to improve with nonoperative treatment. Hospitalization was 35% longer in the group treated nonoperatively.

Risk factors that predict operative mortality include concurrent medical comorbidity, preoperative shock, and long-standing perforation (>48 hours) (44). If these factors are absent, ulcer operation may be performed with predictably low mortality and acceptable morbidity. If one or more risk factors are present, the risk of death increases progressively. Patients with zero, one, two, or three risk factors have been reported to have mortality rates of 0%, 10%, 46%, and 100%, respectively (44). In a recent multivariate analysis, age >65 years, American Society of Anesthesiologists (ASA) stage III or IV, and a delay of surgery beyond 24 hours after onset of symptoms predicted mortality (45). When all three risk factors were present, mortality was 61%.

Operative treatment of perforated duodenal ulcer has four goals: patient safety, peritoneal debridement, closure of the perforation, and alteration of the ulcer diathesis so that the risk of recurrent ulceration is minimized. For most patients peritoneal cleansing can be achieved by either laparoscopy or laparotomy. Laparoscopic closure of duodenal perforation is usually confined to those with a solitary prepyloric ulcer located anteriorly (45). Most reports of laparoscopic repair have employed either omental patching or fibrin glue repair. Perforated ulcers with larger defects or those with destruction of the proximal duodenum or penetration into adjacent organs require laparotomy and resectional therapy.

Laparoscopic repair of duodenal perforation and open repair have been compared in two prospective trials (46,47). Laparoscopic repair requires significantly longer operative time (Table 31-5). Postoperative analgesic requirements are less with laparoscopy. No significant differences were noted between these techniques in duration of nasogastric suction, intravenous infusion, hospital stay, time to resumption of oral diet, reoperation rate, morbidity, or mortality.

TABLE 31-5

COMPARISON OF LAPAROSCOPIC AND OPEN REPAIR OF PERFORATED DUODENAL ULCER

Mortality	Similar
Morbidity	Similar
Analgesics requirements	Less for laparoscopy
Operative time	Shorter for laparotomy
Duration of NG suction	Similar
Duration of IV infusion	Similar
Time to oral intake	Similar
Hospital stay	Similar
Reoperation rate	Similar

Omental patch closure of perforated duodenal ulcer alone is not adequate treatment. Because the underlying ulcer diathesis is not altered, simple patch closure is followed by an ulcer recurrence rate of 61% at a mean of 20 months (48). *H. pylori* eradication following omental patching reduces ulcer recurrence to <5%.

Complications are more frequent and more severe when large duodenal defects or penetration into other organs require resectional therapy. Postoperative morbidity has been reported in 9% of patients with small anterior perforations and in 22% to 34% of those with complicated defects (45).

Postoperative Hemorrhage

Unrecognized injury to the spleen is the most common cause of postoperative hemorrhage after operations on the stomach or duodenum. Splenic hemorrhage occurs as a result of capsular injury from traction on splenic attachments or from inappropriately placed retractors. Failure to properly ligate short gastric vessels during dissection of the greater curvature of the stomach can also lead to splenic hemorrhage. In several series of splenectomy, inadvertent injury during upper abdominal surgery is among the most common indications for splenectomy. In addition to the dangers of hypovolemia, splenectomy increases the incidence of pancreatic fistula, pancreatitis, and septic complications, including subphrenic abscess. Following vagotomy, vessels in proximity to the esophagus may be the source of bleeding.

Intraluminal hemorrhage most commonly represents suture line bleeding from submucosal arterioles and veins. Gastric lavage with warmed saline via the nasogastric tube is used to clear the stomach of clots as a prelude to endoscopy. Endoscopic hemostasis, similar in technique to that described for bleeding ulcers, is usually successful. Uncontrolled hemorrhage is an indication for reoperation.

Gastric Outlet Obstruction

Gastric outlet obstruction and small bowel obstruction are relatively frequent following gastric resection, occurring in 3% to 5% of cases. The major cause of anastomotic obstruction in the early postoperative period is inflammation adjacent to the anastomosis, secondary to subclinical suture line leakage or ischemia. Chronic gastric outlet obstruction is often the consequence of perianastomotic ulceration with resultant cicatrization. Pain is not usually prominent in gastric outlet obstruction. Recurrent vomiting or persistently elevated nasogastric tube output suggests the diagnosis. Fiberoptic endoscopy should be used when gastric outlet obstruction is considered to evaluate anastomotic patency. If the patient has a Billroth II anastomosis, the patency of each limb must be evaluated. An open anastomosis favors delay in reoperation and support of nutritional needs with parenteral alimentation.

Mechanical small bowel obstruction may occur following Billroth II gastrojejunostomy, performed either retrocolic or antecolic. When gastrojejunostomy is performed in a retrocolic position, obstruction may be due to occlusion of the anastomosis by the transverse mesocolon (Fig. 31-5).

The stomach may retract upward, resulting in pinching of one or both jejunal limbs by a relatively unyielding mesentery. This complication may be avoided by suturing the transverse mesentery to the stomach at least 2 cm superior to the anastomosis. The exposure for this maneuver is best

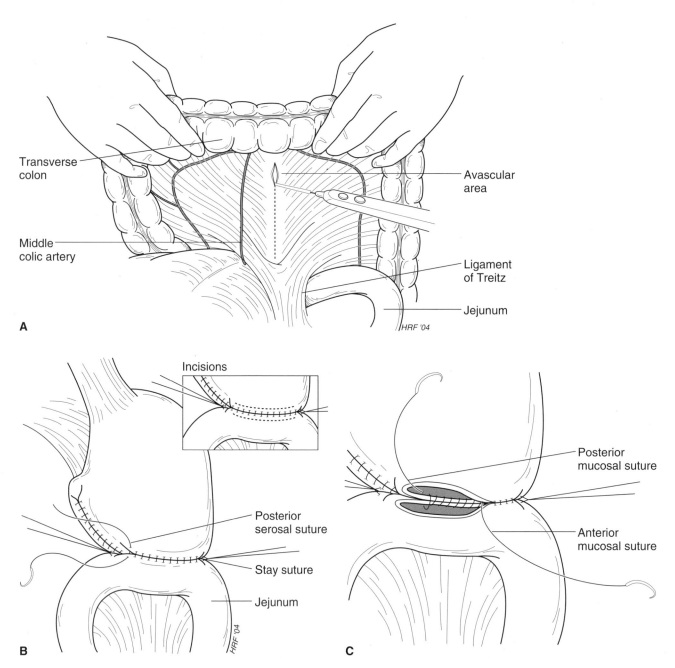

Figure 31-5 Construction of gastrojejunostomy. **A:** The transverse colon is retracted upward, and the vascular arcades within the transverse mesocolon are identified. An avascular area to the left of the middle colic vessels is chosen as the site for incision. An incision large enough to deliver the jejunum to the stomach is created. **B:** Interrupted 3-O seromuscular sutures are placed and tied. Electrocautery is used to create equal length incisions in the stomach and jejunum. **C:** A continuous mucosal suture of absorbable material is begun posterior and is continued along the anterior portion of the anastomosis.

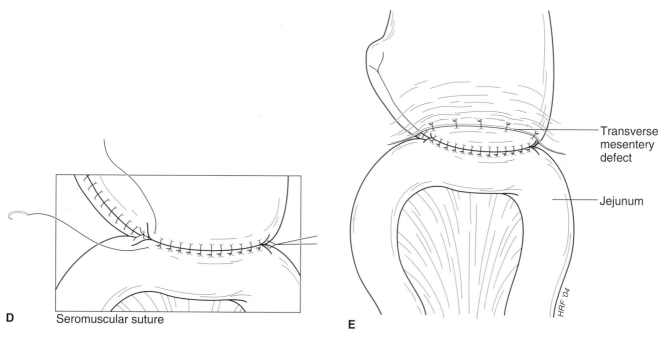

Figure 31-5 (*continued*) **D:** Interrupted seromuscular sutures are used to complete the anterior portion of the double layer of anastomosis. **E:** The completed gastrojejunal anastomosis should be positioned beneath the transverse mesocolon to prevent angulation or obstruction of the efferent or afferent jejunal limbs. The mesenteric defect is secured through the gastric wall with interrupted sutures.

achieved inferior to the transverse colon. Volvulus of the proximal or distal limbs of the gastrojejunostomy is possible following Billroth II reconstruction, more commonly when the anastomosis is antecolic.

The afferent loop syndrome is a condition caused by partial obstruction of the proximal limb of a gastrojejunostomy. Obstruction may be caused by kinking or torsion of the anastomosis, obstruction by the transverse mesentery, internal hernia, or recurrent ulceration (Fig. 31-6). Partial obstruction results in intermittent dilatation of the duodenum and proximal jejunum, with periodic release of pancreatic and biliary secretion into the stomach. Afferent loop obstruction occurring in the immediate postoperative period causes severe and unrelenting epigastric pain. Acute afferent loop obstruction is a surgical emergency because, if unrelieved, obstruction can cause duodenal stump leakage. The dilated loop can be visualized on abdominal CT scan; the obstructed limb will not contain orally ingested contrast. Mechanical stasis in the duodenum may cause elevation in serum amylase values and may be confused with postoperative pancreatitis. Acute afferent loop obstruction requires urgent reoperation because of the possibility of perforation.

Jejunogastric intussusception is an unusual cause of gastric outlet obstruction, occurring in <1% of cases (49). In more than three-fourths of patients, the efferent limb is the source of the intussusception. Urgent endoscopy reveals a friable, bluish mass originating from the orifice of the efferent limb. Abdominal CT scan demonstrates a mass within the stomach with a layered, onion skin-like appearance. Urgent operative reduction of the intussusception is indicated due to the potential for ischemic necrosis of the intussusceptum.

Postsurgical Gastroparesis

Postsurgical gastroparesis is a chronic complication of gastric surgery characterized by disruption of the normal mechanisms of gastric motility (50). Affected patients have postprandial pain, nausea, and vomiting; most have difficulty maintaining adequate oral nutrition. The incidence of motility disturbances following gastric surgery is poorly defined; abnormalities in gastric emptying have been recorded in 30% of patients following truncal vagotomy and Roux-en-Y gastrectomy (50–52).

The pathogenesis of postsurgical gastroparesis is unknown. Lack of vagal tone, abnormalities of neuromuscular coordination, disordered smooth muscle function, and motor abnormalities of the Roux-en-Y limb have been postulated but remain unproven. Histologic examination of the dysfunctional stomach usually reveals no abnormality (50).

The diagnosis of postsurgical gastroparesis requires the absence of anatomic obstruction, including anastomotic stricture and efferent limb obstruction (Table 31-6). Fiberoptic endoscopy of the gastric remnant is a strict

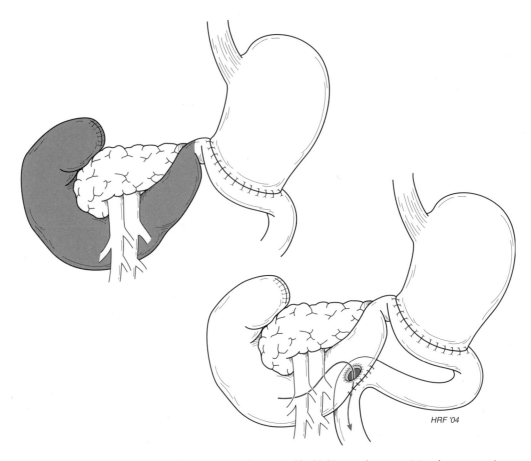

Figure 31-6 Afferent loop obstruction can be caused by kinking at the gastrojejunal anastomosis.

requirement. Contrast studies of the small intestine are useful to exclude distal obstruction or generalized intestinal hypomotility. Radionuclide solid phase gastric emptying studies are used to evaluate gastric function and to provide a quantitative measure of the effectiveness of medical therapy.

Endocrine disturbances can cause disordered gastric emptying. Hypothyroidism and diabetes mellitus are prominent examples. A variety of diseases, including amyloidosis, scleroderma, muscular dystrophy, myasthenia gravis, and psoriasis, can alter gastric emptying. Medications

---

TABLE 31-6

REQUIREMENTS FOR DIAGNOSIS OF POSTSURGICAL GASTROPARESIS

1. Prior history of gastric resection, usually with vagotomy
2. Upper endoscopy to exclude anastomotic obstruction, efferent limb obstruction, jejunogastric intussusception
3. Exclusion of hypothyroidism, diabetes mellitus
4. Exclusion of medical disorders such as scleroderma, amyloidosis, muscular dystrophy
5. Contrast study of small intestine
6. Solid phase gastric emptying study

---

that affect gastric emptying should be discontinued, including narcotics, anticholinergics, and L-dopa. Patients should receive a prolonged trial of prokinetic drug therapy.

Patients who meet these criteria and fail to respond to aggressive medical management are candidates for operative treatment. Total or near-total gastrectomy with Roux-en-Y gastrojejunostomy has been reported as a treatment for postsurgical gastroparesis (50). At a mean follow-up of 56 months, 78% of patients reported symptomatic improvement. For 7% of patients there had been no change in their condition, and for 15% symptoms had worsened. No postoperative deaths were reported for 52 patients. Postoperative complications were noted in 29%, with wound infection, prolonged ileus, and pneumonia the most frequent.

Duodenal Fistula

Duodenal fistula may be a complication of gastric resection, particularly when the duodenum is closed and gastrojejunal reconstruction performed. The duodenal stump may dehisce at the site of closure, an end fistula, or the duodenum may perforate laterally, causing a lateral fistula. Duodenal fistulas are particularly morbid because of the high fluid volume lost and because of the escape of pancreatic and biliary secretions into the peritoneal cavity. Once fistulization has occurred, attempts at immediate operative closure are futile. Initial management is concerned with treatment of sepsis, control of intraperitoneal leakage, and skin protection at any site of external drainage. Parenteral alimentation is necessary to maintain a positive nitrogen balance in the weeks required for spontaneous closure or reoperation. When distal obstruction exists in the afferent jejunal limb, spontaneous fistula closure will not occur.

If spontaneous closure does not occur within 6 weeks, operative repair is justified. If a portion of the duodenum is missing or nonviable, duodenal reconstruction is required. The most widely accepted method is construction of a Roux-en-Y jejunal segment to close the duodenal defect via a functional side-to-end duodenojejunostomy.

Avulsion of the Sphincter of Oddi

Operative injury to the ampulla of Vater is a serious but rare event during gastric resection. Injury to this area is possible during any operation on the duodenum but is most frequent in the presence of scarring or inflammation that causes secondary shortening of the duodenal bulb (53). The injury occurs during dissection between the duodenum and pancreas prior to duodenal transection. Most injuries can be recognized by the sudden appearance of bile in the operative field. Postoperatively, the injury causes collection of bile and pancreatic secretions in the subhepatic space (Fig. 31-7). If disconnection

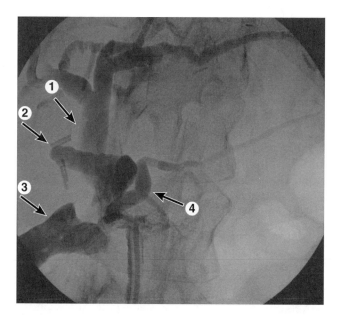

Figure 31-7 Avulsion of the ampulla of Vater demonstrated by percutaneous transhepatic cholangiography (PTC). Injection of the PTC catheter demonstrates free flow of contrast into the subhepatic space. The common biliary-pancreatic channel also provides a pancreatogram. Severe inflammatory changes in the subhepatic space were treated by external drainage and parenteral hyperalimentation. The patient ultimately required pancreaticoduodenectomy for correction of the defect. 1: common bile duct; 2: cystic duct stump; 3: subhepatic collection; 4: pancreatic duct.

of the ampulla is recognized intraoperatively, the duodenal stump may be mobilized further and brought over the ampulla. The ampulla or the individual bile and pancreatic ducts may then be reimplanted. A Roux-en-Y limb of jejunum may also be created for this purpose. When discovered postoperatively, inflammatory changes make ductal reimplantation impractical and pancreaticoduodenectomy becomes necessary.

Dumping

The term *dumping* defines a postoperative syndrome with both gastrointestinal and vasomotor components. The cause of dumping relates to the unregulated entry of ingested food into the proximal small bowel after vagotomy and either resection or division of the pyloric sphincter (Table 31-7). Early dumping symptoms occur within 1 hour of a meal and include nausea, epigastric discomfort, and palpitations. Severely symptomatic patients may also have dizziness or syncope. Late dumping symptoms follow a meal by 1 to 3 hours and may include reactive hypoglycemia.

Although 5% to 10% of patients experience mild dumping symptoms in the early postoperative period, minor dietary alterations and the passage of time bring improvement in approximately 60% (54). The somatostatin analogue octreotide has been reported to improve dumping symptoms when 50 to 100 µg is administered subcutaneously prior to a meal. The beneficial effects of octreotide on vasomotor symptoms of dumping are due to pressor effects of the compound on splanchnic vessels and inhibition of the release of vasoactive peptides from the gut. Octreotide also decreases peak plasma insulin levels and slows intestinal transit. The systemic effects of octreotide include blunting changes in pulse, systolic blood pressure, and packed red cell volume during early dumping and preventing decreases in serum glucose concentration during late dumping.

Cancer in the Gastric Remnant

A growing number of reports suggest that gastric cancer is more likely to develop in individuals who have undergone

TABLE 31-7

FEATURES OF EARLY DUMPING SYNDROME

Cardiovascular	Gastrointestinal
Tachycardia	Nausea
Palpitations	Colic and cramping
Dizziness	Abdominal pain
Syncope	Diarrhea
Sweating	
Flushing	

previous partial gastrectomy. The clearest risk factor for the development of gastric cancer after gastrectomy is the time interval following surgery. A decreased risk of gastric cancer has been observed during the first 15 years after gastrectomy. Cancer reduction is likely due to the removal of at-risk mucosa from the distal stomach. In contrast, patients from 15 to 20 years after gastric resection for ulcer disease have a relative risk for gastric cancer that is three to five times that of the age-matched and sex-matched general population (55,56).

The molecular mechanisms that underlie development of neoplasia in the remnant stomach are unknown. Decreased luminal pH, permitting bacterial overgrowth with increased production of *N*-nitroso carcinogens, and reflux of bile acids into the stomach have been postulated to promote cancer development. The effects of each are unproven. Vagotomy does not appear to promote cancer development. A Swedish population-based study of 7,198 vagotomized patients followed for 9 to 18 years did not reveal increased risk (57). Prognosis is usually guarded because many gastric remnant cancers are diagnosed at an advanced stage (58,59). Reported 5-year survival ranges from 7% to 33%.

GASTRIC CANCER

In the United States, gastric cancer remains among the top ten causes of cancer-related deaths for both men and women. Although the incidence of gastric cancer has declined in the United States, approximately 22,000 new cases of gastric cancer were reported in 2000 (60).

Pathogenesis

Gastric cancer risk is increased in stomachs that contain polyps. Risk is related to polyp histology, size, and number. Hyperplastic gastric polyps are considered to have no neoplastic potential. In contrast, adenomatous polyps have a definite risk for development of malignancy (61). The risk is greatest for polyps >2 cm in diameter. Multiple adenomatous polyps further increase the risk of cancer. Although nitrites in the diet have been demonstrated to have a role in gastric carcinogenesis in animals, specific human dietary constituents that promote tumor formation have not been identified.

Long-term infestation with the organism *H. pylori* appears to predispose to subsequent development of gastric carcinoma. *H. pylori* is unequivocally associated with the development of chronic gastritis, and regions of the world with high rates of gastric adenocarcinoma also have a high prevalence of *H. pylori* infection. Childhood acquisition of *H. pylori* infection appears to be linked to the subsequent development of premalignant lesions and invasive cancer. In the United States, seropositivity for *H. pylori* increases the risk for cancer development approximately threefold,

and in Japanese American males in Hawaii, *H. pylori*-positive subjects demonstrate a sixfold increase in incidence (62,63). *H. pylori* infection is associated with development of adenocarcinoma of both major histologic types and with tumors arising in the body or antrum of the stomach. *H. pylori* infection is not a significant risk factor for cancers of the gastroesophageal junction; these tumors are frequently associated with mucosal abnormalities of Barrett esophagus. However, infection with *H. pylori* alone cannot explain the development of gastric cancer. In North America approximately 50% of adults older than 50 are seropositive for *H. pylori*, yet only a small fraction develop gastric cancer.

Diagnosis

The most common symptoms of gastric cancer are not specific and include pain, anorexia, and weight loss. These symptoms resemble those of a number of nonneoplastic gastroduodenal diseases, especially benign peptic ulcer. Fiberoptic endoscopy is the definitive diagnostic method when gastric cancer is suspected, and only gastric biopsy can definitively differentiate benign from malignant gastric ulcers. Accuracy of diagnosis can exceed 95% if multiple biopsy specimens are obtained.

Cross-sectional imaging, most commonly CT, has been used to assess extragastric spread. When performed with ingestion of oral contrast, CT reliably demonstrates infiltration of the gastric wall by tumor, gastric ulceration, and hepatic metastasis. The technique is less specific with regard to invasion of adjacent organs and in assessing for presence of lymphatic metastases.

Endoscopic ultrasound is useful to characterize subepithelial lesions that may be confused with gastric cancer. Ultrasound-directed biopsy of submucosal tumors is possible. Endoscopic ultrasound can assess the depth of gastric wall penetration by gastric cancer and demonstrates good correlation with intraoperative assessment and histologic findings. Perigastric lymph nodes involved with tumor are reliably identified and may be biopsied with ultrasound guidance. Because endoscopic ultrasound has a limited depth of tissue penetration, hepatic metastases are not detectable; this limitation hinders complete preoperative staging of gastric cancer patients.

Surgical Therapy

Surgical resection is the only curative treatment for gastric cancer, but in the United States advanced disease at the time of diagnosis prevents curative resection for most patients. The surgical objectives in gastric cancer are to attempt cure in patients with localized tumor and to provide palliation that is both effective and safe for patients with advanced malignancy. Operative treatment of gastric adenocarcinoma has focused on the detection of metastatic disease, the limits of gastric resection for potentially curable lesions, the extent of perigastric lymphadenectomy, the role of splenectomy, and the management of directly involved adjacent organs.

Laparoscopy

The ability of cross-sectional imaging to detect metastatic disease is limited when tumor involves the surface of the liver, the omentum, and the peritoneal surfaces. These are common sites for gastric cancer metastasis that are amenable to laparoscopic examination. In a recent prospective study, diagnostic laparoscopy was superior to preoperative CT or percutaneous ultrasound in detection of peritoneal, hepatic, or lymphatic metastasis (64). Diagnostic laparoscopy can be combined with laparoscopic ultrasound. Preoperative endoscopic ultrasound and laparoscopic ultrasound are complimentary techniques. When combined, a 100% sensitivity in detecting inoperable tumors has been reported (65).

Detection of incurable lesions is important because the mean life expectancy of affected patients is 3 to 9 months. In 25% to 30% of patients laparoscopy will detect distant disease that precludes curative resection (66,67). The shortened hospitalization following laparoscopy and reduced operative trauma relative to laparotomy are obvious benefits to individuals with shortened life expectancy. Most patients with metastasis can be treated without the need for palliative surgical resection. In one recent study no patients deemed incurable by laparoscopy required subsequent operation (68).

Resection

Over the past decade the surgical treatment of gastric cancer has diverged, with minimally invasive approaches for early cancers and increasingly radical operations for advanced tumors. The greatest experience with early gastric cancer has been reported by Japanese surgeons. The Japanese Gastric Cancer Association defines early gastric cancer as a tumor in which invasion is restricted to the mucosa or submucosa regardless of the presence or absence of lymph node metastasis (69). The presence of lymphatic metastasis cannot be correctly judged by macroscopic findings but is crucially important in prognosis. For tumors confined to the mucosa, lymphatic metastasis is present in 1% to 3% of cases; with submucosal involvement the rate of nodal positivity increases to between 14% and 20% (70,71).

Endoscopic mucosal resection has been reported for well-differentiated mucosal tumors of <3 cm without ulceration. In a series of 445 patients, 5% experienced postoperative bleeding or perforation (72). In 17% histologic examination revealed submucosal invasion necessitating further operative treatment. Additional analysis, which suggests underdiagnosis of tumor invasion in 45% and missed lymphatic metastasis in 9%, urges caution in acceptance of this technique (73).

Laparoscopic gastrectomy has also been reported for treatment of gastric malignancy, with purported advantages of reduced pain, shorter hospitalization, and improved quality of life (74). Long-term cancer control rates for laparoscopic gastrectomy have not yet been reported by controlled clinical trial, however.

The extent of gastric resection is determined by the need to obtain a resection margin free of microscopic disease. Gastric cancer frequently demonstrates intramural spread due to the extensive intramural capillary and lymphatic network within the stomach. Microscopic involvement of the resection margin by tumor cells is associated with decreased survival (75). Patients with histologically positive margins of resection are at highest risk to develop recurrent disease, with positive margins strongly correlated with development of anastomotic recurrence. Retrospective studies suggest that a 6-cm distance from the tumor mass to the point of resection is associated with the lowest rate of anastomotic recurrence. Larger margins have not improved survival.

Advancements in operative technique and in postoperative physiologic support have improved results of major gastric resection during the past three decades. Increasingly radical gastric operations can be performed with acceptable morbidity and low mortality. The risk of postoperative mortality is very clearly related to age, with several reports indicating a twofold to fivefold increase in mortality for patients older than 70 (76). Although mortality risk is not significantly different for subtotal gastrectomy and total gastrectomy in patients younger than 70, for older patients total gastrectomy doubles mortality. Mortality rates for total gastrectomy now range from 2% to 7% (77,78).

Because gastric cancer metastasizes so frequently to lymph nodes, radical extirpation of perigastric lymph nodes has been advocated as a therapeutic maneuver (79). The therapeutic benefit of extended lymphadenectomy in the treatment of gastric adenocarcinoma was derived initially from retrospective experiences and remains controversial. The first favorable experience was reported by the Japanese Research Society for Gastric Cancer (80,81). In the original Japanese system, resections were characterized as follows:

> R1—resection of stomach, omentum, and perigastric lymph nodes;
>
> R2—resection of stomach, omentum, and en bloc removal of the superior leaf of the transverse mesocolon, the pancreatic capsule, and lymph nodes along the branches of the celiac artery and in the infraduodenal and supraduodenal areas;
>
> R3—resection of the above structures, plus lymph nodes along the aorta and esophagus, along with the spleen, the tail of the pancreas, and skeletonization of vessels in the portahepatis.

The current Japanese classification system is based on anatomical location of lymph nodes. Upper abdominal nodes are grouped into four levels (N1–N4) relative to the location of the primary tumor. The extent of lymphadenectomy corresponds to the level of nodal dissection, with higher levels of dissection involving nodes at greater remove from the primary tumor.

Only retrospective studies of extended perigastric lymphadenectomy have been reported from Japan. Stage for stage, initial reports suggested an improvement of 10% for patients treated with R2 or R3 operations (80–83). The benefits of extended lymphadenectomy have not been confirmed in observational studies from centers outside Japan. Randomized trials have also failed to demonstrate a survival advantage for extended lymphadenectomy when entire patient populations were analyzed (84–88).

An effect of extended lymphadenectomy that may mitigate survival advantage is "upstaging" of tumors. As additional lymph nodes are removed, additional micrometastatic disease is discovered. Patients are consequently placed in higher stage categories with more accurate, although worse, prognosis (89). Patients who do not undergo extended lymphadenectomy have micrometastases, which are undetected and, because of progressive tumor growth and recurrence, will decrease the survivorship of the staging group to which they are assigned.

The safety of extended lymphadenectomy is controversial. Reports from a national Japanese registry indicate a contemporary mortality of <1% (90). Similarly, low mortality risks have been reported from multi-institutional trials in Italy and Germany (89,91). In contrast, reports from the United States, Britain, and the Netherlands have indicated increased short-term morbidity and in-hospital mortality (85–89).

Histologically positive lymph nodes may be present in the splenic hilum and along the splenic artery, and splenectomy has been routinely practiced in some centers, especially in Japan. Splenectomy has not been demonstrated to improve survival for similarly staged patients (92,93). Splenectomy has a clearly adverse effect on postoperative morbidity and mortality. Septic complications due to pancreatic fistula and abscess formation are the major causes of morbidity. Splenectomy is not indicated unless the tumor directly invades the spleen or involves splenic hilar lymph nodes.

Resection of the tail of the pancreas does not improve survival. In a large British trial both morbidity and mortality were doubled when distal pancreatectomy was part of the operation (87). Similar results have been reported in smaller observational series. Pancreatectomy is indicated only if there is direct invasion of the distal pancreas by the primary tumor. Resection of adjacent organs, most commonly the distal pancreas or transverse colon, may be required for local control if direct invasion is present. In these patients operative morbidity is increased and long-term survival approximates 25% (94).

Total gastrectomy is performed almost exclusively in the context of gastric cancer. This procedure is indicated for gastric tumors at the esophagogastric junction, in the proximal stomach, and along the proximal lesser curvature. For patients with carcinoma of the gastric cardia, esophagectomy has no survival advantage when added to total gastrectomy if tumor resection can be achieved (95). Moreover, addition of esophagectomy is associated with significantly higher morbidity.

The most important complication of total gastrectomy is anastomotic leak at the esophagojejunal anastomosis (Fig. 31-8). In two randomized trials, anastomotic failure was observed in 7% and 11% of patients who underwent total gastrectomy (96,97). Anastomotic leak may be heralded by unexplained tachycardia without fever or leukocytosis. Water-soluble contrast radiography should be used to confirm leakage (Fig. 31-9). Intraluminal suction decompression and perianastomotic drainage may be used to create a controlled fistula with expectant fistula closure. Severe surrounding inflammation usually prohibits direct operative repair. Anastomotic dehiscence contributes substantially to the reported operative mortality of total gastrectomy (96,97).

The performance of total gastrectomy creates a substantial postoperative nutritional challenge. Reconstruction with a variety of small intestinal pouch configurations has been reported in observational series (98,99). No controlled data currently exist to prefer pouch reconstruction to simple Roux-Y esophagojejunostomy.

MORBID OBESITY

Obesity is epidemic in the United States. An estimated 20% of Americans are obese, a proportion that has risen annually for each of the past 10 years. Obesity is a major public health problem in Canada, Western Europe, and New Zealand, and many nonwestern countries are also reporting an increasing prevalence of obesity.

Degrees of obesity are quantified on the basis of body mass index (BMI), expressed as weight in kg per (height in meters)^2. An optimal BMI of 20 to 25 kg per m^2 has been determined actuarially with an initial sample size of approximately 20,000 individuals and life table analysis of 4.2 million individuals followed for 17 years (100). A BMI >40 kg per m^2 defines morbid obesity. A BMI of 35 kg per m^2 may be accepted as morbid obesity in the presence of obesity-related complications such as diabetes mellitus. Approximately 4 million Americans have a BMI between 35 and 40 kg per m^2; another 1.5 million have a BMI >40 kg per m^2.

Severe obesity is classified as "morbid" because of the strong association with secondary obesity-related diseases. Morbid obesity is associated with increased risk of hypertension, noninsulin-dependent diabetes mellitus,

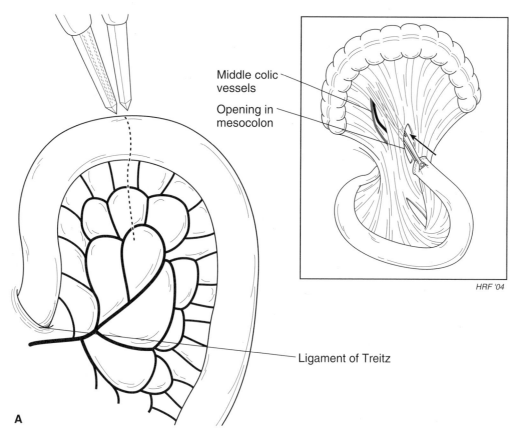

Middle colic
vessels

Opening in
mesocolon

Ligament of Treitz

HRF '04

A

Figure 31-8 Creation of a stapled esophagojejunostomy. **A:** The proximal jejunum is divided creating a Roux limb. An opening is made in the transverse mesocolon to the left of the middle colic vessels. The distal end of the transected jejunum is passed retrocolically to the area of the distal esophagus.

hypertrophic cardiomyopathy, dyslipidemia, pulmonary insufficiency, sleep apnea, and several types of cancer (Table 31-8). Socioeconomic impairment and psychosocial disorders are also increased in morbidly obese individuals. Morbid obesity has an increased risk of premature mortality.

Weight loss reduces the risks of obesity-related comorbidities. For obese patients weight reduction by as little as 5% to 10% of initial weight produces measurable improvements in glucose intolerance, hypertension, and lipid abnormalities.

Behavioral interventions and dietary modification are sometimes effective in moderate obesity. These measures are ineffective in morbid obesity, with recidivism rates of 95% within 1 year. To date no pharmacologic agents have been developed that are both effective and safe for the treatment of obesity. In 1991 a National Institutes of Health Consensus Development Panel recommended operative intervention for morbidly obese individuals (BMI >40 kg per m^2) on the basis that weight reduction by nonsurgical techniques was seldom achieved. The panel also recommended consideration of surgery for less severely obese individuals (BMI 35 to 40 kg per m^2)

with comorbid conditions such as diabetes mellitus or sleep apnea.

Postoperative success requires careful patient selection. In addition to the presence of severe obesity as defined above, the patient must provide evidence of failure to lose weight under medical supervision and the motivation and emotional reserve necessary to undergo the surgical procedure and subsequent lifestyle changes. Comorbid conditions should be sought and treated. Psychiatric evaluation is often useful.

Contemporary bariatric procedures all involve a degree of gastric restriction (Fig. 31-10). Roux-en-Y gastric bypass, the most common procedure in North America, involves creating a small pouch of the proximal stomach, drained via a segment of the proximal jejunum. In this procedure the distal stomach and duodenum are bypassed. Gastric restriction is augmented by malabsorption in the biliopancreatic diversion procedure. The latter procedure has been further modified with duodenal switch.

The small volume of the gastric reservoir limits oral intake, and the major factor causing weight loss after bariatric procedures is reduced caloric ingestion. In gastric bypass the small outlet from the gastric pouch may also

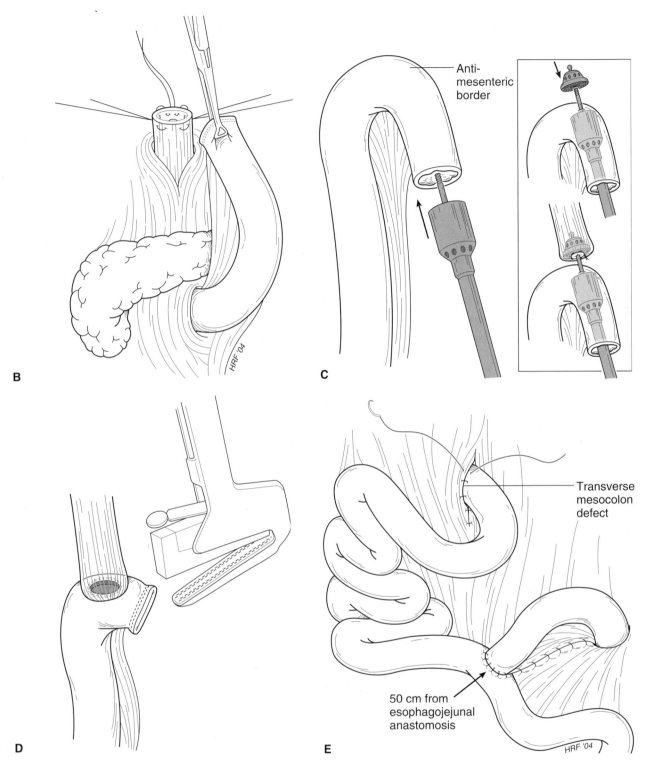

Figure 31-8 (*continued*)   **B:** The jejunal limb is approximated to the esophagus without angulation or tension. The stapled jejunal closure is excised to allow introduction of an EEA-type stapling device. **C:** An EEA stapling device is introduced into the opened end of the Roux-en-Y limb and positioned along the antimesenteric border of the jejunum. The anvil is reattached. The anvil is inserted into the distal esophagus, and a previously placed purse string suture is tied. When the EEA device is fired, an end-to-side esophagojejunal anastomosis is created. **D:** After withdrawal of the EEA stapler, the open end of the jejunal limb is closed with an application of a TA stapler. With the surgeon's guidance, a nasogastric tube is placed across the anastomosis. Anastomotic integrity is insured by observing for bubbles in a saline-filled operative field as the anesthesiologist insufflates air through the nasogastric tube. The jejunum is occluded to permit anastomotic distention. **E:** Intestinal continuity is restored through an end-to-side enteroenterostomy 50 cm distal to the esophagojejunal anastomosis. The mesenteric defect in the transverse mesocolon is approximated to the jejunal limb with interrupted sutures.

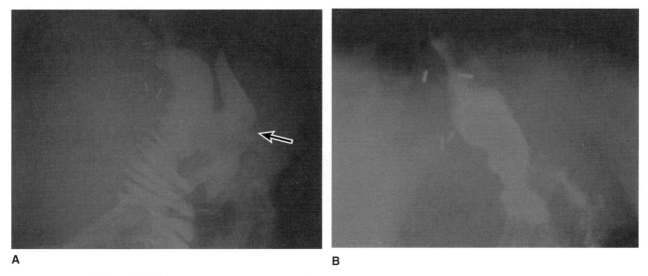

A   B

Figure 31-9 Water-soluble contrast study demonstrating a contained leak at an esophagojejunal anastomosis (*arrow*).

retard gastric emptying. In each of the illustrated procedures the dumping syndrome may occur, inhibiting ingestion of calorie-dense foods. Biliopancreatic diversion is designed to induce malabsorption to further augment the effects of gastric restriction. Bile and pancreatic secretions do not mix with food until the terminal ileum, limiting the time and mucosal surface area for digestion and absorption.

A broad experience has accumulated with the surgical treatment of morbid obesity. Three randomized studies and numerous nonrandomized studies have been published since 1986 that examine the efficacy of gastric bypass. The reports prior to 2000 relate to procedures performed via laparotomy. At 24 months after operation, a mean of 60%

TABLE 31-8

OBESITY-RELATED HEALTH SEQUELAE

Hypertension
Accelerated atherosclerosis
Hypertrophic cardiomyopathy
Dyslipidemia
Diabetes mellitus
Alveolar hypoventilation
Sleep apnea
Hepatic steatosis
Deep vein thrombosis
Venous stasis ulcers
Pulmonary embolism
Gastroesophageal reflux
Hernias
Degenerative joint disease
Female urinary incontinence
Female hirsutism
Amenorrhea
Intertrigenous dermatitis
Carcinoma of uterus, breast, prostate, and colon

of excess weight is lost. For most patients weight loss is maximal between 1 and 2 years postoperatively, with a mean 13-pound regain between 2 and 5 years and stability thereafter (101). A recent report of biliopancreatic diversion demonstrated average excess weight loss of 75% (102). Follow-up ranged from 1 to 21 years.

Surgically induced weight loss is effective in reducing cardiovascular risk. At 2 years surgically treated patients demonstrated significant improvements in hypertension, diabetes mellitus, hyperinsulinemia, hypertriglyceridemia, and levels of high-density lipoprotein cholesterol. A 32-fold reduction in diabetic risk factors was observed at 2 years (103). This effect was persistent. At 8-year follow-up the incidence of diabetes was five times lower in the surgical group relative to unoperated controls.

Relative to nonobese subjects, systolic and diastolic blood pressure are increased in obesity. Left ventricular mass and wall thickness are increased; ejection fraction and diastolic function are decreased in obese subjects. One year after surgery each of these parameters is improved. The greater the weight loss, the greater the reduction in left ventricular mass and the greater the improvement in diastolic function.

Pulmonary function is improved with surgical weight reduction. The percentage of patients reporting physical inactivity is decreased by two-thirds. Sleep apnea, present in 23% of surgically treated patients preoperatively, was observed in 8% after 2 years (105). No change in frequency of sleep apnea was observed in the control group.

Questionnaire data suggest that weight reduction has beneficial economic consequences. Workdays lost to illness or disability are reduced in years 2 to 5 following surgery. Quality of life instruments record improvement in psychosocial scales. The larger the weight loss, the greater the improvement.

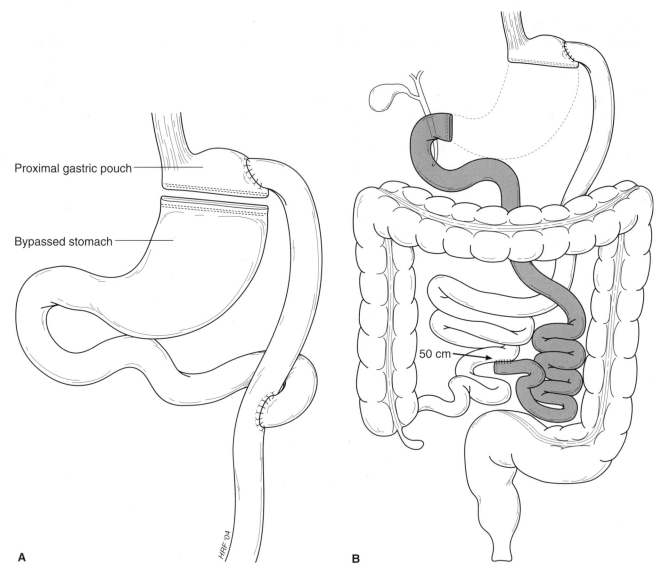

Proximal gastric pouch

Bypassed stomach

50 cm

A

B

HRF '04

Figure 31-10 **A:** Configuration of Roux-en-Y gastric bypass. In this configuration the stomach is divided. The Roux limb is anastomosed along the lesser curvature. **B:** Biliopancreatic diversion. This operation consists of dividing the small bowel 250 cm proximal to the ileocecal valve. A proximal segment of divided small intestine is anastomosed to the distal limb 50 cm proximal to the ileocecal valve. The distal small bowel is anastomosed to the stomach as a Roux limb. Digestion occurs in the common limb of intestine.

Intraoperative Management

Specially designed operating tables are required for bariatric surgery. Standard operating room tables have a maximum weight limit of 200 kg, while those developed specifically for bariatric procedures are capable of holding 450 kg. Because most bariatric procedures require tilting of the table, efforts must be made to assure that the patient does not slip on its surface. A so-called "bean bag," a soft pad filled with thousands of small plastic pellets, is useful for this purpose. The bean bag is molded to the patient's body and, with application of suction, firmly conforms to the patient's contour.

Pressure sores and neural injuries are more common in obese surgical patients, especially diabetics and the super obese. Injuries to the ulnar nerve and the lateral femoral cutaneous nerve are most common. In most instances injury caused by malpositioning or stretch is neuropraxic and reversible. Padded protection of pressure areas is crucial.

Intraoperative blood pressure measurements will be falsely increased if an inappropriately small blood pressure cuff is used. The cuff bladder should ideally encircle the entire arm, but it must be at least of 75% of arm circumference. Accurate noninvasive blood pressure measurements may be obtained from the ankle or wrist. Invasive arterial monitoring should be used in the super obese.

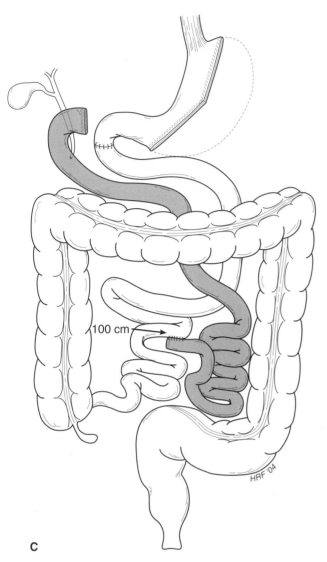

C

Figure 31-10 (continued) **C:** Biliopancreatic diversion modified by duodenal switch. The stomach is resected, producing early satiety but leaving a normal pylorus. The first portion of the duodenum is divided. The jejunum is divided 250 cm proximal to the ileocecal valve, and the distal end at this point of division is anastomosed to the proximal segment of duodenum. The remaining duodenum and proximal small bowel are anastomosed to the ileum 100 cm proximal to the ileocecal valve.

Pneumoperitoneum used during laparoscopy may adversely affect systemic circulation in obese patients, and use of the Trendelenburg position may exacerbate circulatory changes. Elevated intra-abdominal pressure increases systemic vascular resistance. For intra-abdominal pressures <10 mm Hg, venous return to the right heart increases due to decreased splanchnic blood pooling. As intra-abdominal pressure increases to >20 mm Hg, inferior vena caval compression decreases venous return and consequently diminishes cardiac output. Renal blood flow decreases when intra-abdominal pressure exceeds 20 mm Hg, and glomerular filtration rate drops. Hypovolemia accentuates these changes at higher intra-abdominal pressures. Both obesity and pneumoperitoneum adversely affect respiratory mechanics.

Postoperative Complications

The largest number of reported experiences with bariatric surgery relate to operations performed by laparotomy. Collectively, these reports illustrate that for Roux-en-Y gastric bypass, 30-day mortality ranges from 0.3% to 2% (104). Overall complication rates range from 20% to 40%. The most frequent acute postoperative complications include deep vein thrombosis (DVT), pulmonary embolism, anastomotic leakage, and wound infection. Late complications include stomal stenosis, staple line dehiscence, and marginal ulceration. Micronutrient deficiencies have also been reported long-term.

Laparoscopic gastric bypass is associated with a postoperative mortality rate of 0% to 1.7%, similar to the rate observed when the operation is performed via laparotomy (105). Laparoscopic bariatric surgery requires advanced laparoscopic skills, and many observers have commented upon an extended "learning curve" not accounted for by current mortality statistics. The range of postoperative complications recorded with open gastric bypass has also been noted for procedures performed laparoscopically.

Deep Venous Thrombosis

Overall, the most common cause of death postoperatively is pulmonary embolism. DVT occurs in approximately 2% of patients treated via open operation or laparoscopically (106). Immobility, venous stasis, and the effects of pneumoperitoneum may contribute to thrombus formation. Physical examination is not diagnostically reliable. Doppler examination is the preferred initial diagnostic test.

Controlled trials are not available establishing a standard of care for DVT prophylaxis in bariatric surgery. Sequential compression stockings and injection of either subcutaneous heparin or low-molecular weight heparin are recommended.

The consequences of pulmonary embolism are more severe in bariatric patients relative to the general population. The hypoventilation syndrome and *cor pulmonale* are increased in obese patients. Both diminish functional cardiac reserve.

Anastomotic Dehiscence

Anastomotic dehiscence or suture line leak has been reported in 1.2% of patients undergoing open gastric bypass (107). This complication occurs in 3% of cases performed laparoscopically but diminishes with surgeon experience (108). The diagnosis of postoperative peritonitis is more difficult in morbidly obese patients. Tachycardia, worsening abdominal or back pain, and hiccups may be the only signs. Concern mandates radiologic investigation with a water-soluble contrast agent. If a leak is confirmed at laparotomy, the defect should be closed if feasible and the upper abdomen should be externally drained. A gastrostomy tube should be placed in the distal, excluded stomach.

Acute gastric distension of the bypassed distal stomach may occur after either open or laparoscopic gastric bypass. Acute distention may be a result of postoperative peritonitis or as a mechanical consequence of an obstructed enteroenterostomy. Continuous abdominal pain, distension, and hiccups are frequently associated signs. Plain abdominal x-rays or CT demonstrate massive gastric dilatation, often with an air-fluid level. Acute gastric distention must be treated emergently because of the potential for ischemic necrosis of the stomach. Percutaneous or operative gastrostomy decompression is therapeutic.

Incisional Hernia

Postoperative incisional hernias are a major problem in open bariatric surgery, occurring in approximately 20% of cases. A prior incisional hernia doubles this risk. Port site incisional hernias have been reported in 0% to 0.5% of patients after laparoscopic gastric bypass, representing the clearest advantage of the laparoscopic approach (105).

Cholelithiasis

Rapid weight loss, by either dietary means or following surgery, is associated with an increased risk of cholelithiasis. Half of patients following bariatric surgery will demonstrate gallbladder sludge; one-third will develop symptomatic gallstones. The use of prophylactic ursodiol for 6 months following gastric bypass reduced the incidence of symptomatic gallstones to 2% (109). Many surgeons have used the high incidence of postoperative cholelithiasis to justify prophylactic cholecystectomy at the time of gastric bypass. No controlled trial exists to support or refute this practice.

Stomal Complications

The gastrojejunal anastomosis that drains the proximal gastric pouch in gastric bypass is intentionally small at 1 cm. Larger stomas do not create enough restriction of food passage and are not associated with adequate weight loss. As a consequence, stomal stenosis is relatively common, occurring in 12% of cases (110). Affected patients develop early satiety, recurrent vomiting, and upper abdominal pain. Thiamine deficiency has been linked to persistent vomiting, with disturbances in vision and gait (111). Stomal stenosis may also cause symptoms of gastroesophageal reflux.

Upper endoscopy is the preferred means of investigation; contrast radiographs are not demonstrative of the degree of stenosis. Most patients with gastrojejunal stenosis after gastric bypass will respond to endoscopic dilatation.

Stomal ulceration may also cause stomal stenosis. The rate of gastrojejunal stomal ulcer approximates 10%. The etiology of stomal ulceration is often multifactorial, including acid secretion by parietal cells in the proximal pouch, ischemia of the jejunal limb, and NSAID use. Failure to heal with proton pump inhibitors and elimination of NSAIDs suggests jejunal ischemia; mucosal biopsies are confirmatory. Prolonged ulceration causes mechanical obstruction because of chronic cicatrization.

Staple line disruption is a complication of gastric bypass techniques in which the stomach is not divided. This complication is suggested by recurrent weight gain after weight loss stabilization. Correction requires reoperation to restaple and divide the stomach. Staple line disruption occurs in 1% of patients.

Nutrient deficiencies are anticipated after Roux-en-Y gastric bypass because the distal stomach and duodenum are bypassed. Defective absorption of vitamin B_{12}, folate, iron, and calcium are sufficiently common to warrant routine postoperative supplementation. Biliopancreatic diversion worsens micronutrient deficiencies because of the more severe anatomic rearrangement. Steatorrhea is universal and high dose calcium supplementation and monthly intramuscular vitamin D are required to prevent metabolic bone disease. Protein malnutrition is the most severe complication of biliopancreatic diversion.

REFERENCES

1. American Cancer Society. Cancer facts and figures. Available at: www.cancer.org.
2. Terry MB, Gaudet MM, Gammon MD. The epidemiology of gastric cancer. *Semin Radiat Oncol* 2002;12:111–127.
3. Martin RC II, Jaques DP, Brennan MF, et al. Extended local resection for advanced gastric cancer: increased survival versus increased morbidity. *Ann Surg* 2002;236:159–165.
4. Schwarz RE, Zagala-Nevarez K. Gastrectomy circumstances that influence early postoperative outcome. *Hepatogastroenterology* 2002;49:1742–1746.
5. Wainess RM, Dimick JB, Upchurch GR, et al. Epidemiology of surgically treated gastric cancer in the United States, 1988–2000. *J Gastrointest Surg* 2003;7:879–883.
6. Laine L, Peterson WL. Bleeding peptic ulcer. *N Engl J Med* 1994; 331:717–727.
7. Silverstein FE, Gilbert DA, Tedesco FJ, et al. The national ASGE survey on upper gastrointestinal bleeding. *Gastrointest Endosc* 1981;27:73–79.
8. Gilbert DA. Epidemiology of upper gastrointestinal bleeding. *Gastrointest Endosc* 1990;36(suppl 5):8–13.
9. Branicki FJ, Boey J, Fok PJ, et al. Bleeding duodenal ulcer—a prospective evaluation of risk factors for rebleeding and death. *Ann Surg* 1990;211:411–418.
10. Mueller X, Rothenbuehler J, Amery A, et al. Factors predisposing to further hemorrhage and mortality after peptic ulcer bleeding. *J Am Coll Surg* 1994;179:457–461.
11. Branicki FJ, Coleman SY, Folk PJ, et al. Bleeding peptic ulcer: a prospective evaluation of risk factors for rebleeding and mortality. *World J Surg* 1990;14:262–270.
12. Larson G, Schmidt T, Gott J, et al. Upper gastrointestinal bleeding: predictors of outcome. *Surgery* 1986;100:765–772.
13. Imhof M, Schroders C, Ohmann C, et al. Impact of early operation on the mortality from bleeding peptic ulcer—ten years' experience. *Dig Surg* 1998;15:308–314.

14. Feldman RA, Eccersley AJ, Hardie JM. Epidemiology of *Helicobacter pylori*: acquisition, transmission, population prevalence and disease-to-infection ratio. *Br Med Bull* 1998;54:39–53.
15. Vaira D, Menegatti M, Miglioli M. What is the role of *Helicobacter pylori* in complicated pepticulcer disease? *Gastroenterology* 1997; 113:S78–S84.
16. El-Omar EM, Penman ID, Ardill JE, et al. *Helicobacter pylori* infection and abnormalities of acid secretion in patients with duodenal ulcer disease. *Gastroenterology* 1995;109:681–691.
17. Aalykke C, Lauritsen JM, Hallas J, et al. *Helicobacter pylori* and risk of ulcer bleeding among users of nonsteroidal anti-inflammatory drugs: a case-control study. *Gastroenterology* 1999;116:1305–1309.
18. Hay JA, Lyubashevsky E, Elashoff J, et al. Upper gastrointestinal hemorrhage clinical guideline—determining the optimal hospital length of stay. *Am J Med* 1996;100:313–322.
19. Jiranek GC, Kozarek RA. A cost-effective approach to the patient with peptic ulcer bleeding. *Surg Clin North Am* 1996;76:83–103.
20. Collins R, Langman M. Treatment with histamine H$_2$ antagonists in acute upper gastrointestinal hemorrhage: implications of randomized trials. *N Engl J Med* 1985;313:660–666.
21. Khuroo MS, Yattoo GN, Javid G, et al. A comparison of omeprazole and placebo for bleeding peptic ulcer. *N Engl J Med* 1997; 336:1054–1058.
22. Peterson WL, Cook DJ. Antisecretory therapy for bleeding peptic ulcer. *JAMA* 1998;280:877–878.
23. Lau JYW, Sung JJY, Lee KKC, et al. Effect of intravenous omeprazole on recurrent bleeding after endoscopic treatment of bleeding peptic ulcers. *N Engl J Med* 2000;343:310–316.
24. Cooper GS, Chak A, Way LE, et al. Early endoscopy in upper gastrointestinal hemorrhage: associations with recurrent bleeding, surgery, and length of hospital stay. *Gastrointest Endosc* 1999;49: 145–152.
25. Laine L, Cohen H, Brodhead J, et al. Prospective evaluation of immediate versus delayed refeeding and prognostic value of endoscopy in patients with upper gastrointestinal hemorrhage. *Gastroenterology* 1992;102:314–316.
26. Lin HJ, Wang K, Perng CL, et al. Natural history of bleeding peptic ulcers with a tightly adherent clot: a prospective observation. *Gastrointest Endosc* 1996;43:470–473.
27. Cook DJ, Guyatt GH, Salena BJ, et al. Endoscopic therapy for acute nonvariceal upper gastrointestinal hemorrhage: a meta-analysis. *Gastroenterology* 1992;102:139–148.
28. Kubba AK, Palmer KR. Role of endoscopic injection therapy in the treatment of bleeding peptic ulcer. *Br J Surg* 1996;83:461–468.
29. Lau JY, Sung JJ, Lam Y, et al. Endoscopic retreatment compared with surgery in patients with recurrent bleeding after initial endoscopic control of bleeding ulcers. *N Engl J Med* 1999; 340:751–756.
30. Hsu P, Lai K, Lin X, et al. When to discharge patients with bleeding peptic ulcers: a prospective study of residual risk of rebleeding. *Gastrointest Endosc* 1996;44:382–387.
31. Brullet E, Campo R, Calvet X, et al. Factors related to the failure of endoscopic injection therapy for bleeding gastric ulcer. *Gut* 1996;39:155–158.
32. Poxon VA, Keighley MRB, Dykes PW, et al. Comparison of minimal and conventional surgery in patients with bleeding peptic ulcer: a multicentre trial. *Br J Surg* 1991;78:1344–1345.
33. Millat B, Hay JM, Valleur P, et al. Emergency surgical treatment for bleeding duodenal ulcer: oversewing plus vagotomy versus gastric resection, a controlled randomized trial. *World J Surg* 1993;17:568–574.
34. Mulholland MW, Debas HT. Chronic duodenal and gastric ulcer. *Surg Clin North Am* 1987;67:489–507.
35. Johnston D, Blackett RL. Recurrent peptic ulcers. *World J Surg* 1987;11:274–282.
36. Millat B, Fingerhut A, Borie F. Surgical treatment of complicated duodenal ulcers: controlled trials. *World J Surg* 2000;24: 299–306.
37. Graham DY, White RH, Moreland LW, et al. Duodenal and gastric ulcer prevention with misoprostol in arthritis patients taking NSAIDs. *Ann Intern Med* 1993;119:257–262.
38. Silverstein FE, Graham DY, Senior JR, et al. Misoprostol reduces serious gastrointestinal complications in patients with rheumatoid arthritis receiving nonsteroidal anti-inflammatory drugs: a randomized, double-blind, placebo-controlled trial. *Ann Intern Med* 1995;123:241–249.
39. Rokkas T, Karameris A, Mavrogeorgis A, et al. Eradication of *Helicobacter pylori* reduces the possibility of rebleeding in peptic ulcer disease. *Gastrointest Endosc* 1995;41:1–4.
40. Jaspersen D, Koerner T, Schorr W, et al. *Helicobacter pylori* eradication reduces the rate of rebleeding in ulcer hemorrhage. *Gastrointest Endosc* 1995;41:5–7.
41. Santander C, Gravalos RG, Cedenilla AG, et al. Maintenance treatment vs Helicobacter pylori eradication in preventing rebleeding of the peptic ulcer disease: a clinical trial and follow up for two years. *Gastroenterology* 1995;108:A208.
42. Maier M, Sohilling D, Dorlars D, et al. Eradication of Helicobacter pylori or H$_2$ blocker maintenance therapy after peptic ulcer bleeding: a prospective randomized trial. *Gastroenterology* 1995;108:A156.
43. Crofts TJ, Park KGM, Steele RJC, et al. A randomized trial of non-operative treatment for perforated peptic ulcer. *N Engl J Med* 1989;320:970.
44. Boey J, Wong J, Ong GB. A prospective study of operative risk factors in perforated duodenal ulcers. *Ann Surg* 1982;195:265.
45. Kujath P, Schwandner O, Bruch H-P. Morbidity and mortality of perforated peptic gastroduodenal ulcer following emergency surgery. *Langenbecks Arch Surg* 2002;387:298–302.
46. Lau WY, Leung KL, Kwong KH, et al. A randomized study comparing laparoscopic versus open repair of perforated peptic ulcer using suture or sutureless technique. *Ann Surg* 1996;224:131.
47. Lau WY, Leung KL, Zhu XL, et al. Laparoscopic repair of perforated peptic ulcer. *Br J Surg* 1995;82:814.
48. Boey J, Lee NW, Koo J, et al. Immediate definitive surgery for perforated duodenal ulcers: a prospective controlled trial. *Ann Surg* 1982;196:338.
49. Ren P, Huang J, Shin J, et al. Jejunojunogastric intussusception: a rare intussusception in an adult patient after gastric surgery. *Gastrointest Endosc* 2002;56(2):296–298.
50. Eckhauser FE, Conrad M, Knol J, et al. Safety and long-term durability of completion gastrectomy in 81 patients with postsurgical gastroparesis syndrome. *Am Surgeon* 1998;64:1–7.
51. McCallum RW, Polpalle SC, Schirmer B. Completion gastrectomy for refractory gastroparesis following surgery for peptic ulcer disease, long-term follow-up with subjective and objective parameters. *Dig Dis Sci* 1991;36(11):1556–1561.
52. Cohen AM, Ottinger LW. Delayed gastric emptying following gastrectomy. *Ann Surg* 1976;184(6):689–696.
53. Rodkey GV. Safe management of the impossible duodenum, risk avoidance in surgery of peptic ulcer. *Arch Surg* 1988;123: 558–562.
54. Eldh J, Kewenter J, Kock NG, et al. Long-term results of surgical treatment for dumping after partial gastrectomy. *Br J Surg* 1974; 61:90–93.
55. Hansson L. Risk of stomach cancer in patients with peptic ulcer disease. *World J Surg* 2000;24:315–320.
56. Tersmette AC, Giardiello FM, Tytgat GNJ, et al. Carcinogenesis after remote peptic ulcer surgery: the long-term prognosis of partial gastrectomy. *Gastroenterology* 1991;101:148–153.
57. Lundegårdh G, Ekbom A, McLaughlin JK, et al. Gastric cancer risk after vagotomy. *Gut* 1994;35:946.
58. Holstein C. Long-term prognosis after partial gastrectomy for gastroduodenal ulcer. *World J Surg* 2000;24:307–314.
59. Safatle-Riberio AV, Riberio U, Reynolds JC. Gastric stump cancer: what is the risk? *Dig Dis* 1998;16:159–168.
60. Boring CC, Squires TS, Tong T. Cancer Statistics 1993. *CA* 1993;43:19.
61. Harju E. Gastric polyposis and malignancy. *Br J Surg* 1986;73: 532–533.
62. Parsonnet J, Friedman GD, Vandersteen DP, et al. Helicobacter pylori infection and the risk of gastric carcinoma. *N Engl J Med* 1991;325:1127–1131.
63. Nomura A, Stemmermann GN, Chyou P-H, et al. Helicobacter pylori infection and gastric carcinoma among Japanese Americans in Hawaii. *N Engl J Med* 1991;325:1132–1136.
64. Stell DA, Canter CR, Stewart I, et al. Prospective comparison of laparoscopy, ultrasonography and computer tomography in the staging of gastric cancer. *Br J Surg* 1996;83:1260–1262.

65. Mortensen MB, Scheel-Hincke JD, Madsen MR, et al. Combined endoscopy ultrasonography and laparoscopic ultrasonography in the pretherapeutic assessment of resectability in patients with upper gastrointestinal malignancies. *Scand J Gastroenteral* 1996; 31:1115–1119.

66. Lowy AM, Mansfield PF, Leach SD, et al. Laparoscopic staging for gastric cancer. *Surgery* 1996;119:611–614.

67. D'Ugo DM, Coppola R, Persiani R, et al. Immediately preoperative laparoscopic staging for gastric cancer. *Surg Endosc* 1996;10: 996–999.

68. Burke EC, Karpeh MS Jr, Conlou KC. Laparoscopy in the management of gastric adenocarcinoma. *Ann Surg* 1997;225:262–267.

69. Adachi Y, Shiraishi N, Kitano S. Modern treatment of early gastric cancer: review of the Japanese experience. *Dig Surg* 2002;19: 333–339.

70. Nakamura K, Morisaki T, Sugitani A, et al. An early gastric carcinoma treatment strategy based on analysis of lymph node metastasis. *Cancer* 1999;85:1500–1505.

71. Kunisaki C, Shimada H, Takahaski M, et al. Prognostic factors in early gastric cancer. *Hepatogastroenterology* 2001;48:294–298.

72. Ono H, Kondo H, Gotoda T, et al. Endoscopic mucosal resection of treatment of early gastric cancer. *Gut* 2001;48:225–229.

73. Korenaga D, Orita H, Mackawa S, et al. Pathological appearance of the stomach after endoscopic mucosal resection for early gastric cancer. *Br J Surg* 1997;84:1563–1566.

74. Cuschieri A. Laparoscopic gastric resection. *Surg Clin North Am* 2000;80(4):1269–1284.

75. Wanebo HJ, Kennedy BJ, Chmiel J, et al. Cancer of the stomach: a patient care study by the American College of Surgeons. *Ann Surg* 1993;218:583–592.

76. Kranenbarg EK, van de Velde CJH. Gastric cancer in the elderly. *Euro J Surg Oncol* 1998;24:384–390.

77. Bittner R, Butters M, Ulrich M, et al. Total gastrectomy: updated operative mortality and long-term survival with particular reference to patients older than 70 years of age. *Ann Surg* 1996;224:37–42.

78. Schwarz R, Karpeh MS, Brennan MF. Factors predicting hospitalization after operation treatment for gastric carcinoma in patients older than 70 years. *J Am Coll Surg* 1997;184:9–15.

79. Shiu MH, Moore E, Sanders M, et al. Influence of the extent of resection on survival after curative treatment of gastric cancer: a retrospective multivariate analysis. *Arch Surg* 1987;122:1347–1351.

80. Maruyama K, Okabayashi K, Kinoshita T. Progress in gastric cancer in Japan and its limit of radicality. *World J Surg* 1987;11:418–425.

81. Noguchi Y, Imada T, Matsumoto A, et al. Radical surgery for gastric cancer: a review of the Japanese experience. *Cancer* 1989; 64:2053–2062.

82. Adachi Y, Kamakura T, Mori M, et al. Role of lymph node dissection and splenectomy in node-positive gastric carcinoma. *Surgery* 1994;116:837–841.

83. Baba H, Maehara Y, Takeuchi H, et al. Effect of lymph node dissection on the prognosis in patients with node-negative early gastric cancer. *Surgery* 1994;117:165–169.

84. Maeta M, Yamashiro H, Saito S, et al. A prospective plot study of extended (D3) and superextended para-aortic lymphadenectomy (D4) in patients with T3 or T4 gastric cancer managed by total gastrectomy. *Surgery* 1999;125:325–331.

85. Robertson CS, Chung SCS, Woods SDS, et al. A prospective randomized trial comparing R1 subtotal gastrectomy with R3 total gastrectomy for antral cancer. *Ann Surg* 1994;220:176–182.

86. Bonekamp JJ, Hermans J, van de Velde CJH. Extended lymph-node dissection for gastric cancer. *New Engl J Med* 1999;340: 908–914.

87. Cushieri A, Fayers P, Fielding J, et al. Postoperative morbidity and mortality after D1 and D2 resections for gastric cancer. *Lancet* 1996;347:995–999.

88. Siewert JR, Bottcher K, Stein HJ, et al. Relevant prognostic factors in gastric cancer: ten-year results of the German gastric cancer study. *Ann Surg* 1998;228:449–461.

89. Kodera Y, Yamamura Y, Shimizu Y, et al. The number of metastatic lymph nodes: a promising prognostic determinant for gastric carcinoma in the latest edition of the TNM classification. *J Am Coll Surg* 1998;187:579–603.

90. Lee JS, Douglass HO. D2 dissection for gastric cancer. *Surg Oncol* 1997;6(4):215–225.

91. Pacelli F, Doglietto GB, Bellantone R, et al. Extensive versus limited lymph node dissection for gastric cancer: a comparative study of 320 patients. *Br J Surg* 1993;80:1153–1156.

92. Stipa S, DiGiorgio A, Ferri M, et al. Results of curative gastrectomy for carcinoma. *J Am Coll Surg* 1994;179:567–572.

93. Otsuji E, Yamaguchi T, Sawai K, et al. End results of simultaneous splenectomy in patients undergoing total gastrectomy for gastric cancer. *Surgery* 1996;120:40–44.

94. Shchepotin IB, Chorny VA, Nauta RJ, et al. Extended surgical resection in T4 gastric cancer. *Am J Surg* 1998;175:123–126.

95. Stein HJ, Feith M, Siewert JR. Cancer of the esophagogastric junction. *Surg Oncol* 2000;9:35–41.

96. Bonenkamp JJ, Songun I, Hermans J, et al. Randomized comparison of morbidity after D1 and D2 dissection for gastric cancer in 996 Dutch patients. *Lancet* 1995;345:745–748.

97. Roder JD, Böttchen K, Siewert JR, et al. Prognostic factors in gastric carcinoma: results of the German gastric carcinoma study 1992. *Cancer* 1993;72:2089–2097.

98. Nakane Y, Okumura S, Akehira K, et al. Jejunal pouch reconstruction after total gastrectomy for cancer: a randomized controlled trial. *Ann Surg* 1995;222(1):27–35.

99. Espat NJ, Karpeh M. Reconstruction following total gastrectomy: a review and summary of the randomized prospective clinical trails. *Surg Oncol* 1999;7:65–69.

100. Deitel M. Surgery for morbid obesity: a review. *Eur J Gastroenterol Hepatol* 1999;11(2):57–61.

101. Pories WJ, Swanson MS, MacDonald KG, et al. Who would have thought it? An operation proves to be the most effective therapy for adult-onset diabetes mellitus. *Ann Surg* 1995;222:339–352.

102. Scopinaro N, Adami GF, Marinari GM, et al. Biliopancreatic diversion. *World J Surg* 1998;22:936–946.

103. Sjöström L. Surgical intervention as a strategy for treatment of obesity. *Endocrinology* 2000;13(2):213–320.

104. Hsu LK, Benotti PN, Dwyer J, et al. Nonsurgical factors that influence the outcome of bariatric surgery: a review. *Psychosom Med* 1998;60:338–346.

105. Schauer PR, Ikramuddin S. Laparoscopic surgery for morbid obesity. *Obes Surg* 2001;81(5):1145–1179.

106. Byrne TK. Complications of surgery for obesity. *Obes Surg* 2001; 81(5):1181–1193.

107. Surgerman HJ. Gastric surgery for morbid obesity. In: Zinner MJ, ed. *Maingot abdominal operations*, 10th ed. Stamford CT: Appleton & Lange; 1997.

108. Wittgrove AC, Clark GW. Laparoscopic gastric bypass, Roux-en-Y-500 patients: technique and results with 3-6 month follow up. *Obes Surg* 2000;10:233–239.

109. Sugerman HJ, Brewer WH, Shiffman ML, et al. A multicenter, placebo-controlled, randomized, double-blinded, prospective trial of prophylactic ursodiol for the prevention of gallstone formation following gastric-bypass induced rapid weight loss. *Am J Surg* 1995;169:91–97.

110. Sanayal AJ, Sugerman HJ, Kellum JM, et al. Stomal complications of gastric bypass: incidence and outcome of therapy. *Am J Gastroenterol* 1992;87:1165–1169.

111. Kramer LD, Locke GE. Wernicke's encephalopathy: complication of gastric plication. *J Clin Gastroenterol* 1987;9:549–552.

Complications of Hepatic Surgery

James A. Knol

■■■ **COMPLICATIONS OF HEPATIC SURGERY 409**
    Intraoperative Complications 409
    Postoperative Complications 415

■■■ **SUMMARY 421**

■■■ **REFERENCES 421**

The liver and its included proximal biliary tree are essential for life. A number of diseases of the liver are amenable to operative intervention and constitute the surgical diseases of the liver (Table 32-1). For some of the diseases surgical therapy is a secondary option, but for malignant neoplastic disease surgery remains an essential treatment modality in any attempt at a cure. The complications associated with these interventions are the substance of this chapter. Surgical complications related to hepatic surgery encompass a wide spectrum (Table 32-2). These complications relate to the liver's high blood flow, glucose homeostasis and protein anabolism, synthesis of clotting factors, clearance and deactivation of toxins, synthesis and drainage of bile, and role in protection from infectious agents entering the portal circulation through the gastrointestinal (GI) tract.

Most hepatic surgery is directed at neoplastic disease. In Western countries most liver resections are performed for metastatic colorectal cancer, with about 20% performed for primary hepatobiliary cancer and 10% for benign disease (1). The indications for operations for these various

diseases will not be covered here, but they do play a role in a discussion of surgical complications. The indications for operation must be appropriate to justify any operation with associated complications.

Knowledge of the potential complications of liver surgery demands that there be preoperative evaluation to balance the risks of these complications and mortality against potential benefits. Over the past 30 years advances in preoperative evaluation and patient selection, anesthetic management, surgical methods, and postoperative care have allowed performance of major liver resections with a decline of mortality from about 30% to <5% at high volume institutions (1). Liver resection continues to be associated with about a 45% morbidity rate, however.

Selection of patients for resection for malignant liver disease requires staging to eliminate patients for whom cure, or significant palliation in the case of neuroendocrine liver metastases, is not possible. Imaging, either spiral computed tomography (CT) or magnetic resonance imaging (MRI), is requisite in determining the extent of tumor in the liver, relationships to the vasculature of the liver (the markers for the liver's anatomy), and whether a resection to remove the tumor will spare adequate parenchyma to allow postoperative survival (residual liver remnant). Imaging for hypervascular tumors such as hepatocellular carcinoma, neuroendocrine metastases, hepatic adenoma, and focal nodular hyperplasia should include an arterial contrast phase and a portal venous contrast phase for optimal detection of disease and to assist in the differential diagnosis of liver masses. In general, if liver tumor appears resectable, biopsy should be avoided, unless the biopsy will change the decision about whether to operate. Biopsy risks dissemination of tumor within the needle tract or to the peritoneal surfaces.

James A. Knol: University of Michigan, Ann Arbor, MI 48109

TABLE 32-1

SURGICAL DISEASES OF THE LIVER

Neoplasm—benign	Hepatic adenoma Focal nodular hyperplasia, symptomatic Hemangioma, symptomatic Biliary cystadenoma Hemangioendothelioma

Neoplasm—malignant	Hepatocellular carcinoma
	Intrahepatic cholangiocarcinoma
	Hilar cholangiocarcinoma
	Gallbladder cancer
	Hepatoblastoma
	Hemangioendothelioma
	Direct invasion by adjacent cancers—
	    stomach, colon, renal, adrenal,
	    vena caval
	Metastases—colorectal and highly
	    selected: neuroendocrine, melanoma,
	    GI stromal tumor, endometrial, breast,
	    stomach

Biliary disease	Intrahepatic or high extrahepatic bile
	    duct stricture
	Intrahepatic bile duct stones
	Intrahepatic bile duct cysts
	    (Caroli disease)
	Biliary fistula

Infection	Pyogenic abscess Echinococcal abscess Amebic abscess

Vascular disease	Hepatic artery aneurysm or
	    pseudoaneurysm
	Biliary-arterial or biliary-venous fistula
	Arterial-portal fistula or arterial-hepatic
	    venous fistula

TABLE 32-2

COMPLICATIONS OF LIVER SURGERY

Liver Surgery

Intraoperative hemorrhage	Postoperative hemorrhage
Intrahepatic hematoma	Postoperative coagulopathy
Liver failure	Perihepatic abscess
Biliary fistula	Biliary stricture
Biloma	Bile peritonitis
Cholangitis	Hepatic abscess
Wound infection	Pneumonia
Hemobilia	Hepatic necrosis
Hepatic artery thrombosis	Portal vein thrombosis
Intraoperative air embolus	Pleural effusion
Ascites	Peritonitis
Gastrointestinal bleeding	

Special to Ablation Procedures

Myoglobinuria	Thermal injury to surrounding structures

Significant factors in the potential to survive operation for a particular patient are the patient's overall health and the extent of comorbid disease. In a recent large series the rate of pulmonary complications was 21% and the rate of cardiovascular complications was 10% (1). Morbidity and mortality for right hepatic lobectomy have been shown to correlate strongly with preoperative APACHE II scores, and they emphasize the need for preoperative assessment and selection of candidates for liver resection (2).

The liver's health is the final major determinant in selection of patients for liver surgery. Cirrhosis increases the mortality associated with any operation and anesthesia, and an operation that decreases the amount of residual functioning liver further increases that risk (3). Signs of severe cirrhosis include jaundice, ascites, and malnutrition, and laboratory correlates include elevated bilirubin above 3 mg/dL, serum albumin <3 gm per dL, and a platelet count <100,000 per µL. CT or MRI may show a relatively small liver with notching of the surface and, often, relative atrophy of the right lobe and hypertrophy of the left lateral segment and caudate lobe. A preliminary discriminator is

the Child–Pugh score; all patients with grade C and most with grade B are not considered satisfactory candidates for operation. A variety of other methods has been proposed to predict which patients with liver disease are candidates for resection and how much of the diseased liver may safely be removed or ablated (4–6). Severe fibrosis, jaundice due to causes other than cirrhosis, steatosis >30%, and a history of chemotherapy, particularly hepatic artery infusion therapy, are other indicators of a damaged liver and increase the risk of resection or ablation (7,8).

Resection planning requires estimation of the postresection functioning liver remnant. Postoperative liver dysfunction is significantly increased in patients with normal liver function when the liver remnant is ≤25% of the initial liver volume (9). In the normal liver there is variation in the proportions of the hepatic segments that comprise the usual anatomic liver resections (Table 32-3) (10). The

TABLE 32-3

INTRAHEPATIC LIVER VOLUME RATIOS BASED ON CT FOR NORMAL LIVERS

Segments	Percent of Total Liver Volume
Right liver	65 ± 7 (49–82)
Left liver	33 ± 7 (17–49)
Segment IV	17 ± 4 (10–29)
Bisegment II+III	16 ± 4 (5–27)
Segment I	2 ± 0 (1–3)

Adapted from Abdalla EK, Denys A, Chevalier P, et al. Total and segmental liver volume variations: implications for liver surgery. *Surgery* 2004;135:414–420.

From Clavien PA, Emond J, Vauthey JN, et al. Protection of the liver during hepatic surgery. *J Gastrointest Surg* 2004;8:313–327.

<table>
<tr><td>

TABLE 32-4

INDICATIONS FOR PREOPERATIVE PORTAL VEIN EMBOLIZATION

Patients with underlying normal liver
    Future liver remnant volume <30%
    Major hepatectomy associated with gastrointestinal procedure
    Resection of bilobar tumors, including a major hepatectomy
Patients with diseased liver
    Cirrhosis
    Severe fibrosis
    Jaundice
    Steatosis >30%
    Chemotherapy
</td></tr>
</table>

experienced liver surgeon can make some estimates on the basis of the imaging studies. However, volumetric analysis should be done in patients with normal liver in whom an extended lobectomy is planned and in patients with damaged livers in whom any resection or ablation equivalent to a single liver segment is anticipated (11). In addition, in patients for whom there is a possibility of preexisting liver damage, biopsy from the area of the potential remnant liver should be considered.

For patients in whom resection or ablation cannot be executed because of the threat of small functioning liver remnant, inducing hypertrophy in the liver that is to be preserved may be attempted. Hypertrophy is most often induced by percutaneous portal vein embolization to the liver that is to be resected, with operation following at 3 to 4 weeks following embolization (12,13). Patients in whom preoperative portal vein embolization should be considered are listed in Table 32-4. High dose focal liver irradiation also induces hypertrophy in the unirradiated liver. Operative portal vein ligation will also cause hypertrophy in the opposite liver lobe but with more complications relative to percutaneous embolization. Finally, planned two-stage hepatectomy for tumor has been reported as a means of resecting all tumor, and avoids a small functioning remnant liver (14).

COMPLICATIONS OF HEPATIC SURGERY

The complications of hepatic surgery can be variously categorized. For the surgeon they are most usefully divided into intraoperative and postoperative complications.

Intraoperative Complications

Intraoperative complications can be lethal during the operation or in the early, intermediate, or late postoperative periods. Decisions made before and during the operation and the conduct of the operation are significant factors in the incidence and severity of intraoperative and postoperative complications. The major complications occurring during operation are bleeding, vascular injury, air embolus, and biliary injury.

Bleeding

Preexisting Bleeding

Preexisting bleeding associated with liver surgery is generally from blunt or penetrating injury or from rupture of a tumor. Rupture of benign tumor resulting in bleeding is almost exclusively due to hepatic adenoma, with only extremely rare case reports of rupture of hepatic hemangiomas, spontaneously or associated with blunt trauma, or from focal nodular hyperplasia. Rupture of malignant tumor with bleeding is almost always due to hepatocellular carcinoma. Bleeding from liver metastases is vanishingly rare.

The principles and methods for dealing with hepatic bleeding from trauma are not this chapter's topic. The approach is based on classification of the injury and is aimed at control of bleeding. Initial maneuvers are four: (a) packing of the liver with pressure, (b) achieving cardiovascular resuscitation with fluid and blood products, (c) maintaining body temperature, and (d) normalizing coagulation as much as possible. Control of bleeding proceeds from less to more invasive, performing the minimum to achieve bleeding control. Removal of devitalized liver tissue and provision of adequate drainage for bile duct disruption are the other major imperatives in the management of traumatic liver injuries (15).

Operation for bleeding after a percutaneous biopsy should be individualized, based on the indications for the biopsy. Bleeding from liver tissue at the site of needle entry can almost always be stopped with pressure, combined with fulguration, or with horizontal mattress suture of the needle entrance site at the liver capsule. If the bleeding is coming from a hemangioma at the liver's surface, where the needle punctured the tumor, bleeding may be stopped with pressure or with a gently placed horizontal mattress suture around the needle entrance site, but it may occasionally require resection of the tumor by enucleation. Bleeding from other tumors can usually be stopped with pressure, cautery (at high settings), argon plasma coagulation, or suture, and rarely requires resection. However, depending on the surgeon's experience, resection may be the preferred route. In some cases arterial bleeding from within the liver may not readily stop with pressure and can result in intrahepatic hematoma. Packing, closing the abdomen, and emergent angiography with embolization are the preferred steps in such a case.

Frequently, a tumor that ruptures into the peritoneal cavity or produces intracapsular hematoma will stop bleeding spontaneously, and operation can be done on an urgent rather than emergent basis. A history of prolonged oral contraceptive use in a woman is a strong predictor of hepatic adenoma, whereas a history of hepatitis B or C or cirrhosis indicates that hepatocellular cancer is likely to be the cause of bleeding. Abnormal laboratory studies, including hepatitis serologies, liver function studies, and α-fetoprotein suggest cirrhosis and hepatocellular cancer. If the situation allows, liver imaging should be done to delineate the tumor causing the bleeding. CT or MRI should be done with contrast, including arterial phase imaging. Tumors that rupture are usually hypervascular and are best demonstrated by arterial phase imaging. Noncontrast scans and contrast scans in the portal venous phase are likely to be confusing if there is intrahepatic or subcapsular hemorrhage, with difficulty distinguishing between tumor and intrahepatic hematoma. Because the tumor's pathology is not likely to be fully certain at operation, the operative approach should be that for a malignant tumor, with preference to formal resection as opposed to enucleation.

Intraoperative Bleeding

Intraoperative bleeding with liver operations, as with all operations, should be kept to a minimum, and a number of measures can be employed to facilitate minimizing blood loss. The extent of blood transfusion has been correlated with postoperative morbidity and mortality in liver surgery (16). Increasing level of blood transfusion has also been inversely correlated with tumor-free survival after liver resection for malignancy, although studies do not rigorously substantiate this conclusion (16–18).

Perihepatic Bleeding

Blood loss that occurs before transecting the liver can be insidiously large—sometimes the major source of blood loss for the operation. Some of this blood loss is under the surgeon's control, but some perihepatic blood loss is due to disease factors.

Technical Factors

Technical factors leading to perihepatic blood loss in liver surgery are listed in Table 32-5.

Experience, knowledge of the anatomy, and a commitment to limited blood loss are important to minimize loss from these sources. Achieving as much exposure as possible, with an appropriately large incision and appropriate retraction, is also important for minimizing blood loss in this stage of the liver operation. Exposure may be particularly difficult in the deep-chested patient, in patients whose liver lies superior to the costal margin, in patients with large tumors, and in patients with large livers. Usually a bilateral subcostal incision is used for major liver resections (Fig. 32-1). This incision can be extended as far as the right midaxillary line and to the anterior axillary line on the left when necessary. Additional exposure can be gained with a midline subxiphoid extension. Rarely needed, but to be used in difficult circumstances, is extension of the line of

TABLE 32-5
SOURCES OF EXTRAHEPATIC BLOOD LOSS

Liver capsule transgression
Diaphragm injury
Major hepatic vein terminus injury
Vena caval injury
Phrenic vein injury
Short hepatic vein injury
Right adrenal vein injury
Right adrenal gland injury
Portal vein injury
Hepatic artery injury

the left subcostal incision across the right costal margin into the chest, with partial division of the diaphragm.

The usual sources of massive intraoperative bleeding and, occasionally, postoperative bleeding are the hepatic veins and the vena cava. Injuries occur at margins of the liver at the mobilization stage or at the margins of or within the liver during transection or during procedures involving the parenchyma of the liver. Bleeding from these vessels during the mobilization stage is almost always technical and avoidable, except in the reoperative setting, where there may be dense scar adjacent to the major vessels, making the dissection and control extremely difficult. Although these veins are relatively tough, avoidance of excessive traction or torsion on the venous structures is necessary to avoid tearing. Suture ligature, suture closure, or vascular staple closure of medium and large tributaries of the cava are more secure than clips and standard ligatures, which have a tendency to brush or roll off during manipulations of the liver and with traction on the vena cava. If a tear develops in the vena cava, or a clamp slips off a large tributary after its division, finger

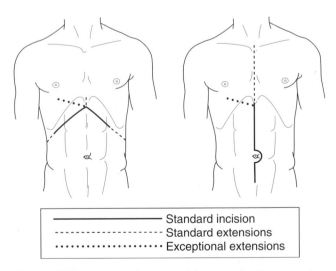

————	Standard incision
- - - - - - - -	Standard extensions
· · · · · · · · ·	Exceptional extensions

Figure 32-1 Incisions for optimal exposure for liver resection. Bilateral subcostal incision is preferred.

occlusion and then serial placement of Babcock or Alice clamps on the vessel across the opening can usually bring a large opening under quick control. The clamps are removed sequentially as the opening is closed with suture.

Portal Hypertension

Some liver operations must be performed in the presence of portal hypertension. The critical areas to be addressed to minimize blood loss are the abdominal wall, intra-abdominal adhesions of the omentum to the abdominal wall and to the area of the liver hilum, the liver hilum and hepatoduodenal ligament, the gastrohepatic ligament, and the retroperitoneum inferior to the liver hilum. Adhesions of omentum to the abdominal wall and to the area of the liver hilum are common routes of portosystemic decompression and are likely to contain large, relatively delicate vessels with blood at pressure above the normal splanchnic venous pressure. These adhesions should be taken down carefully between clamps. Large variceal vessels are often present in the gastrohepatic ligament, which should also be taken down between clamps, remembering to evaluate for the presence of a replaced left hepatic artery crossing the ligament. Large collaterals may be found in the retroperitoneum adjacent or anterior to the infrahepatic vena cava, with the feeding vessels occasionally coming from the liver hilum. Particularly when portal hypertension is associated with portal vein thrombosis there will be large fragile collateral vessels in the hepatoduodenal ligament (representing "recanalization of the portal vein"). Attachments between the diaphragm and the liver are much less likely to have collaterals as a manifestation of portosystemic shunting.

Reoperative Surgery

Reoperative liver surgery is usually associated with increased perihepatic blood loss because of the density of liver adhesions to the diaphragm, retroperitoneum, and right adrenal gland. There is difficulty staying out of the liver and out of the diaphragm and adrenal gland when attempting to dissect those structures one from the other. Judicious use of the cautery and good exposure can minimize blood loss. Special care should be exercised when approaching the liver hilum and the regions of the vena cava and the termini of the hepatic veins.

Hepatic Bleeding

Transection of liver tissue can be associated with significant blood loss. Mortality from intraoperative bleeding continues to be reported, but rarely, although blood loss with major resections often requires one to three transfusions either intraoperatively or postoperatively. In recent series transfusion outliers continue to be to ten units of blood loss or more (3,16).

Control of minor bleeding points on the raw liver surface is best addressed with pressure or cautery during liver transection. Major bleeding points are best controlled with

suture technique. Where there is a side opening in a vessel, such as where a branch has been avulsed, it is preferable to directly close the opening in the vessel with fine suture rather than to include the entire vessel in a mass suture ligature. An end-bleeding vessel that has retracted into the liver parenchyma can be controlled with a figure-8 or horizontal mattress suture into the surrounding parenchyma, tied only tight enough to occlude the vessel. Control of the cut liver edge with large mattress sutures is also a helpful way to control bleeding in situations where those sutures will not occlude important blood inflow, bile drainage, or hepatic venous drainage of the liver remnant and where the sutures are placed relatively close to the liver edge. A similar effect can be achieved using a stapler to divide the liver parenchyma where the liver thickness will accommodate its use (3 cm in normal liver). Because liver bleeding is frequently from low-pressure vessels, control of bleeding with packing is commonly used for brief periods during an operation, but packing can be prolonged for up to 72 hours and can be very useful in the case of an unstable patient or a patient with coagulopathy. Hemostatic agents, such as crystallized collagen or coagulating liquids or sprays, cautery at high settings, and the argon plasma coagulator are all useful methods for dealing with oozing bleeding from the raw liver surface. Sewing omentum or peritoneum over the raw surface has not proven effective in stopping bleeding (19).

Factors that are associated with large operative blood loss are listed in Table 32-6. As many of these factors as possible should be controlled to minimize bleeding. Control of blood loss while transecting the liver can usually be achieved to a remarkable extent. This control involves both liver blood flow control and the use of transection methods that improve exposure of vessels.

Liver Blood Flow Control to Minimize Blood Loss

Inflow occlusion is the primary method by which blood flow control is achieved. There are a variety of methods of performing inflow occlusion. General inflow occlusion is exemplified by the Pringle maneuver, which clamps the

TABLE 32-6

FACTORS IN BLOOD LOSS DURING LIVER TRANSECTION

Unsatisfactory exposure
High central venous pressure
Large tumor
Large liver
Close proximity of tumor to large intrahepatic vessels
Coagulopathy
Inexperienced surgeon
Inexperienced surgical assistants
Improper equipment
Inappropriate operative approach

hepatoduodenal ligament at the foramen of Winslow. More selective means include occlusion of portal flow to a particular portal segment using ultrasound-guided placement of a balloon catheter or dissecting and occluding by ligature or stapling the portal triad to only the particular portion of the liver to be resected. The potential for accessory arterial inflow must be recognized, particularly a replaced or accessory left hepatic artery crossing the gastrohepatic ligament. Because blood loss from the hepatic veins and their tributaries will still occur with inflow occlusion, maintaining a relatively low central venous pressure will help in limiting blood loss during transection (20,21).

Partial vascular exclusion can be performed on a part of the liver and can very effectively limit blood loss, as long as dissection remains within the excluded portion. This method is particularly applicable in the liver with cirrhosis or in other conditions in which the functioning residual liver is small or compromised and when the added insult of warm ischemia could be hazardous. For selective inflow occlusion, facility with intraoperative ultrasound is essential for identifying the appropriate pedicle to be occluded and the position of that pedicle.

Blood loss during liver transection can be nearly completely eliminated by total vascular exclusion, comprising complete inflow and outflow vascular occlusion of the liver. The blood that is lost is only that within vessels in the liver. Total vascular exclusion is accomplished by (a) establishing inflow occlusion, remembering that accessory hepatic arteries may be present; (b) occluding the infrahepatic vena cava; and (c) occluding the suprahepatic vena cava. A method that excludes the right adrenal vein and lumbar veins requires mobilizing the right lobe of the liver, establishing a window posterior to the suprahepatic vena cava, dividing peritoneal attachments between the caudate lobe and the left aspect of the vena cava to mobilize the caudate lobe anteriorly, and then placing an infrahepatic clamp with its tip in the window behind the suprahepatic vena cava. A major consideration with total hepatic vascular exclusion is that cardiac venous return may be compromised, resulting in hypotension when total vascular exclusion is implemented. Hypotension can usually be avoided if the central venous pressure is raised to about 12 mm Hg prior to placing the vena cava clamps. An advantage of this method is that resection or dissection in the liver around the junction of the major hepatic veins can be more safely performed; injuries to those veins can be repaired in a relatively bloodless field. Disadvantages include the need to push up the central venous pressure, the more extensive dissection that must be done to place the clamps, and the possibility that a greater warm ischemic injury may occur to the residual liver segment than would occur with inflow occlusion alone (22).

Liver Transection Methods to Minimize Blood Loss

Early liver surgery made use of the finger-fracture technique, in which the liver parenchyma was crushed between the fingers, leaving behind the more fibrous vessels and bile ducts for control by ligature, clips, staples, or heat coagulation-sealing. Finger-fracture, although still occasionally useful, and the most rapid way of transecting liver short of sharp transection, tends to tear the hepatic venous structures because they contain less connective tissue in the wall. The technique may tear the smaller vascular and biliary structures before they can be controlled and is less effective in livers that have developed fibrosis.

Several methods are commonly in use to transect liver in a way that permits encountered nonparenchymal structures to be controlled. The clamp-crush technique uses an instrument, usually with multiple small teeth—such as a vascular clamp—to crush the parenchyma in small bites. The crushed parenchyma is subsequently washed/aspirated away, and the exposed vascular and biliary structures are ligated. The cavitron ultrasonic aspirator (CUSA) technique uses high-energy ultrasound transmitted to a suction tip through a special handpiece. Hydrodissection uses a fine high-pressure water jet to disrupt the parenchyma. With the CUSA and hydrodissection, the disrupted parenchyma is immediately aspirated through the handpiece, exposing the more fibrous vessels and bile ducts. These latter two techniques are less efficient in fibrotic and cirrhotic livers. Recently, with the development of techniques for laparoscopic liver resection, the harmonic scalpel and linear cutting staplers have shown applicability in selected circumstances (23). These modern techniques are much more effective in maintaining a bloodless field during liver transection compared to finger-fracture. With a bloodless field and exposure of structures, these methods permit recognition of the internal liver anatomy during transection, leading to less chance of misdirection during liver transection.

Mapping of the position of the major vessels within the liver by intraoperative ultrasound can significantly affect blood loss associated with liver transection. Major resections approach the central or right hepatic veins, which, because they are not generally occluded during liver transection, can be a major source of blood loss if injured. Maintaining a centimeter or two distance from these vessels, when possible, avoids avulsion of small and medium-sized tributaries, which tends to occur when the dissection is carried immediately adjacent to these large veins. Ultrasound mapping can direct the desired plane for resection.

Cryoablation

Two sources of intraoperative bleeding that are not common to other liver operations occur with cryoablation. The major source of blood loss as a complication of liver cryoablation is cracking of the liver parenchyma at the margins of the ice-ball as it thaws. Intraparenchymal bleeding adjacent to the thawed ice-ball is not a common problem. If the ice-ball is at the surface of the liver, during the freezing phase, because water expands as it freezes, the capsule or surface will often fracture. When the ice-ball thaws, there is a risk of bleeding at these fractures. The liver can also be avulsed from the ice-ball if care is not taken, resulting in vessel tears. Care in handling the frozen and postfrozen portion of the liver, observation until the surface has thawed before closing the abdomen, and the use of surface-coating hemostatic agents are preventative measures. Treatment for the bleeding includes packing, correction of coagulopathy, procoagulation agents, and judicious suture placement.

The other source of intraoperative bleeding after cryoablation is through the cryoprobe tract after the probe is withdrawn. Two measures prevent bleeding through this tract. The first, and most important, is to avoid placing the initial needle and guidewire for the dilator and sheath through, or in close proximity to, large vessels. The second is to slide the sheath back into the tract over the probe before withdrawing the probe, then to withdraw the probe, and then to pack the tract with small particles of Gelfoam while gradually withdrawing the sheath.

Vascular Injury

Arterial and Portal Venous Injury

A normal liver can survive permanent interruption of arterial inflow if there is normal flow through the portal vein and there is no additional hepatocellular injury due to associated prolonged warm ischemia or decreased splanchnic blood flow secondary to hypotension or due to the use of vasopressors. If the attachments of the liver to the diaphragm and the retroperitoneum remain intact, collateral arterial flow has been demonstrated within 24 hours of ligation of the main arterial inflow. In >85% of instances, either the right or the left hepatic artery can be ligated and there will be establishment of intrahepatic arterial collateral to the dearterialized side immediately or within days (24).

A normal liver can also usually withstand portal vein interruption if arterial flow remains intact and there is no hypotension, decreased splanchnic arterial blood flow, or hepatocellular injury from warm ischemia. However, occlusion of both arterial and venous blood supplies leads to rapid hepatic necrosis and acute liver failure. Already diseased liver may not tolerate decreased blood flow from interruption of either portal or hepatic arterial sources.

Intraoperative complete liver devascularization is a technical issue. Care in dissection in the subhepatic area, continual checking of orientation when dissecting in the area of the liver hilum, and identification of the principal arteries by palpation for pulses in the hepatoduodenal ligament will help prevent hilar vascular injuries. The principles of dissecting the arteries from "large and known to the smaller and nonpalpable" and from anterior inferior left to superior and right will also help to prevent injury to arterial structures. Use of intraoperative ultrasound in the hilum can help define the location of the portal vein in the difficult hilum. The portal vein, in addition, has a very consistent posterior position in the hepatoduodenal ligament, unlike the arteries, which are variable in position and course.

If division of the portal vein or arterial supply, or both, in the hepatoduodenal ligament is discovered intraoperatively, salvage requires immediate revascularization. For the surgeon inexperienced in vascular reconstruction, assistance of a liver transplant surgeon or vascular surgeon should be immediately enlisted. The portal vein should be repaired first, because that repair is done more easily; the portal vein is posterior, and its repair after the arterial repair would put the arterial repair at risk. The portal vein normally supplies more blood to the hepatocytes (60% to 70%) than does the artery. End-to-end repair can often be done, particularly if the duodenum is kocherized, but vein graft may be required. Internal jugular vein, external iliac vein, or spiraled saphenous vein constructed around a mandrel can be used. Externally supported polytetrafluoroethylene (PTFE) graft has been used but is not the first choice. The anastomosis is usually performed with a running fine polypropylene monofilament suture, tied with a slack loop equal to 50% to 100% greater than the diameter of the nondistended portal vein. Arterial repair should be performed with a spatulated repair using fine polypropylene suture. Reversed saphenous vein can be used for graft if necessary. Additional mobility of the proximal artery can be obtained in some cases by dividing the gastroduodenal artery. Ideally, the patient should be heparinized for the repair and started on aspirin intraoperatively or postoperatively.

Injury of the Glisson sheath-encased portal trinity within the liver can occur. Injury at this level is difficult to treat because there is often combined injury to the portal vein, the accompanying artery, and the accompanying bile duct. The most deleterious injury is likely to be the bile duct injury, and its management is outlined below. The best course is usually to suture-repair or ligate the injured vessels and observe briefly to determine how much liver is affected, leaving the bile duct initially unrepaired. If little liver appears devascularized, nothing further need be done with regard to the vessels (although the bile duct injury could still be serious). If a large amount of liver appears devascularized, further attempts should be made to repair the vessels, especially the portal vein. Resection may be advisable, if feasible, based on subsequent residual functioning liver volume. Once a decision had been made with regard to salvage or resection, bile duct repair, by suture or biliary enteric anastomosis, or liver resection should be performed.

When there is irretrievable liver devascularization, the only option may be emergency liver transplant. Bleeding should be controlled as much as possible, and contact with a transplant center and with a liver transplant surgeon at that center should be carried out immediately. Survival for anhepatic patients is usually <24 hours.

Maintenance of venous drainage from the residual liver remnant also demands planning and continued intraoperative attention. Liver tissue without venous drainage will not remain viable. Protection of venous drainage includes evaluation for the course of the major hepatic veins, crossing them with resection only in a planned fashion, evaluation for accessory hepatic veins, which may allow partial lobe resections, and/or taking of a major hepatic vein. In extreme cases vein grafts can be used to replace resected segments of major veins (25). Care for venous drainage must always include not occluding residual hepatic veins with ill-placed sutures into the hepatic parenchyma in an attempt to control bleeding.

Biliary Injury

Extrahepatic Bile Duct Injury

Injury to the extrahepatic bile ducts associated with liver surgery can be irreparable and the etiology of mortality due to acute hepatic failure. The bile ducts, particularly at the hilar plate, are more easily disrupted than the vessels and are usually more difficult to dissect individually at that level. There is some variation in the branching pattern, such that in a small percentage of cases there is a tributary from the right liver draining into the left main duct. Less frequently there may be a tributary from the left liver draining into the right duct (26). Ligation or injury to the remaining bile ducts after a major resection may not always be apparent, so that great care should be exercised in identifying and dissecting the bile ducts at the hilum. With lobectomy or trisegmentectomy, if there is distance between tumor and the hilum it is safer to dissect the bile ducts in a Glissonian fashion—that is, to dissect into the liver substance slightly away from the liver hilum outside the Glisson capsule and to divide the particular duct somewhat away from the actual bile duct bifurcation (27). Even if the vessels are divided at the hilum, division of the bile duct can be delayed until the liver parenchyma is divided at the hilum, when the branching pattern can be demonstrated as the parenchyma is dissected away. This approach is also useful in dissection for hilar cholangiocarcinoma, where later division of the bile duct may allow for more margin on the tumor.

If injury occurs to an extrahepatic bile duct and the injury is minor, such as a tear in the wall less than half the circumference, the injury can be repaired with fine absorbable suture, best done under magnification. If there is major injury, with loss of >50% of the wall, complete division, or loss of length, such injuries should be repaired by anastomosis to a jejunal Roux-en-Y limb, with spatulation of the bile duct to achieve a large circumference anastomosis. Stents are usually not left across the anastomosis, except with very small anastomoses.

Intrahepatic Bile Duct Injury

Operative injury to intrahepatic bile ducts occurs almost exclusively when operation is carried out with disregard for the liver's internal anatomy. The biliary drainage to a segment or segments of liver may be occluded or divided within the liver. With incision into or through the liver, intrahepatic biliary injury will occur if a line of division of the liver crosses the plane of biliary drainage without removing the portion of liver that is served by that biliary drainage. Intrahepatic biliary injury can also occur with placement of probes for cryoablation or radiofrequency ablation, with placement of catheters into the liver for biliary drainage or abscess drainage, or with needle liver biopsy.

If the bile ducts in the isolated segment are completely occluded, and provided that the bile within the isolated segment remains sterile, the result is that the isolated segment of liver will atrophy. However, if the segment of liver associated with an obstructed bile duct is an important component of the functioning liver remnant, the patient may experience postoperative liver failure. If the bile within an isolated bile duct is not sterile, a liver abscess is likely to result. If a bile duct in an isolated segment is not adequately occluded, more so with incision through the liver than with needle or probe bile duct injury, a persistent bile leak from the surface of the liver is likely.

Avoidance of bile duct injury is the best practice and is based on knowledge of liver internal anatomy, demonstrated by intraoperative ultrasound. Successful primary repair of intrahepatic bile ducts may be possible when the ducts are of relatively large caliber (≥3-mm diameter) and the injury does not involve >50% of the circumference of the bile duct. In larger intrahepatic ducts with >50% circumference injury, bile drainage should be established into a Roux-en-Y limb of intestine. Stenting of injured intrahepatic bile ducts may be used to achieve temporary but not permanent drainage.

Air Embolism

Air embolism is a risk during procedures involving division of the hepatic parenchyma. Because of relatively low pressure, with any opening in the hepatic veins there is the risk of air being drawn into the vein and blood flow carrying that air through the right heart and into the pulmonary arteries. The air, if voluminous enough, can cause blockage of pulmonary artery blood flow. More feared is air that crosses an atrial septal defect and passes into the arterial circulation to the coronary arteries or the cerebral circulation, with potentially devastating effects. In practice, the risk of air embolism is not very great during open operations on the liver because patients are maintained on positive pressure ventilation during general anesthesia. The central venous pressure is therefore always greater than zero, and blood exits the openings in the veins rather than air being drawn in. The veins are very thin-walled and collapse to a great degree when central venous pressure drops. Operating in the reverse-Trendelenburg position does decrease central venous pressure, but usually not so far as to result in air embolism. If there is significant blood loss and decreasing central venous pressure, considering moving into a flat position is prudent.

The risk of CO_2 embolus is much more significant with laparoscopic liver surgery because the pressure of the CO_2 within the peritoneal cavity is usually higher than the central venous pressure. Although reports of air embolus occurring with laparoscopic procedures on other organs exist, none exist for laparoscopic liver resection. A single study addressing this issue did not cause any significant or planned openings into a major hepatic vein or the suprahepatic vena cava; so while the complication is possible, its incidence is unknown (28).

Treatment for air embolus intraoperatively includes placement of the patient in Trendelenburg position, aspiration of air through a central line, use of 100% inspired oxygen, restoration of central venous pressure, and closure or occlusion of the opening through which the air entered the circulation. Although recommended with air embolus, turning the patient on the left side is not usually feasible intraoperatively.

Diaphragmatic Injury

Occasionally when resecting liver for tumor, a portion of the diaphragm must be resected. With care, injury to the lung can be avoided, although infrequently the lung is adherent to the process at the diaphragm. If no injury to the lung occurs, there usually is no compromise in respiratory function during the operation. Lung volume can be compromised if large amounts of fluid fill the pleural space, leaving decreased chest volume for lung expansion, or if the opening in the diaphragm is so small that air entering the pleural space is entrapped, causing a tension pneumothorax.

There is usually no problem with leaving the diaphragm open until after the liver resection is completed. The diaphragmatic repair rarely requires prosthetic replacement. The opening should be repaired using two layers of permanent suture, the first with interrupted horizontal mattress technique. Clot and fluid should be evacuated from the pleural space before and during the repair. Usually a chest tube is not required, if residual air is aspirated from the chest cavity with a catheter through the defect while the anesthetist supplies forced inspiration. The catheter is withdrawn on suction as the last mattress suture is tied. A second layer of running suture is then placed.

Postoperative Complications

Liver Failure

Fulminant Hepatic Failure

Fulminant hepatic failure is defined as the development of hepatic encephalopathy within 8 weeks of the patient being healthy. The most common cause of fulminant hepatic failure following liver resection is a small functioning liver remnant. Other etiologies include liver devascularization, interruption of venous drainage from the liver, excessive liver warm ischemia, major bile duct obstruction, halogenated anesthetic agents, viral infections with hepatitis B, and reactions to certain drugs. The hallmark of postoperative liver failure is a persistently rising bilirubin. Coagulopathy usually is a later manifestation of fulminant hepatic failure. Currently there is no treatment for postoperative fulminant liver failure, although bioartificial liver methods have been used in trials as bridges to transplant (29).

Small Functioning Remnant Liver

Acute liver failure following liver surgery is most commonly due to small functioning remnant liver. Small functioning remnant liver encompasses all conditions in which the patient is left with an insufficient amount of satisfactorily functioning liver cell volume, whether from a true small-volume residual with normal liver tissue, due to an intermediate-sized but less well functioning volume of liver, or due to a large volume of poorly functioning liver. The decision about how much liver may be removed when doing liver resection or ablation is based on the anatomic extent of the pathology that is being treated and the associated liver anatomy. A critical determination in the decision to resect or ablate is whether enough functioning hepatocyte volume will remain to permit survival. Liver regeneration can replace the removed liver to a varying extent, depending on the liver's health, but it does not do so instantaneously. In a normal liver full regenerative replacement after a major liver resection occurs in about 6 months. Damaged liver regenerates less rapidly and probably less fully. A guideline has been that in the normal liver, a liver remnant of 25% to 30% of the initial liver volume is compatible with survival; with Child A cirrhosis a liver remnant of 60% to 70% of the initial liver volume is compatible with survival; and with intermediate levels of liver injury, such as with fatty liver, a liver remnant of 50% to 55% of the initial liver volume is compatible with survival.

There have been a number of reports, some prospective, more retrospective, looking at more quantitative ways of predicting how much liver can be taken (or how much must be left behind) when doing liver resection or ablation. Evaluation of liver characteristics such as appearance, density, ultrasound transmission, and fibrous or excessively soft nature of the liver tissue when transecting can assist in assessment of basic liver health. Preoperative or intraoperative biopsy of the portion of the liver that is to be preserved can occasionally help in the decision about how much liver remnant must remain. The surgeon must make the decision in the operating room based on experience and on all the combined factors, including the preoperative planning imaging and function tests.

The amount of residual functioning liver volume is also influenced by technical factors resulting from the operation: injury to the liver by warm ischemia, adequacy of vascular supply to the remaining liver volume, venous drainage from the remaining liver volume, and biliary drainage.

Warm Ischemia

Warm ischemia is associated with injury to liver cells. Warm ischemia causes a postoperative rise in transaminases, which usually peak at about 48 hours; this increase is proportional to the length of the warm ischemia. Most liver surgeons use inflow occlusion to decrease blood loss during resection, and they often use it when doing intraoperative liver ablations. Limiting the duration of each individual event of liver inflow occlusion seems to decrease the postoperative transaminase rise, but this practice demands multiple periods of reperfusion and prolongs the time of transection, and it sometimes increases blood loss. Recently there has been a trend toward "ischemic preconditioning," using an initial 10-minute period of warm ischemia followed by a 10-minute period of reperfusion, after which a continuous longer stretch of warm ischemia seems to cause less liver cell injury than the same duration of warm ischemia without the "ischemic preconditioning" (30). The benefits are greatest in younger patients, for longer duration hepatic inflow occlusions, for resections in which <50% of the liver is resected, and when there is liver steatosis. It has also been reported that warm ischemia is better tolerated with only inflow occlusion as compared to total hepatic vascular exclusion. It is postulated that there is some liver cell perfusion retrograde via the hepatic veins when there is inflow occlusion without outflow occlusion (22).

The tolerated length of warm ischemia is related to the residual functioning liver volume, but few data directly correlate those two parameters. For a right hepatic lobectomy in a normal liver (averaging about 65% resection), warm ischemia is tolerated for 60 minutes without intermittent reperfusion (31). With cirrhosis, warm ischemia can be tolerated up to 30 minutes. However, most liver surgeons who operate frequently on cirrhotic livers maintain inflow occlusion for only 15 to 20 minutes, interspersed with periods of 5 to 10 minutes of reperfusion.

Liver Devascularization

Fulminant hepatic failure will occur rapidly with total devascularization of a normal liver and occurs with less than total devascularization of a cirrhotic or otherwise damaged liver. Intraoperatively recognized devascularization is discussed above. Unrecognized devascularization can occur intraoperatively, and postoperative portal venous or hepatic artery thrombosis can occur due to operative injury or to a hypercoaguable state. Avoidance of devascularization postoperatively includes respectful handling of the hilar blood vessels during operation and investigation of any suspected hypercoaguable states preoperatively so that appropriate postoperative prophylaxis may be implemented. Thrombosis of major hepatic arteries or portal vein postoperatively may be detected by power Doppler ultrasound, arterial and portal venous phase CT, or MRI. With early detection of hepatic artery or portal vein thrombosis and evidence of compromised liver function, treatment

with catheter-directed thrombolysis, operative thrombectomy, and/or vascular repair may be lifesaving (32).

Subacute Liver Failure

Subacute hepatic failure is defined as the onset of hepatic coma at >8 weeks from a healthy state. Etiologies associated with liver operations include small functioning liver remnant, hepatitis B from transfusion or reactivation associated with the operation (33), and partial bile duct obstruction, caused by unrelieved choledocholithiasis, hepatolithiasis, or progressive stricture due to ischemia or thermal injury. Acute postoperative high-grade obstruction of the biliary drainage of the residual liver mass will usually result in rapid liver failure, but ischemic and thermal bile duct injury cause a more gradual onset of jaundice and liver failure. Biliary injury and its consequences will be discussed more fully below.

Chronic Liver Failure

Chronic hepatic failure related to liver operations is very uncommon and results from low-grade biliary obstruction due to injury, untreated stricture, or partially obstructing stones leading to secondary biliary cirrhosis. Where blood is screened, this problem may rarely arise from hepatitis B or C infection.

Biliary Complications

Biloma

An intra-abdominal collection of bile, or biloma, occurs in about 3% of patients after major liver resection, and to a lesser extent after minor liver resection or with drainage of liver abscess (1). Partial excision or enucleation of a biliary cystadenoma also has a moderate risk of biloma. Biloma can be lessened by meticulous detection and closure of all sites of bile drainage on the raw surface of the liver. Placing drains at the time of operation does not lessen bile leak-associated complications, but drainage with a closed system is more likely to convert a biloma to a biliary fistula.

Symptoms and signs of uninfected biloma may be minimal. There may be right upper quadrant or epigastric discomfort and tenderness, rarely a palpable mass, and often a minor rise in serum bilirubin. Diagnosis is by ultrasonography or CT, combined with diagnostic aspiration of bilious fluid. Treatment is tube drainage, which is usually possible percutaneously. Persistent bile drainage indicates a biliary fistula.

Bile Peritonitis

Bile peritonitis results from bile accessing the general peritoneal cavity rather than being walled off into a discrete collection. Bile peritonitis is usually associated with insidious onset of symptoms, including ileus, malaise, abdominal distention, and, eventually, peritoneal signs. The initial peritonitis is chemical, but often bacteria are present and infectious peritonitis subsequently develops. Making the diagnosis of bile peritonitis requires an awareness of the subtlety of initial symptoms and signs and an abdominal ultrasound or CT demonstrating intra-abdominal fluid, confirmed by aspiration of bile. Appropriate placement of closed suction drains following liver operations can usually prevent bile peritonitis. The drains should be left in place for 3 to 4 days to allow any bile leakage to become manifest. Drain fluid should be checked for bilirubin level before retrieving the drain, removing the drain only when the drain fluid bilirubin level is <3 mg per dL with a normal serum bilirubin or when drain fluid bilirubin is similar to serum bilirubin when serum bilirubin is elevated.

Treatment of bile peritonitis requires drainage of the leaking bile. Treatment often also requires decompression of the biliary tree by endobiliary stent or percutaneous transhepatic biliary drain. In cases where the leaking biliary system is not in continuity with the main biliary tree, draining the main bile ducts will not be effective in decreasing the bile leak (see the following section, "Biliary Fistula"). Although drainage of biliary ascites may be possible percutaneously, effective drainage may require laparotomy, evacuation of bile, irrigation of the abdomen, and directed placement of drains.

Biliary Fistula

Postoperative biliary fistula is most frequently a biliary-cutaneous fistula, as represented by bile drainage through an operatively placed drain. A biliary-cutaneous fistula can also occur through a drain site after removal of the drain or through the operative wound or laparoscopic port sites or, occasionally, will erode through the diaphragm into a bronchus or into a gastrointestinal viscus. Such eroding fistulas are almost always associated with infected bile. Persistent biliary fistula is almost always associated with a bile duct that has no free-flowing drainage to the intestine. Such situations include bile drainage from an excluded biliary system (Fig. 32-2) or from a source proximal to an obstructed bile duct. Etiologies of bile duct obstruction include iatrogenic occlusion (clip, ligature, thermal injury), bile duct stone, bile duct hematoma, tumor involving the bile duct or compressing the bile duct, bile duct parasite, inflammatory-associated stenosis, or ischemic or radiation-associated stricture.

Postoperative bile fistula, if confined to a drain, should not be treated by early drain withdrawal (34). The drain should be left in place long enough to allow formation of a fibrous tract around the drain—4 to 6 weeks, or longer if the patient is malnourished or on steroids. If bile leakage continues, the etiology of the drainage is one of the conditions listed above, or the drain may be lying immediately on the leak point, preventing healing. The safest course with persistent bile drainage is to perform a radiocontrast drain injection study, with gravity or very gently injected instillation of contrast to determine: (a) if the drain is

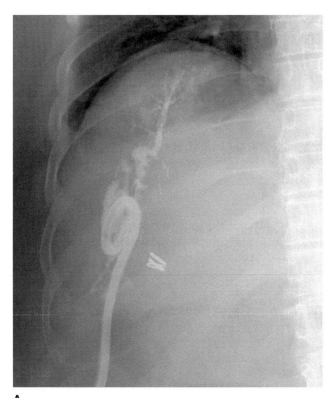 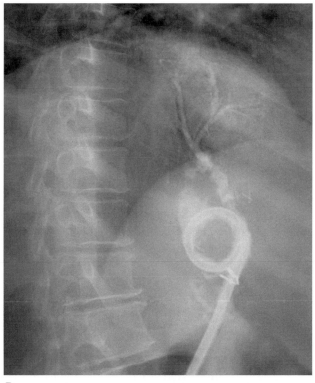

A   **B**

Figure 32-2 Isolated bile duct after nonanatomic liver resection. **A:** anteroposterior view; **B:** lateral view.

immediately against the opening in the biliary tree, (b) if there is an isolated biliary segment, and (c) if there is distal obstruction of the visualized biliary tree. With the first circumstance, withdrawal of the drain beyond the point of contact with the biliary tree will permit scar to close the opening in the biliary tree, and usually the bile leak will resolve, after which the drain can be gradually withdrawn.

When an isolated segment of bile duct is found, the problem is more difficult. By this point the bile may have become contaminated with bacteria. Although withdrawal of the drain after a drain tract has formed may result in closure of the fistula, there is also a chance that fistula will recur or that cholangitis or liver abscess, or both, will result. Measures that have been successful for treatment of the isolated biliary segment include injection with tetracycline or with fibrin glue. In cases in which treatment by these measures fails, reoperation with resection of the isolated biliary segment may be required. If the bile duct draining the isolated segment is large and a 1-cm or larger mucosa-to-mucosa anastomosis can be created, a Roux-en-Y biliary-enteric reconstruction is an option.

When distal obstruction of the biliary tree is responsible for persistent biliary fistula, the focus of treatment should be directed to the distal stricture, the successful treatment of which usually allows resolution of the fistula (35).

If the bile drainage is not through a drain, investigation should begin with CT, looking for parahepatic fluid collection, intrahepatic fluid collection, and biliary tract dilation denoting biliary obstruction. Extrahepatic fluid should be sampled by image-guided needle aspiration and drained if purulent or bilious. The treatment of the drain is then as outlined above. If there is evidence of distal biliary obstruction, further evaluation with magnetic resonance cholangiopancreatography (MRCP), percutaneous transhepatic cholangiography, or endoscopic retrograde cholangiography is indicated. Percutaneous or endobiliary stent placement might be indicated for temporary relief of the obstruction to promote resolution of the fistula.

Biliary Stricture or Obstruction

Biliary stricture following operation or surgical intervention may result from mechanical injury by a scalpel, biopsy needle, ablation probe, or drainage catheter; from thermal injury with cautery, laser, radiofrequency ablation, cryoablation, or laser probe ablation; from ischemia due to devascularization of the bile duct (Fig. 32-3); or from chemical injury with hypertonic saline or formalin or other chemical scolicidal solution in the treatment of echinococcal cyst. Avoidance of bile duct stricture should always be the goal because treatment may be very complicated and is never uniformly successful, and the potential complications associated with bile duct stricture can be devastating. The first and major step in avoidance of bile duct strictures is recognition of the variety of mechanisms that can cause these problems and care in the use of such modalities. Although the normal intrahepatic bile duct is usually not

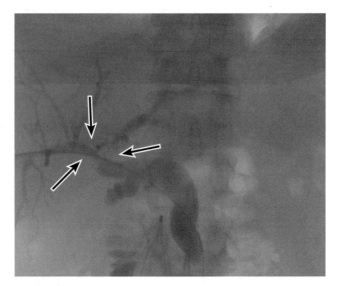

Figure 32-3 Ischemic bile duct injury after ligation of hepatic arterial blood supply. The arrows outline the area of ischemic stricture.

visible with the intraoperative ultrasound, the portal vein that accompanies it is visible, and approach to the portal vein branch is approach to the bile duct.

The results of bile duct stricture are varied and depend on whether there is complete or partial obstruction and on the proportion of liver that is involved. High-grade stricture obstructing bile egress from the entire liver is associated with jaundice and, if unalleviated, liver failure. In situations in which the bile is sterile and the liver parenchyma is relatively normal, high-grade stricture of bile ducts proximal to the main bile duct may prove innocuous. The liver subserved by the obstructed bile duct will atrophy, and the liver with normal bile duct drainage will hypertrophy. If the portion of liver subserved by the obstructed bile duct is small, the damage in the sterile situation is likely to be insignificant. Even with up to 50% of the liver substance obstructed, in the absence of infection, early symptoms or signs are unlikely. Intrahepatic stone formation is unlikely, because at a pressure of 40 mm Hg bile formation in the associated hepatocytes stops and the components necessary to form stones are absent. Although serum alkaline phosphatase will be elevated in such a situation, the bilirubin will often rise only mildly. The two potential complications are (a) infection of the bile in the obstructed biliary tree, with resulting cholangitis or liver abscess, or both, and (b) increased risk of cholangiocarcinoma associated with chronically obstructed bile ducts.

Less than high-grade obstruction is more likely to be associated with intrahepatic duct stone formation. Whether there is an increased risk of cholangitis with intrahepatic duct stone formation is unknown. Intrahepatic bile duct stone formation is likely to worsen the effects of a low-grade stricture, potentially converting it to the equivalent of a high-grade stricture.

Low-grade stricture of the main bile duct or of the drainage to many portions of the liver is likely to result in secondary biliary cirrhosis. The progress to secondary biliary cirrhosis may be occult, the risk of the occurrence denoted only by an elevated alkaline phosphatase. Liver biopsy may be the only method to determine whether cirrhosis has developed. Because the occurrence of secondary biliary cirrhosis is variable, persistently elevated alkaline phosphatase should prompt investigation by imaging studies looking for intrahepatic bile duct dilation.

Early treatment of bile duct stricture is important before atrophy or secondary biliary cirrhosis occurs and consists of reestablishment of free, low-pressure drainage from the affected bile ducts. Such drainage, to be effective long-term, uniformly requires biliary-enteric reconstruction, with a mucosa-to-mucosa large diameter anastomosis >1 cm. Intrahepatic bile duct stones should be removed, even with great effort, because their presence, in addition to serving as an obstruction to bile flow, can cause injury to the mucosa of the bile duct, leading to further stricture. The presence of stones combined with a biliary-enteric anastomosis is associated with a high incidence of cholangitis.

Other treatments for stricture are temporary, and include plastic external, internal, or internal/external drains/stents. Stents have a limited lifetime (usually <16 weeks) because of buildup of bile salts and proteinaceous material on the plastic with occlusion and reobstruction and/or cholangitis. Internal expandable metal stents have a longer lifetime, but have a maximal useful effectiveness with benign strictures of about 5 years (36) and cannot be changed. For strictures that cannot be adequately treated with biliary-enteric anastomosis, consideration should be given to resection of the affected portion of the liver, if an adequate liver remnant can be left. Such a resection avoids the risk of recurrent cholangitis and liver abscess and the more distant risk of cholangiocarcinoma. Unfortunately, in some circumstances, satisfactory treatment of extensive bile duct strictures is not possible and liver transplantation is the only remaining option.

Hemobilia

Hemobilia, bleeding into the bile ducts, can occur after liver resection from direct trauma, such as with core needle biopsy during a procedure on the liver, abscess eroding into both bile duct and adjacent vessel, communication of bile duct and vessel within a postoperative hematoma, arterial pseudoaneurysm rupturing into a bile duct, or injury to both bile duct and a vessel due to radiofrequency ablation, cryoablation, or laser ablation of a liver lesion. Etiologies also include bleeding from tumor within bile ducts, such as hepatocellular carcinoma or bile duct malignancies.

Manifestations are most commonly right upper quadrant pain, jaundice, and hematemesis, but they also include occult unexplained blood loss, melena or hematochezia, hyperbilirubinemia, and acute pancreatitis. With significant hemobilia, the feeding vessel is more often an artery than a portal vein branch or a hepatic vein branch. Arterial pressure is more likely to cause continued bleeding despite increased biliary pressures associated with the formation of clot in the bile ducts.

Diagnosis is made by a combination of studies in correlation with symptoms: finding blood in the stool or hematemesis, without a lesion to explain the bleeding in the gastrointestinal tract on endoscopy; by observing blood coming from the papilla of Vater on upper endoscopy; by biliary dilation on ultrasound or CT with high-density material within the bile ducts; by demonstration of irregular filling defects in the bile ducts on cholangiography; with demonstration of entry of contrast into a vessel on cholangiography; and by demonstration of hepatic artery pseudoaneurysm or contrast entering the biliary tree on visceral angiography. Resolution is often spontaneous. Treatment of persistent or massive hemobilia by hepatic artery embolization is effective. Quite infrequently, hepatic artery ligation or hepatic resection of the affected area of liver is required.

Infection

Cholangitis

Cholangitis is an infrequent early complication of liver resection. If there is no free bile drainage postoperatively after liver surgery and if the biliary tree has been seeded with organisms, cholangitis is likely to occur. Appropriate antibiotics should be administered postoperatively for 5 to 10 days when there is an established preoperative infection. Most critical in treating and avoiding cholangitis is the intraoperative establishment and postoperative maintenance of adequate biliary drainage. At operation that goal includes assessment of biliary drainage, removal of obstructing debris such as stones, and constructing a generous anastomosis whenever possible. Treatment of early postoperative cholangitis is with antibiotics and institution of free biliary drainage.

Cholangitis may occur at months to years after liver surgery, usually resulting from restricted drainage of contaminated bile. Table 32-7 lists the most common etiologies.

TABLE 32-7

ETIOLOGIES OF CHOLANGITIS AFTER LIVER SURGERY

Common bile duct stones
Benign biliary stricture
Malignant biliary stricture
Biliary-enteric anastomotic stricture
Biliary-enteric stent
Percutaneous transhepatic biliary drain
Percutaneous transhepatic cholangiography
Endoscopic retrograde cholangiography
Biliary-enteric fistula
Common bile duct parasites
Recurrent pyogenic cholangitis

Investigation should include determination of serum alkaline phosphatase levels. Evaluation also requires imaging—first, of the biliary tree to assess for site(s) of stricture and for the presence of biliary stones; second, of the surrounding structures to detect extrinsic tissue causing biliary obstruction, such as intrahepatic or extrahepatic tumor, lymphadenopathy, pseudocyst, or abscess; and, third, of the liver to survey for hepatic abscess and for partial liver atrophy. Ultrasonography should serve as an initial screen. If cholangitis is suspected, CT or MRI/MRCP should be performed.

Treatment implements biliary drainage. The long-term solution is to obtain adequate and permanent biliary drainage. Because of the variety of etiologies, there is no single solution. Occasionally, symptoms and signs of cholangitis will occur in some individuals without evidence of inadequate biliary drainage. In these individuals supportive treatment is all that can be offered, but reevaluation should be carried out at intervals if symptoms and signs continue.

Intrahepatic Abscess

Intrahepatic abscess may result as a complication of liver surgery when there is cholangitis, when there is focal bile duct obstruction with the obstructed bile duct becoming secondarily infected, or when an intrahepatic hematoma becomes secondarily infected. If limited in number and >2 to 3 cm in size, hepatic abscesses may be drained percutaneously and treated with antibiotics. Smaller abscesses will often resolve with antibiotic treatment alone. Investigation for obstructed bile ducts should be undertaken whenever hepatic abscess occurs, but treatment should not await this evaluation. When there is no resolution of the abscess or there is occurrence of additional abscesses, reevaluation should be considered. Occasionally, ultrasound-guided operative drainage is required.

Parahepatic Abscess

Parahepatic abscess occurs postoperatively in about 7% of patients after liver resection (1). The usual associated factors are infected biloma or infected hematoma. Meticulous hemostasis, closure of any sites of bile leakage, and avoidance of postoperative coagulopathy are the primary means of preventing parahepatic abscess. Placement of closed suction drains, maintained for only a limited time postoperatively, may decrease the incidence of infected biloma as the source of parahepatic abscess. Treatment of parahepatic abscess is drainage and antibiotics, similar to the treatment of other postoperative intra-abdominal abscesses.

Renal Failure

Renal failure as a complication of liver surgery may have a number of etiologies, including hypotension due to blood loss or sepsis, toxic injury from nephrotoxic drugs, inadequate fluid administration or excessive fluid loss with diuretic use, or, uncommonly, hepatorenal syndrome in patients with cirrhosis or liver failure. Characteristic of the hepatorenal syndrome are a urine sodium concentration of <10 mEq per L, high urine osmolality, and high urine-to-plasma ratios of creatinine. The diagnosis and treatment of the common causes of renal failure are those employed in the postoperative setting and are not unique to liver surgery. Hepatorenal syndrome has no well-established mechanism, although elevation of various cytokines, including endothelin-1, and decreases in certain prostaglandins have been implicated. Hepatorenal syndrome is invariably lethal after liver surgery unless treated by liver transplantation.

GI Bleeding

Gastrointestinal bleeding after liver surgery in the noncirrhotic patient occurs in 1% to 2% of patients (1) and is predominantly due to gastric erosions or ulceration associated with postoperative sepsis. Stress ulceration can largely be avoided with agents that maintain the postoperative gastric pH >5, such as H_2-blockers or proton pump inhibitors. Other etiologies include postoperative coagulopathy and hemobilia. In patients with cirrhosis with portal hypertension, bleeding may also occur from esophagogastric varices or from portal gastropathy.

Ascites

Ascites is not uncommon following major liver resection (>50% of the preoperative functional liver volume resected) in patients without cirrhosis and with any operation in patients with cirrhosis. Factors in the formation of ascites include a decrease in serum colloid osmotic pressure and an increase in portal venous pressure. Serum albumin, the major determinant of serum colloid osmotic pressure, is usually severely depressed after major liver resection—to as low as 1.6 g per dL, with recovery over several weeks to months. With liver resection of >30%, there is an increase in portal venous pressure (37,38).

Complications of ascites include ascitic leak from incisions. Pressure phenomena may occur, including abdominal pain due to the distention, early satiety and vomiting due to compression of the stomach and intestines, and abdominal compartment syndrome. Infected ascites, secondary to contamination through drain tracts, incisions, or from paracenteses, may also occur.

In patients with cirrhosis and in those with major liver resection, immediate postoperative treatment with spironolactone and avoidance of high postoperative central venous pressure (which is a partial determinant of portal venous pressure) may help to decrease the rate of formation of ascites. Infusion of albumin to increase colloid osmotic pressure, combined with use of loop diuretics shortly thereafter, may help to decrease ascites, although mobilization of ascites is notoriously difficult. Development of abdominal compartment syndrome due to ascites requires immediate large-volume paracentesis. Drains in patients with ascites should be avoided and, if placed, should be removed early and the tract closed to prevent ascitic leak. Drains in the presence of ascites and leaks have a high association with infection. Paracentesis, when necessary, should be image-guided to prevent injury to intestine and subsequent infection of ascites. Rarely, peritoneovenous shunt or transjugular intrahepatic portosystemic shunt (TIPS) may be required to treat intractable ascites. Although TIPS may be applicable after a minor liver resection in a patient with cirrhosis, TIPS may lead to liver failure following a major liver resection because of diversion of blood flow from the liver remnant.

SUMMARY

Liver surgery and procedures can be done safely at institutions where high volumes of such surgery are performed. Safety involves experience with patient evaluation, selection for procedures, performance of the operations and procedures, and periprocedure care. Safety also involves recognition of possible complications associated with procedures, avoidance whenever possible, and expeditious treatment of complications when they occur.

REFERENCES

1. Jarnagin WR, Gonen M, Fong Y, et al. Improvement in perioperative outcome after hepatic resection. *Ann Surg* 2002;236:397–407.
2. Gagner M, Franco D, Vons C, et al. Analysis of morbidity and mortality rates in right hepatectomy with the preoperative APACHE II score. *Surgery* 1991;110:487–492.
3. Belghiti J, Hiramatsu K, Benoist S, et al. Seven hundred forty-seven hepatectomies in the 1990s: an update to evaluate the actual risk of liver resection. *J Am Coll Surg* 2000;191:38–46.
4. Hashimoto M, Watanabe G. Hepatic parenchymal cell volume and the indocyanine green tolerance test. *J Surg Res* 2000;92:222–227.
5. Wakbayashi H, Ishimura K, Izuishi K, et al. Evaluation of liver function for hepatic resection for hepatocellular carcinoma in the liver with damaged parenchyma. *J Surg Res* 2004;116:248–252.
6. Hemming AL, Ballinger S, Greig PD, et al. The hippurate ratio as an indicator of functional hepatic reserve for resection of hepatocellular carcinoma in cirrhotic patients. *J Gastrointest Surg* 2001;5:316–321.
7. Selzner M, Clavien PA. Fatty liver in liver transplantation and surgery. *Semin Liver Dis* 2001;21:105–113.
8. Clavien PA, Emond J, Vauthey JN, et al. Protection of the liver during hepatic surgery. *J Gastrointest Surg* 2004;8:313–327.
9. Shoup M, Gonen M, D'Angelica M, et al. Volumetric analysis predicts hepatic dysfunction in patients undergoing major liver resection. *J Gastrointest Surg* 2003;7:325–330.
10. Abdalla EK, Denys A, Chevalier P, et al. Total and segmental liver volume variations: implications for liver surgery. *Surgery* 2004;135:414–420.
11. Vauthey JN, Chaoui A, Do KA, et al. Standardized measurement of the future liver remnant prior to extended liver resection: methodology and clinical associations. *Surgery* 2000;127:512–519.
12. Azoulay D, Castaing D, Smail A, et al. Resection of nonresectable liver metastases from colorectal cancer after percutaneous portal vein embolization. *Ann Surg* 2000;231:480–486.
13. Wakabayashi H, Ishimura K, Okano K, et al. Application of preoperative portal vein embolization before major hepatic resection in patients with normal or abnormal liver parenchyma. *Surgery* 2002;131:26–33.
14. Adam R, Laurent A, Azoulay D, et al. Two-stage hepatectomy: a planned strategy to treat irresectable liver tumors. *Ann Surg* 2000;232:777–785.
15. Wisner DH, Hoyt DB. Trauma. Definitive care phase: abdominal trauma. In: Greenfield LJ, ed. *Surgery: scientific principles and practice*, 3rd ed. Philadelphia, PA: Lippincott Williams & Wilkins; 2001:334–353.
16. Kooby DA, Stockman J, Ben-Porat L, et al. Influence of transfusions on perioperative and long-term outcome in patients following hepatic resection for colorectal metastases. *Ann Surg* 2003;237:860–870.
17. Yamamoto J, Kosuge T, Takayama T, et al. Perioperative blood transfusion promotes recurrence of hepatocellular carcinoma after hepatectomy. *Surgery* 1994;115:303–309.
18. Stephenson KR, Steinberg SM, Hughes KS, et al. Perioperative blood transfusions are associated with decreased time to recurrence and decreased survival after resection of colorectal liver metastases. *Ann Surg* 1988;208:679–687.
19. Paquet JC, Dziri C, Hay JM, et al. Prevention of deep abdominal complications with omentoplasty on the raw surface after hepatic resection. *Am J Surg* 2000;179:103–109.
20. Chen H, Merchant NB, Didolkar MS. Hepatic resection using intermittent vascular inflow occlusion and low central venous pressure anesthesia improves morbidity and mortality. *J Gastrointest Surg* 2000;4:162–167.
21. Smyrniotis V, Kostopanagiotou G, Theodoraki K, et al. The role of central venous pressure and type of vascular control in blood loss during major liver resections. *Am J Surg* 2004;187:398–402.
22. Sato T, Kurokawa T, Kusano T, et al. Uptake of indocyanine green by hepatocytes under inflow occlusion of the liver. *J Surg Res* 2002;105:81–85.
23. Kaneko H, Otsuka Y, Takagi S, et al. Hepatic resection using stapling devices. *Am J Surg* 2004;187:280–284.
24. Cohan AM, Higgins J, Waltman AC, et al. Effect of ligation of variant hepatic arterial structures on the completeness of regional chemotherapy infusion. *Am J Surg* 1987;153:378–380.
25. Sano K, Makuuchi M, Miki K, et al. Evaluation of hepatic venous congestion: proposed indication criteria for hepatic vein reconstruction. *Ann Surg* 2002;236:241–247.
26. Le Foie CC. *Etudes anatomiques et chirurgicales*. New York: Masson Publishing; 1957.
27. Figueras J, Lopez-Ben S, Llado L, et al. Hilar dissection versus the "Glissonean" approach and stapling of the pedicle for major hepatectomies: a prospective, randomized trial. *Ann Surg* 2003;238:111–119.
28. Ricciardi R, Anwaruddin S, Schaffer BK, et al. Elevated intrahepatic pressures and decreased hepatic tissue blood flow prevent gas embolus during limited laparoscopic liver resions. *Surg Endosc* 2001;15:729–733.
29. Demetriou AA, Brown RS, Busuttil RW, et al. Prospective, randomized, multicenter, controlled trial of a bioartificial liver in treating acute liver failure. *Ann Surg* 2004;239:660–670.
30. Clavien PA, Selzner M, Rudiger HA, et al. A prospective randomized study in 100 consecutive patients undergoing major liver resection with versus without ischemic preconditioning. *Ann Surg* 2003;238:843–852.
31. Elias D, Lasser P, Debaene B, et al. Intermittent vascular exclusion of the liver (without vena cava clamping) during major hepatectomy. *Br J Surg* 1995;82:1535–1539.
32. Stange BJ, Glanemann M, Nuessler NC, et al. Hepatic artery thrombosis after adult liver transplantation. *Liver Transpl* 2003;9:612–620.

33. Kubo S, Nishiguchi S, Hamba H, et al. Reactivation of viral replication after liver resection in patients infected with hepatitis B virus. *Ann Surg* 2001;233:139–145.

34. Reed DN, Vitale GC, Wrightson WR, et al. Decreasing mortality of bile leaks after elective hepatic surgery. *Am J Surg* 2003; 185:316–318.

35. Bhattacharjya S, Puleston J, Davidson BR, et al. Outcome of early endoscopic biliary drainage in the management of bile leaks after hepatic resection. *Gastrointest Endosc* 2003;57:526–530.

36. Dumonceau JM, Deviere J, Delhaye M, et al. Plastic and metal stents for postoperative benign bile duct strictures: the best and the worst. *Gastrointest Endosc* 1998;47:8–17.

37. Nagasue N, Yukaya H, Ogawa Y, et al. Portal pressure following partial to extensive hepatic resection in patients with and without cirrhosis of the liver. *Ann Chir Gynaecol* 1983;72(1): 18–22.

38. Kanematsu T, Takenaka K, Furuta T, et al. Acute portal hypertension associated with liver resection. Analysis of early postoperative death. *Arch Surg* 1985;120(11):1303–1305.

Complications of Biliary Surgery

33

Lisa M. Colletti

■ **INTRODUCTION 423**

■ **COMPLICATIONS OF CHOLECYSTECTOMY 423**
Mechanism of Bile Duct Injury 424
Risk Factors for Biliary Injury 425
Classification of Biliary Injuries 426
Clinical Presentation of Biliary Injuries 427
Diagnosis of Postoperative Biliary Injuries 428
Management of Biliary Injuries 429
Repair of Bismuth-Strasberg A–E Injuries 435
Long-term Results 440
Unsuspected Gallbladder Cancer 443

■ **COMPLICATIONS OF BILIARY STONE DISEASE 445**
Surgical Treatment of Common Bile Duct Stones 448
Choledochoduodenostomy and
    Choledochojejunostomy 448

■ **COMPLICATIONS OF BILE DUCT RESECTION 450**
Complications of Biliary Resection 450
Primary Sclerosing Cholangitis 453

■ **REFERENCES 458**

INTRODUCTION

Most complications following surgical procedures on the biliary system are related to iatrogenic injury. They include

Lisa M. Colletti: University of Michigan, Ann Arbor, MI 48109

bile leak, bile duct obstruction or stricture, and infection. The most common biliary operation is cholecystectomy, now usually performed laparoscopically. Other surgical procedures on the biliary tree include those performed for the treatment of retained or recurrent common bile duct stones or benign or malignant biliary strictures.

COMPLICATIONS OF CHOLECYSTECTOMY

Symptomatic gallstones are a common clinical problem. In the Western world the prevalence of gallstone is 5% to 22% and increases with age (1,2). Ten percent to 40% of gallstones are symptomatic, and over 500,000 cholecystectomies are performed in the United States each year. One percent to 2% of cholecystectomies are for acalculous cholecystitis.

Presentations of gallstones include biliary colic, acute cholecystitis, chronic cholecystitis, biliary pancreatitis, and choledocholithiasis. Biliary dyskinesia may also be an indication for cholecystectomy, as is carcinoma of the gallbladder, usually in combination with a portal lymphadenectomy and hepatic resection of segments IVb and V.

Complications of laparoscopic and open cholecystectomy can be classified as major, typically involving injury to the common bile duct or common hepatic duct, or minor, usually evidenced as a bile leak with ensuing bile peritonitis or biloma. Nonspecific complications related to laparoscopy, such as injury to intra-abdominal structures during port placement or deep venous thrombosis due to venous stasis from the pneumoperitoneum-induced increases in intra-abdominal pressure, will not be considered in this chapter.

Compared to open cholecystectomy, laparoscopic cholecystectomy is associated with less postoperative pain, shorter hospital stay, earlier return to work, and better cosmetic outcome (3). Laparoscopic cholecystectomy has been used for the treatment of complicated gallstone disease, such as acute cholecystitis and gallstone pancreatitis, and has become the standard management for biliary colic. Safety and efficacy have been demonstrated in high-risk patients, such as the elderly and pregnant women (4,5).

Laparoscopic cholecystectomy is associated with a higher incidence of biliary injuries relative to the open procedure. Roslyn et al. reported the results of over 42,000 open cholecystectomies performed in the United States in 1989; the incidence of biliary injury in this series was 0.2% (6). In a similar study performed in 1980, the incidence of major bile duct injury after open cholecystectomy was 0.3% (7). In recent studies the rate of biliary injury with laparoscopic cholecystectomy was 0.5% to 0.9%. This incidence has not improved despite the fact that most surgeons are now past the "learning curve" (8,9). In a large study by Adamsen et al., 7,654 patients undergoing laparoscopic cholecystectomy between 1991 and 1994 were reviewed (10). Fifty-seven cases of major bile duct injury were noted (0.74%). One hundred and thirty-two patients (2.1%) had postoperative bile leaks without major bile duct injury. Of these leaks, 71% were cystic duct leaks, 17% were leaks from the gallbladder bed, and 11% were from an unidentified source. Most large studies now suggest that the incidence of major bile duct injury after open cholecystectomy is 0.1% to 0.2%, compared to 0.5% to 0.8% after laparoscopic cholecystectomy (11–13). A review of recent literature pertaining to laparoscopic cholecystectomy concluded that bile duct injury during this procedure occurs 2.5 to 4 times more frequently than with the open technique (7).

Mechanism of Bile Duct Injury

The mechanism of biliary injury during laparoscopic cholecystectomy is well-described (13,14). Misidentification of anatomy is the root cause. The most common scenario was initially described by Davidoff et al. as the "classic" injury (14). In this case the common bile duct is mistaken as the cystic duct. The common bile duct is clipped and divided. Further traction on the gallbladder leads to a second, higher injury with division of the common hepatic duct, often near the bifurcation. This second division of the duct is often described in the operative note as a second cystic duct or an accessory duct. In some cases the right hepatic artery is also injured during this process.

If the proximal hepatic duct is not occluded during this dissection, a bile leak will develop and the patient will present early in the postoperative period with biliary ascites or bile peritonitis. Complete transection of the biliary tree removes any possibility of nonoperative management with endoscopic or radiologic techniques and mandates surgical reconstruction of the biliary tree. In one series this particular complication was reported in 24 of 38 patients (63%) presenting with a biliary injury following laparoscopic cholecystectomy (15).

Other less common mechanisms of injury include "tenting," in which the common bile duct is pulled laterally while the cystic duct is being clipped and is inadvertently caught in the clip, narrowing the common bile duct; thermal injuries due to inappropriate use of cautery; excessive application of clips to control bleeding in the triangle of Calot; and injury to an aberrant or low-inserting right hepatic duct (15) (Table 33-1).

Two methods have been described for accurate cystic duct identification (13). The first, or "infundibular," method, involves dissection of the cystic duct along its anterior and posterior aspects in the triangle of Calot. Confirmation of the anatomy is noted by seeing a "flair" as the cystic duct widens to become the infundibulum of the gallbladder neck. Unfortunately, in one study of 27 common bile duct injuries, the infundibular technique was used in 80% of the cases (16). In acute cholecystitis the cystic duct is often hidden behind an inflamed gallbladder neck. Other factors that may contribute to a hidden cystic duct include large impacted stones, a short or absent cystic duct, and adhesions between the gallbladder neck and the common duct, such that the cystic duct is obscured.

An alternative way to correctly identify the cystic duct is the "critical view" technique (7,13,16). In this method, the triangle of Calot is completely cleared of fibrous and fatty tissues, so that only the cystic duct and artery are visible. After this dissection, the base of segment IV of the liver is visible. If this view is not achieved, the dissection is stopped and a cholangiogram is obtained to define the anatomy or the procedure is converted to open.

Bile duct injury during laparoscopic cholecystectomy is best avoided if the surgeon maintains a low threshold for conversion to an open technique in any case where the anatomy cannot be precisely identified (8). Postoperative

---

TABLE 33-1

MECHANISMS OF BILIARY INJURY DURING LAPAROSCOPIC CHOLECYSTECTOMY

Misidentification of anatomic structures
- Common bile duct misidentified as the cystic duct
- Aberrant right hepatic duct mistaken for the cystic duct

Technical mechanisms
- Inadequately occluded cystic duct
- Use of cautery too close to portal structures
- Tenting of cystic duct during dissection and/or application of clips
- Overuse of clips to control bleeding
- Improper or overrigorous portal dissection

recognition of a biliary injury contributes to increased morbidity due to the development of bile peritonitis and associated increase in scarring around the porta hepatis. Richardson et al. reported a higher incidence of intraoperative identification of biliary injuries relative to prior studies and suggested that earlier recognition and repair resulted in improved outcome (11). The earlier identification in this study was related to a high overall conversion to an open procedure (13.9%) and the selective use of intraoperative cholangiography (8.8% of procedures) (11).

Risk Factors for Biliary Injury

Surgeon Skill and Experience

Early studies suggested that there is a "learning curve" for laparoscopic cholecystectomy and that complication rates would decrease over time. Unfortunately, the complication rate has not declined to the extent that was initially expected (7). More recent studies have suggested that surgeons trained in laparoscopic cholecystectomy during residency have lower complication rates because they are not "at risk" during their learning curve period (17).

Local Operative Risk Factors

Increased frequency of injury with laparoscopic cholecystectomy has been noted with more difficult procedures (7). Acute inflammation, chronic inflammation with dense scarring, bleeding that obscures the operative field, and significant amounts of periportal fat have all been noted to contribute to the occurrence of injury. An increased frequency of biliary injury in association with laparoscopic cholecystectomy for acute cholecystitis has been noted in several series (7). Laparoscopic procedures are more likely to be difficult because of scarring or inflammation when the patient is male, elderly, or has had repeated attacks of pain. These factors are additive. A prior attack of acute cholecystitis also increases risk (18).

Aberrant Anatomy

Anatomic variation is common and is a well-recognized risk of biliary surgery. The biliary anomaly that is most likely to be involved in a ductal injury during laparoscopic cholecystectomy is an aberrant right hepatic duct (7). Many guidelines have been suggested to avoid ductal injuries, including recommendations on the direction of traction on the gallbladder, use of intraoperative cholangiography, and the need to identify (or not identify) the cystic duct-common bile duct junction (7). The key is to conclusively identify the cystic structures before clipping and dividing them; since these are the only structures that are to be divided, they are the only structures that need to be conclusively identified.

Routine Cholangiography

The usual indication for intraoperative cholangiography is identification of stones within the biliary tree (Table 33-2). Routine cholangiography has also been recommended to avoid ductal injury (7,19,20). In a recent retrospective nationwide cohort analysis of Medicare patients, the risk of biliary injury was significantly increased if intraoperative cholangiography was not used (19). After controlling for patient-related and surgeon-related factors, the risk of common bile duct injury was 71% higher when cholangiography was not performed (19). Other studies have suggested that the use of intraoperative cholangiography, although not preventing bile duct injury, results in earlier injury identification and therefore limits morbidity (11,17,21–24). However, other studies suggest that routine intraoperative cholangiography does not prevent biliary injury, nor does it result in earlier identification (25). These studies illustrate that abnormal cholangiograms in the setting of a biliary injury may be misinterpreted (7). A recent study of 2,043 laparoscopic cholecystectomies advocated the use of selective cholangiography and suggested that the cost and morbidity associated with the use of routine intraoperative cholangiography could not be justified (18).

Despite recent reports that the routine use of cholangiography decreases the incidence of biliary injury (19,20,26,27), many surgeons believe that routine cholangiography is time-consuming, expensive, and unnecessary for the detection of asymptomatic choledocholithiasis (28). In fact, one group reported a 0.4% incidence of bile duct injury attributable to intraoperative cholangiography (29). If one excludes the possible prevention or detection of low-frequency events such as bile duct injury, then selective use of intraoperative cholangiography is more cost-effective (28).

TABLE 33-2

INDICATIONS FOR SELECTIVE OPERATIVE CHOLANGIOGRAPHY

Preoperative Indications
- Recent history of acute biliary pancreatitis
- Recent history of jaundice
- Recent history of cholangitis
- Abnormal preoperative ultrasound demonstrating a dilated common bile duct or a defect (stone) in the common bile duct
- Evidence of common bile duct obstruction on HIDA scan
- Increased serum bilirubin
- Increased serum alkaline phosphatase
- Increased serum amylase

Intraoperative Indications
- Dilated extrahepatic bile ducts
- Unusual anatomy or inability to discern anatomy
- Concern or suspicion of bile duct injury

Intraoperative cholangiograms may be misinterpreted. The usual misinterpretation is due to visualization of only the extrahepatic biliary tree, without filling the intrahepatic portions. In many of these cases the proximal extrahepatic biliary tree has been clipped, therefore preventing flow of contrast into the liver. Failure to visualize the intrahepatic ducts must be interpreted as abnormal until proven otherwise. This finding is an indication to convert to an open procedure.

A potential alternative to intraoperative cholangiography is intraoperative ultrasonography. This technique offers the advantages of cholangiography but is noninvasive, repeatable, fast, and inexpensive. A recent study comparing intraoperative cholangiography to intraoperative ultrasonography indicated that intraoperative ultrasonography was associated with significantly fewer common bile duct injuries and postoperative bile leaks and was a superior technique for detection of common bile duct stones (30).

Classification of Biliary Injuries

Major bile duct injuries during laparoscopic cholecystectomy tend to occur higher in the liver hilum and are more complex than those associated with open cholecystectomy. The Bismuth-Strasberg classification of these injuries has been disseminated (Fig. 33-1) (7).

Type A: Bile leak from a minor duct still in continuity with the common duct. Type A injuries are generally cystic duct stump leaks or leaks from accessory ducts (Luschka) in the gallbladder bed. A cystic duct stump leak may be due to inaccurate clip placement, perforation proximal to the clip, cystic duct necrosis, or clip dislodgment due to increased intrabiliary pressure secondary to a retained common bile duct stone. Accessory ducts provide a second route for bile drainage, while aberrant ducts are typically the only route for drainage of a portion of the liver. Accessory ducts can be ligated without consequence, but aberrant ducts cannot.

Type B: Occlusion of a part of the biliary tree. This circumstance most commonly occurs when an aberrant right hepatic duct is injured. This aberrant duct often looks like the cystic duct; if the anatomy is misinterpreted, the aberrant duct can be divided. When this type of aberrant duct is occluded, it is a Type B injury; when it is transected without occlusion, it is a Type C injury (see below). The difference in classification reflects differences in presentation and management of the two injuries. Type B injuries are often asymptomatic or present late with abdominal pain or cholangitis involving the occluded liver segment. Normally, the liver behind a Type B injury will atrophy and the remaining liver will hypertrophy. Type C injuries cause intraperitoneal bile collections.

Type C: Bile leak from a duct not in communication with the common duct. As noted above, this injury is almost

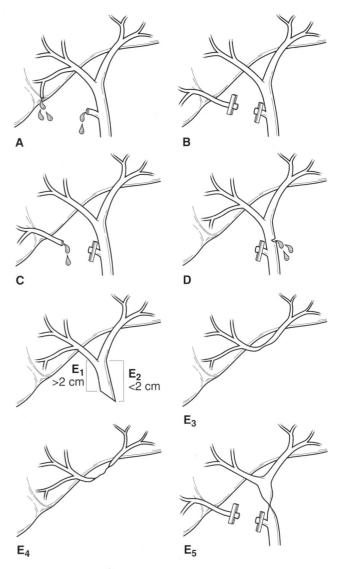

Figure 33-1   Bismuth-Strasberg classification of biliary injuries following laparoscopic cholecystectomy.

always related to transection of an aberrant right hepatic duct with intraperitoneal bile leak.

Type D: Lateral injury to the extrahepatic bile ducts. Analogous to a Type A injury, all hepatic parenchyma remains in communication with the biliary tree and duodenum. The consequences of a Type D injury are generally greater than a Type A injury and often require additional surgery for repair, as they commonly result in a stricture of the main biliary tree. Type D injuries may involve the common bile duct, common hepatic duct, right hepatic duct, or left hepatic duct.

Type E: Circumferential injury of the major bile ducts. These are subclassified below (Bismuth Class 1–5) (Figs. 33-2–33-6). In Type E injuries, the hepatic parenchyma is separated from the lower biliary tree and duodenum. This may be due to ductal stricturing or resection or division of the duct.

Type E1: Circumferential injury to the common duct >2 cm from the bifurcation.

Type E2: Circumferential injury to the common duct <2 cm from the bifurcation.

Type E3: Circumferential injury to the common duct at the bifurcation.

Type E4: Injury to the right or left hepatic duct.

Type E5: Combined injury to the common duct and an aberrant right hepatic duct.

In a series of 300 cases the incidence of Type A injuries was 22.9%; 85% of the Type A injuries were cystic duct stump leaks. The incidence of Type B, C, and D injuries was low—0.37%, 3%, and 8.9%, respectively. Type E injury was by far the most common at 64.8%. Type E injuries that could be further classified were evenly distributed among Types E1–4; only two type E5 injuries were identified. In most series the most common injury is Type A, usually representing 33% to 65% of biliary injuries (7).

Clinical Presentation of Biliary Injuries

When bile duct injuries are not recognized intraoperatively, presenting symptoms typically include abdominal pain, jaundice, and fever (31). These symptoms may be related to an ongoing bile leak, with biloma, biliary ascites, or peritonitis, or a biliary stricture with subsequent obstructive jaundice and cholangitis (32).

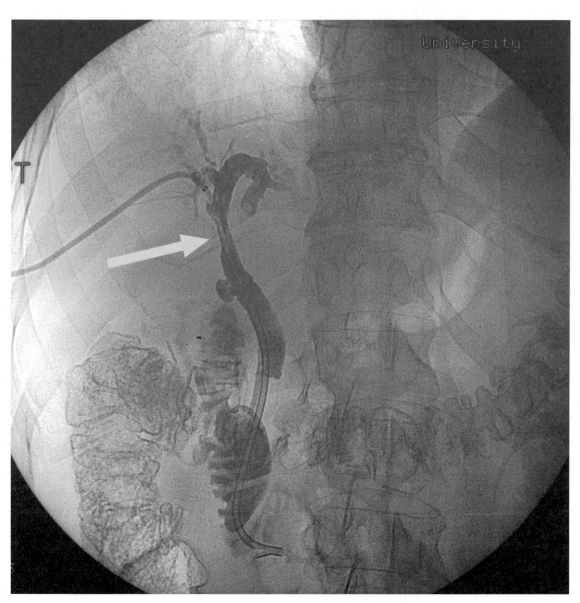

Figure 33-2 Percutaneous transhepatic cholangiogram of a common hepatic duct stricture following an open cholecystectomy. Arrow indicates area of stricture. This is a Bismuth-Strasberg E2 injury.

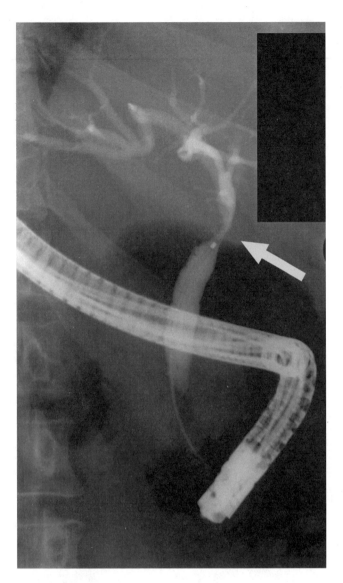

Figure 33-3 Endoscopic retrograde cholangiopancreaticography of a common hepatic duct stricture following a laparoscopic cholecystectomy. Arrow points to area of stricture. This is a Bismuth-Strasberg E2 stricture.

Type A injuries typically present in the first week after surgery, although they have been reported as late as 2 to 3 weeks postoperatively. Type A injuries are usually not detected intraoperatively, although occasionally bile leakage has been noted from the gallbladder bed at the time of surgery (33,34). There are two common presentations for Type A injuries. Approximately two-thirds of patients develop abdominal pain, abdominal distention, fever, and other signs of sepsis related to a localized collection of bile or bile peritonitis. The remaining patients present with an external bile leak via one of the port sites. A few patients will present with only vague symptoms, such as anorexia. Clinical jaundice only occasionally occurs with a Type A injury, although hyperbilirubinemia in the range of 2 to 3 mg per dL is common, as is an increase in alkaline phosphatase (35).

Jaundice is a common presentation with Type E injuries. Type E injuries are sometimes detected at the time of operation, and this is becoming more common (36). Bile leakage or an abnormality seen on intraoperative cholangiography usually precipitates intraoperative recognition. Most Type E injuries are noted within 2 to 3 weeks of the initial operation. About 50% of cases present with a combination of abdominal pain and jaundice (14,33,37,38). Painless jaundice may be the sole manifestation of injury in a late presentation, occurring about 25% of the time (14,33,37,38). Other patients present with pain, fever, jaundice, and sepsis, while a very few patients will develop an external bile leak (14,33,37,38).

Diagnosis of Postoperative Biliary Injuries

A number of investigators have presented algorithms for the diagnosis and management of biliary injuries (13,33,35). Six main investigative tools are used: computed tomography (CT), ultrasound (US), hepatobiliary scintigraphy, endoscopic retrograde cholangiopancreatography (ERCP), fistulography, and percutaneous transhepatic cholangiography (PTC). Many approaches are possible, and several of these techniques, such as PTC and ERCP, also offer therapeutic alternatives.

The initial goals should be to establish a diagnosis, drain bilomas or abscesses, and determine the nature and extent of the injury to the biliary tree. CT and US coupled with percutaneous aspiration and drain placement are used to detect and treat intraperitoneal bile collections. The main role of hepatobiliary scintigraphy is to document the presence of continued bile leak. ERCP and PTC provide more exact anatomical details of the biliary tree and the site of injury, and they can also decompress or dilate the biliary tree.

For a patient presenting with abdominal pain, fever, and signs of sepsis, but without jaundice, CT or US should be the first test to investigate whether or not a fluid collection is present. If a collection is noted, a drain should be placed. If the drainage is bilious, hepatobiliary scintigraphy will determine whether or not there is a continuing leak. If a leak is documented, ERCP can be used to demonstrate the leak's anatomy and location. For Type A injuries a sphincterotomy and stent placement can be used to treat the leak. If a more serious injury is noted, the anatomy will be delineated and further treatment can be planned. Although this approach is less direct than going immediately to ERCP, ERCP is avoided for those patients in whom the leak has stopped. Although the morbidity for a diagnostic ERCP is low, when combined with sphincterotomy the procedure has a complication rate of 7% to 11% and a mortality rate of 0.6% to 1.5% (35,39,40) (Fig. 33-7).

If a patient presents with clinical jaundice or an external bile leak, beginning the investigation with an ERCP is the most appropriate maneuver. For patients with suspected

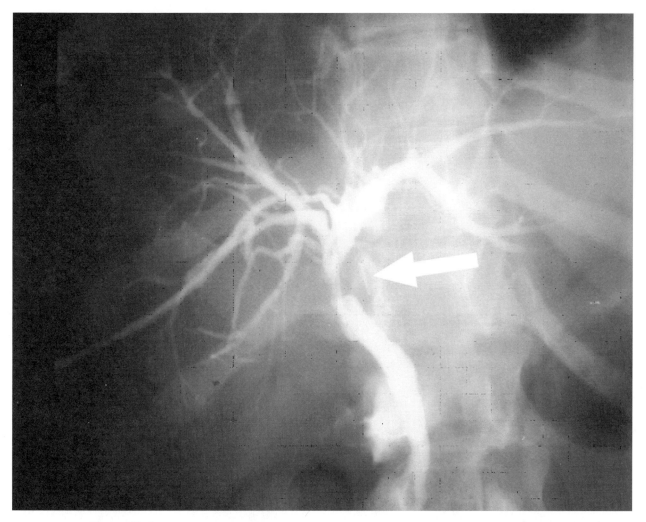

Figure 33-4 Percutaneous transhepatic cholangiogram of a common hepatic duct stricture following a laparoscopic cholecystectomy. Arrow indicates area of stricture. This is a Bismuth-Strasberg E2 injury.

vascular injuries, angiography is the test of choice to define the hepatic arterial and portal venous anatomy. For more significant biliary injuries, particularly those involving a complete transection or complete obstruction of the biliary tree, PTC may be required for precise delineation of the site and nature of the injury, as well as for a detailed outline of the biliary anatomy. For evaluation of longer standing injuries, the above algorithms are also useful. In addition, CT scanning is useful for delineating lobar atrophy or hypertrophy associated with long-standing ductal obstruction or vascular injury (13).

Management of Biliary Injuries

Conversion to an open procedure should not be considered a complication of laparoscopic cholecystectomy, particularly when significant inflammatory changes are present in the porta hepatis or there is difficulty in defining the biliary or arterial anatomy. In most cases biliary injuries are not recognized during laparoscopic cholecystectomy, regardless of the nature of the injury (14,15,21,36,37). Failure to recognize the injury at the time of initial operation and the high incidence of bile leak in the early postoperative period, with attendant sepsis and periportal inflammation, make management of these patients challenging (14,15,21,36,37). It is generally recommended that patients with a suspected major biliary injury not undergo urgent, immediate operation (14,15,21,36,37). Rather, optimal management occurs when the patient is completely evaluated prior to operative management. Most patients will require surgical reconstruction with hepaticojejunostomy; fewer patients have injuries that are amenable to primary repair. Typically, primary repair is done if the injury is recognized at the time of initial laparoscopic cholecystectomy (31). Approximately 15% to 20% of patients will require balloon dilation postoperatively for biliary strictures (31). All these patients have a life-long risk of recurrent biliary stricture and should have life-long follow-up (31).

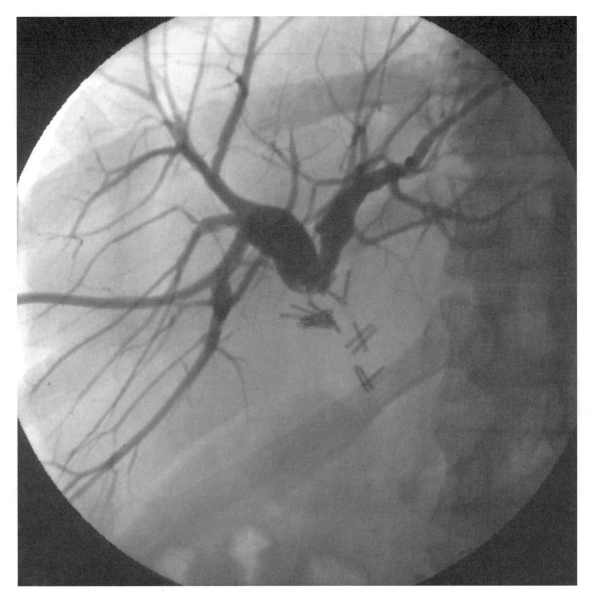

Figure 33-5   Endoscopic retrograde cholangiopancreatography of a combined common bile duct and common hepatic duct injury following a laparoscopic cholecystectomy. This is a Bismuth-Strasberg E3 injury.

Management of Injuries Recognized at Initial Operation

Any suspicion of biliary injury during laparoscopic cholecystectomy is an indication for conversion to an open procedure, with sufficient dissection and intraoperative cholangiography either to determine that an injury has not occurred or to define the injury's site, nature, and extent (13). This circumstance usually represents an injury to the main ducts; Type A injuries are rarely noted intraoperatively. Typically, the injury is suspected because of intraoperative leakage of bile or an abnormal cholangiogram. An intraoperative bile leak is almost always an indication for conversion to an open procedure.

Although early repair of these injuries is advantageous, repair may be difficult and may require dissection and suturing techniques with which many surgeons are not familiar. The keys to successful repair include the ability to dissect the hepatic ducts up into the hilum—up to and above the bifurcation if necessary—and the ability to perform a tension-free mucosa-to-mucosa anastomosis between the biliary system and a loop of small intestine, while maintaining an intact biliary blood supply. Duct-to-duct repairs should be reserved for clean transactions, with no tissue loss and no evidence or risk of thermal injury (7). The advantage of an end-to-end repair includes simplicity and preservation of duct length. This advantage is mitigated by the 50% stricture rate during follow-up, which

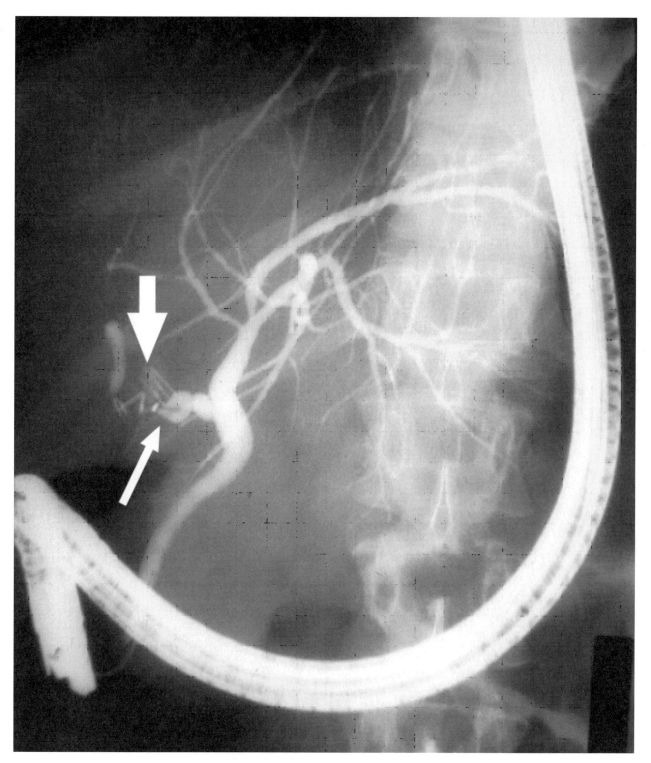

Figure 33-6 Endoscopic retrograde cholangiopancreaticography demonstrating a right hepatic duct injury following a laparoscopic cholecystectomy. The small arrow points to the clipped cystic duct arising from the right hepatic duct. The large arrow points to clipped right hepatic duct. This is a Bismuth-Strasberg E4 injury.

usually requires operative revision (13,41–44). The standard operative management for biliary strictures is to perform a tension-free, mucosa-to-mucosa biliary-enteric anastomosis (45,46). For surgeons who are not familiar with these techniques, placement of right upper quadrant

drains and referral to a hepatobiliary surgeon is a safer approach.

The management of patients sustaining a bile duct injury during laparoscopic cholecystectomy includes surgical, radiologic, and endoscopic techniques. Initially, it is

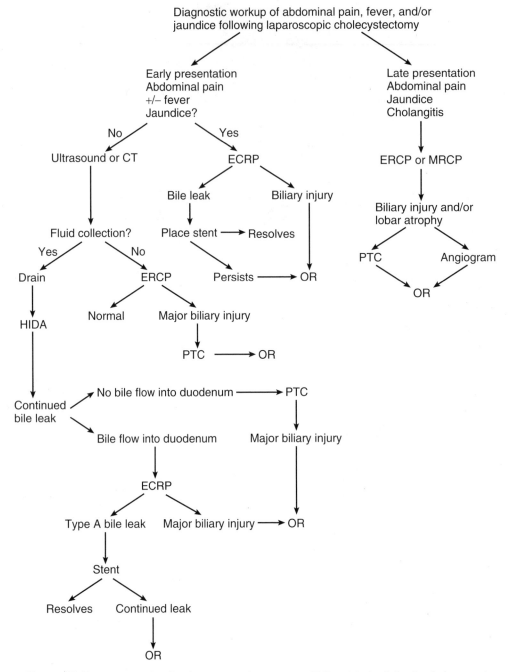

Figure 33-7 Algorithm for the diagnosis and treatment of biliary injuries following laparoscopic cholecystectomy. CT, computed tomography; ERCP, endoscopic retrograde cholangiopancreatography; MRCP, magnetic resonance cholangiopancreatography; PTC, percutaneous transhepatic cholangiography.

important to control bile leak. Although ERCP is occasionally useful for this purpose, if the ducts are completely transected PTC is the procedure of choice. PTC may confirm the injury's exact location and nature and define the anatomy of the proximal biliary tree. This information is useful in planning operative reconstruction. Preoperative placement of PTC tubes also aids in the intraoperative identification of bile ducts. Additional bile collections are usually managed by placement of percutaneous intra-abdominal drains under CT or US guidance. Successful drainage will usually allow the patient to be discharged home for a period of weeks to months to allow time for the periportal inflammation to subside, facilitating subsequent operative reconstruction.

The preferred method for repairing most injuries is a Roux-en-Y hepaticojejunostomy, as the majority of injuries involve a transection and resection of a portion of the bile duct, precluding end-to-end repair (14,15,21,36,37,47–51).

If a major biliary injury is recognized early and the local conditions are acceptable, a single-staged repair with a Roux-en-Y hepaticojejunostomy is the procedure of choice (41–43). In one study (44) repairs were performed a median of 2 days after referral, with a mean length of stay of 11 days, compared to 32 days with a delayed approach by the same group. Eighty-nine percent of these patients had no need for reintervention on follow-up, 9% required a single episode of balloon dilation, and 2% required reoperation (44). Another recent study supports this approach, even with complex Strasberg Class E injuries, but this strategy can be used only in stable patients without ongoing sepsis (52). When bile peritonitis or sepsis exists, external biliary drainage is the preferred approach to bring local and systemic infection under control, prior to consideration of operative repair (41–43). Mortality in the immediate perioperative period, prior to attempts at repair, is typically caused by uncontrolled sepsis and multiorgan system failure and ranges from 2% to 3% (32).

Although most patients will require an operative repair, selected patients have been successfully managed using endoscopic or radiologic techniques (14,15,21,32,36,37). In some cases biliary strictures may be amenable to percutaneous balloon dilation (Figs. 33-8–33-10). In one series of 89 patients, 28 (31%) were managed with balloon dilation (32). In this study balloon dilation had a short-term success rate of 64%, with a mean follow-up of 27.8 months (32). This technique can sometimes be successful after a previous attempt at operative repair. The long-term durability of this approach is not yet known (21,53).

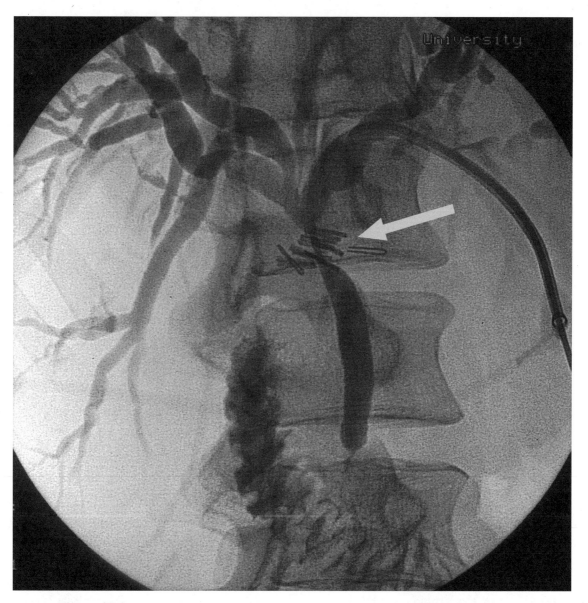

Figure 33-8   Percutaneous transhepatic cholangiogram of a common hepatic duct stricture (*arrow*) following laparoscopic cholecystectomy. This stricture did not become symptomatic for 12 months following the original laparoscopic procedure. This is a Bismuth-Strasberg E3 stricture.

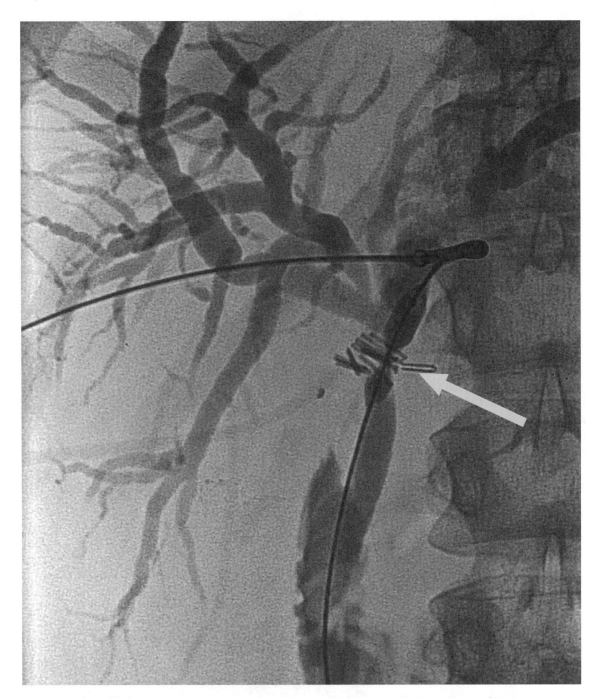

Figure 33-9   Percutaneous transhepatic cholangiogram of attempted balloon dilation of the stricture illustrated in Figure 33-8. Arrow points to balloon crossing stricture.

Stewart and Way analyzed the treatment of 88 patients who sustained a major bile duct injury during laparoscopic cholecystectomy (53). Four factors were found to play a major role in the success or failure of treatment: performance of preoperative cholangiography in order to define the site of injury and biliary anatomy, the choice of surgical repair, details of the operative technique, and the experience of the surgeon performing the repair (53). The importance of delineation of the biliary anatomy preoperatively

is clear: 96% of procedures that were performed in which cholangiograms were not obtained prior to surgery were not successful, and 69% of the procedures in which the cholangiographic data was incomplete prior to operation were unsuccessful (53). With preoperative cholangiographic data, repairs were successful in 84% of cases (53). The type of operative approach is also a significant factor for a successful repair. A primary end-to-end ductal repair was never successful when there was a complete bile duct transection;

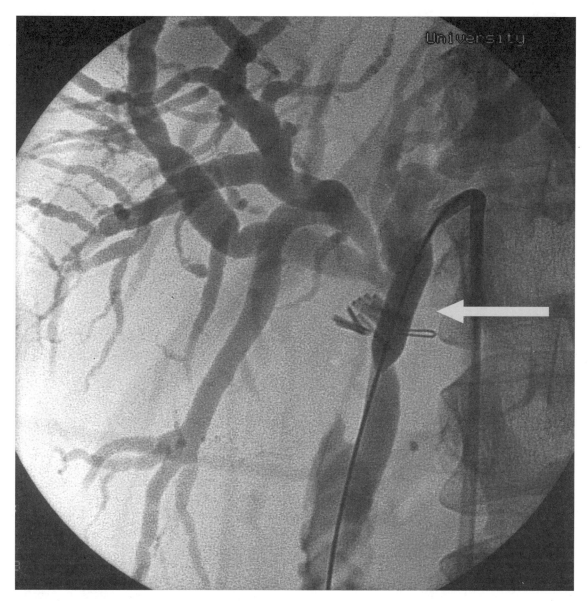

Figure 33-10   Percutaneous tranhepatic cholangiogram of attempted balloon dilation of the stricture illustrated in Figure 33-8. Arrow points to the balloon crossing the stricture, which is now completely inflated.

in this setting, 63% of Roux-en-Y hepaticojejunostomies were successful (21,53).

The surgeon's experience is critical. When the primary surgeon performed the repair, it was successful in only 17% of cases. In contrast, when an experienced surgeon at a tertiary care referral center performed the repair, there was a 94% success rate (21,53). Recent studies support the contention that these repairs should be performed at referral centers with experienced hepatobiliary surgeons in order to optimize outcome (54).

Repair of Bismuth-Strasberg A–E Injuries

Type A: These bile leaks can usually be resolved with decompression of the biliary system via endoscopic sphincterotomy and stenting. Stenting of ampulla Vater

reduces intrabiliary pressure and results in preferential drainage of bile into the duodenum, allowing the leak to seal. In a series of 15 patients, cholangiography demonstrated a cystic duct stump leak in 11 patients and leakage from the gallbladder bed in 4 patients (55). Residual common bile duct stones were noted and removed endoscopically in four of these patients. In this series treatment was either sphincterotomy alone or sphincterotomy with stent placement; in all cases bile leaks stopped and surgical intervention was not required.

Type B: These injuries may remain asymptomatic or present years after the initial operation. The usual presentation is pain or cholangitis (56). For patients who are symptomatic, hepaticojejunostomy or partial hepatic resections are the treatment options. Often a satisfactory biliary reconstruction is not feasible, due to small duct caliber and atrophy of the involved hepatic lobe or segment (13). Hepatic resection is recommended when biliary-enteric anastomosis is not possible (7). In patients who are asymptomatic, treatment is not recommended—particularly when the affected section of the liver is small or if the injury is remote and the involved segment of liver has significantly atrophied.

Type C: This circumstance is usually due to an aberrant right hepatic duct transection. In cases where a fistula is present from a nonligated duct, an ERCP is often interpreted as normal. HIDA scanning may be helpful in making this diagnosis. Preoperative PTC catheter placement is helpful for locating the injured ducts and then to demonstrate the relationship of the involved segment to the remainder of the biliary tree. PTC catheters may facilitate drainage of subhepatic bile collections and help control bile leak. Treatment requires drainage of the leaking bile and either biliary-enteric anastomosis, ligation of the transected duct, or resection of the involved segments of liver. If the duct is very small, <2 mm, a biliary-enteric anastomosis is unlikely to be successful, and ligation or hepatic resection is recommended.

Long-term results of repair to right segmental duct injuries are poorer than results for repair of injuries to the main biliary tree, with higher rates of recurrent stricture formation and cholangitis (13). Although many experts recommend ligation, as opposed to reconstruction, of small segmental ducts, this is possible only when the duct has not been instrumented; in the latter setting an attempt at Roux-en-Y hepaticojejunostomy is appropriate. Although hepatic resection may be used to treat an isolated biliary stricture, this approach should be taken only when patients are having significant symptoms of recurrent pain and cholangitis, have failed at least one attempt at biliary-enteric anastomosis, and other options for management have been exhausted (13).

Type D: This injury is likely more common than reported, as it is often repaired locally at the time of initial operation or shortly thereafter, and referral to a tertiary center is not necessary. Suture repair of the duct over a T-tube is the usual approach to this injury, and whether the T-tube is brought out via the repair site or via a separate stab incision depends on the nature of the injury. When the nature and length of the injury are similar to an intentional choledochotomy, there is no reason to create a second opening in the duct. In settings where the injury is not recent or clean or where there is concern about a potential thermal component to the injury, a second stab incision is recommended. In some cases, when the duct is very small, external drainage and biliary stenting via ERCP may be considered as an alternative to operative repair.

Type E: Some strictures and partial clip occlusions of the biliary tree may be treated with balloon dilation and stents

either via ERCP or PTC techniques. Operation is required for failure of this therapy and in all cases of ductal disruption. The preferred operative approach is hepaticojejunostomy. Many series recommend preoperative placement of transhepatic catheters to facilitate ductal identification at operation (14,36,53,57). The use of postoperative stents is controversial. There is no evidence that postoperative stents help with a large caliber, mucosa-to-mucosa anastomosis; they have been recommended in the setting of small ducts (32).

For E1 and some E2 injuries, the common hepatic duct itself may be used (Fig. 33-11). For higher injuries and for E5 injuries, repair requires anastomosis with several ducts. In some cases anastomosis of several ducts, prior to anastomosis with the jejunum, is appropriate (13,58). For injuries involving both the hepatic confluence and a right segmental duct, reconstruction can be very difficult due to the fact that widely separated ducts must be reconstructed and the small caliber right segmental ducts often have only a short extrahepatic segment.

In performing hepaticojejunostomy, an anterior longitudinal opening should be created in the bile duct and a long side-to-side anastomosis performed. In many cases the extrahepatic portion of the left hepatic duct is an excellent choice for repair of proximal strictures or injuries. One can lower this duct by dividing the hepatic plate as described by Couinaud and recommended by Blumgart and Hepp (Figs. 33-12 and 33-13) (13,58,59). The advantage of this technique, particularly for high injuries, is that it minimizes posterior dissection of the ducts and decreases the chances of devascularization. The location of the left hepatic duct at the base of segment IV and its investing fascia protect it from iatrogenic injury and the inflammatory reaction related to bile leakage and infection. In addition, the duct has a rich blood supply in contrast to the tenuous axial blood supply of the common hepatic and common bile ducts. The generous length of the left hepatic duct also permits a relatively wide anastomosis, regardless of ductal caliber. This feature is particularly suitable for E2 and E3 injuries. The right duct is more often problematic due to its relatively short length.

Some investigators have advocated partial segment IV resection in order to completely expose the upper portions of the biliary tree (60). In this case a partial resection of segment IV is performed in order to expose healthy, nonscarred, noninflamed, nonischemic bile ducts (60). Resection of a 2 cm by 2 cm portion of segment IV between the gallbladder bed and round ligament will expose the intrahepatic portions of the right and left hepatic ducts. This maneuver is typically necessary in Strasberg E3 and E4 injuries. One recent study documented a restenosis rate of 9% for repairs using the Hepp-Couinaud technique (59). In a similar study using the Hepp-Couinaud approach, 95% of patients had an excellent or good result an average of 4.6 years following surgery (51). When the Hepp-Couinaud technique was not

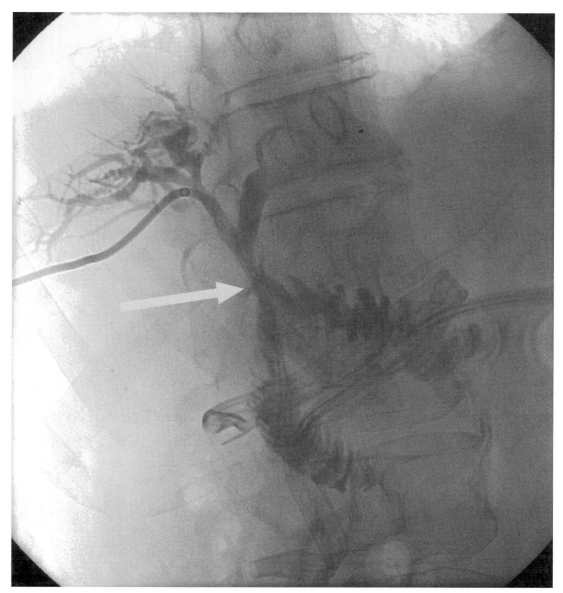

Figure 33-11 Percutaneous tranhepatic cholangiogram following reconstruction of the common hepatic duct stricture illustrated in Figure 33-2 with a hepaticojejunostomy. The arrow indicates the site of the hepaticojejunostomy.

used, four of four patients with E3 and E4 injuries were symptomatic at follow-up and required additional surgical intervention (31).

Optimal timing for reconstruction depends on the patient's condition. If the patient is referred immediately after injury, operation can be performed immediately. More commonly, the patient is referred after at least one attempt at repair has been unsuccessful or after a prolonged period of external drainage. In these cases it is best to wait until the patient has stabilized, all bile collections have been drained, and the injury's anatomy has been well-defined. Concomitant bile leak, perianastomotic infection, and inflammation are all unfavorable conditions for immediate repair. The final extent of injury and stricture develops over time as fibrotic scar tissue replaces the ischemic ductal tissue.

Risk factors for a poor outcome after repair of a biliary injury include failed attempts at repair prior to referral, proximal location of the injury or stricture (E3 or E4), and transanastomotic stenting (51). In one series all patients who failed an attempt at biliary reconstruction became symptomatic at greater than one year after repair, emphasizing the importance of long-term follow-up in these patients. In a recent series reporting long-term outcome of bile duct injuries following laparoscopic cholecystectomy, 25 patients were evaluated (61). There were no deaths. At one-year follow-up, there was a 92% success rate. However, the mid-to-long range (1 to 5 years) results were less favorable, demonstrating a 68% success rate. Eight patients developed a recurrent biliary stricture an average of 3.3 years after the original repair. Two risk factors for restenosis were identified: repair at a nonreferral center and

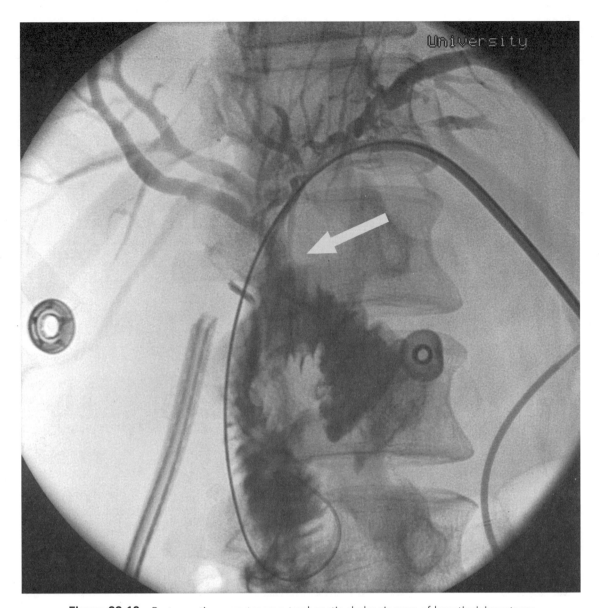

Figure 33-12   Postoperative percutaneous tranhepatic cholangiogram of hepaticojejunostomy that was performed to treat the stricture illustrated in Figure 33-8, which failed a trial of balloon dilation. Arrow points to area of biliary-enteric anastomosis.

repair at a stage with active inflammation. Elevation of serum alkaline phosphatase to >400 IU per L six months postoperatively also correlated with long-term failure.

Proximal biliary injuries can sometimes separate the right anterior and right posterior ducts; it is critically important to identify and drain all such ducts or segments (62). If this is not achieved, serious complications will ensue, including recurrent cholangitis or persistent bile leakage. Investigators have advocated the selective use of segmental hepatic resection in cases of high biliary injury in order to avoid anastamosing small ducts to the bowel. This approach avoids the potential long-term complications of biliary stricture formation and recurrent cholangitis (63).

Concomitant Vascular Injury

Due to the proximity of the biliary structures and hepatic vasculature, concomitant vascular injury in the context of a biliary duct injury is not uncommon. The consequences of vascular injury to the liver are twofold: immediate hepatic parenchymal compromise and delayed biliary stricturing. Postoperative biliary strictures have been shown to be influenced by the status of the biliary blood supply (64,65). Patients with vascular compromise or injury related to laparoscopic cholecystectomy have a 50% anastomotic failure rate (47,66). These studies suggest a correlation between late failure of biliary-enteric anastomosis and the presence of an unrecognized hepatic

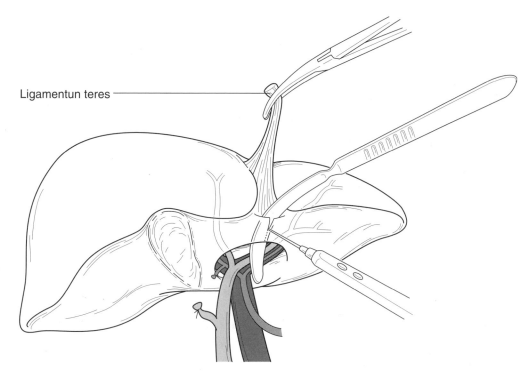

Ligamentun teres

Figure 33-13   Liver split technique for the Hepp-Couinaud approach to biliary reconstruction.

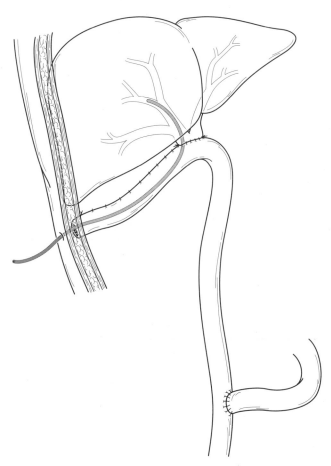

Figure 33-14   Small bowel access loop for potential instrumentation of the biliary tree following hepaticojejunostomy.

arterial injury. Strictures secondary to arterial insufficiency may develop over a longer period of time than technical failures resulting from a suboptimal anastomosis or other mechanisms of injury, such as a thermal injury (66).

Some patients who have undergone primary management for a bile duct injury require a second intervention due to the development of an anastomotic stricture (Fig. 33-14). Since ischemia may play a role in the development of anastomotic strictures, evaluation of the hepatic arterial system is an important component of the preoperative evaluation of these patients (46,47). The arterial supply to the biliary tree arises from segmental hepatic arteries, with communication via the hilar plate arterial plexus. This coaxial arterial supply is particularly important in lower-level injuries; the hepatic arterial supply is usually adequate in the area of the confluence and above. The common hepatic duct normally receives its blood supply from above, and after transection the distal cut end must receive its blood supply from vessels traveling up the common bile duct (67,68).

Concomitant vascular injury should be suspected in cases where significant hemorrhage was noted at the time of cholecystectomy or there is a significant increase in hepatic transaminases after cholecystectomy. Either of these situations should initiate an angiogram. A recent study of 18 cases of failed initial repair of a bile duct injury demonstrated a coexisting arterial injury in 11 patients (61%) (66). There was a significant association of a proximal bile duct injury (Strasberg E3 or E4) and the presence of an arterial injury.

Postoperative Stents

Retrospective series suggest that a successful outcome is more likely if postoperative stenting for 3 to 6 months occurs until liver functions have normalized and the bile duct has healed without stricture (69). This approach has been advocated for very small ducts. Once stents have been removed and recovery is complete, liver function studies should be followed every 3 months for the first year and annually for life (69).

Endoscopic or radiologic interventions with cholangioplasty and the insertion of metallic, expandable stents or Teflon-coated stents to treat biliary strictures have been described. The role of these interventions is still being defined. Teflon-coated stents frequently become clogged with biliary debris and require exchange. Despite this drawback, a recent report demonstrated successful use of this modality in 16 of 20 patients (80%) with benign biliary strictures randomized to stenting (70). The follow-up in this series was >5 years.

Metallic stents have the advantage of larger internal diameter and permit ingrowth of the biliary mucosa, which may reduce stent occlusion. In a study of 25 patients with benign biliary strictures treated with radiologically inserted expandable metal stents, 8 with common duct stenosis and 17 with strictured hepaticojejunostomy, success was achieved in 2 of 8 patients with a common duct stricture and 16 of 17 patients with an anastomotic stricture (71). Mean follow-up was 55 months. This technique is best suited for recurrent anastomotic strictures and for patients with significant comorbidities in whom surgical intervention is excessively risky (72).

Long-term Results

Although recent surgical series cite good short-term results (15,31,32,37), it is known from older studies of open cholecystectomy injury that there is a progressive restenosis rate. Two-thirds of restenoses occur in the first two years, with restenosis described at late as 10 years following repair (46,49,73,74). The restenosis rate varies from 5% to 28% (46). The restenosis rate for repairs of laparoscopic injuries may be higher than with open cholecystectomy, likely related to the increased complexity of laparoscopic injuries (46,49,73,74). Several series also describe the need for hepatic resection or hepatic transplantation after multiple failed repairs (15,38).

Whether the results of bile duct injury repairs after open cholecystectomy are translatable to outcomes for repairs of injuries after laparoscopic cholecystectomy is unclear. A number of series report the long-term results of bile duct strictures occurring prior to the laparoscopic era. In most series successful outcomes are reported in 80% to 95% of patients (57,75). Laparoscopically related injuries tend to be higher in the porta hepatis, often at the confluence of the right and left hepatic ducts, and involve a complete transection of the duct, often with resection of a portion of the biliary tree (7,17,38). In addition, severe periportal inflammation and scarring due to the attendant bile leak usually accompanies these injuries (7,17,38). The high percentage of failed operations performed prior to referral to a tertiary center may also result in poorer outcomes.

The current management of iatrogenic biliary strictures uses a combined modality approach, including preoperative placement of transhepatic catheters, operative hepaticojejunostomy for reconstruction, and interventional radiologic balloon dilation for both primary and recurrent anastomotic strictures (64) (Figs. 33-15 and 33-16). In a recent series totaling 89 patients with laparoscopic bile duct injuries, 28 (31%) were managed with balloon dilation, with a short-term success rate of 64%, at a mean follow-up of 27.8 months (32). Fifty-eight patients (64%) in this study underwent surgical reconstruction with a Roux-en-Y hepaticojejunstomy and transhepatic stenting (32). The success rate for surgical intervention was 92%, at a mean follow-up of 33.4 months (32).

The importance of long-term follow-up is clear. In a series reported by Pitt et al., only 68% of recurrent strictures developed by the third postoperative year (75).

Late Complications

Secondary biliary cirrhosis is well described in the setting of benign biliary obstruction (46). Chronic extrahepatic biliary obstruction leads to dilation of the biliary tree and eventually to the proliferation of biliary ductules within the portal triads. With continued obstruction to bile flow, fibrosis of the portal tracts ensues and may eventually lead to cirrhosis. The time to the onset of biliary cirrhosis is variable and likely depends on the degree of obstruction and the occurrence and frequency of cholangitis.

The ability of biliary decompression to alter or reverse the course of secondary biliary cirrhosis and hepatic destruction is uncertain. Relief of the biliary obstruction can reverse fibrosis without cirrhosis. Once cirrhosis has begun, the lesion does not appear to be reversible (76). The development of secondary biliary cirrhosis is accompanied by the hemodynamic derangements associated with other forms of cirrhosis, including portal hypertension, variceal hemorrhage, ascites, and encephalopathy.

In one series, 37.5% of patients were noted to have histologic evidence of moderate to marked hepatic fibrosis on liver biopsy and 25% were noted to have evidence of evolving cirrhosis (69). Of the patients with fibrosis and evolving cirrhosis, mean time to definitive repair was over a year, significantly longer than patients without histologic changes; mean time for these patients was just under 3 months (69). In another study, a delay in referral led to evidence of hepatic fibrosis in 31% of patients (77). For patients with histologic abnormalities on preoperative hepatic biopsy, follow-up postoperative liver biopsy should also be obtained at one year to exclude progression of disease (69). Close

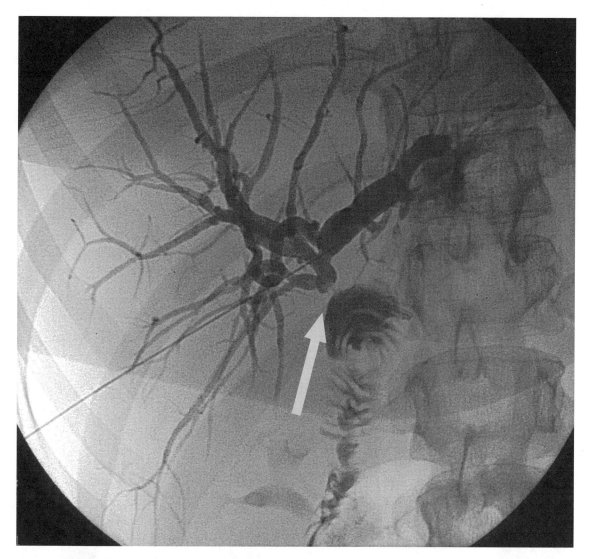

Figure 33-15   Percutaneous tranhepatic cholangiogram of a strictured hepaticojejunostomy. The hepaticojejunostomy was originally performed to treat a bile duct injury after a laparoscopic cholecystectomy. Arrow illustrates the strictured biliary-enteric anastomosis. This stricture is now a Bismuth-Strasberg E3 injury.

observation of these patients is essential to detect the late development of biliary strictures and to avoid the development of secondary biliary cirrhosis (78).

If patient referral is significantly delayed, following unsuccessful attempts at repair, these patients often develop malnutrition, secondary biliary cirrhosis, and portal hypertension (45). Patients presenting with established liver disease are more likely to have undergone more than one repair and to have experienced major infection. The presence of portal hypertension and liver disease increases mortality from 3.2% to 27% in the immediate postoperative period (45,79).

Although the risk of developing biliary cirrhosis and end-stage liver disease is directly related to persistent biliary obstruction and recurrent cholangitis from failed reconstruction, the need for liver transplantation from bile duct injury, even in association with hepatic arterial injury, is an unlikely outcome, as long as a satisfactory reconstruction of the proximal biliary tree can eventually be achieved.

Complications in High-risk Settings

Early in laparoscopic experience, pregnancy, cirrhosis, obesity, acute cholecystitis, and prior surgery were all considered relative or absolute contraindications to laparoscopic cholecystectomy. As experience with this procedure has grown, there are now few contraindications to the laparoscopic approach. However, using a laparoscopic technique in a high-risk setting not only results in a higher conversion rate but may also be associated with a higher complication rate. A low threshold for conversion to open has been shown to minimize the risk of complications in higher risk settings (80).

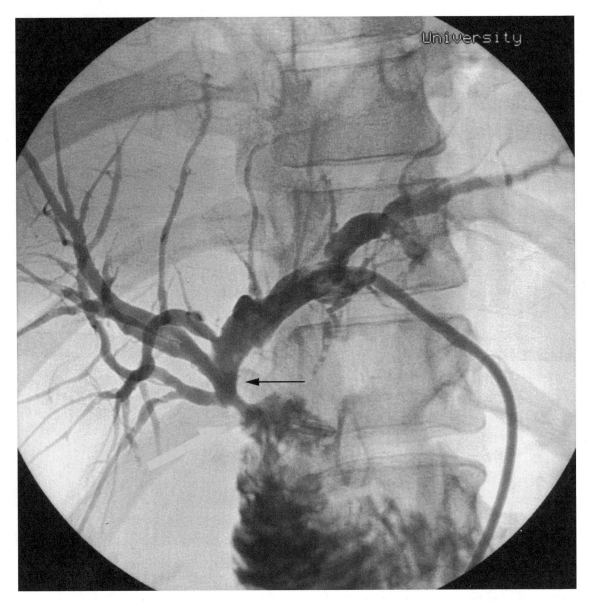

Figure 33-16 Percutaneous tranhepatic cholangiogram of the strictured biliary-enteric anastomosis illustrated in Figure 33-15 following balloon dilation. Arrow indicates area of prior stricture.

Acute Cholecystitis

In a recent large study of 1,000 patients in whom laparoscopic cholecystectomy was attempted, 4.8% required conversion to open, with the most common reason for conversion being an inability to define anatomy in the setting of acute cholecystitis (81). Other risk factors for conversion to an open procedure included male gender; previous abdominal surgery; history of jaundice, obesity, or leukocytosis; and suspicion of common bile duct stones (81). Other studies also support the increased need for conversion to open in the setting of acute cholecystitis. In one study laparoscopic cholecystectomy was performed for acute cholecystitis in 12.6% of patients, with conversion to open occurring 29.4% of the time, compared to 8.2% in patients undergoing laparoscopic cholecystectomy for other indications (10).

Gangrenous Cholecystitis

Gangrenous cholecystitis may be present in up to 30% of cases of acute cholecystitis. Although gangrenous cholecystitis is considered an indication for emergent operation, precise diagnosis of this condition is difficult. Elderly and critically ill patients are at higher risk for developing gangrenous cholecystitis. The conversion rates to open cholecystectomy in the setting of gangrenous cholecystitis approximates 50% and overall morbidity and risk of biliary injury are increased (82).

Acute acalculous cholecystitis is associated with a higher rate of gangrenous cholecystitis. Morbidity includes gallbladder perforation. Free perforation is associated with a mortality rate of 30% and an overall morbidity rate of 70% (83). This situation is also associated with empyema of the gallbladder, which also has a significant complication rate, with up to 50% of patients having at least one postoperative complication (83). Infectious complications are particularly prevalent and include pneumonia, wound infection, and intra-abdominal abscess formation (83). Patients with empyema of the gallbladder may be stabilized by placement of a percutaneous cholecystostomy tube.

Biliary Fistula

Cholecystocholedochal fistulas (Mirizzi Syndrome, Type II) are demonstrated in approximately 1% of patients undergoing cholecystectomy, and biliary-enteric fistulas are found in a similar proportion. A rate of 3% has been reported in American Indians (84). Acquired and congenital absence of the cystic duct has also been reported (84,85). Mirizzi Syndrome, Type I (stone impacted at the cystic duct/common duct junction causing obstructive jaundice) is rarely encountered (84). These problems increase the risk of injury during laparoscopic cholecystectomy, and their management almost always requires conversion to the open technique.

Cirrhosis

Gallstone disease in patients with cirrhosis is a diagnostic and therapeutic challenge. The incidence of gallstones in the setting of cirrhosis is as high as 46%, compared to 5% to 22% in the general population (86,87). Most cirrhotic patients with gallstones remain asymptomatic and do not require surgical intervention. Surgical treatment in these patients has a high mortality, with most deaths in patients with Child's Class C risk status. Patients with Child's A or B cirrhosis have lower morbidity and mortality following surgery, although still higher than the general population.

The role of laparoscopic cholecystectomy in this patient population is being defined. For patients with Child's A or B cirrhosis, laparoscopic cholecystectomy is the procedure of choice (88). In one study of Child's A and B cirrhotics undergoing laparoscopic cholecystectomy there were no operative deaths (88). For elective cases, conversion to open occurred in 5%; for urgent operations, conversion occurred in 36% (88). The conversion rate for elective procedures in this series was similar to that of the general population (88). The morbidity rate was 23% to 36% for urgent operations and 16% for elective operations (88). Morbidity for Child's B patients was 43%, compared to 17% for Child's A patients (88), both significantly higher than the general population. Complications were more frequent in patients with ascites. Particular care should be taken in trocar placement in order to avoid venous collaterals, as they may be a source of major intraoperative hemorrhage. A recent study confirms these results and demonstrates a lower complication rate for elective laparoscopic cholecystectomy relative to open cholecystectomy in Child's A and B cirrhotics (89).

Unretrieved Stones in the Peritoneal Cavity

The laparoscopic approach makes retrieval of dropped stones difficult. Gallbladder perforation during laparoscopic cholecystectomy is not uncommon. Most surgeons do not believe that conversion to an open procedure is justified to retrieve lost stones. A number of reports have suggested, however, that unretrieved stones can cause abscess, inflammation, fibrosis, adhesions, cutaneous sinuses, small bowel obstruction, or generalized sepsis (90). In a series of 856 patients, lost stones were noted in 106 cases (12%) (90). Of these, only 5 patients had any sequelae, all of which were minor. These authors concluded that in the majority of patients, unretrieved stones are of no consequence. In another study of 1,059 patients, spillage occurred in 29% of cases (91). Stone and bile spillage was associated with a statistically significant increase in the incidence of fever and intra-abdominal abscess, compared to cases without spills (91). However, the overall risk of serious complication was again low (91).

As many stones should be retrieved as possible, without converting to an open procedure, and the abdomen should be irrigated copiously prior to completing the procedure (90) (Table 33-3). In cases where an intra-abdominal abscess develops due to loss of intraperitoneal stones, percutaneous drainage will not be effective if the inciting stones are not removed (91). Risk factors for stone spillage include male gender, increased age, and obesity (91). Acute cholecystitis does not appear to be a risk factor.

Unsuspected Gallbladder Cancer

When either laparoscopic or open cholecystectomy is performed, there is a chance that gallbladder cancer will be discovered postoperatively. The incidence of unsuspected gallbladder cancer is low, ranging from 0.35% to 0.40% (92,93). The most common presenting symptom for gallbladder cancer is right upper quadrant pain, followed by weight loss. Jaundice is relatively uncommon, related to compression of the common bile duct, and indicates poor prognosis. Gallstones are present with gallbladder cancer in 65% to 70% of cases (94).

TABLE 33-3

SPILLAGE OF BILE AND STONES DURING LAPAROSCOPIC CHOLECYSTECTOMY

- Retrieve as many stones as possible, without converting to a open cholecystectomy.
- Irrigate abdomen copiously to remove as much bile and as many stones as possible.
- Culture bile as a guide to antibiotic therapy.
- In the presence of infected bile, conversion to open cholecystectomy may be considered.

Gallbladder cancer is a highly lethal disease unless discovered incidentally or at an early stage (Tis or T1) (93). Although several reports have suggested an increased rate of port site or peritoneal seeding after laparoscopic cholecystectomy in the setting of gallbladder cancer (92,93,95), a recent multicenter evaluation demonstrated that the prognosis of unsuspected gallbladder cancer was no worse after laparoscopic than after open cholecystectomy (93,96). Survival correlates with stage of disease and with bile spillage during the first operation. Release of tumor cells inevitably occurs during cholecystectomy if the tumor is located on the hepatic surface during resection of the gallbladder from the liver bed. This factor may explain peritoneal tumor seeding that is sometimes seen in the absence of bile spillage. For either open or laparoscopic procedures, additional surgery is not recommended for patients with early (T1) cancers.

During laparoscopic cholecystectomy, the gallbladder should be opened immediately after extraction to detect a possible malignancy. If a malignancy is suspected, a frozen section should be obtained. If gallbladder cancer is pathologically confirmed, the abdomen should be irrigated with a large volume of saline in an attempt to prevent implantation of malignant cells. Additional surgery is not recommended until the final pathology report to obtain accurate staging, as it is often difficult to determine depth of invasion based on frozen section. Delay of definitive surgical therapy does not have an adverse effect on prognosis (97).

Trocar Site Recurrence

Some authors recommend the routine use of a plastic retrieval bag to extract the gallbladder from the abdomen to avoid the rare possibility of tumor seeding at trocar sites. On the basis of the exceedingly low incidence of gallbladder cancer, this practice is probably not justified. The significance of port site implantation may be overestimated. Recent articles report that the incidence of abdominal wall implantation does not increase with laparoscopy but is more likely a manifestation of this malignancy's aggressiveness (98). Port site recurrence is related to intraoperative gallbladder perforation (99); in one study patients with intraoperative gallbladder perforation had a 40% incidence of port site recurrence, compared to a 9% incidence without gallbladder perforation. In many cases port site recurrence is an indicator of systemic disease and the majority of patients have other sites of disseminated disease (99).

Glandular cells have been shown on 40% of the laparoscopic instruments during cholecystectomy and in the filtrate of the carbon dioxide exhaust gas (100,101). Cellular dissemination likely occurs when the gallbladder wall is macroscopically perforated during operative cholangiography and when grasping instruments microscopically breach the gallbladder wall (100). Other studies also suggest that pneumoperitoneum increases tumor implantation at trocar sites and tumor growth within the peritoneum (102,103).

Recommended Treatment

Patients with invasion confined to the mucosa (pTis, pT1a) do not need further intervention after cholecystectomy (104,105) (Table 33-4). For T1b, T2, or T3 lesions, surgical therapy includes resection of the gallbladder bed (resection of segments IVb and V) and portal lymphadenectomy (99,104–106) (Fig. 33-17). For patients who have undergone laparoscopic cholecystectomy prior to radical resection, port site excision is also recommended (105). Resection of the extrahepatic biliary tree is also sometimes indicated if there is direct involvement of this area (94,99,105). More radical resections may be undertaken in order to achieve microscopically negative margins, which significantly improve prognosis.

A recent study compared the prognosis of gallbladder cancer in the prelaparoscopic era (1985–1988) to that in the laparoscopic era (1992–1995). The 3-year survival for localized disease in the prelaparoscopic period was 29%, compared to 34% in the laparoscopic period (107). The data were corrected for whether the cancer-bearing gallbladder was laparoscopically manipulated or not, and no statistically significant differences in survival remained (107). Another study demonstrated that the 5-year survival after laparoscopic cholecystectomy for undiagnosed gallbladder cancer was 92% for patients with a pT1 lesion and 59% for a pT2 lesion; in older studies the 5-year survival rate after open cholecystectomy for an unsuspected gallbladder cancer ranges from 90% to 100% for pT1 lesions and 40% to 65% for pT2 lesions, suggesting that laparoscopic cholecystectomy has not had a detrimental effect on survival (97).

When polypoid lesions of the gallbladder are solitary, have a diameter >20 mm, are sessile in appearance, and demonstrate rapid growth, an open procedure should be performed and the possibility of segmental hepatic resection (segments IVb and V) with a portal lymphadenectomy should be considered.

TABLE 33-4

PATHOLOGIC TNM CLASSIFICATION OF GALLBLADDER TUMORS

pTis	Carcinoma *In Situ*
pT1	Tumor invades lamina propria or muscle layer
pT1a	Tumor invades lamina propria
pT1b	Tumor invades muscle layer
pT2	Tumor invades perimuscular connective tissue; no extension beyond serosa or into liver
pT3	Tumor perforates serosa (visceral peritoneum) or directly invades into one adjacent organ or both (extension 2 cm or less into the liver)
pT4	Tumor extends >2 cm into the liver and/or into two or more adjacent organs (stomach, duodenum, colon, pancreas, omentum, extrahepatic bile ducts; any distant involvement of liver)

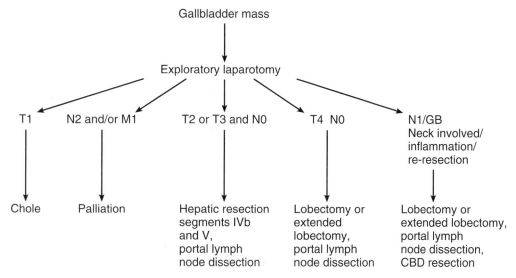

Figure 33-17   Algorithm for the treatment of gallbladder cancer.

Complications Following Treatment of Gallbladder Cancer

Curative resection with negative margins, complete gross resection of tumor, and negative lymph nodes are the most important prognostic factors following surgical treatment of gallbladder cancer (94). Complications occur in 33% of patients and include bile leak, major wound infection, and intra-abdominal bleeding. Operative mortality is approximately 5%. Complications are increased in patients undergoing common bile duct resection (106). Survival of patients with negative nodes is significantly better than for those with positive nodes (5-year survival of 58% vs. 0%). Long-term survival overall is associated with male gender, absence of gallstones, absence of jaundice, and curative resection. Histologic absence of perineural invasion is also important (108).

COMPLICATIONS OF BILIARY STONE DISEASE

Six percent to 20% of patients with symptomatic gallstones have concurrent common bile duct stones; most of these are unsuspected (1,2,109,110). Common bile duct stones can be removed using a variety of techniques, including preoperative or postoperative ERCP extraction, percutaneous transhepatic cholangiographic techniques, conversion of laparoscopic cholecystectomy to open operation, or laparoscopic removal.

Recurrent common bile duct stones are those that form entirely after cholecystectomy. Most recurrent common bile duct stones are brown and are usually associated with biliary infection, particularly *E. coli*. Bile infection precedes brown stone formation and, together with bile stasis, facilitates stone growth. Although recurrent common bile duct stones are primarily brown stones, two other types may also develop: (a) nonbrown stones containing suture material and (b) stones associated with a long cystic duct remnant (111). The formation of brown stones is facilitated if a biliary stricture is present. Increased age is also a major risk factor for the development of recurrent stones.

Common bile duct exploration can be performed laparoscopically, using either a transcystic technique or via choledochotomy (Fig. 33-18). If stones are <15 mm, a transcystic approach may be employed (112). Stones >15 mm are an indication for choledochotomy, and stones >25 mm usually require conversion to an open procedure (112). If the initial transcystic approach does not allow satisfactory removal of large stones or fragments, a choledochotomy is indicated. Choledochoscopy allows direct visualization of the duct system. A completion cholangiogram should always be performed after all stone extraction is complete. If there are concerns about the possibility of retained stones, a T-tube may be inserted either via the cystic duct stump or via the choledochotomy (112).

In a recent study common bile duct stones were identified by cholangiogram in 8.7% of 1,572 patients undergoing laparoscopic cholecystectomy (112). Thirty-one percent of these stones were unsuspected preoperatively. All these patients underwent laparoscopic common bile duct exploration, with successful stone extraction in 83.8% of cases. Eight percent of patients were converted to an open procedure. Overall mortality rate was 1.5%, and major complications occurred in 9.6% of patients, including dislodgment of T-tubes, pulmonary embolus, subhepatic abscess, subhepatic hematoma, and missed common bile duct stones.

A recent multicenter, prospective, randomized study suggests that there is benefit, on the basis of cost and length of stay, to a single staged laparoscopic procedure, including laparoscopic common bile duct exploration

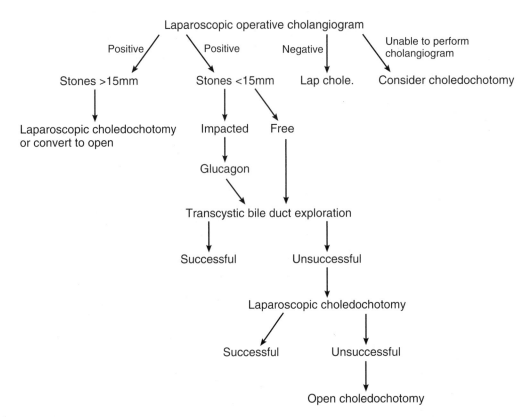

Figure 33-18   Algorithm for the approach and treatment of gallstones discovered during laparoscopic cholecystectomy.

and stone extraction (113). In this study, postoperative ERCP stone extraction was recommended for failed laparoscopic stone removal (113). Another study comparing laparoscopic bile duct exploration to ERCP stone extraction similarly concluded that the laparoscopic approach resulted in a significantly lower length of stay, cost, and complication rate (110).

Endoscopic Stone Extraction

ERCP is an accepted modality for preoperative removal of common bile duct stones; it is also an acceptable alternative to laparoscopic stone extraction. The current rate for ERCP cannulation is 89% to 100%, with subsequent stone extraction success rate of 86% to 100%, a morbidity of 2.5% to 11%, and a mortality of 0% to 1.2% (39,114–118). Morbidity includes pancreatitis, perforation of the bile or pancreatic ducts or duodenum, retained common bile duct stones, bleeding, cholangitis, sepsis, and the development of ampullary stenosis (110,116–118).

ERCP may be used for common bile duct stone extraction in three scenarios: (a) selective preoperative ERCP, (b) intraoperative ERCP, and (c) postoperative ERCP. With few exceptions, patients with both gallstones and common bile duct stones should undergo removal of the common bile duct stones and cholecystectomy, regardless of the

treatment algorithm chosen. Even in patients with significant comorbidity, endoscopic stone extraction alone results in a higher incidence of recurrent symptoms compared to patients also undergoing cholecystectomy; a 25% to 40% incidence of recurrent symptoms has been reported at 24 months requiring subsequent operation for biliary complications (119–121). Cholangitis is the most common recurrent symptom (119).

The goal of selective preoperative ERCP is the removal of common bile duct stones from patients with the greatest likelihood of choledocholithiasis. If the stones are successfully cleared endoscopically, the patient proceeds to laparoscopic cholecystectomy. If the ERCP is unsuccessful, the patient proceeds to definitive surgery, either open or laparoscopic, depending on the surgeon's skills and locally available resources. Preoperative predictors of choledocholithiasis include jaundice, increased serum bilirubin, increased serum alkaline phosphatase, a dilated common bile duct on ultrasound or other preoperative imaging studies, visualized common bile duct stones on preoperative imaging studies, elevated serum amylase, and pancreatitis (114) (Table 33-5). Visualization of a common bile duct stone on ultrasound has a very high predictive value for the presence of stones (114) (Fig. 33-19). In contrast, pancreatitis or an elevated serum amylase are poor predictors for the presence of choledocholithiasis (114).

PREOPERATIVE PREDICTIVE FACTORS FOR COMMON BILE DUCT STONES

Clinical jaundice
Increased serum bilirubin
Increased serum alkaline phosphatase
Increased serum amylase
Dilated common bile duct on ultrasound or other preoperative imaging studies
Visualized common bile duct stones on preoperative imaging studies
Clinical pancreatitis

The rationale for intraoperative ERCP is that the patient is not subjected to the possible failure of postoperative ERCP. If intraoperative ERCP is unsuccessful, the surgeon proceeds to open common bile duct exploration, sparing the patient the need for a second operative procedure and a second anesthetic. However, this approach has substantial logistical problems.

Postoperative ERCP is commonly used for patients with stones demonstrated on an intraoperative cholangiography. There is an obvious risk to this approach, because if the ERCP fails, the patient will need to be returned to the operating room for common bile duct exploration. Table 33-6 lists risk factors for unsuccessful ERCP stone extraction.

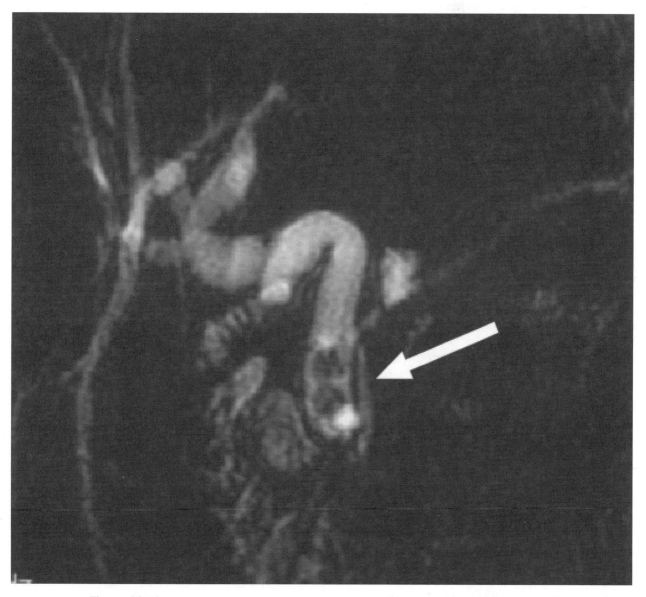

Figure 33-19 Magnetic resonance cholangiopancreatography (MRCP) demonstrating common bile duct stones. Arrow points to two stones in distal common bile duct.

TABLE 33-6

RISK FACTORS FOR UNSUCCESSFUL ERCP STONE EXTRACTION

Stone size >25 mm
Stone diameter greater than duct diameter
Intrahepatic stones
Multiple, tightly packed stones
Impacted stones
Common bile duct stricture
Duodenal diverticulum
Difficult anatomy (Billroth II, Roux-en-Y)

Studies suggest that 60% of stones identified on routine intraoperative cholangiogram will clear with stenting (122). Although most small stones pass spontaneously, no prospective data support a policy of expectant management of retained common bile duct stones.

For patients who are severely ill with ascending cholangitis, unresolved pancreatitis, or severe comorbid illnesses, ERCP with stone extraction is the recommended preoperative approach (110). Acute cholangitis is a serious complication, occurring in 6% to 9% of patients with symptomatic gallstone disease (119). Prior to the advent of endoscopic approaches, open common bile duct exploration was the standard of care for this problem, with a mortality rate of 10% to 40% (119). The use of ERCP in this setting has significantly decreased the mortality rate to the range of 0.4% to 7% (119). For patients who are acutely ill with cholangitis due to common bile duct stones, the overall success rate for ERCP cannulation is 95% (119). In this setting, 84% of patients have been noted to have stones, and biliary decompression was achieved in all patients (119). Complications included acute pancreatitis and postsphincterotomy bleeding. The overall complication rate was 6.6% (119). The mortality rate was 1.6%.

Delayed ERCP in patients with severe cholangitis results in increased mortality and morbidity (123). For severely ill patients, endoscopic biliary drainage can be accomplished by sphincterotomy, followed by stone clearance during that session, or by placement of a biliary endoprosthesis. In hemodynamically unstable septic patients or in those with multiple large stones, temporary drainage without sphincterotomy followed by elective stone extraction may be a safer approach (123). Biliary drainage for the control of sepsis is the important component of this algorithm. After patients are stabilized and sepsis controlled, elective laparoscopic cholecystectomy is recommended. In one study following this algorithm, the conversion rate to open cholecystectomy was relatively high at 9.8% (119). The main reason for conversion was dense adhesions around the triangle of Calot due to prior cholangitis. For surgeons who are not skilled at laparoscopic bile duct exploration, endoscopic sphincterotomy for biliary drainage and stone removal, followed by interval laparoscopic cholecystectomy, is a safe and effective technique for managing common bile duct stones, particularly in the setting of cholangitis (119).

Surgical Treatment of Common Bile Duct Stones

Sphincterotomy

Sphincterotomy can be performed surgically and has been used to treat a number of conditions, including common bile duct stones and papillary stenosis. It was originally thought that sphincterotomy prevented recurrent stone formation by facilitating the passage of stone fragments, biliary sludge, or clots that could function as a nuclei for further stone formation. Recent reports suggest that both surgical and endoscopic sphincterotomy are risk factors for long-term stone recurrence (111,124). One to 10 years after cholecystectomy, brown stones occur with increased frequency in patients who have undergone sphincterotomy or sphincteroplasty (111). Although sphincterotomy or sphincteroplasty facilitates the passage of small stones, long-term damage to the sphincter mechanism can lead to contamination of the common bile duct due to reflux of duodenal contents. Bile cultures are positive in the postoperative period more frequently in patients who have undergone sphincterotomy than control patients who have not undergone sphincterotomy. A 7.4% incidence of bile duct cancer has been observed in patients who have previously undergone a transduodenal sphincteroplasty (125), perhaps related to the presence of chronic cholangitis.

Choledochoduodenostomy and Choledochojejunostomy

Choledochoduodenostomy and Roux-en-Y choledochojejunostomy are definitive operative treatments for patients with retained or recurrent common bile duct stones. Both procedures have been advocated for patients with a high probability of stone retention and recurrent stone formation. Indications include difficulty in extracting stones; the presence of soft friable stones; retained, recurrent, or impacted stones; a dilated common bile duct with or without associated ampullary stenosis; multiple intrahepatic stones; or multiple common duct stones.

Choledochoduodenostomy is easier to perform (126). Roux-en-Y choledochojejunostomy is more difficult to perform and precludes later endoscopic evaluation and treatment. Both short-term and long-term risks of cholangitis are similar for choledochoduodenostomy and choledochojejunostomy. The mortality rates for both procedures are similar, approximating 1.5% to 6%. Perioperative complications include wound infection, biliary leak or fistula, pancreatitis, gastrointestinal hemorrhage, and intra-abdominal abscess, and they occur at a rate of 18% to 21% (126).

Choledochoduodenostomy has a long-term risk of cholangitis that ranges from 0% to 12%; this complication is usually associated with stricture formation at the anastomosis (126) (Fig. 33-20). Stricture may be minimized by performing a mucosa-to-mucosa anastomosis of at least 14 mm in length. Following Roux-en-Y choledochojejunostomy, a similar rate of cholangitis is seen, most commonly due to residual intrahepatic stones (126). Choledochojejunostomy is recommended when there has been a prior bile duct repair, a difficult or recurrent biliary stricture, or when the duodenum is scarred, obstructed, or cannot be safely mobilized for an anastomosis.

Hepatolithiasis

Intrahepatic stones are common in Southeast Asia and Taiwan; they are relatively uncommon in the United States.

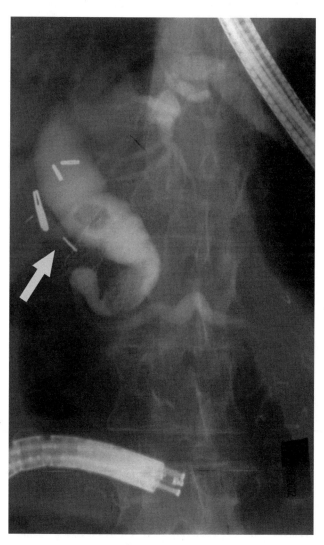

Figure 33-20 Endoscopic retrograde cholangiopancreaticography of a strictured choledochoduodenostomy with stone above stricture. Arrow points to stone.

Surgical procedures for removal of intrahepatic stones include lithotomy by extended choledochotomy, transhepatic cholangiolithotomy, and hepatic resection. Hepatic resection has been combined with percutaneous transhepatic cholangioscopic lithotomy (PTCSL) (127). The complication rate with hepatic resection ranges from 10% to 40% and is related to wound infection, intra-abdominal or hepatic abscesses, bile leak, cholangitis, and sepsis. Operative mortality is reported at 2% to 3% (127–132). The complication rate for PTCSL is 14% to 22% and includes hemobilia, extreme pain, nausea and vomiting, cholangitis, and sepsis (127). Hemobilia is a serious complication that can be associated with massive hemorrhage and death (127). Additional procedures that are recommended for biliary obstruction include transduodenal sphincteroplasty, choledochoduodenostomy, and Roux-en-Y hepaticojejunostomy.

Seventy-five percent of patients with hepatolithiasis have associated biliary stricture (130), and these are the main causes of treatment failures. During treatment it is important to address all biliary strictures, either operatively or with balloon dilation. Many operations include more than one procedure. If strictures are limited to one lobe, hepatic resection can be beneficial. For patients undergoing hepatectomy, liver resection is often also combined with some type of biliary-enteric anastomosis and instrumentation to deal with additional stones and strictures in the remaining liver. For strictures that are not amenable to surgical treatment, balloon dilation can be helpful, although it is less durable, with a restenosis rate of 45% at 5 to 7 years (128).

Retained and recurrent intrahepatic stones are the main long-term complications related to surgical treatment of hepatolithiasis. Of 566 patients who underwent operation, 13.6% had retained stones postoperatively (128). The incidence of retained stones has decreased to 10% to 30% with the use of intraoperative fiberoptic cholangioscopy (133); this technique is superior to intraoperative cholangiography. Postoperative cholangiography and cholangioscopy should be performed routinely in order to detect residual stones (128). Additional stones may then be removed percutaneously or fragmented with lithotripsy (128). Intrahepatic strictures, a dislodged T-tube or tortuous tract, and duodenal fistula were the primary causes of failed attempts to remove stones percutaneously postoperatively. Operative mortality has been reported at 4.6% (128).

Percutaneous removal of intrahepatic stones is an adjunct to operative intervention. Of 48 patients undergoing this modality, 83% had complete stone clearance. Reasons for failure included intrahepatic strictures with retained stones, retained intrahepatic stones associated with liver abscess, and retained intrahepatic stones associated with biliary cirrhosis and complicated by hemobilia and septic shock (128). Recurrent stone formation after complete clearance is 28% and 40% at 4 and 10 years, respectively (128).

Complications are increased in patients with retained stones relative to those with complete clearance, with a significantly increased incidence of repeat operation for recurrent cholangitis or liver abscess, development of secondary biliary cirrhosis, and cholangiocarcinoma. Patients with retained stones have a higher long-term mortality rate than patients with complete stone clearance—23.6% versus 7.6%, respectively. Surgical mortality related to acute cholangitis from hepatolithiasis is high (129).

Hepatolithiasis can also be accompanied by the development of secondary biliary cirrhosis or cholangiocarcinoma (128). Secondary biliary cirrhosis may be further complicated by portal hypertension, bleeding due to varices, hypersplenism with associated pancytopenia, ascites, encephalopathy, and liver failure. Patients who develop biliary cirrhosis are often not acceptable surgical candidates. The percutaneous approach remains reasonable in this group, although with increased risk of bleeding and sepsis. The late development of cholangiocarcinoma is well-described (128,131), with an incidence of 2.5% to 10%. Cancer is thought to be related to prolonged inflammation of the biliary epithelium related to retained stones and the metabolic activity of bacteria in the biliary tree (128).

Stents

Recently, the use of expandable metallic stents as part of the treatment for recurrent biliary strictures has been advocated (134) (Table 33-7). Compared to repeated placement of external stents, the use of a metallic internal stent decreases stone recurrence, decreases the frequency of recurrent cholangitis, simplifies additional procedures, and is more convenient (134). Complications related to stent placement include biliary pleuritis, biliary peritonitis, hepatic artery aneurysm formation, hemobilia, intrahepatic arterial bleeding, subphrenic abscess, and sepsis and are reported to occur at a rate of 8% to 10% (134). The long-term effects of metallic stents on the biliary wall and epithelium are unknown. The most common causes of stent occlusion include recurrent stones, sludge, and epithelial hyperplasia. Stent occlusion rates are increased in the setting of pyogenic cholangitis.

TABLE 33-7

RECOMMENDATIONS FOR USE OF METALLIC STENTS

Failure of surgical intervention(s) with recurrent stones and/or strictures
Failure of previous dilation/stenting procedures
No evidence of cholangiocarcinoma
No history of pyogenic cholangitis
Refractory disease

COMPLICATIONS OF BILE DUCT RESECTION

Bile duct resections are performed for benign strictures, sclerosing cholangitis, choledochal cysts, benign neoplasms, or other less common problems. The main indication for biliary resection is malignancy of the biliary tree.

Benign biliary strictures include congenital and acquired strictures, with the vast majority of benign strictures being iatrogenic in nature. Blumgart has classified benign biliary strictures as congenital, post-traumatic, postradiotherapy, postoperative, and postinflammatory (58). Choledochal cysts, choledocholithiasis, chronic pancreatitis, biliary tract infections, peptic ulcer disease, subhepatic abscess, and primary sclerosing cholangitis (PSC) are etiologies for benign biliary strictures. The location and the extent of the stricture are important factors in choosing treatment options and in predicting outcome (Fig. 33-21). Following resection, reconstruction with a Roux-en-Y choledochojejunostomy or hepaticojejunostomy remains the treatment of choice. In selected situations, biliary bypass with either of the above procedures or choledochoduodenostomy is another treatment option. Several recent reports suggest that endoscopic management is also feasible, particularly in patients who are poor operative risks.

Complications of Biliary Resection

Typical presenting symptoms include jaundice, cholangitis, biliary fistulas, and bile peritonitis. Complicated presentations include right upper quadrant, hepatic, or subhepatic abscess formation or major vascular injury.

Mid-to-low level strictures (Type I and II) are generally repaired via hepaticojejunostomy (Table 33-8). High and diffuse strictures require the Hepp-Couinaud approach for repair.

TABLE 33-8

MODIFICATION OF BISMUTH CLASSIFICATION OF BILIARY STRICTURES

Type I	Papillary Stricture
Type II	Common bile duct stricture with common hepatic duct >2 cm in length
Type III	Common bile duct stricture with common hepatic duct <2 cm in length
Type IV	Common hepatic duct stricture with intact confluence
Type V	Stricture of the confluence with separation of the main ducts
Type VI	Stricture of an intrahepatic duct and of the common hepatic duct
Type VII	Stricture of an intrahepatic duct
Type VIII	Diffuse strictures of the biliary tree

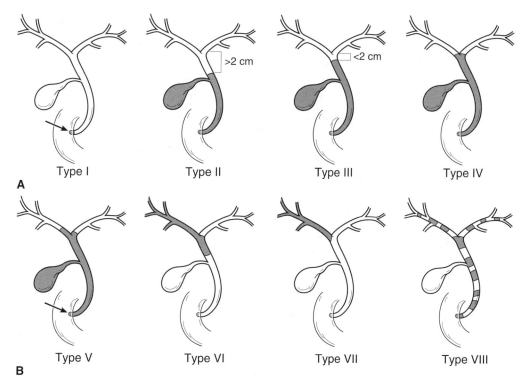

A

B

Figure 33-21 Classification of benign biliary strictures (see also Table 33-8).

Hepatic resection is the treatment of choice when ducts of a suitable size are not available for a biliary-enteric anastomosis and in cases of significant hepatic atrophy or fibrosis. This circumstance is most commonly seen for biliary strictures that are associated with vascular injury.

For postoperative papillary strictures (Type I), a repeat papillotomy (surgical or endoscopic) can be considered if the common bile duct is <2 cm in diameter, there is no biliary infection, and the stricture does not extend to involve the supraampullary portion of the bile duct. For failure of repeat papillotomy, biliary-enteric anastomosis is recommended (Table 33-9). Type II strictures are treated with hepaticojejunostomy. For Type III and IV strictures, Hepp-Couinaud hepaticojejunostomy to the left hepatic duct is the procedure of choice. Type V strictures are difficult to treat, particularly if the confluence cannot be

reconstructed. In this case, separate anastomosis of the right and left hepatic ducts to a single jejunal limb is appropriate. For Type VI strictures, hepatic resection of the affected segments or lobe with hepaticojejunostomy to the remaining duct is the recommended approach. Similarly, hepatic resection alone is the appropriate treatment for Type VII strictures. Type VIII strictures represent the most challenging problem. For these patients, attempts at percutaneous dilation may provide temporary palliation. Surgical treatment is usually limited to hepatic transplantation.

Early postoperative complications of these procedures include external biliary fistula and bile peritonitis, usually related to an anastomotic leak. If this complication occurs, percutaneous drainage of bile collections is the preferred approach, avoiding reoperation. If reoperation is required, it should not be combined with any attempts at biliary repair. Additional early complications include retained stones, pancreatic fistula, acute pancreatitis, and cholangitis. Late complications are primarily related to restenosis of the anastomosis with attendant risks for secondary biliary cirrhosis (Fig. 33-22). Long-term results and complications are related to the age and comorbidities of the patient and local biliary factors, specifically the site of the stricture, the number of previous attempts at repair, portal hypertension, cirrhosis, infection, and the surgeon's experience (135).

In a 21-year experience with the treatment of benign biliary strictures, postoperative mortality and morbidity rates were 2.6% and 20.1%, respectively, in general agreement with other series (135–140). Good results were

TABLE 33-9

PRINCIPLES FOR BILIARY-ENTERIC ANASTOMOSES

- Exposure of healthy bile duct
- Mucosa-to-mucosa anastomosis
- Tension-free anastomosis
- Single layer anastomosis
- Absorbable suture
- Watertight
- Minimal leakage of bile
- Placement of drains to evacuate any leakage of bile

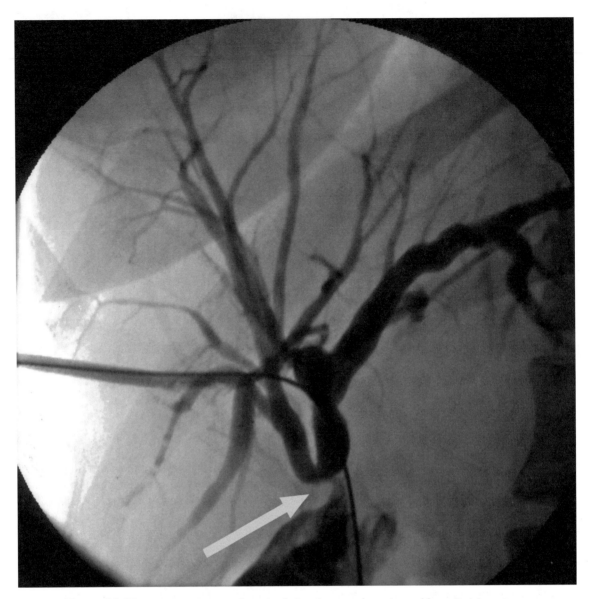

Figure 33-22 Percutaneous transhepatic cholangiogram of a strictured hepaticojejunostomy. This biliary-enteric anastomosis was originally performed following resection of a choledochal cyst. Arrow points to area of strictured biliary-enteric anastomosis. This is a Type IV stricture.

defined as the absence of cholestasis and infection, a moderate result was classified as sporadic and transient episodes of cholestasis and infection (once a year), and an unsatisfactory result was persistence of cholestasis, with or without infection. Unsatisfactory postoperative results are often related to liver failure due to secondary biliary cirrhosis.

The most important factor for postoperative morbidity is the presence of underlying cirrhosis and portal hypertension, resulting in an increased risk for perioperative bleeding and liver failure (136–140). In most series, postoperative morbidity ranges between 15% to 35% (136–140). Prior operations and repeated attempts at reconstruction also increase the risk of morbidity (136,137). Risk factors for recurrence of stricture include previous attempts at repair, age over 30, repair other than a Roux-en-Y, anastomotic

stenting of <1 month for complex, high-risk repairs, and a complex preoperative clinical course, particularly the presence of cirrhosis, portal hypertension, or liver abscess (138). Other risk factors for a poor outcome include the presence of a major vascular injury, active sepsis in the right upper quadrant, and the need for hepatic resection (64). The main reason for development of postoperative cholangitis is anastomotic narrowing, but other factors, such as intrahepatic strictures and excluded bile ducts, biliary calculi or debris, a short or poorly constructed Roux-en-Y loop, or conditions predisposing to bacterial overgrowth, such as the presence of foreign bodies or silk sutures, can contribute as well (139) (Table 33-10).

Overall, most series report a success rate at 7 years in the range of 75% to 93% (136–139). Late mortality from

TABLE 33-10

RISK FACTORS FOR RECURRENT BILIARY STRICTURE

Previous attempts at repair
Age >30
Repair other than a Roux-en-Y approach
Anastomotic stenting of <1 month for complex, high-risk repairs
Cirrhosis
Portal hypertension
Liver abscess
Major vascular injury
Active right upper quadrant sepsis
Hepatic resection

secondary biliary cirrhosis ranges from 0% to 6% in most recent series (136–140). In a series of 51 patients (136), 92% had a low anastomosis and 8% underwent a Hepp-Couinaud procedure. Postoperative complications were seen in 33% and there was a mortality rate of 2%. During an average 7.6-year follow-up period there was an 18% rate of restenosis requiring reoperation.

Endoscopic Dilation

Several recent studies suggest that percutaneous transhepatic biliary dilation can be successful in the treatment of biliary-enteric anastomotic strictures (64,141,142). In one study percutaneous transhepatic dilation was successful in 93% of anastomotic strictures and in 50% of patients with primary strictures, with a minimum follow-up of 2 years (64). Although the long-term results of some techniques are yet to be determined, a combination of surgical and interventional techniques is promising (143,144).

Operative Stenting

Stents are not recommended for wide anastomoses without residual pathology (135,145). In situations where a technically unsatisfactory anastomosis is performed in the absence of normal mucosa in the proximal biliary tree, and particularly when residual disease is noted, placement of a stent is recommended (135). Stents are not removed until serum liver function studies have normalized and healing and scarring are complete.

Nonoperative Placement of Metallic Stents

Although self-expanding metallic stents are quite useful in the treatment of inoperable malignant biliary strictures (146,147), their use in the treatment of benign strictures is controversial. One recent study (148) examined the results of the use of self-expanding metallic stents for the treatment of benign biliary strictures with a mean follow-up of 86 months. The authors concluded that surgical repair

should remain the mainstay of treatment for benign biliary strictures, with metallic stents reserved for patients who are poor surgical candidates and who have intrahepatic biliary strictures or after multiple unsuccessful attempts at operative repair (148). Most of the patients in this series developed recurrent cholangitis and stent obstruction and required reintervention. Ductal mucosal hyperplasia develops in response to stents and is a contributing factor to stent obstruction. The incorporation of the stent into the biliary wall can cause severe inflammation, which can complicate stent removal if this becomes necessary. The mean stent patency interval in this series was 30.6 months (148). In addition, there are concerns that chronic inflammation and obstruction may predispose to the development of cholangiocarcinoma. Although the risk of cholangiocarcinoma is well documented in association with PSC, it has not been previously documented in the context of other benign strictures (148).

Primary Sclerosing Cholangitis

Primary sclerosing cholangitis (PSC) is an idiopathic chronic inflammatory disease that results in multifocal intrahepatic and extrahepatic biliary strictures, chronic cholestasis, and eventual cirrhosis (Fig. 33-23). PSC is associated with the presence of ulcerative colitis. Symptoms of PSC include jaundice, fatigue, pruritis, and steatorrhea and are similar to other cholestatic diseases.

Approximately 50% of patients will eventually develop cirrhosis and liver failure (149). Hepatic transplantation is the preferred treatment once cirrhosis develops. There is a significant risk of developing cholangiocarcinoma in patients with long-standing PSC, and due to the difficulty in diagnosing cholangiocarcinoma in the setting of PSC, some experts advocate early transplantation (150). For patients with PSC, cholangiocarcinoma occurs at a rate of 10% to 15% over 5 years. In autopsy studies this rate is somewhat higher at 15% to 20%. One study suggests that cholangiocarcinoma is more common in patients with PSC and ulcerative colitis and concurrent colorectal neoplasia. Conversely, patients with both PSC and long-standing ulcerative colitis also have an increased risk of colorectal neoplasia relative to patients with ulcerative colitis alone (150).

Treatment options for PSC include primary immunosuppressive therapy, endoscopic and percutaneous dilation with or without stenting, and a variety of biliary surgical procedures (151–154). In properly selected patients, good results have been reported after extrahepatic biliary resection or bypass, with long-term improvement in jaundice and survival in noncirrhotic patients (151–154). In contrast, the results of less extensive biliary operations have been poor, and concerns have been raised about the wisdom of performing any extrahepatic biliary operations in a patient who may eventually require liver transplantation (151–154). Although PSC involves both the intrahepatic

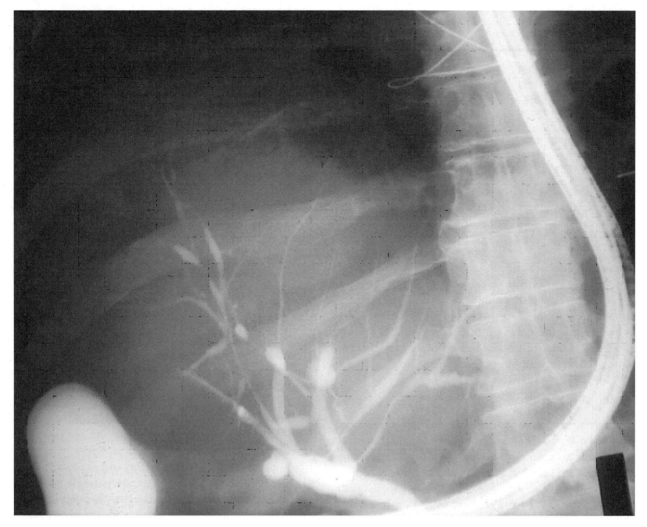

Figure 33-23 Endoscopic retrograde cholangiopancreaticography demonstrating primary sclerosing cholangitis.

and extrahepatic bile ducts in most patients, the hepatic duct bifurcation is often the most severely involved region (151). Therefore, the surgical approach must usually include resection of this area, with dilation of intrahepatic bile ducts and long-term stenting.

In a retrospective review of 146 patients over 15 years, patients with dominant extrahepatic and hilar strictures were managed with biliary resection, endoscopic dilation, and long-term percutaneous stenting; patients with end-stage liver disease underwent hepatic transplantation (151). Fifty patients underwent resection, with a 6% mortality rate. Operative mortality was 20% in patients with cirrhosis and 2.5% in those without cirrhosis. The postoperative complication rate was 32%, with cholangitis being the most common problem, followed by hemobilia related to the transhepatic stenting, sepsis, and liver failure.

Because endoscopic and percutaneous techniques avoid operation prior to potential hepatic transplant, these techniques have become popular in the management of PSC. In one study endoscopic biliary dilation and percutaneous

stenting was performed in 60 patients (151). Thirty-five patients were dilated a mean of 3.2 times. In four patients the initial attempt at dilation was unsuccessful, and no further dilations were attempted. The overall complication rate was 14%, with mild pancreatitis being most common. No mortality was related to endoscopic dilation. Nineteen patients were managed with long-term percutaneous stenting, and two deaths occurred in this group (10.5%). The overall complication rate for endoscopic dilation and long-term percutaneous stenting was 42%, with cholangitis, hemobilia, sepsis, and liver failure occurring most commonly.

The treatment of choice for patients with cirrhosis is liver transplantation. An increased incidence of redevelopment of PSC in the transplanted liver occurs, with need for retransplantation in some patients. Operative time is significantly shorter in patients who have not undergone prior biliary tract operation, but prior operation does not increase operative blood loss or mortality. The 3-year survival after hepatic transplantation now approximates 85% (155).

When these four treatment options are compared, patients without cirrhosis do well in response to extrahepatic biliary resection, with 5-year survivals of 85% and 10-year survivals of 68%. Transplant-free survival rate after biliary resection at 10 years is only 31%. For noncirrhotic patients undergoing endoscopic biliary dilation, 5-year survival is 58%, which is significantly lower than that for the biliary resection group. Similarly, for patients undergoing percutaneous stenting, the 5-year survival for noncirrhotic patients is 63% (156). In summary, overall and transplant-free survival after extrahepatic biliary resection is significantly longer in noncirrhotic patients than after nonoperative biliary drainage.

Although the prognosis for cholangiocarcinoma remains poor, surgical resection offers the only chance for prolonged survival. Many patients are not candidates for curative resection but still require biliary decompression for palliation. Painless jaundice is the most frequent presenting symptom in these patients; accompanying pruritis is also a common manifestation.

Classification of Biliary Tumors

The standard classification of biliary tumors is the Bismuth-Corlette classification (Table 33-11, Fig. 33-24). Some groups have simplified the classification of biliary tumors into intrahepatic, perihilar, and distal. Intrahepatic tumors are defined as those confined to the liver, not involving the extrahepatic biliary tree, and not presenting with jaundice. Intrahepatic tumors generally require hepatic resection for surgical treatment. Perihilar tumors involve the extrahepatic biliary tree, including the bifurcation, and require resection of the biliary tree, sometimes in combination with hepatic resection. Distal tumors involve the extrahepatic biliary tree, usually spare the confluence, are often located in the intrapancreatic portion of the bile duct, and generally require pancreaticoduodenectomy for surgical resection.

Although cholangiocarcinoma is considered a slow-growing tumor, it has a propensity for local extension, most importantly the portal vein and hepatic artery. Local extension coupled with spread along the perineural tissues and in the subepithelium of the bile duct pose significant obstacles to obtaining histologically negative surgical margins (Fig. 33-25).

TABLE 33-11

CLASSIFICATION OF KLATSKIN TUMORS

Type I	Limited to the Confluence
Type II	Tumor involves the confluence with extension up the right or left duct, sparing the opposite duct
Type III	Tumor involves the segmental branches of either the right or the left duct, sparing the opposite side
Type IV	Tumor extends into the segmental branches of both the right and left ducts

Although patients usually present with jaundice, occasionally unilateral or segmental biliary obstruction may result in hepatic atrophy without the development of frank jaundice. Compensatory hypertrophy of the opposite lobe may accompany the development of lobar atrophy. This growth can result in significant distortion of portal anatomy, with rotation of the vascular structures, placing the portal vein in a more superficial position and making this structure more prone to injury during dissection. Any resection that leaves only residual atrophic hepatic parenchyma places the patient at risk for postoperative hepatic failure (Figs. 33-26 and 33-27).

Outcomes and Complications

An aggressive approach to cholangiocarcinoma, with the goal of negative margins, is the most important predictor of survival (157). In most large series surgical exploration is attempted in 70% to 85% of patients, with 10% to 22% of those patients undergoing exploration only, 13% to 18% receiving a palliative surgical procedure, and the remaining 40% to 65% undergoing curative resection (158). Despite curative resection, long-term survival in these patients is only 25% to 32%. The inclusion of hepatic resection and pancreaticoduodenectomy increases long-term survival in some series (158). Surgical treatment with intent for cure often requires a major hepatic resection combined with extrahepatic biliary resection. Recent literature suggests that these radical surgical procedures can be performed safely (157,158).

The recommended operative approach involves en bloc resection of the common bile duct, cystic duct, gallbladder,

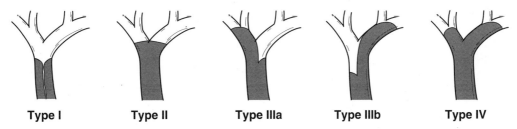

Type I   Type II   Type IIIa   Type IIIb   Type IV

Figure 33-24   Classification of malignant biliary strictures (see also Table 33-11).

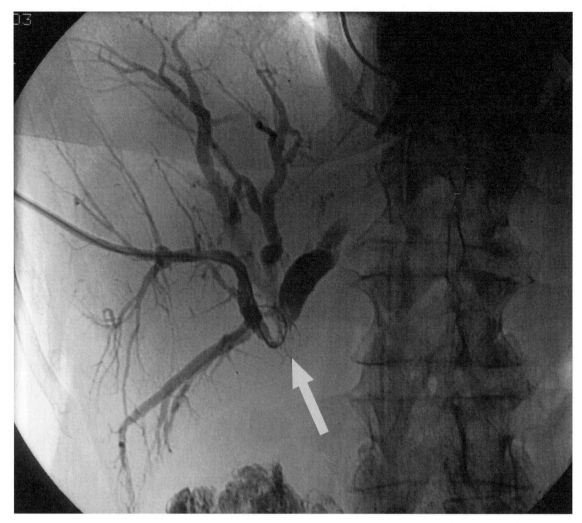

Figure 33-25 Percutaneous transhepatic cholangiogram demonstrating an unresectable cholangiocarcinoma at the bifurcation of the right and left hepatic ducts (Klatskin tumor). Arrow illustrates tumor location.

and common hepatic duct, including the confluence, if involved. The proximal bile duct is transected as far above the grossly visible tumor in the hilum as possible, and the entire specimen is sent for frozen section. If the margins are positive, additional ductal resection with frozen section is performed until margins are microscopically negative or the limits of resection are obtained. Bismuth I and II tumors are amendable to extrahepatic biliary resection; the addition of vascular resection to this procedure does not improve long-term survival (159). For Type III tumors, extensive extrahepatic biliary resection should be combined with hepatic resection, with a goal of a tumor-free margin. Although the morbidity and mortality rates for these types of resection are high, survival rates have improved with this approach (159).

In a study of 88 consecutive patients with cholangiocarcinoma, 67% underwent major resection with curative intent (157). Unresectable patients were usually treated with endoscopic or percutaneous placement of metallic

stents for palliation (157). A hilar lesion with extension into the secondary biliary radicals was the most common reason for unresectability in tumors without evidence of distant metastatic disease. Tumor differentiation and location did not correlate with survival (157). Complete resection with negative margins was the only positive predictor of survival, and survival times were directly related to the tumor stage in these patients. Five-year survival for Stage I and II disease is 14% to 33%, while for Stage III disease and above, survival decreases to 0% to 25% (157,158). Survival after palliative operations is usually <1 year (157,158). Unresectable patients palliated nonoperatively have a significantly increased survival relative to unresectable patients treated operatively (157). Perioperative mortality was 9.3%, and morbidity in this series was 29%, with abscess, biliary leak, hemorrhage, and myocardial infarction occurring most frequently (157).

With the simplified categorization of biliary tumors into intrahepatic, perihilar, and distal, morbidity and mortality

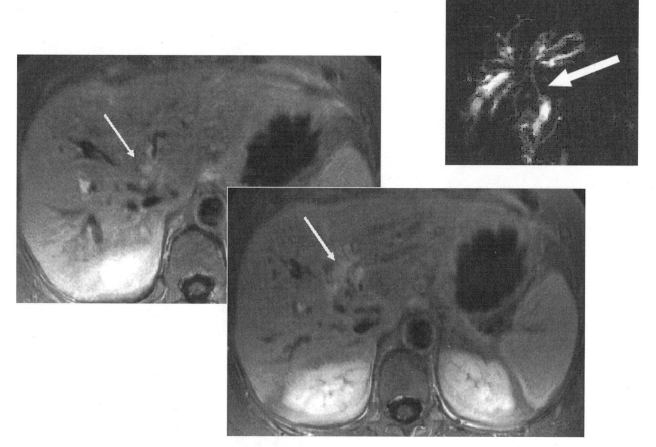

Figure 33-26 MRCP demonstrating a cholangiocarcinoma. Large arrow illustrates malignant stricture at and involving the bifurcation of the hepatic ducts. Small arrows demonstrate areas of tumor within the liver parenchyma.

following surgical resection are intrahepatic: mortality—6%, morbidity—22%, perihilar: mortality—4%, morbidity—47%, and distal: mortality—1%, morbidity—33% (160). Wound infection is the most common complication, followed by cholangitis and pancreatic or biliary fistula. Complications are not significantly different by site, although delayed gastric emptying and postoperative fistulas were more common in patients with distal tumors (160). Multivariate analysis shows that negative microscopic margins, preoperative serum albumin, and postoperative sepsis are important predictors of survival (160).

Most series report a relatively high complication rate following surgical treatments for cholangiocarcinoma, often up to 65%, with mortality rates of 9% to 14% (157,159). The most common acute complications include bile leak, biloma, hemobilia, hepatic or intra-abdominal abscess, hemorrhage, cholangitis, biliary fistula, pulmonary complications, and liver failure (157–159,161) (Table 33-12). Long-term complications included cholangitis and biliary obstruction, usually from tumor recurrence, which is noted in 37% of patients at a mean of 15 months postoperatively (157). Local recurrence is more common than distant. Nonsurgical stenting is palliative for local tumor recurrence after resection. Liver transplantation

for cholangiocarcinoma has a 50% tumor recurrence rate in the first year posttransplant.

Prolonged survival with this disease is associated with tumor resectability. Some investigators have found that tumor location is an important determinant for survival, but other investigators have not found this variable to be important. Tumor histology has been related to outcome in some, but not in all, studies (157–159,161,162,163). Tumor location in the distal one-third of the biliary system, tumor histology, papillary histology, and resectability appear to be the most important variables in predicting a favorable outcome (157–159,161,162,163). The papillary

TABLE 33-12

RISK FACTORS OF RESECTION OF HILAR CHOLANGIOCARCINOMA

Preoperative albumin <3.5 g/L
Extended liver resection
Vascular resection

From Gerhards MF, van Gulik TM, de Wit L, et al. Evaluation of morbidity and mortality after resection for hilar cholangiocarcinoma—a single center experience. *Surgery* 2000;127:395–404, with permission.

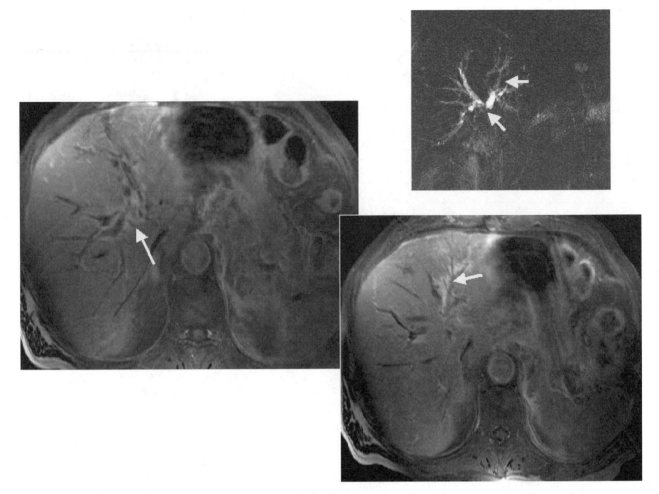

Figure 33-27   MRCP demonstrating a cholangiocarcinoma. Arrows demonstrate areas of tumor.

variant is most common in the distal biliary tree, while sclerosing histology predominates in the more proximal biliary tree, particularly in the region of the hilum. In addition, microscopically negative margins are a very important predictor of survival. Since cholangiocarcinoma has a propensity to spread proximally and distally within the biliary tree, it is often difficult to achieve microscopically negative margins. Positive biliary margins have been reported in 28% to 89% of cases following perihilar resection (160,164). It has been suggested that neoadjuvant chemoradiation may improve the ability to achieve negative microscopic margins after surgery, but postoperative chemotherapy and radiation therapy has not been shown to improve overall survival (160,164).

Palliation

Nonoperative palliation usually includes percutaneous or endoscopic placement of stents. In one report, while stenting was possible in 73%, adequate relief of jaundice occurred in only 41% of these patients (165). Complications in this series included cholangitis, pancreatitis, and bleeding from the papillotomy site (165). Other methods include placement of bilateral metallic stents (166). This technique had an 88% success rate and an equal probability for the relief of jaundice.

REFERENCES

1. Couse NF, Delaney CP, Gorey TF. Evolving management of biliary tract disease. In: Nyhus LM, ed. *Surgery annual.* Norwalk, CT: Appleton & Lange; 1993:231–253.
2. Herman R. The spectrum of biliary stone disease. *Am J Surg* 1991;161:171–173.
3. McMahon AJ, Russell IT, Baxter JN, et al. Laparoscopic versus mini-laparotomy cholecystectomy: a randomized trial. *Lancet* 1994;1:135–138.
4. Cosenza CA, Saffari B, Jabbour N, et al. Surgical management of biliary gallstone disease during pregnancy. *Am J Surg* 1999;178: 545–548.
5. Lo C, Lai ECS, Fan S, et al. Laparoscopic cholecystectomy for acute cholecystitis in the elderly. *World J Surg* 1996;20:983–987.
6. Roslyn JJ, Pinns GS, Hughes EF. Open cholecystectomy: a contemporary analysis of 42,474 patients. *Ann Surg* 1993;218: 129–137.
7. Strasberg SM, Hertl M, Soper NJ. An analysis of the problem of biliary injury during laparoscopic cholecystectomy. *J Am Coll Surg* 1995;180:101–125.

8. Deziel DJ, Millikan KW, Econonou SG, et al. Complications of laparoscopic cholecystectomy: a national survey of 4,292 hospitals and an analysis of 77,604 cases. *Am J Surg* 1993;165:9–14.
9. Wherry DC, Rob CG, Marohn MR, et al. An external audit of laparoscopic cholecystectomy in the steady state performed in medical treatment facilities of the Department of Defense. *Ann Surg* 1994;220:626–634.
10. Adamsen S, Hansen OH, Funch-Jensen P, et al. Bile duct injury during laparoscopic cholecystectomy: a prospective nationwide series. *J Am Coll Surg* 1997;184:571–578.
11. Richardson MC, Bell G, Fullarton GM. Incidence and nature of bile duct injuries following laparscopic cholecystectomy: an audit of 5,913 cases. *Br J Surg* 1996;83:1356–1360.
12. Gouma DJ, Go PM. Bile duct injury during laparoscopic cholecystectomy and conventional cholecystectomy. *J Am Coll Surg* 1994;178:229–233.
13. Chapman WC, Abecassis M, Jarnigan W, et al. Bile duct injuries 12 years after the introduction of laparoscopic cholecystectomy. *J Gastrointest Surg* 2003;7:412–416.
14. Davidoff AM, Pappas TN, Murray EA, et al. Mechanisms of major biliary injury during laparoscopic cholecystectomy. *Ann Surg* 1992;215:196–202.
15. Branum G, Schmitt C, Baille J, et al. Management of major biliary complications after laparoscopic cholecystectomy. *Ann Surg* 1993;217:532–541.
16. Strasberg SM, Eagon CJ, Drebin JA. The "hidden cystic duct syndrome" and the infundibular technique of laparoscopic cholecystectomy—the danger of the false infundibulum. *J Am Coll Surg* 2000;191:661–667.
17. Archer SB, Brown DW, Smith CD, et al. Bile duct injury during laparoscopic cholecystectomy. Results of a national survey. *Ann Surg* 2001;234:549–559.
18. Barkun JS, Barkun AM, Meakins JL. Laparoscopic versus open cholecystectomy: the Canadian experience. *Am J Surg* 1993;165:455–458.
19. Flum DR, Dellinger EP, Cheadle A, et al. Intraoperative cholangiography and risk of common bile duct injury during cholecystectomy. *JAMA* 2003;289:1639–1644.
20. Flum DR, Flowers C, Veenstra DL. A cost-effectiveness analysis of intraoperative cholangiography in the prevention of bile duct injury during laparoscopic cholecystectomy. *J Am Coll Surg* 2003;196:385–393.
21. Woods MS, Traverso LW, Kozarck RA, et al. Characteristics of biliary tract complications during laparoscopic cholecystectomy: a multi-institutional study. *Am J Surg* 1994;167:27–34.
22. Deziel DJ. Complications of cholecystectomy: incidence, clinical manifestations, and diagnosis. *Surg Clin North Am* 1994;74:809–823.
23. Wright KD, Wellwood JM. Bile duct injury during laparoscopic cholecystectomy without operative cholangiography. *Br J Surg* 1998;85:191–194.
24. Fletcher DR. Biliary injury at laparoscopic cholecystectomy: recognition and prevention. *Aust NZ J Surg* 1993;63:673–677.
25. Snow LL, Weinstein LS, Hannon JK, et al. Evaluation of operative cholangiography in 2043 patients undergoing laparoscopic cholecystectomy. *Surg Endosc* 2001;15:14–20.
26. Fletcher DR, Hobbs MS, Tan P, et al. Complications of cholecystectomy: risks of the laparoscopic approach and protective effects of operative cholangiography: a population-based study. *Ann Surg* 1999;229:449–457.
27. Vezakis A, Davides D, Ammori BJ, et al. Intraoperative cholangiography during laparoscopic cholecystectomy. *Surg Endosc* 2000;14:1118–1122.
28. Soper NJ, Denegan DL. Routine versus selective intra-operative cholangiography during laparoscopic cholecystectomy. *World J Surg* 1992;16:1133–1140.
29. Ohtani T, Kawal C, Shirai Y, et al. Intraoperative ultrasonography versus cholangiography during laparoscopic cholecystectomy: A prospective comparative study. *J Am Coll Surg* 1997;185:274–282.
30. Biffl WL, Moore EE, Offner PJ, et al. Routine intraoperative laparoscopic ultrasonography with selective cholangiography reduces bile duct complications during laparoscopic cholecystectomy. *J Am Coll Surg* 2001;193:272–280.
31. Bauer TW, Morris JB, Lowenstein A, et al. The consequences of a major bile duct injury during laparoscopic cholecystectomy. *J Gastrointest Surg* 1998;2:61–66.
32. Lillemoe KD, Martin SA, Cameron JL, et al. Major bile duct injuries during laparoscopic cholecystectomy: follow-up after combined surgical and radiological management. *Ann Surg* 1997;225:459–471.
33. Ferguson CM, Rattner DW, Warshaw AL. Bile duct injury in laparoscopic cholecystectomy. *Surg Laparosc Endosc* 1992;2:1–7.
34. Kozarek RA, Traverso LW. Endoscopic stent placement for cystic duct leaks after laparoscopic cholecystectomy. *Gastrointest Endosc* 1991;37:71–72.
35. Vitale GC, Stephens G, Wieman TJ, et al. Use of endoscopic retrograde cholangiography in the management of biliary complications after laparoscopic cholecystectomy. *Surgery* 1993;114:806–814.
36. Soper NJ, Flye MW, Brunt LM, et al. Diagnosis and management of biliary complications of laparoscopic cholecystectomy. *Am J Surg* 1993;165:663–669.
37. Asbun HF, Rossi RL, Lowell JA, et al. Bile duct injury during laparoscopic cholecystectomy: mechanism of injury, prevention, and management. *World J Surg* 1993;17:547–552.
38. Roy AF, Rassi RB, Lapointe RW, et al. Bile duct injury during laparoscopic cholecystectomy. *Can J Surg* 1993;36:509–516.
39. Cotton PB, Lehman G, Vennes J, et al. Endoscopic sphincterotomy complications and their management: an attempt at consensus. *Gastrointest Endosc* 1991;37:383–393.
40. Sherman S, Ruffolo TA, Hawes RH, et al. Complications of endoscopic sphincterotomy. A prospective series with emphasis on the increased risk associated with sphincter of Odi dysfunction and non-dilated ducts. *Gastroenterology* 1991;101:1068–1075.
41. Tsalis KG, Christoforidis EC, Dimitriadis CA, et al. Management of bile duct injury during and after laparoscopic cholecystectomy. *Surg Endosc* 2003;17:31–37.
42. Keulemans YC, Bergman JJ, de Wit TH, et al. Improvement in the management of bile duct injuries? *J Am Coll Surg* 1998;187:246–254.
43. Topal B, Aerts R, Penninckx F. The outcome of major biliary tract injury with leakage in laparoscopic cholecystectomy. *Surg Endosc* 1999;13:53–56.
44. Wudel LJ, Wright KJ, Pinson CW, et al. Bile duct injury following laparoscopic cholecystectomy. *Am Surg* 2001;67:557–564.
45. Blumgart LH, Kelley CJ, Benjamin IS. Benign bile duct stricture following cholecystectomy: critical factors in management. *Br. J Surg* 1984;71:836–843.
46. Lillemoe KD, Pitt HA, Cameron JL. Current management of benign bile duct strictures. *Adv Surg* 1992;25:119–175.
47. Gupta N, Solomon H, Fairchild R, et al. Management and outcome of patients with combined bile duct and hepatic artery injuries. *Arch Surg* 1998;133:176–181.
48. Majno PE, Pretu R, Mentha G, et al. Operative injury to the hepatic artery. Consequences of a biliary-enteric anastomosis and principles for rational management. *Arch Surg* 1996;131:211–215.
49. Lillemoe KD, Melton GB, Cameron JL, et al. Post-operative bile duct strictures: management and outcome in the 1990's. *Ann Surg* 2000;232:430–441.
50. Johnson SR, Keohler A, Pennington LK, et al. Long-term results of surgical repair of bile duct injuries following laparoscopic cholecystectomy. *Surgery* 2000;128:668–677.
51. Murr MM, Gigot JF, Nagorney DM, et al. Long-term results of biliary reconstruction after laparoscopic bile duct injuries. *Arch Surg* 1999;134:604–610.
52. Mercado MA, Chan C, Orozco H, et al. Acute bile duct injury. *Surg Endosc* 2003;17:1351–1355.
53. Stewart L, Way LW. Bile duct injuries during laparoscopic cholecystectomy. *Arch Surg* 1995;130:1123–1129.
54. Flum DR, Cheadle A, Prela C, et al. Bile duct injury during cholecystectomy and survival in Medicare beneficiaries. *JAMA* 2003;290:2168–2173.
55. Christoforidis E, Goulimaris I, Tsalis K, et al. The endoscopic management of persistent bile leakage after laparoscopic cholecystectomy. *Surg Endosc* 2002;16:843–846.

56. Christensen RA, van Sonnenberg E, Nemcek AA, et al. Inadvertent ligation of the aberrant right hepatic duct at cholecystectomy: radiologic diagnosis and therapy. *Radiology* 1992; 183:549–553.

57. Tochi A, Costa G, Lepre L, et al. The long-term outcome of hepaticojejunostomy in the treatment of benign bile duct strictures. *Ann Surg* 1996;224:162–167.

58. Blumgart LH. Benign biliary strictures. In: Blumgart LH, ed. *Surgery of the liver and biliary tract. I.* Edinburgh: Churchill Livingston; 1998:721–752.

59. Hepp J. Hepaticojejunostomy using the left biliary trunk for iatrogenic biliary lesions: the French connection. *World J Surg* 1985;9:507–511.

60. Mercado MA, Orozco H, de la Garza L, et al. Biliary duct injury: partial segment IV resection for intrahepatic reconstruction of biliary lesions. *Arch Surg* 1999;134:1008–1010.

61. Huang CS, Lein HH, Tai FC, et al. Long-term results of major bile duct injury associated with laparoscopic cholecystectomy. *Surg Endosc* 2003;17:1362–1367.

62. Jarnigan WR, Blumgart LH. Operative repair of bile duct injuries involving the confluence. *Arch Surg* 1999;134:769–775.

63. Lichtenstein S, Moorman DW, Malatesta JQ, et al. The role of hepatic resection in the management of bile duct injuries following laparoscopic cholecystectomy. *Am Surg* 2000;66: 372–377.

64. Millis JM, Tompkins RK, Zinner MJ, et al. Management of bile duct strictures: an evolving strategy. *Arch Surg* 1992;127:1077–1084.

65. Blumgart LH, Kelly CJ, Benjamin IS. Benign bile duct stricture following cholecystectomy: critical factors in management. *Br J Surg* 1984;71:836–843.

66. Koffron A, Ferrario M, Parsons W, et al. Failed primary management of iatrogenic biliary injury: incidence and significance of concomitant hepatic arterial disruption. *Surgery* 2001;130: 722–731.

67. Terblanche J, Worhtley CS, Krige JE. High or low hepaticojejunostomy for bile duct strictures? *Surgery* 1990;108:828–834.

68. Northover JM, Terblanche J. A new look at the arterial blood supply of the bile duct in man and its surgical implications. *Br J Surg* 1979;66:379–384.

69. Johnson SR, Koehler A, Pennington LK, et al. Long-term results of surgical repair of bile duct injuries following laparoscopic cholecystectomy. *Surgery* 2000;128:668–677.

70. Tocchi A, Mazzoni G, Liotta G, et al. Management of benign biliary strictures: biliary enteric anastomosis vs endoscopic stenting. *Arch Surg* 2000;135:153–157.

71. Bonnel D, Ligoury C, Lefebvre J, et al. Placement of metallic stents for treatment of post-operative biliary strictures: long-term outcome in 25 patients. *Am J Roentgenol* 1997;169:1517–1522.

72. Mercado MA, Chan D, Orozco H, et al. To stent or not to stent bilioenteric anastomosis after iatrogenic injury: a dilemma not answered? *Arch Surg* 2002;137:60–63.

73. Moraca RJ, Lee FT, Ryan JA, et al. Long-term biliary function after reconstruction of major bile duct injuries with hepaticoduodenostomy or hepaticojejunostomy. *Arch Surg* 2002;137:889–894.

74. Johnson SR, Koehler A, Pennington LK, et al. Long-term results of surgical repair of bile duct injuries following laparscopic cholecystectomy. *Surgery* 2000;128:668–677.

75. Pitt HA, Miyamoto T, Parapatis SK, et al. Factors influencing outcome in patients with post-operative biliary strictures. *Am J Surg* 1982;144:14–21.

76. Friedman SL. Hepatic fibrosis. In: Schiff ER, Sorrell MF, Maddrey WC, eds. *Diseases of the liver,* 8th ed. Philadelphia: Lippincott–Raven Publishers; 1999:371–386.

77. Moosa AR, Easter DW, van Sonnenber E, et al. Laparoscopic injuries to the bile duct. A cause for concern. *Ann Surg* 1992; 215:203–208.

78. Savader SJ, Lillemoe KD, Prescott CA, et al. Laparoscopic cholecystectomy-related bile duct injuries: a health and financial disaster. *Ann Surg* 1997;225:268–273.

79. Chapman WC, Halevy A, Blumgart LH, et al. Post-cholecystectomy bile duct strictures. *Arch Surg* 1995;130:597–604.

80. Molloy M, Sorrell MJ, Bower RH, et al. Patterns of morbidity and resource consumption associated with laparoscopic cholecystectomy in a VA medical center. *J Surg Res* 1999;81:15–20.

81. Kama NA, Doganay M, Dolapci M, et al. Risk factors resulting in conversion of laparoscopic cholecystectomy to open surgery. *Surg Endosc* 2001;15:965–968.

82. Merriam LT, Sannaan SA, Dawes LG, et al. Gangrenous cholecystitis: analysis of risk factors and experience with laparoscopic cholecystectomy. *Surgery* 1999;126:680–686.

83. Barie PS, Fischer E. Acute acalculous cholecystitis. *J Am Coll Surg* 1995;180:232–244.

84. Dorrance HR, Lingam MK, Hair A, et al. Acquired abnormalities of the biliary tract from chronic gallstone disease. *J Am Coll Surg* 1999;189:269–273.

85. Redaelli CA, Buchler MW, Schilling MK, et al. High coincidence of Mirizzi syndrome and gallbladder carcinoma. *Surgery* 1997;121: 58–63.

86. Iber FL, Caruso G, Polepalle C, et al. Increasing prevalence of gallstones in male veterans with alcoholic cirrhosis. *Am J Gastroenterol* 1990;85:1593–1596.

87. Diehl AK. Epidemiology and natural history of gallstone disease. *Gastroenterol Clin North Am* 1991;20:1–19.

88. Friel CM, Stack J, Forse RA, et al. Laparoscopic cholecystectomy in patients with hepatic cirrhosis: a five year experience. *J Gastrointest Surg* 1999;3:286–291.

89. Poggio JL, Rowland CM, Gores GJ, et al. A comparison of laparoscopic and open cholecystectomy in patients with compensated cirrhosis and symptomatic gallstone disease. *Surgery* 2000;127: 405–411.

90. Memon MA, Deeik RK, Maffi TR, et al. The outcome of unretrieved gallstones in the peritoneal cavity during laparoscopic cholecystectomy. *Surg Endosc* 1999;13:848–857.

91. Rice DC, Memom MA, Jamison RL, et al. Long-term consequences of intraoperative spillage of bile and gallstones during laparoscopic cholecystectomy. *J Gastrointest Surg* 1997;1:85–91.

92. Paolucci V, Schaeff B, Schneider M, et al. Tumor seeding following laparoscopy: international survey. *World J Surg* 1999;23: 898–997.

93. Sarli L, Contini S, Sansebastiano G, et al. Does laparoscopic cholecystectomy worsen the prognosis of unsuspected gallbladder cancer? *Arch Surg* 2000;135:1340–1344.

94. Behari A, Sikora SS, Wagholikar GD, et al. Longterm survival after extended resections in patients with gallbladder cancer. *J Am Coll Surg* 2003;196:82–88.

95. Othani T, Takano Y, Shiray Y, et al. Early intraperitoneal dissemination after radical resection of unsuspected gallbladder carcinoma following laparoscopic cholecystectomy. *Surg Laparosc Endosc* 1998;8:58–62.

96. Suzuki K, Kimura T, Ogawa H. Is laparoscopic cholecystectomy hazardous for gallbladder cancer? *Surgery* 1998;123:311–314.

97. Suzuki K, Kimura T, Ogawa H. Long-term prognosis of gallbladder cancer diagnosed after laparoscopic cholecystectomy. *Surg Endosc* 2000;14:712–716.

98. Ricardo AE, Feig BW, Ellis LM, et al. Gallbladder cancer and trocar site recurrence. *Am J Surg* 1997;174:619–623.

99. Tsukada K, Hatakeyama K, Kurosaki I, et al. Outcome of radical surgery for carcinoma of the gallbladder according to the TNM stage. *Surgery* 1996;120:816–821.

100. Double M, King G, Thomas WM, et al. The movement of mucosal cells of the gallbladder within the peritoneal cavity during laparoscopic cholecystectomy. *Surg Endosc* 1996;10:1092–1094.

101. Champault G, Taffinder N, Ziol M, et al. Cells are present in the smoke created during laparoscopic cholecystectomy. *Br J Surg* 1997;84:993–995.

102. Wu JS, Brasfield EB, Guo LW, et al. Implantation of colon cancer at trocar sites is increased by low pressure pneumoperitoneum. *Surgery* 1997;122:1–7.

103. Fligelstone L, Rhodes M, Flook D, et al. Tumour inoculation during laparoscopy. *Lancet* 1993;342:368–369.

104. Kapoor VK, Benjamin IS. Resectional surgery for gallbladder cancer. *Br J Surg* 1998;85:145–146.

105. Yoshida T, Matsumoto T, Sasaki A, et al. Laparoscopic cholecystectomy in the treatment of patients with gallbladder cancer. *J Am Coll Surg* 2000;191:158–163.

106. Bartlett DL, Fong Y, Fortner JG, et al. Long-term results after resection for gallbladder cancer: implications for staging and management. *Ann Surg* 1996;224:639–646.

107. Whalen GF, Bird I, Tanski W, et al. Laparoscopic cholecystectomy does not demonstrably decrease survival of patients with serendipitously treated gallbladder cancer. *J Am Coll Surg* 2001;192:189–195.
108. Chijiiwa K, Nakano K, Ueda J, et al. Surgical treatment of patients with T2 gallbladder carcinoma invading the subserosal layer. *J Am Coll Surg* 2001;192:600–607.
109. Houdart R, Perniceni T, Darne B, et al. Predicting common duct lithiasis: determination and prospective validation of a model predicting low risk. *Am J Surg* 1995;170:38–43.
110. Heili MJ, Wintz NK, Fowler DL. Choledocholithiasis: endoscopic versus laparoscopic management. *Am Surg* 1999;65:135–138.
111. Cetta F. Do surgical and endoscopic sphincterotomy prevent or facilitate recurrent common duct stone formation? *Arch Surg* 1993;128:329–336.
112. Snow LL, Weinstein LS, Hannon JK, et al. Management of bile duct stones in 1572 patients undergoing laparoscopic cholecystectomy. *Am Surg* 1999;65:530–547.
113. Cuschiere AAA, Croce E, Faggioni A, et al. EAES ductal stone study. *Surg Endosc* 1996;10:1130–1135.
114. Park AE, Mastrangelo MJ. Endoscopic retrograde cholangiopancreatography in the management of choledocholithiasis. *Surg Endosc* 2000;14:219–226.
115. Lambert ME, Betts CD, Hill J, et al. Endoscopic sphincterotomy: the whole truth. *Br J Surg* 1991;78:473–476.
116. Arregui ME, Cavis CJ, Arquash AM, et al. Laparoscopic cholecystectomy combined with endoscopic sphincterotomy and stone extraction or laparoscopic choledochoscopy and electrohydraulic lithotripsy for management of cholelithiasis and choledocholithiasis. *Surg Endosc* 1992;6:10–15.
117. Carr-Locke DL. Acute gallstone pancreatitis and endoscopic therapy. *Endoscopy* 1990;22:180–183.
118. Cotton PB. Endoscopic management of bile duct stones (apples and oranges). *Gut* 1984;25:587–597.
119. Tung-Ping Poon R, Liu CL, Lo CM, et al. Management of gallstone cholangitis in the era of laparoscopic cholecystectomy. *Arch Surg* 2001;136:11–16.
120. Suc B, Escat J, Cherquai D, et al. Surgery vs. endoscopy as the primary treatment in symptomatic patients with suspected common bile duct stones. *Arch Surg* 1998;133:702–708.
121. Trias M, Targarona EM, Ros E, et al. Prospective evaluation of a minimally invasive approach for treatment of bile duct calculi in the high-risk patient. *Surg Endosc* 1997;11:632–635.
122. Fitzgibbons RJ Jr, Deeik RK, Martinez-Serna T. Eight years experience with the use of a transcystic common bile duct duodenal double-lumen catheter for the treatment of choledocholithiasis. *Surgery* 1998;124:699–705.
123. Boender J, Nix GA, de Ridder MA, et al. Endoscopic sphincterotomy and biliary drainage in patients with cholangitis due to common bile duct stones. *Am J Gastroenterol* 1995;90:233–238.
124. Cetta F. The possible role of sphincteroplasty and surgical sphincterotomy in the pathogenesis of recurrent common duct brown stones. *HBP Surg* 1991;4:261–270.
125. Hakamada K, Sasaki M, Endoh M, et al. Late development of bile duct cancer after sphincteroplasty: a ten- to twenty-two-year follow-up study. *Surgery* 1997;121:488–492.
126. Panis Y, Fagniez PL, Brisser D, et al. Long term results of choledochoduodenostomy versus choledochojejunostomy for choledocholithiasis. *Surg Gynecol Obstet* 1993;176:33–37.
127. Otani K, Shimizu S, Chijiiwa K, et al. Comparison of treatments for hepatolithiasis: hepatic resection versus cholangioscopic lithotomy. *J Am Coll Surg* 1999;189:177–182.
128. Jan YY, Chen MF, Wang CS, et al. Surgical treatment of hepatolithiasis: long-term results. *Surgery* 1996;120:509–514.
129. Fan ST, Lai ELS, Mok FPT, et al. Acute cholangitis secondary to hepatolithiasis. *Arch Surg* 1991;126:1027–1031.
130. Nakayama F, Soloway RD, Nakama T, et al. Hepatolithiasis in East Asia: retrospective study. *Dig Dis Sci* 1986;31:21–26.
131. Chen MF, Jan YY, Wang CS, et al. A reappraisal of cholangiocarcinoma in patients with hepatolithiasis. *Cancer* 1993;71:2461–2465.
132. Chijiiwa K, Kameoka N, Komura M, et al. Hepatic resection for hepatolithiasis and long-term results. *J Am Coll Surg* 1995;180:43–48.
133. Sheen PC, Ker CG. Postoperative choledochofiberscopy. In: Okuda K, ed. *Intrahepatic calculi*. New York: Liss; 1984:303–319.
134. Jeng KS, Sheen IS, Yang FS. Are expandable metallic stents better than conventional methods for treating difficult intrahepatic biliary strictures with recurrent hepatolithiasis? *Arch Surg* 1999;134:267–273.
135. Frattaroli FM, Reggio D, Guadalaxara A, et al. Benign biliary strictures: a review of 21 years of experience. *J Am Coll Surg* 1996;183:506–513.
136. Rothlin MA, Lopfe M, Schlumpf R, et al. Long-term results of hepaticojejunostomy for benign lesions of the bile ducts. *Am J Surg* 1998;175:22–26.
137. Schweizer WP, Matthews JB, Baer HU, et al. Combined surgical and interventional radiological approach for complex benign biliary tract obstruction. *Br J Surg* 1991;78:599–563.
138. Csendes A, Diaz C, Burdiles P, et al. Indications and results of hepaticojejunostomy in benign strictures of the biliary tract. *Hepato-Gastroenterol* 1992;39:333–336.
139. Matthews JB, Bauer HU, Schweizer WP, et al. Recurrent cholangitis with and without anastomotic stricture after biliary-enteric bypass. *Arch Surg* 1993;128:269–272.
140. Nealon WH, Urrutia F. Long-term follow-up after bilioenteric anastomosis for benign bile duct stricture. *Ann Surg* 1996;6:639–648.
141. Hutson DG, Russell E, Yrizarry J, et al. Percutaneous dilation of biliary strictures through the afferent limb of a modified Roux-en-Y choledochojejunostomy or hepaticojejunostomy. *Am J Surg* 1998;175:108–113.
142. Smith MT, Sherman S, Lehman GA. Endoscopic management of benign strictures of the biliary tree. *Endoscopy* 1995;27:253–266.
143. Lee MJ, Mueller PR, Saini S, et al. Percutaneous dilation of benign biliary strictures: single session therapy with general anesthesia. *Am J Roentgenol* 1991;157:1263–1266.
144. Perry LJ, Stokes KR, Lewis DW, et al. Biliary intervention by means of percutaneous puncture of the antecolic jejunal loop. *Radiology* 1995;195:163–167.
145. Raute M, Podlegh P, Jaschke W, et al. Management of bile duct injuries and strictures following cholecystectomy. *World J Surg* 1993;17:553–562.
146. Neuhaus H, Hagenmueller F, Griebel M, et al. Percutaneous cholangioscopic or transpapillary insertion of self-expandable biliary metal stents. *Gastrointest Endosc* 1991;37:31–37.
147. Adam A, Chetty N, Roddie M, et al. Self-expandable stainless steel endoprothesis for treatment of malignant bile duct obstruction. *Am J Roentgenol* 1991;156:321–325.
148. Lopez RR, Cosenza CA, Lois J, et al. Long-term results of metallic stents for benign biliary strictures. *Arch Surg* 2001;136:664–669.
149. Wiesner RH, Gramlosch PM, Dickson ER, et al. Primary sclerosing cholangitis: natural history, prognostic factors, and survival analysis. *Hepatol* 1989;10:430–436.
150. Broome U, Lofberg R, Veress B, et al. Primary sclerosing cholangitis and ulcerative colitis: evidence for increased neoplastic potential. *Hepatol* 1995;22:1404–1408.
151. Ahrendt SA, Pitt HA, Kalloo AN, et al. Primary sclerosing cholangitis: resect, dilate, or transplant? *Ann Surg* 1998;227:412–423.
152. Cameron JL, Pitt HA, Zinner MJ, et al. Resection of hepatic duct bifurcation and transhepatic stenting for sclerosing cholangitis. *Ann Surg* 1988;207:614–622.
153. Pitt HA, Thompson HH, Tompkins RK, et al. Primary sclerosing cholangitis: results of an aggressive surgical approach. *Ann Surg* 1982;196:259–268.
154. Myburgh JA. Surgical biliary drainage in primary sclerosing cholangitis: the role of the Hepp-Couinaud approach. *Arch Surg* 1994;129:1057–1062.
155. Lee YM, Kaplan MM. Primary sclerosing cholangitis. *N Engl J Med* 1995;332:924–933.
156. Bismuth H, Nakache R, Diamond T. Management strategies in resection for hilar cholangiocarcinoma. *Ann Surg* 1992;215:31–38.
157. Washburn WK, Lewis WD, Jenkins RL. Aggressive surgical resection for cholangiocarcinoma. *Arch Surg* 1995;130:270–276.
158. Johnson SR, Kelly BS, Pennington LJ, et al. A single center experience with extrahepatic cholangiocarcinomas. *Surgery* 2001;130:584–592.

159. Gerhards MF, van Gulik TM, de Wit, LT, et al. Evaluation of morbidity and mortality after resection for hilar cholangiocarcinoma—a single center experience. *Surgery* 2000;127:395–404.
160. Nakeed A, Pitt HA, Sohn TA, et al. Cholangiocarcinoma: a spectrum of intrahepatic, perihilar, and distal tumors. *Ann Surg* 1996; 224:463–475.
161. Capussotti L, Muratore A, Polastri R, et al. Liver resection for hilar cholangiocarcinoma: in-hospital mortality and longterm survival. *J Am Coll Surg* 2002;195:641–647.
162. Chalasani N, Baluyut A, Ismail A, et al. Cholangiocarcinoma in patients with primary sclerosing cholangitis: a multicenter case-control study. *Hepatol* 2000;31:7–11.

163. Chung C, Bautista N, O'Connell TX. Prognosis and treatment of bile duct carcinoma. *Am Surg* 1998;64:921–925.
164. McMasters KM, Tuttle TM, Leach SD, et al. Neoadjuvant chemoradiation for extrahepatic cholangiocarcinoma. *Am J Surg* 1997;174: 605–609.
165. Liu CL, Lo CM, Lai EC, et al. Endoscopic retrograde cholangiopancreatography and endoscopic endoprosthesis insertion in patients with Klatskin tumors. *Arch Surg* 1998;133:293–296.
166. Dumas R, Demuth N, Buckley M, et al. Endoscopic bilateral metal stent placement for malignant hilar stenoses: identification of optimal technique. *Gastrointest Endosc* 2000;51: 334–338.

Complications of Pancreatic Surgery

34

Diane M. Simeone

■■■ INTRODUCTION 463

■■■ COMPLICATIONS OF OPERATIVE
PROCEDURES 463
  Drainage of Pancreatic Pseudocysts 463
  Drainage of Infected Pancreatic Necrosis 466
  Longitudinal Pancreaticojejunostomy 468
  Pancreaticoduodenectomy 469
  Complications of Distal and Subtotal
    Pancreatectomy 472
  Complications of Total Pancreatectomy 473

■■■ REFERENCES 474

INTRODUCTION

Surgical diseases of the pancreas are often more difficult to treat than those of other abdominal viscera. The pancreas lies hidden within the recesses of the retroperitoneum and during laparotomy is not easily visualized without extensive mobilization and dissection. The difficult location of the pancreas gland, with its intimate association with other vital structures that surround it, add to the complexity of pancreatic surgery. Resection of the pancreas is considered a major operative procedure that can be associated with significant morbidity and mortality. This chapter will discuss complications of operative procedures involving the pancreas, as well as management strategies to address specific complications.

Diane M. Simeone: University of Michigan, Ann Arbor, MI 48019

COMPLICATIONS OF OPERATIVE PROCEDURES

Drainage of Pancreatic Pseudocysts

A pancreatic pseudocyst is a localized collection of pancreatic juice enclosed by a wall of fibrous or granulation tissue, arising as a consequence of acute or chronic pancreatitis, neoplastic obstruction of the pancreatic duct, or pancreatic trauma. It is important to differentiate pseudocysts from acute fluid collections that form early in the course of acute pancreatitis, which can occur in up to 40% of cases. These acute fluid collections lack a wall of fibrous or granulation tissue and are likely a serous reaction to pancreatic inflammation. Most resolve spontaneously without any directed intervention. The development of a pancreatic pseudocyst should be suspected in any patient with a bout of acute pancreatitis who has prolonged recovery from the acute episode. A computed tomography (CT) scan can be performed to confirm the presence of pancreatic inflammation.

Previously, surgical dogma was to treat any pseudocyst that lasted longer than 6 weeks because they were believed to have a low likelihood of resolution and a high frequency of complications. The advent of more routine use of CT scanning in the 1970s allowed a more precise documentation of the natural history of pancreatic pseudocysts. Two large reports in the early 1990s (1,2) documented the safety of conservative management of asymptomatic pancreatic pseudocysts using careful clinical and radiographic follow-up, with intervention limited to patients with persistent symptoms related to the pseudocyst (pain, impaired gastric emptying) or pseudocyst-related complications. Pseudocyst-related complications include infection, hemorrhage, rupture, and obstruction of the gastrointestinal tract.

TABLE 34-1

SURGICAL OPTIONS TO TREAT PSEUDOCYSTS

Internal drainage
Cystgastrostomy
Cystjejunostomy
Cystduodenostomy
Pseudocyst excision
External drainage

Surgical options for the management of pancreatic pseudocysts include internal drainage, pseudocyst excision, and external drainage (Table 34-1). With all these options a frozen section biopsy of the wall of the pseudocyst should be included as part of the operative procedure to exclude the possibility of a cystic neoplasm, which has an epithelial lining. If the cyst has an epithelial lining, it probably represents a neoplastic cyst (or, in rare situations, a simple cyst or duplication cyst). Neoplastic cysts should be excised.

Internal Drainage Procedures

Internal drainage is the preferred surgical approach to uncomplicated pseudocysts requiring operative intervention. Most cyst walls will mature within 6 weeks of the onset of symptoms. Enteric drainage of the pseudocyst into the stomach, duodenum, or jejunum is possible, with the choice of drainage procedure based on the pseudocyst's location.

Cystgastrostomy

Cystgastrostomy should be performed when the pseudocyst is firmly adherent to the posterior wall of the stomach (Fig. 34-1). Cystgastrostomy is a faster and less technically demanding procedure than drainage into duodenum or jejunum. An exception to this approach may be made with giant (>15 cm) pseudocysts. A higher failure rate with cystgastrostomy has been noted in these patients, most likely because cystgastrostomy does not provide dependent drainage of the large cyst cavity (3). A cystjejunostomy may be more appropriate in this setting. Important components of the operation include (a) ensuring that the pseudocyst is adherent to the stomach to minimize risk of leakage at the anastomosis—this should be evident by anterior displacement of the stomach's back wall and confirmed by needle aspiration; (b) creation of a wide, 4- to 5-cm opening between the pseudocyst and posterior wall of the stomach to facilitate drainage; (c) removal of all debris in the pseudocyst cavity; and (d) ensuring hemostasis by performing a continuous, locking closure of the suture line.

Cystjejunostomy

Cystjejunostomy is a versatile technique that can be used to internally drain pseudocysts that are located in a variety

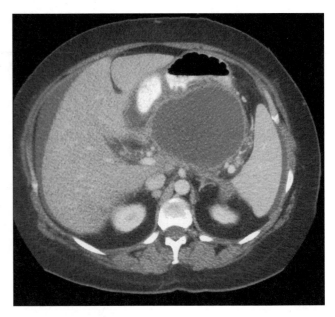

Figure 34-1 Large pancreatic pseudocyst adherent to the posterior wall of the stomach.

of locations due to the jejunal limb's mobility. For cysts drained into the jejunum, a Roux-en-Y limb of 60 cm in length is used. A two-layer anastomosis is performed to the most dependent part of the cyst so that drainage will be complete and to facilitate rapid obliteration of the cyst cavity.

Cystduodenostomy

Cystduodenostomy is performed infrequently, and its use is limited to pseudocysts in the head or uncinate process of the pancreas that lie within 1 cm of the duodenal lumen. The procedure can be associated with significant morbidity if an anastomotic leak and resultant duodenal fistula ensues, and therefore it is a less desirable procedure.

Laparoscopic Management of Pancreatic Pseudocysts

There are no large published series on the use of laparoscopy to treat pancreatic pseudocysts. Several small series have reported good results and minimal morbidity with laparoscopic cystgastrostomy or cystjejunostomy (4–6). At present, this approach should be limited to surgeons highly experienced in advanced laparoscopic techniques. The frequency of a laparoscopic approach to pseudocyst treatment will likely increase in the future.

Alternatives to Surgical Therapy

Percutaneous Drainage

Percutaneous drainage of pancreatic pseudocysts has been reported as an alternative to surgical treatment for over two decades. Simple percutaneous aspiration may be indicated to sample pseudocyst fluid if there is a clinical concern of pseudocyst infection. Aspiration without drain placement as primary therapy to treat pancreatic pseudocysts has a low success rate and is not advocated. Many groups have supported percutaneous catheter drainage for treatment of symptomatic pseudocysts as an alternative to surgical drainage, with initial reports touting a 70% to 90% success rate (7–9). There has not been a randomized, prospective study comparing the results of percutaneous drainage to operative drainage of pseudocysts. Several retrospective studies examining the long-term results of percutaneous catheter drainage have reported less favorable long-term results, with long-term success rates ranging from 21% to 60% (10–12). Percutaneous catheter drainage may be a useful technique for treatment of infected pancreatic pseudocysts if there is otherwise no indication for laparotomy. Complications associated with percutaneous catheter drainage include creation of a pancreatic fistula and inability to completely evacuate a cyst, both of which may ultimately require operative intervention. The likelihood of a persistent pancreatic fistula is increased in patients in whom the pseudocyst has a direct communication with the pancreatic duct (13).

Endoscopic Drainage

Endoscopic approaches have also been reported as treatment options for patients with pancreatic pseudocysts. One approach, transmural drainage, has been used for pseudocysts adherent to the wall of either the duodenum or stomach. Two prerequisites are necessary before attempting this form of treatment: bulging due to the cyst should be obvious on upper endoscopy and the distance between the cyst and lumen should not exceed 1 cm (14). Using the Seldinger technique, the cyst is cannulated with a guidewire, followed by stent placement. A second endoscopic approach, transpapillary (transampullary) drainage, has been used in selected patients to drain pseudocysts directly into the pancreatic duct. To use this approach, the pseudocyst must directly communicate with the pancreatic duct. A stent is placed and left for 6 to 8 weeks or until CT examination demonstrates resolution of the pseudocyst. Although the reported success rates with both approaches are favorable, there is a relatively high bleeding and perforation rate (15,16).

Complications of Surgical Drainage

Mortality

The mortality rate following internal drainage procedures ranges from 0% to 13%, with several recent series reporting a 0% mortality rate (11–13).

Recurrence

The recurrence rate following internal drainage of pseudocysts ranges from 0% to 15% (11–13). Pseudocysts might recur following internal drainage for several reasons. If an inadequately sized opening (<4 cm) has been created

between the stomach, jejunum, or duodenum and the pseudocyst cavity, a pseudocyst may recur. This is a technical complication that should easily be avoided. Inadequate drainage of multiple pseudocysts may be a cause of persistent abdominal pain or recurrence. Additionally, a cyst may recur if it is a cystic neoplasm that was mistaken for a pseudocyst, highlighting the need to send a frozen section of the pseudocyst wall to confirm the absence of an epithelial lining.

Bleeding

Hemorrhage occurs following internal drainage of pancreatic pseudocysts in 2% to 16% of patients (2,11,12). Hemorrhage following an internal drainage procedure may be due to bleeding at a suture line, and if bleeding occurs in the immediate postoperative period it should be treated by reexploration. Alternatively, patients may have erosion of a pancreatic pseudocyst into adjacent vessels, which can result in massive hemorrhage. The splenic artery is most commonly involved (45%), followed by the gastroduodenal (18%) and pancreaticoduodenal (18%) arteries (17). In this setting selective visceral angiography should be performed, with angiographic embolization using coils or pledgets usually resulting in definitive therapy (18,19) (Fig. 34-2). Surgery should be reserved for patients who are hemodynamically unstable or who have failed embolization procedures. Peripancreatic inflammation and postoperative changes may make operative control difficult. Initial control of bleeding may be obtained by digital compression of the bleeding vessel or by packing of the pseudocyst. Surgical approaches for definitive treatment include proximal and distal arterial ligation combined with intracystic suture ligation, distal pancreatectomy and splenectomy for bleeding

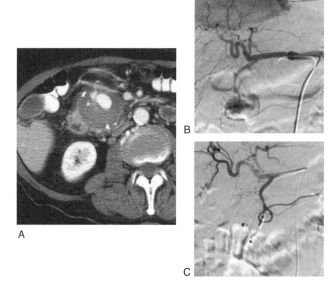

Figure 34-2 **A:** CT scan of a pancreatic pseudocyst with intravenous contrast within the pseudocyst, demonstrating active hemorrhage. **B:** Visceral angiogram documenting a pseudoaneurysm of the gastroduodenal artery. **C:** Postembolization angiogram depicting successful coil embolization of the pseudoaneurysm images are too small, especially the one on the right.

arising from the body and tail of the pancreas, or in rare cases, pancreaticoduodenectomy (18–20).

External Drainage

External drainage of pancreatic pseudocysts is indicated for pseudocysts that are found to be grossly infected or that do not have a mature wall sufficient for anastomosis at the time of exploration. External drainage is performed by opening the pseudocyst, evacuating its contents, and inserting a soft, silastic catheter into the pseudocyst cavity. A pancreaticocutaneous fistula may develop following the external drainage procedure. In most cases these fistulas will close spontaneously.

Special Consideration—Multiple Pseudocysts

Multiple pseudocysts that require treatment may occasionally be present. Although pancreatic resection is an option (especially if the pseudocysts are located in the gland's tail), internal drainage is the preferred treatment. This can be performed by converting multiple cysts into one large cyst to be used for a single anastomosis cystjejunostomy or by combined treatment with cystgastrostomy and cystjejunostomy. In these cases the surgeon should ensure that all cysts have been drained, using intraoperative ultrasound if needed.

Drainage of Infected Pancreatic Necrosis

Although most cases of acute pancreatitis are mild and self-limiting, necrotizing pancreatitis develops in about 15% of patients, with infection of pancreatic and peripancreatic necrosis representing the most important risk factor for a fatal outcome. Infection of pancreatic necrosis typically occurs in the second or third week after the onset of the disease and should be suspected in any patient with a severe bout of acute pancreatitis who develops multisystem organ dysfunction or systemic signs of sepsis, or both. In such patients a dynamic CT scan with intravenous contrast should be obtained to determine if there is pancreatic necrosis, evidenced by areas of nonperfusion. If there are signs of infection, such as presence of extraluminal gas, surgical exploration and debridement are indicated (Fig. 34-3). Otherwise, if infection of necrosis is clinically suspected, patients should undergo CT-guided fine needle aspiration (FNA) with Gram stain and bacteriologic cultures. Infection of pancreatic necrosis as proven by FNA is regarded as an indication for surgical debridement. The use of surgical debridement for sterile pancreatic necrosis remains controversial (21–23).

Operative Technique

Infected pancreatic necrosis is an absolute indication for an operative necrosectomy. Several approaches have been

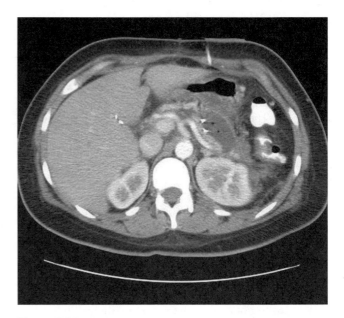

Figure 34-3 A CT scan in a patient with necrotizing pancreatitis with evidence of extraluminal gas.

advocated, including debridement with immediate closure over drains (with or without continuous lavage of the lesser sac), debridement with open or semiopen packing, and staged debridement with closure over drains (21–25). Many investigators favor the technique of repeated operative necrosectomy with closure over drains (26). A recent CT scan is used to guide surgical exploration to ensure that all areas of necrosis or fluid accumulation are explored. Upon entering the abdomen, the lesser sac may be entered through the gastrocolic ligament or through the transverse mesocolon. Peripancreatic necrotic tissue should be removed bluntly. Forceful or sharp dissection should be avoided, as this may result in bleeding or injury to the bowel. A sample of the necrotic tissue should be sent for bacteriologic analysis. If fluid collections or necrosis extend to the pararenal or retrocolic spaces, these should be opened and debrided. Extensive irrigation is then performed. If all necrotic debris has been removed, the abdomen may be closed over drains. If necrotic or questionably viable tissue remains adherent, repeated operative evaluation should be carried out within 48 hours and further necrosectomy performed as outlined. This is repeated as necessary until all necrotic tissue is removed and the abdomen is closed over drains. Soft silastic drains rather than firm sump drains should be used to minimize the risk of pressure injury to blood vessels and the bowel. Repeated exploration may be facilitated by use of zipper placement, which allows easy rapid entry into the abdomen and prevents loss of abdominal domain (26).

Mortality

In patients with infected pancreatic necrosis managed without surgery, the mortality rate approaches 100%. The mortality rate in several recent series for patients who undergo operative treatment of infected pancreatic necrosis ranges from 6% to 25% (24–26); however, morbidity rates remain high. The management of patients with infected pancreatic necrosis is challenging, as these patients often require prolonged ICU care and lengthy hospital stays. Despite this, encouraging data from long-term follow-up of patients who have recovered from pancreatic debridement reveal that most of these patients are able to return to normal activity and have a good quality of life (27).

Hemorrhage

Hemorrhage requiring some form of active intervention following pancreatic debridement is reported to occur in 5% to 20% of patients (22,25,26). Hemorrhage can occur during the operative procedure or postoperatively and may be secondary to general oozing from the debridement bed or due to direct injury to nearby vascular structures, including the splenic and portal veins, or the splenic, superior mesenteric, inferior pancreatic, or middle colic arteries. Gentle blunt dissection during debridement and care to place drains away from major vessels are important in decreasing the risk of hemorrhage. Direct surgical control in this setting is the standard approach, but angiographic embolization is another option in selected patients.

Recurrent Intra-abdominal Abscess

Recurrent intra-abdominal abscess is reported to develop in 13% to 26% of patients following necrosectomy (24–26). Many of these patients can be successfully managed by simple, CT-guided percutaneous drainage, with only a few patients requiring reoperative drainage. In one series using a strategy of planned reoperative necrosectomy with final closure over drains, the incidence of postoperative intra-abdominal abscess was increased in patients who underwent fewer reoperative necrosectomies, highlighting the importance of complete removal of all infected necrotic tissue (26). The development of an intra-abdominal abscess does not appear to have an effect on survival; mortality in these patients was similar to other patients.

Fistulas

Pancreatic and gastrointestinal tract fistulas are common complications of surgical treatment of necrotizing pancreatitis. The pathogenesis of fistula formation in this setting appears to be multifactorial. Perhaps the most common factor in the development of fistulas is pancreatic parenchymal necrosis, which results in disruption of pancreatic ducts with extravasation of pancreatic juice into the retroperitoneum. Although this is clearly important in the development of pancreatic fistulas, the enzymatic juices and inflammatory mediators produced as part of the necrotizing process may

also cause vascular thrombosis with resultant ischemia, which can lead to segmental necrosis of bowel. Extravasated secretions may also directly result in necrosis of adjacent segments of the gastrointestinal tract. Alternatively, the development of fistulas may be iatrogenic, due to trauma to the surface of organs of the gastrointestinal tract, either secondary to debridement, repeated packing, or pressure necrosis from an adjacent drain.

The incidence of pancreatic fistulas ranges from 19% to 53% (25,26,28). Diagnosis is based on persistent drainage with high amylase concentration from drains left in the lesser sac or by endoscopic retrograde cholangiopancreatography (ERCP) (Fig. 34-4). The vast majority of these fistulas can be successfully managed conservatively with drains left in the surgical site, which are gradually advanced out. It is unclear whether octreotide facilitates fistula closure in these patients. In the small percentage of patients who have a persistent, high-output fistula that fails to close with conservative management, operative treatment of the fistula is required. Operative treatment may require a pancreaticojejunostomy or distal pancreatectomy.

Gastrointestinal fistulas, when they occur, can be difficult to manage, with the likelihood of spontaneous closure dependent on the fistula site (Table 34-2). Fistulas are defined by a contrast study showing direct communication with the underlying organ. In one report, two of two gastric fistulas, three of five duodenal fistulas, three of four enteric fistulas, and one of eight colonic fistulas closed spontaneously (28). The remaining fistulas required operative closure. Repair of duodenal fistulas may be managed by Roux-en-Y duodenojejunostomy or, if necessary, by a pyloric exclusion procedure that consists of pyloric stapling with a gastrojejunostomy. Enteric fistulas are usually corrected by segmental resection. Colonic fistulas may occasionally be treated with segmental resection, but they frequently require proximal diversion.

TABLE 34-2

MANAGEMENT OF GASTROINTESTINAL FISTULAS AFTER NECROSECTOMY

	Number	Spontaneous Closure	Operative Treatment Required
Colonic	8	3	5
Duodenal	5	2	3
Enteric	4[a]	3	0
Gastric	2	2	0

[a]One patient died of multisystem organ failure with a persistent, controlled fistula. Data from Tsiotos GG, Smith CD, Sarr MG. Incidence and management of pancreatic and enteric fistulas after surgical management of severe necrotizing pancreatitis. *Arch Surg* 1995;130:48–52.

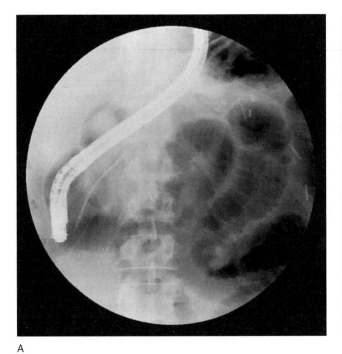

A

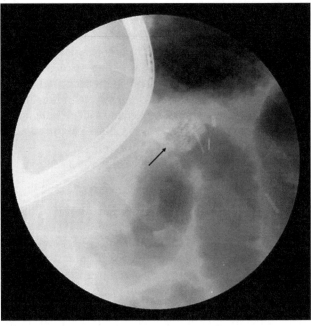

B

Figure 34-4 An ERCP of a patient 3 weeks after an operative debridement for necrotizing pancreatitis demonstrating a pancreatic fistula (*arrow*). **A:** Depicts early pancreatic ductal injection. **B:** the extravasation of contrast outlines the fistula.

Longitudinal Pancreaticojejunostomy

Longitudinal pancreaticojejunostomy, or the Puestow procedure, is performed to treat intractable pain in patients with chronic pancreatitis who have pancreatic ductal dilatation (Fig. 34-5). In patients with chronic pancreatitis, damage to acinar cells results in release of proteolytic enzymes into the duct, which induces protein plug formation and stone development. This process promotes ductal obstruction and hypertension, which is thought to lead to increased pain. The rationale for this operation is to relieve the ductal hypertension, and hence pain.

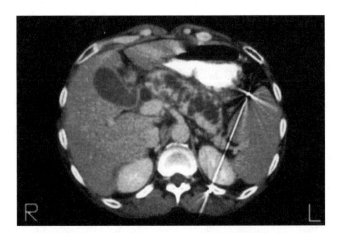

Figure 34-5 A CT scan in a patient with chronic pancreatitis with a history of intractable abdominal pain. A markedly dilated pancreatic duct is evident, making this patient a good candidate for a lateral pancreaticojejunostomy (Puestow procedure).

Operative Technique

A lateral (longitudinal) pancreaticojejunostomy is the most effective drainage procedure. Treatment involves a longitudinal incision in the pancreas through the anterior wall of the main pancreatic duct. The duct can usually be palpated as a soft, compressable area in an otherwise firm gland. Needle aspiration of clear fluid can confirm identification of the duct. If there is any difficulty in duct identification, intraoperative ultrasound can be used. A Roux-en-Y limb of jejunum is then sutured to the opened duct along its length so that pancreatic juice drains directly into the intestine. Ductal stones and debris are removed if present. Several large series have evaluated this procedure's success rate, which ranges from 60% to 90% (29–31). Factors contributing to success of the operation are duct size (>8 mm) and a lengthy (>6 cm) pancreatic-jejunal anastomosis that extends from the pancreatic tail to a point 1 cm from the duodenum.

Mortality

Lateral pancreaticojejunostomy is a relatively safe procedure, with most series reporting operative mortality rates of <5% and an associated complication rate of 10% to 25% (29–31). Long-term mortality has been reported to be much higher—in some series as much as 50% at 5 years (31). Continued alcoholism has been an important contributing factor to this high rate of mortality.

Recurrent/Persistent Pain

Most patients remain pain-free or have significantly improved pain following the operative procedure. Recurrent or persistent pain following a lateral pancreaticojejunostomy warrants investigation to exclude other potential sources of pain, including peptic ulcer disease and biliary stricture. If other disease processes are excluded, an ERCP or magnetic resonance cholangiopancreatography (MRCP) should be performed to examine the patency of the pancreaticojejunal anastomosis and to ensure that there are no undrained segments of the pancreatic duct. If the anastomosis is occluded or if residual undrained segments are identified, redrainage can provide satisfactory pain relief (32).

Endocrine and Exocrine Insufficiency

An immediate change in insulin requirement is uncommon after pancreaticojejunostomy, as resection of pancreatic tissue is not performed. In one series of patients followed for 10 years after pancreaticojejunostomy, approximately 20% of patients experienced worsening of diabetes, which was likely a result of continued gland (and islet) destruction due to the inflammatory process (33). Although ductal drainage does not improve established pancreatic endocrine or exocrine insufficiency, some reports suggest that the progression of pancreatic dysfunction may be slowed in patients who undergo a drainage procedure. A study by Nealon and Thompson used a 5-point grading system to measure severity of pancreatitis (ERCP findings, oral glucose testing, and three different measures of exocrine function). In patients with mild to moderate chronic pancreatitis who underwent ductal decompression, only 13% progressed to severe chronic pancreatitis, as opposed to a control group in which 78% progressed to severe disease (34).

Pancreatic Fistula

Postoperative pancreatic fistulas following lateral pancreaticojejunostomy are uncommon, most likely because the gland is quite firm and easily holds sutures. These fistulas usually close spontaneously with closed suction drainage.

Pancreaticoduodenectomy

Pancreaticoduodenectomy, as described by Whipple in 1935, is the standard surgical treatment for pancreatic adenocarcinoma. The operation is also performed for other pancreatic neoplasms, such as cystic neoplasms, intraductal papillary mucinous neoplasms, islet cell tumors, sarcomas or other rare tumors involving the pancreatic head, metastatic lesions involving the pancreatic head, and tumors of the distal bile duct, ampulla, and duodenum, as well for chronic pancreatitis with symptomatic disease involving primarily the pancreatic head. The procedure is rarely performed for massive injury of the head of the pancreas involving the duodenum, distal common bile duct, or portal vein. As performed today, pancreaticoduodenectomy involves removal of the pancreatic head, the duodenum, the gallbladder, and the distal common bile duct, with or without the removal of the gastric antrum. Reconstruction after pancreaticoduodenectomy requires anastomosis of the proximal jejunum to the pancreatic remnant, bile duct, and gastrojejunostomy (or duodenojejunostomy if a pylorus-preserving technique is used).

Mortality

Since the advent of pancreaticoduodenectomy (Whipple procedure) to treat adenocarcinoma of the pancreatic head, outcomes following pancreaticoduodenectomy have improved substantially. Previously, operative mortality rates as high as 20% were not uncommon. Recently, better results have been reported, with operative mortality rates well below 5% at many large academic centers. One case series of 650 consecutive patients undergoing pancreaticoduodenectomy described a mortality rate of 1.7% (35), and other studies with >100 patients have reported no postoperative deaths (36,37). The reasons for the decline in operative mortality rates are likely multifactorial, including refinements in operative technique as well as improvements in perioperative care. However, large population-based studies still demonstrate that mortality rates remain high at many smaller hospitals. In fact, of all procedures analyzed in a large study examining volume-related differences in mortality for 14 different procedures, the greatest volume-related differences in mortality were observed with pancreatic resection, with adjusted mortality rates at very low volume hospitals (<1 case per year) of 16.3% versus 3.8% at very high volume hospitals (>16 cases per year) (Fig. 34-6) (38). Although a number of initiatives are underway to better understand the reasons for these differences and how this issue can be addressed from a national healthcare perspective, current data support performance of pancreaticoduodenectomies in high volume centers.

Pancreatic Fistula

Pancreatic fistulas, usually resulting from an anastomotic leak, are an important cause of morbidity and mortality following pancreaticoduodenectomy. In the setting of pancreaticoduodenal resection, a pancreatic fistula is generally defined as the persistent drainage of 50 ml or more of amylase-rich fluid on or after postoperative day 3 through 10 (39). The incidence of pancreatic anastomotic leak varies from 5% to 25% in most series (40–43). An increased rate of fistula formation has been associated with pancreatic glands with a soft consistency. Because pancreatic fistula formation has been identified as such a common problem after pancreaticoduodenectomy, variations in technique for managing the pancreatic remnant as well as the utility of treatment with perioperative octreotide have been studied.

In an effort to decrease the pancreatic fistula rate following pancreaticoduodenectomy, a variety of technical modifications in handling of the pancreatic remnant has been evaluated. A meta-analysis of the published literature from 1965 to 1980 revealed that pancreatic fistula formation

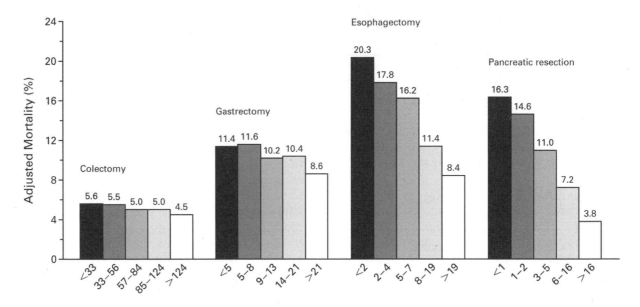

Figure 34-6   Adjusted in-hospital or 30-day mortality among Medicare patients (1994 through 1999), according to quintile of total hospitalization volume for resections of gastrointestinal cancer. [From Birkmeyer JD, Stukel TA, Siewers AE, et al. Surgeon volume and operative mortality in the United States. *N Engl J Med* 2003 Nov 27;349(22):2117–2127, with permission.]

was statistically more frequent after simple suture ligation of the pancreatic remnant than after pancreaticojejunostomy (44). This was corroborated by a more recently published trial by Tran et al. randomizing patients undergoing pancreaticoduodenectomy for periampullary or pancreatic adenocarcinoma to pancreaticojejunostomy (*n* = 8) or obliteration of the pancreatic duct without anastomosis (*n* = 86) (45). Occlusion of the pancreatic duct resulted in significantly higher rates of pancreatic fistula (17% versus 5%) and pancreatic endocrine insufficiency. Other studies have examined the effects of different methods of pancreatic-jejunal reconstruction on pancreatic fistula formation. One prospective study in patients undergoing pancreaticoduodenectomy for periampullary tumors compared two methods of reconstruction: an end-to-end, invaginating anastomosis (*n* = 46) to an end-to-side (duct-to-mucosa, using a stent) anastomosis (*n* = 47) (46). The end-to-end, invaginating technique was associated with a trend toward a higher fistula rate compared to the end-to-side technique using stents (15% vs. 4%, *p* = 0.09). No differences in overall postoperative morbidity or mortality were observed between the two groups. No studies directly address the effect of stent placement as an individual factor in pancreatic fistula formation.

Another option for drainage of the pancreatic remnant is pancreaticogastrostomy. The potential use of this technique was initially based on several retrospective series reporting lower fistula rates with pancreaticogastrostomy versus pancreaticojejunostomy. In a randomized prospective trial by Yeo et al. evaluating 146 patients undergoing

pancreaticoduodenectomy, patients were randomized intraoperatively to either pancreaticogastrostomy (*n* = 73) or pancreaticojejunostomy (*n* = 72) (47). Pancreaticojejunostomy was performed in two layers without stents in either an end-to-side or end-to-end fashion at the surgeon's discretion. Pancreaticogastrostomy was performed by anastomosing the pancreatic remnant to the posterior gastric wall. The incidence of pancreatic fistula was 11% for pancreaticojejunostomy and 12% for pancreaticogastrostomy reconstructions. This trial demonstrated that pancreaticogastrostomy is a safe and viable option for pancreatic-enteric reconstruction, with similar perioperative morbidity and mortality.

The effectiveness of perioperative octreotide in patients undergoing elective pancreatic resection was initially investigated in several prospective, randomized European trials (48–51). A subsequent meta-analysis of the European trials found that the use of octreotide significantly reduced the rate of pancreatic fistula formation (10.7% for octreotide vs. 23.4% for placebo) (52). However, there were inherent limitations in extrapolating the data from these studies to validate use of prophylactic octreotide in patients undergoing pancreaticoduodenectomy. First, the trials examined all types of pancreatic resections, including pancreaticoduodenectomy, distal pancreatectomy, and enucleation. It is certainly possible that the fistula rates vary based on the type of resection and therefore may not necessarily be applicable for pancreaticoduodenectomy. Second, the rates of pancreatic fistula reported in these studies were much higher than rates reported at major institutions in the United States, which might amplify the benefit of octreotide observed in these studies (53). To address these issues, Lowy et al. (54) evaluated the use of perioperative octreotide specifically in patients undergoing pancreaticoduodenectomy for malignant disease. No significant differences were found in pancreatic fistula rates, mortality, or length of hospitalization between the two groups. In a similar study by Yeo et al. in pancreatic cancer patients, no differences were found in pancreatic fistula rate in patients treated with octreotide versus placebo (55). Multivariate analysis revealed that soft pancreatic gland consistency was an independent predictor of the development of a pancreatic fistula. Overall, these studies demonstrate that routine use of perioperative octreotide for patients undergoing pancreaticoduodenectomy cannot be justified based on the available data. Further studies are needed to determine if perioperative octreotide is of benefit in specific patient groups that undergo pancreaticoduodenectomy—that is, soft versus firm glands—or patients with malignant versus benign disease.

Pancreatic fistulas that develop following pancreaticoduodenectomy can usually be managed conservatively if there is no evidence of abdominal sepsis. The presence of a pancreatic fistula should be suspected in a postoperative patient who develops clinical evidence of intra-abdominal sepsis. Isolated fluid collections should be drained, percutaneously if possible, and they usually heal spontaneously if adequately drained. Octreotide is often used to treat established pancreatic anastomotic leaks that require percutaneous drainage.

Anastomotic Leak at Biliary-enteric Anastomosis

Development of an anastomotic leak at the biliary-enteric anastomosis is reported from several large series to occur in 1% to 8% of pancreaticoduodenectomies (41–43,56). A biliary leak may be evident if an intraoperatively placed drain develops bilious output, or it may require evaluation with a cholangiogram or fistulogram. A small bile leak that is adequately drained often seals spontaneously. In more persistent cases, biliary anastomotic leaks may require a transhepatic catheter to allow for external biliary drainage.

Delayed Gastric Emptying

Delayed gastric emptying is a frequent and significant postoperative problem following pancreaticoduodenectomy. In most series, delayed gastric emptying, defined as the need for postoperative nasogastric decompression for >10 days, has a reported incidence ranging from 20% to 40% (57,58). Although not life-threatening, delayed gastric emptying results in a significant prolongation of hospital stay and contributes to increased hospitalization costs. The etiology of delayed gastric emptying following pancreaticoduodenectomy is uncertain, but possible etiologies include decreased motilin levels, removal of the duodenal pacemaker, and disruption of gastroduodenal

neural connections. Erythromycin, a motilin agonist, has been found to improve gastric emptying of both solids and liquids when administered intravenously during the postoperative period. To test the potential role of erythromycin in gastric emptying following pancreaticoduodenectomy, a prospective, randomized trial was performed in which patients received either 200 mg of intravenous erythromycin or placebo from the third to tenth postoperative days, and on the tenth postoperative day dual phase gastric emptying studies were performed (57). The erythromycin group had a significantly reduced incidence of delayed gastric emptying (19% vs. 30%), with measurable improvements in gastric emptying studies, supporting the use of erythromycin to decrease early delayed gastric emptying after pancreaticoduodenectomy.

Hyperbilirubinemia and Preoperative Biliary Drainage

The effect of preoperative hyperbilirubinemia on mortality risk with pancreaticoduodenectomy remains controversial. Although quite a few studies examining various other surgical procedures have shown that preoperative jaundice is associated with increased mortality risk, the literature describing the effect of preoperative hyperbilirubinemia on mortality following pancreaticoduodenectomy is unclear. Although several studies did not report an effect of preoperative hyperbilirubinemia on perioperative mortality (59–62), other studies have identified hyperbilirubinemia as a risk factor for mortality after pancreaticoduodenectomy (63–66). In a retrospective analysis of 279 patients by Braasch and Gray, patients with serum bilirubin >20 mg per 100 mL had significant higher mortality rates (6/28, 22%) than patients with lower bilirubin levels (29/251, 11.5%), suggesting that the mortality rate may well be associated with the severity of hyperbilirubinemia.

Although some controversy does remain as to whether preoperative hyperbilirubinemia contributes to mortality, it is not clear that preoperative biliary drainage can decrease risk. Results from a number of prospective trials and retrospective analyses have not shown a reduction in operative mortality by preoperative biliary drainage (66–70). A number of studies have sought to address the issue of whether preoperative biliary drainage affects outcomes following pancreaticoduodenectomy. Patients who had preoperative biliary stents experienced significantly increased rates of wound infection (increased from an average of 4% to 10%), with mixed results regarding the effect of preoperative stenting on pancreatic fistula formation. No differences were observed between stented and unstented groups in incidence of intra-abdominal abscess or other major complications. Overall, the preponderance of data does not suggest benefit or detriment of preoperative biliary drainage procedures with regard to perioperative mortality. Preoperative biliary drainage demonstrates an increased risk of wound infection and may increase the risk of pancreatic fistula formation. In general, preoperative biliary drainage is relatively safe but should be reserved for patients with intolerable jaundice in which definitive surgical treatment is delayed.

Surgical Technique

In the classic pancreaticoduodenectomy, as described by Whipple (71), an antrectomy was performed, whereas in the pylorus-preserving modification the duodenum is transected 2 to 3 cm distal to the pylorus. The rationale for the more extensive gastric resection in the standard Whipple procedure was that it was a better oncologic operation and would reduce the acid burden and subsequent incidence of marginal ulceration. Pylorus preservation (PPPD), on the other hand, has been touted as maintaining more normal gastrointestinal physiology in terms of acid production, gastric reservoir and emptying functions, and hormone secretion.

A number of studies have been performed to compare the outcomes of the standard versus the pylorus-preserving procedures. Several reports have shown no difference in survival between patients with periampullary tumors treated with PPPD versus standard pancreaticoduodenectomy (72–74). In one of the reports (72), a randomized trial of 77 patients compared the clinical results of classic pancreaticoduodenectomy versus PPPD. The PPPD group had a significantly shorter operative time and reduced blood loss. The incidence of delayed gastric emptying was identical in both groups. A similar incidence of delayed gastric emptying with standard versus PPPD has been verified in other studies (75,76). Postoperative nutritional parameters remain normal in most patients regardless of which procedure is performed. There were no differences in tumor recurrence or long-term survival (58,73). The published data do not indicate a significant advantage of the PPPD compared to standard pancreaticoduodenectomy, and the procedure chosen can be at the surgeon's discretion.

Complications of Distal and Subtotal Pancreatectomy

Distal pancreatectomy (50% to 60% of the gland) is performed for a variety of benign and malignant conditions. Indications include chronic pancreatitis, cystic neoplasms, intraductal papillary mucinous tumors (IPMTs), pancreatic adenocarcinoma, neuroendocrine tumors, pancreatic pseudocysts, and resection en bloc for management of tumors arising from nearby organs, such as stomach or kidney. Subtotal pancreatectomy (80% to 95% of the gland) may be required for neoplastic disease processes requiring a more extensive resection. Although commonly performed in the past, subtotal resection of the pancreas is rarely indicated for the treatment of intractable pain due to diffuse chronic pancreatitis when the pancreatic duct is not

dilated. In both distal and subtotal pancreatectomy, the spleen is typically removed because of the extensive collaterals that exist between the splenic vessels and the body and tail of the pancreas. If the transection of the pancreas is carried out to the left of the portal and superior mesenteric vessels, this constitutes a <60% resection, whereas resection at the level of the portal vein and superior mesenteric vessels constitutes a 60% to 70% resection and resection to the right of the vessels mandates an 80% or greater resection (Fig. 34-7).

Pancreatic Fistula Formation

Pancreatic fistulas in patients undergoing distal pancreatectomy are reported to occur in 5% to 25% of cases (41,77–79). Surgeons have tried to determine the optimal management strategy for the residual transected pancreatic parenchyma and the divided pancreatic duct. Commonly used techniques for management of the transected parenchyma include oversewing of the remnant or staple closure (usually with a TA-55 stapler), with or without direct ductal ligation. In two large series there was no difference in pancreatic leak rates between patients whose stumps were sutured versus stapled (77,80). However, in a study by Bilimoria et al., the incidence of pancreatic leak was found to be significantly decreased (9.6% vs. 34%, p <0.001) when the pancreatic duct was identified and ligated, independent of whether the remnant was sutured or stapled closed. On the basis of these data, every effort should be made to directly ligate the pancreatic duct following parenchymal transection, irrespective of the technique employed for stump closure. So far no studies have adequately addressed the role for routine use of octreotide after elective distal pancreatectomy.

Endocrine Insufficiency

Diabetes may be a complication of distal pancreatectomy or subtotal pancreatectomy in patients operated on for chronic pancreatitis if a major portion of the gland is removed. In an otherwise normal pancreas, as much as 80% of the pancreas may be removed without the development of diabetes. However, in the setting of diffuse parenchymal disease, as in chronic pancreatitis, resection of as little as 50% of the gland may cause diabetes or may worsen diabetes in chronic pancreatitis patients who have antecedent glucose intolerance before surgical resection. In several large series of distal pancreatectomy, the overall reported incidence of new onset, insulin-dependent diabetes mellitus following distal pancreatectomy was approximately 8% (78,79). In patients with chronic pancreatitis, the risk is reported to range from 12% to 46% (81–83).

Exocrine Insufficiency

Like diabetes, exocrine insufficiency following distal or subtotal pancreatectomy is predominately a complication

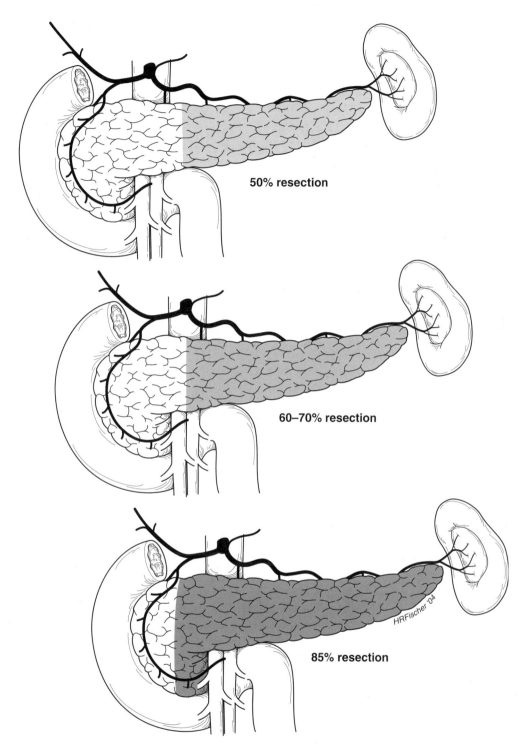

Figure 34-7 Level of parenchymal transection for 50%, 60% to 70%, and 85% distal pancreatectomy.

that occurs in patients with chronic pancreatitis. Exocrine insufficiency occurs in about one-third of patients with a diagnosis of chronic pancreatitis before surgical intervention and has been reported to be present in 55% of post-surgical patients (81). Exocrine insufficiency is not considered a serious complication of pancreatic surgery and can usually be easily treated by oral pancreatic enzyme supplementation.

Complications of Total Pancreatectomy

Total pancreatectomy is an operation that is not commonly performed because of the profound metabolic consequences of complete removal of the gland. It is an operation that should be considered only in a patient who will be able to deal with the difficult-to-manage diabetes that usually follows the procedure. Conditions for which total pancreatectomy may be performed include pancreatic neoplasms, such as multifocal or extensive IPMTs, multifocal neuroendocrine tumors, and chronic pancreatitis complicated by diffuse gland involvement and severe, unremitting pain. Total pancreatectomy was a popular operation for adenocarcinoma of the pancreas in the 1970s because the long-term survival following pancreaticoduodenectomy was relatively poor. However, the results from total pancreatectomy in this group of patients was not improved (84), and little data currently supports the use of total pancreatectomy in this setting.

Mortality

Over time, the mortality rate for total pancreatectomy has demonstrated the same improvement as that observed with pancreaticoduodenectomy. Although it was not uncommon for mortality rates following total pancreatectomy to be as high as 26% to 28% in older series, reports from several series over the last decade list operative mortality rates ranging from 3% to 5% in experienced hands (84,85).

Endocrine Insufficiency

The most significant complication encountered in patients who undergo total pancreatectomy is endocrine insufficiency. Pancreatogenic diabetes is characterized by (a) absence of the major glucoregulatory hormones insulin and glucagon, (b) instability, and (c) frequent hypoglycemia, with the latter parameters improving with rigorous home glucose monitoring. Dresler et al. (86) reported on the metabolic consequences of total pancreactectomy in 49 patients, with a third of patients followed for >48 months. Although patients became diabetic and experienced alterations in lifestyle, most patients were able to resume a reasonable functional status and level of activity. Only 1 of the 49 patients died from metabolic complications due to their surgical procedures, while no other patients had serious sequelae from their diabetes. At the time of the report, no patients had developed clinically overt diabetic microvascular or macrovascular disease. Other reports have demonstrated good performance status in patients following total pancreatectomy, with intermittent hypoglycemia being the most frequent complication (87). For patients with severe, unremitting pain due to chronic pancreatitis, an alternative approach is total pancreatectomy with either autologous islet cell transplantation or transplantation of a pancreatic allograft. In highly specialized centers this approach has demonstrated promising results (88,89).

REFERENCES

1. Yeo CJ, Bastidas JA, Lynch-Nyhan A, et al. The natural history of pancreatic pseudocysts documented by computed tomography. *Surg Gynecol Obstet* 1990;170:411–417.
2. Vitas GJ, Sarr MG. Selected management of pancreatic pseudocysts: operative versus expectant management. *Surgery* 1992;111:123–130.
3. Johnson LB, Rattner DW, Warshaw AL. The effect of size of giant pancreatic pseudocysts on the outcome of internal drainage procedures. *Surg Gynecol Obstet* 1991;173:171–174.
4. Siperstein A. Laparoendoscopic approach to pancreatic pseudocysts. *Semin Laparosc Surg* 2001;8:218–222.
5. Mori T, Abe N, Sugiyama M. Laparoscopic pancreatic cystgastrostomy. *J Hepato Biliary Pancreat Surg* 2002;9:548–554.
6. Bhattacharya D, Ammori BJ. Minimally invasive approaches to management of pancreatic pseudocyst: review of the literature. *Surg Laparosc Endosc Percutan Tech* 2003;13:141–148.
7. von Sonnenberg E, Wittich G, Casola G. Percutaneous drainage of infected and noninfected pancreatic pseudocysts: experience in 101 cases. *Radiology* 1989;170:757–761.
8. Adams D, Anderson M. Percutaneous catheter drainage compared with internal drainage in the management of pancreatic pseudocysts. *Ann Surg* 1992;215:571–578.
9. D'Egidio A, Schein M. Percutaneous drainage of pancreatic pseudocysts: a prospective study. *World J Surg* 1991;16:141–146.
10. Criado E, DeStefano AA, Weiner TM, et al. Long term result of percutaneous catheter drainage of pancreatic pseudocysts. *Surg Gynecol Obstet* 1992;175:293–298.
11. Spivak H, Galloway JR, Amerson JR, et al. Management of pancreatic pseudocysts. *J Am Coll Surg* 1998;186:507–511.
12. Heider R, Meyer AA, Galanko JA, et al. Percutaneous drainage of pancreatic pseudocysts is associated with a higher failure rate than surgical treatment in unselected patients. *Ann Surg* 1999;229:781.
13. Nealon WH, Walser E. Main pancreatic ductal anatomy can direct choice of modality for treating pancreatic pseudocysts (surgery versus percutaneous drainage). *Ann Surg* 2002;235:751–758.
14. Sahel J. Endoscopic drainage of pancreatic cysts. *Endoscopy* 1991;23:181.
15. De Palma GD, Galloro G, Puzziello A, et al. Endoscopic drainage of pancreatic pseudocysts: a long-term follow-up study of 49 patients. *Hepato-Gastroenterol* 2002;49:1113–1115.
16. Binmoeller KF, Seifert H, Walter A, et al. Transpapillary and transmural drainage of pancreatic pseudocysts. *Gastrointest Endosc* 1995;42:219.
17. Lillemoe K, Yeo CJ. Management of complications of pancreatitis. *Curr Prob Surg* 1998;35:33–51.
18. Carr JA, Cho JS, Shepard AD, et al. Visceral pseudoaneurysms due to pancreatic pseudocysts: rare but lethal complications of pancreatitis. *J Vasc Surg* 2000;32:722–730.
19. Steckman ML, Dooley MC, Jaques PF, et al. Major gastrointestinal hemorrhage from peripancreatic blood vessels in pancreatitis: treatment by embolotherapy. *Dig Dis Sci* 1984;29:486–497.
20. Bresler L, Boissel P, Grosdidier J. Major hemorrhage from pancreatic pseudocysts and pseudoaneurysms caused by chronic pancreatitis: surgical therapy. *World J Surg* 1991;15:649–653.
21. Bradley EL, Allen K. A prospective longitudinal study of observation versus surgical intervention in the management of necrotizing pancreatitis. *Am J Surg* 1991;161:19–25.
22. Buchler MW, Gloor B, Muller CA, et al. Acute necrotizing pancreatitis: treatment strategy according to status of infection. *Ann Surg* 2000;232:619–626.
23. Warshaw AL. Pancreatic necrosis: to debride or not to debride—that is the question. *Ann Surg* 2000;232:627–629.
24. Branum G, Galloway J, Hirchowitz W, et al. Pancreatic necrosis: results of necrosectomy, packing, and ultimate closure over drains. *Ann Surg* 1998;227:870–877.
25. Fernandez-del Castillo C, Rattner DW, Makary MA, et al. Debridement and closed packing for the treatment of necrotizing pancreatitis. *Ann Surg* 1998;228:676–684.
26. Tsiotos GG, Luque-de Leon E, Soreide JA, et al. Management of necrotizing pancreatitis by repeated operative necrosectomy using a zipper technique. *Am J Surg* 1998;175:91–98.
27. Broome AH, Eisen GM, Harland RC, et al. Quality of life after treatment for pancreatitis. *Ann Surg* 1996;223:665–672.
28. Tsiotos GG, Smith CD, Sarr MG. Incidence and management of pancreatic and enteric fistulas after surgical management of severe necrotizing pancreatitis. *Arch Surg* 1995;130:48–52.

29. Bradley EL. Long-term results of pancreaticojejunostomy in patients with chronic pancreatitis. *Am J Surg* 1987;153:207–213.

30. Ihse I, Borch K, Larsson J. Chronic pancreatitis: results of operation for relief of pain. *World J Surg* 1990;14:53–58.

31. Prinz RA, Greenlee HB. Pancreatic duct drainage in 100 patients with chronic pancreatitis. *Ann Surg* 1981;194:313–320.

32. Prinz RA, Aranha GV, Greenlee HB. Redrainage of the pancreatic duct in chronic pancreatitis. *Am J Surg* 1986;151:150–156.

33. Taylor RH, et al. Ductal drainage or resection for chronic pancreatitis. *Am J Surg* 1981;141:28.

34. Nealon WH, Thompson JC. Progressive loss of pancreatic function in chronic pancreatitis is delayed by main duct decompression: a longitudinal prospective analysis of the modified Puestow procedure. *Ann Surg* 1993;217:458–468.

35. Yeo CJ, Cameron JL, Sohn TA, et al. Six hundred fifty consecutive pancreaticoduodenectomies in the 1990's: pathology, complications, outcomes. *Ann Surg* 1997;226:248–260.

36. Trede M, Schwall G, Saeger H-D. Survival after pancreaticoduodenectomy: 118 consecutive resections without a mortality. *Ann Surg* 1990;211:447–458.

37. Cameron JL, Pitt HA, Yeo CJ, et al. One hundred and forty five consecutive pancreaticoduodenectomies without mortality. *Ann Surg* 1993;217:430–438.

38. Birkmeyer JD, Siewers AE, Finlayson EV, et al. Hospital volume and surgical mortality in the United States. *N Engl J Med* 2002;346(15):1128–1137.

39. Yeo CJ, Cameron JL, Lillemoe KD, et al. Does prophylactic octreotide decrease the rates of pancreatic fistula and other complications after pancreaticoduodenectomy? *Ann Surg* 2000;232: 419–429.

40. Adam U, Makowiec F, Riediger H, et al. Risk factors after pancreatic head resection. *Am J Surg* 2004;187:201–208.

41. Balcom JH, Rattner DW, Warshaw AL, et al. Ten-year experience with 733 pancreatic resections. *Arch Surg* 2001;136:391–398.

42. Gouma DJ, van Geenen RCI, van Gulik TM, et al. Rates of complications and death after pancreaticoduodenectomy: risk factors and the impact of hospital volume. *Ann Surg* 2000;232:786–795.

43. Sohn TA, Yeo CJ, Cameron JL. Resected adenocarcinoma of the pancreas—616 patients: results, outcomes, and prognostic indicators. *J Gastrointest Surg* 2000;4:567–579.

44. Bartoli FG, Arnone GB, Ravera G, et al. Pancreatic fistula and relative mortality in malignant disease after pancreaticoduodenectomy. Review and statistical meta-analysis regarding 15 years of literature. *Anticancer Res* 1991;11:1831–1848.

45. Tran K, van Eijck C, Di Carlo V, et al. Occlusion of the pancreatic duct versus pancreaticoduodenectomy: a prospective randomized trial. *Ann Surg* 2002;236:422–428.

46. Chou FF, Sheen-Chen SM, Chen YS, et al. Postoperative morbidity and mortality of pancreaticoduodenectomy for periampullary cancer. *Eur J Surg* 1996;162:477–481.

47. Yeo CJ, Cameron JL, Maher MM, et al. A prospective randomized trial of pancreatico-gastrostomy and pancreatico-jejunostomy after pancreaticoduodenectomy. *Ann Surg* 1995;225:580–588.

48. Buchler M, Friess H, Klempa I, et al. Role of octreotide in the prevention of postoperative complications following pancreatic resection. *Am J Surg* 1992;163:125–130.

49. Pederzoli P, Bassi C, Falconi M, et al. Efficacy of octreotide in the prevention of complications following pancreatic resection: Italian Study Group. *Br J Surg* 1994;81:265–269.

50. Montorsi M, Zago M, Mosca F, et al. Efficacy of octreotide in the prevention of pancreatic fistula after elective pancreatic resections: a prospective, controlled, randomized clinical trial. *Surgery* 1995;117:26–31.

51. Friess H, Beger HG, Sulkowski U, et al. Randomized controlled multicentre study of the prevention of complications by octreotide in patients undergoing surgery for chronic pancreatitis. *Br J Surg* 1995;82:1270–1273.

52. Rosenberg L, MacNeil P, Turcotte L. Economic evaluation of the use of octreotide for prevention of complications following pancreatic resection. *J Gastrointest Surg* 1999;3:225–232.

53. Yeo CJ. Does prophylactic octreotide benefit patients undergoing elective pancreatic resection? *J Gastrointest Surg* 1999;3:223–224.

54. Lowy AM, Lee JE, Pisters PWT, et al. Prospective randomized trial of octreotide to prevent pancreatic fistula after pancreaticoduodenectomy for malignant disease. *Ann Surg* 1997;226:632–641.

55. Yeo CJ, Cameron JL, Lillemoe KD, et al. Does prophylactic octreotide decrease the rates of pancreatic fistula and other complications after pancreaticoduodenectomy? Results of a prospective randomized placebo-controlled trial. *Ann Surg* 2000;232: 419–429.

56. Miedema BW, Sarr MG, Van Heerden JA, et al. Complications following pancreaticoduodenectomy. Current management. *Arch Surg* 1992;127:945–949.

57. Yeo CJ, Barry MK, Sauter PK, et al. Erythromycin accelerates gastric emptying after pancreaticoduodenectomy. A prospective randomized placebo-controlled trial. *Ann Surg* 1993;218: 229–238.

58. Spanknebel K, Conlon K. Advances in the surgical management of pancreatic cancer. *Cancer J* 2001;7:312–323.

59. Sohn TA, Yeo CJ, Cameron JL, et al. Do preoperative biliary stents increase postpancreaticoduodenectomy complications? *J Gastrointest Surg* 2000;4:258–268.

60. Pisters PW, Hudec WA, Hess KR, et al. Effect of preoperative biliary decompression on pancreaticoduodenectomy-associated mortality in 300 consecutive patients. *Ann Surg* 2001;234:47–55.

61. Bakkevold KE, Kambestad B. Morbidity and mortality after radical and palliative pancreatic cancer surgery. Risk factors influencing short-term results. *Ann Surg* 1993;217(4):356–368.

62. Hodul P, Creech S, Pickleman J, et al. The effect of preoperative biliary stenting on postoperative complications after pancreaticoduodenectomy. *Am J Surg* 2003;186:420–425.

63. Braasch JW, Gray BN. Considerations that lower pancreaticoduodenectomy mortality. *Am J Surg* 1977;133:480–484.

64. Andren-Sandberg A, Ihse I. Factors influencing survival after total pancreatectomy in patients with pancreatic cancer. *Ann Surg* 1983;198:605–610.

65. Bottger TC, Junginger T. Factors influencing morbidity and mortality after pancreaticoduodenectomy: critical analysis of 221 resections. *World J Surg* 1999;23:164–171.

66. Povoski SP, Karpeh MS, Conlon KC, et al. Preoperative biliary drainage: impact on intraoperative bile cultures and infectious morbidity and mortality after pancreaticoduodenectomy. *J Gastrointest Surg* 1999;3:496–505.

67. Pitt HA, Gomes AS, Lois JF, et al. Does preoperative percutaneous biliary drainage reduce operative risk or increase hospital cost? *Ann Surg* 1985;201:545–553.

68. Trede M, Schwall G. The complications of pancreatectomy. *Ann Surg* 1988;207:39–47.

69. Heslin MJ, Brooks AD, Hochwald SN, et al. A preoperative biliary stent is associated with increased complications after pancreatoduodenectomy. *Arch Surg* 1998;133:149–154.

70. Ceuterick M, Gelin M, Rickaert F, et al. Pancreaticoduodenal resection for pancreatic or periampullary tumors—a ten year experience. *Hepato-Gastroenterol* 1989;36:467–473.

71. Whipple A. Present day surgery of the pancreas. *N Engl J Med* 1942;226:515–518.

72. Seiler CA, Wagner M, Sadowski C, et al. Randomized prospective trial of pylorus-preserving vs. classic duodenopancreatectomy (Whipple procedure): initial clinical results. *J Gastrointest Surg* 2000;4:443–452.

73. Mosca F, Giulianotti PC, Balestracci T, et al. Long-term survival in pancreatic cancer: pylorus preserving versus Whipple pancreaticoduodenectomy. *Surgery* 1997;122:553–566.

74. Patel AG, Toyama MT, Kusske AM, et al. Pylorus-preserving Whipple resection for pancreatic cancer: is it any better? *Arch Surg* 1995;130:838–843.

75. Crist DW, Sitzmann JV, Cameron JL. Improved hospital morbidity, mortality, and survival after the Whipple procedure. *Ann Surg* 1987;206:358–365.

76. van Berge Henegouwen MI, van Gulik TM, DeWit LT, et al. Delayed gastric emptying after standard pancreaticoduodenectomy versus pylorus-preserving pancreaticoduodenectomy: an analysis of 200 consecutive patients. *J Am Coll Surg* 1997;185: 373–379.

77. Bilimoria MM, Cormier JN, Mun JE, et al. Pancreatic leak after left pancreatectomy following main pancreatic duct ligation. *Br J Surg* 2003;90:190–196.

78. Fahey BN, Frey CF, Ho HS, et al. Morbidity, mortality, and technical factors of distal pancreactectomy. *Am J Surg* 2002;183: 237–241.

79. Lillemoe KD, Kaushal S, Cameron JL, et al. Distal pancreatectomy: indications and outcomes in 235 patients. *Ann Surg* 1999;229:693–700.

80. Cogbill TH, Moore EE, Morris JA, et al. Distal pancreatectomy for trauma: a multicenter experience. *J Trauma* 1991;31:1600–1606.

81. Sohn TA, Campbell KA, Pitt HA, et al. Quality of life and long-term survival after surgery for chronic pancreatitis. *J Gastrointest Surg* 2000;4:355–365.

82. Hutchins RR, Hart RS, Pacifico M, et al. Long-term results of distal pancreatectomy for chronic pancreatitis in 90 patients. *Ann Surg* 2002;236:612–618.

83. Slezak LA, Anderson DK. Pancreatic resection: effects on glucose metabolism. *World J Surg* 2001;25:452–460.

84. Karpoff HM, Klimstra DS, Brennan MF, et al. Results of total pancreatectomy for adenocarcinoma of the pancreas. *Arch Surg* 2001;136:44–47.

85. Fleming WR, Williamson RC. Role of total pancreatectomy in the treatment of patients with end-stage chronic pancreatitis. *Br J Surg* 1995;82:1409–1412.

86. Dresler CM, Fortner JG, McDermott K, et al. Metabolic consequences of (regional) total pancreatectomy. *Ann Surg* 1991;214:131–140.

87. Assan R, Alexandre JH, Tiengo A, et al. Survival and rehabilitation after total pancreatectomy: a follow-up of 36 patients. *Diabet Metab* 1985;11:303–309.

88. Rilo R, Ahmad SA, D'Alessio SA, et al. Total pancreatectomy and autologous islet transplantation a means to treat severe chronic pancreatitis. *J Gastrointest Surg* 2003;7:978–989.

89. Gruessner RW, Sutherland DE, Dunn DL, et al. Transplant options for patients undergoing total pancreatectomy for chronic pancreatitis. *J Am Coll Surg* 2004;198:559–567.

Complications of Intestinal Surgery: Small Bowel

35

Arden M. Morris

■ **PREOPERATIVE RISK MODIFICATION 479**

■ **TECHNICAL ISSUES 479**

Exploration 480
Anastomosis 480
Mesenteric Defects 480
Adhesion Prevention 480
Ileus 480

■ **SPECIFIC INTESTINAL DISORDERS REQUIRING INTERVENTION 481**

Short Bowel Syndrome 481
Crohn Disease 482
Irradiated Bowel 484
Intussusception 486
Neoplasms of the Small Bowel 486
Hemorrhage 488
Ischemia 489
Small Intestinal Bypass 490
Hypomotility 490
Ileostomy Complications 491
Jejunostomy Tube Complications 494

■ **SUMMARY 495**

■ **REFERENCES 495**

Arden M. Morris: University of Michigan, Ann Arbor, MI 48109

The small bowel integrates digestive and barrier functions, resulting in a metabolic engine that is the body's largest barrier to the outside world. Yet it remains remarkably resistant to infection, toxins, and neoplastic growth. Digestive functions, including secretion of hormones, enzymes, and electrolytes into the bowel lumen, confer resistance to infection and injury. Physical, immunologic, and physiologic barriers provide key defenses against infection and malignant transformation of cells. In fact, although it comprises 90% of the entire gastrointestinal surface area, the small intestine produces <5% of gut tumors (1). Thus, the need for operative intervention for intestinal failure is frequently a result of previous operation rather than of treatment of an intrinsic small bowel problem.

This chapter reviews the complications of surgical treatment of intestinal failure. Fleming and Remington defined intestinal failure as "the reduction in functioning gut mass below the amount necessary for adequate digestion and absorption of food" (2). This simple definition focuses on the intestine's functional role, clarifying the pathophysiology of numerous possible underlying mechanisms of failure resulting from even more numerous possible disease states (Table 35-1).

Acute intestinal failure, such as failure due to postoperative ileus, is usually limited. Subacute or chronic failure results in slowly escalating debilitation due to associated malnutrition. Wound healing slows and stops without adequate amino acid, carbohydrate, fat, and vitamin and mineral substrates. Immunity is broadly suppressed, including

TABLE 35-1

UNDERLYING ETIOLOGIES OF INTESTINAL FAILURE

Etiology of Failure	Mechanism	Specific Disease Examples
Mechanical obstruction		
	Extrinsic compression	Peritoneal adhesions, incarcerated hernia, extraluminal mass
	Stricture	Crohn disease, ischemia
	Torsion	Postoperative, congenital malrotation
	Obstruction	Tumor, stool, gallstone, bezoar
Dysmotility		
	Ileus	Postoperative, narcotic use, inflammation, distal obstruction
	Neuromuscular disorder	Acquired or congenital visceral myopathy, enteric neuropathy
Hemorrhage		
	Vascular	Ateriovenous malformations, vascular-enteric fistula formation, ulceration
	Tumor erosion	Adenocarcinoma, carcinoid, lymphoma, gastrointestinal stromal tumor
	Other erosion	Meckel diverticulum
Necrosis		
	Chronic ischemia	Atherosclerotic disease, radiation enteritis
	Acute ischemia	Thromboembolic disease, mesenteric torsion
Leak of intestinal contents (fistula, abscess, peritonitis)		
	Iatrogenic injury	Unrecognized intraoperative injury, technical failure during anastomosis, ischemia
	Anastomotic breakdown	Inflammation, infection, malnutrition, immunosuppression
	Spontaneous	Ischemia, Crohn disease, postradiation, distal obstruction, tumor erosion, ischemia, foreign body
Nutritional deficits		
	Malabsorption	Previous ileal resection, Crohn disease, radiation enteritis, sprue, infectious diarrhea, bacterial overgrowth
	Short bowel syndrome	Postoperative, Crohn disease, radiation enteritis, ischemic bowel

neutrophil, T-cell, and antibody function. Patients with unintentional weight loss of >10% to 15% of baseline body weight or with a serum albumin level <3.0 are severely malnourished. Prior to elective surgery, such patients benefit from preoperative parenteral nutritional supplementation to reduce the perioperative risk of infection or nonhealing (3). Longer-term markers like serum albumin are useful for prognostication, while shorter-term markers such as prealbumin or retinol binding protein can assist with day-to-day assessment of nutritional repletion.

Medical therapy for intestinal failure aims to reduce the severity of malnutrition, avoid complications, and maximize quality of life (4). Prevention of bowel edema due to excessive saline administration, limitation of intestinal electrolyte losses due to ingestion of hypotonic fluids, and monitoring serum and urine electrolytes frequently are important steps in management. An elemental or low

residue diet and pharmacological agents to slow intestinal transit time can be helpful. The value of exogenous trophic factors is less clear.

If nonoperative management fails, operative intervention can sometimes reestablish nutritional function and relieve underlying pathology (Table 35-2). Restoration of the intestine's nutritional role may be an anatomic, physiologic, or combined exercise; for example, placement of a colon interposition graft to interrupt peristalsis for patients with rapid small bowel transit uses an anatomic alteration to correct a physiologic problem. The surgical dictum holds that avoidable perioperative complications arise as a result of technical or, more commonly, judgment errors. Errors are prevented or limited by clear goals, careful technique, and appropriate alternative strategies. However, many less controllable factors can have an impact on short-term and long-term complications, such as patient age, functional status, underlying disease, and severity of illness. Therefore,

TABLE 35-2

THERAPEUTIC GOALS OF INTESTINAL SURGERY

Restore nutritional role of small bowel
    Adequate length
    Adequate lumen
    Adequate absorption

Relieve pathology
    Obstruction
    Bleeding
    Infection
    Ischemia

Prevent postoperative complications
    Sepsis
    Obstruction

consideration of specific preoperative and intraoperative measures to reduce risk is critical.

PREOPERATIVE RISK MODIFICATION

Prudent planning for operation must include preoperative care designed to prevent complications. For example, preoperative optimization of respiratory and hemodynamic parameters limits perioperative morbidity and mortality. In a randomized trial of normal preparation versus preoperative breathing exercises among upper abdominal surgery patients at significant risk, the postoperative pulmonary complication rate decreased from 60% to 19% (5). Subsequent studies demonstrate even better results among abdominal surgery patients with preoperative incentive spirometry training and chest physiotherapy (6).

Similarly, intervention for previously unrecognized cardiac arrhythmias or poorly controlled hypertension reduces perioperative risk of circulatory embarrassment (7,8). A recent meta-analysis demonstrated significant mortality reduction among high-risk patients who received *early* optimization of hemodynamic parameters

and oxygen delivery but no such benefit after organ failure had occurred (9).

Recognition of barriers to healing is another part of the preoperative risk management process. The association between severe malnutrition and increased risk for postoperative complications or death is well established (Table 35-3) (10,11). The severely nutritionally depleted patient can benefit substantially from 7 to 10 days of preoperative hyperalimentation. Comorbid diseases associated with impaired microcirculation, such as renal failure and diabetes, also inhibit mechanisms of healing and merit scrupulous preoperative medical control. Glucocorticoids interfere with virtually every step in the phases of wound healing. Cumulative data suggest that retinoids (12) and transforming growth factor β (13) counter the steroid effect on collagen metabolism, but neither has been incorporated effectively into regular practice. In a multivariate analysis of a large retrospective cohort, long-term steroid use was the only variable associated with a significantly higher rate of serious complications after anastomosis among Crohn patients (14). In contrast, a recent retrospective study of outcomes after bowel resection (15) reported that high-dose and low-dose steroid-dependent Crohn patients had perioperative morbidity rates nearly identical to one another and to nonsteroid dependent patients. Little is known of the healing impact or operative risk of newer immunosuppressive medications for Crohn disease, such as infliximab, a recombinant anti–TNF-α antibody. However, an early prospective study funded by the manufacturer indicated minimal operative risks beyond those already faced by Crohn disease patients (16).

TECHNICAL ISSUES

Evidence-based recommendations for intraoperative technique to prevent postoperative complications largely rest upon Halsted's early tenets to handle tissue gently, employ aseptic technique, avoid closure under tension, and close wounds completely whenever possible. Limiting intra-abdominal dissection to that required for adequate

TABLE 35-3

IMPACT OF NUTRITIONAL STATUS ON POSTOPERATIVE COMPLICATIONS AMONG INTESTINAL FAILURE PATIENTS

Degree of Malnutrition	% Weight Loss over 3 Months	Serum Albumin	Postoperative Complication Risk (%)
Mild	5–10	2.8–3.4	20–30
Moderate	10–20	2.1–2.7	30–45
Severe	>20	≤2.0	40–60

exposure and handling tissue gently helps to prevent serosal injury and limit blood loss, thereby restricting adhesion formation (17,18). Massive adhesions and herniations can lead to loss of abdominal domain, a vexing intraoperative problem that may require use of mesh or relaxing incisions to close without tension.

Exploration

During exploratory laparotomy of a nonhostile abdomen, initial evaluation of the small bowel consists of examination from the ligament of Treitz to the cecum. Serosal injuries should be repaired when identified. Other incidental lesions may be addressed after correcting the preoperative issue. Incidentally identified tumors should be excised. Frozen section examination can be useful to determine benign versus malignant features and to ascertain clear margins. Meckel diverticuli should be excised except in moribund patients, according to long-term population-based data (19). Anecdotally, incidental appendectomy has fallen into disfavor. Although cumulative data suggest prohibitive risk among patients who are >50 years old, are immunosuppressed, are medically unstable, or have prosthetic material or previous diagnosis of Crohn disease, many studies support performing incidental appendectomy on patients <30 years old (20–23). Resisting the urge to "tidy up" the abdomen is generally appropriate, limiting the operation to the problem at hand.

Anastomosis

Much has been written and little resolved about anastomotic technique; stapled versus sutured, single layer versus double layer, type of suture material, and impact of diversion are all open controversies. The goal of enteric anastomosis is to prevent leakage, promote healing, preserve bowel length, and prevent stricture formation. An effective anastomosis requires adequate mobilization, perfusion, apposition, and inversion of the mucosal edges into the bowel lumen. Healing depends on approximation of the collagen-containing submucosal layer. Inadequate perfusion or tension across the anastomosis may cause early leakage or late stricture formation.

Anastomotic leakage is a potentially disastrous complication, running the gamut from a contained self-limited event to sepsis and abdominal catastrophe (24–26). Investigations into the frequency of leakage after stapled versus sewn anastomoses are contradictory; available data support the superiority of each and of neither (27,28), possibly reflecting a difference in patient populations.

Anastomotic strictures form as a result of ischemia, tension, or infection due to previous anastomotic failure. Technical choices are fairly forgiving but may also play a role; in a randomized controlled trial of esophagogastrostomy anastomoses, a double-layer closure led to significantly more stricture formation than single-layer (29).

Much of the remaining research addressing anastomosis is limited to the colon and rectal literature, which has limited application to small bowel issues. The principles of a safe anastomosis can be observed using a variety of techniques.

Mesenteric Defects

Literature addressing closure of mesenteric defects is also scarce. Customarily, an absorbable suture incorporating only the peritoneal leaves of divided mesentery is run from the apex of the defect toward the bowel. With the advent of laparoscopic colon resection, the utility of mesenteric closure has been questioned and the technique simply abandoned by some. However, many surgeons elect to close defects small enough to potentially incarcerate the bowel.

Adhesion Prevention

Placement of a bioresorbable adhesion barrier over abdominal contents prior to anterior wall closure can limit or even prevent postoperative abdominal wall adhesion formation (30,31). This is an especially useful exercise for patients with Crohn disease, temporary ileostomy, or other indications for a future laparotomy. Wrapping a fresh anastomosis in such an adhesion barrier results in a higher leak rate and is discouraged (32).

Ileus

Postoperative ileus is a predictable but poorly understood phenomenon that generally lasts 3 to 5 days and is managed expectantly. If the ileus is prolonged >7 days in a patient with previously normal motility, an early mechanical obstruction or possible enteric leak should be considered (33–35). Timing of reoperation becomes especially relevant during the 2 to 6 week postoperative window, when extensive adhesions and inflammation create a significant technical challenge increasing the risk of bleeding, fistula, abscess, and abdominal sepsis (36).

Previous surgical treatment plays a major role in the development of intestinal failure. In an extensive review of the literature, Tera and Aberg (37) determined that 1.6% of abdominal operations result in a reoperation and 34% to 43% of reoperations result in mortality, a number confirmed by more recent studies (24–26,36). The two most common reasons for return to the operating room are peritonitis (32% of reoperative cases) and ileus or obstruction (25% of cases). Other series (38,39) determined that adhesions after a previous operation accounted for more than half of episodes of small bowel obstruction; however, most episodes were successfully managed with nasogastric tube decompression. Thirteen percent to 38% of obstructed patients ultimately return to the operating room after 6 to 8 days of unsuccessful decompression, and the risk increases with each subsequent operation.

SPECIFIC INTESTINAL DISORDERS REQUIRING INTERVENTION

Although the potential complications of intestinal surgery are myriad, they tend to be closely related and even overlapping (Fig. 35-1). Many underlying diseases predispose to particular postoperative issues. This section examines the complications that arise most frequently after operative intervention for specific underlying diseases or conditions.

Short Bowel Syndrome

Short bowel syndrome describes a constellation of symptoms, including malnutrition, weight loss, steatorrhea, and diarrhea, resulting from inadequate absorptive gut surface area. The disorder may follow massive intestinal resection for ischemia, infection, mesenteric desmoid tumors, or other diseases. It may be the cumulative effect of sequential excisions or the functional result of proximal fistula formation. Although individual variation and adaptation can occur, most patients with <100 cm total bowel or <150 cm without the ileocecal valve will not survive with enteric nutrition alone.

In addition to the expected complications of malnutrition, other associated complications include cholelithiasis, nephrolithiasis, and gastric hypersecretion. Symptomatic cholelithiasis develops in 20% to 40% of patients and is most frequent in those dependent on parenteral nutrition. In reviews of the topic, Thompson recommends considering prophylactic gallbladder excision prior to the development of hepatic changes, dense adhesion formation, and medical complications of malnutrition (40,41). Nephrolithiasis arises in about 25% of patients with some retained colon, due to increased colonic oxalate absorption and excretion through the urinary system. Calcium oxalate stone formation

may be prevented by careful diet management and cholesterol binding medication (42). Gastric hypersecretion after massive bowel resection is poorly understood and usually temporary but can lead to profound peptic ulcer disease requiring long-term use of proton pump inhibitors (43).

Enormous advances in the prevention and management of short bowel syndrome have been made in the past two decades. The best strategy is clearly prevention, especially when future abdominal operations are anticipated. In cases of viable but obstructed bowel, limiting the extent of resection and performing stricturoplasty have become standards of care. Measurement of remaining bowel is easily performed before closing the abdomen (Fig. 35-2), and facilitates diagnosis of related disorders and planning of future therapy.

Effective medical treatment for short bowel syndrome improves absorption of nutrients and slows intestinal transit time. Postoperative mucosal hyperplasia occurs over a period of 6 to 12 months. Early reports suggested that glutamine and growth hormones enhance mucosal adaptation, but these data have not been replicated in well-designed subsequent studies (44–46). An elemental, high-carbohydrate, low-fat diet may have a trophic effect and improve absorption (45). Agents that slow bowel transit are staples of therapy. Loperamide decreases intestinal motility and secretion and has been shown to increase sphincter pressure (47); however, it is metabolized via the enterohepatic circulation. Codeine or tincture of opium may be necessary if the patient is sufficiently impaired. Octreotide may prove useful if transit is too rapid or the intestine is too short for absorption of oral antisecretory medication.

Operative treatment of short bowel syndrome consists of procedures to relieve obstruction, increase bowel surface area, and slow transit time. Relief of obstruction is usually achieved by stricturoplasty and is most relevant in the

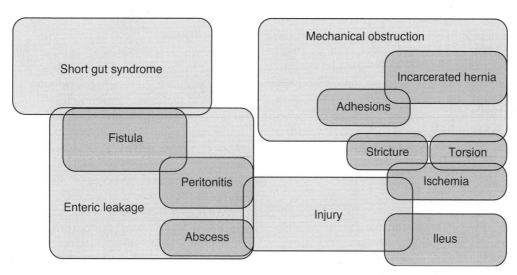

Figure 35-1 Schematic association of common postoperative complications.

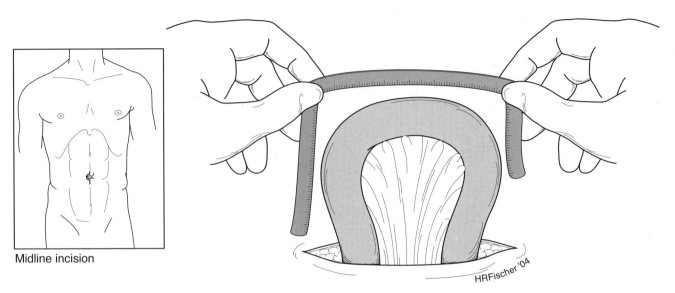

Midline incision

Figure 35-2 Measuring the small bowel (short gut).

Crohn disease patient. The most useful method for increasing the absorptive surface is reintroduction of defunctionalized bowel into the enteral stream. However, although reapproximation of the small intestine and colon improves surface area and provides a trophic effect, it can also lead to increased diarrhea and stone formation. Tapering and lengthening procedures improve absorption and motility and have been most extensively used in pediatric patients (48,49). Transit slowing procedures historically include formation of valves and sphincters. Creation of an antiperistaltic segment has had variable efficacy, possibly due to inconsistent technique, low patient numbers, and lack of standardized follow-up and outcome measurements. Interposition of a colonic segment has shown promising results in some reports but has led to obstruction and failure in others (40,41,50).

Refractory short bowel disease, whether anatomic or physiologic, requires nutritional support and consideration of transplantation. Hyperalimentation has become increasingly sophisticated since its introduction in 1968, but it is associated with many inherent potential complications. For patients in whom hyperalimentation has been fraught with complications, intestinal transplantation may be an option. Several studies now indicate outcomes approximating those of lifelong total parenteral nutrition if the transplant can be accomplished before the onset of hepatic cirrhosis (51–53).

Crohn Disease

Crohn disease is a chronic, segmental, transmural, T helper cell-mediated disease that can arise anywhere in the gastrointestinal tract and various extraintestinal organs. Symptomatic hallmarks include diarrhea, weight loss, and abdominal pain. Seventy percent of Crohn patients overall and 84% of those with ileocecal disease require surgical intervention at some time (54). Solid data are limited on the impact of preoperative immunosuppressive medication on postoperative complication rates among Crohn patients. As previously indicated, steroid use has been associated with greater risk in some large retrospective series (14,55) but not others (15,56). Preoperative treatment with nonsteroid immunosuppressives has actually been associated with better postoperative outcomes (16,56).

Acute or chronic obstruction, fistula or abscess formation, and complications of previous operations are the most common indications for operation. Short bowel syndrome, fistula formation, and development of an abdomen so rife with adhesions that it must be considered frankly hostile are among the many potential complications of operating in this setting.

Malabsorption

Malabsorption and diarrhea, intimately related manifestations of Crohn disease, may result in a functional short bowel syndrome, but they are also caused by an anatomically short gut due to multiple resections. Micronutrient malnutrition depends on the anatomic site and length of bowel resection. Cyanocobalamine (vitamin B_{12}) is the most common deficiency and occurs predictably after resection of 50 to 60 cm of terminal ileum. Folate deficiency results from resection or disease of the proximal jejunum. Diminished vitamin D absorption may occur with reduced absorption of bile salts, and contributes to calcium deficiency and osteoporosis.

Iatrogenic short bowel syndrome is one of the most notorious and challenging complications of operating for Crohn disease. Short bowel syndrome is of particular concern

TABLE 35-4

MANAGEMENT OF ENTEROCUTANEOUS FISTULAE

	Quantity/ 24 hr	Management		Likelihood of Spontaneous Resolution	Mortality
		Early	Late		
Low output	<200 cc	Bowel rest, nutrition repletion, skin protection, appropriate drainage	After 30–40 days: Consider curettage of tract, instillation of noxious substance or fibrin glue, or resection of tract with primary closure	Moderate	5%
Medium output	200–500 cc	Bowel rest, TPN, skin or wound protection, drainage of sepsis	Sepsis: Consider diversion with delayed repair versus resection		
High output	>500 cc	Diversion, TPN, skin or wound protection including consideration of vacuum-assisted closure, drainage of sepsis	After 40–90 days or resolution of sepsis: Resection with temporary diversion	None	35%–50%

TPN, total parenteral nutrition.

among Crohn patients due to their common presentation with terminal ileal disease, necessitating ileocecal valve resection. Patients are subject to inadequate nutrition for healing and health maintenance, dehydration, and exacerbation of diarrhea, which can be debilitating to quality of life. Stricturoplasty for preserving bowel length in Crohn disease patients is essential to long-term outcome and is reviewed in detail below.

Fistula Formation

Spontaneous intra-abdominal abscesses and fistulae form in 20% to 40% of Crohn patients and are a fundamental characteristic of the disease. Postoperative fistula formation occurs in about 10% to 15% of patients in the 30-day perioperative period (14,55) but in >20% over the ensuing 5 years (57). Either may be identified preoperatively based on symptoms and radiologic studies or identified incidentally while examining the bowel. Appropriate therapy is based on the clinical situation. Lichtenstein's review of medical therapy highlights encouraging early results with use of infliximab but acknowledges frequent need for surgical intervention (58). Treatment of symptomatic fistulae includes resection of the fistulizing bowel and tract, with simple closure of the involved nondiseased viscus. No intervention is warranted for spontaneous, asymptomatic enteroenteric fistula formation (59).

Management of an enterocutaneous fistula is based on symptoms, duration, and, most importantly, output (Table 35-4). Preliminary therapeutic goals are treatment of sepsis, skin protection, accurate output measurement, and ascertainment of adequate nutrition. Spontaneous closure is possible, depending primarily on the cause, location, related infection, and nutritional status (Table 35-5). Proximal fistulae are associated with a higher daily output

and nutritional deficiency (a functional short gut); distal fistulae are more likely to have a lower output and to heal spontaneously. Low to moderate output enterocutaneous fistulae (<200 cc per day and 200 to 400 cc per day, respectively) may be managed by observation, consideration of bowel rest, and parenteral nutrition if indicated. Some authors advocate curettage of the fistula tract, with or without fibrin glue insertion, or instillation of a noxious substance to facilitate scar formation, such as phenol. Reported outcomes are highly variable and based on small series with poorly quantified follow-up.

Obstruction

Intestinal obstruction in the Crohn patient generally begins as an acute inflammatory process, best controlled by immunosuppressive medication if possible. If medical therapy is ineffective after 7 to 10 days or if acute obstruction repeatedly recurs, operative resection or bypass should be considered (60,61). There is no need to resect beyond macroscopically noninvolved bowel, and a conservative approach to resection has decreased the incidence of postoperative short bowel syndrome in recent years. Recording

TABLE 35-5

FACTORS PREVENTING SPONTANEOUS FISTULA CLOSURE

Sepsis
Distal obstruction
Radiation injury
Mucosal eversion at the skin level
High output/proximal fistula
Poor nutrition

the measured bowel length in the operative note will help with future treatment planning (Fig. 35-2).

In contrast to the inflammation, adhesions, and abscesses observed in an acute Crohn disease obstruction, chronic obstruction is primarily a fibrotic process. Strictures may be detected preoperatively based on computed tomography (CT) or small bowel contrast studies, or fibrosis may be identified during the intraoperative bowel examination. At these sites the small bowel appears and feels thickened and firm. Proximal bowel may appear distended, with a smooth edematous or thickened wall. If access to the lumen has already been obtained, a balloon catheter distended to 2.5 cm may be pulled from the ligament of Treitz to the cecum to assess the luminal diameter. Sometimes even areas of intestine that appear normal externally will reveal a narrow lumen with extensive internal fibrotic strands.

Short strictures can be dilated with the catheter balloon. Longer strictures, or those with extensive fibrosis, are best managed by resection or stricturoplasty (Fig. 35-3). The judgment for resection versus preservation with stricturoplasty is based on the length, proximity, and overall number of strictures and on the length of remaining short bowel. The risk of stricture recurrence is high. At least 30% of Crohn patients operated on for acute disease will require at least one additional operation for obstruction.

Adhesion formation is another potential source of postoperative obstruction. Placement of a hyaluronic acid–based adhesion barrier prior to wound closure can greatly facilitate future avoidance of enterotomy in the patient destined for multiple operations (30,32). Additionally,

preliminary evidence supports the role of newer anti–TNF-α antibody medication in reducing postoperative adhesions and inflammation in Crohn patients (62).

Recurrence

Perhaps the most common complication of operating for Crohn disease is Crohn recurrence. Asymptomatic endoscopic evidence of disease has been reported as early as 3 months postoperatively and up to 75% of patients within the first postoperative year (63,64). Data regarding the influence of endoscopically identified disease on development of symptoms requiring operation are inconclusive. The extent of resection does not appear to have an impact on recurrence; although macroscopic disease should be removed, the presence of residual microscopic disease has no correlation with symptomatic recurrence. Inconsistent data have made clear identification of risk factors difficult (57,65) (Table 35-6). Prophylaxis against recurrence using medical therapy has been disappointing overall, but several well-designed studies of newer medications are currently underway.

Irradiated Bowel

Many complications resulting from radiation injury to the small bowel are reminiscent of Crohn disease, such as stricture (obstruction), chronic bleeding, diarrhea, malabsorption, fistula formation, and abdominal pain. One may infer from the broad variety of interventions designed to slow motility and enhance absorption that surgical therapy

---

TABLE 35-6
RISK FACTORS FOR POSTOPERATIVE RECURRENCE OF CROHN DISEASE

	Factor	Impact on Clinical Recurrence
Patient-related factors	Age	Mild increase in recurrence.
	Gender	No impact on recurrence.
	Smoking	Independent risk factor for recurrence with odds ratio = 2–4 compared to nonsmokers. Odds are especially high among women who smoke.
Disease-related factors	Location of disease	Data have suggested increased recurrence with ileocolonic disease, but are inconclusive.
	Duration of disease	No impact on recurrence.
Surgical factors	Margin	Histologic evidence of residual Crohn disease has no impact on recurrence.
	Anastomotic method	No impact on recurrence.
	Diversion of the fecal stream	Specific toxins or antigens in the feces have not been identified, but lack of diversion and reversal of diversion appear associated with higher recurrence rates.

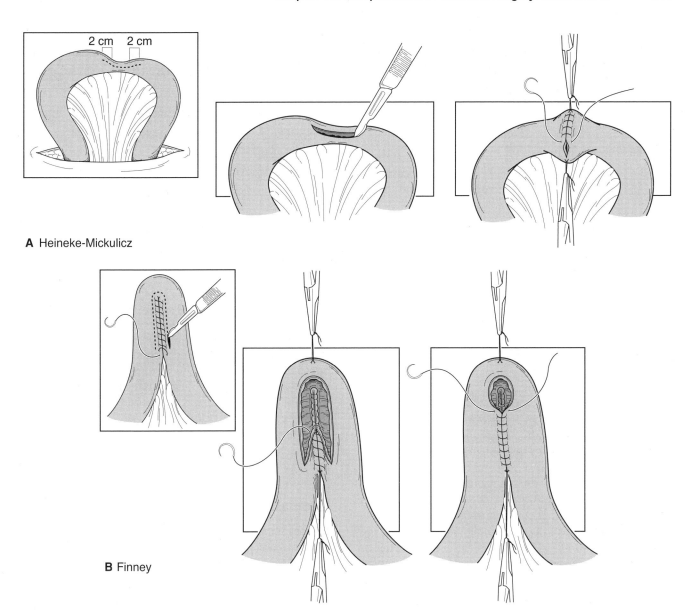

A Heineke-Mickulicz

B Finney

Figure 35-3 Bowel-preserving techniques for management of intestinal strictures. **A:** Heineke-Mickulicz stricturoplasty. A longitudinal incision is created sharply in the antimesenteric wall to 2 cm beyond the proximal and distal boundaries of the stricture. Two 3-0 silk stay sutures are placed on either side of the incision at the midpoint and retracted to reorient the incision to transverse. A single layer of full-thickness 3-0 silk interrupted sutures is placed to reapproximate the bowel edges in the new transverse orientation. **B:** Finney stricturoplasty. The Finney technique is advised for very long (≥25 cm) strictures of the small bowel. A longitudinal incision is created sharply in the antimesenteric wall. A stay suture placed at the apical midpoint is retraced to facilitate an upside-down U orientation. The inner edge is sutured to itself longitudinally from the luminal side to become a new posterior wall, with the previous distal-most bowel now abutting the proximal-most bowel. Similarly, the outer edge of the U is closed with simple interrupted full-thickness suture to become the new anterior wall.

has limited efficacy. However, a symptom-directed operation may be unavoidable, and in this setting the extreme fragility of irradiated bowel must be respected. Resection and bypass are the foundations of surgical therapy. Complication rates are high, with anastomotic leakage rates up to nearly 60%, probably due to compromised perfusion (66). Although the value of resection versus bypass has been debated, bypass is associated with lower short-term complication and mortality rates (Table 35-7). Longer-term issues arising from bypass include ongoing fibrotic stricture formation, bacterial overgrowth, and issues of chronic mucosal damage (67). In one small series, Dietz et al. reported encouraging results using stricturoplasty for long-segment radiation-associated obstruction (68). The importance of cautious consideration of operative goals and alternative strategies is widely recognized. Because radiation damage and

TABLE 35-7

POSTOPERATIVE MORTALITY AFTER INTERVENTION FOR IRRADIATED INTESTINE

Source	Bypass		Resection	
	n	Mortality (%)	*n*	Mortality (%)
Joelsson and Raf (96)	–	–	19	16
Swan et al. (97)	28	7	17	53
Schmitt and Symmonds (98)	20	0	65	9
Lillemoe et al. (99)	11	0	6	17
Wobbes et al. (66)	20	10	7	57
Galland and Spencer (100)	2	0	18	44
Total	81	5	132	23

obstructive symptoms can continue to manifest, sometimes over decades, preserving bowel length even in the initial operation is recommended.

Intussusception

Intussusception, or telescoping of the bowel, is a rare event usually identified by symptoms of bowel obstruction and a CT scan revealing an asymmetrical target sign (Fig. 35-4). In contrast to the pediatric patient, intussusception in the adult is more frequently due to an anatomic leadpoint abnormality, such as a tumor, and thus traditionally treated by exploratory celiotomy and probable resection (69). Potential complications of such intervention are postoperative ileus, bleeding, infection, damage to nearby structures, and adhesion formation. Delay in operation for incarcerated intussuscepted bowel can lead to ischemic necrosis. However, an interesting artifact of

improved CT technology has led to a new possible complication of surgery for diagnosis of intussusception: unnecessary exploratory laparotomy. High-resolution circular CT has become so rapid, and images are so clear, that bowel seen end-on may be captured during peristalsis, potentially resulting in a diagnosis of intussusception that does not actually require intervention. A large single institution review identified intussusception length of <3.5 cm to be a reliable predictor of a self-limiting process (70). So far, no prospective test of criteria for nonoperative intussusception has been performed.

Neoplasms of the Small Bowel

Tumors of the small bowel are rare and tend to be diagnosed at advanced stages due to nonspecific symptoms and difficult access. The most common presenting symptoms are pain, anemia, and weight loss. About half of tumors are found in

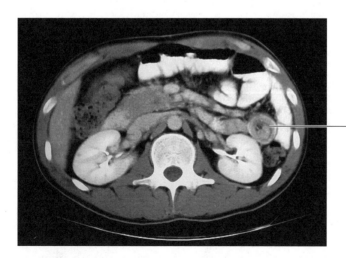

Asymmetrical target sign

Figure 35-4 Computed tomography scan revealing an asymmetrical target sign previously considered the *sine qua non* of small bowel intussusception. This asymptomatic patient was referred for further evaluation of incidentally identified "intussusception."

TABLE 35-8

NEOPLASMS OF THE SMALL INTESTINE: INCIDENCE AND PROGNOSIS

Tumor Type	Incidence (%)	Examples of Associated Syndromes	1-Year survival (%)	5-Year Survival (%)
Benign				
Leiomyoma	75	Spontaneous		
Adenoma	17	Familial adenomatous polyposis		
Hamartoma	8	Peutz-Jaegers, Cronkite-Canada		
Hemangioma	<1	Osler-Webber-Rendu		
Lymphangioma	<1	Spontaneous		
Other	<1			
Total benign	12/54 (22)		67	50
Malignant				
Adenocarcinoma	33	Familial adenomatous polyposis		
Carcinoid tumor	17	Multiple endocrine neoplasia I, von Hippel-Lindau, Neurofibromatosis-1		
Gastrointestinal stromal tumor	17	Spontaneous		
Nonhodgkins lymphoma	12	Spontaneous		
Melanoma	9	Dysplastic Naevus syndrome		
Other	12			
Total malignant	42/54 (78)		43	21

From Naef M, Buhlmann M, Baer HU. Small bowel tumors: diagnosis, therapy and prognostic factors. *Langenbecks Arch Surg* 1999;384(2):176–180, with permission.

the jejunum; the rest are evenly split between the duodenum and the ileum. The resectability rate is high; however, 1-year and 5-year survival rates are less encouraging (Table 35-8). In a 10-year series, Naef et al. reported that 71% of all small bowel tumors were malignant and 62% had already metastasized at the time of diagnosis (71). Major postoperative complications occurred in 24% of patients; 4% required reoperation for anastomotic leaks and 4% died.

Benign Neoplasms

Benign neoplasms of the small bowel are uncommon and are typically discovered incidentally during laparotomy for another purpose. Although all may occur sporadically, many are associated with specific underlying diseases. For example, hamartomas are associated with Peutz-Jaegers syndrome and Cronkite-Canada syndrome, hemangiomas are associated with Osler-Weber-Rendu syndrome, and adenomas are associated with familial adenomatous polyposis syndrome. Resection of symptomatic tumors or tumors that are dysplastic by definition (adenoma) can be performed endoscopically through an enterotomy that should then be closed transversely or by limited local excision with end-to-end anastomosis. Resection of isolated asymptomatic benign lesions is reasonable in the setting of intra-abdominal examination. However, resection of numerous asymptomatic benign tumors is not warranted due to the limited benefit and additive complication risk of each enterotomy.

Adenocarcinoma

Adenocarcinoma is the most common malignancy of the small intestine, accounting for about one-third of cases. It may occur sporadically or in association with a defined polyposis syndrome. Adenomas and adenocarcinomas of the small bowel are not associated with particularly high complication rates; however, lesions due to underlying Gardner syndrome may have associated desmoid tissue. Desmoid tumors, a histologically benign but behaviorally malignant process, are a cause for grave concern. They are composed of fibroblasts growing in thick, white plaques that gradually surround, contract, and compress viscera and vessels. Desmoid tumors are akin to biological cement, inexorably filling the peritoneal cavities of these unfortunate patients. No real cure or prevention has been identified, although estrogen and nonsteroidal anti-inflammatory medications have shown limited efficacy. Because the trauma of operating appears to stimulate growth, operative intervention should be undertaken cautiously.

Carcinoid Tumor

Carcinoid tumors are neuroendocrine tumors that are associated with a number of family cancer syndromes. Patients typically present with complaints of vague abdominal pain and weight loss. Carcinoid tumors generally produce such symptoms due to ischemia from mesenteric microvasular invasion, desmoplasia, and lymphedema from metastatases to draining lymph nodes. Fibrosis can extend to the root of the mesenteric vessels, creating a major technical challenge to resection and potentially mandating bypass to avoid massive intestinal devascularization from resection.

Carcinoid syndrome occurs in about 10% of patients with midgut carcinoids and frequently indicates hepatic involvement. A carcinoid syndrome "attack" is mediated by neurotransmitters, hormones, and peptides released by the tumor cells. The humoral products stimulate vasomotor changes, bronchospasm, gastrointestinal hypermotility, and hypotension.

Carcinoid crisis is a potentially fatal carcinoid syndrome attack, with pronounced changes in blood pressure, diarrhea, confusion, bronchoconstriction, cardiac arrhythmia, and hyperthermia. Carcinoid crisis may occur spontaneously while inducing anesthesia, while handling tumor in the operating room, or during hepatic arterial embolization or chemotherapy treatment. Octreotide and histamine blockers, as well as supportive care, must be administered immediately.

Gastrointestinal Stromal Tumor (GIST)

Gastrointestinal stromal tumors (GISTs) have captured scientist and clinician attention in recent years due to major advances in understanding the pathophysiology and treatment. Previously, these tumors were often miscategorized as sarcomas, but they are now believed to derive from the interstitial cells of Cajal, the intrinsic pacemaker cells of the gut. Complications arising from resection are predictable: anastomotic leakage, stricture formation, adhesions. When malignant, these cells tend to metastasize hematogenously and to recur either locally (possibly due to inadequate margins) or in the liver.

Exogenous Tumors

Endometriomas are benign collections of endometrial tissue that have spread outside the female reproductive anatomy. They can result in adhesion formation, ill-defined abdominal pain, and obstruction, and they can even erode through the bowel wall, resulting in bleeding into the lumen. In general, endometriomas can be treated medically and tend to recede during the postmenopausal period.

Intraperitoneal metastases from nonintestinal sites are reminiscent of desmoid tumors and are best diagnosed by CT or positive emission tomography (PET) scan. Such lesions portend a dismal prognosis; operation for minimal gain that confers substantial risk should be avoided. However, palliative intervention such as enteroenteric bypass or simple gastrostomy drainage may be indicated.

Hemorrhage

Intestinal hemorrhage between the duodenal bulb and the ileocecal valve accounts for only 3% to 5% of bleeding from the gastrointestinal tract (72), but it may be caused by a greater variety of lesions than in the entire remaining bowel (Table 35-9). Prevention of complications of surgery for intestinal hemorrhage is based upon timely diagnosis, appropriate diagnostic testing, and judgment about the advantages of resection versus observation.

Identification of an intestinal bleeding source can be difficult due to its infrequent and usually intermittent occurrence, the length of the small intestine, and the paucity of sensitive tests. Traditionally, after upper and lower endoscopy, evaluation of a suspected small intestine bleeding source begins with a small bowel series, which is diagnostic in only 5% to 10% of cases (73,74). The technetium-99 labeled red blood cell scan is a more sensitive diagnostic test and carries few risks beyond time delay. Additionally, as long as no transfusion is required, the tagged cells will remain positive for 12 to 24 hours, permitting delayed testing. Although this test can help diagnose blood loss within the small intestine, pooled blood can be deceptive. Localization of the exact bleeding site is difficult unless the site has specific anatomic features, as in the duodenum or terminal ileum.

Angiography can help to localize a lesion bleeding at ≥0.5 mL per minute but is <50% sensitive if bleeding has slowed or stopped. Moreover, a major advantage of angiography—its therapeutic value—is limited in the small intestine's small, branching arcades.

Exploratory surgery also has therapeutic value. Because many of the causative lesions are flat or small and thus hard to palpate, exploration is best accompanied by diagnostic endoscopy of the small bowel. Intraoperative enteroscopy, termed "push enteroscopy," requires the advancement of a colonoscope or sometimes a specialized enteroscope under direct visualization with mechanical assistance. Localization of the bleeding site is possible in 38% to 75% of cases, and many lesions can be treated endoscopically (75).

An exciting new development in diagnosis of obscure sources of small bowel blood loss is capsule endoscopy. A small wireless endoscopic capsule is swallowed and takes two pictures of the lumen per second. Recording devices worn by the patient capture images and track the route of the capsule for localization. Two recent small head-to-head studies showed up to a twofold increased sensitivity over push endoscopy for diagnosis of small bowel lesions (76,77).

Timing of the operation requires judicious planning. After the initial presentation many vascular lesions demonstrate no further bleeding. Angioectasias represent 80% of bleeding lesions in patients over 60 but only rebleed in 10% of cases (78). In contrast, small bowel tumors—the most common source of small intestinal bleeding in patients younger than age 50—are best resected unless too numerous or diffusely distributed. Briskly bleeding lesions also must be addressed, preferably before extensive transfusion is required.

TABLE 35-9
ETIOLOGIES OF SMALL INTESTINAL BLEEDING

Causes of Intestinal Bleeding	Location	Features
Vascular lesions		
Angiodysplasias or vascular ectasias	Throughout, but most concentrated in the right colon	Mucosal and submucosal dilated arterial vessels.
Telangiectasias	Throughout the intestine	Full-thickness dilated vessels, diffuse.
Arteriovenous malformations	Throughout	Thick-walled arteries and veins without intervening capillaries.
Vascular anomalies		
Small bowel varices	Duodenum, proximal jejunum	Associated with prehepatic portal hypertension.
Aortoenteric fistula	Duodenum, ileum	Herald bleeding followed by massive hemorrhage.
Dieulafoy lesion	Fundus, duodenum, jejunum	Painless, massive bleeding.
Vasculidities		
Collagen-vascular diseases		Large and small arterial compromise.
Venulitis		Mucosal edema, malabsorption, ulcerations.
Radiation damage		Mucosal edema and ulcerations.
Ulcerations		
Crohn disease	Throughout	Transmural ulceration; bleeding is usually indolent.
Gastrinomas	Duodenum, jejunum	
Infection associated	Throughout	
Medication induced	Throughout	
Meckel diverticulum	100 cm proximal to the ileocecal valve	Ulceration and brisk bleeding due to ectopic gastric mucosa within the diverticulum.
Pseudo-diverticula	Jejunum	Mesenteric border of the intestine; unlikely to be a source of blood loss but may bleed massively.
Small bowel tumors (see above)		

Ischemia

Intestinal ischemia in adults is generally the result of thromboembolic disease, small vessel disease such as collagen-vascular disease, or a complication of previous operation. Diagnosis of intestinal ischemia can be difficult and is based on symptoms and an examination consistent with impending peritonitis. The traditional admonition of "pain out of proportion to physical examination" is most easily appreciated with hindsight. Useful serology studies include the leukocyte count, lactate level, and bicarbonate level. Thromboembolic disease, chronic mesenteric ischemia, and small vessel disease are explored in more detail in another chapter. Nonvascular reasons for a low flow state, such as reduced cardiac output, usually compromise the colon prior to affecting the small bowel.

The most common etiology of postoperative intestinal ischemia is an incarcerated or strangulated small bowel hernia. The diagnosis is relatively straightforward among nonobese patients with a ventral hernia. Ultrasound or CT scan can help to make the diagnosis in the patient whose examination is obscured by a thicker abdominal wall. An incarcerated intraperitoneal hernia can sometimes be appreciated on CT scan, particularly if a clear transition point in the small bowel lumen is seen. Mesenteric torsion is another source of intestinal ischemia. In adults, mesenteric torsion is usually a complication of the anastomotic alignment and is easily avoided by purposefully orienting the mesenteric edges during anastomosis or stoma formation.

Intraoperatively, questions regarding viability of bowel or an anastomosis can be resolved by obtaining a Doppler signal at the antimesenteric border. Alternatively, intravenous injection of 1 mg of fluoroscein dye followed by use of a Wood lamp can delineate inadequately perfused bowel. In addition, prudent use of a follow-up second look operation can help elucidate ongoing ischemia or nonviable resection margins.

Small Intestinal Bypass

Defunctionalization of some portion of the small intestine can occur due to enteroenteric fistula, but it is more commonly the result of operative intervention. Surgical bypass is categorized as therapeutic for weight loss or palliative for obstruction. Although intestinal bypass for either purpose carries similar operative risks, the underlying disease process has a major impact on long-term outcome. Several late complications of defunctionalized bowel or "blind loops" have been identified. Bacterial overgrowth due to reduced or absent peristalsis and diversion of digestive juices can lead to formation of metabolites toxic to the intestinal mucosa, poor nutrient absorption, intractable diarrhea, and resultant mechanical trauma. Diagnosis is usually based on symptoms of diarrhea, bloating, fever, and malaise and on a positive hydrogen breath test (79). Intermittent treatment with metronidazole helps to reestablish normal flora and control symptoms. Micronutrient malnutrition can lead to osteoporosis, night blindness, skin rashes, calculi formation, anemia, and immunopathy. Prevention is effected by careful attention to vitamin, mineral, and electrolyte replacement.

Therapeutic Intestinal Bypass for Weight Loss

Although intestinal surgery generally is founded on improving the availability of nutrition, the unique aim of a bariatric intestinal bypass is to reduce nutritional volume. In the United States, bariatric surgery is enjoying renewed popularity and is now the most common electively performed abdominal operation (80,81). Early complications of bariatric surgery generally fall within the same categories as complications of palliative bypass, and anastomotic leak is independently predictive of perioperative mortality (82). In previous decades, profound late complications of jejuno-ileal bypass, especially hepatic cirrhosis, led to a moratorium on the procedure (83–85). More recently, creation of a common intestinal channel >50 cm in length has helped to mitigate protein-calorie malnutrition (85). Flow of bile and pancreatic fluid through the defunctionalized limb has reduced bacterial overgrowth and resultant diarrhea, fever, and malaise. Close postoperative attention to vitamin supplementation, prevention of electrolyte disturbances, and adequate protein intake have helped to ameliorate sequellae of micronutrient depletion and malnutrition.

Palliative Bypass for Obstruction

Intestinal bypass is an important alternative strategy when resection is not feasible—for example, in the setting of short bowel, previous radiation, matted bowel or mesenteric fibrosis, or widely disseminated tumor. The primary goal of palliative surgical bypass is relief of obstructive pain. Secondary goals are prevention of perforation and peritonitis and reestablishment of anatomic continuity. The patient's preferences and a realistic assessment of the prognosis must be carefully considered preoperatively. For example, a patient with slowly advancing obstruction due to mesenteric fibrosis or longstanding radiation damage potentially could have many remaining years with a satisfactory quality of life. Alternatively, a moribund patient who is not expected to recover may be best served by a less invasive procedure for decompression. The underlying disease process affects tissue quality and perfusion, which have a direct impact on intraoperative risks of unplanned enterotomy and anastomotic leakage. Late complications include malnutrition, bacterial overgrowth, and renal and biliary calculi formation.

Hypomotility

Intestinal motility is mediated by an assortment of peptides, hormones, and extrinsic and intrinsic neural pathways. Transient hypomotility secondary to postoperative ileus, narcotic use, bowel edema, or systemic inflammation is best managed supportively, with decompression, fluid replacement, and removal of the offending source if possible. Longer-term hypomotility can be iatrogenic as a result of surgically disrupted pathways, for example, postvagotomy or intestinal bypass, or intrinsic as in the setting of connective tissue disorders, or visceral neuropathy or myopathy.

Chronic Intestinal Pseudo-obstruction

Intestinal pseudo-obstruction is manifested by abdominal distension, nausea, vomiting, and pain and can be difficult to distinguish clinically from mechanical obstruction. An incorrect presumption of mechanical obstruction leading to operation can result in combined functional and mechanical obstruction, an even more challenging clinical situation. The etiology of pseudo-obstruction is generally an underlying autoimmune connective tissue disorder, such as systemic lupus erythematosis, scleroderma, or amyloidosis. The prognosis is directly related to progress of the underlying disease. Treatment is based on avoidance of laparotomy, use of promotility agents, and supportive care (86). Anaerobic bacterial overgrowth can lead to steatorrhea and may require treatment with antibiotics. Chronic pain due to distension may become severe enough to warrant creation of a venting enterostomy. Correction of electrolyte derangements, especially magnesium, can also resolve the symptoms.

Visceral Myopathy/Neuropathy

Pseudo-obstructed patients with no clear underlying connective tissue abnormality are thought to have an abnormality of the enteric smooth muscle or (less frequently) intrinsic nervous system (87). Numerous case series report such ill-defined syndromes, which tend to be familial and progressive and to extend to other visceral or even skeletal muscle systems. Supportive care includes hyperalimentation and medication for vague but frequently severe pain. Promotility agents have not proven useful. Surgical intervention is generally ineffective, leaving patients vulnerable to all of the risks but none of the advantages of laparotomy. However, patients unable to tolerate long-term hyperalimentation may benefit from consideration of small intestinal transplantation.

Ileostomy Complications

Ileostomies are usually created at the end of an operative case after the abdomen has been closed and the senior surgeon may have stepped back from the table. Although ileostomy formation seems simple enough, the technical complication rate is not trivial. In 1952, Brooke made a major contribution to reduction of ileostomy complications by proposing immediate maturation (eversion) of the ileostomy end (88). However, in an actuarial analysis with a decade of yearly follow-up, Leong et al. found that ileostomy complications still approached 76% among ulcerative colitis patients (89). Complications of end or loop ileostomy formation can be immediately obvious or can continue to accrue over years (Table 35-10). Although much of the surgical dogma is now disputed, specific technical issues merit special attention. Additionally, volume replacement and treatment with a bulking agent and antidiarrheal medication can prevent the numerous sequellae of dehydration.

Brooke Ileostomy

The most important initial steps in stoma creation and prevention of complications are appropriate siting, aligning the abdominal wall tunnel through the rectus abdominus muscle, and eversion of an adequate length of intestine (Fig. 35-5).

The proposed site should be flat, within the patient's view, and away from scars, skin folds, or bony prominences. Optimally this site is located through the rectus sheath at one-third of the distance between the umbilicus and the anterior superior iliac spine. In obese patients the stoma site should be shifted upward for visualization. An inappropriate site may lead to poor appliance fit, leakage, and sometimes profound dermatitis.

A circular incision of 2-cm diameter is created sharply, and fat is divided to the anterior fascial sheath. The tract should be aligned by retracting the skin and fascia to the midline. A poorly aligned tract can cause obstruction, edema, and ischemia. A cruciate incision is created in the anterior sheath using Bovie electrocautery. A muscle-splitting incision through the rectus muscle should preserve the epigastric vessels and expose the posterior fascia for the next cruciate incision. The tract should be bluntly dilated to about a two-finger width for withdrawal of the mobilized terminal ileum.

Vigorous clearing of mesentery from the ileal end can result in ischemia and is generally unnecessary. Adequate mobilization for eversion is crucial at this step, especially if weight gain is anticipated. Inadequate mobilization can lead to tension on the mesentery and ischemia. Additionally, a poorly everted stoma may retract and stenose, resulting in poor appliance fit, leakage, dermatitis, skin ulcerations, and obstruction. Repair of a retracted, stenotic stoma frequently requires laparotomy.

Small bowel obstruction, the most common complication of ileostomy formation after skin breakdown, is most often caused by intra-abdominal adhesions. Other reasons for bowel obstruction include fibrinous food bolus, parastomal herniation, intra-abdominal torsion, and recurrent Crohn disease. Closing the lateral space or suturing the mesentery to the abdominal wall appears to have no impact on the long-term obstruction rate (89).

Parastomal herniation is essentially a ventral herniation. The actuarial risk is about 16%, and risk factors are identical to those of other incisional hernias: age, obesity,

TABLE 35-10

COMPLICATIONS OF ILEOSTOMY FORMATION AND CLOSURE

	Early Complications	Late Complications
Both loop and end ileostomies	Poor location Poor orifice size Ischemic necrosis Dehydration Bowel obstruction Parastomal abscess Dermatitis	Prolapse Parastomal herniation Peristomal fistula formation Bowel obstruction Dermatitis
End ileostomy		Retraction Stenosis Variceal bleeding

Loop ileostomy	Erroneous closure of the proximal end	Closure-related:
		  Bowel obstruction
		  Anastomotic leakage
		  Stricture formation

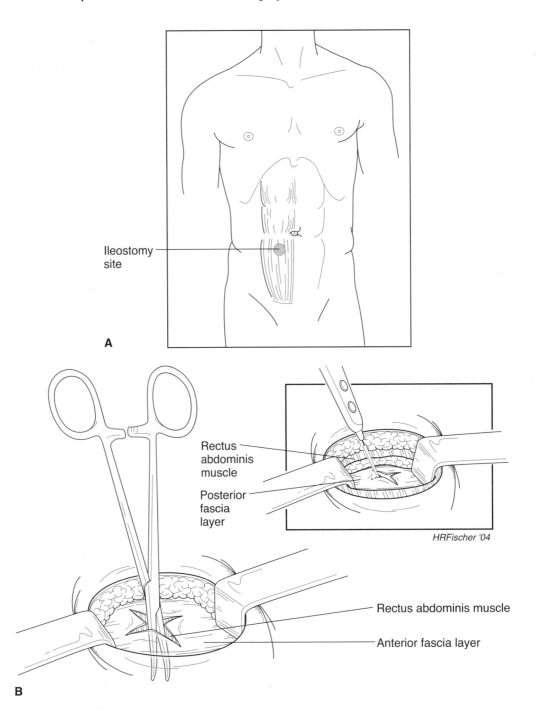

Ileostomy site

Rectus abdominis muscle

Posterior fascia layer

HRFischer '04

Rectus abdominis muscle

Anterior fascia layer

A

B

Figure 35-5 Brooke ileostomy formation. **(A)** Ileostomy site. **(B)** Muscle splitting incision.

pulmonary disease, steroid dependence, and a history of hernias. A customized truss can provide symptom relief. Repair should be postponed until there is a compelling reason; results are usually discouraging. Rubin et al. reported a 76% recurrence rate with primary fascia repair, a 33% recurrence rate with stoma relocation, and an overall operative complication rate of 62% (90). On the basis of these data, the authors recommended stoma relocation as the initial repair strategy, followed by mesh placement for recurrent hernia.

Peristomal fistulae develop in about 7% of patients, most of whom have Crohn disease. Tacking suture through the dermis only, thus avoiding a tract through the epidermis, and a well-fitted stoma appliance that limits skin pressure may help to limit this problem.

Ileostomy construction can form an additional communication between the portal and systemic venous systems. Bleeding varices can potentially develop in cirrhotic patients. Temporizing measures include oversewing the

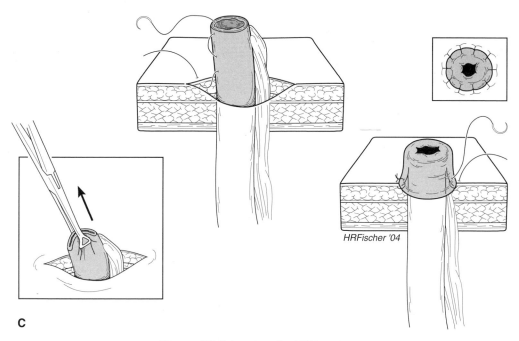

Figure 35-5 (*continued*) **(C)** Eversion.

bleeding site, cauterization or sclerosis, or even disconnecting and reanastomosing the mucocutaneous junction. Longer-term management requires changing the portal flow or curing the cirrhosis with a liver transplant.

Loop Ileostomy

A loop ileostomy is created for ease of closure, thus intended to be temporary. Although the loop ileostomy is associated with many of the same short-term complications as the end ileostomy, a few notable differences exist. Furthermore, closure of the ileostomy summons a whole different group of potential complications.

Loop ileostomy formation begins with the same principles as an end ileostomy (Fig. 35-6). Certainty that there is no twist in the bowel and mesentery is essential prior to orientation of the stoma limbs. Placing the distal limb in

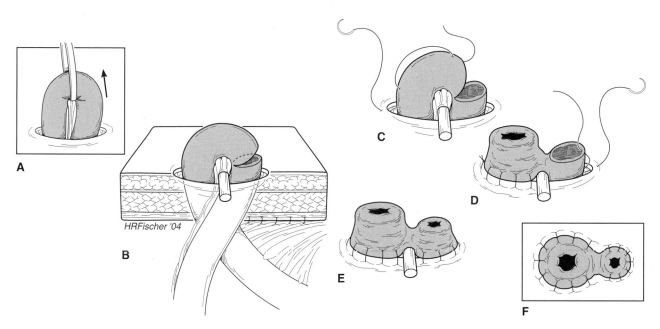

Figure 35-6 Loop ileostomy formation. **(A)** Delivery of intestine through the stoma incision; **(B)** proper orientation of the bowel: no bowel torsion and distal limb inferior; **(C)** mechanical prevention of reduction prior to healing; **(D)** eversion of both limbs in a Brooke fashion; **(E)** and **(F)** final loop ileostomy appearance.

the dependent position is standard technique and can be helpful for future operative planning. If the loop ileostomy is to be converted to an end ileostomy, appropriate orientation can help to prevent closing off the wrong (proximal) limb. Wrapping the intestinal loop in an adhesion barrier prior to delivery through the fascia can greatly facilitate future stoma closure.

Loop ileostomies are more prone to prolapse, which can be quite distressing to the patient. Fortunately, adverse sequelae are rare. Incarcerated prolapse is usually reducible with the application of granulated sugar. Data are inconclusive on the effectiveness of fixing the mesentery to the fascia to prevent prolapse.

Complications of ileostomy closure center on obstruction and leakage. Because the distal limb may be substantially narrowed, a side-to-side closure is best. In a randomized trial of stapled versus sutured closure, Hasegawa et al. determined

that a stapled closure was associated with 80% fewer postoperative bowel obstructions (28). However, hospital stay, readmission rates, and reoperative rates were the same.

Jejunostomy Tube Complications

Feeding jejunostomy tube placement has been an adjunct to a variety of abdominal operations, but it is associated with respective major complication and mortality rates of 4% to 10% and 1.4% to 3.2% (91–94). The classic method for jejunostomy placement has been a sizeable tube through an imbricated tract (Fig. 35-7) at least 30 cm beyond the ligament of Treitz, with sutures to the abdominal wall to prevent kinking or torsion.

A primary indication for jejunostomy over gastrostomy has been a perception of reduced risk of aspiration. Fox et al. retrospectively reviewed gastrostomy and jejunostomy tube

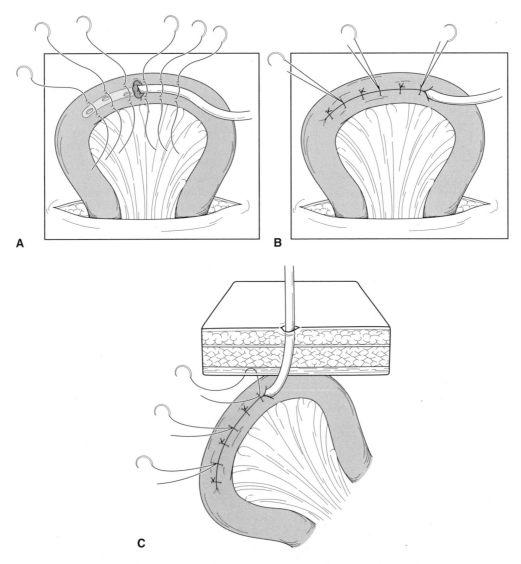

A

B

C

Figure 35-7 Witzelling a jejunal feeding tube. **(A)** Placement of sutures longitudinally in the seromuscular layer; **(B)** imbrication of the tube; **(C)** prevention of torsion or kinking by fixing the bowel to the abdominal wall.

placements and reported aspiration in 4 of 69 patients with a gastrostomy tube compared to 2 of 86 patients with a jejunostomy tube (95). In contrast, Weltz et al. found a substantially reduced rate of aspiration with feeding by jejunostomy tube compared to feeding by nasogastric tube (93).

Leakage, torsion, and erosion with perforation of viscera occur infrequently but consistently. The traditional jejunostomy tube may soon be outmoded by newer enthusiasm for percutaneous, laparoscopic, and needle catheter placement. However, no clearly superior method has been established.

SUMMARY

In summary, intestinal surgery is performed for an enormous variety of underlying diseases. Complications that arise as a result of technical errors can be associated broadly with obstruction or anastomotic leakage. Careful postoperative attention to the patient will permit an earlier diagnosis, which usually allows more effective intervention. Complications that arise as a result of judgment errors may be more specific to the underlying disease or operation. Prevention of judgment errors rests on a timely and thorough preoperative evaluation and on a treatment plan based on specific features of the underlying disease. Optimization of the patient's preoperative nutritional status, appropriate timing of surgery, and appreciation of alternative treatment strategies are keys to the prevention and management of complications.

REFERENCES

1. Ashley SW, Wells SA, Jr. Tumors of the small intestine. *Semin Oncol* 1988;15(2):116–128.
2. Fleming CR, Remington M. Intestinal failure. In: Hill GL, ed. *Nutrition and the surgical patient.* New York: Churchill Livingstone; 1981: 219–235.
3. The Veterans Affairs Total Parenteral Nutrition Cooperative Study Group. Perioperative total parenteral nutrition in surgical patients. *N Engl J Med* 1991;325(8):525–532.
4. Nightingale JM. The medical management of intestinal failure: methods to reduce the severity. *Proc Nutr Soc* 2003;62(3):703–710.
5. Roukema JA, Carol EJ, Prins JG. The prevention of pulmonary complications after upper abdominal surgery in patients with noncompromised pulmonary status. *Arch Surg* 1988;123(1):30–34.
6. Hall JC, Tarala RA, Tapper J, et al. Prevention of respiratory complications after abdominal surgery: a randomised clinical trial. *Br Med J* 1996;312(7024):148–152; discussion 152–153.
7. Eagle KA, Berger PB, Calkins H, et al. ACC/AHA guideline update for perioperative cardiovascular evaluation for noncardiac surgery—executive summary: a report of the American College of Cardiology/American Heart Association Task Force on Practice Guidelines (Committee to Update the 1996 Guidelines on Perioperative Cardiovascular Evaluation for Noncardiac Surgery). *J Am Coll Cardiol* 2002;39(3):542–553.
8. Potyk D, Raudaskoski P. Preoperative cardiac evaluation for elective noncardiac surgery. *Arch Fam Med* 1998;7(2):164–173.
9. Kern JW, Shoemaker WC. Meta-analysis of hemodynamic optimization in high-risk patients. *Crit Care Med* 2002;30(8):1686–1692.
10. Giner M, Laviano A, Meguid MM, et al. In 1995 a correlation between malnutrition and poor outcome in critically ill patients still exists. *Nutrition* 1996;12(1):23–29.
11. Middleton MH, Nazarenko G, Nivison-Smith I, et al. Prevalence of malnutrition and 12-month incidence of mortality in two Sydney teaching hospitals. *Intern Med J* 2001;31(8):455–461.
12. Anstead GM. Steroids, retinoids, and wound healing. *Adv Wound Care* 1998;11(6):277–285.
13. Slavin J, Unemori E, Hunt TK, et al. Transforming growth factor beta (TGF-beta) and dexamethasone have direct opposing effects on collagen metabolism in low passage human dermal fibroblasts *in vitro. Growth Factors* 1994;11(3):205–213.
14. Post S, Betzler M, von Ditfurth B, et al. Risks of intestinal anastomoses in Crohn's disease. *Ann Surg* 1991;213(1):37–42.
15. Bruewer M, Utech M, Rijcken EJ, et al. Preoperative steroid administration: effect on morbidity among patients undergoing intestinal bowel resection for Crohns disease. *World J Surg* 2003;27(12):1306–1310.
16. Marchal L, D'haens G, Van aasche G, et al. The risk of post-operative complications associated with infliximab therapy for Crohn's disease: a controlled cohort study. *Aliment Pharmacol Ther* 2004;19:749–754.
17. Holmdahl L, Risberg B, Beck DE, et al. Adhesions: pathogenesis and prevention-panel discussion and summary. *Eur J Surg* 1997;163(Suppl. 577):56–62.
18. Thompson J. Pathogenesis and prevention of adhesion formation. *Dig Surg* 1998;15(2):153–157.
19. Cullen JJ, Kelly KA, Moir CR III, et al. Surgical management of Meckel's diverticulum. An epidemiologic, population-based study. *Ann Surg* 1994;220(4):564–568; discussion 568–569.
20. Fisher KS, Ross DS. Guidelines for therapeutic decision in incidental appendectomy. *Surg Gynecol Obstet* 1990;171(1):95–98.
21. Snyder TE, Selanders JR, Strom PR, et al. Incidental appendectomy—yes or no? A retrospective case study and review of the literature. *Infect Dis Obstet Gynecol* 1998;6(1):30–37.
22. Strom PR, Turkleson ML, Stone HH. Safety of incidental appendectomy. *Am J Surg* 1983;145(6):819–822.
23. Warren JL, Penberthy LT, Addiss DG, et al. Appendectomy incidental to cholecystectomy among elderly Medicare beneficiaries. *Surg Gynecol Obstet* 1993;177(3):288–294.
24. van Goor H, Hulsebos RG, Bleichrodt RP. Complications of planned relaparotomy in patients with severe general peritonitis. *Eur J Surg* 1997;163(1):61–66.
25. Golub R, Golub RW, Cantu R Jr, et al. A multivariate analysis of factors contributing to leakage of intestinal anastomoses. *J Am Coll Surg* 1997;184(4):364–372.
26. Ching SS, Muralikrishnan VP, Whiteley GS. Relaparotomy: a five-year review of indications and outcome. *Int J Clin Pract* 2003;57(4):333–337.
27. Brundage SI, Jurkovich GJ, Grossman DC, et al. Stapled versus sutured gastrointestinal anastomoses in the trauma patient. *J Trauma* 1999;47(3):500–507; discussion 507–508.
28. Hasegawa H, Radley S, Morton DG, et al. Stapled versus sutured closure of loop ileostomy: a randomized controlled trial. *Ann Surg* 2000;231(2):202–204.
29. Zieren HU, Muller JM, Pichlmaier H. Prospective randomized study of one-or two-layer anastomosis following oesophageal resection and cervical oesophagogastrostomy. *Br J Surg* 1993;80(5):608–611.
30. Vrijland WW, Tseng LN, Eijkman HJ, et al. Fewer intraperitoneal adhesions with use of hyaluronic acid-carboxymethylcellulose membrane: a randomized clinical trial. *Ann Surg* 2002;235(2):193–199.
31. Becker JM, Dayton MT, Fazio VW, et al. Prevention of postoperative abdominal adhesions by a sodium hyaluronate-based bioresorbable membrane: a prospective, randomized, double-blind multicenter study. *J Am Coll Surg* 1996;183(4):297–306.
32. Beck DE, Cohen Z, Fleshman JW, et al. A prospective, randomized, multicenter, controlled study of the safety of Seprafilm adhesion barrier in abdominopelvic surgery of the intestine. *Dis Colon Rectum* 2003;46(10):1310–1319.
33. Seror D, Feigin E, Szold A, et al. How conservatively can postoperative small bowel obstruction be treated? *Am J Surg* 1993;165(1):121–125; discussion 125–126.
34. Shih SC, Jeng KS, Lin SC, et al. Adhesive small bowel obstruction: how long can patients tolerate conservative treatment? *World J Gastroenterol* 2003;9(3):603–605.

35. Fevang BT, Jensen D, Svanes K, et al. Early operation or conservative management of patients with small bowel obstruction? *Eur J Surg* 2002;168(8−9):475–481.

36. Zer M, Dux S, Dintsman M. The timing of relaparotomy and its influence on prognosis. A 10 year survey. *Am J Surg* 1980;139(3): 338–343.

37. Tera H, Aberg C. Relaparotomy. A ten-year series. *Acta Chir Scand* 1975;141(7):637–644.

38. Ellozy SH, Harris MT, Bauer JJ, et al. Early postoperative small-bowel obstruction: a prospective evaluation in 242 consecutive abdominal operations. *Dis Colon Rectum* 2002;45(9):1214–1217.

39. Fraser SA, Shrier I, Miller G, et al. Immediate postlaparotomy small bowel obstruction: a 16-year retrospective analysis. *Am Surg* 2002;68(9):780–782.

40. Thompson JS. Surgical considerations in the short bowel syndrome. *Surg Gynecol Obstet* 1993;176(1):89–101.

41. Thompson JS, Edgar J. Poth memorial lecture. Surgical aspects of the short-bowel syndrome. *Am J Surg* 1995;170(6):532–536.

42. Nightingale JM, Lennard-Jones JE, Gertner DJ, et al. Colonic preservation reduces need for parenteral therapy, increases incidence of renal stones, but does not change high prevalence of gall stones in patients with a short bowel. *Gut* 1992;33(11): 1493–1497.

43. Tang SJ, Nieto JM, Jensen DM, et al. The novel use of an intravenous proton pump inhibitor in a patient with short bowel syndrome. *J Clin Gastroenterol* 2002;34(1):62–63.

44. Scolapio JS, Camilleri M, Fleming CR, et al. Effect of growth hormone, glutamine, and diet on adaptation in short-bowel syndrome: a randomized, controlled study. *Gastroenterology* 1997; 113(4):1074–1081.

45. Scolapio JS. Effect of growth hormone and glutamine on the short bowel: five years later. *Gut* 2000;47(2):164.

46. Szkudlarek J, Jeppesen PB, Mortensen PB. Effect of high dose growth hormone with glutamine and no change in diet on intestinal absorption in short bowel patients: a randomised, double blind, crossover, placebo controlled study. *Gut* 2000;47(2): 199–205.

47. Hallgren T, Fasth S, Delbro DS, et al. Loperamide improves anal sphincter function and continence after restorative proctocolectomy. *Dig Dis Sci* 1994;39(12):2612–2618.

48. Bianchi A. Intestinal loop lengthening a technique for increasing small intestinal length. *J Pediatr Surg* 1980;15(2):145–151.

49. Bianchi A. Experience with longitudinal intestinal lengthening and tailoring. *Eur J Pediatr Surg* 1999;9(4):256–259.

50. Thompson JS. Strategies for preserving intestinal length in the short-bowel syndrome. *Dis Colon Rectum* 1987;30(3):208–213.

51. Sudan DL, Kaufman SS, Shaw BW Jr, et al. Isolated intestinal transplantation for intestinal failure. *Am J Gastroenterol* 2000; 95(6):1506–1515.

52. Abu-Elmagd K, Reyes J, Bond G, et al. Clinical intestinal transplantation: a decade of experience at a single center. *Ann Surg* 2001;234(3):404–416; discussion 416–417.

53. Abu-Elmagd K, Bond G. Gut failure and abdominal visceral transplantation. *Proc Nutr Soc* 2003;62(3):727–737.

54. Bernell O, Lapidus A, Hellers G. Risk factors for surgery and recurrence in 907 patients with primary ileocaecal Crohn's disease. *Br J Surg* 2000;87(12):1697–1701.

55. Yamamoto T, Allan RN, Keighley MR. Risk factors for intraabdominal sepsis after surgery in Crohn's disease. *Dis Colon Rectum* 2000;43(8):1141–1145.

56. Tay GS, Binion DG, Eastwood D, et al. Multivariate analysis suggests improved perioperative outcome in Crohn's disease patients receiving immunomodulator therapy after segmental resection and/or strictureplasty. *Surgery* 2003;134(4):565–572; discussion 572–573.

57. Borley NR, Mortensen NJ, Jewell DP. Preventing postoperative recurrence of Crohn's disease. *Br J Surg* 1997;84(11):1493–1502.

58. Lichtenstein GR. Treatment of fistulizing Crohn's disease. *Gastroenterology* 2000;119(4):1132–1147.

59. Broe PJ, Bayless TM, Cameron JL. Crohn's disease: are enteroenteral fistulas an indication for surgery? *Surgery* 1982;91(3): 249–253.

60. Wullstein C, Gross E. Laparoscopic compared with conventional treatment of acute adhesive small bowel obstruction. *Br J Surg* 2003;90(9):1147–1151.

61. Yamamoto T, Keighley MR. Long-term results of strictureplasty for ileocolonic anastomotic recurrence in Crohn's disease. *J Gastrointest Surg* 1999;3(5):555–560.

62. Kurtovic J, Segal I. Recent advances in biological therapy for inflammatory bowel disease. *Trop Gastroenterol* 2004;25(1):9–14.

63. de Jong E, van Dullemen HM, Slors JF, et al. Correlation between early recurrence and reoperation after ileocolonic resection in Crohn's disease: a prospective study. *J Am Coll Surg* 1996;182(6): 503–508.

64. Tytgat GN, Mulder CJ, Brummelkamp WH. Endoscopic lesions in Crohn's disease early after ileocecal resection. *Endoscopy* 1988; 20(5):260–262.

65. Williams JG, Wong WD, Rothenberger DA, et al. Recurrence of Crohn's disease after resection. *Br J Surg* 1991;78(1):10–19.

66. Wobbes T, Verschueren RC, Lubbers EJ, et al. Surgical aspects of radiation enteritis of the small bowel. *Dis Colon Rectum* 1984; 27(2):89–92.

67. Swan RW. Stagnant loop syndrome resulting from small-bowel irradiation injury and intestinal by-pass. *Gynecol Oncol* 1974; 2(4):441–445.

68. Dietz DW, Remzi FH, Fazio VW. Strictureplasty for obstructing small-bowel lesions in diffuse radiation enteritis—successful outcome in five patients. *Dis Colon Rectum* 2001;44(12):1772–1777.

69. Agha FP. Intussusception in adults. *Am J Roentgenol* 1986;146(3): 527–531.

70. Lvoff N, Breiman RS, Coakley FV, et al. Distinguishing features of self-limiting adult small-bowel intussusception identified at CT. *Radiology* 2003;227(1):68–72.

71. Naef M, Buhlmann M, Baer HU. Small bowel tumors: diagnosis, therapy and prognostic factors. *Langenbecks Arch Surg* 1999; 384(2):176–180.

72. Netterville RE, Hardy JD, Martin RS, Jr. Small bowel hemorrhage. *Ann Surg* 1968;167(6):949–957.

73. Rabe FE, Becker GJ, Besozzi MJ, et al. Efficacy study of the small-bowel examination. *Radiology* 1981;140(1):47–50.

74. Lewis BS. Small intestinal bleeding. *Gastroenterol Clin North Am* 2000;29(1):67–95, vi.

75. Zuckerman GR, Prakash C, Askin MP, et al. AGA technical review on the evaluation and management of occult and obscure gastrointestinal bleeding. *Gastroenterology* 2000;118(1):201–221.

76. Mata A, Bordas JM, Feu F, et al. Wireless capsule endoscopy in patients with obscure gastrointestinal bleeding: a comparative study with push enteroscopy. *Aliment Pharmacol Ther* 2004; 20(2):189–194.

77. Mylonaki M, Fritscher-Ravens A, Swain P. Wireless capsule endoscopy: a comparison with push enteroscopy in patients with gastroscopy and colonoscopy negative gastrointestinal bleeding. *Gut* 2003;52(8):1122–1126.

78. Lewis B, Goldfarb N. Review article: the advent of capsule endoscopy—not-so-futuristic approach to obscure gastrointestinal bleeding. *Aliment Pharmacol Ther* 2003;17(9):1085–1096.

79. Riordan SM, McIver CJ, Walker BM, et al. The lactulose breath hydrogen test and small intestinal bacterial overgrowth. *Am J Gastroenterol* 1996;91(9):1795–1803.

80. Livingston EH. Procedure incidence and in-hospital complication rates of bariatric surgery in the United States. *Am J Surg* 2004;188(2):105–110.

81. Pope GD, Birkmeyer JD, Finlayson SR. National trends in utilization and in-hospital outcomes of bariatric surgery. *J Gastrointest Surg* 2002;6(6):855–860; discussion 861.

82. Fernandez AZ Jr, Demaria EJ, Tichansky DS, et al. Multivariate analysis of risk factors for death following gastric bypass for treatment of morbid obesity. *Ann Surg* 2004;239(5):698–702; discussion 702–703.

83. Backman L, Hallberg D. Some somatic complications after small intestinal bypass operations for obesity. Possible factors of significance in the incidence. *Acta Chir Scand* 1975;141(8):790–800.

84. Dean P, Joshi S, Kaminski DL. Long-term outcome of reversal of small intestinal bypass operations. *Am J Surg* 1990;159(1): 118–123; discussion 123–124.

85. Sugerman HJ, Kellum JM, DeMaria EJ. Conversion of proximal to distal gastric bypass for superobesity. *J Gastrointest Surg* 1997;1(6):517–525.

86. Hirsh EH, Brandenburg D, Hersh T Jr, et al. Chronic intestinal pseudo-obstruction. *J Clin Gastroenterol* 1981;3(3):247–254.

87. Mann SD, Debinski HS, Kamm MA. Clinical characteristics of chronic idiopathic intestinal pseudo-obstruction in adults. *Gut* 1997;41(5):675–681.

88. Brooke BN. The management of an ileostomy, including its complications. *Lancet* 1952;2(3):102–104.

89. Leong AP, Londono-Schimmer EE, Phillips RK. Life-table analysis of stomal complications following ileostomy. *Br J Surg* 1994; 81(5):727–729.

90. Rubin MS, Schoetz DJ Jr, Matthews JB. Parastomal hernia. Is stoma relocation superior to fascial repair? *Arch Surg* 1994; 129(4):413–418; discussion 418–419.

91. Holmes JH, Brundage SI, Yuen P, et al. Complications of surgical feeding jejunostomy in trauma patients. *J Trauma* 1999;47(6): 1009–1012.

92. Sonawane RN, Thombare MM, Kumar A, et al. Technical complications of feeding jejunostomy: a critical analysis. *Trop Gastroenterol* 1997;18(3):127–128.

93. Weltz CR, Morris JB, Mullen JL. Surgical jejunostomy in aspiration risk patients. *Ann Surg* 1992;215(2):140–145.

94. Simon T, Fink X. Recent experience with percutaneous endoscopic gastrostomy/jejunostomy (PEG/J) for enteral nutrition. *Surg Endosc* 2000;14(5):436–438.

95. Fox KA, Mularski RA, Sarfati MR, et al. Aspiration pneumonia following surgically placed feeding tubes. *Am J Surg* 1995; 170(6):564–566; discussion 566–567.

96. Joelsson I, Raf L. Late injuries of the small intestine following radiotherapy for uterine carcinoma. *Acta Chir Scand* 1973; 139(2):194–200.

97. Swan RW, Fowler WC Jr, Boronow RC. Surgical management of radiation injury to the small intestine. *Surg Gynecol Obstet* 1976; 142(3):325–327.

98. Schmitt EH III, Symmonds RE. Surgical treatment of radiation induced injuries of the intestine. *Surg Gynecol Obstet* 1981; 153(6):896–900.

99. Lillemoe KD, Brigham RA, Harmon JW, et al. Surgical management of small-bowel radiation enteritis. *Arch Surg* 1983;118(8): 905–907.

100. Galland RB, Spencer J. Natural history and surgical management of radiation enteritis. *Br J Surg* 1987;74(8):742–747.

Complications of Appendectomy and Colon and Rectal Surgery

36

Emina H. Huang

▰▰▰ **APPENDECTOMY 498**
Pathophysiology 498
Clinical Diagnosis 499
Complications of Appendicitis 499
Special Considerations 500
Complications of Colorectal Surgery 500
Postoperative Complications 504
Total Proctocolectomy with Ileal Pouch
    Anal Anastomosis 511
Stoma Complications 513

▰▰▰ **COMPLICATIONS OF ANORECTAL
PROCEDURES 514**
Hemorrhoidectomy 514
Anal Fissure 516
Anorectal Abscesses 518
Fistula-in-Ano 519

▰▰▰ **REFERENCES 520**

Emina H. Huang: University of Michigan, Ann Arbor, MI 48109

APPENDECTOMY

Appendicitis is the most common cause of acute pain in the abdomen, requiring surgical intervention, and must be considered in any patient complaining of abdominal pain. The lifetime incidence of acute appendicitis is 6.7% to 20%, with the lifetime incidence of appendectomy of 12% for men and 23% for women (1). The presentation of appendicitis is often confusing and may cause delayed diagnosis, especially in patient populations in which other changes in physiology, such as pregnancy or extremes in age, may exist. Since the accepted pathophysiology of appendicitis contributes directly to presentation, diagnosis, and complications, understanding of this process helps to promote early intervention and, therefore, avoidance of complications.

Pathophysiology

Obstruction of the appendiceal lumen, due to a range of etiologies that includes lymphoid hyperplasia, parasites, malignancy, and fecolith, is the primary cause of appendicitis. Although fecolith is considered the most common cause of appendicitis, the presence of a fecolith is demonstrated in only 30% to 50% of cases (2). Obstruction leads to stasis, with mucus accumulation, and increasing intraluminal pressure. Bacteria overgrow, and pus accumulates. The integrity of the appendiceal serosa is challenged, with obstruction of lymphatic drainage and edema. The classical presentation of diffuse abdominal pain, followed by localized peritonitis in acute appendicitis, results.

With time, venous obstruction with bacterial invasion into the wall ensues, causing suppurative appendicitis. Once venous thrombosis and arterial compromise occur, gangrenous appendicitis, with focal areas of perforation, allows bacteria, pus, and fecal matter to escape into the peritoneal cavity, and the patient develops perforated appendicitis. If intra-abdominal mechanisms are unable to effectively contain the process, generalized peritonitis may ensue.

Clinical Diagnosis

The classic history of pain—first diffuse, then localizing to the right lower quadrant of the abdomen—associated with fever is obtained in only half of patients (3). Associated symptoms of anorexia and vomiting may be absent. Therefore, clinical suspicion must be maintained in patients still possessing an appendix when history or physical examination is atypical. These factors are particularly prominent in infants, who are unable to give a history, and in the elderly, where comorbidities, as well as operative delay, may contribute to complications.

Recent advances in radiologic imaging have contributed to earlier intervention for appendicitis. Although there may be institutional (4) differences in approach to abdominal pain, ultrasound or computed tomography (CT) can often clarify the challenging, and at times confusing, clinical picture. The radiologic literature quotes sensitivities as high as 92% (5) when these studies are used as adjuncts to history and physical examination. These studies may contribute to earlier operation while decreasing the incidence of negative appendectomy.

Operative Approach

Recent advances in minimal access surgical techniques, antimicrobial agents, and imaging have allowed for options in the treatment of appendicitis. Although few would disagree with a right lower quadrant incision in a thin, young man with a classical history, the approach is not as clear in most patients. In patients with physical examination that is difficult to interpret, radiologic imaging may provide data allowing delay in operative intervention, as when the appendix is surrounded by a well-defined abscess collection amenable to percutaneous drainage. Imaging may push the patient more quickly toward appendectomy or may provide another, nonoperative, diagnosis. Appropriate use of targeted antimicrobial agents (6) for prevention of postoperative complications is warranted and may be beneficial for minimizing symptoms in those with complicated

appendicitis (7). The laparoscopic approach to appendectomy allows improved visualization of other disease processes and smaller incisions and may promote surgical intervention (8).

Complications of Appendicitis

Complications at Presentation

Peritonitis is a common complication of appendicitis, and it implies that the pathophysiologic process has progressed, with associated ischemia, mucosal ulceration, transmural necrosis, and leakage of bacteria and fecal material. Peritonitis may be localized if the surrounding organs—usually the small bowel, colon, omentum or colonic epiploicae—contain the perforation. In the absence of this protective host response, generalized peritonitis may occur. Generalized peritonitis is more common in children, who possess a less generous omentum. Though localized peritonitis may occur in patients with a periappendiceal abscess due to perforated appendicitis, generalized peritonitis may also occur if the abscess loses its containment.

Associated sepsis is due to mixed colonic flora, including anaerobic Bacteroides, aerobic *Escherichia coli*, and streptococci. Antimicrobial treatment should be targeted to these organisms.

When a patient presents in a delayed fashion several days after the onset of symptoms, a contained perforation with abscess is suspected. Although classic teaching is that operative drainage with or without appendectomy is necessary, this approach is associated with a high morbidity of 18% to 50% (9,10). Radiologic imaging in the form of ultrasound or CT confirms the diagnosis and facilitates management. Small (<3 cm) abscesses respond to bowel rest and intravenous antibiotics, while larger abscesses require percutaneous drainage. With this approach an initial failure rate of 12% necessitates urgent appendectomy, which has a complication rate of 12% (11). Because recurrent appendicitis occurs with an incidence of 8% to 14% following resolution of the acute episode, the question of delayed interval appendectomy arises. Although the risk of recurrence is low, additional pathology may be identified in the appendix or cecum. However, most patients in whom interval appendectomy is performed have a tiny, scarred, fibrotic appendix lacking a lumen, and therefore they are not at risk for appendicitis. A barium enema helps to determine whether other pathology exists and to demonstrate patency of the appendiceal lumen to assist with the decision on interval appendectomy. A patent lumen or other pathology favors a decision for interval appendectomy, while a sclerosed lumen without other pathology will defer operation.

Postoperative Complications

The most common postoperative complication of appendicitis is wound infection. Like much of the morbidity of appendicitis, this complication's incidence is correlated with the pathology's severity. In patients with nonperforated appendicitis the incidence of wound infection is <10%; wound infection increases with perforated appendicitis to 15% to 20% and is highest with diffuse peritonitis (35%) (12). The offending organisms are colonic bacteria, especially *Bacteroides fragilis* and *E. coli*. Meta-analytical reviews regarding antimicrobial agents suggest that use of antibiotics is superior to placebo in the prevention of wound infection (6). Wounds in patients with perforated appendicitis should be left to delayed primary closure or to healing by secondary intention.

If the patient does not resolve fever postoperatively and the wound is excluded as a source of infection, an intra-abdominal abscess should be suspected. The most common locations for abscesses are the iliac fossa, the pericecal area, and the pelvis. Both CT and ultrasound are useful imaging techniques for diagnosis, and both provide a guide for drainage. Pelvic collections may be drained transrectally by the placement of a mushroom catheter or Foley catheter using palpation or ultrasound guidance to create a controlled fistula. When drainage and symptoms cease, the drains are downsized and then removed.

Continued feculent drainage heralds a fecal fistula. Usually, a fecal fistula is the result of a necrotic appendiceal stump or cecum. A fecal fistula may also suggest a new diagnosis of Crohn disease. Imaging studies should be used to ensure that drainage is adequate and to determine the source of the fistula. A low output fistula should close in the absence of distal obstruction, neoplasia, radiation, or inflammatory bowel disease.

Special Considerations

Pregnancy

The gravid uterus alters both the presentation and the morbidity of appendicitis. The increasing size of the uterus displaces the appendix out of its usual pelvic position, into the mid and upper abdomen. Nausea and vomiting, which often accompany early pregnancy, further confuse the picture. Ultrasound is key to determine the viability of the pregnancy and to diagnose appendicitis. CT and magnetic resonance imaging (MRI) have been used, but fear of radiation to a fetus and unknown effects of MRI have made these modalities less popular.

Since miscarriage is associated with appendicitis, early diagnosis and therapy are critical. The incidence of miscarriage is 10% in the absence of perforation, but it increases to 30% in the presence of perforation (13). Concerns about the laparoscopic approach, including decreased uterine blood flow, fetal hypotension and hypoxia, and acidosis due to CO_2, do not seem to be major issues; however, current information is retrospective in nature. Additionally, the complications that have been reported with laparoscopy have also been associated with appendicitis, general anesthesia,

and the open surgical procedure (14). Beyond the age of 28 weeks, pneumoperitoneum is difficult to establish, and thus an open approach, with appropriate monitoring and positioning, is recommended.

Elderly

Although people older than 70 constitute only 5% to 10% of patients with appendicitis, morbidity and mortality within this age group is disproportionately elevated. These patients may have significant comorbidities, which, with atypical and delayed presentations, contribute to an incidence of perforation as high as 70% (15,16). Often, the admitting diagnosis is incorrect and elderly patients are given incorrect diagnoses, such as diverticulitis and bowel obstruction, which delay operative intervention (17). Recent advances in imaging and laparoscopy have facilitated the diagnosis and treatment of appendicitis. However, adoption of these modalities has not yet influenced results in the elderly, with consistently elevated rates of perforation and morbidity (18).

Tumors of the Appendix

Carcinoid tumor is the most common neoplasm of the appendix. Many carcinoid tumors are discovered incidentally and often only as a histopathologic finding. Therapy depends on size and histologic features. The appendiceal location accounts for 50% of gastrointestinal carcinoids (19). There are no reported cases of metastatic disease in carcinoid tumors <1.5 cm in size; metastatic potential increases to 30% in tumors >2 cm. Ileocolectomy is indicated for tumors >2 cm, for those with evidence of lymphovascular invasion, and for tumors of intermediate size in younger patients.

Mucocele of the appendix is caused by either benign or malignant disease. In the benign form, mucus accumulates distal to an obstruction of the appendiceal lumen. The malignant form is due to mucous cystadenocarcinoma, a tumor which usually does not metastasize but which produces mucus. If the malignant form ruptures, intraperitoneal tumor causes pseudomyxoma peritonei. The large amounts of gelatinous material may cause mechanical obstruction, with debulking and chemotherapy necessary for symptomatic relief. For the benign form of disease, appendectomy is sufficient. For the malignant form, ileocolectomy is recommended.

Adenocarcinoma of the appendix is rare and presents either as appendicitis or as ruptured, disseminated disease. Removal of associated lymph node bearing tissue necessitates ileocolectomy.

Complications of Colorectal Surgery

Surgical procedures for diseases of the colon and rectum are among the most common procedures performed. With advances in imaging technology, both radiologic and endoscopic, visualization and access to the colon and rectum for diagnosis and therapy has improved. The principles of surgical management for the disease processes, whether benign or malignant, remain steadfast.

Segmental colonic or colorectal resection with a continent reconstruction mandates knowledge of the physiology, anatomy, and microbiology of the colon and of the disease process for which the operation is required. The indications for intervention in colonic processes are the same as indications elsewhere in the abdomen—that is, bleeding, perforation, obstruction, malignancy, infection, and failure of medical management. A deeper understanding of these processes will contribute to improved outcomes and avoidance of complications.

Relative to other intra-abdominal organs, the physiology of the colon and rectum has been less studied. Though principally regarded as an organ for storage and elimination of feces, complex interconnecting pathways between the colorectum, neuroendocrine system, newly described peptides, dietary factors, and genetics continue to emerge, influencing both symptoms and management. The colon is one-quarter to one-fifth the length of the small intestine, and its absorptive function serves to remove sodium, water, and bile acids from the intestinal effluent. Colonocytes secrete bicarbonate and potassium against a concentration gradient. The storage and elimination functions of the colon and rectum are vital in dysmotility syndromes such as slow transit constipation and fecal incontinence.

The relative ease of access to the colon and rectum has implications for health care screening, diagnosis, and treatment. Recommendations for screening studies (20) of the aging population and recent data on the limitations of fecal occult blood testing and flexible sigmoidoscopy (21) have increased the need for colonoscopy. Complementary imaging modalities, including barium enema and the newer "virtual colonoscopy" (22), may help diagnosis. Currently, endoscopy is standard in that this modality allows for visual diagnosis, biopsy, polypectomy, management of bleeding, marking of lesions, surveillance of previously identified lesions, placement of stents for obstructing lesions, and detection and removal of foreign bodies.

Understanding of the microbiology of the colon and its contribution to morbidity remains paramount. The past 60 years of progress in colorectal surgery are in large part attributable to improvement in postoperative septic complications. Principles include mechanical preparation followed by antimicrobial reduction in the bacterial load. Debate continues on the necessity of the preparation; the mode, method, and duration of antimicrobial delivery; and the consideration of host factors.

Once the abdomen is entered and a segmental resection is initiated, the goals of safe dissection with creation of a tension-free anastomosis possessing adequate blood supply require an appreciation of both the disease process and the pertinent anatomy. Malignant processes mandate tumor-free margins, while inflammatory diseases require margins that facilitate reconstruction and avoid recurrence. Involvement in either type of disease process may cause visible or palpable loss of the normal anatomic relationships of structures such as ureters, spleen, or pancreas. Preoperative planning to improve visualization of a nonreconstructive, staged operative plan may be required.

Usually tumors of the cecum or ascending colon may be managed with an ileocolectomy, resecting the distal ileum, ascending colon, and proximal transverse colon, with ligation of the accompanying ileocolic, right colic, and the right branch of the middle colic vessels. Lesions involving the transverse colon are removed with a transverse colectomy; one or both of the flexures may also require mobilization or resection to facilitate oncologic principles of a tension-free, well-vascularized anastomosis. Lesions of the splenic flexure and descending colon require wide mobilization, especially if the sigmoid colon is diseased or suboptimal for anastomosis. The sigmoid colon, which may be involved with diverticular complications or malignancy, may have a foreshortened, inflamed mesentery, and thus splenic flexure mobilization may be required to ease anastomosis from the descending colon to the rectum. Minimal access approaches, with a myriad of variations dependent on training, experience, and comfort levels, have contributed to possible complications.

Brief summaries of disease processes for which colorectal resection is necessary follow, with discussion of the complications that are common to all the disease processes for which segmental colon or rectal resection is required. Unique complications of the ileal pouch-anal anastomosis will then be outlined, followed by complications distinct to procedures in which an anastomosis is not created—that is, to permanent stoma formation.

Diverticular Disease

Although initial reports early in the twentieth century described an incidence of diverticulosis in the 5% to 10% range (23), current estimates describe an occurrence as high as 65% in those older than 85. These reports indicate that sigmoid diverticular disease is an acquired condition, which is now more readily detectable, with an increased prevalence in Western populations.

The condition referred to as "sigmoid diverticulosis" is a misnomer, as these diverticula represent a herniation of the mucosa and submucosa through the muscular layer of the bowel wall and not true diverticula, which contain all layers of the bowel wall. Diverticula form at points in the colon wall where the vasa recta penetrate the circular muscle layer in their journey to the mucosal surface. Therefore, diverticula tend to form between the antimesenteric tenia and the mesenteric tenia and not between the two antimesenteric tenia.

Segmentation of the colon with increased intraluminal pressures develops in response to a chronic low-fiber diet.

These pressures are most elevated in the sigmoid colon. Theories on the pathogenesis include the possibility that a connective tissue disorder allows the development of diverticula in the absence of increased luminal pressures (24). Another theory relates to the control the rectosigmoid junction exerts on the aboral progression of peristalsis. This theory states that the rectosigmoid junction normally relaxes in response to a fecal bolus but that age, low fiber consumption, and constipation contribute to an area of low-grade resistance that fails to relax sufficiently (25).

Although diverticulosis is quite common, only 10% to 30% of patients will actually become symptomatic (26) from diverticulitis, obstruction, or bleeding. Approximately 30% of patients with diverticular disease will eventually require operative intervention (27). Although most patients will respond to antibiotic treatment during their first attack, success dwindles to <10% by the third attack (28). Up to 20% of patients presenting with diverticulitis are younger than 50. The literature on management of these patients is mixed. Some studies find that nearly 80% of these patients eventually require operative resection, while others believe that the same management and follow-up is mandated as that which applies to those patients over 50. Special categories of patients include those who are immunosuppressed or with a fistula. Immunosuppressed patients are best served by elective resection following a well-documented episode of diverticulitis, since immunosuppression impairs their ability to localize the inflammatory process and thus recurrent disease may be more severe. Patients with fistulas, commonly colovesical or colovaginal, benefit from elective resection with takedown of the fistula. In individuals with major comorbities and minor symptoms, chronic oral antibiotic administration may sometimes be more prudent.

Multiple classification schemes have been developed to help categorize acute inflammatory episodes. The most quoted is the Hinchey classification (29). In the absence of generalized peritonitis, stage I and II presentations may be treated with antimicrobial agents and percutaneous drainage as needed, allowing a less urgent procedure with bowel preparation and without the need for a stoma. However, the more severe presentations of purulent peritonitis (stage III) or fecal peritonitis (stage IV) mandate emergent resection of the perforated sigmoid colon with a stoma.

Lower gastrointestinal hemorrhage due to diverticuli will often cease spontaneously (30) and presents one of the most difficult diagnostic dilemmas within surgery. Angiodysplasia is more common on the right side of the colon. Exclusion of both an anorectal source of bleeding and an upper gastrointestinal cause is necessary. Once these sources have been excluded, colonoscopy is the next step. In an unprepared state, jet irrigation aids visualization and offers options for therapeutics. The opportunity for therapeutic embolization and localization exists with angiography. Prior to operative resection, localization is required to ensure a successful segmental resection.

Ulcerative Colitis

In the United States this enigmatic disease has an incidence of 5 to 15 per 100,000 (31). The causative agent or provoking elements for ulcerative colitis have not been identified. Familial tendencies do exist.

The disease is limited to the colon and rectum, with minimal and reversible involvement of the terminal ileum, called "backwash ileitis." Ulcerative colitis is limited to the mucosa and presents with diarrhea and bleeding. Abdominal pain, tenesmus, and fever may accompany disease episodes. The diagnosis is suggested colonoscopically by ulcerated mucosa and islands of regenerating tissue (pseudopolyps), beginning at the rectum and extending proximally. With chronic disease, the mucosa may develop a granular appearance lacking haustral folds. Endoscopic biopsy usually reveals cryptitis and crypt abscesses. Medical therapy targets inflammation with steroids and aminosalicylates.

Indications for surgery include toxic megacolon, perforation, bleeding, growth retardation in children and, most commonly, intractability to medical therapy. One of the most serious complications of extensive or long-standing ulcerative colitis is the development of colon or rectal carcinoma. Early in the disease process, the risk is <5%. With increased duration of disease, risk rises to 50% and 75%, respectively, after 30 and 40 years (32).

In the elective setting the choice of operative procedure should involve the patient's informed choice. Total proctocolectomy with ileostomy is the standard against which other operations are measured. Total abdominal colectomy with ileostomy and the Hartmann procedure or mucus fistula may be performed in the emergent setting. In appropriate patients with a disease-free rectum, colectomy with an ileorectal anastomosis may be appropriate, with surveillance of the rectal stump. Proctocolectomy with Kock continent ileostomy may be constructed; many patients require revision of a slipped nipple valve (30% to 50%). Modifications of this procedure may allow increased valve longevity and are currently under investigation. Modifications of the pelvic pouch procedure were first described in 1978 and have become the most popular curative reconstruction. Usually created with a diverting loop ileostomy, which may itself become the source of complication, this procedure removes the diseased tissue and allows for maintenance of continence.

Crohn Disease

In 1932, Crohn, Ginzburg, and Oppenheimer used the term regional ileitis to describe a form of subacute or chronic inflammatory bowel disease. In the United States the incidence is approximately 5 per 100,000. The etiology is unknown. Crohn disease is not limited to the colorectum but instead may involve the gastrointestinal tract anywhere from mouth to anus. The entity is characterized by skip lesions, fistulas, transmural inflammation with creeping of fat on the bowel wall, stricturing, and fibrosis. The presentation is commonly one of abdominal pain, diarrhea, and weight loss. Ileocolic disease is the most common, but Crohn colitis may be the only manifestation in up to 45% of patients (33). Disease limited to the anorectum occurs in 5% of patients.

The natural history of Crohn disease is one of exacerbation and remission. Forty percent to 70% of patients with Crohn disease require at least one operation (34). Sadly, the recurrence rate for another procedure is 10% to 20% per year. Since the disease cannot be cured either medically or surgically, the role of surgery is to relieve deleterious symptoms, to prevent or treat carcinoma, and to facilitate an improved quality of life if medical treatment has failed or has induced harmful side effects.

For intractable Crohn colitis, proctocolectomy with ileostomy is the standard of treatment. For limited disease, segmental colectomy or total abdominal colectomy is possible, provided that grossly normal bowel is available for anastomosis.

Familial Adenomatous Polyposis

Familial adenomatous polyposis (FAP) is an autosomal dominant disease characterized by the development of multiple polyps in the colon. The disease is caused by a deletion mutation in chromosome 5q21 at the adenomatous polyposis coli (APC) gene, which normally acts as a tumor suppressor. Relatively common, with an incidence of 1 in 7,000 to 10,000, spontaneous mutations do occur and represent 15% to 20% of patients.

The average age of diagnosis in patients without known kindred is 36 years. However, the age at which adenomas appear is much younger, about 25. Due to the loss of the APC tumor suppressor gene, progression to malignancy is aggressive, with an average age of 39 for the development of colorectal malignancy (35). These patients have a host of extracolonic manifestations that contribute to morbidity and mortality.

Since transformation to malignancy is assured by age 40 and because a completely ablative form of medical therapy does not currently exist, total proctocolectomy is recommended. Total proctocolectomy has been combined with ileostomy, ileal pouch reconstruction, or ileorectal anastomosis. Genetic analysis may permit the identification of patients at risk for extraintestinal manifestations and may predict those who may be responsive to medical management.

Rectal Prolapse

Rectal prolapse is an intussusception of the full thickness of the rectal wall through the anal sphincter. The fact that there are many procedures to treat this entity suggests that little is understood about its pathogenesis. Patients complain that a mass protrudes from the anal opening, often in the act of straining. Frequently the prolapse is accompanied by bleeding, mucus discharge, and incontinence.

The other disease process that may be confused with rectal prolapse is rectal mucosal or hemorrhoidal prolapse. In contrast to rectal prolapse, where mucosal folds are circular, in hemorrhoidal prolapse folds are orientated radially. Evaluation of this disorder includes colonoscopy, to exclude a tumor as the lead point for the intussusception, and cinedefecography, to evaluate the patient for internal prolapse. Evaluation of constipation is important if this is an accompanying complaint.

Since pathophysiology is poorly understood, a variety of procedures are available for treating this entity. The most popular perineal approaches include those of Altemeier and Delorme, while the choices for the abdominal approaches include sutured rectopexy, the Ripstein procedure, anterior resection, abdominal rectopexy, and sigmoid resection, with laparoscopic options available for the abdominal approaches. Variations in recurrence rates have been reported and may influence the choice of procedure.

Ischemic Colitis

The most common form of gastrointestinal ischemia is ischemic colitis. Its true incidence is unknown, but fortunately it is uncommon. Ischemic colitis classically presents with abdominal pain, diarrhea, and blood per rectum. Abdominal pain is sudden in origin, with low volume hematochezia. Other symptoms include fever, hypotension, tachycardia, and abdominal distension.

The etiology is believed due to "watershed" areas of colonic blood supply, including the splenic flexure, known as the "Griffith point," and the rectosigmoid, known as the "Sudek critical point." Ischemia on the right side of the colon has also been reported. A precipitating cause is uncommon, and most commonly the condition is attributed to a low-flow state. The classification of ischemic colitis includes (a) transient ischemia (80% to 90%), (b) recurrent ischemia (5%), (c) chronic ischemia, including stricture (2%), and (d) gangrenous ischemia (10% to 20%) (36). The transient form is associated with mucosal edema, congestion, superficial ulceration, and submucosal hemorrhage and petechia. Changes are limited to the mucosa and submucosa, consisting of an inflammatory response with superficial sloughing of the mucosa. Plain films may demonstrate "thumbprinting" caused by submucosal hemorrhage. Strictures from ischemic colitis are due to a partial-thickness injury involving the mucosa and muscular layers, resulting in fibrosis and narrowing of the lumen.

Diagnosis requires a gentle colonoscopy. If ischemia is not documented, colonoscopy may identify inflammatory bowel disease or malignancy. Areas of gray and green or black mucosa indicate transmural injury.

Treatment of ischemic colitis depends on the degree of injury. With early diagnosis of mild cases, bowel rest with adjunctive intravenous antibiotics is beneficial.

Optimization of blood flow to prevent further ischemia is mandatory. More severe cases, with peritonitis, perforation, sepsis, clinical deterioration despite medical therapy, or gangrene, require colectomy. In the acute setting anastomosis may be unsafe, and diversion or a second-look operation is indicated.

Colorectal Carcinoma

Recent cancer statistics show that colorectal cancer remains the third most common cause of cancer death in the United States (37). In 2003 approximately 147,000 new cases of colorectal cancer were diagnosed, with approximately 55,100 deaths. In North America there is a 6% lifetime risk with a 50% mortality rate, accounting for 11% of all cancer deaths.

The adenoma-to-carcinoma sequence (35) with the associated local genetic changes is widely accepted as the model by which a benign lesion in the colon is transformed into a malignancy. Recent investigation into heritable cancer family syndromes has increased the understanding of tumorigenesis. Syndromes with well understood genetics include FAP and hereditary nonpolyposis colon cancer (HNPCC). Of these, FAP is the most understood. The FAP syndrome demonstrates autosomal dominant inheritance due to a deletion of 5q21 that, although most often traced to a known kindred, may also present as a new mutation in 15% to 20% of index patients. This syndrome, found with an incidence of 1 in 7,000 to 10,000, is characterized by the presence of hundreds to thousands of colonic polyps forming first during the teen years. Often asymptomatic until their early adult years, affected individuals will develop invasive cancer during the third to fourth decade of life. Associated abnormalities may present in the retina, skin, stomach, duodenum, thyroid, and liver. Neoplastic manifestation includes gastric, duodenal, and endocrine adenomas, as well as periampullary duodenal carcinomas, papillary thyroid cancers, and hepatoblastomas.

HNPCC, or Lynch syndrome, accounts for 5% of new colorectal cancers. This syndrome, also inherited in an autosomal dominant fashion, is characterized by the presence of colon cancer at an age <45, a propensity for right-sided lesions, and an excess of synchronous and metachronous cancers. Lynch syndrome type I is site specific for the colon, while patients with the type II syndrome are at risk for developing other neoplasms such as gastric, small intestinal, upper urologic tract, ovarian, and endometrial cancers. The genetic defects responsible for these syndromes are involved with DNA mismatch repair genes, principally hMLH1, hMSH2, hPMS1, and hPMS2.

Though less clearly defined, both forms of inflammatory bowel disease, ulcerative colitis and Crohn disease, are associated with an increased propensity for malignant transformation. The genetics of inheritance of both of these diseases is poorly understood, and some kindreds have both diseases. Whether genetic susceptibility added to an environmental insult is cocausally involved has yet to be clarified. In both disease processes up to a 200-fold increase in malignant transformation is documented. In ulcerative colitis this transformation increases with both the duration and severity of the disease. In Crohn colitis, stricturing, which may be a protean manifestation, may eventuate in malignancy.

Detection of those with colorectal cancer during a period when surgical cure is possible is a goal. Recommendations for screening colonoscopy are derived from the knowledge that most cancers develop from benign polyps. Few contraindications to colonoscopy exist, and the technique allows access to the entire colon, with the ability to both diagnose and manage abnormalities.

Once cancer is diagnosed, preoperative evaluation includes a screen for metastatic disease. The standard recommendation for screening includes CT of the abdomen. For extraperitoneal rectal cancer, preoperative staging includes the addition of transrectal ultrasound, or endorectal MRI. Transrectal ultrasound is performed to determine depth of invasion and to detect enlarged perirectal lymph nodes. Additionally, transrectal ultrasound defines the relationship of the tumor to the anal sphincter and other extraperitoneal structures. This information is invaluable for determining whether definitive local treatment is an option and whether preoperative chemoradiation therapy may be beneficial. If preoperative staging for either colon or rectal cancers reveals the presence of metastatic disease, palliative options are considered.

Since surgical resection is the only curative treatment for colon cancer, segmental colectomy, including the tumor, adequate margins, segmented blood supply, and draining lymph nodes is the mainstay of treatment. Early on, the widespread adoption of laparoscopic approaches for the management of colon cancer was associated with an alarming rate of trocar site tumor infiltration. Currently, a trial sponsored by the National Cancer Institute examining the safety of a laparoscopic approach has been closed to accrual and is in the third year of follow-up (38). Early results and data submitted by others suggest that technical factors contributed to this phenomenon and that care regarding manipulation of the specimen may alleviate this complication in the future.

Postoperative Complications

Ileus

Postoperative ileus is a form of temporary bowel motor dysfunction that follows operative procedures in the abdomen. This reflex is caused by excitation of the splanchnic sympathetic nerves that occurs during manipulation of the bowel, but it may also be associated with surgery or trauma to other organs. The stomach recovers from this state within several hours, while the small bowel requires 1 to 2 days and the colon 2 to 3 days. Recovery that includes coordinated motor function may require up to 5 days. With the relatively short period of ileus after localized procedures, a nasogastric tube is usually not necessary for elective procedures. Although the auscultation of bowel sounds or resumption of appetite have been used to herald the resolution of ileus, the passage of flatus is the only true indicator that colonic ileus has resolved. An ileus lasting for longer periods may be associated with peritonitis or hematoma.

Prolonged ileus may be difficult to distinguish from mechanical small bowel obstruction. Although differentiation based on the quality of bowel sounds and the association of abdominal pain may be helpful, postoperatively the distinction may be quite challenging. A treatment algorithm includes continued supportive care with documentation and management of infection, including leak or abscess. CT is helpful in assessing the possibility of intra-abdominal abscess and to determine whether the patient has an ileus or a mechanical small bowel obstruction (39). If no other intervention is necessary, supportive care with nasogastric decompression is all that is necessary. In the absence of progressive symptoms, nutritional support may be instituted. Most partial mechanical small bowel obstructions resolve in 1 week with this plan; if no improvement is noted by 3 weeks, consideration must be given to exploration. Because adhesions may be very dense at this time, an alternative is continued supportive care in the outpatient environment.

Leak

Anastomotic healing occurs as a function of the patient's general condition, and, importantly, of local factors such as blood supply, tension, and the health of the bowel utilized. The mesentery should provide appropriate vasculature to the bowel, with clearance of no greater than 5 mm from the cut edge. If there is doubt, Doppler examination and transillumination are useful tools to aid in determination of blood supply. Too much tension on the anastomosis may cause disruption and compromise of the blood supply. Thin, healthy bowel is preferred to thickened, inflamed, or edematous bowel.

At times the presentation may be subtle, but the consequences are severe. The risk of mortality increases ten times relative to that of an uncomplicated operation. Among the most significant factors associated with loss of anastomotic integrity is the location of the anastomosis. In large series intra-abdominal leak rates range from 1% to 5%, while those in the pelvis exhibit a 5% to 30% rate of leakage. The closer the anastomosis is to the anal verge, the higher the probability of leakage. Several studies have noted that anastomoses distal to 7 cm from the anal verge are at highest risk for leakage (40). Historically, leakage occurred in >30% of low pelvic anastomoses (41). Contemporary rates are <10% (41). The improvement may be due to the practice of air insufflation at the time of creation of the anastomosis to verify the absence of a leak, or due to

improved stapling devices. Diversion of stool in the form of an ostomy does not prevent leak.

Typically, anastomotic leak is discovered 5 to 7 days after surgery (Fig. 36-1). Hindsight usually reveals earlier signs that should make the surgeon more suspicious of a leak, including fever, leukocytosis, localized or generalized tenderness, generalized ileus with abdominal distention, and tachycardia. CT is helpful to determine whether there is an associated abscess. In cases where leak is suspected, a gentle gastrograffin enema may assist the diagnosis.

Once recognized, aggressive management of the anastomotic leak is mandatory. Patients with generalized peritonitis require exploration. At exploration, proximal diversion with dismantling of the anastomosis and fecal diversion is the goal. In the case of a distal left-sided anastomosis, the inflammatory response may be so intense as to impair safe recognition of the anastomosis. In these cases prudent management includes proximal diversion with lavage of the peritoneal cavity and placement of drains near the anastomosis.

If the patient has low-grade sepsis and the leak is subtle enough to require a contrast study to demonstrate, and there is no concurrent abscess, close observation with intravenous antibiotics and bowel rest is initiated. If there is failure of improvement, exploration is necessary.

Abscess

An intra-abdominal abscess may be the presenting sign of acute inflammatory conditions such as appendicitis, diverticulitis, perforated colon cancer, or Crohn disease. In the case of elective colorectal surgery, postoperative intra-abdominal abscess is due to a break in technique. Due to spillage of enteric or colonic contents, especially into a hematoma or other devitalized tissues, or as evidence of an anastomotic leak, abscess should be suspected if other sources of sepsis have been eliminated. Unless a mass is palpable through the abdominal wall or rectum, CT is the surest means to determine the presence of an abscess. Though ultrasound may document the amount and location of fluid, there are no specific sonographic characteristics to distinguish free postoperative fluid from an abscess cavity.

If an abscess is amenable to guided drainage, either by palpation or imaging technology, drainage is effected. Abscesses are usually identified when reentry into the abdomen may be difficult or hazardous, and thus the optimal management may involve the assistance of an interventional radiologist. To treat bacteremia, continuation of antibiotics is indicated.

Fistula

Fecal fistula may be the expression of an intra-abdominal abscess. CT scanning is necessary to identify the abscess and to direct appropriate drain placement. Antibiotics and supportive care are initiated. In the absence of distal obstruction, foreign body, radiation, or inflammatory bowel

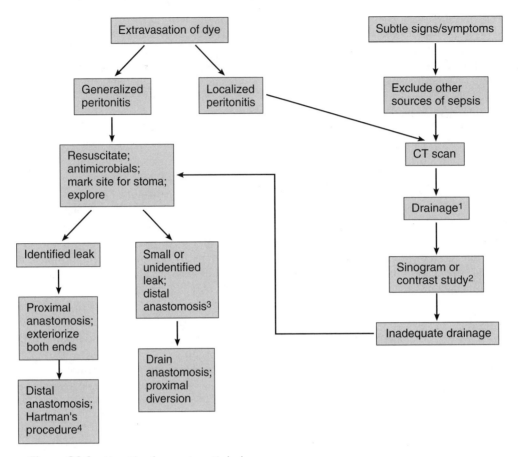

Figure 36-1   Algorithm for anastomotic leak.
[1] Drainage may usually be accomplished percutaneously, but it may be accomplished either transrectally or by open laparotomy if necessary.
[2] If the abscess is associated with an anastomotic leak, a fistulogram or contrast study may be helpful to determine the location, size, and so on, which may be helpful to determine subsequent management.
[3,4] In the case of low or distal anastomoses, the inflammatory response may be so intense that dismantling the anastomosis may be difficult. In these particular instances lavage, wide drainage, and proximal diversion is the most appropriate operative approach.

disease, most fistula resolve. Low output distal colonic fistula do not routinely require parenteral nutrition. Fistulas originating from proximal small bowel or proximal colonic sources may require this additional supportive care. Fistulas that do not resolve or recur may require additional intervention such as fibrin glue or revisional surgery once the acute inflammation has subsided.

Presacral Hemorrhage

Preservation of the presacral fascia is paramount to preventing this complication, which occurs during rectal mobilization. If a presacral vein is torn, bleeding is brisk but may be controlled with suture, bone wax, or cautery. Massive hemorrhage occurs in patients who have basivertebral connections to the presacral vein. This anatomy is encountered in approximately 15% of individuals (42). Occlusion with the index finger or balloon tamponade is necessary for temporary arrest of the hemorrhage; permanent hemostasis is possible by driving a thumbtack through the sacrum.

Anastomotic Hemorrhage

The incidence of anastomotic hemorrhage is low, with an incidence of 0.5% to 1% (43). Whether the anastomosis was created with staples or sutures does not influence incidence. Proper staple height and appropriate suture tension—that is, just enough to approximate but not so tight as to cause ischemic necrosis—is a learned skill. Intraoperatively, excessive use of cautery is to be avoided since metal in staples may transmit electrical energy of the cautery device to the bowel. Instead, meticulously placed sutures are used to arrest bleeding.

Gastrointestinal hemorrhage in the early postoperative period is challenging to manage. The patient requires supportive care, with the usual resuscitative and diagnostic maneuvers to exclude upper gastrointestinal hemorrhage. Distal anastomoses may be viewed endoscopically and controlled with injections of dilute epinephrine or short bursts of cautery. The manipulation may increase the incidence of anastomotic leakage. Alternatively, angiographic control may be effected, with the same risk. More proximal anastomoses may require exploration for control. If suture reinforcement is not effective or if the bleeding point is not obvious, dismantling the anastomosis with resection and reanastomosis may be required.

Splenic Injury

Splenic injury occurs during procedures on the colorectum (0.8%) and in those in which the splenic flexure is mobilized (3%) (44). The injury is usually small, involving a capsular tear at the anterior or medial surface of the spleen's inferior pole. The injury is caused by disrupting the normal splenic attachments or by traction on the greater omentum. In the case of the injury caused by traction on the greater omentum, the injury may extend to the splenic hilum.

To avoid such injuries, the distal greater omentum should be mobilized prior to initiation of splenic flexure mobilization. Placing an operator between the legs of a patient in stirrups facilitates exposure in open laparotomy. Visualization of the splenic flexure laparoscopically may also help to prevent injury, since the ribcage often shelters the spleen, and thus during open surgery a large incision with cephalad and superficial retraction is necessary.

Techniques to preserve the spleen are numerous (Fig. 36-2). Pressure, topical hemostatic agents (including thrombin and gelfoam), and cautery placed on an elevated setting may aid hemostasis for small injuries. For larger injuries the spleen must be mobilized so that it becomes nearly a midline organ. If the hilar vasculature has been injured and cannot be controlled without devitalizing a portion of the spleen, a partial splenectomy may be indicated. For larger parenchymatous injuries an absorbable mesh may be used to wrap the spleen to facilitate tamponade.

Should these measures fail, a splenectomy is indicated. The lifelong risk of postsplenectomy infection is nontrivial. Protective vaccination should include encapsulated bacteria such as *Streptococcus pneumoniae* (pneumococcus), *Hemophilus influenzae* (type B), and *Neisseria meningi-*

tidis. Pneumococcus is the most common and is associated with a mortality rate of 60%. The vaccination for pneumococcus (Pneumovax, Merck, Sharp & Dohme, West Point, NY) utilizes a 23-valent polysaccharide capsular vaccine, which is 90% effective in adults older than 55. The reimmunization schedule is every 5 to 10 years. Vaccination for *H. influenzae* is now administered to most children. Immunity from the initial vaccination series may not be sufficient in the asplenic host, and repeat vaccination or determination of effective titers may be necessary. Vaccination for meningococcus is unnecessary for the asplenic patient, except when traveling to an area with increased risk.

Ureteral Injury

Altered rectosigmoid anatomy with inflammation, radiation, previous surgery, or malignancy is associated with iatrogenic ureteral injury. For colorectal surgery an incidence of 0.3% to 10% has been reported (45). Only a fraction of ureteral injuries is noted at the time of surgery. Recognition of injury is critical, since immediate repair results in improved healing. Delayed recognition is associated with significant morbidity and increases the incidence of nephrectomy sevenfold (46).

In colonic operations the left ureter is more commonly injured than the right. The abdominal ureter originates at the renal pelvis and travels superficial to the psoas muscle. As the ureter enters the pelvis, it crosses the bifurcation of the iliac arteries, passing posteriorly and inferiorly along the pelvis to the levator muscles before entering the posterior bladder. In women the distal ureter passes in the ureterosacral ligament behind the ovary and continues inferiorly in the broad ligament. In colorectal procedures several types of injuries may occur: crush, partial or complete transaction, ligation, or devascularization.

These injuries occur in association with ligation of the inferior mesenteric vessels, division of the lateral rectal stalks, and surgery in the cul-de-sac or sacral promontory or during reperitonealization. Intraoperatively, if the surgeon

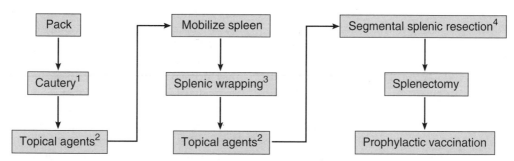

Figure 36-2 Algorithm for intraoperative splenic capsular tear.
¹ Cautery placed on a high setting may be used to achieve hemostasis.
² Topical agents such as thrombin with gelfoam may be used in addition to the above measures.
³ Use of the omentum or polyglycolic mesh may facilitate hemostasis.
⁴ Preservation of a portion of the spleen in the absence of central arterial supply may not maintain immunocompetency.

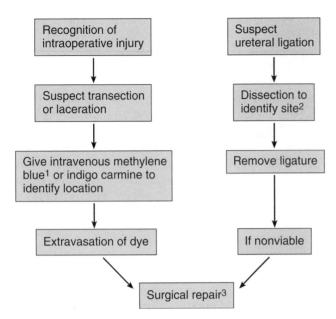

Figure 36-3 Algorithm for intraoperative ureteral injury. If the ureteral injury is confirmed and urologic consultation is available, the consultation would greatly facilitate repair and follow-up. [1] Administration of methylene blue causes the urine to have a blue color and may transiently decrease oxygenation as measured by pulse oximetry. Indigo carmine is not associated with this transient decrement. [2] If the ureter is not able to be clearly delineated, cystotomy with passage of a ureteral catheter proximally may aid in the identification. [3] Proper surgical repair depends on the injury's area and extent. Proximal to the pelvic rim, a ureteroureterostomy may be used. To facilitate a tension-free repair, not only is the ureter mobilized, but also both the bladder and the kidney may be mobilized. The repair should be spatulated, sutured with absorbable monofilament suture over a stent, and drained. Injuries to the ureter within 5 cm of the bladder may be repaired with a ureteroneocystostomy. To minimize the tension on this repair, a psoas hitch or Boari flap may be indicated. Finally, if the injury is extensive, a transureteroureterostomy may be used to effect repair. However, this may compromise a normal ureter on the opposite side.

is suspicious of ureteral injury or is unable to identify the ureter, administration of indigo carmine (2 vials) or methylene blue may be helpful (Fig. 36-3). Unfortunately, these maneuvers do not aid in the identification of a ureteral ligation but only a transection injury. If transection is suspected, a retrograde study, either with contrast or via cystoscopy with stent placement, may identify the injury.

If an injury is identified, a surgeon with familiarity, skill, and judgment with repair is necessary. Ideally, an urologist is requested to perform the repair. The principles involved in repair include debridement of devitalized tissues, a tension-free anastomosis that is spatulated and repaired with fine, absorbable, monofilament sutures over a stent, with drainage. For most injuries, ureteroureterostomy is sufficient. With significant tissue loss, the kidney, bladder, and ureter may require additional mobilization and advanced reconstruction, including a psoas hitch, Boari flap, ureteroneocystotomy, or transureteroureterostomy (Fig. 36-4).

Although preoperative ureteral stenting in situations in which a difficult dissection is anticipated has not been shown to decrease the incidence of injury, stenting may facilitate identification of injuries (47). A small number of complications have been documented, including failure to pass the stents, hematuria, and reflex anuria upon stent removal. To ease identification of the ureters during laparoscopic procedures, lighted stents have been used, but they may cause thermal injury.

Bladder Dysfunction

This complication of procedures on the rectum is multifactorial. Injury to the parasympathetic nerves that innervate the detrusor muscle or to the sympathetic nerves that innervate the bladder neck, trigone, and urethra during the pelvic dissection may be contributory. Postoperative distension, prostatic hypertrophy, packing, and pain may all contribute.

Bladder dysfunction occurs in 20% to 30% of patients following rectal dissection (48). Leaving the Foley catheter in place for a minimum of 4 days allows for some of the immediate operative edema, pain, and diuresis to resolve. A trial of voiding should then be initiated. The patient who is maintained on medication for prostatic hypertrophy should reinitiate this medication for 48 hours prior to an attempt at spontaneous voiding. If the patient develops frequency, especially of small amounts of urine, the catheter is replaced and the trial of void is reinitiated in a few days. Failing these measures, with intermittent catheterization most patients improve with time, suggesting that nerve recovery or recovery from postoperative edema is mechanistic. In a minority of patients prostatic hypertrophy is revealed and may require urologic management.

Sexual Dysfunction

Injuries to the sympathetic and parasympathetic nerves in the pelvis cause sexual dysfunction. Sexual dysfunction ranges from 15% to 60% (49,50). The neurologic input for erection arises from the parasympathetic nervi erigentes, while sympathetic input is required for ejaculation. Women experience less frequent dysfunction. The contributory factors for both men and women are multifactorial, including age, preoperative libido, the availability of a partner, and radiation.

Preservation of the main nerve trunks is possible and may decrease the incidence of sexual dysfunction. The sacral nerve roots 2, 3, and 4 may be injured during posterior rectal mobilization just above the sacral promontory. The nerves may be seen in the filmy plane of dissection just deep to the proximal mesorectum. The pelvic plexus may also be injured during ligation of the rectal stalks.

Sexual dysfunction may spontaneously improve over the 6-month to 12-month period following proctectomy. Sildenafil (Viagra) improves erectile dysfunction in nearly 80% of these patients and greatly alleviates this source of postoperative morbidity (51).

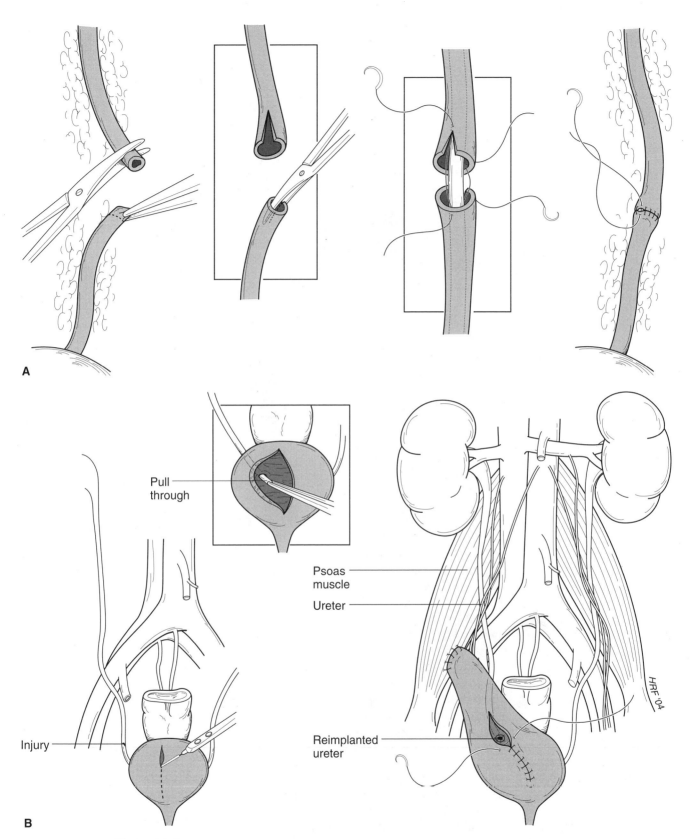

Figure 36-4 Surgical options for repair of ureteral injury. **A:** Ureteroureterostomy. The repair is completed in a tension-free manner. The ends are spatulated, and monofilament absorbable suture is used to effect the repair over a stent. The area is drained. **B:** Psoas hitch. In the pelvis, if the ureter is injured, the ureter may be reimplanted into the bladder and tension on the repair alleviated by approximation of the superior bladder to the psoas tendon.

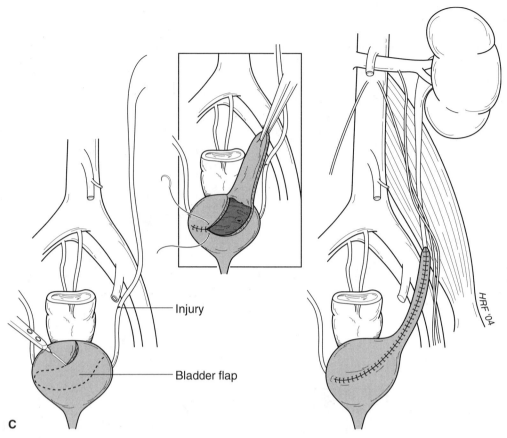

Injury

Bladder flap

C

Figure 36-4 (*continued*)   **C:** Boari flap. The bladder flap is spiraled and approximated to the psoas, with ureteroneocystostomy.

Incontinence

The increased emphasis on anal sphincter–sparing procedures has resulted in fecal incontinence as a complication. Currently, at least 80% of procedures for lesions in the middle and lower third of the rectum are completed such that restoration of continuity is possible (52). The incidence of this complication may reach 20% to 50% (53,54).

The etiology of this dysfunction is multifactorial. Certainly, the introduction of stapling devices through the anus may injure the sphincter, while rectal mobilization may lead to denervation of the pelvic muscles. Clustering of bowel movements, incomplete evacuation, soiling, and urgency are troublesome symptoms. In the adult the absence of the rectal reservoir, with the addition of postoperative chemoradiation, may overcome the sphincter mechanism, leading essentially to an anal colostomy.

To combat this disabling lifestyle issue, alternative techniques have been proposed. In 1986 both Parc et al. (55) and Lazorthes et al. (56) reported colonic J-pouch construction. Composed similarly to the ileal J-pouch, but with limbs of 5 to 6 cm, the technique has improved results compared to straight coloanal anastomosis. Another modification is the coloplasty, first reported by Maurer et al. (57). This technique creates an 8 to 10 cm longitudinal incision in the proximal colon 3 cm above the anastomosis,

which is sutured horizontally. Like the colonic J-pouch, results from this technique show improvement in early postoperative function, and, since only a single limb of bowel is used, difficulties with a fatty mesentery or a narrow male pelvis may be avoided. Currently, small series report that these techniques have nearly equivalent short-term and long-term functional results.

If incontinence is present preoperatively, the creation of a coloanal anastomosis is not indicated. The additional challenges to the continence mechanism may be impossible for the patient to manage, and the local irritation and lifestyle changes may be painful and inhibitory. The importance of preoperative counseling is critical to a consensual outcome.

Femoral and Peroneal Neuropathies

Femoral neuropathies are usually due to self-retaining retractors. An incidence of 0.7% has been reported following colon resection (58). Injury occurs as the femoral nerve, the largest branch of the lumbar plexus, passes through the psoas major muscle. Either direct retraction of the psoas muscle with the nerve or impingement of the nerve against the lateral abdominal wall causes injury. Patients at risk are those who are thin, short, or who have minimal rectus muscles. Neuropathy can be avoided by appropriate placement of retractor blades so that only the anterior and lateral abdominal walls are mobilized.

The patient presents with weakness of the quadriceps femoris, hypoesthesia of the anteromedial thigh, and decreased or absent patellar tendon reflex. Early in the postoperative period, the signs and symptoms of injury may not be obvious in the patient with an epidural catheter for pain control. Prognosis for recovery is good. Physical therapy should be initiated, with the expectation that >90% of patients will recover (59,60).

Peroneal nerve injury is due to positioning. During distal colonic and rectal procedures, with modified lithotomy position for access and with placement of the legs in stirrups, the calves may be subjected to prolonged lateral pressure. The peroneal nerve is at risk as it courses from the posterior aspect of the knee passing laterally around the head of the fibula. Pressure, if there must be any, should be medially placed. Ideally, pressure would be on the heels, and all other portions of the lower leg should be adequately cushioned and free from compression.

The clinical presentation of peroneal nerve injury is footdrop. The rapid test to document intactness is dorsiflexion of the great toe. Fortunately, without preexisting neuropathy, prognosis for this injury is excellent.

Wound Infection

Modern antimicrobial prophylaxis combined with colonic lavage and oral antibiotics has decreased the incidence of this complication. For elective colorectal surgery, a bowel preparation consisting of some type of purgative followed by oral antimicrobials is the standard of care. Popularized by Nichols and Holmes (61) and Condon and Ulnalp (62), this approach has recently been challenged (63). The original basis for bowel preparation was a decrease in wound infection rate to <10%.

Although wound infections are morbid, they are not usually the cause of mortality. To prevent wound infections, the condition of host tissues, including surgical trauma, level and type of contamination, and host defenses, must all be optimized. Antimicrobials must be present early to aid in host defense, but they cannot overcome large amounts of fecal contamination or a greatly compromised host.

Total Proctocolectomy with Ileal Pouch Anal Anastomosis

Primarily indicated for FAP and for ulcerative colitis, this operative approach, which eliminates most of the disease and preserves the anal sphincter, has gained popularity since the 1980s. Success with this procedure involves selection of appropriate patients. Although variations in pouch exist, the most popular reconstruction involves the J-pouch, created of terminal ileal limbs. Complications are due to the pouch, the accompanying rectal dissection, and the protective loop ileostomy.

Inadequate Pouch Length

The possibility always exists that the pouch will not be long enough to reach deep into the pelvis for anastomosis. This event is met with much angst but may be predictable based on preoperative assessment. Based on body habitus, those at increased risk for this difficulty may be identified, and the possibility should always be discussed in the preoperative consent process (64). Patients at risk include extremely tall individuals, those with a narrow pelvis, and the obese.

Intraoperatively, prior to initiating proctectomy an estimate of whether the pouch will reach may be gleaned by grasping the most dependent portion of the ileum and determining whether it will reach 5 to 6 cm inferior to the symphysis pubis. To maximize mesenteric length, the ileal mesentery should be mobilized so that it is free of the duodenum and pancreas. The peritoneum overlying the superior mesenteric artery may be divided on both the superficial and deep surfaces of the mesentery. Either the ileocolic or the superior mesenteric artery may be divided where there are numerous collaterals to the small bowel, usually more proximally than distally. A distal arcade may also be divided, as long as there is sufficient collateral flow. An additional centimeter or two may be gained in the construction of an S-pouch rather than a J-pouch due to the spout at the distal end. If it appears that a pouch will not reach the anal area and the distal colonic and rectal disease is not severe, an end ileostomy with a planned return when the patient is optimized may be prudent.

Small Bowel Obstruction

Bowel obstruction occurs with a frequency between 10% and 20% following restorative proctocolectomy. Approximately half of all patients do not require operative intervention. Those who require operation often have adhesions near the ileostomy site. Studies to document integrity of the pouch, followed by ileostomy closure with management of the cause of the obstruction, are prudent.

To minimize the risk of adhesions, a multicenter trial involving colorectal surgeons with the use of Seprafilm (Genzyme, Framingham, MA) was reported in 1996 (65). Nearly 200 patients undergoing restorative proctocolectomy with diverting loop ileostomy were randomized to standard care or placement of membrane. At the time of ileostomy closure 12 weeks later, laparoscopy was used to rank the incidence, extent, and severity of adhesion formation. Placement of the membrane significantly decreased the density of adhesions.

Leak

Anastomotic leakage following an ileal pouch-anal anastomosis procedure occurs in up to 12% of patients (66,67) Leakage may lead to significant morbidity, including localized or generalized peritonitis, abscess formation, fistulas, anastomotic stricture, and a dysfunctional pouch. The presence of an asymptomatic leak may be documented by a contrast study obtained prior to ileostomy closure. If present, closure is deferred for several months, prior to which another contrast study documenting resolution is necessary.

The construction of a diverting ileostomy during proctocolectomy is controversial. Many surgeons divert all patients. Diversion does not prevent leak, but it eliminates some symptoms and sequelae should a leak develop. Most agree that a breach in anastomotic integrity, undue tension, intraoperative instability, and high dose immunosuppression are indications for diversion. Some centers manage elective patients without diversion (68,69).

In some cases a small, persistent, asymptomatic sinus is seen. These may be managed expectantly, or the tract may be curetted. Usually, the tract will heal. If the tract does not heal, there should be suspicion of Crohn disease.

Pouch-vaginal Fistula

This type of fistula occurs with an incidence of 4% to 16% after proctocolectomy and is associated with significant morbidity. Seen early after restorative proctocolectomy, fistula is usually due to an infectious anastomotic source. Patients complain of pain, fever, and purulent vaginal discharge. Careful examination should be completed with attention given to the vaginal septum.

If the examination fails to reveal signs of infection of fistula but clinical suspicion remains, a careful water-soluble contrast enema is requested, completed by a radiologist familiar with restorative proctocolectomy. If the patient has signs of systemic illness, hospitalization with intravenous antibiotics and drainage of the associated abscess cavity is prudent.

Repairs take several forms. If the pouch is neither scarred nor inflamed, advancement of a pouch-based flap is usually the first approach. If this procedure is difficult, concomitant loop ileostomy may be required. If there is significant scarring or inflammation of the distal pouch, consideration should be given to an anal advancement procedure. If there is circumferential scarring, transanal or abdominal approaches to readvance the pouch, with reestablishment of a diverting stoma, may be necessary. In these cases the patient must be advised that pouch excision may eventuate. In cases where the pouch was completed for a diagnosis of ulcerative colitis, this complication may indicate a true diagnosis of Crohn disease. Overall, approximately half of the patients will achieve healing, with 25% having persistent fistulas and 22% requiring pouch excision (70).

Pelvic Abscess

The incidence of pelvic abscess following restorative proctocolectomy is approximately 5%. The etiology is usually contamination of the presacral space during the dissection or a leak of the pouch-anal anastomosis. Presenting complaints include pelvic or low back pain, accompanied by fever and leukocytosis.

CT is helpful for diagnosis and to plan the therapeutic strategy. CT-guided drainage may be possible. If the patient has a diverting ileostomy, the stoma should be left in place until the septic process has resolved. Unfortunately, pelvic sepsis is strongly associated with pouch dysfunction and is responsible for nearly half of the cases requiring pouch excision (71). If the ileostomy has been closed or no ileostomy had been made, strong consideration for establishment of an ileostomy should be given. Entry into the abdomen allows for irrigation and drain placement.

Stricture

Strictures at the anastomosis are common but usually not problematic. In approximately 5% to 15% of patients, significant stricturing occurs (72,73). Strictures may be palpable prior to ileostomy closure and may be manually dilated. Lewis et al. (74) identified some contributory factors, including use of a small-diameter stapling gun, construction of a W-pouch, defunctioning ileostomy, and anastomotic dehiscence with pelvic abscess. For strictures in which dilation is not possible or has failed, investigators have described a technique for pouch advancement (75).

Pouchitis

Pouchitis represents acute or chronic inflammation of the ileal reservoir. Although it is common in patients with ulcerative colitis, pouchitis is essentially absent in those who have had restorative proctocolectomy for FAP. Pathogenesis is poorly understood and includes bacterial stasis, ischemia, recurrent ulcerative colitis, and fatty acid deficiency. Other theories include overproduction of nitric oxide and free radical production (76). The incidence of pouchitis is not related to the type of pouch created. The prevalence of acute pouchitis varies from 10% to 60% (77). However, 5% to 15% of patients suffer from chronic pouchitis, although only 1% to 3% of the patients require pouch excision (78).

Symptoms of pouchitis include bleeding, increased stool frequency, abdominal discomfort, and fever. In addition to these clinical symptoms, endoscopic findings include mucosal edema, granularity, friability, loss of vascular pattern, mucous exudates, and ulceration, with histologic evidence of acute leukocyte infiltration and ulceration. Initial treatment includes administration of metronidazole. Alternatives include ciprofloxacin, erythromycin, and tetracycline. Topical anti-inflammatory agents, including steroid enemas, mesalamine enemas, and suppositories, may be attempted. If there is no response, oral agents may be used to supplement local measures. Unfortunately, this strategy returns patients to the regimens they so wanted to leave behind. Oral bismuth or other immunosuppressants, including azathioprine, may be successful in aborting symptoms. Ultimately, if the condition persists, pouchitis may necessitate pouch excision.

Poor Pouch Function

Although >85% of patients are pleased with pouch activity, a minority will have poor pouch function. The incidence of total failure requiring pouch excision, with the establishment of permanent ileostomy, is 3% to 10% (79). The most common causes leading to pouch failure include pelvic sepsis, pouch fistulization, and Crohn disease (80).

Stoma Complications

Despite recent advances in surgical technique, stomas are still a necessary part of general surgical practice. Although many complications are avoidable with good surgical technique and enterostomal nursing, a significant number of patients will have problems ranging from a mild skin irritation to parastomal hernia.

Dermatitis

Dermatitis is very common (>30%), with most cases occurring during the first year after stoma formation (81). Contact dermatitis may take two forms: due to the stomal effluent or due to the pouch, its solvents, or adhesives. Effluent dermatitis is an inflammation or excoriation of the skin due to leakage of the stoma output. More common in patients with an ileostomy or urostomy, approximately 20% of colostomy patients will have this type of dermatitis (82). Gut enzymes and bile are irritating to the skin and damage the keratinized surface. Some aspects may be corrected with patient education by teaching patients to cut a correctly sized aperture to avoid improper placement or pancaking. Pancaking refers to lack of air in the appliance, which creates negative pressure and causes the appliance's plastic sides to stick together, thus preventing stool from passing freely into the appliance. Other causes of effluent dermatitis include an overfull appliance, an appliance that is left on too long, or an excessively liquid output.

Other etiologies relate to preoperative and intraoperative management. For example, a poor stoma site leading to poor visualization of the appliance or an inadequate seal may contribute to leakage. Similarly, the creation of a stoma that lacks an adequate spout will cause leakage deep to the appliance. Ideally, ileostomies should be created with a 2-cm to 3-cm spout and should be everted. Techniques to enhance eversion include circumferential suture placement prior to tying down. The mesentery of the end of the ileum must provide good blood supply without tension; lack of these factors contributes to retraction.

Allergic contact dermatitis is caused by an antigenic response to a stomal product. A systematic review of possible etiologic agents is necessary so that a nonoffending substitute product may be identified.

Enterostomal nurses are instrumental for the preoperative siting, education, and continued support of these patients. Their input has been documented to improve the lives of ostomates (83,84).

Prolapse

Though alarming to the patient when prolapse initially occurs, there is usually no functional significance (Fig. 36-5). An overgenerous fascial defect contributes to the pathophysiology. Prolapse is more common with loop than with end stomas and is more common with colostomies than with ileostomies. In the acute setting osmotic therapy with table sugar may shrink an incarcerated prolapse sufficiently to allow reduction (85). The long-term prolapse rate for all types of stomas is approximately 11% to 12% (86,87).

Simple prolapse may be repaired by mobilizing the mucocutaneous junction and resecting the redundant bowel through a local incision. Recurrence may require laparotomy and resiting of the stoma. For patients in whom a full laparotomy is ill-advised with prolapse from either a loop or transverse colostomy, a procedure that strips the redundant mucosa with plication of the bowel from the apex to the mucocutaneous junction may be performed (88).

Retraction

Stomal retraction occurs as a result of the failure to mobilize sufficient bowel and its mesentery to avoid tension. Retraction occurs in 1% to 6% of colostomies (89,90) and 3% to 17% of ileostomies (81). Retraction permits the

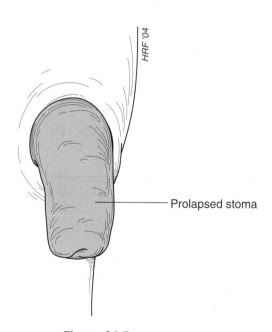

HRF '04

———— Prolapsed stoma

Figure 36-5 Stomal prolapse.

stomal effluent to seep underneath the appliance and may result in pouch loosening.

Although local procedures may be sufficient for the management of retraction, laparotomy is often necessary. For left-sided end colostomies, mobilization of the splenic flexure may be required to produce a tension-free muco-cutaneous apposition. If the mesentery is providing tension, the use of the "end-loop" or "divided loop" stoma, in which the stapled ends are left in place, with opening and maturation of only the stapled proximal end, may provide additional centimeters of length.

Necrosis

Early postoperative necrosis is secondary to vascular insufficiency at the distal edge of the stoma, either due to arterial insufficiency or venous congestion. This complication is caused by mesenteric ischemia with overtrimming of the mesentery from end of the bowel, inadequate proximal mobilization, or too tight a fascial opening. Immediately postoperatively, a normal stoma may appear dusky due to venous engorgement or stomal edema; this appearance should evolve to a bright pink color as these processes resolve. Necrosis is more likely in patients who are obese and in those who have undergone an emergent procedure, encompassing 1% to 10% of colostomies and 1% to 5% of ileostomies (91).

If necrosis is suspected, the immediate question relates to the depth and extent of necrosis. This determination is facilitated by the placement of a clear glass or plastic tube inside the stoma and shining a pen flashlight down the barrel. If necrosis extends to the level of the fascia, reoperation is necessary to prevent tension, retraction, stricture, or passage of fecal material into the peritoneal cavity.

Stenosis

Stomal stenosis occurs in 2% to 10% of end ileostomies and colostomies (89). The stricturing of Crohn disease may increase stomal stenosis (87). At the minimum, stenosis may cause loud passage of air and bowel content into the appliance, and at worst, it may cause obstruction.

For colostomies, stricture almost always occurs at the skin level. Since most colostomies are now matured at the time of creation, stricture is the result of necrosis of the distal stoma. Minor stricture may be managed by daily manual dilation. Long length narrowing, especially when due to ischemia, tension, or Crohn disease, requires laparotomy for complete mobilization.

Parastomal Hernia

Parastomal hernias are challenging problems, occurring in up to 37% of colostomies and 16% of ileostomies (81). Paracolostomy hernias are more frequent than paraileostomy hernias. Similar to other types of incisional

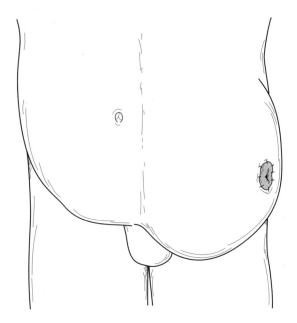

Figure 36-6 Parastoma hernia associated with nonprotruding stoma may be associated with obstruction, peristomal skin care, and pouching difficulty.

hernias, parastomal hernias are more common in patients with obesity, malnutrition, steroid dependency, or wound infection. Bringing the stoma through the rectus muscle, rather than lateral to the rectus sheath, is helpful in preventing hernia (92) (Fig. 36-6).

Indications for repair include difficulty with appliance application, pain, incarceration or strangulation, poor location, or an association with other stoma-related problems such as stricture. Options to repair the hernia locally include application of mesh. Newer options for mesh repair or reinforcement include porcine collagen, which is resistant to absorption, permitting a scaffold for native collagen, resisting infection and an inflammatory response.

The recurrence rate of parastomal hernia is quite high, ranging from 33% to 50% after relocation (93), 50% to 100% after fascial repair, and 50% after prosthetic repair. Additionally, after relocation nearly half of patients will develop an incisional hernia. If mesh is used to reinforce a repair and its characteristics do not include infection resistance, care should be taken to avoid contamination.

COMPLICATIONS OF ANORECTAL PROCEDURES

Hemorrhoidectomy

Vascular "cushions" consisting of bundles of submucosa with an arteriovenous network, smooth muscle, and elastic and connective tissue are present in every patient. The term "hemorrhoids" usually refers to pathologic conditions associated with these "cushions." Primary internal hemorrhoids lie in constant positions, right anterior, right posterior, and left lateral. External hemorrhoids are distal to the dentate line, while internal hemorrhoids are proximal to the dentate line.

The National Center for Health Statistics reports a prevalence of 4.4%. One-third of affected individuals seek physician assistance for symptoms. The majority has other anorectal diseases, ranging from pruritus ani, fissures, fistulas, skin tags, and neoplasms. Most patients will not require a major procedure for the management of symptoms and will instead be treated effectively with modifications in lifestyle or simple office procedures.

Symptoms are related to bleeding and prolapse. Bleeding is usually bright red and associated with defecation. Since internal hemorrhoids are located proximal to the dentate line, the bleeding is painless. Although usually intermittent and minimal, at times the bleeding may be spontaneous and profuse. Acute, severe pain may occur when an external hemorrhoid undergoes thrombosis, since external hemorrhoids exist in an area where sensation and discrimination are present.

The most popular approach for the management for grades III and IV disease in the United States is the Ferguson closed hemorrhoidectomy. However, due to significant postoperative pain, other approaches have been investigated, including the use of lasers and the harmonic scalpel. A handheld device similar to the end-to-end anastomotic stapler may be used to perform a mucosectomy of the area proximal to the dentate line. This approach essentially fixes the proximal tissues and may even assist with mild external hemorrhoidal disease.

Early Complications of Hemorrhoidectomy

Bleeding

Bleeding that occurs in the recovery room is due to technical error, most commonly the result of inadequate ligation of the vascular pedicle. If the source is visible on bedside inspection, suture ligation may be utilized to control hemorrhage. If the source is not easily identified, or if discomfort is excessive, insertion of a Foley catheter with the balloon inflated to tamponade the hemorrhage as the operating room is prepared is the most prudent approach.

Pain

The moderate degree of anal pain and rectal spasm that accompanies hemorrhoidectomy has been sufficient to cause many patients to avoid this procedure, even when clinically indicated. Pain is not only challenging to manage but contributes to urinary retention and fecal impaction. Multiple approaches have been used to minimize this expected outcome. Ketorolac tromethamine has been given intravenously, with subsequent recommendations for the outpatient intake of anti-inflammatory agents. In the belief that low-grade infection may contribute to pain, metronidazole has been

given intravenously, with follow-up outpatient dosing for 3 to 7 days. Although initially noted to have positive responses, later studies reveal no efficacy (94). Perioperative application of 0.2% glyceryl trinitrate ointment, in an effort to increase blood flow and relax the sphincter muscles, has also been attempted, with mixed success (95). Even postoperative pain pumps placed directly into the anal canal have received some attention (96).

The use of laser energy and ultrasound energy (harmonic scalpel) instead of scalpel, sutures, and diathermy has not consistently improved symptoms. Mucosectomy for prolapsed hemorrhoidal tissue in the form of a circular stapler is a recent alternative. Although this additional technique met with initial criticism due to early complications such as bleeding, perforation, and later stricture and incontinence, it may be effective for patients with appropriate indications (97,98).

Severe anal pain may be a sign of a perianal hematoma. The dressing should be removed and the wound inspected. Undue tension in the closure is the most likely cause of discomfort; it is better to leave a wound open than to close it with excessive tension.

Urinary Retention

Urinary retention occurs with an incidence from 3% to 20% (99,100). This complication's etiology is multifactorial. Contributing factors include prostatic hypertrophy fluid overload, rectal pain and spasm, high ligation of the hemorrhoidal pedicle, heavy suture material, tight packing, bulky dressings, anticholinergics, and narcotics (99). Anorectal surgery may decrease parasympathetic input to the detrusor muscle, while pain may increase sympathetic input to the urethral sphincter, both contributing to spasm.

Intraoperative fluids should be limited to avoid perioperative bladder distension. Patients are asked to void prior to entry into the operating room, where intravenous fluids are limited to 500 cc or less. Patients who receive a local anesthetic with sedation have a decreased incidence of this complication.

If the patient is unable to void, the subject should undergo catheterization. If residual is >500 cc, the catheter should be left in place, with a trial of voiding in 24 hours. With a residual <500 cc, the catheter should be removed, and a trial of voiding reinitiated.

Fecal Impaction

Fecal impaction is serious, though rare, occurring in 0.4% of patients after hemorrhoidectomy (101). Most patients dread their first posthemorrhoidectomy bowel movement due to the anticipated discomfort. They must be warned that constipation that evolves into impaction is even more uncomfortable. Constipation should be prevented. Laxatives, stool softeners, oral fiber, adequate hydration, and activity are necessary to promote bowel function. Narcotics and anticholinergics should be avoided.

Impaction may be difficult to diagnose postoperatively. Perineal discomfort, lack of bowel function, or overflow diarrhea are dominant symptoms. Discomfort out of proportion to operative trauma is a common finding. If rectal examination is possible, the fecal bolus is palpable. A high enema given with a red rubber catheter may be all that is required to allow stool egress. In cases when discomfort is severe and disimpaction is not possible, evacuation in the operating room with the assistance of anesthesia may be necessary.

Late Complications of Hemorrhoidectomy

Anal Tags
After hemorrhoidectomy the anal area becomes edematous. Occasionally, external thrombosed hemorrhoids may occur and in the resolution a skin tag is left. Tags may also simply be a manifestation of wound healing. Nuisance skin tags may cause discomfort to the patient if they impair local hygiene. If the symptoms are sufficient, tags may be excised.

Stricture
Removal of an excessive amount of mucosa, especially anoderm, is responsible for anal stricture. Acute management of hemorrhoids with extirpation of all the edematous, inflamed, or thrombosed tissue may lead to inadequate elastic anal tissue, which, as healing progresses, leads to a fibrous scar. This complication may result in the elective setting as well, and adequate anodermal bridges are necessary to preserve sufficient tissue to prevent its occurrence. Indicators to help prevent this complication include tension-free placement of a large sized Hill-Ferguson retractor and at least 1-cm bridges between each excised area.

If stricture is a long-term outcome of the procedure, postoperative dilation, ensuring the passage of stool, and maintained physician observation is necessary. If stricturing ensues and is epithelialized and fixed, anoplasty is indicated.

Anoplasty involves mobilization of perianal skin to cover a defect in the anal canal. If the stricturing process involves the sphincter, a careful lateral sphincterotomy may be indicated as well. Anoplasty flaps take many shapes, including V-Y, Y-V, house, and rotational flaps. The stricture's length and depth, along with the local tissue availability, dictate which flap is preferred (Fig. 36-7).

Mucosal Prolapse and Ectropion
Inadequate removal of redundant mucosa at the time of hemorrhoidectomy contributes to prolapsing mucosa. Patients will recall a wet lump of tissue discharging mucous that requires manual reduction. The wet perianal tissue contributes to local pruritus. Rubber band ligation may effectively deal with this complication.

An ectropion results when rectal mucosa descends and heals outside the anal canal. Ectropion may result from mobilization of the rectal mucosa and fixing the mucosa to the anoderm. Like mucosal prolapse, the "wet anus" produces mucus that contributes to discomfort and pruritus.

If the ectropion is evident in a limited area, the mucosa may be excised, with suture fixation of the remaining distal rectal edge to the proximal sphincter. If the ectropion is more pronounced, an anoplasty may be indicated.

Incontinence
Anal sensation may be impaired in up to 50% of patients after hemorrhoidectomy, but by 6 weeks the majority resolve their symptoms (102). Classically, hemorrhoidectomy removes vascular tissue superficial to the sphincter muscles. The elderly are especially at risk for this complication. Careful preoperative questioning is necessary to discern preexisting incontinence, although the symptoms may be mild. Appropriate tailoring of the procedure and medical management is necessary to avoid more severe incontinence. If incontinence occurs, sphincteroplasty may be required.

Anal Fissure

A fissure is a painful linear tear or ulcer in the anal canal, distal to the dentate line that may extend to the anal margin. Primary fissures are most often due to a change in bowel habits and are located posteriorly, with 10% in women and 1% in men located anteriorly. Secondary fissures are due to inflammatory bowel disease, sexually transmitted diseases, neoplasms, or trauma and are located laterally. The current theory of pathophysiology relates the development of fissures to ischemia.

Acute fissures are superficial, show little induration, and have sharply defined borders with a smooth base. Chronic fissures exhibit the triad of (a) sentinel skin tag, (b) anal ulcer, and (c) hypertrophic anal papilla. Induration and inflammation causes undermining, and the fibers of the internal anal sphincter may become visible.

The usual presentation is pain with defecation, which may be accompanied by bright red blood on the toilet paper or on the surface of the stool. Pain, with accompanying spasm, may last for hours after a bowel movement. Fear of repeated pain promotes constipation, which is often a factor contributing to the initial development of the fissure.

At least 85% of acute fissures will respond to medical management (103,104). Relief of constipation and management of spasm with a high-fiber diet, stool softeners, sitz baths, and mild analgesics are foremost in the nonoperative approach. Due to the belief that ischemia contributes to the generation of anal fissure, 0.2% glyceryl trinitrate ointment, which promotes blood flow, has been used in the management of both acute and chronic fissures. A high level of recurrence, with headaches as a side effect of treatment, has limited utility.

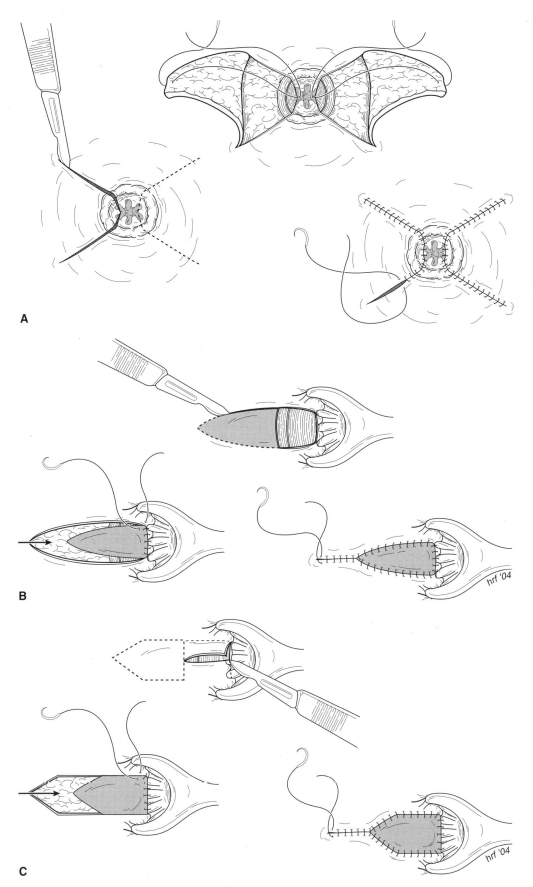

Figure 36-7 Anoplasty for stricture/stenosis. **A:** Bilateral V-flaps advance into the anal canal. **B:** V-Y flap may be repeated bilaterally. **C:** House flaps are a modification of the V-Y flap, may be repeated on the contralateral side, and may advance additional anoderm into the canal.

Complications of Internal Sphincterotomy

Abscess

The incidence of abscess following the closed internal sphincterotomy is <1%, nearly always associated with an anal fistula (105). As with other abscesses and fistulas related to cryptoglandular disease, principles of treatment include drainage of the abscess and management of the fistula.

Recurrence/Nonhealing Wound

Following lateral internal sphincterotomy, the recurrence rate ranges from 0% to 12% (106,107). Recent literature suggests a failure rate of <5%. When failure of sphincterotomy is documented, an ultrasound and anal manometry are indicated prior to performance of a second lateral sphincterotomy on the opposite side. If the initial sphincterotomy is anatomically correct and fears of incontinence are present, treatment with botulinum toxin is indicated. The possibility of another process, particularly Crohn disease, must be explored.

Incontinence

The length of internal sphincter that may be safely divided to treat patients with anal fissure and the closed versus open approach to sphincterotomy continue to be debated. Although most symptoms are due to incontinence to flatus, which usually resolves, there is persistence of fecal incontinence of 1% to 2%. When the length of sphincter divided is examined by ultrasound, more sphincter may have been transected than was intended (108). With short follow-up, a 0.5-cm open sphincterotomy yielded only a 3% incidence of postprocedural incontinence to fluid and flatus (109). Others have suggested tailoring the length of sphincter divided, depending on the length of the fissure, with no incidence of incontinence of feces or stool leakage (110).

Assessment of continence is critical for determining management options. In patients with decreased continence, the management algorithm may include the use of botulinum toxin injection prior to lateral sphincterotomy. If performed, the sphincterotomy should be conservative and a higher rate of recurrence may be expected. Those who fail to heal also require investigation for occult fissure-associated diseases such as Crohn disease, tuberculosis, syphilis, leukemia, and HIV infection.

Anorectal Abscesses

Anorectal abscess is a common surgical emergency. In the acute phase the abscess produces signs of inflammation: erythema, pain, heat, and loss of function, seen at or near the anal verge. However, an intersphincteric abscess may not be visible at this level and may require examination under anesthesia both for diagnosis and management. Likewise, a deep ischiorectal abscess may be difficult to detect on preliminary physical examination, especially in the immunocompromised host.

The presence of an abscess mandates surgical drainage. Although drainage may often be accomplished in the office, large abscesses, pain without an appreciable source, significant cellulitis, or an uncooperative patient may require examination and drainage in the operating room. The drainage site is selected over the area of greatest fluctuance, close to, but not into, the sphincter complex. The intersphincteric abscess may require internal drainage, including creation of a small defect in the internal sphincter cephalad to the sphincter complex.

Complications of Abscess Drainage

Incomplete Drainage

The major cause of recurrent anorectal abscesses is inadequate drainage. Most causes are due to cryptoglandular disease, and drainage is necessary. If the origin cannot be ascribed to an anorectal source, extra-anal sources include hidradenitis suppuritiva or pilonidal disease. Chrabot et al. (111) reported that >70% of patients with recurrent abscesses have fistula, with 30% of these patients having undergone a prior procedure.

Horseshoe abscesses present a special challenge and can present recurrently if the opposite arm of the abscess is incompletely drained. Horseshoe abscesses may occur in three planes: the intersphincteric plane, the ischioanal plane, or the supralevator plane. Classically, the horseshoe originates from the posterior midline and enters the deep postanal space with arms extending anteriorly. The opposite configuration may also occur. Entrance into the deep postanal space and drainage, consisting of counterincisions placed radially, allow egress of pus and rapid healing of the tracts.

Intersphincteric abscess may present without external signs of inflammation in patients who have symptoms of an abscess. These patients often will not permit digital rectal examination and will require an examination under anesthesia. Once the abscess is identified it is unroofed to the level of the dentate line, allowing drainage of the offending crypt. The edges of the wound are sutured for hemostasis, which also permits continued drainage.

Necrotizing Perineal Infections

In fewer than 1% of cases, anorectal suppuration may be the cause of necrotizing perineal infection (112). Patients particularly at risk include those with immunocompromise, including diabetes, renal insufficiency, and inflammatory bowel disease. In these high-risk groups necrosis can occur in the absence of an obvious source of infection, and systemic toxicity can be severe.

Aggressive resuscitation is required with parenteral antibiotics and extensive debridement. Return trips to the operating room may be necessary to remove devitalized tissue. The anorectal fistulous origin must be identified and appropriately managed.

Fistula

Although not truly a complication, a fistula remains in 30% to 70% of patients presenting with an abscess. The abscess is the distal expression of the fistula.

Fistula-in-Ano

An abscess is usually due to a cryptoglandular infection from anal duct obstruction. Approximately half do not heal but eventuate into a fistula. A fistula is an abnormal connection between two epithelial structures—in this case the mucosa of the anal canal and the skin. Other causes of fistulas include inflammatory bowel disease, anorectal malignancy, actinomycosis, trauma, sexually transmitted diseases, and pelvic sepsis.

Although most fistulas stem from an original intersphincteric source (56%), other fistulas are trans-sphincteric (21%), suprasphincteric (4%), or extrasphincteric (3%). Patients present with intermittent pain, which may herald bloody or purulent discharge. An external opening is usually identified, but the internal opening may not be obvious on routine office anoscopy.

Intraoperative techniques for identification of the internal opening include the instillation of methylene blue, or hydrogen peroxide. Complex fistulas may require ultrasound, CT, or MRI to determine the pathway of the tract and the possible source.

Management is individualized, but the goals are to eradicate the infection and the source, prevent recurrence, and maintain continence. Although the surest method for abolishing the infection is to perform a fistulotomy, this technique also divides the most muscle and may contribute to incontinence. Anterior fistulas, especially in women, may require alternative management, including seton placement, mucosal advancement flaps, or sphincteroplasty, to achieve the goals outlined above.

Complications of Surgery for Fistula-in-Ano

Recurrence After Fistulotomy

After fistulotomy, recurrence is noted in 4% to 10% of cases (113). The most common cause of recurrence is failure to identify the primary internal opening. Other factors include complex fistulas with horseshoe or upward extensions, prior surgery, and failure of adequate fistulotomy for fear of causing incontinence. Crohn disease may also contribute to recurrence. Management of acute suppuration, followed by adjunctive imaging, using ultrasound or MRI, is helpful to define the tract and the offending anal gland.

Incontinence After Fistulotomy

The incidence rates for incontinence following fistulotomy are quite broad, 10% to 50% (114). Although most agree that severance of the anorectal ring results in incontinence, the question of how much muscle may be safely divided is still unanswered and may depend on age, gender, previous anorectal or local procedures (an episiotomy, for example), and location (anterior vs. posterior). Since the anterior quadrant lacks the puborectalis muscle and women possess shorter sphincter complexes, special care should be taken when fistulotomy would mandate trans-sphincteric muscle division in this area.

When decreased continence is a consideration, staged management of the tract is most prudent. For example, a noncutting seton may be placed, and later, after the inflammation has largely subsided, a return to delineate the anatomy with the performance of a mucosal advancement flap would be judicious.

Other Options

Although fistulotomy has the highest rate of cure, the complexity of fistulous disease with the possibility of altered continence has led to other avenues for management. Common contemporary intermediaries include seton placement, mucosal advancement flap, and instillation of fibrin glue.

A seton has several purposes, including drainage, stimulation of fibrosis, and delineation of the muscle beneath. The use of a cutting seton, which stimulates fibrosis while gradually cutting through the underlying muscle, results in a variable degree of incontinence and can be quite uncomfortable (115–117). Current utilization favors use of a seton as a drain, maintained for months, allowing acute inflammation to resolve prior to pursuing other methods of management.

Rectal advancement flaps are useful when concerns exist about incontinence and perineal wound healing, especially when fistulas are complex, associated with Crohn disease, anovaginal, or rectovaginal. With a success rate of 70% to 85% (118–120), this approach is quite attractive. Subtle differences in operative technique, varied definition of incontinence, and variable duration of follow-up render outcome data difficult to interpret.

Fibrin glue can be applied without division of sphincter muscle. The technique is simple and can be repeated. Most series report a success rate of 60% to 70% (121–123).

Few studies have been completed using these techniques serially or simultaneously. For complex fistulas, drainage perpetuated by a seton, followed by advancement flap with fibrin glue prior to consideration of a proctectomy, is warranted. Although rare, malignancy is reported to arise in the chronic fistulous tracts and must be considered. If the anorectum becomes a noncompliant, incontinent organ, proctectomy with an end colostomy may be the best option to restore control and hygiene to the suffering patient.

REFERENCES

1. Addiss DG, Shaffer N, Fowler BS, et al. The epidemiology of appendicitis and appendectomy in the United States. *Am J Epidemiol* 1990;132:920–925.
2. Miller WT Jr, Greenson TJ, Miller WT. The solitary teardrop: sign of appendicolith. *Am J Roentgenol* 1988;151(6):1252.
3. Lewis FR, Holcroft JW, Boey J, et al. Appendicitis: a critical review of the diagnosis and treatment in 1000 cases. *Arch Surg* 1975; 110:677–684.
4. Kieran JA, Curet MJ. Institutional variations in the management of patients with acute appendicitis. *J Gastrointest Surg* 2001;7(4): 523–528.
5. Peck J, Peck A, Peck C, et al. The clinical role of noncontrast helical computed tomography in the diagnosis of acute appendicitis. *Am J Surg* 2000;180:133–136.
6. Andersen BR, Kallehave FL. Antibiotics versus placebo for prevention of postoperative infection after appendicectomy. In *The Cochrane Library*, Issue 3. Oxford: Update Software; 2003.
7. Taylor E, Dev V, Shah D, et al. Complicated appendicitis: is there a minimum intravenous antibiotic requirement? A prospective randomized trial. *Am Surg* 2000;66(9):887–890.
8. McGreevy MD, Finlayson SRG, Alvarado R, et al. Laparoscopy may be lowering the threshold to operate on patients with suspected appendicitis. *Surg Endosc* 2002;16:1046–1049.
9. Gale ME, Birnbaum S, Stephen GG, et al. CT appearance of appendicitis and its local complications. *J Comput Assist Tomogr* 1985;9:34–37.
10. Oliak D, Yamini D, Udani VM, et al. Initial nonoperative management for perappendiceal abscess. *Dis Colon Rectum* 2001; 44(7):936–941.
11. Bagi P, Dueholm S. Nonoperative management of the ultrasonically evaluated appendiceal mass. *Surgery* 1987;101:602–605.
12. Lemieur TP, Rodriguez JL, Jacobs DM, et al. Wound management in perforated appendicitis. *Am Surg* 1999;65:339–443.
13. Fisher KS, Ross DS. Guidelines for therapeutic decision in incidental appendectomy. *Surg Gynecol Obstet* 1990;171:95–98.
14. Fatum M, Rojansky N. Laparoscopic surgery during pregnancy. *Obstet Gynecol Surv* 2001;56(1):50–59.
15. Hardin D. Acute appendicitis: review and update. *Am Fam Physician* 1999;60:2027–2036.
16. Yamini D, Hernan V, Bongard F, et al. Perforated appendicitis: is it truly a surgical urgency? *Am Surg* 1998;64:970–975.
17. Storm-Dickerson TL, Horattas MC. What have we learned over the past 20 years about appendicitis in the elderly? *Am J Surg* 2003;185:198–201.
18. Hui TT, Major KM, Avital I, et al. Outcome of elderly patients with appendicitis. *Arch Surg* 2002;137:995–1000.
19. Stinner B, Kisker O, Zielke A. Surgical management for carcinoids tumors of small bowel, appendix, colon and rectum. *World J Surg* 1996;170:606–608.
20. Winawer S, Fletcher R, Rex D, et al. Colorectal cancer screening and surveillance: clinical guidelines and rationale—update based on new evidence. *Gastroenterology* 2003;124:544–560.
21. Autier P, Boyle P, Buyse M, et al. Is FOB screening really the answer for lowering mortality in colorectal cancer? *Recent Results Cancer Res* 2003;163:254–263.
22. Yee J, Akerkar GA, Hung RK, et al. Colorectal neopolasia: performance characteristics of CT colography for detection in 300 patients. *Radiology* 2001;219:685–692.
23. Painter NS, Burkitt DP. Diverticular disease of the colon: a 20th century problem. *Clin Gastroenterol* 1975;4:3.
24. Ryan P. Two kinds of diverticular disease. *Ann R Coll Surg Engl* 1991;73:73–79.
25. Mann CV. Problems in diverticular disease. *Proctology* 1979;1: 20–25.
26. Horner JL. Natural history of diverticulosis of the colon. *Am J Dig Dis* 1958;3:343–350.
27. Ulin AW, Pearce AE, Weinstein SF. Diverticular disease of the colon: surgical perspectives in the past decade. *Dis Colon Rectum* 1981;24:276–281.
28. Wong WD, Wexner SD, Lowry A, et al. Practice parameters for the treatment of sigmoid diverticulitis: supporting documentation. The Standards Task Force of the The American Society of Colon and Rectal Surgeons. *Dis Colon Rectum* 2000;43:289–297.
29. Hinchey EJ, Schaal PGH, Richards GK. Treatment of perforated disease of the colon. *Adv Surg* 1978;12:86–109.
30. Forde KA, Treat MR. Colonoscopy for lower gastrointestinal bleeding. In: Dent TL, Strudel SF, Turcotte JG et al., eds. *Surgical endoscopy*, Chicago, IL: Yearbook Medical Publishers; 1988: 261–275.
31. Garland CF, Lilienfeld AM, Mendeloff AI, et al. Incidence rates of ulcerative colitis and Crohn's disease in fifteen areas of the United States. *Gastroenterology* 1981;81:1115–1124.
32. Devroede G. Risk of cancer in inflammatory bowel disease. In: Winawer SJ, Schottenfeld D, Sherlock P, eds. *Colorectal cancer: prevention, epidemiology and screening*, New York: Raven Press; 1980:325–334.
33. Ritchie JK. The results of surgery for large bowel Crohn's disease. *Ann R Coll Surg Engl* 1990;72:155–157.
34. Sacher DB. Maintenance strategies in Crohn's disease. *Hosp Pract* 1996;15:99–106.
35. Fearon ER, Vogelstein B. A genetic model for colorectal tumorigenesis. *Cell* 1990;61(5):759–767.
36. Gandhi SK, Hanson MM, Vernava AM, et al. Ischemic colitis. *Dis Colon Rectum* 1996;39:88–100.
37. Jemal A, Murray T, Samuels A, et al. Cancer statistics. *CA Cancer J Clin* 2003;53(1):5–26.
38. Weeks JC, Nelson H, Gelber S, et al. Short-term quality-of-life outcomes following laparoscopic-assisted colectomy vs open colectomy for colon cancer: a randomized trial. *JAMA* 2002; 287(3):321–328.
39. Frager DH, Baer JW, Rothpearl A, et al. Distinction between postoperative ileus and mechanical small-bowel obstruction: value of CT compared with clinical and other radiographic findings. *Am J Roentgenol* 1995;164(4):891–894.
40. Pollard CW, Nivatvongs S, Rojanasakul A, et al. Carcinoma of the rectum. Profiles of intraoperative and early postoperative complications. *Dis Colon Rectum* 1994;37:866–874.
41. Vignali A, Fazio VW, Lavery IC, et al. Factors associated with the occurrence of leaks in stapled rectal anastomoses: a review of 1014 patients. *J Am Coll Surg* 1997;185:105–113.
42. Wang O, Shi W, Zhaw Y. New concepts in severe presacral hemorrhage during proctectomy. *Arch Surg* 1985;120:1015–1020.
43. Dochetry JG, McGregor JR, Akyol AM, et al. Comparison of manually constructed and stapled anastomoses in colorectal surgery. *Ann Surg* 1995;221:176–184.
44. Langevin JM, Rothenberger DA, Goldberg SM. Accidental splenic injury during surgical treatment of the colon and rectum. *Surg Gynecol Obstet* 1984;159:139–144.
45. Fry DE, Milhalen L, Harbeecht R. Iatrogenic ureteral injury. *Arch Surg* 1983;118:454.
46. McGinty DM, Mendez R. Traumatic ureteral injuries with delayed recognition. *Urology* 1977;10:115–117.
47. Bothwell WN, Bleicher RJ, Dent TL. Prophylactic ureteral catheterization in colon surgery. A five-year review. *Dis Colon Rectum* 1994;37:330–334.
48. Janu NC, Bokey EL, Chapuis PH, et al. Bladder dysfunction following anterior resection for carcinoma of the rectum. *Dis Colon Rectum* 1986;29:182–183.
49. Walsh PC, Schlegel PN. Radical pelvic surgery with preservation of sexual function. *Ann Surg* 1988;208:391–400.
50. Hojo K, Sawada T, Moriya Y. An analysis of survival and voiding, sexual function after wide iliopelvic lymphadenectomy in patients with carcinoma of the rectum, compared with conventional lymphadenectomy. *Dis Colon Rectum* 1989;32:128–133.
51. Lindsay I, George B, Kettlewell M, et al. Randomised, double-blind, placebo-controlled trial of sildenofil (Viagra) for erectile dysfunction after rectal excision for cancer and inflammatory bowel disease. *Dis Colon Rectum* 2002;45(6):727–732.
52. Kuvshinoff B, Maghfoor I, et al. Miedema distal margin requirements after preoperative chemoradiotherapy for distal rectal carcinomas: are </= 1 cm distal margins sufficient? *Ann Surg Onc* 2000;8(2):163–169.
53. Rasmussen OO, Peterson IK, Christianson J. Anorectal function following low anterior resection. *Colorectal Dis* 2003;5(3):258–261.

54. Ikeuchi H, Kasunoki M, Shoji Y, et al. Clinicophysiological results after sphincter-preserving resection for rectal carcinoma. *Int J Colorectal Dis* 1996;11:172–176.

55. Parc R, Tiret E, Frileau P, et al. Resection and colo-anal anastomosis with colonic reservoir for rectal carcinoma. *Br J Surg* 1986;73:139–141.

56. Lazorthes F, Fages P, Chiotasso P, et al. Resection of the rectum with construction of a colonic reservoir and colo-anal anastomosis for carcinoma of the rectum. *Br J Surg* 1986;73:136–138.

57. Maurer CA, Z'graggen K, Mettler D, et al. Experimental study of neorectal physiology after formation of a transverse coloplasty pouch. *Br J Surg* 1999;86:1451–1458.

58. Brasch RC, Bufo AJ, Kreienberg PF, et al. Femoral neuropathy secondary to the use of self-retaining retractor. Report of three cases and review of the literature. *Dis Colon Rectum* 1995;38:1115–1118.

59. Goldman JA, Feldberg D, Dicker D, et al. Femoral neuropathy subsequent to abdominal hysterectomy: a comprehensive study. *Eur J Obstet Gynecol Reprod Biol* 1985;20:385–392.

60. Dillavou ED, Anderson LR, Bernert RA, et al. Lower extremity iatrogenic nerve injury due to compression during intraabdominal surgery. *Am J Surg* 1997;173(6):504–508.

61. Nichols RL, Holmes JWC. Prophylactic and therapeutic antibiotics in colon and rectal surgery. *Perspect Colon Rectal Surg* 1990;3(1):183–195.

62. Ulnalp K, Condon RE. Antibiotics prophylaxis for scheduled operative procedures. *Surg Clin North Am* 1992;6:613–625.

63. Wille-Jorgensen P, Guenaga KF, Castro AA, et al. Clinical value of preoperative mechanical bowel cleansing in elective colorectal surgery: a systematic review. *Dis Colon Rectum* 2003;46(8):1013–1018.

64. Browning SM, Nivatvongs S. Intraoperative abandonment of ileal pouch-anal anastomosis: the Mayo clinic experience. *J Am Coll Surg* 1998;41:A27.

65. Becker JM, Dayton MT, Fazio VW, et al. Prevention of postoperative abdominal adhesions by a sodium hyaluronate-based bioresorbable membrane: a prospective, randomized, double-blind multicenter study. *J Am Chem Soc* 1996;183(4):406–407.

66. Fazio VW, Ziv Y, Church JM, et al. Ileal pouch-anal anastomosis complications and function in 1005 patients. *Ann Surg* 1995;222(2):120–127.

67. Grobler SP, Hosie KB, Keighley MR. Randomized trial of loop ileostomy in restorative proctocolectomy. *Br J Surg* 1992;79:903–906.

68. Sagar PM, Lewis W, Holdsworth PJ, et al. One-stage restorative proctocolectomy without temporary defunctioning ileostomy. *Dis Colon Rectum* 1992;35:582–588.

69. Sugarman HJ, Sugarman EL, Meador JG, et al. Ileal pouch anal anastomosis without ileal diversion. *Ann Surg* 2000;232(4):530–541.

70. Shah NS, Remzi F, Massmann A, et al. Management and treatment outcome of pouch-vaginal fistulas following restorative proctocolectomy. *Dis Colon Rectum* 2003;46(7):911–917.

71. Fazio VW, Wu JS, Lavery IC. Repeat ileal pouch-anal anastomosis to salvage septic complications of pelvic pouches. *Ann Surg* 1998;228(4):588–597.

72. Senapati A, Tibbs CJ, Ritchie JK, et al. Stenosis of the pouch anal anastomosis following restorative proctocolectomy. *Int J Colorectal Dis* 1996;11:57–59.

73. Fazio VW, Ziv Y, Church JM, et al. Ileal pouch-anal anastomoses: complications and function in 1005 patients. *Ann Surg* 1995;222:120–127.

74. Lewis WG, Kuzu A, Sagar PM, et al. Stricture at the pouch-anal anastomosis after restorative proctocolectomy. *Dis Colon Rectum* 1994;37:120–125.

75. Fazio VW, Tjandra JJ. Pouch advancement and neoileoanal anastomosis for anastomotic stricture and anovaginal fistula complicating restorative proctocolectomy. *Br J Surg* 1992;79:694–696.

76. Kuhbacher T, Schreiber S, Runkel N. Pouchitis: pathophysiology and treatment. *Int J Colorect Dis* 1998;13:196–207.

77. Stein RB, Lichtenstein GR. Complications after ileal pouch-anal anastomosis. *Semin Gastroinest Dis* 2000;11(1):2–9.

78. Stahlberg D, Gullberg K, Liljeqvist L, et al. Pouchitis following pelvic pouch operation for ulcerative colitis. Incidence, cumulative risk, and risk factors. *Dis Colon Rectum* 1996;39:1012–1018.

79. MacRae HM, McLeod RS, Cohen Z, et al. Risk factors for pelvic pouch failure. *Dis Colon Rectum* 1997;40:257–262.

80. Breen EM, Schoetz DJ, Marcello PW, et al. Functional results after perineal complications of ileal pouch-anal anastomosis. *Dis Colon Rectum* 1998;41(6):691–695.

81. Leong APK, Londono-Schimmer EE, Phillips RKS. Life-table analysis of stomal complications following ileostomy. *Br J Surg* 1994;81:727–729.

82. Collett K. Practical aspects of stoma management. *Nurs Stand* 2002;17(8):45–52.

83. Duchesne JC, Wang YZ, Weintraub SL, et al. Stoma complications: a multivariate analysis. *Am Surg* 2002;68(11):961–966.

84. Bass EM, Del Pino A, Tao A, et al. Does preoperative stoma marking and education by the enterostomal therapist affect outcome? *Dis Colon Rectum* 1997;40(4):440–442.

85. Myers JO, Rothenberger DA. Sugar in the reduction of incarcerated prolapsed bowel: report of two cases. *Dis Colon Rectum* 1991;34:416–418.

86. Williams NS, Nasmyth DG, Jones D, et al. Defunctioning stomas: a prospective controlled trial comparing loop ileostomy with loop transverse colostomy. *Br J Surg* 1986;72:566–570.

87. Carlsen E, Bergen A. Technical aspects and complication of end ileostomies. *World J Surg* 1995;19:632–636.

88. Abulafi AM, Sherman JW, Fiddian RV. Delorme operation for prolapsed colostomy. *Br J Surg* 1989;76:1321–1322.

89. Shellito PC. Complications of abdominal stoma surgery. *Dis Colon Rectum* 1998;41(12):1562–1572.

90. Doberneck RC. Revision and closure of the colostomy. *Surg Clin North Am* 1991;71(1):193–201.

91. Leenan LP, Kyuypers JH. Some factors influencing the outcome of stoma surgery. *Dis Colon Rectum* 1989;32:500–504.

92. Sjodahl R, Anderberg B, Bolin T. Parastomal hernia in relation to site of the abdominal stoma. *Br J Surg* 1988;75:339–341.

93. Rubin MS, Schoetz DJ, Matthew JB. Parastomal hernia: is stoma relocation superior to fascial repair? *Arch Surg* 1994;129:413–418.

94. Balfour L, Stojkovic SG, Botterill ID, et al. A randomized, double-blind trial of the effect of metronidazole on pain after closed hemorrhoidectomy. *Dis Colon Rectum* 2002;45:1186–1190.

95. Hwang DY, Yoon SG, Kin HS, et al. Effect of 0.2 percent glyceryl trinitrate ointment on wound healing after a hemorrhoidectomy. *Dis Colon Rectum* 2003;46(7):950–954.

96. Goldstein ET, Williamson PR, Lach SW. Subcutaneous morphine pump for postoperative hemorrhoidectomy pain management. *Dis Colon Rectum* 1993;36(5):439–446.

97. Balasubramanian S, Kaiser AM. Management options for symptomatic hemorrhoids. *Curr Gastroenterol Rep* 2003;5(5):431–437.

98. Dixon MR, Stamos MJ, Grant SR, et al. Stapled hemorrhoidectomy: a review of our early experience. *Am Surg* 2003;69(10):862–865.

99. Bailey HR, Ferguson JA. Prevention of urinary retention by fluid restriction following anorectal operations. *Dis Colon Rectum* 1976;19:250–252.

100. Bleday R, Pena JP, Rothenberger DA. Symptomatic hemorrhoids; current incidence and complications of operative therapy. *Dis Colon Rectum* 1992;35:477.

101. Buls JG, Goldberg SM. Modern management of hemorrhoids. *Surg Clin North Am* 1978;58:469–478.

102. Roe AM, Bartolo DCC, Vellacort KD, et al. Submucosal versus ligation excision hemorrhoidectomy: a comparison of anal sensation, anal sphincter manometry, and postoperative pain and function. *Br J Surg* 1987;74:948–951.

103. Jensen SL. Treatment of first episodes of acute anal fissure: prospective randomized study of lignocaine ointment versus hydrocortisone ointment or warm sitz baths plus bran. *Br Med J* 1986;292:1167–1169.

104. Lund JN, Armitage NC, Scholefield JH. Use of glyceryl trinitrate ointment in the treatment of anal fissure. *Br J Surg* 1996;83:776–777.

105. Oh C, Divino CM, Steinhagen RM. Anal fissure: 20-year experience. *Dis Colon Rectum* 1995;38(4):378–382.

106. Romano G, Rotondano G, Santangelo M, et al. A critical appraisal of pathogenesis and morbidity of surgical treatment of chronic anal fissure. *J Am Coll Surg* 1994;178:600–604.

107. Hiltunen KM, Metikainen M. Closed lateral subcutaneous sphinctertomy under local anesthesia in the treatment of chronic anal fissure. *Ann Chir Gynaecol* 1991;80:353–356.

108. Sultan AH, Kamm MA, Nicholls RJ, et al. Prospective study of the extent of internal anal sphincter division during lateral sphincterotomy. *Dis Colon Rectum* 1994;37(10):1031–1033.

109. Garcia G, Sutton C, Mansoori S, et al. Results following conservative lateral sphincterotomy for the treatment of chronic anal fissures. *Colorectal Dis* 2003;5:311–314.

110. Littlejohn DR, Newstead GL. Tailored lateral sphincterotomy for anal fissure. *Dis Colon Rectum* 1997;40(12):1439–1442.

111. Chrabot CM, Prasad ML, Abcarian H. Recurrent anorectal abscesses. *Dis Colon Rectum* 1983;24:105–108.

112. Huber J, Kissack AS, Simonton CT. Necrotizing soft tissue infection from rectal abscess. *Dis Colon Rectum* 1983;26:507–511.

113. Lilius HG. Fistula-in-ano, an investigation of human fetal anal ducts and intramuscular glands and a clinical study of 150 patients. *Acta Chir Scand Suppl* 1968;383:1–88.

114. Joy H, Williams JG. The outcome of surgery for high anal fistulas. *Colorectal Dis* 2002;4(4):254–261.

115. Pearl RK, Andrews JR, Orsay CP, et al. Role of seton in the management of anorectal fistulas. *Dis Colon Rectum* 1993;36(6):573–579.

116. Van Tets WF, Kuijpers JH. Seton treatment of perianal fistula with high anal or rectal opening. *Br J Surg* 1995;82:895–897.

117. Garcia-Aguilar J, Belmonte C, Wong WD, et al. Anal fistula surgery: factors associated with recurrence and incontinence. *Dis Colon Rectum* 1996;39:723–729.

118. Kodner IF, Mazor A, Shemesh EI, et al. Endorectal advancement flap repair of rectovaginal and other complicated anorectal fistulas. *Surgery* 1993;114:682–690.

119. Makowiec F, Jehle EC, Becker HD, et al. Clinical course after transanal advancement flap repair of perianal fistula in patients with Crohn's disease. *Br J Surg* 1995;82:603–606.

120. Hyman N. Endoanal advancement flap repair for complex anorectal fistulas. *Am J Surg* 1999;178:337–340.

121. Venkatesh KS, Ramanujam P. Fibrin glue application in the treatment of recurrent anorectal fistulas. *Dis Colon Rectum* 1998;42(9):1136–1139.

122. Park JJ, Cintron JR, Orsay CO, et al. Repair of chronic anorectal fistulae using commercial fibrin sealant. *Arch Surg* 2000;135:166–169.

123. Sentovich SM. Fibrin glue for anal fistulas. *Dis Colon Rectum* 2003;46(4):498–502.

Complications of Abdominal Wall and Hernia Operations

37

Michael G. Franz

■ **COMPLICATIONS OF ABDOMINAL WALL AND HERNIA SURGERY 523**
Laparotomy Incisions 524
Myofascial Dehiscence and Evisceration 526
Preoperative Risk Factors for Hernia Operations 529
Modification of Preoperative Risk Factors 529
Autologous Tissue Repairs 531
Incisional Hernias 538
Autologous Tissue Repairs 538

■ **REFERENCES 544**

COMPLICATIONS OF ABDOMINAL WALL AND HERNIA SURGERY

The abdominal wall is a complex soft tissue structure that functions to maintain upright posture, allow movement of the torso, and protect the enclosed peritoneal organs. It is composed of skin, subcutaneous tissues, fascia, muscles, peritoneum, and associated blood vessels and nerves. All abdominal operations require wounding of the abdominal wall, making it a common site of surgical morbidity.

Hernias are openings in the abdominal wall that can result in the abnormal movement of intra-abdominal organs

and structures across the defects. Hernias are clinically disabling when they become painful or limit function of the abdominal wall. Hernias can also become surgically dangerous when intra-abdominal organs become incarcerated or strangulated within the defects, leading to bowel obstruction and organ infarction. Understanding the pathology of hernias requires a thorough understanding of abdominal wall physiology, as the two subjects are intimately connected.

Abdominal wall hernia repairs are among the most common major surgical procedures performed in the United States, with approximately one million cases annually. Nearly 700,000 operations are for inguinal hernias, with an additional 100,000 procedures for umbilical, epigastric, Spigelian, and flank hernia repairs (1,2). Together, these constitute the bulk of the primary abdominal wall hernias that occur spontaneously. An additional 90,000 incisional hernia repairs are performed each year in the United States. Incisional hernias are iatrogenic complications of abdominal operations. The operative volume establishes primary and secondary hernias as a common problem for general surgeons and their patients.

The history of hernia repairs and failures is, in many ways, the history of general surgery itself. The era of modern general surgery is full of descriptions of techniques for the ideal hernia repair. From the original local autologous tissue reconstructions to more modern alloplastic implantations, the common goal has been a safe and efficient operation that yields the lowest hernia recurrence rate. The best operation is the one tailored to each patient's unique

Michael G. Franz: University of Michigan, Ann Arbor, MI 48109 problem based on a thorough understanding of abdominal wall anatomy and physiology.

Laparotomy Incisions

Exposure

The ideal laparotomy incision provides exposure for the safe and effective examination and surgical therapy of intra-abdominal organs and structures. The size of the incision is dictated by the need for a therapeutic operation and should not be compromised for cosmetic reasons. It has never been shown that the length of a celiotomy incision worsens surgical outcomes in the medium or long term. Similarly, it has never been shown that the length of an incision affects the rate of healing. The main proven benefits measured following minimally invasive procedures are earlier return to usual activity, lower wound infection rates, less pain, and less scarring. Safe exposure should never be compromised to achieve the benefits of minimized incisions since the benefits do not outweigh the risk of complications associated with inadequate access to diseased organs.

An incision's location is equal in importance to its size. A misplaced incision of the abdominal wall may compromise exposure and access. Examples include celiotomy incisions placed too high on the abdominal wall, leading to difficulty mobilizing the lower bowel mesenteries and increasing the risk of ureteral injury, and incisions placed too low, increasing the risk of inadvertent injuries to structures of the upper abdomen, including the bile duct, esophagus, or spleen. Preoperative imaging studies are useful in planning the most effective abdominal wall site for laparotomy. When using computed tomography (CT) scans, the umbilicus provides a useful abdominal wall surface landmark for counting 5 mm or 10 mm image slices and measuring the optimum location for incision.

Recommended abdominal incisions for specific operations are discussed in dedicated chapters elsewhere. General principles may be applied to all laparotomy incisions. Midline celiotomy incisions are usually used for emergency access and exposure, such as following blunt or penetrating trauma to the abdomen, especially when a definitive diagnosis has not been made. The midline incision is the most versatile in terms of access to the entire peritoneum and may easily be extended cephalad or caudad. Elective procedures of the colon and small bowel are also usually best performed through midline incisions to preserve lateral anterior abdominal wall integrity in the event of a concurrent or future ileostomy or colostomy. The liver, biliary tract, pancreas, and spleen are safely and completely exposed through bilateral subcostal incisions. Most surgeons apply upper midline incisions for access and exposure of the stomach and intra-abdominal esophagus. Intrathoracic extension of this incision can improve proximal exposure.

Wound bursting strength in cadavers is twice as great for transverse as for midline incisions when sutures are placed 1 cm from the wound edge (3). However, when a midline incision is closed using a "wide-bite" with a through-and-through rectus muscle mass closure technique, wound bursting strength was 150% to 200% of the transverse incision closure. The predominant mechanism of failure in burst-tested cadaver incisions is suture cutting through tissue. Retrospective studies suggest that the rate of dehiscence is higher in midline incisions than in transverse incisions of the abdominal wall. Critics of midline incisions interpret the data to show that midline incisions are nonanatomic and cut across aponeurotic fibers, as opposed to transverse incisions that cut parallel to these fibers. Contraction and loading of the abdominal wall tends to pull the midline incision apart but brings the edges of transverse incisions together. Furthermore, it is thought that sutures in a midline incision tear out more easily than in the transverse wound because ripping in the former occurs parallel to dominant collagen bundles. However, available prospective controlled trials have not substantiated the belief that transverse incisions suffer fewer dehiscences than midline incisions.

Closure

Clinical studies of acute wound failure report three principles in achieving low wound dehiscence rates: wide tissue bites, short stitch intervals, and nonstrangulating tension on the suture. Fundamental to the development of an ideal technique of laparotomy incision closure is an appreciation of the fact that the abdominal wall incision may lengthen by 30% as a patient begins to load the abdominal wall or if the abdomen becomes distended postoperatively (4). The stitch interval must therefore elongate with the incision; if the tissue bite is small, there is an increased chance for the suture to tear through tissue. The length of suture used to close a celiotomy incision has been normalized to wound length and defined as a suture length to wound length ratio (SL:WL). The lowest wound dehiscence rates occurred using a SL:WL ratio of 4:1, where 1 dehiscence developed in 1,505 prospective and continuous cases (0.07%). A 1-cm stitch interval with 1-cm tissue bites achieves the 4:1 SL:WL ratio. (Fig. 37-1). A similar study found that the SL:WL ratio used during closure of the abdominal wall at the original operation was also a risk factor for incisional hernia formation. This observation affirms developing theories that the majority of incision hernias are derived from undetected or occult fascial dehiscences. The preponderance of data supports the use of a running, mass closure with a SL:WL ratio of 4:1 or greater (3).

Suture tension that raises the interstitial pressure in the center of the incision above capillary perfusion pressure (30 mm to 40 mm Hg) may cause fascial necrosis. In animal studies this situation has increased the risk of acute wound failure. Ideal suture tension should approximate fascia while maintaining the perfusion of healing tissue. A short, 1-cm stitch interval with a moderate tension load should prevent omentum or intestine from protruding through the suture line.

Unplanned Visceral Injury

Abdominal organs may be injured when the peritoneum is opened. The risk of visceral injury during laparotomy is increased by the presence of previous abdominal wall scars, adhesions, and distended organs. The risk of visceral injury can be reduced by incising the abdominal wall in layers, carefully identifying component structures and layers, retracting as needed, and identifying the peritoneum. In the presence of dense scars or adhesions, sharp dissection is usually recommended until potential planes between organs and the peritoneum are identified. Often, a lateral dissection must be pursued away from the midline scar until the uninjured peritoneum is identified and more safely and easily opened.

Retractors may also cause unintended organ injury. Great vigilance must be used in the safe application of handheld and self-retaining abdominal retractors. In a normal peritoneum, each retractor should be placed under direct vision and the deep edge palpated to ensure safe placement without undue tension on organs. In a reoperative peritoneum with dense adhesions, great care must be used to prevent torque injuries caused by retractors pulling on adhered structures. Following removal of retractors, abdominal organs should routinely be examined for injury. Retractor injury is not always obvious at the time of abdominal wall closure, and the first sign of injury may be delayed hemorrhage or intestinal perforation during the convalescent period.

Sutures may penetrate the intestines during closure of the abdominal wall and can result in bowel obstruction and fistulization. This is most easily avoided by maintaining careful anatomic identification of abdominal wall and visceral structures at the end of the case. Communication with the anesthesiologist is helpful to maintain adequate levels of abdominal wall relaxation to complete the optimum closure. Prospective studies of abdominal wall closure techniques suggest that the optimum depth of a fascial stitch is 1 cm into normal fascia (4). Deeper fascial stitches, such as those placed as retention sutures, increase the risk of bowel injury. Distended organs also increase the risk for injury.

Retained Instrument

A retained instrument, sponge, or needle is a technical error that can occur during laparotomy. The complication occurs most often during emergency procedures or when operating in two or more widely separated fields and when using packs for hemostasis (5). Retained gauze causes abscess formation. Retained instruments or needles may penetrate viscera and cause an abscess, fistula, or obstruction.

The retention of needles is best avoided by the compulsive reapplication of needles to needle drivers and by accounting for every needle when an empty driver is returned. In most hospitals all instruments and needles are counted.

The incidence of retained gauze sponges may be reduced by using only large laparotomy pads when operating in the abdomen. Sponge stick or peanut dissectors should be avoided. Large gauze pads are more easily palpated during a careful manual search of the peritoneal cavity. The surgeons should vigilantly account for the placement and removal of all laparotomy pads. Surgeons should routinely examine all locations where gauze pads might have been placed, such as behind the liver or spleen. The nursing sponge count needs to be correct. An incomplete closing count requires a reexamination of the peritoneal cavity and retrieval of the missing sponge. If the final count remains incomplete, an intraoperative radiograph should be performed to prove without any doubt that no radiopaque marker remains in the abdomen.

Despite systematic approaches and a correct count, a gauze pad or even an instrument might be left. If this situation is detected in the postoperative period, the surgeon should first inform the patient or the patient's family, or both, of the presence of the foreign body and then recommend its removal at the safest interval.

Incisional Pain

Clinical experience suggests that some abdominal wall incisions are more painful than others in the perioperative period. Methods for measuring incisional pain include the use of pain analog scales and narcotic analgesic requirements. Respiratory splinting due to abdominal wall incisional pain and narcotic therapy both predispose to reduced pulmonary tidal volumes and atelectasis. Urinary retention and delayed gastrointestinal function may also follow increased narcotic usage due to abdominal wall pain. It is generally believed that pain is greatest following vertical midline and paramedian incisions because they are subject to the greatest distractive forces during recovery. Abdominal wall flexion and extension and lateral traction from the oblique musculature are the primary sources of vertical laparotomy wound motion. Less pain is reported following transverse and oblique abdominal wall incisions, especially retroperitoneal flank incisions. In these incisions the normal abdominal wall load forces are distributed parallel to the abdominal wall wounds, thereby minimizing distractive wound-load vectors. Many surgeons believe that a transverse incision minimizes respiratory dysfunction in patients with pulmonary disease. A definitive study of pain associated with abdominal wall incisions is difficult to control and has not been done.

Abdominal Wall Wound Infections

Abdominal wall wound infections may be categorized as superficial, deep, or organ space, depending on the anatomic location of the infected wounded tissue. Most serious are deep laparotomy wound infections. The best-characterized invasive organisms include hemolytic streptococci, staphylococci, clostridia, and synergistic combinations of gramnegative rods and anaerobes (streptococci or bacteroides). The invasive infections frequently cause intense pain and tenderness. Patients developing these signs and symptoms as early as the second postoperative day must be followed closely for progression to abdominal wall crepitus and signs of toxemia. Streptococcal erysipelas and clostridium cellulitis often respond well to β-lactam antibiotics such as penicillin. All other invasive infections require urgent surgical debridement of destroyed tissue and intravenous antibiotics directed toward the offending organism or organisms. Repeated debridements may be required until the infection is controlled.

Debridement of abdominal wall infections may result in full-thickness defects exposing the peritoneum. These are difficult surgical circumstances requiring a variety of approaches to effect successful abdominal wall wound management. Traditionally, a temporary alloplastic implant like polypropylene mesh has been used to bridge the myofascial defect. Alloplastic materials may, however, behave as foreign bodies within a contaminated field and become chronically infected. In addition, a high incidence of bowel fistulization has been reported using meshed alloplastics. It is ideal if a large omentum or existing preperitoneal tissue protects peritoneal organs before alloplastic implantation of a contaminated or infected field. Alloplastics like polypropylene have also been successfully used for serial temporary closure of the abdominal wall. This approach involves intensive care unit level sedation or a return to the operating room every 2 to 3 days for wound debridement and "reefing" of the alloplastic bridge closure to reduce the implant surface area. Ultimately, closure with autologous ventral abdominal wall myofascia is achieved.

Another approach to temporary closure of infected and/or contaminated abdominal wall defects has been the use of absorbable implants such as polyglycolic acid polymer mesh. These materials may also fistulize to bowel and always result in a large incisional hernia that presents a set of significant secondary surgical problems and complications. Small series and case reports have cited the successful management of infected or contaminated abdominal wall defects using newer biologic patch implants. Sheets of biomaterials derived from porcine submucosa or cadaveric dermis have some of the mechanical properties of an ideal abdominal wall soft tissue implant. In addition, early evidence suggests that some biomaterials may act as an extracellular matrix scaffold. The grafts are repopulated with host abdominal wall cells like repair fibroblasts and become vascularized so that wound infections may clear and long-term abdominal wall wound mechanical integrity is maintained. Larger prospective studies are required to determine the safety and efficacy of newer abdominal wall implants.

Most abdominal wall wound infections are confined to the subcutaneous fat as cellulitis. There infections manifest as increasing wound pain and tenderness on postoperative days 5 through 7 when a normal wound inflammatory response should be resolving. Subcutaneous tissue necrosis also predisposes to abscess formation following cautery, mass ligature, or creation of ischemic suture lines. The incidence of subcutaneous abscesses appears to be higher in obese patients.

Once diagnosed, especially in the presence of fever and an elevated white blood cell count, a superficial wound should be opened through the skin and all pus should be drained. Antibiotics are usually not necessary unless the abscess is associated with an invasive soft tissue infection or an adjacent prosthesis, or both. These wounds should be lightly packed with moistened gauze two to three times a day until normal granulation tissue appears and wound contraction begins.

Multifilament, nonabsorbable sutures may harbor bacteria and predispose a wound to stitch abscess and sinuses. A recurrent stitch abscess diagnosed months or years after an operation should be treated by excision of the offending stitch. Waiting may result in spontaneous expulsion of the stitch, or the wound may be operatively reexplored under controlled conditions.

Myofascial Dehiscence and Evisceration

The reported incidence of fascial dehiscence (acute wound failure) ranges from 0.2% to 10% (3,6). The Veterans Affairs National Surgical Quality Improvement Program (NSQIP) maintains the largest prospective database of perioperative surgical risk factors and outcomes in the United States (7). An analysis of 34,809 laparotomies performed between 1996 and 2000 revealed a 3.3% incidence of fascial dehiscence. This was the largest series of fascial dehiscence ever reported. A review of the fascial dehiscence literature shows that the rates of reported fascial dehiscence are higher in prospective studies than in retrospective reviews. The Veterans Affairs NSQIP study confirmed that deep wound space infection is the greatest risk factor for fascial dehiscence. It is probable that some cases of deep space infections following laparotomy are derived from apparent or evolving gastrointestinal fistulas. Other significant perioperative risk factors included failure to wean from the ventilator and emergency procedures.

Acute myofascial wound failure occurs for one of four fundamental reasons: a suture breaks, a knot unties, a loose or excessive stitch interval that allows the protrusion of viscera, or suture pulls through the fascia. Contemporary data suggest that tissue tearing is the predominant cause of dehiscence and that in the absence of recognized risk factors the primary mechanism is an inadequate tissue bite with the suture needle (3).

Myofascial dehiscence or the mechanical separation of coapted fascial wound edges follows two major scenarios. The first form of fascial dehiscence occurs without a wound infection. The classic clinical finding is the sudden soaking of dressings and sheets with serosanguinous fluid on postoperative day 3 to 7. This sign is reported to occur in 23% to 84% of cases of documented dehiscence (3). Patients and their nurses often report a "gush" of "watermelon" colored fluid. When the area of the dehiscence is small, evisceration may not occur as the inflamed viscera adhere to each other and to the parietal peritoneum.

It is also now known that many fascial dehiscences are occult, remaining clinically undetected. One study found that 94% of incisional hernias resulted from clinically occult fascial dehiscences of laparotomy wounds that had occurred by postoperative day 30. The mechanically intact overlying skin wound prevented earlier diagnosis. In larger area dehiscences small bowel and omentum may cross the myofascial closure and be visibly apparent.

The second most frequently encountered scenario involves myofascial infection in the deep wound space. The associated tissue inflammation and necrosis predisposes to fascial failure and the "pulling through" of sutures and wound edge separation. In this circumstance the wound infection must be treated with added caution due to the anatomic defect. There is an increased risk for enterocutaneous fistulas when debriding necrotic tissue in the deep space of an infected celiotomy wound. When clinically appropriate, a small area dehiscence may be managed with gentle moist irrigation and nonadherent dressings until covered with granulation tissue. Epidermal closure may be accelerated with a split-thickness skin graft if necessary. An incisional hernia is inevitable with this approach and will present a set of surgical problems at a later date. When the defect is large enough to threaten evisceration, the acute abdominal defect may require mechanical reinforcement or replacement with an implant.

In the presence of infection many surgeons use absorbable material like polyglycolic acid polymer mesh. This approach will also result in the development of a ventral incisional hernia, but it is less likely to cause a chronic, foreign body abscess. In very large ventral defects, rapidly absorbable meshes may mechanically fail 2 to 3 weeks after implantation, placing adherent bowel at risk for shear injuries. Polypropylene woven mesh implants maintain greater breaking and tensile strength but have an increased risk of mesh infection. Both polyglycolic acid polymer and polypropylene mesh are associated with a risk for fistulization to the bowel. Every effort should therefore be made to interpose omentum or preperitoneal fat between the mesh implants and viscera. Newer patch implants derived from porcine submucosa or cadaveric dermis may provide an effective alternative, although no large clinical series are reported. The strategy with biomaterials is to provide the mechanical integrity of an alloplastic implant while avoiding the risk of chronic foreign body–induced inflammation and infection.

Biomaterial allografts are revascularized when engrafted and evolve into a neofascial layer. Extruded polytetrafluorethylene (PTFE) mesh patches are microporous on the peritoneal surface, resulting in lower visceral adhesions and fistulas. This same micromechanical design, however, limits both fibroblast and inflammatory cell ingrowth and results in a slightly greater risk for implant associated infections. PTFE probably should not be used for permanent repair in the setting of acute dehiscence, given the contaminated nature of these wounds.

Many series report mortality rates of 15% to 50% following dehiscence and evisceration (3). It is not clear if this alarmingly high mortality is the result of the clinical risk factors leading to dehiscence, the surgical and medical interventions required following dehiscence, or a combination of both. Too often dehiscences associated with deep space wound infections are not clearly separated from those occurring in the absence of an infection. Another frequent criticism of studies of fascial dehiscence is that they include large numbers of patients at extremely low risk for acute fascial wound failure.

The most frequently reported systemic risk factors for acute fascial wound failure include severe malnutrition, shock, obesity, uremia, and liver failure. Local wound factors include mechanical loading of the abdominal wall due to ileus or mechanical ventilation, ascites, and deep wound infection (3). There is no proof that midline laparotomy incisions are more likely to result in evisceration than transverse or oblique incisions. The best prospective studies of acute abdominal wall wound failure note that midline celiotomy incisions are more likely to be used in multiply injured, septic, or cancer patients.

Systems used to predict acute wound failure have focused on patient characteristics. One case-control study empirically documented risk factors associated with fascial dehiscence as: Age >65, wound infection, pulmonary disease, hemodynamic instability, ostomy within the incision, low serum albumin, sepsis, obesity, uremia, hyperalimentation, malignancy, ascites, steroid use, and hypertension. Patients with three to five of these characteristics were at a significantly increased risk for acute wound failure. All patients with eight or more characteristics developed disrupted wounds (8) (Table 37-1).

The use of absorbable versus permanent suture material has never been shown to affect wound dehiscence rates. Similarly, it has not been definitively shown that using

TABLE 37-1

RISK FACTORS FOR MYOFASCIAL DEHISCENCE

Systemic	Local
Malnutrition	Abdominal distention from ileus
Shock	Prolonged ventilation
Obesity	Deep wound infection
Steroids and antiproliferative drugs	Ascites
Uremia	Poor surgical technique
Liver failure	Ischemia
Age >65	Ostomy near incision
Malignancy	

continuous versus interrupted technique affects the incidence of dehiscence (3). One large prospective series did report that the use of a continuous suturing technique with an SL:WL ratio of 4:1 resulted in the lowest incidence of incisional hernia formation over a 10-year follow-up period (4). This closure is achieved by taking a 1-cm bite back from the fascial edge and making 1 cm of progress with each stitch. The ideal continuous suture length results in a coil around the fascial closure that expands with the wound as the patient recovers. This coil minimizes high loads at the fascial-stitch interface, decreasing the incidence of sutures "pulling through" (Fig. 37-1). The only

obvious disadvantage of the continuous suture technique is that if the single suture fails, the entire wound is at risk.

Some surgeons use retention sutures passing through all layers of the abdominal wall to prevent evisceration of patients at increased risk for dehiscence. Available series find that this technique may prevent clinically disastrous evisceration but does not lower the incidence of fascial dehiscence. Most surgeons believe that the ischemic and traumatic effects of external retention sutures on the skin outweigh the limited effect on outcomes of high-risk abdominal wall closures. A frequently applied alternative is the technique of placing interrupted internal retention sutures during the continuous closure of a celiotomy incision, although no definitive outcomes data are available.

If dehiscence is clinically suspected based on the sudden appearance of serosanguinous fluid on dressings in the early postoperative period, patients should be returned to the operating room for careful wound examination and immediate reclosure. Bedside probing does not have the sensitivity or specificity needed to diagnose fascial dehiscence. If the patient is not a candidate for operative intervention, frequent moist dressing changes with nonadherent dressings may be employed, accepting the evolution of an incisional hernia. If the nonoperative path is chosen, it must be confirmed that there is no incarceration, obstruction, or strangulation of bowel (Fig. 37-2). Remarkably, the results of reclosure are usually good. It is likely that healing of the second closure is accelerated due to the presence in the second wound of the cellular and molecular elements of tissue repair. Classic wound studies showed long ago that

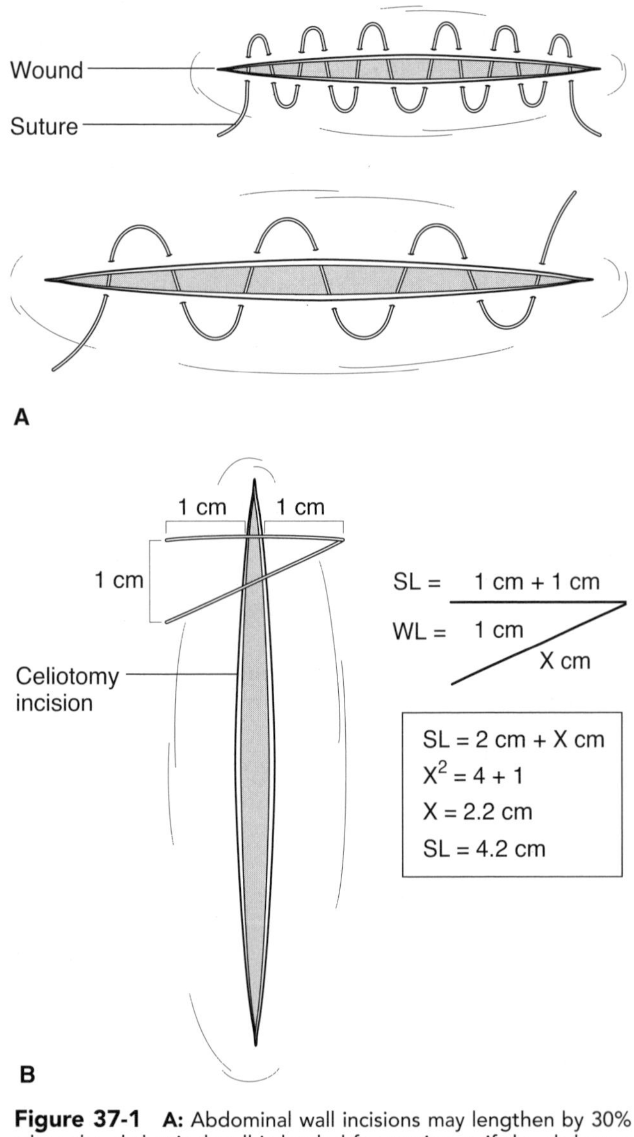

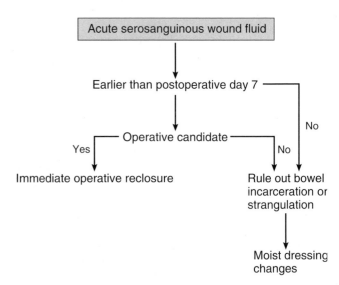

Figure 37-2   If fascial dehiscence is suspected, most patients should be returned to the operating room for careful wound examination and immediate reclosure. Bedside probing does not have the sensitivity or specificity to diagnose fascial dehiscence. If the patient is not a candidate for operative intervention, frequent moist dressing changes with nonadherent dressings may be used, accepting the inevitability of an incisional hernia. When the nonoperative path is chosen, it must be confirmed that there is no incarceration, obstruction, or strangulation of bowel.

Figure 37-1   **A:** Abdominal wall incisions may lengthen by 30% when the abdominal wall is loaded for motion or if the abdomen becomes distended postoperatively. The ideal stitch interval should elongate with the incision so that the suture does not tear through the fascia. **B:** The ideal length of suture to close a celiotomy incision has been normalized to the wound length and defined as the suture length to wound length ratio (SL:WL). The lowest wound dehiscence rates occurred using a SL:WL ratio of 4:1. A 1-cm stitch interval with 1-cm tissue bites achieves the 4:1 SL:WL ratio.

delayed reclosure of incisions results in the accelerated recovery of wound tensile strength (9,10).

Preoperative Risk Factors for Hernia Operations

Prospective, randomized controlled trials of hernia operations describe both mechanical and biologic preoperative risk factors for hernia recurrence following repair. Study of incisional hernia repair found that recurrent herniation within 3 years of the operation was significantly more likely to occur in men with symptoms of prostatism or bladder outlet obstruction and in patients with a history of an abdominal aortic aneurysm (6). Presumably, prostatism contributes to the higher rate of hernia recurrence because of repetitive Valsalva maneuvers or loading of the repaired abdominal wall that occurs with urination. Patients who develop abdominal aortic aneurysms express abnormal tissue collagen isoforms and metalloproteinase levels. The aberrant structural collagen and increased turnover catalyzed by tissue proteinases result in defective wound repair (11,12).

Another established risk factor for recurrent herniation is operating upon an already recurrent hernia. The incidence of recurrent herniation following repair increases with each subsequent repair (6,13). The reported recurrence rate following primary inguinal hernia repair is around 1%, while the recurrence rate following the repair of multiply recurrent hernias is 12 times that frequency. A prospective, randomized, controlled trial of incisional hernia repair established a 24% recurrence rate with the use of an alloplastic mesh implant and a 54% recurrence rate following a primary repair using *in situ* local autologous tissues after the initial hernia repair (6). Many less well-controlled studies and large clinical experiences report a 50% or greater hernia recurrence rate after the second hernia repair and 60% recurrence rates after the third. Preclinical wound healing data suggest that part of the explanation for increased recurrent hernia rates following each repair is the selection of a defective, chronic wound.

Since incisional hernias are iatrogenic, they are associated with a unique set of preoperative risk factors. It was long held in the surgical wound healing literature that incisional hernias were a late event, developing years after celiotomy closure. Small series and class II data suggested that abnormal progression through all the phases of wound healing (inflammation, fibroplasias, and scar maturation) ultimately resulted in wound breakdown and herniation (14). Biochemical measurements suggested defects in collagen isoform structure and tissue proteinase expression as a late phenomenon.

A more recent and provocative hypothesis suggests that most incisional hernias occur as the result of very early occult abdominal wall wound dehiscence (15). Prospectively, at the time of celiotomy closure in 149 patients, metal clips were placed along the border of the myofascial incision and the skin closed as usual. Plain film abdominal x-rays were then performed on postoperative day 30. Eighteen (12%) of the patients developed clinically obvious incisional hernias during the 43-month follow-up, as demonstrated by separation of the metallic markers on postoperative x-ray. Of the 18 patients who developed incisional hernias, 17 (94%) demonstrated 12 mm or greater fascial clip separation by postoperative day 30. By contrast, only 1 of the remaining 131 patients who did not develop 12 mm fascial separation by postoperative day 30 developed a hernia. This simple, but well-done study indicates a much higher rate of occult primary celiotomy wound failure—in the vicinity of 11% to 15%. The high incidence appears to be due to the lag phase in the recovery of wound tensile strength following injury.

The wound infection rate appears to be higher following abdominal wall hernia repair than for other clean cases, although the mechanism is unclear (16). One possibility is that patients with significant comorbid conditions are at risk for both hernia formation and wound infection. A Veterans Affairs NSQIP study found a 4.3% wound infection rate and 15.1% hernia recurrence rate. The expected clean surgical wound infection rate for nonhernia cases is closer to 1%. Multiple logistic and linear regression analyses have documented that coronary artery disease, chronic obstructive pulmonary disease, low serum albumin, and steroid use are independent risk factors for wound infection and prolonged hospital stay.

Modification of Preoperative Risk Factors

On the basis of prospective, randomized, controlled trials of hernia repair, it is prudent to screen prospective hernia repair patients for signs and symptoms of prostatism (6). By logical extension, questions should be asked during the preoperative evaluation about other symptoms leading to chronic Valsalva maneuvers or loading of the abdominal wall. Increased difficulties having bowel movements or a chronic cough are common examples. Important colorectal pathology is often diagnosed during workups for hernias. When time permits, a urologic or gastrointestinal evaluation may be indicated prior to hernia surgery to diagnose and treat occult processes and to potentially improve the results of repair.

Most biologic risk factors are more difficult to correct. Patients with abdominal aortic aneurysms express defective tissue repair pathways that cannot be treated today (17,18). Operating during periods of profound shock is often unavoidable when a life is at stake. All efforts should be directed toward correcting hemodynamics and using optimum surgical technique. Cessation of cigarette smoking has been shown to improve skin healing, but it is not clear that cessation affects rates of abdominal wall wound failure (19). It is likely that cigarette smoking impedes tissue repair pathways dependent on oxygen delivery and that associated chronic coughs overload abdominal wall closure. Obesity has never been shown to cause a wound healing defect.

However, increased mechanical forces are likely to contribute to abdominal wall wound failure. Class II data show an increased incidence of incisional hernia formation in obese patients (20). Efforts to lose weight prior to hernia repair surgery should improve outcomes, although this belief has never been definitively proven. Reduced weight reduces fascial wound load forces and also provides locally mobile skin to assure fascial wound coverage.

Inguinal Hernias

Inguinal hernia repair is the most common abdominal wall operation and the most frequent elective procedure performed by general surgeons (Fig. 37-3). Comparing the results of different operative approaches to hernia repair is difficult. There is no agreed-upon definition of hernia recurrence, typically the most cited outcome measure. Most hernia surgeons support the appearance of any new hernia on the operative side as the definition of a recurrence. Distinguishing a new hernia from a recurrent hernia through an existing repair is often inexact. The other possibility is that an adjacent defect went undetected and a persistent hernia manifests in the postoperative period. The length of follow-up also affects the quality of hernia repair outcome databases. Recurrence rates increase with increased length of follow-up. Recurrence rates also increase when dedicated, expert postoperative examinations are used for assessment (21).

The original operations designed for inguinal hernia repair all depended on loco-regional tissue transfers. The advantages of these approaches include simple operations without the need for prostheses and the reliable healing of well vascularized tissues. The problems associated with local tissue repairs include biomechanical limitations (closing "under tension") and the use of abnormal tissue that demonstrated a tendency to herniate. Although proponents of each technique report very low personal recurrence rates, prospectively controlled series report recurrence rates of 6% to 11% when general surgeons use these techniques outside of dedicated centers (22). When analyzed this way, recurrent inguinal hernias occur in decreasing incidence following femoral hernia repair (49%), direct inguinal hernia repair (21%), and indirect inguinal hernia repair (9%), respectively.

The posterior wall of the inguinal canal is composed of the transversalis muscle, its aponeurosis, and the transversalis fascia that together insert on Cooper ligament. In the inferior abdominal wall there is a weak area in the groin where overlying myofascia do not reinforce this posterior layer. This area of the posterior, inferior abdominal wall is often referred to as the myopectineal orifice. The area is defined by the rectus muscle medially, the internal oblique and transversalis muscles superiorly, the iliopsoas muscle

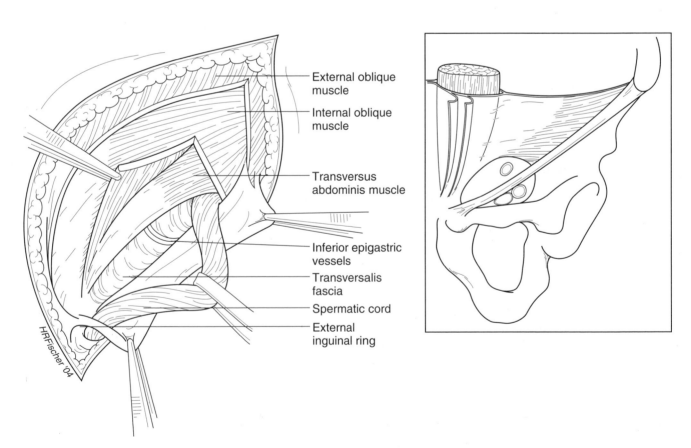

External oblique muscle

Internal oblique muscle

Transversus abdominis muscle

Inferior epigastric vessels

Transversalis fascia

Spermatic cord

External inguinal ring

Figure 37-3 Normal anatomy of the left inguinal canal.

laterally, and the pubis inferiorly. The myopectineal orifice is crossed by the inguinal ligament and traversed by the spermatic cord and femoral vessels. All groin hernias begin as weaknesses within the myopectineal orifice. The transversalis fascia deteriorates, resulting in peritoneal protrusion. Inguinal hernias are surgically treated by repairing all or part of the myopectineal orifice directly using autologous tissue or by implanting a prosthesis to augment or replace the defective transversalis fascia.

A method of classifying inguinal hernias is needed in order to standardize the operations performed and to quantify surgical outcomes. One frequently used classification system for inguinal hernias was devised by Nyhus (Table 37-2). Type I inguinal hernias occur most commonly in infants and children where the internal ring is normal in size and structure and the Hesselbach triangle is normal as well. The mechanism of herniation is a patent processus vaginalis of variable length from the internal ring. Type II inguinal hernias are indirect defects where the internal ring is now enlarged with some impingement on the deep inferior epigastric vessels but without defects within the Hesselbach triangle. Examination of the inguinal canal's medial floor may be performed through the dilated internal ring, confirming its integrity. Type III inguinal hernias involve defects in the posterior wall (floor) of the inguinal canal and have been classified into three subtypes: direct, indirect, and femoral. Type IIIA defects are direct inguinal hernias without protrusion through the internal ring. Type IIIB defects are indirect and occur through a much-dilated internal ring with significant impingement and deterioration of the inguinal floor medial to the inferior epigastric vessels with or without a scrotal component to the hernia. The distortion of the internal ring may occur without displacement of the inferior epigastric vessels. The hernia may have both direct and indirect components, resulting in a pantaloon hernia surrounding the inferior epigastric vessels. Femoral

TABLE 37-2

CLASSIFICATION OF INGUINAL HERNIAS

Type I indirect inguinal hernia
    Internal ring is normal

Type II indirect inguinal hernia
    Internal ring is dilated, but the posterior inguinal wall is intact

Type III posterior inguinal wall defects
    Direct inguinal hernia
    Indirect inguinal hernia with dilated internal ring and
        attenuated medial transversalis fascia of the Hesselbach
            triangle
    Femoral hernias

Type IV recurrent inguinal hernias
    Direct
    Indirect
    Femoral
    Combined

hernias are classified as type IIIC. Type IV inguinal hernias are recurrent.

Prospective nonrandomized data and many large reviews suggest that recurrence rates should be lower for type I and type II inguinal hernia repairs. These include simple and complex internal ringplasties following high ligation of an indirect hernia sac. Surgical experience supports the concept that the most difficult inguinal hernias to repair are types III and IV. These include indirect and direct hernias with significant posterior inguinal canal wall deterioration, femoral hernias, and recurrent inguinal hernias.

Autologous Tissue Repairs

Shouldice Repair

The Shouldice Clinic near Toronto, Ontario, Canada has performed >250,000 inguinal hernia repairs since its inception in 1945. The Shouldice Clinic promotes a holistic concept of hernia surgery that includes preoperative preparation and education, an extensive inguinal floor dissection, and closely supervised early postoperative convalescence. Numerous reports have been published in the surgical literature, with some lack of consistency, demonstrating the provincial complexities of this procedure. The Shouldice Clinic reports medium- and long-term total hernia recurrence rates of approximately 1% (22). These outstanding results have never been duplicated outside of the Shouldice Clinic or in a well-controlled and powered, prospective, randomized trial of inguinal hernia repair.

Shouldice pioneered early postoperative ambulation without increased complications, a fundamental principle of modern surgery. Hospital stays following inguinal herniorrhaphy were reduced from 21 to 3 days. General or spinal anesthetics were converted to local infiltration of anesthetic to promote earlier ambulation and return to usual activity. Fine silk sutures were found to be associated with an increased risk of suture abscess and were exchanged for less reactive monofilaments like fine wire. Groin wound infection rates were also reduced by staging bilateral inguinal hernia repairs 2 days apart, which also facilitates the use of local anesthetics.

The successful approach of the Shouldice Clinic and the Shouldice technique may be extended to all types of management for inguinal hernias. In addition to an open technique using local anesthetics and encouraging early ambulation, the Shouldice Clinic applies other general principles to their management of inguinal hernias. Weight reduction is a frequently overlooked preoperative preparation that may make hernia repair technically more successful. Most series of herniorrhaphy outcomes suggest that increased weight increases the risk of hernia recurrence. Weight loss improves the effectiveness of the local anesthetic technique and improves anatomic dissections for bilateral and recurrent hernias. They also believe that the postoperative load placed across the repair is more

TABLE 37-3

SHOULDICE CLINIC PRINCIPLES OF INGUINAL HERNIORRHAPHY

Weight reduction
Open technique with complete anatomic dissection
Use of local anesthetics
Autologous tissue repairs
Early return to usual activity

conducive for hernia repair scar formation. A 3-day supervised convalescence is followed by a return to normal activity as comfort permits. The maximum convalescence period is 4 weeks for patients involved in strenuous activity (Table 37-3).

Local anesthetic infiltration is used in association with conscious sedation (diazepam and meperidine). Awake procedures using local anesthesia reduce cardiac and pulmonary complications, especially in elderly patient populations. The incidence of deep venous thrombosis, pulmonary embolism, and pulmonary atelectasis is well below 1%. The Shouldice series mortality is <0.01%.

A complete dissection of all groin anatomy, normal and abnormal, is performed. Prior to opening the external oblique fascia, the inferior edge of the inguinal ligament is examined in the thigh to rule out a femoral hernia component. The external oblique aponeurosis is incised and opened from the external ring to 3 cm lateral to the internal ring. The lateral dissection rules out an unsuspected Spigelian or interstitial hernia. The ilioinguinal and iliohypogastric nerves are identified, isolated, and preserved without injury if possible. The cremasteric muscle fibers are then incised longitudinally, and the spermatic cord with any associated indirect hernia is freed from its sheath. Cremasteric fibers are then excised to facilitate accurate transversalis fascia to fascia repair. Part of the proximal stump of the cremasteric fibers is used during reconstruction of the internal ring. The inferomedial stump of the excised cremasteric fiber is included in the repair of the inguinal floor in order to suspend the testicle. Some concern has been raised about testicular dependency following the extensive cremasteric dissection and excision.

The internal ring is thoroughly dissected. The peritoneum is identified and completely dissected back along the spermatic cord. Most males have protrusion of preperitoneal fat at the superolateral quadrant of the internal ring, which is usually not the source of hernia symptoms unless it extends significantly (2 cm) down the spermatic cord. The incidence of sliding hernias in the Shouldice series is about 1%. Great care should be used to recognize a sliding viscus component at the internal ring, to work distally to proximally to separate it from the spermatic cord, and to protect the sliding organ's blood supply. If the indirect hernia sac is transected at the internal ring, some authors recommend leaving the distal end of the sac *in situ* to avoid spermatic cord injury and to reduce the risk of an ischemic testicle or testicular atrophy. Others advocate dissection of the remnant sac from the spermatic cord to eliminate the possibility of hydrocele. Most series report an incidence of testicular atrophy of <0.1%. The Shouldice experience also suggests that ligation of indirect hernia sacs is not mandatory. In their view complete reduction of the hernia sac with meticulous reconstruction of the internal ring minimizes recurrence rates.

The Shouldice technique requires incision and opening of the posterior wall of the inguinal canal (the canal floor), which is comprised mainly of transversalis fascia. Any direct hernias thus encountered are carefully reduced. If opening of a direct hernia sac is required, it is performed from the lateral edge to avoid injury to potential medial wall bladder components. Finally, the inferior preperitoneal space is explored beneath the inferolateral transversalis flap to rule out a femoral hernia component.

The Shouldice repair incorporates an indirect and direct reconstruction in all instances, overlapping inguinal floor muscle and fascia in what is described as their natural sequence. Continuous monofilament permanent sutures are used on the posterior wall. A continuous suturing technique is advocated to evenly distribute tension and to leave no gaps. The Shouldice Clinic preference is 34-gauge or 32-gauge stainless steel wire because it is inert in tissues, provides maximum breaking strength for its caliber (tensile strength), and well-placed knots maintain integrity. Two disadvantages of steel wire include a tendency to kink and break if mishandled and the risk of laceration to surgeons and assistants. One continuous suture with two opposing lines of repair is then used to repair the inguinal floor. The first layers approximate transversalis fascia and peritoneum running from medially to laterally, and the second layer approximates muscle and aponeurotic fibers from the internal oblique and transversalis muscles down to the inguinal ligament. Relaxing incisions on the ipsilateral rectus sheath are seldom required but are recommended if necessary prior to the initiation of the first half of the suture line. Two more lines of running suture are then placed to reinforce the repair. This time, starting just medial to the internal ring, the external oblique aponeurosis is plicated toward the pubic crest and then reversed back to the internal ring. The external oblique aponeurosis is then closed in a continuous manner, recreating the external ring.

Femoral hernias are a common site and cause of recurrence following hernia repair, which is the reason for advocating that the femoral sheath be routinely examined and even explored during suprainguinal herniorrhaphy. In the Shouldice series 1 in 400 inguinal hernia repairs recurred as a femoral hernia. Most operative modifications applied to reduce the incidence of recurrent femoral hernias involve opening of the posterior wall of the inguinal canal (transversalis fascia) and closing the space medial to the femoral outlet (the femoral ring) using Cooper ligament. Conversely, when only a femoral hernia was suspected on clinical grounds, simultaneous significant suprainguinal pathology was detected at operation in 87% of males and 63% of females in the Shouldice series (22). This observation reinforces the need for careful and complete suprainguinal and infrainguinal examination during all inguinal hernia repairs in order to minimize recurrence rates.

The incidence of recurrent hernia increases with each subsequent repair (6,23,24), most likely due to tissue loss and scarring. Highest recurrence rates (12%) are reported following repairs of multiply recurrent inguinal hernias. Because recurrent wound failure appears to select abnormal scar and fascia expressing a tissue repair defect, the implantation of prosthetic material has been advocated. The interval between the first and second operations should be at least 6 months to allow optimum recovery of the tissue to be used again for repair. When the inguinal ligament was intact, an autologous tissue repair was possible in 91% of the cases of recurrent hernia repair in the Shouldice experience. For the remaining 9% of patients, the groin defect was described as too extensive or the groin tissue as too friable and inelastic to allow autologous tissue repair. In these cases an alloplastic prosthetic implant in the preperitoneal space was used. When the bowel was covered with peritoneum, polypropylene mesh was used. When the bowel was exposed, a microporous PTFE patch was used. With a minimum follow-up of 18 months, the reported recurrence rate was 2.2% (22).

Cooper Ligament Repair

The first reported use of the Cooper ligament (the superior pubic ligament) in hernia repair was to treat femoral hernias by suturing the inguinal ligament down to it, obliterating the femoral sheath space (21). Later, McVay popularized the technique by recommending a rectus sheath-relaxing incision and transfer of the transversalis abdominus aponeurosis and muscle and transversalis fascia down to the Cooper ligament in order to repair the inguinal canal's posterior wall. This maneuver requires opening the floor of the inguinal canal and exploring the preperitoneal space. This added dissection is also believed to reduce the incidence of missed hernias, especially femoral hernias.

In most descriptions the ilioinguinal nerve is preserved. If the nerve is traumatized during groin dissection, many experts recommend ligation and division of the nerve to reduce the incidence of postoperative chronic pain syndromes. The spermatic cord is fully mobilized in the inguinal canal. No dissection is performed medial to the pubic tubercle in order to avoid injury to the external pudendal blood supply and to preserve collateral circulation to the testicles. Starting laterally, the anterior surfaces of the femoral artery and vein are cleared and the anterior femoral fascia is identified. Working medial to the femoral

vein, fat and lymphatics are dissected free from the femoral canal and any femoral sac is reduced. The tendinous portion of the transversus abdominis aponeurotic arch is then identified, and a relaxing incision is placed at the point of fusion of the external oblique muscles and the rectus sheath. This starts at the pubic tubercle and then extends superiorly by 6 to 8 cm. The remainder of the repair can be performed with the patient in the Trendelenburg position to minimize intestinal injuries. In independent, noncontrolled, or randomized series, recurrence rates of 2% have been reported by high-volume surgeons who limit their practice to herniorrhaphy (21).

The disadvantages of the Copper ligament (McVay) repair include the more extensive dissection and reported prolonged recovery period. Some authors have argued that the tension placed on the posterior wall repair is suboptimal as well and that vascular injuries are more common with the McVay repair. Proponents of this procedure recommend relaxing incisions and careful dissections around the femoral vessels to achieve a reliable procedure with low recurrence rates and minimal morbidity.

Alloplastic Tissue Implants

Billroth wrote in 1878, "If we could artificially produce tissues of the density and toughness of fascia and tendon, the secret of the radical cure of hernia would be discovered" (25). In addition to replacing defective soft tissue, alloplastic implants are believed to reduce the chance for "missed" hernia. Recurrent hernias often result from simultaneous inguinal defects that were missed at the time of the initial herniorrhaphy. Covering the entire myopectineal orifice with a prosthesis should reduce the incidence of missed simultaneous hernia. Finally, replacing or augmenting abnormal inguinal soft tissue may prevent the development of future hernias.

Today, various prosthetic meshes are available for hernia repair. Knitted polypropylene mesh is used most commonly. This material induces a rapid and reliable fibroblastic response and is efficiently incorporated into the abdominal wall. Alloplastic meshes, however, tend to stiffen over time and induce disorganized scar tissue. Polyethylene meshes (Mersilene) are more pliable than most polypropylene meshes and are more popular in Europe. PTFE meshes are extruded with a microporous surface to allow abdominal wall fibroblast and macrophage ingrowth for abdominal wall incorporation and immune surveillance, while at the same time minimizing adherence to the bowel and other intra-abdominal viscera.

The term "tension-free" hernioplasty was first published by Lichtenstein et al. in 1986 (26,27). That report described an onlay technique using sutured alloplastic mesh. What was most significant about this approach was that the mesh was not used as reinforcement to an antecedent autologous tissue reconstruction but defined the repair itself. No attempt is made to use abnormal autologous groin tissues in the reconstruction. The initial report from this non-controlled or randomized, single experience cited 1,000 consecutive repairs with no recurrences over 5 years.

Mesh Plugs

Another surgical concept developed to replace or augment biologically defective groin tissue and achieve tension appropriate repairs was mesh-plugging herniorrhaphy (Fig. 37-4). This was first described by Lichtenstein and Shore in 1974 for the treatment of recurrent or femoral hernias (28). In this operation the hernia sac is dissected and reduced to the level of the myofascial hernia ring. The sac neck is then dissected from the hernia ring, and the hernia is invaginated without ligation or excision. A sheet of alloplastic mesh (usually knitted polypropylene) approximately 2 cm × 20 cm is rolled into a cylindrical shape that best fits the defect. The plug is inserted into the preperitoneal space until the outer edge is flush with the hernia defect margin and secured into place with circumferential interrupted sutures. Single institution series with minimum follow-up of 1 year report recurrence rates of <5%. Proponents of the technique argue that it is simple to learn and safe. The minimum dissection required lowers the incidence of inguinal nerve and adjacent organ injury. In addition, the absence of extensive groin dissection and opening of the inguinal floor prevents iatrogenic injury to the structures of the inguinal canal. A common modification of the mesh-plug technique includes the addition of a sheet mesh onlay onto the floor of the inguinal canal following implantation of the mesh plug. Proponents of this technique believe this repair can be done without suture anchors, again lowering the risk of inguinal nerve and adjacent organ injury, with equal medium-term results. The mesh plug and mesh plug combined with a mesh sheet onlay appear most amenable to Nyhus types I and II (indirect) inguinal hernia repairs and to easily definable recurrent inguinal hernias.

Preperitoneal Inguinal Hernia Repair

The posterior approach to the inguinal canal and iliopubic tract repair using a prosthetic buttress has reported success in both complicated primary and recurrent inguinal hernias (Nyhus types III and IV) (29,30). Procedures to repair the iliopubic tract using a posterior approach have several immediate advantages. Primary among these is operation for recurrent hernia, where dissection can be carried out through unscarred and undistorted preperitoneal tissue planes. All defects within the myopectineal orifice can be reduced and repaired via the same incision. These principles have now been adapted to minimally invasive technologies. The preperitoneal space can be entered and developed using two or three 5-mm or 10-mm incisions and an identical repair completed laparoscopically.

An open approach to the preperitoneal space is typically completed using a transverse lower abdominal wall incision placed approximately 4 cm superior to the pubic symphysis. The incision is slightly higher than that used for anterior inguinal herniorrhaphies. The external ring is identified so that an estimation of the location of the internal ring may be made. The posterior approach to the floor of the inguinal canal requires that the abdominal wall incision be fashioned above the internal ring. The transversalis fascia is incised transversely, and the preperitoneal space is carefully developed with blunt dissection. It is usually unnecessary to ligate and divide the deep inferior epigastric vessels in order to achieve adequate exposure. The inferior epigastric vessels can be inadvertently injured at the lateral margin of this incision. Care must be used to avoid unintended opening of the peritoneum and entry into the peritoneal cavity. Examination of the posterior wall of the inguinal canal allows for diagnosis and reduction of hernia defects. Most direct hernia sacs are easily reduced and inverted. A large direct hernia sac may be invaginated using a pursestring suture carefully placed in the transversalis fascia or aponeurosis. Injury to the adjacent bladder should be avoided, especially if a decision is made to excise a direct hernia sac. In performing an autologous tissue repair, the superior transversalis fascia and aponeurosis of the transversalis arch are typically sewn to the iliopubic tract to close the direct defect. Medially, the suture may also be passed through both the Cooper ligament and the medial iliopubic tract for reinforcement.

If there is an indirect hernia, the sac is reduced with careful traction and a high ligation is performed. If dissection of a large indirect hernia sac is difficult, abdominal organs are reduced and the sac may be transected at its neck and closed with a pursestring suture. The distal sac is left open to minimize the incidence of postoperative hydrocele. An internal ringplasty is then performed.

Femoral hernias may also be gently reduced via the preperitoneal approach. If there is an incarcerated femoral hernia, it might be released by incising the insertion of the iliopubic tract to the Cooper ligament at the medial border of the femoral ring. Once reduced, the femoral sheath defect is obliterated using sutures between the iliopubic tract and the Cooper ligament. On rare occasion, a counter incision in the upper thigh over an incarcerated femoral hernia may be necessary to affect a safe release from restricting fascia. This should, however, be an uncommon maneuver.

Hemostasis is especially important following the preperitoneal approach. A relatively larger potential space exists for hematoma accumulation following the preperitoneal dissection. However, the tamponading effect of the peritoneal sac and preperitoneum once it is returned to its normal anatomic location makes the incidence of significant postoperative bleeding very uncommon following the preperitoneal approach. Investigators have reported a lower incidence of testicular atrophy and chronic neuropathic pain following the posterior preperitoneal approach to

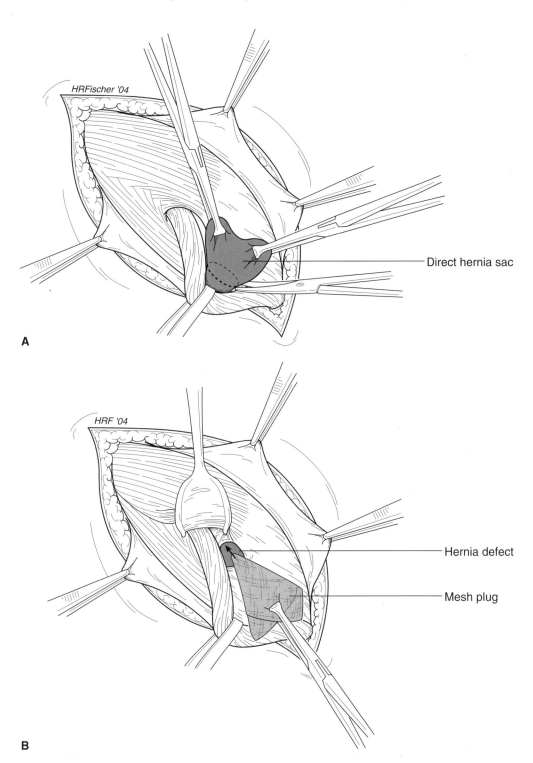

A

Direct hernia sac

B

Hernia defect

Mesh plug

Figure 37-4 Mesh-plug inguinal herniorrhaphy starts with a careful dissection of the limits of the hernia sac (**A**), reduction of the hernia sac to the preperitoneal space and the sizing of a cone-shaped mesh-plug (**B**), and anchoring of the seated mesh plug to the surrounding transversalis fascia with several interrupted sutures.

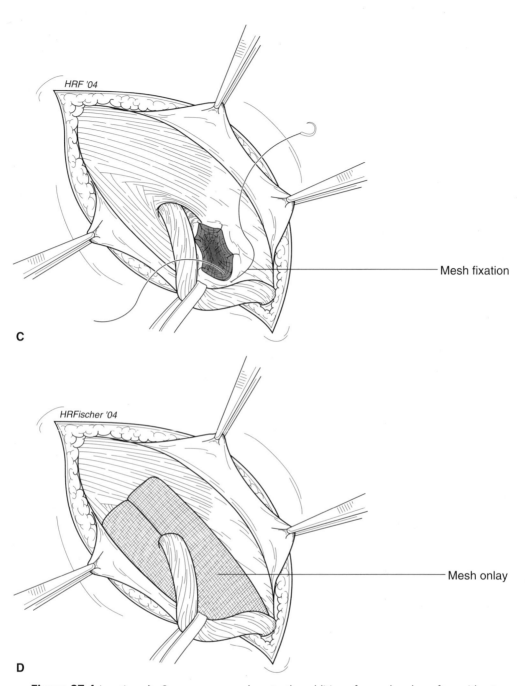

HRF '04

C

Mesh fixation

HRFischer '04

D

Mesh onlay

Figure 37-4 (*continued*) Some surgeons advocate the addition of a mesh onlay, often without sutures or tacks, to reinforce the plug and to protect against herniation through adjacent tissue within the floor of the inguinal canal (**C, D**).

inguinal hernias (29), believed to be the result of sparing injury to the inguinal nerve supply that courses lateral and anterior to this operative field. Reported hernia recurrence rates average 3% to 6%.

The preperitoneal posterior repair of recurrent inguinal hernias is usually "buttressed" with an approximately 5 cm × 12 cm rectangle of polypropylene mesh that is anchored to the Cooper ligament and the transversalis fascia superior to the previous repair. The preperitoneal position of the mesh implant imparts a mechanical advantage to the radial load forces of the abdominal wall.

Laparoscopic Inguinal Herniorrhaphy

Various laparoscopic techniques for repairing inguinal hernia are the newest developments in the long history of hernia surgery. Proponents of laparoscopic approaches to inguinal herniorrhaphy argue that they are the most anatomically appropriate. The advantages are a clear, up-close videoscopic examination of the posterior inguinal floor, simultaneous examination of the three major sites of inguinal herniation (internal ring, Hesselbach triangle, and femoral triangle), and the most mechanically advantageous repair. Following reduction of hernia contents, reinforcement of all myopectineal defects is completed in the preperitoneal position. Placement of a mesh prosthesis posterior to the inguinal floor is such that distractive forces originating in the peritoneum tend to secure the prosthesis in place.

The most commonly reported technique for laparoscopic inguinal hernia repair is the totally extraperitoneal preperitoneal approach (TEPPA) (Fig. 37-5). Like most laparoscopy, TEPPA herniorrhaphy requires a general anesthetic. The operation begins with dissection and development of a preperitoneal space. This dissection is typically achieved through an infraumbilical incision with subsequent incision of the anterior rectus sheath and lateral retraction of the rectus muscle. A balloon dissector may be directed toward the pubic symphysis and inflated slowly to create this operating space. Some surgeons omit using a balloon dissector and create the preperitoneal space using finger or hemostat dissection.

Great care must be exercised to avoid inadvertent entry into the peritoneal space, which obviates the advantages of the TEPPA approach. The most obvious advantage of the TEPPA approach is the ability to stay out of the peritoneal cavity and reduce the chance of injury to abdominal organs. The preperitoneal space is fairly avascular, with occasional small vessels traversing between the transversalis fascia and the reflected peritoneum. If a balloon dissector is used, it may remain inflated for several minutes to tamponade these crossing vessels. Significant hematomas can form in the preperitoneal space, especially in older patients with more areolar tissue planes.

An adequate dissection should extend just beyond the midline, below the Cooper ligament (6 to 8 cm below the inguinal ligament), well above the transversus abdominis aponeurotic arch and widely beyond the internal ring. Experts report that an inadequate dissection of the peritoneum away from the posterior inguinal wall is the most common reason for recurrent hernias following TEPPA repairs.

An appropriately sized piece of alloplastic mesh (approximately 12 cm × 6 cm) is delivered via the endoscopic portsite into the preperitoneal space to reinforce the posterior wall of the inguinal canal. Debate exists on whether it is necessary to secure this mesh in place with either sutures or tacks. It is also unclear whether it is necessary to split the mesh and encircle the spermatic cord through a "keyhole." Proponents argue that a minimum of mesh anchors placed into the transversalis fascia and encircling of the spermatic cord through a slit mesh results in lower hernia recurrence rates. Opponents suggest that anchoring the mesh and the additional dissection of the spermatic cord increases the incidence of postoperative chronic pain. No definitive reports have resolved these technical issues.

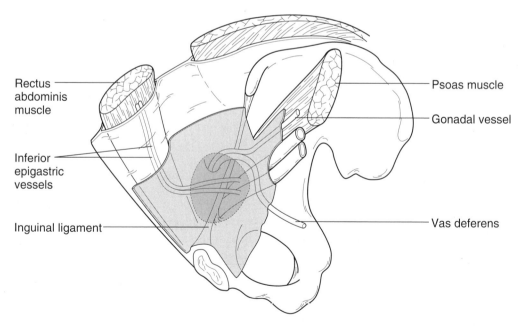

Figure 37-5 The totally extraperitoneal preperitoneal approach (TEPPA) during laparoscopic inguinal hernia repair requires the development of the preperitoneal space of the lower abdominal wall. This allows a posterior approach to the potential and real defects of the inguinal canal. Important nearby structures are illustrated, including the vas deferens, iliac vessels, inferior epigastric vessels, rectus muscle, and inguinal ligament. Mesh delivered into this preperitoneal space may be secured in place by the radial pressure of the peritoneal sac following desufflation. This finding has led to the successful development of TEPPA inguinal hernia repairs without the need for suture or tack fixation. It is believed that this modification lowers the incidence of chronic pain syndromes due to nerve injuries.

The TEPPA repair can result in recurrence rates equivalent to open herniorrhaphy, without significant wounding of the anterior abdominal wall and, therefore, with a lower wound complication rate. There is a slightly earlier return to usual activities following TEPPA inguinal herniorrhaphy. The incidence of neuropathic pain following laparoscopic inguinal hernia repairs is minimized if anchoring tacks or sutures, or both, are placed above the inguinal ligament and away from the course of the ilioinguinal, iliofemoral, and hypogastric nerves (31).

The transabdominal preperitoneal (TAPP) approach for laparoscopic inguinal hernia repair was described before the TEPPA technique was developed. The TAPP approach is intrabdominal and has a higher risk of abdominal organ injury. The hernia dissection is somewhat easier because the space is greater. The preperitoneal space is ultimately exposed with this approach as well. It is important to incise completely through the peritoneum and preperitoneum posterior to the inguinal floor until the areolar space of Bogros is entered between the transversalis fascia and the peritoneum. If not, dissection in the amorphous preperitoneal fat and fascia may lead to bleeding and confusion about inguinal anatomy.

Complications unique to the laparoscopic approach to inguinal herniorrhaphy include trocar injuries and problems with insufflation. The operating space for the TEPPA procedure is a much smaller volume than for intraperitoneal laparoscopic operations. Operating ports should always be placed under direct vision so that injury to adjacent structures and organs may be avoided. Blunt, radially dilating ports have lower incidences of adjacent organ injury and lower abdominal wall complications than bladed laparoscopic ports. Occasionally, insufflation of the preperitoneal space will result in unexpected pneumoperitoneum. This occurrence suggests the presence of a defect in the peritoneum. If a defect in the peritoneum is identified, the hole should be closed with sutures or clips, taking care to protect against injury to intra-abdominal organs. Preperitoneal insufflation may induce the same hemodynamic changes observed during intra-abdominal laparoscopic procedures, usually the result of reduced venous return. One distressing effect of preperitoneal insufflation is the appearance of scrotal dissection and pneumoscrotum. This development is almost uniformly self-limiting, and patients should be reassured.

Autologous Tissue Transfers

Recurrent hernias often occur because of the failure of collagenous tissues to obliterate the course of a hernia. When sufficient collagenous material is not present, it may be necessary to transfer such tissue into the operative field. Frequently used techniques include harvest and implantation of free tensor fascia lata and the tensor fascia lata myocutaneous flap. Tensor fascia lata free grafts are ideal for small area defects under medium to low abdominal

wall loads. The risk of using tensor fascia lata is mechanical failure parallel to the line of collagen bundles and the requirement for lateral thigh wounds to harvest the grafts. Alloplastic implants like polypropylene or polyethylene have higher tensile strengths but have a higher incidence of bowel fistulization and foreign body infections.

Strangulated Hernias

If the preoperative evaluation raises any concern for a strangulated viscus, a transperitoneal approach to the involved bowel should be strongly considered. Transperitoneal exposure of the unaffected intestine at the hernia ring improves the control of the gangrenous bowel segment. The iliopubic tract repair may follow intestinal resection and anastamosis.

Incisional Hernias

Incisional hernia is the most common indication for reoperation in abdominal surgery patients (32). Many recurrent inguinal hernias are also incisional hernias. Incisional hernias are unique because they are the only abdominal wall hernias considered iatrogenic. Because the reported incidence of acute fascial dehiscence is 0.5% and the incidence of primary incisional hernia formation is 11%, it is clear that many incisional hernias go unrecognized in the early postoperative period (6,13).

Fascial wound healing achieves only 60% to 80% of unwounded fascial strength after 6 weeks (19). Collagen deposition and fiber orientation along lines of stress occur during this interval. Nine to 12 months pass before fascial scar approaches uninjured breaking strength. For this reason most patients should be cautioned to avoid overloading their abdominal wall for at least 6 weeks following celiotomy. A common practice is to resume near-normal activity and abdominal wall loads 2 weeks following fascial closure, with great care to load the abdominal wound only as comfort permits. Patients should be educated about the biology of wound repair and the need to restrict sudden loads of their ventral wounds.

Success of incisional hernia repair depends on basic surgical principles. These precepts include the incorporation of normal fascial tissue brought together under an appropriate abdominal wall load and the avoidance of the risk factors for recurrent herniation.

Autologous Tissue Repairs

Historically, incisional hernia repairs made use of local, autologous abdominal wall tissue to correct abdominal wall defects. Most often this amounted to no more than reclosure of a laparotomy incision. The reoperative nature of incisional herniorrhaphy increases the risk of unplanned visceral injuries due to the requirement for adhesiolysis and enterolysis. Blood loss may also be increased, depending on the extent of the adhesiolysis. Many prospective series have documented the extremely high incisional hernia recurrence rate following repair with local, autologous tissue (24% to 54%) (3,6,33).

Recent large reviews have also found an increased risk of wound infection following incisional hernia repair (16). The risk factors for incisional hernia formation and the risk factors for wound infections are often the same. These risks include malnutrition, advanced age, chronic pulmonary disease, and polypharmacy. Wounds following incisional hernia repair are at increased risk for infection due to technical factors like prolonged operations, hematoma formation, devascularized or ischemic tissue, bowel injury, and the presence of foreign material such as previously placed mesh (Table 37-4).

A prospective, randomized, and controlled study of incisional hernia repair concluded that mesh implantation is required to achieve the lowest recurrent hernia rate (6). In practice, alloplastic mesh implantation is not always a clinical option or the patient's preference, and even with mesh implantation the recurrent incisional hernia rate was 24% in one well-done study. For all these reasons autologous tissue closures are still often recommended and undertaken.

The size of the fascial defect and the quality of the fascia should guide the selection of the hernia repair. The skin and subcutaneous tissue are dissected away from the hernia sac, but great care should be used to preserve the blood supply to the overlying skin. Viable skin provides the most important coverage for the underlying hernia repair, by whatever method. Healthy fascia should be identified back from the fascial hernia ring on both ventral and peritoneal surfaces. A minimum of 3 cm of fascial exposure for suture placement appears to be the consensus.

If a fascial defect is so large as to preclude incisional hernia repair by simple reclosure, a number of other repairs using autologous tissue have been described. Simplest among these is the use of internal retention sutures. Other variations of local myofascial relaxing incisions are used. During the Keel procedure, vertical relaxing incisions are placed along the lateral edge of the anterior rectus sheath, allowing medial advancement of the medial edge of the

TABLE 37-4

RISK FACTORS FOR WOUND INFECTION FOLLOWING INCISIONAL HERNIA REPAIR

Operative time
Devascularized tissue
Hematoma formation
Foreign material (mesh)
Bowel or bladder injury
Malnutrition
Advanced age
Chronic disease
Polypharmacy

anterior rectus sheath. This approach is especially useful in upper midline abdominal wall hernias, where a stout posterior rectus sheath protects against further iatrogenic injury (34). For midline defects in the lower abdomen, the lower section of rectus muscle and enveloping fascia may be mobilized off the pubis and reapproximated to the contralateral bone.

More recently, abdominal wall component separation techniques have been described in an effort to reconstruct large abdominal wall defects. Fundamentally, these operations include the elevation of long, lateral skin flaps to identify the underlying myofascial anatomy and to release the fascia from its dermal attachments. Next, the full length of the external oblique muscle is incised, usually from the costal margin to the pubis. Great care is used to preserve the integrity of the underlying internal oblique and transversalis muscles. The external oblique incision is typically placed approximately 1 cm lateral to the lateral edge of the rectus sheath. This maneuver often provides 4 to 6 cm of medial advancement of the rectus sheath. Anterior rectus sheath or posterior rectus sheath relaxing incisions may be added to increase the advancement distance of the midline. All variations of abdominal wall component separations increase the risk for bleeding and hematoma/seroma formation. Prolonged subcutaneous drainage is also frequently indicated. The risk for overlying skin necrosis is increased because of the necessity for long skin flaps.

Alloplastic Tissue Implants

The implantation of alloplastic tissue prostheses was introduced to incisional herniorrhaphy in an attempt to reduce the unacceptably high incisional hernia recurrence rates when using local, autologous tissue for reclosure (Fig. 37-6). Prospective, randomized studies found that an independent risk factor for recurrent incisional hernia is the technique of primary tissue repair without the use of a mesh implant (6). Alloplastic implants are, however, associated with a characteristic set of complications. First among these complications is mesh-associated infection and foreign body inflammatory reaction. It is not clear from the largest series that mesh implantation in the groin is associated with a higher wound infection rate. The rate of wound infection after the repair of incisional hernias is, however, significant after inguinal hernia repair (35). Other series report a higher incidence of chronic pain following mesh implantation, although this may depend on the technique used (36–38).

The most commonly used mesh materials are knitted monofilament polypropylene (Marlex), woven polypropylene (Prolene), woven polyester (Mersilene), expanded or extruded polytetrafluoroethylene (ePTFE, Gore-Tex), knitted polyglycolic acid (Vicryl), and knitted polygalactic acid (Dexon). Polypropylene meshes are the most widely used in the United States, while polyester mesh remains popular in Europe (39,40). PTFE gained popularity because of its

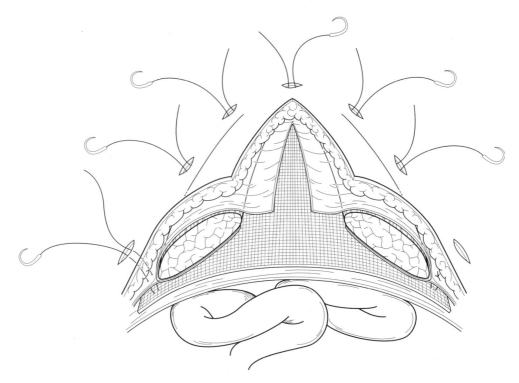

Figure 37-6 The best available evidence suggests that an alloplastic "under-lay" technique results in the lowest recurrence rates following incisional hernia repairs. Anatomically, retrofascial/retromuscular, preperitoneal, and intraperitoneal mesh fixation is described. Circumferential, transfascial, or transabdominal fixation sutures are frequently used following the repair of large incisional hernias or when using the laparoscopic technique.

reported reduced tissue reactivity and adhesion formation, although concerns have been raised about seroma formation and mesh infection rates. Most authors conclude that absorbable mesh should not be used for permanent abdominal wall reconstruction because of the universal development of recurrent incisional hernias and an increased risk for bowel fistulization (41).

Serious complications have been observed in a small percentage of patients after incisional hernia repairs with alloplastic mesh implantation. The most important serious problems are mesh-associated infection, chronic skin sinus tract formation, erosion into adjacent structures, including bowel, and chronically exposed or extruded mesh (42,43). Mesh placement in the presence of heavy contamination was reported to be associated with a >50% acute wound failure rate (dehiscence) and 22% enteric fistulization rate.

Recurrent Hernia

A prospective, randomized study of incisional hernia repair found that risk factors for recurrent hernias included primary reclosure without the use of mesh, postoperative prostatism, and a history of abdominal aortic aneurysm (6). These findings point to potential mechanisms for recurrent incisional herniation. The first two conditions highlight the importance of increased mechanical loads on

the abdominal wall hernia recurrence. The history of aortic aneurysm disease suggests biological risk factors for hernia recurrence, such as the elevated expression of tissue metalloproteinase. In a single, small, uncontrolled series the use of internal retention sutures has been reported to reduce incisional hernia recurrence rates to 3% (44).

Typically, recurrent incisional hernias are small in area or volume as the result of a limited disruption, usually between the alloplastic mesh and the fascia. Often, a simple repair can be undertaken, directed to the area of this defect (Fig. 37-7). When mesh failure occurs, it is almost always at the mesh:fascia interface rather than mesh material failure.

Infection increases the risk of hernia recurrence. Deep wound infections prolong inflammation and impede collagen deposition. Elective repair should therefore not be attempted if any signs of infection exist, such as a stitch abscess or sinus or overlying skin excoriation. Foreign materials associated with infections should be removed and the overlying skin healed prior to hernia repairs.

The application of high tension loads during hernia repair is a risk factor for recurrence. Tension is an especially difficult problem during the repair of multiply recurrent hernias where extensive scar tissue usually is present, limiting compliance of the abdominal wall. Wound tension is exacerbated in giant ventral hernias when the fascial ring encroaches on other immobile structures like the iliac crest

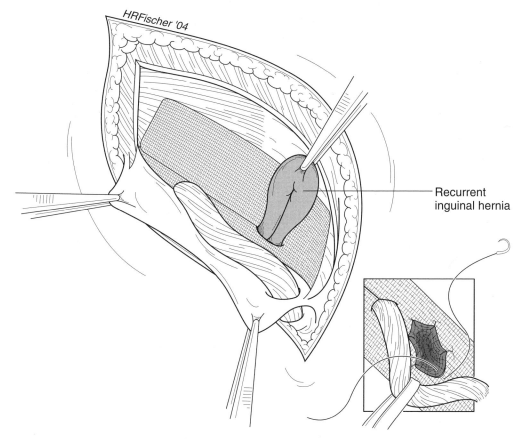

Figure 37-7 When detected early, recurrent incisional hernias are usually of a small area or volume as the result of a limited disruption. The mechanism of recurrent incisional hernia formation includes a failure of tissue repair at the interface between the alloplastic mesh implant and the native fascia. Often, a limited salvage repair can be undertaken, directed to the area of this defect.

or latissimus and/or paraspinous muscles. During repair of recurrent incisional hernias, great care must be taken to maintain the integrity of chronic wound tissue and to optimize tissue perfusion.

The use of autologous local tissues is often preferred during ventral hernia repair. A common situation occurs when infected alloplastic mesh is removed. The autologous tissues may be mobilized by several approaches to the components of the abdominal wall. One commonly employed technique is to carefully incise the external oblique muscle and fascia 1 to 2 cm lateral to the rectus sheath. Anterior or posterior rectus sheath relaxing incisions may also be used to further mobilize abdominal wall components for autologous closure. One or both sides of the abdominal wall may not be amenable to component separation because of previous existing defects such as stoma sites. Extensive reconstructions of the abdominal wall should be planned in collaboration with a plastic surgeon.

Giant Ventral Hernias

Patients with massive incisional hernias usually present with functional loss of the abdominal wall and substantial protrusion of abdominal viscera. Such hernias are frequently associated with chronic abdominal pain, chronic back pain, and erosion of overlying skin. Severe skin lymphedema may ensue. Peritoneal volume (abdominal domain) is gradually lost as abdominal viscera remain herniated. Massive ventral hernias with significant loss of abdominal domain also can cause diaphragmatic dysfunction and intestinal circulatory congestion (45).

The technique of serial preoperative therapeutic pneumoperitoneum to reestablish abdominal domain offers one approach to the problem of peritoneal volume loss (45). This method has lost popularity with the increased use of "tension-free" mesh repair. Because the incidence of primary and recurrent incisional hernias remains so high and the complications associated with alloplastic mesh implantation have not been solved, there is renewed interest in serial abdominal pneumoperitoneum and other techniques for the development of autologous tissue sources to repair these difficult wounds (46,47).

Compulsive preparation for operation is mandatory in patients with giant incisional hernias. All skin erosions should be treated prior to elective repair in order to reduce the risk of subsequent infection. Pulmonary function should be optimized, including smoking cessation. Smoking is also a recognized impediment to wound healing. Weight loss is encouraged and medically supported. A multidisciplinary plan involving both general and plastic surgeons is often applied.

Visceral Injuries

The bowel may be injured during the opening or high ligation of an indirect hernia sac. The complication is minimized by careful dissection and the identification of groin structures and by inspection for sliding components. The bladder may be injured during opening of a lower midline incisional hernia or the medial extent of a direct inguinal hernia. If the bladder is injured, it should be repaired and continuously drained with an indwelling catheter until a cystogram provides proof of healing.

Entercutaneous fistulas are usually associated with complex abdominal wall defects and large hernias. The presence of knitted or woven polypropylene or polyethylene meshes appears to increase the risk for delayed enteric fistulization. The presence of mesh during reoperative incisonal hernia repair increases the risk of unintended bowel injury due to the presence of dense adhesions (42). Management should be directed toward control of the fistula and metabolic support of the patient. Once the fistula has been controlled, 6 to 8 weeks should be allowed to pass to permit spontaneous closure. If closure does not occur, this period of time will allow surrounding tissue inflammation and infection to improve in anticipation of definitive repair. When operative closure of an enteric fistula is planned in association with a recurrent hernia repair, preoperative diagnostic staging should be done to precisely identify the fistula's anatomy. Every effort should be made to repair the abdominal wall defect with autologous tissue, such as a local advancement flap or free tensor fascia lata.

Vascular Injuries

Inadvertent injury to an aberrant inferior epigastric or obturator artery may occur during lower abdominal wall hernia repairs. Inferior epigastric injuries may result in significant hemorrhage. Another source of inferior epigastric artery injury is the placement of lower abdominal wall ports for laparoscopic hernia operations. Open inguinal floor repairs, such as the Cooper ligament repair and laparoscopic inguinal hernia repairs, place the femoral vessels at risk for injury. A stitch in the femoral vein should be removed and hemostasis achieved prior to proceeding.

Nerve Injuries

Three nerves are exposed to injury during inguinal hernia repairs—the ilioinguinal, genitofemoral, and iliohypogastric nerves (Fig. 37-8). The ilioinguinal and genitofemoral nerves are adjacent to the spermatic cord and the iliohypogastric runs within the internal oblique muscle of the lower abdominal wall. Nerve transection usually results in self-limiting groin or inner thigh anesthesia. Nerve injury is presumably the mechanism for cases of disabling postoperative pain. Recent prospective studies report a 29% incidence of chronic pain following inguinal herniorrhaphy (36,38). For these reasons great care should be exercised during dissections and repairs to not include the nerves in suture lines or at mesh or tack sites. If pain develops after an initial recovery period, a deep space abscess or dehiscence should be considered. Without either of these two complications, most pain resolves with supportive measures only.

Postherniorrhaphy neuralgia can become a disabling condition. It is important to determine whether the patient had pain prior to hernia repair, whether postoperative pain is the same in character as the preoperative pain, and when inguinodynia began. Most postherniorrhaphy neuralgia is the result of perineural fibrosis, a normal biological process following operation. Available studies suggest that mesh-associated inguinodynia is not an independent entity and that evidence does not support clinical references to mesh-induced chronic pain syndrome.

The most common mechanism of inguinal nerve injury is failure to identify and protect the three major groin nerves exposed during herniorrhaphy. Limited dissection without the identification of all major structures of the inguinal canal increases the risk of nerve injury and therefore of chronic inguinodynia. The external ring should not be closed too tightly to prevent exposure of the ilioinguinal nerve to the suture line of the external oblique fascial closure. The ilioinguinal nerve should not be extensively mobilized from the cremasteric layer in order to minimize injury to its neurolemmal sheath. During the dissection of the subcutaneous adipose tissue, early surface branches of the ilioinguinal and/or iliohypogastric nerves should be spared. Deep stapling or tacking should be avoided during laparoscopic inguinal hernia repair in order to prevent entrapment of the iliohypogastric, genital (medial to the internal ring), and ilioinguinal (lateral to the internal ring) nerves.

When conservative measures fail for at least 6 months, surgical therapy of neuralgia may be considered. Surgery is usually required for perineural fibrosis, nerve entrapment by suture, staple, or prosthetic device, and neuroma formation. The triggering or aggravation of neuropathic pain by walking or during hyperextension of the hip and alleviation by rest and flexion of the thigh suggest that traction of the involved nerve due to its adherence to the aponeurotic tissue of the groin is an important mechanism. Surgical therapy of postherniorrhaphy inguinodynia is most likely to be successful if the three involved nerves are resected. Neurolysis is not recommended. The approach to the lower abdominal wall is preperitoneal via a lower midline or high inguinal incision. The entire lengths of the nerves should be resected as proximally as possible to include the

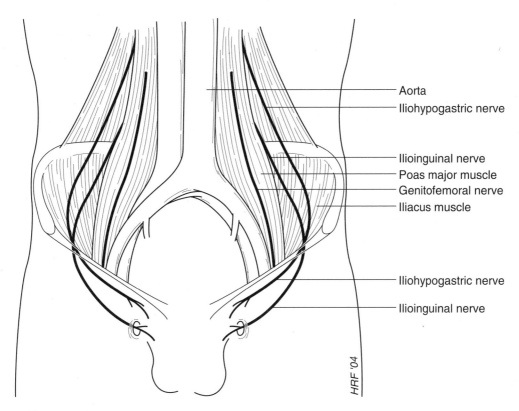

Figure 37-8 The ilioinguinal, genitofemoral, and iliohypogastric nerves are exposed to injury during inguinal hernia repairs. The ilioinguinal and genitofemoral nerves are encountered posteriorly during a preperitoneal inguinal hernia repair or within the spermatic cord. The iliohypogastric nerve courses within the internal oblique muscle of the lower abdominal wall and is especially at risk for injury when tacks are placed below the inguinal ligament during a laparoscopic inguinal hernia repair.

involved segment and the numerous neural communications that exist between the three nerves. The transected proximal nerve ends are ligated and embedded into the internal oblique muscle layer to reduce the incidence of neuroma formation. Any suture, staple, or alloplastic mesh material encountered along the length of the nerves is also excised. The complete removal of mesh does not appear to be necessary.

Testicular Infarct

Severe testicular pain, swelling, and tenderness may occur after inguinal hernia repair, especially if the spermatic cord is skeletonized of muscle and fat or divided. Orchiectomy is sometimes required to resolve this complication. If obliteration of the internal ring is anticipated, such as during the repair of a multiply recurrent inguinal hernia, consent for orchiectomy may be obtained. During the dissection of fat and muscle from the spermatic cord, great care should be used in preserving the testicular artery and vein.

Scrotal Hematoma

Hematoma in the scrotum arises from small vessels within the cremasteric muscles. In the loose, areolar tissue of the scrotum, tamponade is minimal. This complication may

be avoided by minimizing dissection of indirect sacs off of the spermatic cord. Only the high point of the indirect sac is mobilized for ligation of the internal ring. When a long indirect sac must be mobilized, as in a sliding hernia, the risk for a scrotal hematoma may be reduced by the use of a scrotal support after operation. Prophylactic drainage does not prevent scrotal hematoma formation.

When a scrotal hematoma occurs, it is usually dispersed between several layers of the repair and the spermatic cord. Needle aspiration is therefore usually not helpful. Effective evacuation would require reopening of the wound and is necessary only for very large and tense hematomas that occur immediately following surgery. Stable or delayed hematomas may be managed with rest, warm and cold compresses, and close observation for continued bleeding or infection, or both.

Chronic Abdominal Wall Wounds

Abdominal wall wounds may lead to chronic clinical complaints, including incisional pain, protrusion, numbness, or unappealing appearance. An underlying visceral abnormality must first be excluded. Questions may be raised about secondary gain, especially in cases of disability claims (48,49). It is often helpful to educate patients about the expected course of surgical recovery, especially as it relates to the phases of wound healing. For example, patients are often concerned about the color or mass of scars. This anxiety may be reduced by explaining that the inflammatory and proliferative phases of tissue repair may last weeks to months. Laparotomy patients may develop a prominent "healing ridge" as fascial scar proliferation maximizes 2 to 6 weeks postoperatively. Some patients complain of numbness below transverse or oblique incisions. This occurs as the result of transected distal spinal nerves and usually becomes unnoticeable after several months.

Chronic pain in a scar may be difficult to explain and treat. Prior to any intervention, an incisional hernia should be excluded by careful examination and noninvasive imaging. An intraperitoneal disorder is unlikely if the symptom is reproduced or aggravated by straining the muscles of the abdominal wall. Rarely, incisional pain is caused by ossification of the scar and relieved by excision of bony tissue. Chronic pain at the epigastrium may be due to injury to the xiphoid process during wound closure. Excision of the xiphoid process often relieves this source of discomfort. Underlying fascial sutures that came close to the skin surface may cause chronic pain, especially in thin patients. Ultimately, suture removal may be required.

Eccentric bulging of the abdominal wall may occur when nerve or arterial supply is severed during surgical incision. Examples include division of the 12th intercostal nerve during flank incision with rib resection.

Wound Hematoma

During ventral hernia repair the fascia is widely exposed and relaxing incisions are made to minimize the hernia ring area and to maximize the use of autologous local tissue transfers. The broad subcutaneous skin dissection predisposes to wound hematoma formation. This potential mandates meticulous hemostasis during operation and closed-suction drainage until discharge stops. Surgical techniques to reduce tissue dead space and the application of pressure dressings may also help reduce hematoma formation.

Pulmonary Complications

Reduction and repair of large hernias may impair pulmonary function by inhibiting coughing due to the incisional pain and by mechanically restricting diaphragmatic excursion. The repair of a giant hernia with the loss of abdominal domain may require prolonged ventilator dependence until incisional pain improves and the peritoneal cavity accommodates its restored contents. The implantation of an allograft mesh is often required to minimize abdominal cavity pressures.

REFERENCES

1. National Center for Health Statistics. *Detailed diagnoses and procedures*. National Hospital Discharge Survey Series 13, No. 122. Atlanta, GA: National Center for Health Statistics Database; 1995.
2. DuBay DA, Franz MG. Acute wound healing: the biology of acute wound failure. *Surg Clin North Am* 2003;83:463–481.
3. Carlson MA. Acute wound failure. Wound healing. *Surg Clin North Am* 2001;77(3):607–635.
4. Jenkins TPN. The burst abdominal wound: a mechanical approach. *Br J Surg* 1976;63:873.
5. Etchells E, O'Neill C, Bernstein M. Patient safety in surgery: error detection and prevention. *World J Surg* 2003;27(8):936–941.
6. Luijendijk RW, Hop WCJ, van den Tol MP, et al. A comparison of suture repair with mesh repair for incisional hernia. *N Engl J Med* 2000;343(6):392–398.
7. Best WR, Khuri SF, Phelan M, et al. Identifying patient preoperative risk factors and postoperative adverse events in administrative databases: results from the Department of Veterans Affairs National Surgical Quality Improvement Program. *J Am Coll Surg* 2002;194(3):257–266.
8. Webster C, Neumayer L, Smout R, et al. Prognostic models of abdominal wound dehiscence after laparotomy. *J Surg Res* 2003;109:130–137.
9. Smith PD, Kuhn MA, Franz MG, et al. Initiating the inflammatory phase of incisional healing prior to tissue injury. *J Surg Res* 2000;92:11–17.
10. Banda MJ, Dwyer KS, Beckmann A. Wound fluid angiogenesis factor stimulates the directed migration of capillary endothelial cells. *J Cell Biochem* 1985;29:183–193.
11. Ayde B, Luna G. Incidence of abdominal wall hernia in aortic surgery. *Am J Surg* 1998;175:400–402.
12. Hall KA, Peters B, Smyth SH, et al. Abdominal wall hernias in patients with abdominal aortic aneurysm versus aortoiliac occlusive disease. *Am J Surg* 1995;170:572.
13. Santora TA, Rosylyn JJ. Incisional hernia. Hernia surgery. *Surg Clin North Am* 1993;73(3):557–570.
14. Peacock EE Jr. Fascia and muscle. In: Peacock EE Jr, ed. *Wound repair*. Philadelphia, PA: WB Saunders; 1984:332–362.
15. Pollock AV, Evans M. Early prediction of late incisional hernias. *Br J Surg* 1989;76:953–954.
16. Dunne JR, Malone DL, Tracy K, et al. Abdominal wall hernias: risk factors for infection and resource utilization. *J Surg Res* 2003;111:78–84.
17. Tilson MD, Seashore MR. Human genetics of the abdominal aortic aneurysm. *Surg Gynecol Obstet* 1984;158:129–132.
18. Lehnert B, Wadouh F. High coincidence of inguinal hernias and abdominal aortic aneurysms. *Ann Vasc Surg* 1992;6:134–137.
19. Leaper DJ, Gottrup F. Surgical wounds. In: Leaper DJ, Harding KG, eds. *Wounds: biology and management*. Oxford: Oxford University Press; 1998:23–40.
20. Manninen MJ, Lavonius M, Perhoniemi VJ. Results of incisional hernia repair: a retrospective study of 172 unselected hernioplasties. *Eur J Surg* 1990;157:29–31.
21. Rutledge RH. The Cooper ligament repair. *Surg Clin North Am* 1993;73(3):471–485.
22. Welsh DRJ, Alexander MAJ. The Shouldice repair. *Surg Clin North Am* 1993;73(3):451–469.
23. Nilsson E, Kald A, Anderberg B. Hernia surgery in a defined population. A prospective three year audit. *Eur J Surg* 1997;163:823–829.
24. Kald A, Nilsson E, Anderberg B, et al. Reoperation as surrogate endpoint in hernia surgery: a three year follow-up of 1565 herniorrhaphies. *Eur J Surg* 1998;164:45–50.
25. Halstead WS. *Surgical papers by William Stewart Halstead*. Baltimore, MD: The Johns Hopkins Press; 1924:1, 271.
26. Lichtenstein IL, Shulman AG. Ambulatory outpatient hernia surgery, including a new concept. *Int Surg* 1986;71:1.

27. Lichtenstein IL, Shulman AG, Anderberg B, et al. The tension-free hernioplasty. *Am J Surg* 1989;157:188.
28. Lichtenstein IL, Shore JM. Simplified repair of femoral and recurrent inguinal hernias by a "plug" technique. *Am J Surg* 1974;128:439–444.
29. Nyhus LM, Condon RE, Harkins HN. Clinical experience with preperitoneal hernia repair for all types of hernia of the groin. *Am J Surg* 1960;100:234.
30. Stoppa R, Petit J, Henry X. Unsutured dacron prosthesis in groin hernias. *Int Surg* 1975;60:411.
31. Ferzli GS, Frezza EE, Pecoraro AM, et al. Prospective randomized study of stapled versus unstapled mesh in laparoscopic preperitoneal inguinal hernia repair. *J Am Coll Surg* 1999;188(5):461–465.
32. Duepree HJ, Senagore AJ, Delaney CP, et al. Does means of access affect the incidence of small bowel obstruction and ventral hernia after bowel resection? Laparoscopy versus laparotomy. *J Am Coll Surg* 2003;197(2):177–181.
33. Clark JL. Ventral incisional hernia recurrence. *J Surg Res* 2001;99:33–39.
34. Pollock AV, Nyhus LM. Incisional hernias. In: Schwartz SI, Ellis H, eds. *Maingot's abdominal operations.* Norwalk, CT: Appleton-Century-Crofts; 1985:335–350.
35. Houck JP, Rypins EB, Sarfeh IJ, et al. Repair of incisional hernia. *Surg Gynecol Obstet* 1989;169:397–399.
36. Bay-Nielson M, Perkins F, Kehlet H. Pain and functional impairment one year after inguinal herniorrhaphy: a nationwide questionnaire study. *Ann Surg* 2001;233:1–7.
37. Evans DS. Value of herniography in the management of occult hernia and chronic groin pain in adults. *Br J Surg* 2001;88(1):153–154.
38. Hair A, Paterson C, Wright D, et al. What effect does the duration of an inguinal hernia have on patient symptoms? *J Am Coll Surg* 2001;193(2):125–129.
39. Chan STF, Esufali ST. Extended indications for polypropylene mesh closure of the abdominal wall. *Br J Surg* 1986;73:3–6.
40. Molloy RG, Moran KT, Waldron RP, et al. Massive incisional hernia: abdominal wall replacement with Marlex mesh. *Br J Surg* 1991;78:242–244.
41. Kyzer S, Kadouri A, Levi A, et al. Repair of fascia with polyglycolic acid mesh cultured with fibroblasts—experimental study. *Eur Surg Res* 1997;29(2):84–92.
42. Kaufman ZS, Engleberg M, Zager M. A late complication of Marlex mesh repair. *Dis Colon Rectum* 1981;24:543–544.
43. Voyles CR, Richardson JD, Bland KI, et al. Emergency abdominal wall reconstruction with polypropylene mesh: short-term benefits versus long-term complications. *Ann Surg* 1981;194:219–223.
44. Sitzmann JV, McFadden DW. The internal retention repair of massive ventral hernia. *Am J Surg* 1989;55:719–723.
45. Stoppa RE. The treatment of complicated groin and incisional hernias. *World J Surg* 1989;13:545–554.
46. Caldirone MW, Romano M, Bozza F, et al. Progressive pneumoperitoneum in management of giant incisional hernias. *Br J Surg* 1990;77:306–308.
47. Raynor RW, Del Geurcio LRM. The place for pneumoperitoneum in the repair of massive hernia. *World J Surg* 1989;13:581–585.
48. Salcedo-Wasicek MC, Thirlby RC. Postoperative course after inguinal herniorrhaphy. A case-controlled comparison of patients receiving workers' compensation vs patients with commercial insurance. *Arch Surg* 1995;103(1):29–32.
49. Barkun JS, Keyser EJ, Wexler MJ, et al. Short-term outcomes in open vs. laparoscopic herniorrhaphy: confounding impact of worker's compensation on convalescence. *J Gastrointest Surg* 1999;3(6):575–582.

Complications of Laparoscopic Surgery

38

Kathleen M. Diehl

■ **EARLY COMPLICATIONS 546**

Access Injury 546

Insufflation 548

■ **INTRAOPERATIVE COMPLICATIONS 550**

Ureteral/Bladder Injury 550

Solid Organ and Visceral Injury 551

Bleeding/Vascular Injury 551

Pneumothorax/Pneumomediastinum/Subcutaneous
    Emphysema 552

Gas Embolism 552

Equipment 552

■ **POSTPROCEDURE COMPLICATIONS 553**

Nausea/Vomiting 553

Pain 553

Port Site Recurrence 553

■ **CONCLUSION 554**

■ **REFERENCES 554**

Laparoscopy can be defined as inserting an illuminated tubular instrument—the laparoscope—through a small incision in the abdominal wall and injecting carbon dioxide into the abdominal cavity for the purpose of diagnosis, biopsy, or performing surgery (1). Although originally used for gynecologic procedures and then cholecystectomy, laparoscopic techniques are increasingly

Kathleen M. Diehl: University of Michigan, Ann Arbor, MI 48109

being applied to major abdominal procedures. As the use of laparoscopic surgery has increased, so has an awareness of the potential complications associated with it. A general knowledge of laparoscopic techniques and the ability to troubleshoot laparoscopic complications will become increasingly important to all aspects of general surgery. This chapter focuses on major complications associated with the use of laparoscopy; complications germane to specific procedures will be discussed in subsequent chapters.

EARLY COMPLICATIONS

Early complications during a laparoscopic case are generally related to difficulty encountered either (a) while obtaining access into the peritoneum, most often related to a trocar injury, or (b) after insufflation of the abdomen due to the establishment of pneumoperitoneum.

Access Injury

Trocar insertion and placement is arguably the most important aspect of a laparoscopic operation (Table 38-1). Proper placement of the trocars sets up the operative field and can establish an ergonomically easy operation with good visualization. Improper placement can create a more difficult operation and may result in patient injury and harm. The incidence of trocar injury is estimated to be 0.1% to 4%, including major vascular injury (0% to 4%) and bowel injury (0.03% to 0.3%) (2). No one method of trocar insertion has been shown to decrease the risk of patient injury. The complication rate of a closed trocar insertion using a Veress needle is reported to be approximately

TABLE 38-1

PRECAUTIONS FOR AVOIDING TROCAR INJURY AND COMPLICATIONS

- Maintain the table height at waist level of the surgeon inserting the trocar
- Place trocars in the midline whenever possible
- Assure adequate abdominal wall relaxation
- Maintain the patient in neutral position during insertion of first trocar
- Exert the minimum pressure necessary during insertion
  - Open skin sufficiently to prevent use of excessive force
- Stop insertion whenever resistance is encountered
- Insufflate under low flow initially until it is ensured that no resistance to flow is encountered
- Insert laparoscopic camera into abdomen as soon as insufflation is sufficient to allow safe visualization
- Maintain upward traction of the abdominal wall fascia
  - During trocar insertion
  - During insufflation of the peritoneum
- Avoid angling trocar toward midline structures
- Inspect the abdomen and trocar site for bleeding after trocar insertion
- During insertion of second and remaining trocars
  - The trocar should be inserted by the surgeon standing on that side of the table
  - Direct placement by illuminating the abdominal wall in order to outline vessels
  - Insert only while visualizing the abdominal wall insertion site
  - Place trocars lateral to rectus sheath whenever possible
- Inspect the trocar site and underlying peritoneum for bleeding after insertion
- Immediate conversion to an open procedure for
  - Free blood visualized in the peritoneum
  - Development of a retroperitoneal hematoma
- At the end of the case
  - Inspect for bleeding by visualizing removal of trocars
  - Remove trocars with the valves closed to decrease herniation of bowel
  - Lift fascia superiorly to decrease adherence of underlying bowel
  - Close the fascia of trocar sites of 10 mm or more

0.01% to 0.52%, and the complication rate for an open technique with placement of a blunt trocar is reported to be 0.01% to 0.36%.

The patients most at risk for trocar-related vascular complications are those who are very thin because there is little space between the abdominal wall and retroperitoneal major vascular structures. Patients with adhesions from prior abdominal operations are at risk for vascular, solid organ, and visceral injury during trocar insertion. In patients with a prior history of abdominal surgery, particularly those in whom preoperative imaging indicates adhesions to the abdominal wall, care should be taken to access the abdomen in an area that is judged to be relatively free of adhesions and to use an open technique in order to avoid underlying bowel or organs adherent to the abdominal wall. Particular care should be taken in patients who report a prior history of surgery with postoperative infection, abscess, or small bowel obstructions, all of which increase the likelihood of adhesions. Review of old operative notes and case histories can help to evaluate the likelihood of adhesions and distorted anatomy. Often abdominal/pelvic computed tomography

(CT) scans are helpful in identifying an area for placement of the initial trocar that is potentially free of adhesions.

Initial access should be obtained through the midline whenever possible or, alternatively, lateral to the rectus muscle in order to avoid injury to the epigastric vessels. The most important aspect of insertion is to maintain controlled insertion of the trocar. An often overlooked aspect of trocar control is the ergonomics of the operating surgeon. As the table height increases relative to the operating surgeon, the tendency is for the surgeon to compensate by abducting his or her arms; this is associated with a loss of control of arm movement. The table should be placed at a height that is comfortable for the surgeon and that allows keeping the arms and shoulders relaxed and the elbows close to the body. This will allow for a smoother, more controlled trocar placement, with better control of the depth of insertion, stopping the thrust when the peritoneum is entered.

Mental visualization of the surrounding structures in the area of trocar insertion should be attempted. Although the position of the aortic bifurcation is usually within

1.25 cm superior or inferior to the iliac crest, this landmark is variable and is affected by factors such as patient position and body mass index (BMI). In obese patients the aortic bifurcation can be superior to the umbilicus. In very thin patients the retroperitoneal vessels are as close as 2.5 cm below the abdominal wall, particularly after general anesthesia and muscular relaxation (3–5). Moving the patient into a Trendelenburg position often rotates the sacral promontory and aorta closer to the umbilicus and the inserting trocar. The origin of the right common iliac artery will most often lie in close proximity to the umbilicus. If the sacral promontory can be palpated, estimation of the position of the left common iliac vein can be made (2,6).

Injury to the epigastric vessels is estimated to occur in 0.7% to 2.5% of laparoscopic cases. The abdomen should be transilluminated in order to outline the abdominal wall vessels, and the same principles outlined for the placement of the original trocar should be followed for the insertion of each remaining trocar. Because the epigastric vessels lie at the lateral portion of the rectus sheath, in an area between 4 and 8 cm from the midline (4,7), an attempt should be made to insert secondary trocars lateral or medial to this area whenever possible. Once the abdomen has been insufflated, the light source from the laparoscope can be used to transilluminate the abdominal wall and the epigastric vessels in order to avoid injury to vessels during trocar placement. A prospective randomized study (8) found that transillumination of epigastric vessels was successful in 84% of normal weight patients, in 61% of patients with a BMI of 25 to 30 kg per m^2, and in only 23% of obese patients with a BMI of >30 kg per m^2. Investigators noted a decreasing ability to identify vessels in patients with darker skin color (69% vs. 42%). In heavier patients the inferior epigastric vessels are more likely to be located lateral to the superficial vessels. In these patients transillumination is helpful in identifying superficial epigastric vessels, while direct visualization is required to identify the inferior vessels.

No randomized controlled studies have confirmed the superiority of initial trocar insertion by Veress needle technique or open blunt trocar placement. No specific type of trocar, including optical trocars, has been found to be superior in eliminating inadvertent injury (2,9–14). Most studies comparing access techniques have been series reviews from individual surgeons or institutions. A recent meta-analysis of randomized, nonrandomized, and cohort studies, or case studies including over 1000 patients (14) allows the best comparison of closed technique, with or without use of a Veress needle, to open blunt port technique. These investigators reported a rate of major complications from open access of 0% to 2% and from needle/trocar access of 0% to 4%—even with meta-analysis, the data were not powerful enough to detect significant differences between the techniques. The authors concluded that there was a trend toward a decrease in major and minor complication rates and a decreased risk of conversion to an open procedure using an open technique. However, an open technique was associated

with an increased risk of abdominal wall hematoma (0.1% to 2% vs. 0% to 0.5%). Of note, these investigators also reported twice the risk of major bowel injury with an open access technique compared to a closed access technique. The only deaths were reported in the closed technique groups and resulted from unrecognized vascular or visceral injury (14). Given the low rate of access complications, the authors estimated that a definitive randomized trial to compare the various access techniques would require 10,000 patients in each study arm, which they rightly concluded was impractical and unlikely to occur. Many reviews in the literature indicate that for a large number of surgeons, general criteria for the use of open technique include a history of previous abdominal surgery or obesity, both for reasons of expediency, and prior experience with complications. It is widely acknowledged, however, that access complications are likely underreported.

One of the most commonly cited complications is bleeding from a vessel injured at the port site. This form of bleeding can be controlled by placement of a suture ligature or by extending the skin incision at the port site to allow direct visualization of the vessel for coagulation or suturing. Visualization of the underlying abdominal wall with the laparoscope can allow safe placement of a transabdominal figure-of-eight or horizontal mattress suture in an attempt to control bleeding. The vessel should be sutured on both sides of the trocar site. If control of bleeding makes keeping an airtight seal around the cannula difficult, the site should be closed and an alternative site should be chosen for trocar placement. Care should be taken to control even minor bleeding, as a postoperative abdominal wall hematoma can lead to a significant drop in hematocrit. General tips for avoiding injury during peritoneal access are listed in Table 38-1. Treatment of vascular, solid organ, or visceral injury will be discussed separately below.

Insufflation

The known consequences of peritoneal insufflation with carbon dioxide (CO_2) are noted in Table 38-2. In addition to these effects, cardiovascular collapse due to bradyarrhythmias, tachyarrhythmias, asystole, venous embolization, acute hemorrhage, pneumothorax, and cardiac tamponade have been reported (15). Insufflation of the abdomen causes an elevation of the diaphragm and increased intra-abdominal and intrathoracic pressures with subsequent pulmonary, hemodynamic, and neurohormonal effects (15–25) (Table 38-2). These effects are proportional to the abdominal pressure used to maintain insufflation, are particularly apparent at the initiation of insufflation, and are aggravated by changes in patient position (19,24,26,27). Trendelenburg position can further accentuate the effects of pneumoperitoneum by causing increasing central venous and pulmonary capillary wedge pressures. A reverse Trendelenburg position can alleviate changes in respiratory compliance due to insufflation of the abdomen (22).

TABLE 38-2

EFFECTS OF CARBON DIOXIDE PNEUMOPERITONEUM

Cardiovascular
    Decreased cardiac contractility
    Systemic vasodilatation with decreased systemic vascular
        resistance
    Increased central venous pressure with decreased venous
        return
    Increased mean arterial pressure
    Increased pulmonary artery pressure
    Increased pulmonary vascular resistance
    Decreased mesenteric and renal blood flow
    Decreased cardiac output
Pulmonary
    Hypercarbia
        Acidosis
    Elevation of the diaphragm
        Increased peak airway pressure
        Decreased respiratory compliance
        Decreased functional residual capacity
        Increased ventilation perfusion mismatch
        Increased shunting
        Increased alveolar-arterial gradient
Vascular
    Venous gas embolism (0.0016%–0.013%)
    Decreased common femoral venous flow
    Lower extremity venous pooling
Neuro-humoral
    Sympathetic stimulation
        Tachycardia
        Vasoconstriction
    Increase in plasma concentrations of:
        Cortisol
        Vasopressin
        Epinephrine
        Norepinephrine
        Renin
Peritoneal irritation

Although pneumoperitoneum is generally well tolerated by healthy patients, the minimal pressure required to achieve adequate exposure in the abdomen should be used, particularly in patients with limited cardiovascular reserve or in elderly patients who depend on cardiac filling to maintain cardiac output. Even though subjects with decreased abdominal wall laxity, such as patients with scleroderma or obesity, may require increased insufflation pressure to maintain adequate pneumoperitoneum, the pressure should be kept at a maximum of 12 mm Hg whenever possible. Although placing the patient in a reverse Trendelenburg position is often helpful for exposing upper abdominal organs, this maneuver can accentuate venous pooling and further decrease venous return (16,26,28).

Carbon dioxide is widely used for insufflation of the abdomen because the gas is inexpensive, soluble in blood, rapidly eliminated by the lungs, and noncombustible (23).

However, CO_2 solubility, and therefore absorption and potential hypercapnia, has side effects that can be additive to those of pressure and diaphragmatic changes due to peritoneal insufflation. The effects of CO_2 insufflation on cardiac output are mixed (Table 38-2). Hypercapnia from CO_2 insufflation can be associated with increased blood pressure, heart rate, and cardiac output. The decreased venous return associated with increased intraperitoneal and intrathoracic pressures associated with insufflation often negate these effects (22).

Insufflation and pneumoperitoneum should always be considered the offending factors when adverse cardiovascular effects are noted intraoperatively, and a return of the patient to the supine position, a decrease of insufflation, and a blood gas to measure the Pa_{CO_2} should be undertaken. One should remember that the measured end-tidal CO_2 may not accurately reflect Pa_{CO_2}, and a low threshold for drawing an arterial blood gas should be maintained if difficulties arise, particularly for patients with underlying cardiopulmonary disease (15,20,23,27).

A prospective randomized trial compared the hemodynamic and pulmonary changes noted perioperatively in laparoscopic cholecystectomy patients to those undergoing open cholecystectomy. Patients most at risk for hemodynamic and pulmonary complications due to pneumoperitoneum were those with an ASA class $\geqslant$I and those with a preoperative $FEF_{75-85\%}$ <900 mL.

Although other causes of cardiovascular collapse, such as vasovagal reaction, cardiac tamponade, or anesthetic drug-related reactions, should be considered when instituting pneumoperitoneum, it must be assumed that acute changes are related to the procedure and changes should be made accordingly. The ABCs of resuscitation should be followed, with confirmation of adequate airway and ventilation and exclusion of venous embolism, tension pneumothorax, or endotracheal tube displacement. Consideration of cardiac and circulation causes should include myocardial arrhythmia or tamponade. Figure 38-1 outlines an algorithm for troubleshooting adverse cardiovascular events during laparoscopic procedures.

Another complication is endotracheal tube migration. In a recent article comparing laparoscopic to open procedures for band gastroplasty, the authors noted that the endotracheal tube moved downward significantly more during laparoscopic procedures than during open procedures (27). The endotracheal tube was noted to shift during 50% of laparoscopic procedures, and the right main bronchus was intubated during 17% of these cases. Tube migration was most often noted at the time of maximal abdominal insufflation (12 mm Hg) or after a change to a reverse Trendelenburg position. The authors noted no significant change in arterial saturation, peak inspiratory pressure, or end-tidal CO_2 during endotracheal tube migration. Although no standardized method of securing the endotracheal tube was used during these procedures, and the cases were performed in an obese patient population, any surgeon making changes in patient

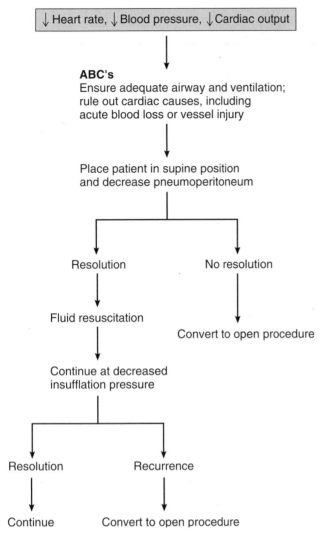

↓ Heart rate, ↓ Blood pressure, ↓ Cardiac output

ABC's
Ensure adequate airway and ventilation; rule out cardiac causes, including acute blood loss or vessel injury

Place patient in supine position and decrease pneumoperitoneum

Resolution   No resolution

Fluid resuscitation

Convert to open procedure

Continue at decreased insufflation pressure

Resolution   Recurrence

Continue   Convert to open procedure

Figure 38-1 Algorithm for troubleshooting adverse cardiovascular events during laparoscopic procedures.

position in the operating room should consider the potential for endotracheal tube displacement during the maneuvers.

INTRAOPERATIVE COMPLICATIONS

Discussed here as intraoperative complications are injury to vessels, solid organs, and viscera. Estimates for specific types of injury are just that—estimates. Most complications are reported from early single institution or surgeon reviews as initial reports of new techniques. It is generally assumed that the complication rates of laparoscopic surgery are underreported.

Ureteral/Bladder Injury

The incidence of bladder injury during laparoscopic procedures is estimated to be 0.02% to 8.3% (29,30), with the

most common site of injury being the bladder dome. The most common operation leading to bladder injury is laparoscopic-assisted hysterectomy, followed by diagnostic laparoscopy. Most injuries are noted intraoperatively. These can be lacerations due to trocar placement or from mobilization of the bladder during pelvic procedures, either directly from instrumentation, or indirectly following dissection of the bladder from inflamed or diseased pelvic organs. Pelvic inflammatory processes, either acute inflammation due to infection or chronic inflammation from malignancy or adhesions, are predisposing factors, both because of limitations to visualization and because of the bladder's decreased mobility.

In addition, bladder injury can occur from electrocautery. Electrocautery injury can present either immediately or in a delayed manner as a result of necrosis. Although direct visualization of the bladder dome before placing secondary trocars is recommended to decrease the risk of bladder injury, bladder identification is possible in only 45% of patients, and the ability to visualize the bladder dome decreases as patient BMI increases (8). Routine placement of a Foley catheter for laparoscopic procedures will keep the bladder decompressed, minimizing the chances of trocar injury. Indications of bladder injury include bleeding or extravasation of urine, the ability to see the Foley catheter within the operative field, hematuria, or pneumaturia noted in the Foley bag. If needed, intravesical instillation of betadyne, methylene blue, or indigo carmine can facilitate inspection for leaks. Delayed presentation of bladder injury is usually accompanied by fever, ileus, abdominal pain and distention, oliguria, increasing creatinine, peritonitis, azotemia, hyponatremia, and urine "ascites." If injury is suspected because of persistent drainage from the wound, surgical drains, vagina, or rectum, the fluid can be sent for creatinine measurement. CT cystography can aid in diagnosis.

If they are noted at the time of operation, bladder lacerations can be repaired primarily, either laparoscopically or by converting to an open procedure. Usually small tears not involving the ureter or bladder neck can be repaired laparoscopically. Although there are reports of laparoscopic closure using staples, this is not currently recommended, both because of the lack of clinical trials attesting to its effectiveness and because of the theoretical risk of permanent foreign bodies in the bladder wall acting as a nidus for calculus formation, of recurrent urinary tract infections, or of interfering with normal contraction of the bladder. Repair should be done in two layers—the underlying mucosa, then overlying muscularis—with absorbable suture. A Foley catheter is left in place for 7 to 10 days, and then cystography is done before removing the catheter. Long-term success rates of repair are approximately 98% (30).

The incidence of ureteral injury during laparoscopic pelvic surgery is estimated at 0.26% to 3%, which is comparable to open procedures (31,32). Injuries can be immediately detected by the extravasation of urine intraoperatively.

However, two-thirds of injuries are detected postoperatively during a work-up for fever and peritonitis. There are reports of delayed recognition up to 2 weeks postoperatively by leakage of urine from a ureterovaginal fistula. Delayed injuries may be due to thermal injury causing delayed necrosis and ureteral breakdown. Most injuries involve the distal ureter, and a common associated risk factor is inflammatory or infectious adhesions limiting visualization during the operation. If suspected intraoperatively, the ureter's integrity can be investigated by injection of indigo carmine or by retrograde ureterocystography.

Distal ureteral injuries can be repaired as a primary end-to-end anastamosis over a stent or by reimplantation of the ureter as a ureteroneocystostomy with a psoas hitch if needed (31). Recently, investigators reported a series of four patients repaired laparoscopically with a primary end-to-end repair over a 7F double-J ureteral stent (33). They reported successful laparoscopic repair with 6 to 33 months of follow-up. These investigators confirmed contralateral ureteral patency via cystoscopy and then aligned the ends of the ureter with absorbable suture. The investigators then passed a ureteral stent and finished the repair using interrupted absorbable suture. Intravenous injection of indigo carmine confirmed the repair's patency. Stents were removed 6 to 8 weeks postoperatively.

Solid Organ and Visceral Injury

The incidence of visceral injury during laparoscopic operations is estimated to be 0.05% to 0.7% and most frequently involves the small bowel, including the duodenum (6,34–36). Common mechanisms of visceral injury include penetrating injury from Veress needle or trocar placement, blunt dissection of tissues, cutting of tissues, cautery, or traction injuries. The most common procedure associated with iatrogenic bowel injury is laparoscopic cholecystectomy, likely because of the procedure's frequency and the number of times it is performed in the setting of inflammation and infection. One review of a single institution experience showed that 83.3% of visceral injuries occurred intraoperatively from the use of electrocautery or from dissection and that >50% of these injuries occurred with laparoscopic surgeons who had >100 laparoscopic cases. In addition, >50% of these injuries were recognized only belatedly.

General rules for avoiding visceral injury include keeping cautery devices within the operative field at all times, using only atraumatic graspers to manipulate bowel, and taking care to handle bowel gently without excessive traction or torsion. Inadvertent injury can occur during the application of stapling devices or clip appliers. It is imperative that both sides of the tissue being stapled or cut are visualized to minimize this complication. If noted at the time of the initial operation, simple small bowel injuries can be repaired using laparoscopic techniques, either by autosuturing devices or staplers or by extending a trocar

incision and suturing extracorporeally. Given the rapid resolution of CO_2 pneumoperitoneum, the recognition of free air on abdominal x-ray over 24 hours postoperatively should raise the suspicion of bowel injury and consideration should be given for reoperation.

Bleeding/Vascular Injury

The incidence of major vascular injury during laparoscopic surgery is estimated to be 0.05% to 4.7%, with an associated mortality rate of 8% to 17%. Vascular injury is the second-leading cause of mortality from laparoscopic procedures, although some authors believe that the incidence has increased with the increased number of complex laparoscopic procedures being performed (3,5,37). It is likely that minor vascular injury, such as injury to mesenteric or omental vessels, or minor lacerations to the liver or spleen, occur much more frequently but can be repaired using clip or stapling devices or hemostatic agents without sequelae and thus are never reported. Injury to mesenteric vessels needs to be closely monitored during the course of the case as mesenteric hematomas can compromise vascular perfusion of the associated bowel. A registry allowing anonymous entries of complications indicated that 76.5% of vascular injuries occurred during access procedures with either Veress needle or trocar insertion. The remaining injuries occurred during the operation, with 17.6% from monopolar cautery.

The locations of the injuries vary. The vena cava was the site of injury in 23.8%, the external iliac vessels in 23.8%, the aorta in 19%, the common iliac vessels in 19%, and the mesenteric vessel in 9.6%. In 88.2% of patients the injury was noted immediately because of hemoperitoneum. In 11.8% of patients the diagnosis was made when a retroperitoneal hematoma was noted at the end of the procedure. This observation underscores the need be alert to the possibility of vascular injury and to inspect the abdomen before ending the procedure, as a slow build-up of a retroperitoneal hematoma can be the first sign of a major vascular injury. There are case reports of delayed recognition of major vascular injury up to several hours after the end of operation. It is speculated that the decreased venous return associated with pneumoperitoneum and compression of abdominal vessels from insufflation conceals the injury and that reversal of these factors at the end of the case results in hemorrhage (38).

Although there are case reports of laparoscopic control of vessel injury using laparoscopic clips or thrombin glue or extending a small incision in order to clamp a vessel or place a suture, most injuries require conversion to an open procedure in order to obtain proximal and distal control of the vessel and repair of the site of injury. In the case of vascular injury due to trocar insertion, the trocar should, if possible, remain in place while the procedure is converted to an open procedure in order to effect some tamponade and to help in identification of the site of injury. Alternatively, pressure can be held on the injury with a laparoscopic sponge during the conversion in order to minimize hemorrhaging. It is inadvisable to use cautery on a bleeding edge from a laparoscopic staple line, as this application can cause a coagulation necrosis proximal to the staple line and worsen bleeding.

Pneumothorax/Pneumomediastinum/Subcutaneous Emphysema

Although rare, subcutaneous extravasation of CO_2 can occur, particularly if the trocar or Veress needle is not in the peritoneum, resulting in insufflation of fascial or subcutaneous planes. Carbon dioxide can then track cephalad and caudad. Although usually self-limiting after removal of the offending trocar, if the subcutaneous emphysema tracks upward, there is a theoretical potential for airway compromise. Tracking of gas to the thorax or mediastinum may result in pneumothorax or pneumomediastinum. Signs of inadvertent extraperitoneal insufflation include increase in airway pressure and an increase in end-tidal CO_2 measurements due to the increased surface area available for gas absorption (15).

Estimates of pneumothorax during laparoscopic surgery range from <1% to 5.8% (23). Pneumothorax is most commonly reported during procedures in the vicinity of the diaphragm, particularly with dissection around the esophageal hiatus during Nissen fundoplication or gastric hernia repair. Signs of pneumothorax include visualization of the lung, bulging of the contralateral diaphragm, decreased lung compliance, increased airway pressures, decreased O_2 saturation, and hypotension. With CO_2 insufflation, one of the first signs of pneumothorax is often increased end-tidal CO_2 measurement. Depending on the patient's stability and the size of the pleural defect, options for treatment include simple aspiration of the pneumothorax, placement of a drain or catheter into the pleural space and out through a trocar site placed to water seal, or placement of a chest tube via thoracostomy. Diaphragmatic repair, if indicated, can be done using laparoscopic suturing techniques before aspiration of the pneumothorax (39).

An interesting study examined the effects of pneumothorax in sheep. The investigators reported a decrease in the electrocardiogram QRS amplitude of precordially placed leads after introduction of as little of 20 mL of CO_2 or Helium (He) into the pleural space and a 50% decrease in QRS amplitude after introduction of 100 mL (40). They postulated that the introduction of gas into the space under the precordial leads caused a decreased conduction of electrical impulses, resulting in decreased amplitude of the complex. There was a 90% resolution of the pneumothorax when CO_2 was used, whereas helium pneumothorax remained unchanged. This ready resolution of CO_2 pneumothorax underscores the need to consider electrocardiogram (EKG) effects when contemplating alternative insufflation gases and that conservative management of asymptomatic pneumothoraces is a viable strategy.

Gas Embolism

Asymptomatic gas embolism has been noted in 6% to 69% of patients observed with transesophageal echocardiography during laparoscopic procedures (15). Serious or symptomatic gas embolism is estimated to occur in approximately 0.0016% to 0.013% of laparoscopic cases (41). The first sign of unrecognized vessel injury can be a gas embolism. Indications of potential gas embolism include a rapid drop in end-tidal CO_2 measurements and patient decompensation with hypotension and bradycardia or tachycardia, sometimes cardiac arrest. Cyanosis of the head and neck (15,42) occurs as gas is trapped in the right ventricle, causing pulmonary outflow obstruction. If decompensation occurs, insufflation should be stopped immediately and the patient rolled into a decubitus position on the left side with the head down in an attempt to move gas to the apex of the right ventricle, thus relieving outflow obstruction until the CO_2 can be absorbed. There should be aggressive fluid support. Support with 100% O_2 and hyperventilation can speed absorption of CO_2. If less aggressive supportive measures fail, emergent use of cardiopulmonary bypass can be used to stabilize the patient.

Equipment

A seldom discussed aspect of laparoscopic surgery is the operating surgeon's dependence on instrument capability and reliability. A failure of the stapling device inherently carries more immediate risk to the patient than the failure of a tie or suture during an open procedure—there is simply not an opportunity to pick up the offending vessel with the forceps. Laparoscopic stapling devices cut and staple through a few cm of tissue at a time and therefore will leave a large bleeding edge if failure of the stapling device occurs. Stapler failure is reported to occur with a frequency of 1% to 1.7%, with primary device failure occurring in 0.3% of cases (43,44). This problem is likely underreported, as most surgeons are likely to isolate the stapler and report failure only during a serious event, such as during the attempt to staple across a large vessel. Most of these failures are reported through an institutional risk management system, not through the journal literature. An institutional review and an analysis of the Food and Drug Administration (FDA) database involving stapler malfunction was done by Deng et al. (44). These investigators discussed 60 reports of linear cutting stapler failure since 1996. Preventable problems included (a) incorporating a previously placed clip in the suture line, (b) use of excessive force in deploying the stapler, leading to overcoming of the stapler lockout mechanism, which would have prevented the stapler from cutting without staples, (c) usage of a previously used stapler cartridge, and (d) entrapment of other vessels in the stapling device.

Injuries due to cautery are estimated to occur in about 0.06% to 0.5% of laparoscopic cases. These injuries are the result of overzealous use of cautery or cauterizing of tissue before adequate visualization is established. The cautery devices, whether mono or bipolar cautery or harmonic instruments, remain heated after use, and one must always keep the tip of the instrument in view of the camera. If the cautery tip moves outside the field of view, iatrogenic injury can occur to whatever structure the instrument encounters. Although unusual, complications from cautery that are due to the instrument rather than error have been reported. A break in the instrument's insulation can allow electrical current to leak to other trocars, instruments, or adjacent viscera. Direct coupling, or "arcing," of current can occur when two metal instruments are close to each other. Although sometimes a useful tool for hemostasis, this can lead to injury to surrounding structures in the vicinity of the metal instruments. In addition, a "capacitive current effect," or the transfer of energy from the active electrode through intact insulation and into adjacent conductive materials such as viscera, can occur when activating the current in the air and not adjacent to the intended tissue (35).

Tips for minimizing cautery injury include routine maintenance and inspection of equipment and instruments, keeping the instruments within camera view at all times, deploying current only with good contact to the tissue intended to be cut or cauterized, and ensuring that all other tissue or structures are not close to, or incorporated into, the instruments. Cautery should be used only in short bursts and with the minimal voltage needed to cauterize or cut tissue, thus allowing the instruments and tissue to cool between applications. In addition, if the expected effect from the voltage level on the generator and the application of instruments is not obtained, an alternative pathway for current should be suspected. An often overlooked potential for injury is the light on the laparoscopic camera. When left close to drapes or against the viscera for prolonged periods, the light source can become heated and injure surrounding viscera or cause patient burns.

POSTPROCEDURE COMPLICATIONS

Nausea/Vomiting

Postoperative nausea is estimated to occur in 20% to 30% of patients in the immediate postoperative period and in up to 60% of patients at some time during their hospital stay after laparoscopic surgery (45). The etiology and treatment of postoperative nausea in laparoscopic surgery is controversial, likely because the causes are multifactorial. Factors associated with postoperative nausea and vomiting include bowel manipulation, pneumoperitoneum, female gender, a history of postoperative nausea, a history of motion sickness, and opioid use (46). There is conflicting evidence on whether neuromuscular blockade reversal agents are associated with postoperative nausea. Propofol is associated with less postoperative nausea and vomiting

than inhalation anesthetics, but it is more difficult to titrate and inadequate anesthesia can be associated with awareness (47,48). The administration of supplemental oxygen perioperatively and supplemental fluids preoperatively and the administration of metoclopramide, dexamathasone, ondansetron, or 5–HT$_3$ receptor antagonists at the end of surgery have been associated with less postoperative nausea in some, but not all, studies (47–52).

Pain

An issue unique to laparoscopic surgery is the 20% to 25% incidence of postoperative shoulder tip pain. This symptom is commonly ascribed to entrapment of gas under the diaphragm or to peritoneal or diaphragmatic irritation or stretching. There is no consensus on effective methods for minimizing its occurrence or for treatment. Intraperitoneal or diaphragmatic instillation of bupivacain has been advocated, but the effects seem to be transient (53,54). Leaving in place a temporary peritoneal drain reduced the intensity of shoulder pain but was found to be less cost-effective than using analgesics, and, given a lack of correlation between postoperative shoulder tip pain and postoperative duration of pneumoperitoneum, this maneuver is unlikely to be adopted into common practice (55,56). A double-blinded study reported heated and humidified CO$_2$ to insufflate the abdomen during awake laparoscopy. Heating and humidifying the gas during insufflation decreased the incidence of shoulder pain from 30% to 10% (57).

Port Site Hernia

Port site hernias occur after 0.14% to 3% of laparoscopic operations and have been associated with small bowel obstruction due to a Richter-type defect (6,14,37). The incidence of port site hernias is correlated to the size of the incision used for trocar placement. Extended port incisions used for extracorporeal anastamosis or specimen extraction in laparoscopic-assisted colon surgeries have a rate of postoperative hernia development similar to open colectomy operations (58). Additional risk factors for port site hernia include a history of diabetes and obesity (58).

The fascia of all port sites of 10 mm or more should be closed (59,60). Not reversing muscle relaxation until after closure of the fascial defects will minimize bowel entrapment and allow for safer fascial closure. Some authors advocate desufflation of the abdomen through a trocar and then removing trocars with the valves closed to minimize this complication. This practice is hard to envision as being helpful and may lead to trocar injury. Removal of infected tissue or specimens through a bag can decrease the incidence of wound infection, which can contribute to this complication.

Port Site Recurrence

The occurrence of port site metastasis in patients undergoing laparoscopic choleycystectomy with unsuspected gallbladder cancer and the reports of port site metastasis after laparoscopic exploration or after resection for other malignancies raised concerns about the safety of laparoscopic oncologic procedures (61). Theories on the cause of port site metastasis include exfoliation of malignant cells by instrument manipulation, tumor contact and malignant cell shedding along port sites due to the removal of tumor through small incisions, increased contact of the tumor with wound surfaces due to abdominal wall movement during the case, aerosolization of tumor cells due to pneumoperitoneum and a "chimney effect" of tumor cells seeding laparoscopic ports during leakage of gas around port sites, direct effects of pneumoperitoneum or CO_2 itself, defects in immune function caused by laparoscopic procedures, and movement of contaminated ports or instruments through incisions (62,63). There is conflicting evidence from *in vitro* and animal models and from clinical reports on the true etiology of port site metastasis (64,65). Port site metastases have been reported when specimens have been removed in endoscopic bags or when wound protection devices were in place and at port sites away from the location where the specimen was removed and in cases where there was no manipulation or excision of tumor (61,66,67). In addition, port site metastases have been reported in thoracoscopic cases when gas insufflation has not been used (65).

More recent reports have called into question whether the incidence of port site metastases is truly more frequent in laparoscopic compared to open cases. Port site metastases occur in approximately 0% to 1.7% of colorectal cancer cases and in 12% to 28% of laparoscopic gallbladder cancer cases (61,65,67−70). This incidence is similar to that seen in open procedures (66). Incisional metastases are estimated to occur in approximately 0.6% to 0.85% of laparotomies for colorectal cancer and in 14% to 32% of patients operated on for gallbladder cancer (64−66,70).

Until more is known about the true etiology of port site metastasis, it is prudent to minimize desufflation episodes during oncologic laparoscopic cases, minimize port site trauma, avoid port site gas leaks, minimize manipulation of the tumor and the contact of ports and instruments with the tumor, and to remove all specimens in an impermeable specimen bag. These steps are technically easy and inexpensive. Although its benefit is debatable (66,71,72), excision of port sites normally requires little loss of abdominal wall, and it therefore seems prudent to excise port and drain sites when there is concern about tumor contamination, particularly in the case of carcinoma of the gallbladder.

CONCLUSION

The ability to apply laparoscopic surgery to a wider variety of patients and procedures has brought potential complications. Attentiveness to the potential complications associated with laparoscopic operations and careful, meticulous attention to potential dangers associated with the operation

are mandatory. Visualization of the operative field and the instruments at all times, associated with good positioning of trocars to prevent arm fatigue, is an important aspect of all laparoscopic operations. In addition, it is important to convert to an open operation whenever there is any question about the ability to continue safely. Conversion to an open procedure should not be considered a complication of the operation but an exercise in good judgment on the part of the surgeon.

REFERENCES

1. *Concise Medical Dictionary*. Oxford: Oxford University Press; 2002.
2. Brill AI, Cohen BM. Fundamentals of peritoneal access. *J Am Assoc Gynecol Laparosc* 2003;10(2):287–297.
3. Chapron CM, Peirre F, Lacroix S, et al. Major vascular injuries during gynecologic laparoscopy. *J Am Coll Surg* 1997;185(5): 476–481.
4. Tomacruz RS, Bristow RE, Montz FJ. Management of pelvic hemorrhage. *Surg Clin North Am* 2001;81(4):925–948.
5. Roviaro GC, Varoli F, Saguatti L, et al. Major vascular injuries in laparoscopic surgery. *Surg Endosc* 2002;16:1192–1196.
6. Philips PA, Amaral JF. Abdominal access complications in laparoscopic surgery. *J Am Coll Surg* 2001;192(4):525–536.
7. Saber AA, Meslemani AM, Davis R, et al. Safety zones for anterior abdominal wall entry during laparoscopy: a CT scan mapping of epigastric vessels. *Ann Surg* 2004;239(2):182–185.
8. Hurd WW, Amesse LS, Gruber JS, et al. Visualization of the epigastric vessels and bladder before laparoscopic trocar placement. *Fertil Steril* 2003;80(1):209–212.
9. Borgatta L, Gruss L, Barad D, et al. Direct trocar insertion vs. Verres needle use for laparoscopic sterilization. *J Reprod Med* 1990;35(9): 891–894.
10. Nezhat FR, Silfen SL, Evans D, et al. Comparison of direct insertion of disposable and standard reusable laparoscopic trocars and previous pneumoperitoneum with Veress needle. *Obstet Gynecol* 1991; 78(1):148–150.
11. Byron JW, Markenson G, Miyazawa K. A randomized comparison of Verres needle and direct trocar insertion for laparoscopy. *Surg, Gynecol Obstet* 1993;177(3):259–262.
12. Bonjer HF, Hazebroek EJ, Kazemier G, et al. Open versus closed establishment of pneumoperitoneum in laparoscopic surgery. *Br J Surg* 1997;84(5):599–602.
13. Yerdel MA, Karayalcin K, Koyuncu A, et al. Direct trocar insertion versus veress needle insertion in laparoscopic cholecystectomy. *Am J Surg* 1999;177:247–249.
14. Merlin TL, Hiller JE, Maddern GJ, et al. Systematic review of the safety and effectiveness of methods used to establish pneumoperitoneum in laparoscopic surgery. *Br J Surg* 2003;90:668–679.
15. Joshi GP. Anesthesia for minimally invasive surgery: laparoscopy, thoracoscopy, hysteroscopy. *Anesthesiol Clin North Am* 2001;19(1): 89–105.
16. Tillman Hein HA, Joshi GP, Ramsay M, et al. Hemodynamic changes during laparoscopic choleycystectomy in patients with severe cardiac disease. *J Clin Anesth* 1997;9:261–265.
17. Cuschieri A. Adverse cardiovascular changes induced by positive pressure pneumoperitoneum. *Surg Endosc* 1998;12:93–94.
18. Jakimowicz J, Stultiens G, Smulders F. Laparoscopic insufflation of the abdomen reduces portal venous flow. *Surg Endosc* 1998;12: 129–132.
19. Joris JL, Chiche J-D, Canivet J-LM, et al. Hemodynamic changes induced by laparoscopy and their endocrine correlates: effects of clonidine. *J Am Coll Cardiol* 1998;32(5):1389–1396.
20. Volpino P, Cangemi V, D' Andrea N, et al. Hemodynamic and pulmonary changes during and after laparoscopic cholecystectomy. *Surg Endosc* 1998;12:119–123.
21. Chekan EG, Pappas TN. Minimally invasive surgery. *Sabiston textbook of surgery*. Townsend: W B Saunders; 2001.
22. O'Malley C, Cunningham AJ. Anesthesia for minimally invasive surgery: laparoscopy, thoracoscopy, hysteroscopy. *Anesthesiol Clin North Am* 2001;19(1):1–19.

23. Tsereteli Z, Terry ML, Bowers SP, et al. Prospective randomized clinical trial comparing nitrous oxide and carbon dioxide pneumoperitoneum for laparoscopic surgery. *J Am Coll Surg* 2002; 195(2):173–180.

24. Zuckerman RS, Heneghan S. The duration of hemodynamic depression during laparoscopic cholecystectomy. *Surg Endosc* 2002;16:1233–1236.

25. Sprung J, Whalley DG, Falcone T, et al. The effects of tidal volume and respiratory rate on oxygenation and respiratory mechanics during laparoscopy in morbidly obese patients. *Anesth Analg* 2003; 97:268–274.

26. Rauh R, Hemmerling TM, Rist M, et al. Influence of pneumoperitoneum and patient positioning on respiratory system compliance. *J Clin Anesth* 2001;13:361–365.

27. Ezri T, Hazin V, Warters D, et al. The endotracheal tube moves more often in obese patients undergoing laparoscopy compared with open abdominal surgery. *Anesth Analg* 2003;96:278–282.

28. Morrison CA, Schreiber MA, Olsen SB, et al. Femoral venous flow dynamics during intraperitoneal and preperitoneal laparoscopic insufflation. *Surg Endosc* 1998;12:1213–1216.

29. Ostrzenski A, Ostrzenska KM. Bladder injury during laparoscopic surgery. *Obstet Gynecol Surv* 1998;53(3):175–180.

30. Armenakas NA, Pareek G, Fracchia JA. Iatgrogenic bladder perforations: longterm followup of 65 patients. *J Am Coll Surg* 2004;198(1): 78–82.

31. Tamussino KF, Lang PFJ, Breinl E. Ureteral complications with operative gynecologic laparoscopy. *Am J Obstet Gynecol* 1998;178(5): 967–970.

32. Miklos JR, Kohli N, Moore RD. Laparoscopic management of urinary incontinence, ureteral and bladder injuries. *Curr Opin Obstet Gynecol* 2001;13:411–417.

33. Tulikangas PK, Gill IS, Falcone T. Laparoscopic repair of ureteral injuries. *J Am Assoc Gynecol Laparosc* 2001;8(2):259–262.

34. El-Banna M, Abdel-Atty M, EI-Meteini M, et al. Management of laparoscopic-related bowel injuries. *Surg Endosc* 2000;14:779–782.

35. Wu M-P, Ou C-S, Chen S-L, et al. Complications and recommended practices for electrosurgery in laparoscopy. *Am J Surg* 2000;179:67–73.

36. Kwon A-H, Inui H, Kamiyama Y. Laparoscopic management of bile duct and bowel injury during laparoscopic choleycystectomy. *World J Surg* 2001;25(7):856–861.

37. Li TC, Richmond M, Cooke ID. Complications of laparoscopic pelvic surgery: recognition, management and prevention. *Hum Reprod Update* 1997;3(4):505–515.

38. Leron E, Piura B, Ohana E, et al. Delayed recognition of major vascular injury during laparoscopy. *Obstet Gynecol* 1998;79:91–93.

39. Potter SR, Kavoussi LR, Jackman SV. Management of diaphragmatic injury during laparoscopic nephrectomy. *J Urol* 2001; 165:1203–1204.

40. Ludemann R, Krystopik R, Jamieson GG, et al. Pneumothorax during laparoscopy. *Surg Endosc* 2003;17:1985–1989.

41. Maktabi MA, Airan MC, Scott-Conner CEH. Anesthesia and Monitoring. *The Sages Manual*. New York: Springer-Verlag; 1999: 15-21

42. Larach SW, Gallaher JT. Complications of laparoscopic surgery for rectal cancer: avoidance and management. *Semin Surg Oncol* 2000;18(3):265−268.

43. Chan D, Bishoff JT, Ratner L, et al. Endovascular gastrointestinal stapler device malfunction during laparoscopic nephrectomy: early recognition and management. *J Urol* 2000;164:319–321.

44. Deng DY, Meng MV, Nguyen HT, et al. Laparoscoic linear cutting stapler failure. *Urology* 2002;60(3):415–420.

45. Bradshaw WA, Gregory BC, Finley C, et al. Frequency of postoperative nausea and vomiting in patients undergoing laparoscopic foregut surgery. *Surg Endosc* 2002;16:777–780.

46. Koivuranta M, Laara E, Snare L, et al. A survey of postoperative nausea and vomiting. *Anesthesia* 1997;52:443–449.

47. Smith I. Anesthesia for laparoscopy with emphasis on outpatient laparoscopy. *Anesthesiol Clin North Am* 2001;19(1):21–41.

48. Apfel CC, Korttila K, Abdalla M, et al. A factorial trial of six interventions for the prevention of postoperative nausea and vomiting. *N Engl J Med* 2004;350(24):2441–2451.

49. Ahmed AB, Hobbs GJ, Curran JP. Randomized, placebo-controlled trial of combination antiemetic prophylaxis for day-case gynaecological laparoscopic surgery. *Br J Anesth* 2000;85(5): 678–682.

50. Goll V, Akca O, Greif R, et al. Ondansetron is no more effective than supplemental intraoperative oxygen for prevention of postoperative nausea and vomiting. *Anesth Analg* 2001;92:112–117.

51. Ali SZ, Taguchi A, Holtmann B, et al. Effect of supplemental preoperative fluid on postoperative nausea and vomiting. *Anesthesia* 2003;58:780–784.

52. Purhonen S, Turunen M, Ruohoaho R-M, et al. Supplemental oxygen does not reduce the incidence of postoperative nausea and vomiting after ambulatory gynecologic laparoscopy. *Ambul Anesth* 2003;96: 91–96.

53. Szem JW, Hydo L, Barie PS. A double-blinded evaluation of intraperitoneal bupivacaine vs saline for the reduction of postoperative pain and nausea after laparoscopic cholecystectomy. *Surg Endosc* 1996;10(1):44–48.

54. Cunniffe MG, McAnena OJ, Dar MA, et al. A prospective randomized trial of intraoperative bupivacaine irrigation for management of shoulder-tip pain following laparoscopy. *Am J Surg* 1998;176:258–261.

55. Draper K, Jefson R, Jongeward R, et al. Duration of postlaparoscopic pneumoperitoneum. *Surg Endosc* 1997;11:809–811.

56. Abbott J, Hawe J, Srivastave P, et al. Intraperitoneal gas drain to reduce pain after laparoscopy: randomized masked trial. *Obstet Gynecol* 2001; 98(1):97–100.

57. Demco L. Effect of heating and humidifying gas on patients undergoing awake laparoscopy. *J Am Assoc Gynecol Laparosc* 2001; 8(2):247–251.

58. Winslow RR, Fleshman JW, Birnbaum EH, et al. Wound complications of laparoscopic vs open colectomy. *Surg Endosc* 2002;16:1420–1425.

59. George JP. Presentation and management of laparoscopic incisional hernia. *J Am Assoc Gynecol Laparosc* 1994;4(2):S12.

60. Lajer H, Widecrantz S, Heisterberg L. Hernias in trocar ports following abdominal laparoscopy. A review. *Acta Obstet Gynecol Scand* 1997;76(5):389–393.

61. Paolucci V, Schaeff B, Schneider M, et al. Tumor seeding following laparoscopy: International survey. *World J Surg* 1999;23(10): 989–997.

62. Tseng LNJ, Berends FJ, Wittich P, et al. Port-site metastases: Impact of local tissue trauma and gas leakage. *Surg Endosc* 1998;12:1377–1380.

63. Curet MJ. Port site metastases. *Am J Surg* 2004;187(6):705–712.

64. Maxwell-Armstrong CA, Robinson MH, Scholefield JH. Laparoscopic colorectal cancer surgery. *Am J Surg* 2000;179: 500–507.

65. Zmora O, Gervaz P, Wexner SD. Trocar site recurrence in laparoscopic surgery for colorectal cancer: Myth or real concern? *Surg Endosc* 2001;15:788–793.

66. Pearlstone DB, Feig BW, Mansfield PF. Port site recurrences after laparoscopy for malignant disease. *Semin Surg Oncol* 1999;16:307–312.

67. Lundberg O. Port site metastases after laparoscopic choleycystectomy. *Eur J Surg* 2000;166(Suppl. 585):27–30.

68. Lacy AM, Delgado S, Garcia-Valdecasas JC, et al. Port site metastases and recurrence after laparoscopic colectomy, a randomized trial. *Surg Endosc* 1998;12:1039–1042.

69. Hartley JE, Mehigan BJ, MacDonald AW, et al. Patterns of recurrence and survival after laparoscopic and conventional resection for colorectal carcinoma. *Ann Surg* 2000;232(2):181–186.

70. Chapman AE, Levitt MD, Hewett P, et al. Laparoscopic-assisted resection of colorectal malignancies: a systematic review. *Ann Surg* 2001; 234(5):590–606.

71. Bartlett DL, Fong Y, Fortner J, et al. Long-term results after resection for gallbladder cancer: implications for staging and management. *Ann Surg* 1996;224(5):639–646.

72. Fong Y, Jarnagin W, Blumgart LH. Gallbladder cancer: comparison of patients presenting initially for definitive operation with those presenting after prior noncurative intervention. *Ann Surg* 2000;232(4):557–569.

Complications of Endocrine and Oncologic Surgery

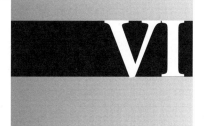

Complications of Adrenal Surgery

39

Paul G. Gauger

■ INTRODUCTION 559

■ THERAPEUTIC GOALS OF
ADRENALECTOMY 559

■ EXPECTED OUTCOMES 560
Primary Hyperaldosteronism 560
Hypercortisolism 563
Pheochromocytoma 564
Adrenocortical Carcinoma 565
Adrenal Incidentaloma 566

■ IDENTIFICATION AND MODIFICATION
OF PREOPERATIVE RISK FACTORS 567
General Risks 567
Hyperaldosteronism 567
Hypercortisolism 567
Pheochromocytoma 568
Adrenocortical Carcinoma 568
Critical Principles of Patient Selection 568
Open Anterior Adrenalectomy 569
Open Posterior Adrenalectomy 571
Open Thoracoabdominal Adrenalectomy 571
Laparoscopic Transperitoneal Adrenalectomy 571
Laparoscopic Posterior Adrenalectomy 571

■ IDENTIFICATION AND MANAGEMENT
OF POSTOPERATIVE COMPLICATIONS 572
Bleeding 572
Glucocorticoid Insufficiency 572
Hernia 572

Hypertension 572
Hypotension 572
Ileus 572
Mineralocorticoid Insufficiency 572
Nelson Syndrome 573
Pneumonia 573
Pneumothorax 573
Subphrenic Abscess 573
Wound Infection 573

■ SUMMARY 573

■ REFERENCES 573

INTRODUCTION

Adrenalectomy is an example of a procedure that has been transformed from an invasive and temporarily disabling operation to one that gives many patients a minimally invasive and less morbid alternative. Yet diverse complications can still ensue. Some complications relate to the disease process being treated and some relate to the specific surgical approach. With proper vigilance and preparation, most complications can be either avoided or managed.

THERAPEUTIC GOALS OF ADRENALECTOMY

Appropriate use of adrenalectomy conceptually applies to (a) patients with clinically or biochemically apparent

Paul G. Gauger: University of Michigan, Ann Arbor, MI 48109

hormonal hyperfunction, (b) patients with a probable or certain malignant adrenal mass, and (c) patients with an adrenal mass of uncertain significance. Patients with hormonal syndromes for whom adrenalectomy is appropriate include those with primary hyperaldosteronism, primary or secondary hypercortisolism, and pheochromocytoma. The goal of adrenalectomy—whether unilateral or bilateral—is to provide long-term relief of the hormonal excess. Resection of an adrenocortical carcinoma is offered in the hope of providing long-term disease-free survival. Resection of a metastatic deposit from another malignancy to the adrenal gland is occasionally indicated if histologic proof is required to determine the type and intensity of adjuvant therapy for the primary cancer or if the adrenal mass is the only measurable residual tumor in a patient for whom removal would be expected to have a beneficial impact. The third category describes patients for whom workup of an incidentally noted adrenal mass has failed to yield conclusive evidence of etiology and in whom the risk of observation is determined to exceed the risk of removal.

EXPECTED OUTCOMES

The outcomes of adrenalectomy may be associated with the surgical approach. Anterior, transabdominal approaches may be complicated by pancreatitis, incidental splenectomy, pneumonia, longer hospitalization, and more prolonged recovery. Posterior approaches often require rib resection and can be complicated by bleeding or pneumothorax. Laparoscopic approaches have been shown to be superior to either of these approaches in terms of length of stay and pain control as well as complication rates (1,2). Many long-term outcomes are determined by the specific adrenal disorder being treated.

Primary Hyperaldosteronism

This chapter will discuss only surgically remediable hyperaldosteronism, which affects approximately two-thirds of all patients with primary hyperaldosteronism. The characterization of primary hyperaldosteronism, as caused by an adrenocortical adenoma, is commonly attributed to Jerome Conn (3). Because of variability in screening practices and diagnostic criteria, Conn syndrome is likely more common than prevalence statistics would suggest (0.05% to 2% of patients evaluated for arterial hypertension) (4). Although most patients have hypokalemia accompanying hypertension, the diagnosis is often more subtle and conventional diagnostic criteria have been expanded.

Primary hyperaldosteronism most often affects patients between 30 and 50 years of age and is more common in females by a ratio of 2:1 (5). Up to 5% of patients evaluated in hypertension clinics have primary hyperaldosteronism. The severity and duration of hypertension are often indistinguishable from essential hypertension, although occasionally blood pressure elevation can be profound. Polyuria and nocturia are common. Symptoms of hypokalemia such as muscle weakness or cramps may be present. Rarely, periodic paralysis can occur as hypokalemia acutely worsens following increased sodium intake or administration of sodium-wasting diuretics.

Evaluation of metabolic and hormonal disturbances is most accurate if the patient has a diet with normal sodium intake (6 to 9 gm per day) and is not taking diuretics, β-blocker agents, angiotensin-converting enzyme inhibitors, or angiotensin II receptor blockers. In this setting, relative hypokalemia, with a potassium of <3.9 mEq per L, and a metabolic alkalosis, with HCO_3^- of >32 mEq per L, are both consistent with the diagnosis. Elevated 24-hour urinary aldosterone secretion is often present. Plasma aldosterone levels are more commonly obtained. Isolated plasma aldosterone levels are not consistently elevated above the upper end of normal. However, in the context of a suppressed plasma renin activity, a ratio of plasma aldosterone/plasma renin activity >25 is highly suggestive of primary hyperaldosteronism (5,6).

Primary hyperaldosteronism is generally caused by either an adenoma (Conn syndrome) or by bilateral hyperplasia of the zona glomerulosa of the adrenals. The classification of primary hyperaldosteronism has expanded to include (a) multiple or bilateral adenomas, or adenomas arising in hyperplastic glands; (b) familial dexamethasone-suppressible hyperaldosteronism; and (c) unilateral hyperplasia. Not all these entities are surgically remediable. As the specific pathophysiology influences the indications for operation and, ultimately, the expected outcomes, it is important to identify the specific condition underlying primary hyperaldosteronism.

Clinical features may be helpful in this regard. The degree of hypertension and hypokalemia is often relatively more severe in Conn syndrome than in idiopathic hyperaldosteronism. In response to an upright position for 2 hours, plasma aldosterone will increase in idiopathic hyperaldosteronism, while it will not with Conn syndrome. Idiopathic hyperaldosteronism is suggested if plasma aldosterone levels are reduced in response to saline loading or captopril administration. Serum 18-OH-corticosterone levels are often elevated in Conn syndrome, while they are not in idiopathic hyperaldosteronism.

Differentiation of Conn syndrome from idiopathic hyperaldosteronism is an imperfect process. The dichotomous concept of the unilateral adrenal mass amenable to surgery versus the bilateral adrenal enlargement amenable to medical therapy is oversimplified and does not account for the full spectrum of disease. Apart from the suggestive clinical factors noted above, anatomic and functional imaging tests are necessary. Cross-sectional imaging performed under appropriate adrenal protocols is quite sensitive in determining the presence of an adrenal mass. The most practical initial imaging test is a computed tomography

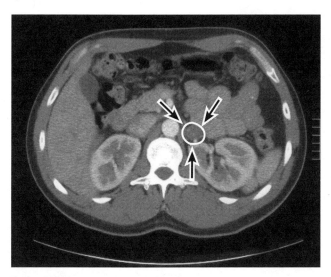

Figure 39-1 Arrows indicate a 2.1-cm left adrenal mass seen on CT scan of a 38-year-old male with primary hyperaldosteronism as determined by hypertension, hypokalemia, and an aldosterone/PRA ratio of 48.

(CT) scan (Fig. 39-1). Magnetic resonance imaging (MRI) scanning is more expensive and adds little information.

If a mass is seen, it may be nonsecreting in the presence of a contralateral microaldosteronoma or a background of bilateral hyperplasia. A unilateral aldosteronoma may arise in the background of microscopic hyperplasia, and yet the patient will be cured by unilateral adrenalectomy (7). Bilateral adrenal adenomatous changes may be hypersecreting on one side only (8).

If a CT scan detects a unilateral adrenal mass and the contralateral adrenal appears normal, the presumption that this represents unilateral disease, curable by unilateral adrenalectomy, is correct >90% of the time. If there is bilateral enlargement, it is necessary to corroborate anatomic data with functional information from dexamethasone suppressed adrenal scintigraphy or selective adrenal venous sampling.

^{131}I labeled noriodocholesterol (NP-59) is a radionuclide capable of imaging cortical adrenal tissue. When administered after 7 days of dexamethasone suppression, NP-59 can image small aldosterone-producing masses by suppressing normal cortical uptake (see Fig. 39-2). Although it is a cumbersome test requiring pharmacologic preparation and many days of imaging, its accuracy has been reported to be from 70% to 94% (9–11). When an aldosteronoma is <1 cm in size, NP-59 scanning is not reliable.

Adrenal venous sampling for aldosterone levels provides the most specific confirmation of a unilateral or bilateral hypersecretory process. Venous sampling is technically demanding, related to the challenge of catheterizing the

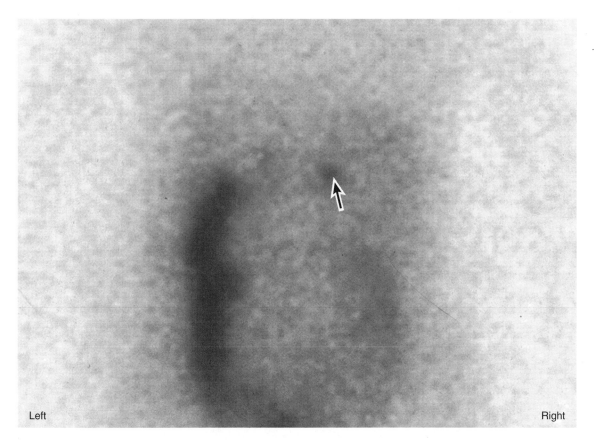

Left   Right

Figure 39-2 Posterior view of a NP-59 adrenal scintigram after 10 days of dexamethasone suppression in a 33-year-old woman with hyperaldosteronism caused by Conn syndrome. The arrow indicates the right adrenal tumor. The remaining activity is excreted into the GI tract.

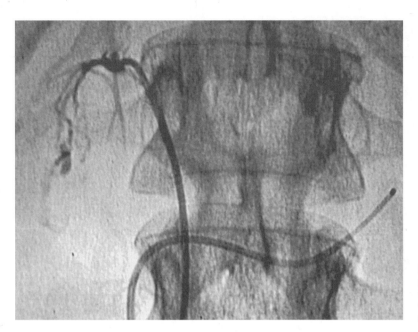

Figure 39-3 Bilateral adrenal vein catheterization (with contrast injection into right central adrenal vein) that was done in the course of selective adrenal venous sampling in a patient with primary hyperaldosteronism.

right central adrenal vein (Fig. 39-3). In addition to aldosterone levels, cortisol levels are sampled to assure proper catheter position. Adrenocorticotropic hormone (ACTH) is infused to equalize stress-induced fluctuations in adrenal output. Although ACTH is usually thought of as a stimulatory hormone for glucocorticoid secretion, it is typical to also observe a brisk response in aldosterone secretion in the abnormal gland (Table 39-1).

Thoughtful patient selection and a thorough preoperative workup are necessary to ensure excellent outcomes. As a general rule, primary hyperaldosteronism caused by an adrenocortical adenoma responds to surgical resection while idiopathic hyperaldosteronism does not. Some patients with idiopathic hyperaldosteronism who have asymmetric hypersecretion of excess aldosterone respond well to surgical resection.

Unilateral adrenalectomy for primary hyperaldosteronism caused by a cortical adenoma nearly always provides rapid resolution of hypokalemia. The response of hypertension can be more variable, from complete response to continued reliance on antihypertensive medications. Hypertension is improved in nearly all patients; 60% are cured and free of antihypertensive medications (12–17). In some series the proportion of cured patients has been as high as 88% (18), likely related to patient selection. Predictors of an unfavorable response include long-standing hypertension, a family history of hypertension, advanced age, and absence of preoperative response to spironolactone administration.

Most patients with idiopathic hyperaldosteronism are treated without operation. Both hypertension and hypokalemia can be controlled with chronic spironolactone

TABLE 39-1

SELECTIVE ADRENAL VENOUS SAMPLING FOR ALDOSTERONE AND CORTISOL LEVELS INDICATING OVERSECRETION OF ALDOSTERONE FROM THE RIGHT ADRENAL GLAND

Aldosterone R / L / IVC (1–16 ng/dL)	Aldo Ratio	Cortisol R / L / IVC (7–22 ug/dL)	A/C ratio R / L / IVC	Ratio of A/C R / L
3860 / 53 / 39	72	89 / 25 / 22	43 / 2.1 / 1.7	20
10, 20, and 30 min post ACTH				
17344 / 504 / 46	34	486 / 390 / 24	36 / 1.3 / 1.9	28
20018 / 714 / 87	28	526 / 401 / 22	38 / 1.8 / 3.9	21
17984 / 540 / 96	33	569 / 437 / 28	31 / 1.2 / 3.3	25

or eplerenone therapy. In the spectrum of disease between these two entities are cortical adenomas arising in a background of hyperplasia. Hyperplasia can occur as an asymmetric disease. If this condition can be determined by preoperative workup, these patients can be offered unilateral adrenalectomy with the expectation of excellent outcomes. Disease-related outcomes are largely independent of specific operative approach, such as anterior adrenalectomy, posterior adrenalectomy, or laparoscopic adrenalectomy.

Hypercortisolism

With the exception of Cushing disease, all conditions resulting from glucocorticoid excess are commonly known as Cushing syndrome. The condition can be classified as either corticotropin-dependent or corticotropin-independent. The former is responsible for >80% of patients with hypercortisolism. Chronic corticotrophin (ACTH) stimulation results in adrenocortical hyperplasia with overproduction of cortisol and other adrenal hormones. The pituitary dependent form (Cushing disease) accounts for 70% of hypercortisolism, while the ectopic ACTH syndrome accounts for 10%, usually from small-cell carcinoma of the lung, carcinoid tumor, medullary thyroid carcinoma, or malignant tumors of the pancreas or thymus. With the exception of iatrogenic steroid excess, corticotropin-independent hypercortisolism implies primary overproduction of cortisol from the adrenal gland(s). This condition usually occurs as a function of a unilateral cortical adenoma, accounting for 10% of patients with hypercortisolism, but it may be caused by primary hyperplasia of both adrenal glands. An adrenal mass accompanied by hypercortisolism may also represent a primary adrenocortical carcinoma.

Although many patients with ectopic ACTH syndrome have advanced malignancies and, accordingly, a poor prognosis, operation is often indicated to remove the source of ACTH overproduction and to simplify medical management. Palliative operation may involve bilateral adrenal resection to treat refractory Cushing syndrome if the secretion of ACTH cannot be adequately controlled. An adrenocortical adenoma is best treated by unilateral adrenalectomy. Cushing syndrome caused by primary adrenal hyperplasia can often be managed medically, but when this fails, bilateral adrenalectomy is indicated.

The clinical presentation of Cushing syndrome usually includes insidious onset of weakness, increased appetite, weight gain, and oligomenorrhea. As the syndrome develops, patients develop centripetal obesity with rounded facies, gradual disappearance of the ears in the frontal profile, fullness of the supraclavicular fat pads, and a "buffalo hump." Skin fragility and bruising are common, as are purple striae on the flanks, abdomen, and limbs. Hirsutism, acne, and facial plethora may occur, as well as hypertension and diabetes.

Diagnosis of Cushing syndrome requires biochemical confirmation. A low-dose dexamethasone suppression test is obtained by administering 1 mg oral dexamethasone at 11 PM followed by an 8 AM serum cortisol determination the next morning. Patients without hypercortisolism should have a cortisol value <5 μm per dL with this test. Urinary free cortisol measurement is also useful.

To establish whether the corticotropin-dependent or corticotropin-independent form is present, it is necessary to measure plasma ACTH at basal levels. If ACTH is normal or elevated, this implies corticotropin-dependent pathophysiology. A high-dose (8 mg) dexamethasone suppression test typically reveals that patients with Cushing disease suppress, while those with ectopic ACTH syndrome do not. Selective venous catheterization of bilateral petrosal venous sinuses during corticotropin-releasing hormone stimulation can confirm pituitary hypersecretion of ACTH. Patients with ectopic ACTH secretion usually have markedly elevated corticotropin levels, often >200 pg per mL. If corticotropin levels are low or undetectable, the suppression of the hypothalamic-pituitary axis is caused by cortisol-secreting adrenal tumor.

Adrenal imaging is useful in the setting of hypercortisolism. Since secondary adrenal stimulation caused by ACTH excess predictably affects both adrenals, imaging is most helpful in the setting of corticotropin-independent Cushing syndrome. CT and MRI scanning of the adrenals can document unilateral or bilateral enlargement. Functional correlation can be provided by 6-iodomethyl-norcholesterol (NP-59) or selenium 75-selenomethyl norcholesterol scintigraphy. Bilateral adrenocortical hyperplasia from corticotropin-dependent disease is indicated by bilateral radionuclide uptake. An adrenocortical adenoma is indicated by unilateral dense uptake concordant with cross-sectional imaging and suppression of contralateral adrenal uptake (Fig. 39-4). This pattern is a very sensitive indication that the hypothalamic-pituitary axis is suppressed and that, consequently, steroids will be required after adrenalectomy. If a patient with Cushing syndrome and a large unilateral mass has no concordant uptake on scintigraphy, concern for adrenocortical carcinoma should be greatly heightened.

The treatment of Cushing disease is usually accomplished by (a) trans-sphenoidal microsurgery to remove pituitary tumor, (b) external or interstitial pituitary irradiation, or (c) pharmacologic therapy. Bilateral adrenalectomy is occasionally indicated (a) if trans-sphenoidal resection is not possible or not successful, (b) if hypercortisolism is rapidly progressive and particularly severe, (c) if palliation of ectopic ACTH syndrome is required, or (d) if the patient has primary adrenal hyperplasia. Up to 50% of patients with pituitary Cushing disease require bilateral adrenalectomy (19). Adrenalectomy can often be accomplished by a laparoscopic approach, and an associated increased quality of life has been documented (20). Recovery is often prolonged and incomplete. Approximately 30% of patients

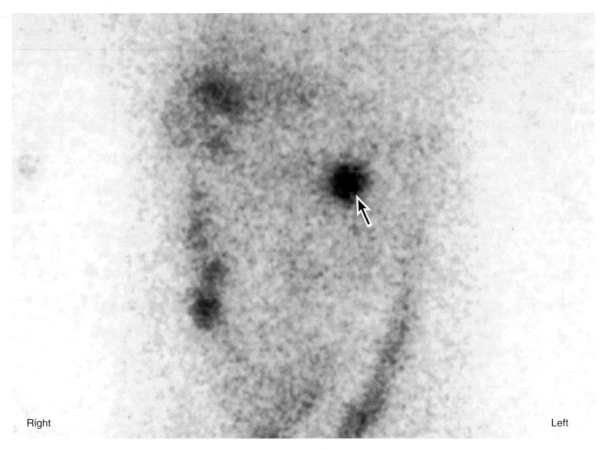

Right   Left

Figure 39-4 Anterior view of NP-59 adrenal scintigraphy in a 16-year-old woman with Cushing syndrome. This imaging pattern was concordant with the 2.4-cm left adrenal mass noted on cross-sectional imaging. Adrenal activity is indicated by the arrow. Note that the contralateral adrenal is not seen and thus its function is not suppressed.

remain hypertensive, 20% continue to have diabetes, and 20% remain obese (21).

Until the last two decades, adrenalectomy in patients with hypercortisolism was associated with significant morbidity (about 30%) and mortality (5% to 10%). In recent series the outcomes have improved appreciably to a range that approaches that of treatment of other adrenal diseases. Approximately 10% of patients will have a complication such as hemorrhage, deep venous thrombosis, pulmonary embolus, respiratory failure, coagulopathy, pneumonia, or wound infection. Complication rates are lowest in patients requiring unilateral adrenalectomy (10% morbidity, 1% mortality) and are improved by the laparoscopic approach. In general, patients requiring unilateral adrenalectomy for a hypersecreting cortical adenoma have better long-term outcomes than patients requiring bilateral adrenalectomy for medically refractory disease. Patients undergoing unilateral adrenalectomy have gradual disappearance of the signs and symptoms of hypercortisolism and have excellent long-term survival. Although the metabolic derangements tend to improve in the months following operation, it may take up to 12 months for some of the physical changes, such as hirsutism, obesity, and acne, to reverse.

If the source of ectopic ACTH syndrome can be localized and safely resected, this is the most effective treatment. Due to the small size of some tumors, such as bronchial tumors or carcinoid tumors, localization is not always possible. In that case palliative pharmacologic treatment with ketoconazole, mitotane, or octreotide is indicated. If this therapy is not effective in controlling hypercortisolemia, bilateral adrenalectomy is indicated. In general, long-term prognosis of patients with ectopic ACTH syndrome is poor. Some patients (bronchial carcinoid or medullary thyroid carcinoma) may live for years with residual neoplasm while others (e.g., with pancreatic carcinoid or lung carcinomas) have short survival.

Pheochromocytoma

Pheochromocytoma is a tumor derived from the adrenal medulla. This tumor's functional nature demands accurate and early preoperative diagnosis. Although pheochromocytoma is present in only 0.1% to 1% of hypertensive patients, the overall incidence is approximately 1 to 2 per 100,000. Despite improved clinical understanding of the syndrome, many patients still go undiagnosed. For patients with pheochromocytoma discovered at autopsy, most have died suddenly from myocardial infarction or cerebrovascular accident, and pheochromocytoma remains a cause of sudden death.

The clinical presentation of pheochromocytoma includes a wide array of symptoms. The most typical are headache, sweating, palpitations, and episodic hypertension. Less common symptoms include nausea, anxiety, abdominal pain, pallor, and exacerbation of hyperglycemia. Hypertension is sustained in approximately 50%. The presentation can occasionally be acute and severe, involving massive catecholamine release from tumor necrosis and leading to critical hypertension and subsequent cardiovascular collapse. Pheochromocytoma must always be considered in the gravid patient with a hypertensive crisis during pregnancy or labor.

The diagnosis requires discriminating clinical suspicion and biochemical confirmation. Serum or urine catecholamine levels are often inaccurate and difficult to interpret. Metabolites of catecholamines (metanephrines, normetanephrines, and vanillylmandelic acid) can be measured in the urine with acceptable sensitivity and specificity. Plasma metanephrine and normetanephrine levels are currently supplanting urinary tests due to excellent sensitivity, very good specificity, and improved patient ease (22).

When biochemical testing supports the diagnosis of pheochromocytoma, evidence of an adrenal tumor is sought, typically, by abdominal CT or MRI scanning (Fig. 39-5). Since 10% of pheochromocytomas are extra-adrenal, additional anatomic and functional imaging may be required. [123]I or ^{131}I metaiodobenzylguanidine (MIBG) is a radionuclide that concentrates in abnormal adrenergic tissue. MIBG can be very useful in defining the presence of

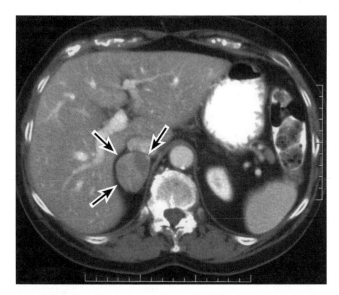

Figure 39-5 CT scan of a 71-year-old woman with intermittent hypertension, pounding chest sensations, headaches, and elevation of plasma metanephrine levels. The arrows indicate a 3.8-cm right adrenal pheochromocytoma.

metastatic or extraadrenal disease. In the patient with clear-cut clinical and biochemical evidence of pheochromocytoma and a unilateral adrenal mass on CT scan, MIBG scanning adds little additional preoperative information (Fig. 39-6) (23).

Although the first resection of a pheochromocytoma was performed in 1926, adrenalectomy remained an operation that was associated with high rates of morbidity and mortality until the introduction of phentolamine for α receptor blockade and norepinephrine for postresection hypotension. Outcomes have improved substantially in the last decades. In large part, complications are related to the hemodynamic pathophysiology associated with the tumor and its removal. The specific surgical approach does not seem to influence outcomes in any important way. Although there was initial worry about the suitability of the laparoscopic approach, due to concerns about the pressure of insufflation, manipulation pressure on the tumor, and incomplete resection, the approach is generally as safe as standard open operation (24–26).

Overall, the risk of recurrence approximates 10%. This number is not based on specific data, and long-term outcomes after resection for pheochromocytoma are influenced by factors such as sporadic or familial disease and clinical evidence of malignancy.

Adrenocortical Carcinoma

Although accounting for a tiny fraction of human malignancies, adrenal cancer remains one of the most malignant of endocrine tumors. Incidence is about 1 to 2 per million population and adrenocortical carcinoma is slightly more common in women (60%) than men (40%). Approximately 40% of patients have metastases at the time of diagnosis and overall 5-year survival is poor (27,28). More than 50% of patients have evidence of associated hormonal overproduction, typically cortisol, occasionally androgens/estrogens, or aldosterone. Tumors may be hormonally silent as well.

Complete surgical resection is the only potentially curative therapy. Adjuvant systemic chemotherapy, adrenolytic agents, and external beam radiotherapy have not met with success. Completeness of resection is the strongest predictor of outcome in this disease. The 5-year actuarial survival following potentially curative resection ranges from 32% to 48% (29). If curative resection requires removal of tumor thrombus in the renal vein or inferior vena cava or extended local resection, this circumstance does not necessarily predict a poor prognosis unless gross residual tumor remains. If patients undergo incomplete initial resection, prognosis is uniformly poor with median survival <1 year (29). Pathologic factors associated with short survival include large tumor size (>12 cm), high histologic grade (≥6 mitotic figures per 10 hpf), and intratumoral hemorrhage (30).

The impact of systemic chemotherapy and agents such as mitotane upon survival is very difficult to ascertain.

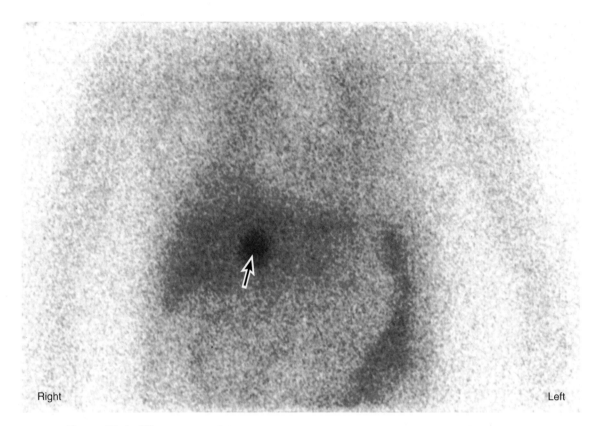

Right   Left

Figure 39-6 ^{123}I MIBG scan of the same patient as in Figure 39-5. Concentration of the radionu-clide in the right adrenal (*arrow*) confirms that the known mass is a pheochromocytoma.

Although many regimens have produced rare complete responses and occasional partial responses, it is difficult to translate these retrospective data into coherent clinical practice.

Approximately 40% of patients develop local recurrence or distant metastases after attempted curative resection, with a mean disease-free interval of 22 months (31). Approximately 40% of patients with recurrence are amenable to reoperation and have a 5-year survival of 50%. Patients who do not undergo resection have a 5-year survival of 8% (31).

Adrenal Incidentaloma

An "incidentaloma" is a mass of the adrenal gland discovered serendipitously that is unrelated to the patient's clinical presentation. With the increase in high resolution cross-sectional imaging of the abdomen, it has become apparent that these tumors are relatively common—up to 4% of patients undergoing abdominal CT and 7% of autopsies (32,33). Most are nonthreatening in nature as nonfunctioning cortical adenomas. However, about 10% of adrenocortical carcinomas are initially discovered as incidental adrenal masses, highlighting the need for appropriate workup (Fig. 39-7). Whenever a mass is discovered, it is compulsory to complete a basic workup to determine (a) whether the mass is associated with hormonal hyperfunction and (b) whether it is an adrenal malignancy, primary, or secondary. All patients should undergo biochemical testing to exclude hyperaldosteronism, hypercortisolism, and pheochromocytoma. The minimum level of testing includes a serum potassium, 24-hour urinary free cortisol or 1 mg dexamethasone suppression test, and measurement of metanephrines in a timed urine collection or in plasma. Further testing, such as levels of aldosterone, plasma renin, ACTH, and dehydroepiandrosterone (DHEA), is obtained if dictated by clinical features. The specific characteristics of cross-sectional imaging often clarify the possibility of malignancy. The tumor's density and the postcontrast density (washout calculation) are very useful in determining which tumors are likely to be lipid rich adenomas and in classifying the remaining tumors as "something else"—often a tumor that will ultimately require therapy.

The workup of an incidentaloma is aimed at segregating lesions into those that should be treated with resection (cortical adenoma causing Conn syndrome or Cushing syndrome, pheochromocytoma, adrenocortical carcinoma) or observation (small benign nonfunctional cortical adenoma). Despite these efforts, many patients fall outside these categories and have an incidentaloma of uncertain significance that requires resection. An example of this dilemma is a patient without evidence of hormonal hyperfunction but with large adrenal masses (>4 cm) that may or may not have atypical imaging characteristics, such

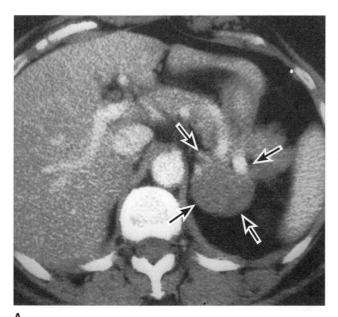
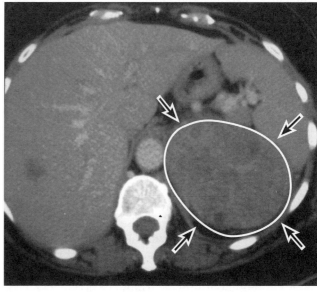

A

B

Figure 39-7 These paired images indicate the importance of the workup of the incidental adrenal mass (*arrows*). Initially, this 64-year-old woman had the CT scan **(A)** performed after a motor vehicle accident. The left adrenal abnormality was ascribed to trauma. Five years later, another CT scan **(B)** revealed a 13-cm left adrenal mass typical for adrenocortical carcinoma as well as small liver metastases.

as an increased density per CT scan or delayed contrast washout.

Avoiding needle biopsy of an adrenal mass may prevent potential complications during workup. With the exception of a patient with a primary malignancy, such as lung, renal cell, breast, or melanoma, whereby a secondary adrenal metastasis is possible, there is no real role for needle biopsy. The test is not sensitive for discrimination of benign and malignant tissue. Needle biopsy can be critically dangerous if the tumor is a pheochromocytoma. If the tumor is an adrenocortical carcinoma, the capsule will be broken, which can lessen the curative potential of subsequent resection.

IDENTIFICATION AND MODIFICATION OF PREOPERATIVE RISK FACTORS

General Risks

As with any major surgical procedure, the patient needs to be assessed for pulmonary and cardiac comorbidities as well as risk for deep venous thrombosis and related pulmonary embolism. Patients with significant limitation of pulmonary function may be guided toward a laparoscopic approach if it is clinically appropriate, since postoperative pain and respiratory impact will be less than with an open approach. Patients with significant CO_2 retention need close monitoring during the insufflation associated with laparoscopy—especially during prolonged procedures.

With the exception of pheochromocytoma or significant intraoperative bleeding, the physiologic challenge of adrenalectomy is moderate. However, it is prudent to institute perioperative β-adrenergic blockade in patients with significant coronary artery disease. Patients with risk factors for postoperative deep venous thrombosis, such as obesity, age >40, malignancy, and previous deep venous thrombosis, should have perioperative prophylaxis. Deep venous thrombosis prophylaxis is a requisite for abdominal laparoscopic procedures as well.

Hyperaldosteronism

Once the diagnosis of primary hyperaldosteronism has been made, it is helpful to start the patient on spironolactone therapy (typical dose 100 mg PO b.i.d.) at least 2 weeks before operation. Therapy is usually effective in controlling blood pressure preoperatively and blunts mineralocorticoid-related electrolyte changes around the time of operation. If a patient is also receiving KCl supplementation, it is important to check the serum potassium level a few days after starting aldactone as potassium requirements may decrease substantially.

Hypercortisolism

There is a generally accepted, but poorly documented, observation that tissue integrity is lessened in Cushing syndrome so that intraoperative blood loss is increased. Many patients with hypercortisolism have diabetes or glucose intolerance. Perioperative attention to this factor is required to provide tight glucose control. The main specific risk of adrenalectomy for hypercortisolism is postoperative hypoadrenalism due to suppression of the hypothalamic/pituitary/adrenal axis. For this reason, preoperative stress dose steroids are given (100 mg hydrocortisone IV immediately preop). Postoperative replacement is usually required.

Pheochromocytoma

Preoperative pharmacologic preparation is mandatory to decrease hemodynamic complications. The minimum period for preparation is 7 to 10 days preoperatively. The most common method is to establish α-adrenergic blockade with phenoxybenzamine and later β-adrenergic blockade with an agent such as propranolol. Phenoxybenzamine should be started at a dose of 10 mg PO t.i.d. and titrated upward until mild orthostatic symptoms occur. Frequent blood pressure and pulse checks should be reported in order to manage dosage increases. A few patients are sensitive to the drug and may be well prepared on as little as 40 mg per day, but some patients can require as much as 400 mg per day. If the patient is on the maximum tolerated dose of phenoxybenzamine and tachycardia is present, propranolol should be started at 10 mg PO t.i.d. Alternative regimens such as calcium channel blockade with nicardipine can be as effective. An arterial line should be placed before operation because with intraoperative manipulation rapid and severe hemodynamic changes may occur.

Adrenocortical Carcinoma

The most important risks are related to hyperfunction and to the tumor's anatomic extent. If hypercortisolism exists, the patient will need perioperative stress dose steroids and ongoing postoperative supplementation. Although many adrenocortical cancers are regionally extensive or have intra-abdominal metastatic disease, aggressive resections are often appropriate. A safe operation to provide for gross total removal without capsular breach should be done.

For right-sided cancers, one must assess whether limited hepatic resection will be required for gross tumor removal and whether the tumor invades the superior pole of the kidney or the renal hilum, indicating the need for en bloc nephrectomy. Native renal function must be considered to determine that this is safe. If there is obliteration of the plane between the tumor and the inferior vena cava, the possibility of caval invasion or intracaval tumor thrombus extension must be considered. The extent of caval tumor should be investigated preoperatively with MRI with venous reconstruction, contrast venography, or intravascular ultrasound. If involvement is extensive, the patient must be prepared for potential thoracoabdominal access or venovenous bypass to facilitate caval resection and reconstruction.

For left-sided tumors, the considerations about possible nephrectomy are identical. The patient should be counseled on potential distal pancreatectomy or partial colectomy. If a splenectomy is potentially required, pneumococcal, meningococcal, and hemophilus influenza B vaccinations should be provided at least 2 weeks before operation.

Critical Principles of Patient Selection

Imprudent patient selection increases complication rates. A number of guiding principles offer the appropriate balance between short-term and long-term outcomes. In general, patients with a benign functioning adrenal tumor, such as cortical adenoma or pheochromocytoma, should be offered laparoscopic adrenalectomy unless specific contraindications exist—for example, prohibitively extensive previous surgery. If the tumor is small and benign but laparoscopic adrenalectomy is contraindicated, a posterior open approach may be appropriate as pain and disability is intermediate between laparoscopic and open anterior adrenalectomy. The posterior approach may also be useful in patients who are exceptionally obese where laparoscopic access is difficult or dangerous. If the tumor is an adrenocortical carcinoma, the patient should be offered open anterior adrenalectomy. If the tumor is exceptionally large and difficulty with exposure and vascular control is anticipated, a thoracoabdominal approach may best suit the situation.

Despite these guidelines, unclassified patients with "incidentalomas" of uncertain significance are not easily categorized as to operative approach. These patients usually require adrenalectomy due to the concern that the mass "might" be cancer. Since adrenocortical carcinomas should not be resected laparoscopically, the quandary is whether all these patients require open adrenalectomy. Thoughtful patient selection is key. Although there is no role for laparoscopic removal of a known or likely adrenocortical carcinoma (34), laparoscopic resection is appropriate for removal of indeterminate incidentalomas that could conceivably be small adrenocortical carcinomas. The rationale for this choice is that the benefits of laparoscopic adrenalectomy are clear and will be provided to many patients while the negative influence of inadvertent laparoscopic removal of adrenocortical carcinoma is not yet fully appreciated and will potentially affect fewer patients.

Criteria that guide patient selection include (a) tumor size, (b) tumor function, and (c) imaging characteristics. With few exceptions, lesions >6 cm in diameter should be removed by open anterior approach. Lesions <4 cm without evidence of hyperfunction may be observed longitudinally with removal reserved for demonstrated growth or change in function. Lesions between 4 cm and 6 cm should be completely resected by laparoscopic approach if (a) there are no contraindications to laparoscopy, (b) there are no suspicious functional characteristics, or (c) there are no suspicious imaging characteristics. Functional characteristics include excess secretion of androgens or cortisol, mixed excess secretion of aldosterone and cortisol, and excess secretion of estrogen secretion in a male. Suspicious cross-sectional imaging characteristics include (a) indistinct borders or unclear relationship to surrounding organs with obliteration of fat planes, (b) unenhanced density >10 Hounsfield units, (c) 15-minute delayed enhancement of contrast washout of <60%, and (d) absence of signal intensity loss on out-of-phase MRI. Nonvisualization on NP-59 scintigraphy, discordant compared to CT, is a concern for malignancy.

Open Anterior Adrenalectomy

An adrenal mass that is potentially an adrenocortical carcinoma should be resected by an open approach. Typically, this is accomplished via a bilateral subcostal or midline incision (Fig. 39-8). Occasionally, very large tumors may require thoracoabdominal access, especially if extensive en bloc resection with control of the inferior vena cava is required (Fig. 39-9). Vascular control may be required for the inferior vena cava, renal vessels, and aorta. Exposure must be adequate to allow en bloc resection of involved contiguous structures such as kidney, liver, spleen, and pancreas. If the

mass is an adrenocortical carcinoma, it is critical to avoid capsular breach and tumor spill. Blunt dissection should be avoided. If the tumor is a large pheochromocytoma, the adage of "dissecting the patient away from the tumor" should be heeded to avoid rough physical manipulation, which can provoke hypertension and intraoperative hemodynamic lability.

For right adrenalectomy, mobilization of the hepatic flexure of the colon and a partial Kocher maneuver is often required. The liver's right lobe is mobilized by dividing the triangular ligament. The lobe must be fully mobilized to a point that the posterior portion of the intrahepatic cava is widely seen. This exposure is necessary to determine the extent of suprahepatic caval involvement. If possible, it is useful to divide the inferior phrenic vascular pedicle to allow the tumor to be retracted slightly caudad as it is separated from the diaphragm. The tumor's lateral margin is mobilized. If there is substantial involvement of the vena cava, there are often large venous collaterals that require ligation. The tumor's inferior margin is separated from the kidney's superior pole. If there is evidence of transcapsular invasion of the renal parenchyma, the inferior margin of the resection is changed to mobilize the kidney en bloc, and the renal hilar vessels are defined.

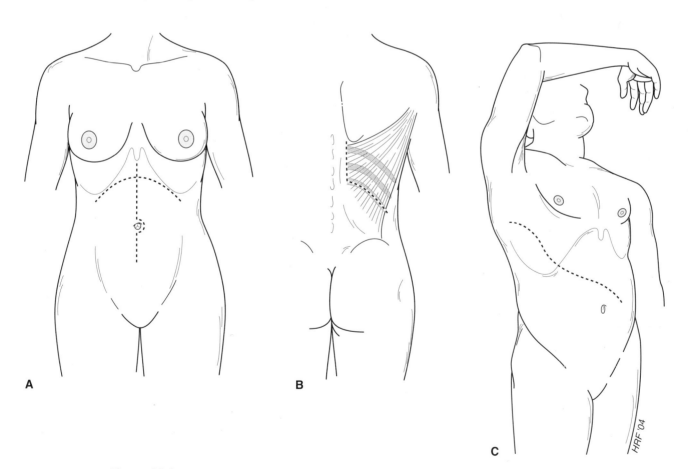

Figure 39-8 Standard incision placement for various open approaches to the adrenal gland: **A:** anterior; **B:** posterior; **C:** thoracoabdominal.

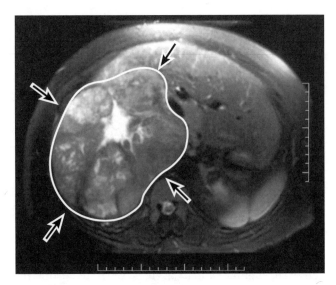

Figure 39-9 MRI of a 51-year-old woman with a 20-cm nonfunctioning low-grade adrenocortical carcinoma (*arrows*). The vena cava is severely compressed but not directly invaded.

If the opportunity arises to expose and divide the central adrenal vein early in the dissection, this vein should be transected. This is not often the case with large malignant masses, and in that circumstance the tumor should be mobilized until the central adrenal vein is the last major point of attachment. If there is transmural venous invasion or significant caval thrombus, partial caval resection may be required. If the resulting caval defect is elliptical, a patch of bovine pericardium or polytetrafluoroethylene (PTFE)

may be used. If the defect is circumferential, a ribbed PTFE interposition graft may be used, with the assistance of venovenous bypass circulation.

Preoperative cross-sectional imaging of large right-sided malignant masses often raises the concern of involvement of the adjacent hepatic parenchyma. If hepatic invasion limits curative resection, the dissection can proceed under Glisson capsule or with a nonanatomic hepatic parenchymal resection.

For open anterior left adrenalectomy, there are two main approaches to expose the adrenal tumor. The first approach involves opening the gastrocolic omentum and reflecting the splenic flexure of the colon caudad. From within the lesser sac, the inferior margin of the pancreas is mobilized and elevated to expose the adrenal tumor (Fig. 39-10). This maneuver is useful if the adrenal gland is located posterior to the pancreatic tail or slightly caudad. This approach may provide inadequate exposure if the adrenal gland is superior to the pancreatic tail. In that case an alternative approach involves dividing the superior and lateral splenic attachments to mobilize the spleen and distal pancreas en bloc via partial medial visceral rotation. It is often possible to expose and divide the central adrenal vein early in the dissection where it joins with the left renal vein. It is helpful to divide the inferior phrenic pedicle to allow some caudad retraction of the tumor. With large tumors, splenectomy may be necessary due to tumor invasion or to provide adequate exposure. An en bloc distal pancreatectomy may also be necessary because of local invasion. Nephrectomy may be required for renal parenchymal invasion or hilar vessel involvement.

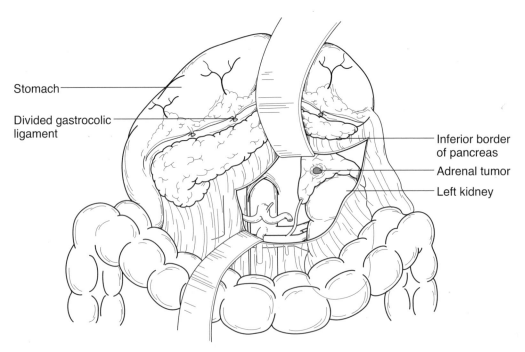

Stomach

Divided gastrocolic ligament

Inferior border of pancreas

Adrenal tumor

Left kidney

Figure 39-10 Infrapancreatic approach to the left adrenal gland after division of the gastrocolic omentum to open the lesser sac.

Open Posterior Adrenalectomy

A direct route to the retroperitoneum can avoid the morbidity associated with major laparotomy. The disadvantage to the posterior approach is the relatively limited exposure and "tight" operating space. A hockey-stick type incision is carried down to the level of the ipsilateral paraspinous muscle and carried obliquely over the course of the 12th rib (Fig. 39-8). The latissimus dorsi fibers are divided and the paraspinous muscle is mobilized medially but not divided. The 12th rib is resected subperiosteally, avoiding the intercostal bundle. It is easy to violate the pleura here and enter the costophrenic sulcus—especially in the medial portion of the field. If the sacrospinous fascia is opened in the most caudad portion of the wound, pleural injury can usually be avoided. If pleural entry occurs, it is straightforward to evacuate the resultant air from the pleura and close this again. A tube thoracostomy is unnecessary if no pulmonary injury is incurred. When the retroperitoneum is entered, the kidney is palpated in the deep medial aspect of the wound and gently pulled caudad to allow the adrenal mass to be exposed. Because of the limited space inside the wound, hemostatic clips are very useful for controlling the inferior phrenic vessels and the central adrenal vein. Because the adrenal gland is anatomically posterior to the inferior vena cava, the central adrenal vein is the last major structure seen and divided when removing the right adrenal gland by this approach. This effect is less pronounced on the left side where the central adrenal vein may be encountered and divided earlier in the dissection.

Open Thoracoabdominal Adrenalectomy

Because of the associated pulmonary morbidity of this approach, it is used only for very large malignant adrenal masses. Although occasionally necessary on the left side, a thoracoabdominal incision is most relevant to large right-sided adrenocortical carcinomas when venous involvement is present. The patient is positioned intermediate between supine and flank orientation with the table flexed (Fig. 39-8). A single incision is made over the 10th rib (11th on the left) and carried obliquely onto the abdomen. The rib is resected subperiosteally. The diaphragm is divided curvilinearly to limit denervation of fibers that are distributed from the central aspect. Superior retraction of the lung and anterior retraction of the right hepatic lobe provides wide exposure for adrenalectomy. Occasionally, this approach on the left may be accomplished without pleural entry. After adrenalectomy, the diaphragm and peritoneum are repaired. A tube thoracostomy is necessary if the pleural cavity is entered.

Laparoscopic Transperitoneal Adrenalectomy

The patient is secured in a beanbag pad in flank position with the table flexed. The arms must be padded and secured in gentle anterior flexion. Typical port placement is along the line of a subcostal incision with the exception of the camera port. It is often useful to place that port out of line with the others toward the umbilicus, which decreases intracorporeal instrument collisions. After a 30-degree surgical telescope is inserted, two additional ports are placed, one on either side, for instrumentation. An additional port is usually necessary for retraction of the right lobe of the liver after it is mobilized. The right lobe of the liver is mobilized by dividing the triangular ligament with an ultrasonic shears. This is done progressively to open the space anterolateral to the adrenal gland until the vena cava is seen. After division of Gerota fascia, blunt dissection between the vena cava and the medial margin of the gland will define the central adrenal vein. This vein is taken between endoscopic clips and divided. If the vein is particularly broad, division may require application of an endoscopic linear stapler. The inferior phrenic pedicle is divided after controlling small vessels with endoscopic clips. The remaining attachments include small arterial branches from the renal artery or aorta, which can be easily controlled with the endoscopic shears. The gland is removed in an endoscopic specimen bag.

For left-sided lesions, the port placement is similar; usually a fourth port is not necessary. After introduction of the 30 degree scope and instruments, the lateral attachments of the spleen are divided with ultrasonic shears. To begin this dissection it may be necessary to take down the splenic flexure of the colon. As the plane is developed, the spleen will begin to fall medially. The plane must be developed posterior to the pancreatic tail to locate the adrenal gland without injuring the pancreas. This dissection must be continued until the adrenal gland is seen, which will be nearly to the level of the aorta. Small glands may be obscured in retroperitoneal fat, especially in males and in patients with Cushing syndrome. Laparoscopic ultrasound can help identify the gland and indicate the proper target for exposure. Once the gland is located, it is circumferentially mobilized with ultrasonic shears. The inferior phrenic pedicle and the central adrenal vein are exposed with blunt dissection. These structures are controlled with endoscopic clips and divided. There is often an anastomotic vein between these two vessels, and it is important to divide these main veins at a level distal to the anastamosis to prevent bleeding. The central adrenal vein is often short, but it is usually not necessary to expose the left renal vein in order to safely divide it.

Laparoscopic Posterior Adrenalectomy

It is possible to provide access to the adrenal tumor's retroperitoneal location without traversing the peritoneal cavity. The patient is placed prone and the table flexed. The surgeon stands on the side of the gland to be resected. The first port is placed inferior to the tip of the 12th rib. The port may be placed by blunt technique or with a direct viewing trocar. The other ports are placed lateral to the paraspinous muscles in the posterior axillary line. After initial port placement, an inflatable balloon dissector is placed and expanded to create an operating space around the adrenal gland. This space is maintained with insufflation. The issues of vascular control are similar to those described above for the laparoscopic transperitoneal approach.

IDENTIFICATION AND MANAGEMENT OF POSTOPERATIVE COMPLICATIONS

Bleeding

Although usually avoided with careful and patient application of surgical technique, significant bleeding can occur with any approach to the adrenal gland. Hemorrhage is often from injury to the renal vein, inferior vena cava, or liver on the right or to the renal vein, splenic vein, or spleen on the left. Major bleeding during right adrenalectomy may be caused by failure to recognize the right hepatic vein or an aberrant central adrenal vein that drains into the right hepatic vein. Often, a hole in the inferior vena cava can be primarily repaired with suture venorrhaphy, but occasionally a patch of bovine pericardium or PTFE may be required to prevent iatrogenic inferior vena cava stenosis.

Glucocorticoid Insufficiency

This problem may occur if hypercortisolism with suppression of the hypophyseal pituitary adrenal axis is not recognized preoperatively and the patient is not adequately supplemented with corticosteroids perioperatively. Insufficiency will also occur after bilateral adrenalectomy if not actively prevented. Glucocorticoid insufficiency should be considered in any patient after adrenalectomy who develops hypotension, hyponatremia, hyperkalemia, hypoglycemia, and acidosis. If suspected, the problem should be treated immediately with intravenous hydrocortisone. Patients should receive 100 mg IV hydrocortisone every 6 hours on the day of the operation. Usually, 200 mg hydrocortisone distributed over postoperative day 1 and 100 mg over postoperative day 2 is adequate. When oral alimentation is established, the dose is converted and weaned to a maintenance dose of approximately 15 to 37.5 mg per day, divided into three doses. Following unilateral adrenalectomy, the recovery of the hypophyseal/pituitary/adrenal axis can be determined with a Cosyntropin stimulation test after approximately 3 months. An alternative strategy may apply to patients in whom the suppression of the hypophyseal/pituitary/adrenal axis is not certain. In this case a Cosyntropin stimulation test may be performed on the morning of postoperative day 1. This is done by administering 250 μg Cortrosyn IV. Cortisol measurements

are obtained at 0, 30, and 60 minutes after administration. A cortisol level ≥ 18 μ per dL indicates sufficient function. If the hypophyseal/pituitary/adrenal axis is intact, the patient will not need supplemental steroids but will still need to be counseled about the critical symptoms and signs of adrenal insufficiency.

Hernia

Incisional hernia can be a long-term complication of any approach to the adrenal gland. Hernia must be distinguished from segmental abdominal muscle relaxation due to denervation resulting from approaches such as the posterior or thoracoabdominal incisions that require rib resection. Although incisional hernia may be related to operative choices and techniques, it also appears to be more likely to occur in patients with hypercortisolism.

Hypertension

Hypertension can be an indication of incomplete resection of a hormonally active tumor. Especially with hyperaldosteronism, the patient may also be left with underlying essential hypertension even after excess aldosterone secretion is addressed. An occasional cause of postoperative hypertension may be inadvertent injury to a renal artery. This injury may not have been an obvious intraoperative event if only a superior polar vessel was ligated.

Hypotension

This complication can follow resection of pheochromocytoma. Hypotension is minimized by adequate preoperative pharmacologic preparation to decrease vasoconstriction and cardiac afterload as well as intraoperative hydration. Decisions about ongoing postoperative invasive blood pressure monitoring can be made in the recovery room. Sometimes vasoactive pressor therapy, including intravenous neosynephrine or norepinephrine, is required until regulatory homeostasis is restored.

Ileus

Ileus may occur with open approaches, such as the anterior and thoracoabdominal, but is less common with posterior and laparoscopic approaches. Ileus combined with fever and evidence of systemic inflammation should raise the suspicion of trocar or cautery injury to intestinal structures.

Mineralocorticoid Insufficiency

Patients generally do not require corticosteroid or electrolyte replacement. Mild postoperative hyperkalemia can be seen in the days following resection of an adrenal tumor causing hyperaldosteronism. A rare patient may experience transient mineralocorticoid deficiency, which can be corrected with oral fludrocortisone 0.1 mg daily. Patients undergoing bilateral adrenalectomy often require 0.1 to 0.2 mg fludrocortisone per day.

Nelson Syndrome

This is a unique complication of bilateral total adrenalectomy for Cushing disease that affects approximately 30% of long-term survivors. Nelson syndrome is characterized by ongoing pituitary enlargement and cutaneous pigmentation related to ACTH hypersecretion. The syndrome can be prevented in some patients by pituitary irradiation.

Pneumonia

Pneumonia is an unusual complication with less invasive approaches, but it can occur in the setting of significant postoperative pulmonary compromise associated with a thoracoabdominal or other extensive open approach. Pulmonary infection is treated as a nosocomial infection with appropriate antibiotic therapy.

Pneumothorax

Pneumothorax is a potential complication of thoracoabdominal or posterior approaches, but it should be considered if any adrenalectomy requires significant dissection around the diaphragmatic crus. If the problem is of significant size and physiologic impact, it needs to be treated with tube thoracostomy. The need for this is usually short-lived unless pulmonary parenchymal injury has occurred.

Subphrenic Abscess

Abscess is a rare complication usually limited to extensive resections of large adrenal tumors or the occasional patient with Cushing syndrome. Abscess can usually be treated with percutaneous radiologic placement of a drain.

Wound Infection

Because of the increased likelihood of this complication in patients with hypercortisolism compared to those with other indications for adrenalectomy, prophylactic antibiotics are indicated.

SUMMARY

Although the advent of laparoscopic adrenalectomy has changed the typical patient experience for most patients undergoing adrenalectomy for any benign tumor into a well tolerated, accelerated recovery, the trend belies the broad spectrum of adrenal diseases and difficult surgical management dilemmas. It is critical for any surgeon caring for these patients to have a broad understanding of adrenal diseases as well as options for treatment. Some of the older techniques are still appropriate for certain patients. It is only with judicious application of any of these techniques to patients that one can prevent complications and improve patient outcomes.

REFERENCES

1. Prinz R. A comparison of laparoscopic and open adrenalectomies. *Arch Surg* 1995;130:489–494.
2. Brunt LM, Doherty GM, Norton JA, et al. Laparoscopic adrenalectomy compared to open adrenalectomy for benign adrenal neoplasms. *J Am Coll Surg* 1996;183:1–10.
3. Conn JW. Primary aldosteronism: a new clinical syndrome. *J Lab Clin Med* 1955;45:3–17.
4. Young WF, Hogan MJ, Klee GG, et al. Primary hyperaldosteronism: diagnosis and treatment. *Mayo Clin Proc* 1990;65:96–110.
5. Blumenfeld JD, Sealey JE, Schlussel Y, et al. Diagnosis and treatment of primary hyperaldosteronism. *Ann Intern Med* 1994;121:877–885.
6. Hiramatsu K, Yamada T, Yukimura Y, et al. A screening test to identify aldosterone-producing adenoma by measuring plasma renin activity. Results in hypertensive patients. *Arch Intern Med* 1981;141:1589–1593.
7. Angelini L, Bezzi M, Chiarot M, et al. Primary hyperaldosteronism caused by monolateral adrenal hyperplasia. *Minerva Chir* 1995;50:131–137.
8. Hollak CE, Prummel MF, Tiel-van Buul MM. Bilateral adrenal tumours in primary aldosteronism: localization of a unilateral aldosteronoma by dexamethasone suppression scan. *J Intern Med* 1991;229:545–548.
9. Ikeda DM, Francis IR, Glazer GM, et al. The detection of adrenal tumors and hyperplasia and patients with primary aldosteronism: comparison of scintigraphy, CT, and MR imaging. *Am J Roentgenol* 1989;153:301–306.
10. Nomura K, Kusakabe K, Maki M, et al. Iodomethylnorcholesterol uptake in an aldosteronoma shown by dexamethasone-suppression scintigraphy: relationship to adenoma size and functional activity. *J Clin Endocrinol Metab* 1990;71:825–830.
11. Gross MD, Shapiro B, Grekin RJ, et al. Scintigraphic localization of adrenal lesions in primary aldosteronism. *Am J Med* 1984;77:839–844.
12. Obara T, Ito Y, Okamoto T, et al. Risk factors associated with postoperative persistent hypertension in patients with primary aldosteronism. *Surgery* 1992;112:987–993.
13. Proye CA, Mulliez EA, Carnaille BM, et al. Essential hypertension: first reason for persistent hypertension after unilateral adrenalectomy for primary hyperaldosteronism? *Surgery* 1998;124:1128–1133.
14. Simon D, Goretzki PE, Lollert A, et al. Persistent hypertension after successful adrenal operation. *Surgery* 1993;114:1189–1195.
15. Weigel RJ, Wells SA, Gunnells JC, et al. Surgical treatment of primary hyperaldosteronism. *Ann Surg* 1994;219:347–352.
16. Siren J, Valimaki M, Huikuri K, et al. Adrenalectomy for primary hyperaldosteronism: long-term follow-up study in 29 patients. *World J Surg* 1998;22:418–421.
17. Lo CY, Tam PC, Kung AW, et al. Primary hyperaldosteronism. Results of surgical treatment. *Ann Surg* 1996;224:125–130.
18. Shen WT, Lim RC, Sipperstein AE, et al. Laparoscopic vs. open adrenalectomy for the treatment of primary hyperaldosteronism. *Arch Surg* 1999;134:628–631.
19. Favia G, Boscaro M, Lumachi F, et al. Role of bilateral adrenalectomy in Cushing's disease. *World J Surg* 1994;18(4):462–466.
20. Hawn MT, Cook D, Deveney C, et al. Quality of life after laparoscopic bilateral adrenalectomy for Cushing's disease. *Surgery* 2002;132:1064–1068.

21. Grabner P, Hauer-Jensen M, Jervell J, et al. Long-term results of treatment of Cushing's disease by adrenalectomy. *Eur J Surg* 1991;157:461–464.

22. Marini M, Fathi M, Vallotton M. Determination of serum metanephrines in the diagnosis of pheochromocytoma. *Ann Endocrinol* 1994;54:337–342.

23. Miskulin J, Shulkin BL, Doherty GM, et al. Is preoperative ^{123}I MIBG scintigraphy routinely necessary before initial adrenalectomy for pheochromocytoma? *Surgery* 2003;134:918–923.

24. Fernandez-Cruz L, Saenz A, Benarroch B, et al. Does hormonal function of the tumor influence the outcome of laparoscopic adrenalectomy? *Surg Endosc* 1996;10:1088–1091.

25. Fernandez-Cruz L, Saenz A, Kuriansky J, et al. Laparoscopic adrenalectomy for pheochromocytoma. *Acta Chir Austriaca* 1999;31:203–206.

26. Gagner M, Breton G, Pharand D, et al. Is laparoscopic adrenalectomy indicated for pheochromocytomas? *Surgery* 1996;120:1076–1080.

27. Icard P, Chapuis Y, Andreassian B, et al. Adrenocortical carcinoma in surgically treated patients. A retrospective study on 156 cases by the French Association of Endocrine Surgery. *Surgery* 1992;112:972–979.

28. Venkatesh S, Hickey RC, Sellin RV, et al. Adrenal cortical carcinoma. *Cancer* 1989;64:765–769.

29. Dackiw APB, Lee JE, Gagel RF, et al. Adrenal cortical carcinoma. *World J Surg* 2001;25:914–926.

30. Harrison LE, Gaudin PB, Brennan MF. Pathologic features of prognostic significance for adrenocortical carcinoma after curative resection. *Arch Surg* 1999;134:181–185.

31. Bellantone R, Ferrante A, Boscherini M, et al. Role of reoperation in recurrence of adrenal cortical carcinoma: results from 188 cases collected in the Italian national registry for adrenal cortical carcinoma. *Surgery* 1997;122:1212–1218.

32. Lee JE, Evans DB, Hickey RC, et al. Unknown primary cancer presenting as an adrenal mass: frequency and implications for diagnostic evaluation of adrenal incidentalomas. *Surgery* 1998;124:1115–1122.

33. Abecassis M, McLoughlin MJ, Langer B, et al. Serendipitous adrenal masses: prevalence, significance, and management. *Am J Surg* 1985;149:783–788.

34. Kebebew E, Sipperstein AE, Clark OH, et al. Results of laparoscopic adrenalectomy for suspected and unsuspected malignant adrenal neoplasms. *Arch Surg* 2002;137:948–953.

Complications of Thyroid and Parathyroid Surgery

40

Gerard M. Doherty

■ INTRODUCTION 575

■ THYROID SURGERY 576
Diagnostic Thyroid Evaluation 576
Therapeutic Thyroidectomy 577
Thyroid Carcinoma 577
Graves Disease 578
Goiter 578

■ POTENTIAL COMPLICATIONS OF THYROIDECTOMY 578

■ NECK HEMATOMA 579

■ HYPOPARATHYROIDISM 579

■ NERVE INJURIES 581

■ AIRWAY MANAGEMENT 583

■ INJURY TO OTHER CERVICAL STRUCTURES 584

■ IATROGENIC HYPERTHYROIDISM OR HYPOTHYROIDISM 585

■ PARATHYROID SURGERY 585

■ INDICATIONS FOR OPERATION IN PATIENTS WITH PRIMARY HYPERPARATHYROIDISM 585

■ INDICATIONS FOR OPERATION IN PATIENTS WITH SECONDARY HYPERPARATHYROIDISM 586

■ CURRENT PROCEDURE STRATEGIES 586
Initial Operation 586
Reoperation 587

■ POTENTIAL COMPLICATIONS OF PARATHYROIDECTOMY 587

■ HYPOPARATHYROIDISM 587

■ NERVE INJURY 587

■ PERSISTENT OR RECURRENT HYPERPARATHYROIDISM 589

■ SUMMARY 591

■ REFERENCES 591

Gerard M. Doherty: University of Michigan, Ann Arbor, MI 48109

INTRODUCTION

Thyroid and parathyroid operations are generally safe procedures with rare life-threatening complications. Although the complications common to any operation, such as bleeding, infection, and anesthetic reactions, can occur, they are all quite unusual. Bleeding during the procedures is limited, and almost never is enough blood lost to require transfusion. Bleeding following the procedure can cause dangerous local effects, but it still rarely requires blood replacement. The neck is a privileged site for wound healing, with a robust blood supply to the skin and soft tissue that can withstand substantial contamination without clinical infection. These procedures are typically performed as ambulatory or overnight hospitalizations, with short (1 to 3 hours) general or regional anesthetic techniques, thus limiting the risk of anesthetic or pulmonary complications and deep venous thrombotic events.

In spite of these features, cervical endocrine surgery is considered a delicate, somewhat risky area of clinical practice. Significant technical complications can occur that can create permanent, life-altering changes in the patient's function. The most common of these are hypoparathyroidism and nerve injury. Other less frequent complications include cervical hematoma and aerodigestive tract damage. Finally, failure of the operative strategy to fulfill its goals, as with persistent hyperparathyroidism, can complicate overall patient care.

THYROID SURGERY

Thyroid operations are performed to manage actual or potential malignancy, thyroid hyperfunction, or thyromegaly producing local symptoms from compression of surrounding structures. The indications and strategies for these procedures will be considered in their clinical contexts.

Diagnostic Thyroid Evaluation

The diagnostic evaluation of a thyroid nodule addresses two issues: (i) Is the nodule or the remaining thyroid hyperfunctional? and (ii) Is the nodule malignant? All patients have a thorough history and physical examination, with a focus on the personal history of thyroid disease and radiation exposure, the family history of thyroid diseases, and the physical features in the neck, including regional adenopathy. An ultrasound evaluation of the thyroid is a part of the physical examination and should accompany all thyroid nodule evaluations. Patients with personal history of therapeutic or accidental (but not, apparently, diagnostic) doses of radiation exposure (>2500 cGy) to the thyroid have an increased risk of both thyroid nodules and thyroid cancer, with a latency of 2 to 4 decades; this information can change the diagnostic scheme and, in particular, leads most surgeons to remove the entire thyroid if any operative procedure is necessary (1,2). A family history of thyroid disease is very common and may include a variety of benign or malignant diagnoses within one family. Often, different family members will have multinodular goiter, papillary thyroid cancer, Graves disease, or Hashimoto thyroiditis in

a variety of first-degree relatives. These families seem to have a predilection to develop any one of several thyroid conditions. In addition, there are specific heritable genetic defects that can predispose to papillary (Familial Adenomatous Polyposis—APC gene) or medullary (Multiple Endocrine Neoplasia Type 2 syndromes—*Ret* proto-oncogene) thyroid cancers. Evidence of these abnormalities should prompt further evaluation and genetic counseling.

Thyroid ultrasound adds very useful information to the evaluation of thyroid nodules (3–5). It can accurately characterize the size, nature (solid vs. cystic), and texture (homogeneous, macrocalcifications or microcalcifications, smooth or irregular margins) of the index nodule, as well as the remainder of the thyroid gland. Since the thyroid gland can be difficult to reproducibly and accurately investigate on physical examination alone, ultrasound is critical. Ultrasound can also be used to guide tissue sampling. Thyroid function tests, specifically including thyroid stimulating hormone (TSH) and tetraiodothyronine (T4) levels, demonstrate the status of the pituitary-thyroid axis and the physiologic appropriateness of thyroid hormone production. Notably, the only clinical situation in which thyroid scintigraphy (nuclear medicine scanning) is currently useful in the diagnostic evaluation of a thyroid nodule is when the patient is hyperthyroid (6,7). It allows distinction between a hyperfunctioning nodule with suppressed surrounding thyroid parenchyma and a neoplastic nodule in Graves disease.

For the most typical patient, one who is euthyroid with a dominant solitary nodule, the mainstay of the diagnostic evaluation is fine needle aspiration cytology (6–11). This procedure is done in the clinic, often under ultrasound guidance, and provides the best information to address whether the nodule is malignant. The potential results are (i) malignant, prompting specific therapy; (ii) benign, prompting interval follow-up evaluation for most patients; (iii) insufficient sample, prompting repeat needle aspiration cytology; and (iv) indeterminate. Indeterminate aspirations imply that there is adequate cellular material for assessment but that the diagnosis is uncertain because of the lesion's nature. This frequently occurs with follicular lesions of the thyroid gland. In this clinical situation the next best step is typically a diagnostic thyroid resection.

The minimum appropriate procedure for assessing the nature of a potentially malignant thyroid lesion is lobectomy and isthmusectomy (12–15). This should include some gross margin of normal thyroid gland between the line of division and the lesion in question. The complications of removing one side of the thyroid gland are similar to the complications of total thyroidectomy, with some important distinctions. First, because a single functional parathyroid gland is sufficient to maintain normal parathyroid control of calcium flux and there are parathyroid glands on each side of the larynx, it is not possible to produce permanent hypoparathyroidism by thyroid lobectomy. Second, although injury to the ipsilateral

TABLE 40-1

THERAPEUTIC THYROIDECTOMY INDICATIONS

Thyroid lobectomy
> Solitary toxic nodule
> Unilateral benign adenoma or cyst producing local symptoms
> Best-prognosis thyroid cancers

Total thyroidectomy
> Most thyroid carcinoma
> Graves disease
> Hashimoto thyroiditis
> Toxic multinodular goiter
> Symptomatic multinodular goiter
> Substernal goiter (most)

TABLE 40-2

CLASSIFICATION OF THYROID CARCINOMA

Cell of Origin	Tumor Type	Subtypes
Follicular cell		
	Papillary	
		Classic
		Follicular variant
		Tall cell
		Diffuse sclerosing
	Follicular	
		Minimally invasive
		Hürthle cell
		Insular
	Anaplastic	
C cell		
	Medullary	
Lymphocyte		
	Lymphoma	

recurrent laryngeal nerve (RLN) can produce permanent voice changes, thyroid lobectomy does not carry a risk of bilateral recurrent nerve injury and consequent airway occlusion. Finally, for most patients who require only unilateral thyroidectomy, there is no need for thyroid hormone replacement therapy, thus eliminating the possibility of iatrogenic hyperthyroidism or hypothyroidism.

Therapeutic Thyroidectomy

Thyroidectomy has a major role in the therapy of several thyroid processes (Table 40-1). For patients with unilateral, symptomatic lesions, thyroid lobectomy can be the therapeutic procedure of choice and carries risks similar to diagnostic lobectomy. For most patients requiring therapeutic thyroidectomy, however, the procedure involves resection of both lobes of the thyroid gland (total thyroidectomy).

Thyroid Carcinoma

Thyroid carcinoma can be categorized based on the cell of origin and the tumor's growth pattern (Table 40-2). The follicular-cell derived thyroid cancers are by far the most common, and the bulk of these (75% or more) are well-differentiated papillary thyroid cancers with an excellent long-term survival. A variety of prognostic scoring systems are available to categorize the probable patient outcome. One of the most used and easiest to apply, because the information is available soon after resection, is the MACIS system (Table 40-3) (16). There is a subgroup of patients that comprises the very best prognosis lesions: women <45 years of age with tumors that measure 10 mm or less in diameter and that are confined entirely to the thyroid gland, with no thyroid capsule invasion or lymph node metastasis. All investigators agree that this group does not benefit from the additional dissection done for a total thyroidectomy and can be treated by thyroid lobectomy (13,14,17,18). For most patients, however, there is some advantage to total thyroidectomy, mainly in improved disease-free survival rather than overall or cause-specific mortality. Improved disease-free survival releases the patient from the need for additional

episodes of care and the associated potential side effects, complications, and time lost. The magnitude of the advantage is more substantial for some groups than others. In general, being older, male, having a larger tumor, and having spread of disease outside of the thyroid gland each individually correlate with having a greater risk of recurrence or

TABLE 40-3

MACIS THYROID CANCER PROGNOSIS CLASSIFICATION SYSTEM

Acronym	Feature	Score
M	Metastasis	Add 3.0 if distant metastasis present
A	Age	Add 3.1 if age <40 y *or* add 0.08 X age
C	Completeness of surgical resection	Add 1.0 if the surgical resection leaves gross tumor in place
I	Invasiveness (local)	Add 1.0 if there is local extrathyroidal invasion by tumor
S	Size	Add 0.3 X tumor size

Patient Total Score	Predicted 20 Year Cause-specific Survival from Mayo Clinic Data	Fraction of Total Group
<6.0	>99%	>80%
6.0–6.9	89%	
7.0–7.9	56%	
>8.0	24%	<5%

From Hay ID, Bergstralh EJ, Goellner JR, et al. Predicting outcome in papillary thyroid carcinoma: development of a reliable prognostic scoring system in a cohort of 1779 patients surgically treated at one institution during 1940 through 1989. *Surgery* 1993;114:1050–1057; discussion 1057–1058, with permission.

death, or both. These patients benefit from total thyroidectomy and further adjuvant therapy with radioiodine and thyroid hormone suppression of TSH (13,19).

For anaplastic cancer and lymphoma, the role of operative intervention is mainly for diagnosis, although it is occasionally for palliative resection (20–23). In these specific situations the tumor is often quite extensive, and so incisional biopsy to supply tissue for pathologic analysis is appropriate (in contrast to diagnostic lobectomy, above). Anaplastic thyroid carcinoma is an extremely aggressive, poorly differentiated tumor derived from thyroid follicular cells. Resection is often not possible, and even when it is feasible it is typically unsuccessful at controlling this rapidly progressive process. Lymphoma is generally treated by radiation and chemotherapy once the diagnosis and cell type is secure.

Graves Disease

Graves disease is an autoimmune condition in which stimulated autoantibodies form against the TSH receptor on thyroid cells. These antibodies stimulate the thyroid gland to grow and to overproduce thyroid hormone. The therapeutic options for Graves disease include radioiodine therapy (by far the most common treatment chosen in the United States), chronic antithyroid medications (propylthiouracil or methimazole), or total thyroidectomy. Total thyroidectomy is a very effective strategy for Graves disease, and it has the advantage of resolving the issue quickly and definitively; repeat treatments are often necessary for radioiodine to eradicate the hyperthyroidism. However, most patients would prefer the radioiodine approach in order to avoid the pain, scar, and potential complications of operation. There are some clinical situations, however, in which radioiodine therapy is contraindicated or less desirable than resection (Table 40-4).

The complications of total thyroidectomy for Graves disease are unique only in the frequent severity of the

hypocalcemia that can follow the operation (24–27). Patients with Graves disease often have significant bone demineralization as an effect of their hyperthyroidism. After operation, they can have an acute drop in serum levels of calcium requiring replacement that is sometimes accompanied by an early fall in serum PTH and subsequent rise of PTH to supernormal levels (temporary secondary hyperparathyroidism). It appears that both a sudden correction of the hyperthyroidism and some insult to the parathyroid glands are necessary since (i) similar hypocalcemia does not follow radioiodine therapy for Graves, when the decrease in hyperthyroidism is much slower and (ii) there is no hypocalcemia after thyroid lobectomy for toxic adenoma when two parathyroid glands have been left undisturbed.

Goiter

Goiter is a general term for an enlarged thyroid and is usually reserved for benign processes that diffusely affect the gland. The gland may be normally active, hyperactive, or hypoactive. The goiter can result from any of several processes, including generalized hyperplasia, multiple hyperplastic nodules, or Hashimoto thyroiditis. The most common indication for resection is local compression of adjacent structures. Patients develop difficulty in swallowing as the most frequent symptom of cervical compression. Pressure on the larynx can cause a "tightening" of the voice, which sounds more high-pitched and constricted in range than usual for the patient; the patient is often more sensitive to this than others. This voice change is from laryngeal compression rather than from effects on the RLN. True hoarseness from nerve compression with vocal cord paralysis is unusual with benign conditions and should raise suspicion of unrecognized malignancy. Enlargement of a substernal goiter is more likely to cause compression of the trachea. Patients may complain of difficulty breathing with exercise, as peak airway flow is limited, or they may develop symptoms when recumbent in a supine position, as the weight of the anterior mediastinal thyroid further compresses the trachea (28,29).

The resection for goiter is planned to relieve the local compressive symptoms. This is generally very successful, although the temporary edema following operation may mask the improvement for several weeks. Resection carries all of the same complication risks as operation for other indications. In addition, operation for Hashimoto thyroiditis can be difficult because of the local inflammation that is inherent in the disease. Most patients with Hashimoto thyroiditis require no therapy beyond thyroid replacement; resection is not routinely necessary.

POTENTIAL COMPLICATIONS OF THYROIDECTOMY

The potential complications of thyroid operations include the immediate complication of cervical hematoma, as well

---

TABLE 40-4

INDICATIONS FOR OPERATIVE THERAPY IN GRAVES DISEASE

Increased radioiodine risk
    Pregnancy
    Desire to become pregnant within 6 months
    Childhood/adolescence

Decreased effectiveness of therapeutic radioiodine
    Large goiter
    Severe thyrotoxicosis requiring rapid control
    Amiodarone-induced thyrotoxicity

Associated conditions
    Coexistent suspicious thyroid nodule
    Coexistent hyperparathyroidism

Patient preference

as the more chronic complications of hypoparathyroidism, nerve injury, and injuries to the aerodigestive tract. Finally, chronic problems can arise from iatrogenic hyperthyroidism or hypothyroidism.

NECK HEMATOMA

A neck hematoma requiring reoperation develops after operation in about 1 of every 150 thyroidectomies (30,31). The hematoma nearly always appears within 6 hours after the completion of the procedure, although with anticoagulation the hematoma can appear up to several days later. This complication is manifested by increasing pain, neck swelling, and often marked anxiety. The hematoma can collect either between the platysma muscle and the sternohyoid muscles (superficial) or deep to the strap muscles along the larynx (deep). The deep hematomas are the more dangerous as they can be sequestered on one side of the larynx, causing a shift and compression of the airway.

Although a minority of patients with postoperative hematomas develop airway compromise requiring emergent evacuation at the bedside, this possibility exists with every neck hematoma. *Patients with a hematoma of the neck should not be left alone until the hematoma has been evacuated.* Medical personnel with the capability of opening the wound to decompress the airway must stay with the patient until the situation is resolved. For most patients, the hematoma is less immediately threatening and the patient can be urgently returned to the operating room, placed under anesthesia, and the hematoma then evacuated and the bleeding controlled. Often no specific bleeding site can be identified at reoperation, although when one is found, the most likely areas are the anterior jugular veins under the platysma flaps, the superior pole vascular pedicle, and the vessels of the ligament of Berry, adjacent to the RLN insertion. Careful hemostasis during the initial operation is justified, with particular attention to these areas, to try to prevent this complication.

The risk of cervical hematoma has led some to question the safety of outpatient thyroidectomy, because there would be some possibility of the hematoma developing after discharge (30,31). The current experience with outpatient thyroid surgery by experts in the field has demonstrated that this can be done safely, although postoperative observation for 6 hours is routine in order to detect this complication prior to facility discharge (P. Logerfo, personal communication).

HYPOPARATHYROIDISM

The parathyroid glands are small, delicate structures that share a blood supply with the thyroid gland. Their diminutive size (normal 30 to 60 mg) and fragile nature make them particularly prone to damage during thyroidectomy.

Patients who have markedly diminished or absent parathyroid function after thyroidectomy have severe hypocalcemia that requires replacement. If permanent, calcium supplements can palliate this complication, but this requires multiple doses each day and uncomfortable symptoms occur if doses are late or missed. In addition, there is cumulative bone damage over time.

The symptoms of hypoparathyroidism are those of severe hypocalcemia. In the earliest phases patients have numbness and tingling in the distal extremities and around the mouth or tongue. With more severe hypocalcemia, patients develop muscle cramping at rest or especially with use. The anxiety that often accompanies these symptoms exacerbates them because the patient hyperventilates. The consequent respiratory alkalosis shifts more calcium intracellularly, lowering the serum level of calcium and worsening the symptoms. Severe tetany can result. Patients can then be limited in their ability to help themselves resolve the episode with calcium supplements, as their hands and forearms are often severely affected by the muscle spasms.

The classic signs of hypocalcemia are the Chvostek sign and the Trousseau sign. The Chvostek sign is generated by tapping gently over the facial nerve in the lateral cheek to demonstrate facial muscle contraction due to increased nerve irritability. This sign is present in some minority of people with a normal serum level of calcium, and so it is not entirely reliable in the diagnosis of hypocalcemia, but it can be helpful in following levels in some people. The Trousseau sign is elicited by placing a sphygmomanometer cuff on the upper arm and inflating to systolic pressure. Within a few minutes the patient develops severe carpal spasm, with flexion of the wrist and fingers and abduction of the thumb. This sign is very uncomfortable for the patient and should not be used clinically. In general, the symptoms of hypocalcemia are much more reliable and useful for patient assessment than the signs.

The acute management of hypocalcemia in the postoperative patient depends on the severity of the hypocalcemia and symptoms. Total serum calcium levels correlate roughly with symptoms but are quite variable among individuals. Some patients can have extremely low total serum levels of calcium with no symptoms, while others can have severe symptoms and signs with nearly normal calcium levels. Ionized calcium measurements correlate better than total serum calcium levels, but there is still variability. Replacement is generally guided by symptoms. For mild hypocalcemia with tingling, oral calcium supplements (calcium carbonate, 500 to 1500 mg PO, b.i.d.-q.i.d.) are often sufficient to resolve the hypocalcemia. Daily doses of calcium above 3,000 mg provide little incremental benefit, however, because of the limits of gastrointestinal absorption of calcium. If supplementation beyond this level is necessary (as it is for most patients with severe hypocalcemia), the addition of supplemental vitamin D (calcitriol 0.25 to 1.0 μg q.i.d.) will increase the gastrointestinal absorption of calcium. Vitamin D requires 48 to 72 hours to have its effect, however, so intravenous calcium supplementation may be needed until then. Anticipation of the need for vitamin D can smooth the patient management considerably by starting it early.

Hypocalcemia that is not controlled by oral supplements and not accompanied by severe symptoms such as muscle cramping is best managed by intravenous calcium administration. Intravenous calcium gluconate is the only option for calcium supplementation. Calcium chloride can cause severe tissue damage if accidental tissue infiltration occurs and should never be used outside of the acute, life-threatening cardiac emergency. Bolus administration of calcium gluconate (supplied in 1,000 mg ampules containing 90 mEq calcium) corrects serum levels of calcium rapidly and safely, although the effect is short-lived. An alternative is to use a calcium gluconate solution (6 ampules calcium gluconate = 6 g calcium gluconate = 540 mEq calcium in 500 mL D5W) infused at 1 mL/kg/h. This provides a steady calcium supplement and can be adjusted to maintain the calcium in the normal range while oral supplements are absorbed.

Temporary hypocalcemia occurs in about 10% of patients after total thyroidectomy, and permanent hypocalcemia occurs in about 1% (Table 40-5) (32–38). The temporary hypocalcemia can be severe, and it requires intravenous and oral supplementation for the duration of the effect. Permanent hypoparathyroidism requires lifelong support with calcium supplements and vitamin D analogs. Missing doses of the supplements will usually produce symptoms of varying severity, which while being manageable, are often quite bothersome for patients. In addition to the discomfort and inconvenience of the supplements, patients develop low-turnover bone disease, which resembles osteomalacia. Although dysmorphic, bone mass is generally preserved or increased in hypoparathyroidism and fracture risk is not apparently increased. Finally, the calcium

and vitamin D supplements with low PTH lead to an increased daily urinary excretion of calcium and significant risk of nephrolithiasis.

The recent availability of pharmacologic PTH for exogenous administration has opened the opportunity to replace PTH in patients with postoperative hypoparathyroidism. The experience with this to date is limited, but early results demonstrate that PTH delivered subcutaneously twice daily can maintain serum calcium levels in the same range as oral calcium and vitamin D supplements and decreases the amount of hypercalciuria (39). Further experience with this strategy will be necessary before the full long-term effects are clear.

Avoidance of permanent hypoparathyroidism is far more desirable than treatment of it. This can be accomplished by preservation of the parathyroid glands on their native blood supply or by autografting of parathyroid tissue to a muscular bed (40). During thyroidectomy the blood supply to each parathyroid gland should be identified and specifically considered during dissection. Every parathyroid gland should be treated as though it were the only remaining gland. The parathyroid glands receive their blood supply via the inferior thyroid artery (Fig. 40-1). During dissection of the thyroid, the inferior thyroid artery branches should be divided distal to the branching of the parathyroid end-arteries. The parathyroid glands can then be moved posteriorly in the neck away from the thyroid to allow safe dissection of the RLN and thyroid attachments to the trachea.

If the parathyroid glands cannot be preserved on their native blood supply, transfer of the gland to a convenient grafting site can maintain function (28,40). For normal parathyroid glands, transfer to the sternocleidomastoid muscle provides a convenient vascular bed for transplant (Fig. 40-2). The parathyroid gland must be reduced to pieces that can survive on the diffusion of nutrients temporarily, while neovascular in-growth occurs over several weeks. This strategy is effective, as is clear from operative series in which

TABLE 40-5

INCIDENCE OF COMPLICATIONS AFTER TOTAL THYROIDECTOMY

Authors, Year	Number of Patients	Transient Nerve Paresis, n (%)	Permanent Nerve Paresis, n (%)	Transient Hypo-parathyroidism, n (%)	Permanent Hypo-parathyroidism, n (%)
Thompson, 1978 (33)	165	NR	0	NR	<2%
Farrar, 1980 (32)	29	NR	1 (3)	2 (7)	4 (14)
Schroder, 1986 (34)	56	1 (2)	0	9 (17)	3 (6)
Clark, 1988 (35)	160	4 (2.5)	3 (2)[a]	NR	1 (0.6)
Ley, 1992 (36)	124	1 (0.8)	1 (0.8)	13 (10)	2 (1.6)
Tartaglia, 2003 (37)	1636	31 (1.9)	15 (0.9)	NR	14 (0.9)
Rosato, 2004 (38)	9599	195 (2)	94 (1)	797 (8.3)	163 (1.7)

NR, not reported.
[a]Each from deliberate sacrifice of the recurrent laryngeal nerve due to tumor involvement.

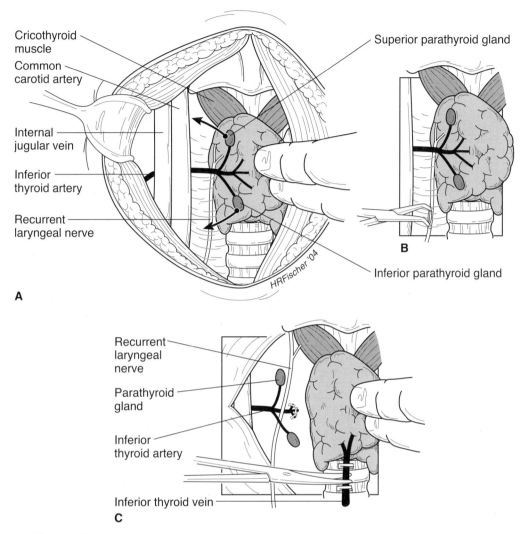

Figure 40-1 Relationship and dissection of the parathyroid gland blood supply and the recurrent laryngeal nerve. **A:** Once the upper pole vessels have been divided and the thyroid lobe has been reflected anteriorly, dissection of the tracheoesophageal groove exposes the blood supply to the parathyroid glands. The glands are usually entrapped under adherent soft tissue stretched across the surface of the thyroid gland. The parathyroid dissection begins along the edge away from its blood supply, and the parathyroid glands are released back toward the carotid artery (*arrows*). **B:** The recurrent laryngeal nerve is identified below the inferior thyroid artery, at or below the level of the lower pole of the thyroid gland. The nerve is predictable in its position at this level, in the groove between the trachea and esophagus (easily identified if a stethoscope or temperature probe is in the lumen). The recurrent laryngeal nerve (RLN) is not tethered by any attachments at this level and so can be dissected with less danger of injury. The nerve dissection then continues superiorly to the inferior thyroid artery. The inferior thyroid artery branches can then be divided with the nerve in full view to ensure the safety of the dissection. **C:** Once the inferior thyroid artery branches have been divided and the thyroid separated from the dense attachments to the trachea near the level of the RLN insertion under the cricopharyngeal muscle, the lower pole vessels can be divided safely.

all parathyroid glands were autografted in order to try to optimize the long-term outcome of normal parathyroid function. All patients became temporarily hypoparathyroid, but all recovered to become dependent fully on their autografts. Although this strategy is effective, it leads to significant short-term morbidity due to the uniform, severe hypocalcemia that occurs before graft function begins. A selective strategy of autografting only the parathyroid glands that are devascularized during dissection is equally effective and more comfortable for most of the patients.

NERVE INJURIES

Several nerves adjacent to the thyroid gland can be deliberately or inadvertently affected during thyroidectomy. These include the RLN immediately adjacent to the thyroid and the vagus nerve, which is slightly more removed but which causes the same symptoms when damaged. The external branch of the superior laryngeal nerve (EBSLN) can be injured during dissection of the upper pole of the thyroid gland, and the sympathetic chain and

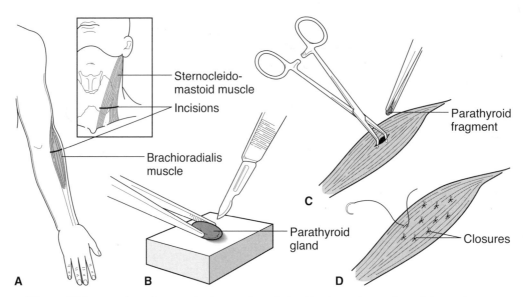

Figure 40-2 Parathyroid autograft. If a parathyroid gland has been devascularized during dissection, the best management is to autograft the gland. In addition, there are certain conditions (e.g., familial parathyroid multiple gland disease or renal osteodystrophy) for which it may be advantageous to remove the parathyroid glands from the native site and autograft them elsewhere. **A:** Normal parathyroid glands can be grafted into the sternocleidomastoid muscle. As a rule, abnormal parathyroid glands should not be autografted back into the neck but rather grafted to a distant location, such as the nondominant forearm. Transverse incisions over the brachioradialis muscle heal much better than longitudinal incisions. **B:** The parathyroid gland is sliced cleanly into pieces 1 to 2 mm in maximum dimension. **C:** Each piece to be grafted is placed into an individual pocket in the selected muscle. **D:** Each pocket is closed with a suture to prevent extrusion of the graft. For abnormal parathyroid glands grafted into the arm, the sites may be marked by using permanent sutures; however, for normal glands grafted in the neck, resorbable sutures are preferable.

stellate ganglion can be injured near the posterior aspect of the upper pole of the gland as well.

Recurrent Laryngeal Nerve

The RLN fibers are a part of the vagus nerve on each side until they branch off in the upper chest and course around the ligamentum arteriosum (left RLN) or the subclavian artery (right RLN) and back along the tracheoesophageal groove on each side. They pass between the thyroid and the larynx and insert in the larynx at the inferior border of the cricopharyngeal muscle. The nerve often branches at about the level of the lower pole of the thyroid and inserts to the larynx as two or more adjacent fibers; there is also an esophageal branch that extends posteriorly from about the level of the thyroid lower pole.

Damage to the RLN causes unilateral paralysis of the muscles that control ipsilateral vocal cord tension. Unilateral RLN injury changes the voice substantially in most patients and also significantly affects the swallowing mechanism. The voice can range from a soft, whispery voice, with the inability to increase the volume at all, to a nearly normal-sounding voice that cannot be raised to a yell. The difference between these is based on the contralateral vocal cord's ability to cross the midline and appose the affected cord. If the cords cannot meet, the voice will be soft and breathy. If the cords can meet, the speaking voice will be more normal in timbre but the affected cord prolapses with increased airway

pressure and the ability to yell is lost. Swallowing is affected also, and the aspiration of liquids is a mark of severe RLN paresis. This improves with time and can be helped by swallowing training.

Bilateral RLN injury causes paralysis of both cords and usually results in a very limited airway lumen at the cords. These patients usually have a normal-sounding speaking voice but severe limitations on inhalation velocity because of upper airway obstruction. They often require reintubation to maintain ventilation.

RLN paresis is usually temporary and resolves over days to months (Table 40-5) (32–38). There is no known method of aiding or speeding recovery. If a unilateral paresis proves to be permanent, palliation of the cord immobility and voice changes can be achieved with vocal cord injection or laryngoplasty. These procedures stiffen and medialize the paralyzed cord in order to allow the contralateral cord to appose the paralyzed cord during speech. If both cords are affected, the palliative procedures are more limited and involve creating an adequate airway for ventilation; improvements in voice quality are not likely, as there is no muscular control of the cord function.

Avoidance of RLN injury is far superior to palliation. Great care must be taken during the dissection of the nerve in order to protect it. In some clinical situations the RLN is sacrificed in order to allow an adequate tumor resection. Absent this unusual circumstance, however, careful dissection can generally preserve cord function. The principles of the dissection are the following:

1. *Avoid dividing any structures in the tracheoesophageal groove until the nerve is definitively identified.* Small branches of the inferior thyroid artery may seem like they can clearly be safely transected; however, the distortion of tumor, retraction, or previous scar may lead the surgeon to mistakenly divide a branch of the RLN. The identifying feature of the RLN is that the more it is dissected, the more it looks like the correct structure. This is based on the morphologic appearance and the anatomic course. The nerve can tolerate manipulation but not cutting. Once cut, repair of the nerve is of unproven benefit.

2. *Identify the nerve low in the neck, well below the inferior thyroid artery, at the level of the lower pole of the thyroid gland or below.* This allows dissection of the nerve at a site where it is not tethered by its attachments to the larynx or its relation to the inferior thyroid artery. Traction injuries to the nerve can occur when the nerve is manipulated near a site of fixation (Fig. 40-1).

3. *Keep the nerve in view during the subsequent dissection of the thyroid away from the larynx.* Once the nerve is identified, the dissection can generally proceed from inferior to superior along the nerve, dividing the inferior thyroid artery branches and preserving the parathyroid glands. This allows careful dissection of the tissues with minimal manipulation of the RLN.

4. *Minimize the use of powered dissection posterior to the thyroid.* Although the electrocautery and high-frequency ultrasonic scalpel are useful tools in dissection, they have some risk of lateral thermal spread, which can damage adjacent tissues. Careful cold dissection and hemostasis with ligatures or clips will avoid this risk. This is particularly important at the entry of the RLN to the larynx, immediately adjacent to the ligament of Berry and its vessels.

The use of nerve stimulators and laryngeal muscle potential monitors has recently been investigated as a tool to try to limit or avoid nerve injuries (41,42). The data do not currently support the routine use of these devices. This may be because they merely help to identify the nerve, while the portion of the operation most likely to produce damage in experienced hands is the dissection of the RLN at the fixed point of the cricopharyngeus. Further investigation may identify specific circumstances in which this technology is helpful.

About 10% of patients have some evidence of RLN paresis after thyroidectomy; however, this resolves in most patients. About 1% or fewer patients have permanent nerve injury when experienced surgeons perform total thyroidectomy (Table 40-5).

External Branch of the Superior Laryngeal Nerve (EBSLN)

This nerve courses adjacent to the superior pole vessels of the thyroid gland before separating to penetrate the cricopharyngeus muscle fascia at its supero-posterior aspect (Fig. 40-3). The nerve supplies motor innervation of the inferior constrictor muscles of the larynx. Damage to this nerve changes the ability of the larynx to control high-pressure phonation, such as high-pitched singing (soprano/falsetto) or yelling (38,43).

To avoid damaging this nerve, the dissection of the upper pole vessels should proceed from a space where the nerve is safely sequestered under the cricopharyngeal fascia to the superior vessels themselves, thus safely separating the nerve from the tissue to be divided (Fig. 40-3).

Sympathetic Chain

Although it is separated from the posterior aspect of the thyroid, the sympathetic chain and stellate ganglion can be damaged during thyroidectomy, producing a Horner syndrome (ipsilateral ptosis, miosis, and anhidrosis). This is probably due to retractor-induced injury, as the sympathetic chain and ganglion itself are out of the operative field. These injuries are nearly always temporary.

AIRWAY MANAGEMENT

Because the thyroid lies directly anterior to the trachea, enlargement of the thyroid or direct invasion of the trachea by tumor can cause airway compromise that can become critical during the induction of anesthesia (44–47). Compression of the trachea can cause loss of airway patency in the supine patient under anesthesia. Once the negative intrathoracic pressure needed to lift the thyroid and keep the trachea patent is lost, it may be difficult or impossible to ventilate the patient with positive pressure. This can be avoided by awake intubation to maintain airway patency.

Compression of the trachea in the neck can narrow the lumen substantially and require placement of a smaller endotracheal tube at intubation. However, the more difficult management issue can be significant lateral deviation of the trachea. Although these patients can usually be ventilated by positive pressure mask ventilation, the shift of the larynx can make it difficult or impossible to access the vocal cords for placement of an endotracheal tube. Intubation over a fiberoptic laryngobronchoscope can be helpful in most patients. However, there are patients who cannot be intubated in spite of all attempts and who require tracheostomy at the outset of the thyroidectomy in order to safely perform the operation. Anticipation of the difficulties that may be faced, the assembly of a team expert in airway management, and the readiness of an experienced surgeon prepared to access the airway operatively is critical to the safe outcome of these occasionally extremely challenging and dangerous situations.

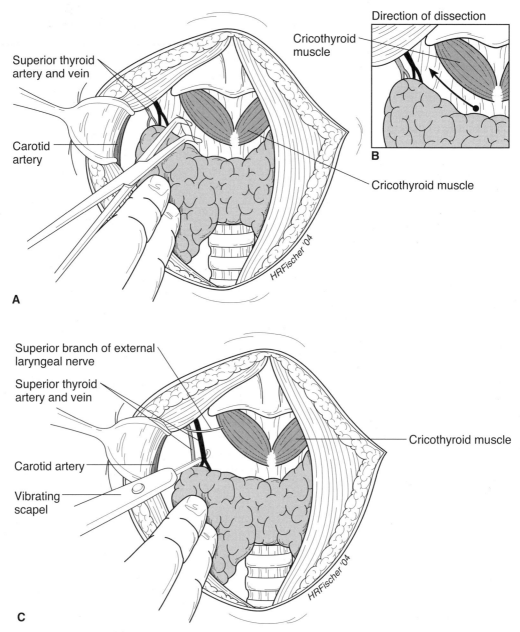

Figure 40-3 Protection of the external branch of the superior laryngeal nerve. **A:** After separation of the lateral border of the thyroid gland from the carotid sheath to expose the lateral portion of the upper pole vessels, the medial aspect of the upper pole is exposed by bluntly entering the avascular space between the thyroid gland and the cricothyroid muscle. This space is safe if dissected directly posteriorly to the anterior surface of the spine. **B:** The dissection is then carried superolaterally between the surfaces of the thyroid gland and the cricothyroid muscle (*arrow*). **C:** This maneuver clears the medial aspect of the superior thyroid vessels, and traction on the thyroid gland inferiorly separates the external branch of the superior laryngeal nerve from these vessels. The vessels can then be safely divided using any technique, including the high-frequency ultrasonic dissector (depicted).

INJURY TO OTHER CERVICAL STRUCTURES

A variety of other structures in the neck are vulnerable to injury during operation, particularly if large tumors extend out of the usual confines of the thyroid gland. The thoracic duct empties into the left internal jugular vein posterior to the clavicular insertion of the sternocleidomastoid muscle. Damage to the thoracic duct can cause a large collection of lymph or chyle in the operative bed. This can heal spontaneously after drainage if the leak is small; however, the leak frequently continues in spite of attempts to allow healing by decreasing output (NPO, total parenteral nutrition, and octreotide injections). If the leak persists for >3 weeks, the thoracic duct can be divided in the left hemithorax using thoracoscopic techniques. This will nearly always allow the leak to heal.

Tracheal injuries can occur, particularly during removal of large invasive tumors. Most tracheal injuries can be repaired primarily with resorbable suture. For defects >10 mm, it may be preferable to patch the trachea with a pedicle of the sternocleidomastoid muscle or to perform a sleeve resection of the affected area. If resected, the cut ends of the trachea are reapproximated with absorbable suture. A drain should be placed to evacuate any air that escapes through the repair. This is less of an issue if the patient is extubated at the completion of the operation, avoiding the effects of positive pressure ventilation on the repair. A tracheostomy is rarely necessary, although if there are other issues concerning airway safety, placement of a temporary tracheostomy may be preferable to prolonged intubation.

Esophageal injuries rarely occur during thyroidectomy. If the esophageal lumen is entered, the operative options include primary repair or closure of the distal lumen and construction of a cervical esophagostomy. Primary repair is generally preferable, unless there is extensive tissue loss or damage.

IATROGENIC HYPERTHYROIDISM OR HYPOTHYROIDISM

After total thyroidectomy, and as a part of the therapy for most thyroid carcinoma, patients receive thyroid hormone replacement therapy (13). As a chronic medication, thyroid hormone is among the most well-tolerated. It has a long half-life, which makes daily dosing adequate and which means that patients do not develop symptoms if they miss or change the timing of doses. The problems with thyroid hormone administration, however, are (i) its long half-life allows adjustment of dosage only once a month or so, making the titration of the proper dose a slow process; (ii) its narrow therapeutic window means that small changes in dosing or medication preparation can change the physiologic effect; and (iii) it is largely protein-bound, so other protein-bound drugs or changes in the proteins themselves can change the effects of a given dose of the drug. Once patients understand that the process of titration can take time, they are usually accepting. Trying to speed the process by making more frequent changes often delays the identification of the appropriate dose by overcorrecting the dose.

The narrow therapeutic window of thyroid hormone efficacy is another aspect that patients should understand. In particular, the effect of changing thyroid hormone preparations from one brand to another or to generic preparations may change the patient's response to the drug. Patients should be encouraged to be consistent about the preparation that they use, or, if a change is unavoidable, to

recheck their TSH levels a month after a change to document the effect. This has been well documented in the medical and lay literature, and most pharmacists are also sensitive to this issue (48–57).

A more frequent problem is the addition or subtraction of some other chronic medication, such as oral contraceptive pills or estrogen replacement therapy, that changes the serum protein binding of the thyroid hormone dose. Patients should be informed of this potential effect and of the need to redocument and adjust thyroid hormone dosing after these changes in other medications.

PARATHYROID SURGERY

Parathyroidectomy is performed frequently for primary hyperparathyroidism and less frequently for secondary or tertiary hyperparathyroidism. The indications for intervention vary with the clinical situation. Although some recent changes in operative strategy have made the operation simpler for many patients, this procedure can still be difficult and surgeons undertaking it must be skilled at recognizing the pathology and correcting it while avoiding the complications of persistent hyperparathyroidism and hypoparathyroidism.

INDICATIONS FOR OPERATION IN PATIENTS WITH PRIMARY HYPERPARATHYROIDISM

Patients with primary hyperparathyroidism can be separated into symptomatic and asymptomatic groups (58). Barring other life-limiting illness, all patients with symptomatic hyperparathyroidism should have operative correction of the disease. The symptoms that can occur include fractures, particularly vertebral compression fractures, renal stones, severe neuromuscular weakness, easy fatigability and loss of stamina, sleep disturbance, depression, memory loss, and pancreatitis. All these issues improve with correction of hyperparathyroidism. The hypertension that occurs more frequently in the hyperparathyroid population probably stops worsening with correction of the disease but does not reliably improve.

Patients with asymptomatic disease can present more complex decision-making (58,59). Management guidelines for patients with asymptomatic hyperparathyroidism from the National Institutes of Health (NIH) recognize risk factors for long duration of disease (age), rate of calcium loss (serum calcium, urine calcium), and end-organ effects (serum creatinine, bone density) (Table 40-6). The patient's risk for the operation and concurrent illnesses must be considered to determine whether the patient is likely to gain benefit from the procedure. These guidelines were designed in an NIH Consensus Conference in 1991 and then revisited and revised in an NIH-sponsored meeting in 2002

TABLE 40-6

INDICATIONS FOR PARATHYROIDECTOMY IN ASYMPTOMATIC HYPERPARATHYROIDISM

Measurement	Guidelines, 1991	Guidelines, 2002
Serum calcium (above ULN)	1–1.6 mg/dL	1.0 mg/dL
24-hour urinary calcium	>400 mg	>400 mg
Creatinine clearance	Reduced by 30%	Not recommended
Serum creatinine	Not recommended	If abnormal
Bone mineral density	Z-score <−2.0 (forearm)	T-score <−2.5 at any site
Age	<50	<50

ULN, upper limits of normal.

(58,59). The most significant change was from Z-score for bone density that was used in 1991 to T-score in 2002. Z-score compares patient bone density to age, gender, and race-matched controls while T-score compares patient bone density to ideal bone mass. T-score correlates better with fracture risk and so is more appropriate in judging the patient's personal risk.

Once the decision to operate is clear, the best strategy for resolution of the hyperparathyroidism can be considered, including decisions on preoperative imaging. Imaging should not be used to determine the diagnosis of hyperparathyroidism or the decision for operation.

INDICATIONS FOR OPERATION IN PATIENTS WITH SECONDARY HYPERPARATHYROIDISM

Secondary and tertiary hyperparathyroidism occur because of chronic parathyroid stimulation by hypocalcemia, usually in patients with chronic renal failure on dialysis. The best management of this is to correct the underlying problem by renal transplant or by dialysis management and vitamin D replacement. These measures can limit the parathyroid abnormality and consequent bone disease in most patients, but if the PTH level is chronically above 1,000 pg per mL, the nonoperative measures are unlikely to resolve the hyperparathyroidism. However, parathyroidectomy can be beneficial in patients who develop severe bone pain, severe itching, soft tissue calcification, or tissue damage from microcalcification (calciphylaxis) (60–62). Because of the secondary nature of the hyperparathyroidism, a full cervical exploration is necessary to identify and manage the disease in all the parathyroid glands. Intraoperative PTH levels may be helpful (61).

Tertiary hyperparathyroidism occurs when chronically stimulated parathyroid tissue becomes autonomous and drives the calcium to supernormal levels. This typically occurs only after renal transplant has corrected the need for dialysis. Usually just one of the parathyroid glands has become autonomous and it is not necessary to resect all the glands.

CURRENT PROCEDURE STRATEGIES

Initial Operation

For patients who have no previous history of parathyroid or thyroid operation, the approach to parathyroidectomy has changed substantially in recent years because of improvements in the ability to identify the abnormal parathyroid glands preoperatively and the ability to measure PTH intraoperatively for immediate feedback regarding adequacy of the resection. Most parathyroid surgeons use some combination of these advances in their approach to parathyroidectomy. Some also incorporate intraoperative localization with an γ radiation probe and nuclear medicine administration at operation, although this has proved less useful than was initially hoped.

The conventional approach to parathyroidectomy has been a full neck exploration with identification of all parathyroid glands and removal of the enlarged ones. This proven approach has a success rate of 95% to 97%. It relies on the surgeon's ability to recognize the abnormal glands by their size. The pitfalls of the approach are failure to identify all the glands, leaving an abnormal gland or glands in place, and the resection of normal functioning glands that can produce hypoparathyroidism.

The newer approaches to parathyroid operation improve upon the previous approach by helping to identify the abnormal gland before operation (giving the surgeon a place to start the exploration) and by providing a physiologic, rather than anatomic, endpoint for the operation (letting the surgeon know when to stop). Although this may theoretically improve the outcome of parathyroidectomy, in practical terms the operation was already very safe and successful. The main benefit has been to make the easy operations easier; most patients with a single adenoma can have it identified by preoperative imaging and resected in a focused operation and avoid further exploration if the PTH level falls appropriately (63,64). The availability of these modalities can help the difficult operations, with multiple or ectopic abnormal glands, but they can still be quite challenging. There are some patient situations in which limited neck exploration for primary hyperparathyroidism is not appropriate because of a high risk of multiple gland disease. These include familial hyperparathyroidism (including the multiple endocrine neoplasia syndromes) and hyperparathyroidism during lithium use.

The most typical way that these modalities are incorporated is called the minimally invasive parathyroidectomy (MIP) or concise parathyroidectomy (63,64). After the decision to operate, technetium sestamibi scanning or cervical ultrasound is used to try to identify the abnormal glands. Each of these modalities is successful in 80% to 90% of patients. If a suspicious gland is identified, the surgeon explores that site in the operating room, often under sedation and local anesthesia or regional nerve blockade. If an abnormal gland is identified, it is resected and the serum PTH level is measured 10 minutes after excision. If the post-excision PTH level falls by 50% from the pre-excision baseline level, the operation is completed. If no abnormal gland is identified at the suspicious site or if the PTH level does not fall adequately, additional exploration to identify all the abnormal glands is done, usually during the same anesthetic; this occurs in about 10% of patients. The technique for these patients, as for those who have no glands identified on preoperative imaging, is similar to the conventional full neck exploration, with one distinction. Because of the available PTH measurements, the operation can be terminated when the PTH level drops by 50%, even if all the parathyroid glands have not been identified.

Reoperation

Reoperation for persistent or recurrent hyperparathyroidism has increased challenges because of the scar from the previous exploration and because there may be specific anatomic reasons (especially ectopic glands outside the neck) that caused the initial operation to fail. For these reasons it is imperative for the surgeon to have localization of the abnormal gland that is as precise as possible before beginning the exploration (64–68). All the information from the previous exploration must be reviewed, including the operative report and pathology report, so that the locations and histologic nature of the identified parathyroid glands can be considered. The patient must also have definitive imaging that correlates with the previous operative information. Most experienced parathyroid surgeons require two concordant preoperative images of the abnormal gland before proceeding with exploration. The most commonly used initial imaging techniques are technetium sestamibi nuclear imaging and cervical ultrasound. If these both identify what appears to be the same gland, no further imaging is needed. If they do not, further studies proceed. Usually noninvasive imaging modalities are used first [computed tomography (CT) scan of the neck and chest, magnetic resonance (MR) scan] and invasive imaging only if needed (selective venous sampling for PTH, arteriography). The sequence of these studies depends on the individual patient findings and local experience and expertise with these studies. Our preferences are led by our experience with CT scan and selective venous sampling.

The reoperation for hyperparathyroidism is conducted in a fashion similar to the initial procedure. The suspicious site is explored, and abnormal tissue is resected. The intraoperative PTH level is used to determine whether that has resolved the hyperparathyroidism and whether any further exploration, or parathyroid autograft, is necessary (64).

The same criteria are used for successful drop in the intraoperative PTH level.

POTENTIAL COMPLICATIONS OF PARATHYROIDECTOMY

Any of the complications that can occur in thyroid operations can occur in parathyroid operations, except for the production of hypothyroidism. In particular, the complications of neck hematoma, nerve injuries, and hypoparathyroidism occur for similar reasons and are managed in similar ways. Persistent hyperparathyroidism is unique to parathyroidectomy.

HYPOPARATHYROIDISM

Hypocalcemia occurs after parathyroidectomy because of either bone remineralization or hypoparathyroidism. If hyperparathyroidism has been corrected in a patient with significant bone disease, the bone remineralization process can remove substantial amounts of calcium from the blood and cause hypocalcemia. This symptomatic process usually resolves within 2 to 4 weeks after parathyroidectomy, but in patients with very severe bone disease it can go on for several months. The only treatment necessary is calcium replacement. If large amounts of calcium are needed, vitamin D can be helpful to aid absorption, as in the treatment of hypoparathyroidism. The serum PTH level is normal or high, responding appropriately to the hypocalcemia (69).

Hypoparathyroidism can occur after resection of all parathyroid tissue, either during an operation for multiple gland parathyroid disease or during a reoperation, before which some parathyroid tissue may have been damaged or resected at the initial procedure. This is an uncommon complication, particularly now that intraoperative PTH measurement can document the presence of functional parathyroid tissue at the completion of the exploration. If, at the end of a difficult or reoperative parathyroidectomy, the PTH level has dropped to unmeasurable levels, the best management is to autograft some of the resected parathyroid tissue, following the same guidelines noted above (Fig. 40-2). Abnormal parathyroid tissue should not be grafted into the neck, however, and so autografting into the nondominant forearm may be more appropriate.

NERVE INJURY

Because of the proximity of the dissection, the same nerves that are at risk during thyroidectomy are at risk during parathyroidectomy. However, because there is rarely a need to divide the upper pole thyroid vessels during parathyroidectomy, the EBSLN is at substantially

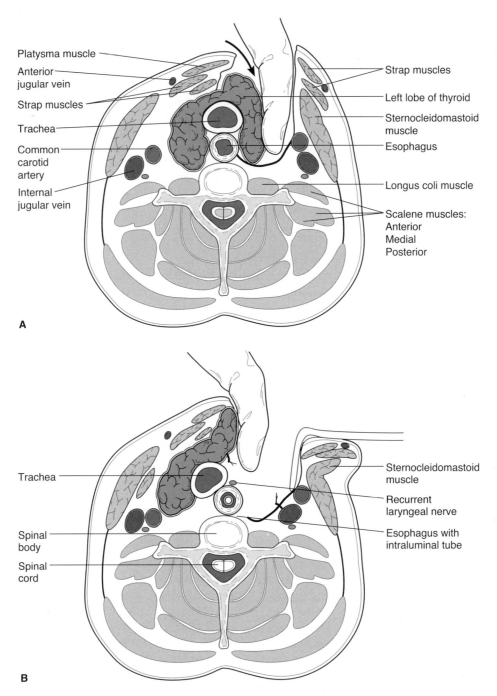

Figure 40-4   Exposure and identification of the parathyroid glands in their normal anatomic positions. **A:** After making subplatysmal flaps and separating the strap muscles in the midline, the elevation of the strap muscle proceeds immediately along the strap muscles and the carotid sheath directly posteriorly to the longus coli muscle. Only after the anterior surface of the longus coli muscle has been exposed medial to the carotid sheath along the length of the thyroid gland is the dissection turned medially. This plane leaves all the tissues likely to contain the parathyroid glands attached to the larynx. **B:** The thyroid gland is rolled anteriorly, rotating the larynx and upper trachea to bring the tracheoesophageal tissues into view. The middle thyroid vein, if it is placed on tension by this maneuver, is divided.

less risk. The RLN can be quite close to the parathyroid glands, and, in fact, it is sometimes enveloped in a groove in an enlarged upper parathyroid gland that extends inferiorly along the esophagus and nerve. The main principle

that is used to protect the RLN during parathyroidectomy is to avoid dividing any structures other than the middle thyroid vein until the parathyroid gland is completely mobilized. Once the gland is attached at only one site by

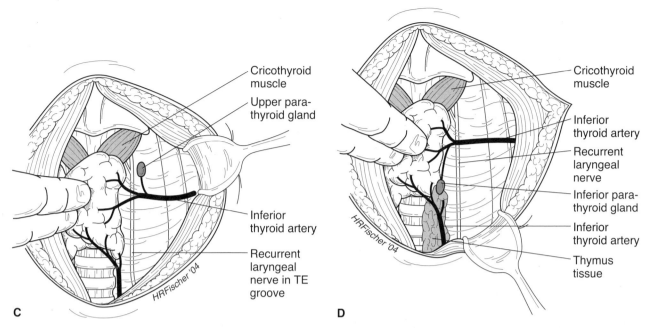

Figure 40-4 (*continued*)   **C:** The upper parathyroid gland is most often identified immediately adjacent to the thyroid gland, posterior to the recurrent laryngeal nerve, and superior to the inferior thyroid artery. However, when enlarged, the gland often grows inferiorly, with the bulk lying deep to, and extending inferior to, the inferior thyroid artery, still posterior to the RLN. The blood supply remains from the upper branches of the inferior thyroid artery, however, and can be identified in the normal position. **D:** The lower pole of the thyroid gland is retracted superiorly to identify the lower parathyroid gland. This is most often immediately adjacent to the thyroid gland, although it can "slide down" within the sheath of the thymus and often resides there. To uncover the parathyroid in this area, the sheath overlying the thymus is opened but the attachments to the thyroid gland are not divided as they provide important traction superiorly. TE, tracheoesophageal.

artery and vein, the nerve cannot be involved and it is safe to divide the vessels. The RLN is often identified during the course of the parathyroid dissection. If there is any question regarding the location of the nerve, the same technique of nerve identification described above is used to protect the nerve from injury (Fig. 40-1).

PERSISTENT OR RECURRENT HYPERPARATHYROIDISM

Persistent hyperparathyroidism is the appearance of hypercalcemia and elevated PTH levels within 6 months after parathyroid exploration. Most often this occurs when the parathyroid adenoma is not identified at exploration or when multiglandular disease is not recognized. Recurrent hyperparathyroidism is the reappearance of hypercalcemia and elevated PTH levels >6 months after exploration. This usually occurs because of unrecognized mild multiglandular disease, when there is an underlying stimulus for the development of more abnormal parathyroid glands (e.g., MEN-1), or if a parathyroid adenoma is incompletely resected or fractured (70). These problems occur in 2% to 4% of patients after operation by experienced hands. Proper performance of the neck exploration and use of the intraoperative PTH assay should minimize the occurrence of this problem (63,64).

To maximize the therapeutic value and minimize the operative risks of parathyroidectomy, the most important factor is thorough and precise dissection technique. The operation, whether performed as a focused exploration beginning at one site or performed as a full parathyroid exploration, must proceed in an organized way. The parathyroid glands are exposed by dissecting the superficial structures of the neck (from the strap muscles out) away from the underlying structures that derive their blood supply from the laryngeal system (Fig. 40-4). Thus, all the tissues attached to the larynx remain attached at the end of the mobilization, so the parathyroid glands and their blood supply are not separated and dropped into an "acquired ectopic" position. Once the tissues have been mobilized, the normal sites for parathyroid glands can be easily explored. Most missed parathyroid adenomas that cause persistent hyperparathyroidism are in normal anatomic sites and were missed at initial operation.

If no parathyroid gland is identified in a corresponding normal site, knowledge of the ectopic sites where parathyroid glands can be guides further exploration (Fig. 40-5). Although ectopic parathyroid adenomas are unusual, they occur frequently enough that no surgeon should undertake this operation without complete familiarity with this anatomy. If no abnormal parathyroid tissue is found after full neck exploration and exploration of all cervically accessible ectopic sites, most

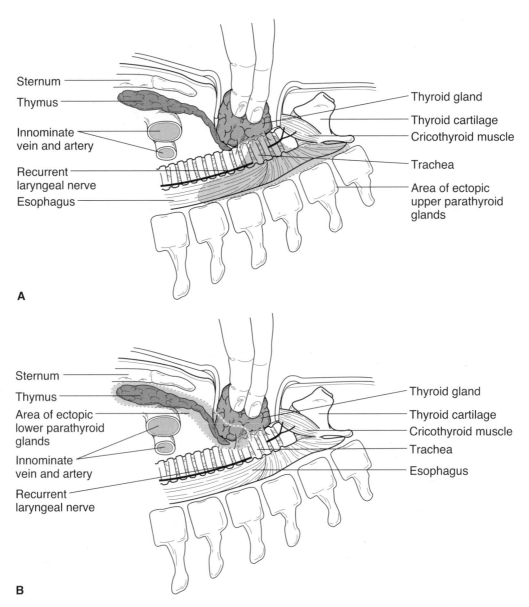

Figure 40-5 Identification of the parathyroid glands in ectopic sites. **A:** The upper parathyroid glands usually remain close to the thyroid; however, if the gland is not present there, it most likely is posterior to the recurrent laryngeal nerve along the esophagus or pharynx (*shaded area*). **B:** The lower parathyroid gland is usually near the lower pole of the thyroid gland; however, it can slide down into the anterior mediastinum within the thymus (*shaded area*). More rarely, the lower parathyroid gland can be in the upper neck along the carotid artery, often with a bit of residual thymus attached there as well.

parathyroid surgeons would close the wound, terminate the operation, and re-evaluate the patient postoperatively. This should include reconfirmation of the diagnosis and imaging to try to identify the abnormal gland. Most surgeons would not perform a trans-sternal mediastinal exploration at the initial operation without localizing studies that indicated a gland there.

Operative strategy at reoperation should include consideration of alternative anatomic approaches that might avoid operating through previous scar. The most common alternative approach is most useful for a posteriorly placed

(usually upper) parathyroid adenoma (Fig. 40-6). This lateral approach takes the operation through fresh tissue lateral to the strap muscles, along the anterior border of the sternocleidomastoid muscle, and only then to the previously operated area medial to the carotid sheath. This sheath is quite durable and tolerates dissection easily, even in reoperation. In addition, this area posteriorly has often been left undissected, thus leaving the posteriorly placed gland unidentified at the initial attempt. This avoids the tedious and sometimes bloody dissection of the strap muscles from the anterior surface of the thyroid gland.

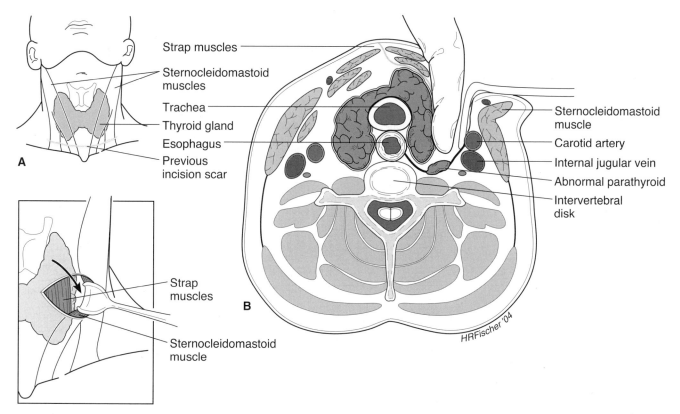

Figure 40-6 The lateral approach to the tracheoesophageal groove. For patients with previous neck explorations who have a posteriorly placed parathyroid gland, a lateral approach can avoid some treacherous dissection. **A:** The neck is usually entered through the old incision or a new, more laterally placed, incision. **B:** A fresh plane is entered between the lateral border of the strap muscles and the medial border of the sternocleidomastoid muscle. The thyroid and strap muscles are then rolled anteriorly as a unit, exposing the esophagus. This is the area where upper parathyroid adenomas are often missed, and dissection in these planes avoids the area of the previous dissection of the strap muscles from the thyroid surface and the thyroid from the recurrent laryngeal nerve.

SUMMARY

In conclusion, operations for diseases of the thyroid and parathyroid glands are quite common. Most of the complications of these procedures are technical in nature, and their risk can be minimized by proper understanding of the indications for operation, the anatomy and pathology of the area, and the proper dissection approach. The management of the complications depends on each complication's severity and temporal nature. For many temporary issues, reassurance alone and explanation of the natural history of the recovery is all that is necessary. The permanent, life-altering nature of some of the complications makes it mandatory, as with all invasive procedures, that the indications for the intervention be very clear.

REFERENCES

1. Schneider AB, Ron E, Lubin J, et al. Dose-response relationships for radiation-induced thyroid cancer and thyroid nodules: evidence for the prolonged effects of radiation on the thyroid. *J Clin Endocrinol Metab* 1993;77:362–369.

2. Antonelli A, Silvano G, Bianchi F, et al. Risk of thyroid nodules in subjects occupationally exposed to radiation: a cross sectional study. *Occup Environ Med* 1995;52:500–504.

3. Kouvaraki MA, Shapiro SE, Fornage BD, et al. Role of preoperative ultrasonography in the surgical management of patients with thyroid cancer. *Surgery* 2003;134:946–954; discussion 954–945.

4. Gimm O, Sutter T, Dralle H. Diagnosis and therapy of sporadic and familial medullary thyroid carcinoma. *J Cancer Res Clin Oncol* 2001;127:156–165.

5. Ito M, Yamashita S, Ashizawa K, et al. Childhood thyroid disease around Chernobyl evaluated by ultrasound examination and fine needle aspiration cytology. *Thyroid* 1995;5:365–368.

6. Jones AJ, Aitman TJ, Edmonds CJ, et al. Comparison of fine-needle aspiration cytology, radioisotopic and ultrasound scanning in the management of thyroid nodules. *Postgrad Med J* 1990;66:914–917.

7. Belfiore A, LaRosa GL, LaPorta GA, et al. Cancer risk in patients with cold thyroid nodules: relevance of iodine intake, sex, age, and multinodularity. *Am J Med* 1992;93:363–369.

8. Layfield LJ, Mohrmann RL, Kopald KH, et al. Use of aspiration cytology and frozen section examination for management of benign and malignant thyroid nodules. *Cancer* 1991;68:130–134.

9. Wool MS. Thyroid nodules: the place of fine-needle aspiration biopsy in management. *Postgrad Med J* 1993;94:111–122.

10. Gharib H. Fine-needle aspiration biopsy of thyroid nodules: advantages, limitations, and effect. *Mayo Clin Proc* 1994;69:44–49.

11. Hamburger JI. Diagnosis of thyroid nodules by fine needle biopsy: use and abuse. *J Clin Endocrinol Metab* 1994;79:335–339.

12. Udelsman R, Westra WH, Donovan PI, et al. Randomized prospective evaluation of frozen-section analysis for follicular neoplasms of the thyroid. *Ann Surg* 2001;233:716–722.

13. Mazzaferri EL. An overview of the management of papillary and follicular thyroid carcinoma. *Thyroid* 1999;9:421–427.

14. Hay ID, Grant CS, Bergstralh EJ, et al. Unilateral total lobectomy: is it sufficient surgical treatment for patients with AMES low-risk papillary thyroid carcinoma? *Surgery* 1998;124: 958–964; discussion 964–966.

15. Chen H, Nicol TL, Zeiger MA, et al. Hurthle cell neoplasms of the thyroid: are there factors predictive of malignancy? *Ann Surg* 1998;227:542–546.

16. Hay ID, Bergstralh EJ, Goellner JR, et al. Predicting outcome in papillary thyroid carcinoma: development of a reliable prognostic scoring system in a cohort of 1779 patients surgically treated at one institution during 1940 through 1989. *Surgery* 1993;114: 1050–1057; discussion 1057–1058.

17. Hay ID, Thompson GB, Grant CS, et al. Papillary thyroid carcinoma managed at the Mayo Clinic during six decades (1940–1999): temporal trends in initial therapy and long-term outcome in 2444 consecutively treated patients. *World J Surg* 2002;26:879–885.

18. Yim JH, Doherty GM. Papillary thyroid cancer. *Curr Treat Opin Oncol* 2000;1:329–338.

19. Hay ID, McConahey WM, Goellner JR. Managing patients with papillary thyroid carcinoma: insights gained from the Mayo Clinic's experience of treating 2,512 consecutive patients during 1940 through 2000. *Trans Am Clin Climatol Assoc* 2002;113: 241–260.

20. McWilliams RR, Giannini C, Hay ID, et al. Management of brain metastases from thyroid carcinoma: a study of 16 pathologically confirmed cases over 25 years. *Cancer* 2003;98:356–362.

21. McIver B, Hay ID, Giuffrida DF, et al. Anaplastic thyroid carcinoma: a 50-year experience at a single institution. *Surgery* 2001;130:1028–1034.

22. Sweeney PJ, Haraf DJ, Recant W, et al. Anaplastic carcinoma of the thyroid. *Ann Oncol* 1996;7:739–744.

23. Kobayashi T, Asakawa H, Umeshita K, et al. Treatment of 37 patients with anaplastic carcinoma of the thyroid. *Head Neck* 1996;18:36–41.

24. Shimizu K, Kumita S, Kitamura Y, et al. Trial of autotransplantation of cryopreserved thyroid tissue for postoperative hypothyroidism in patients with Graves' disease.[see comment]. *J Am Coll Surg* 2002;194:14–22.

25. Thomusch O, Machens A, Sekulla C, et al. Multivariate analysis of risk factors for postoperative complications in benign goiter surgery: prospective multicenter study in Germany. *World J Surg* 2000;24:1335–1341.

26. Cobin RH. Thyroid carcinoma and Graves' disease. *Endocr Pract* 2000;6:264–267.

27. Gann DS, Paone JF. Delayed hypocalcemia after thyroidectomy for Graves' disease is prevented by parathyroid autotransplantation. *Ann Surg* 1979;190:508.

28. Thomusch O, Machens A, Sekulla C, et al. The impact of surgical technique on postoperative hypoparathyroidism in bilateral thyroid surgery: a multivariate analysis of 5846 consecutive patients. *Surgery* 2003;133:180–185.

29. Moley JF, Lairmore TC, Doherty GM, et al. Preservation of the recurrent laryngeal nerves in thyroid and parathyroid reoperations. *Surgery* 1999;126:673–677; discussion 677–679.

30. Burkey SH, van Heerden JA, Thompson GB, et al. Reexploration for symptomatic hematomas after cervical exploration. *Surgery* 2001;130:914–920.

31. Abbas G, Dubner S, Heller KS. Re-operation for bleeding after thyroidectomy and parathyroidectomy. *Head Neck* 2001;23:544–546.

32. Farrar WB, Cooperman M, James AG. Surgical management of papillary and follicular carcinoma of the thyroid. *Ann Surg* 1980;192:701–704.

33. Thompson NW, Nishiyama RH, Harness JK. Thyroid carcinoma: current controversies. *Curr Probl Surg* 1978;15:1–67.

34. Schroder DM, Chambous A, France CJ. Operative strategy for thyroid cancer. Is total thyroidectomy worth the price? *Cancer* 1986;58:2320.

35. Clark OH, Levin K, Zeng QH, et al. Thyroid cancer: the case for total thyroidectomy. *Eur J Cancer Clin Oncol* 1988;24:305–313.

36. Ley PB, Roberts JW, Symmonds RE Jr, et al. Safety and efficacy of total thyroidectomy for differentiated thyroid carcinoma: a 20-year review. *Am Surg* 1993;59:110–114.

37. Tartaglia F, Sgueglia M, Muhaya A, et al. Complications in total thyroidectomy: our experience and a number of considerations. *Chir Ital* 2003;55:499–510.

38. Rosato L, Avenia N, Bernante P, et al. Complications of thyroid surgery: analysis of a multicentric study on 14,934 patients operated on in Italy over 5 years. *World J Surg* 2004;28:271–276.

39. Winer KK, Ko CW, Reynolds JC, et al. Long-term treatment of hypoparathyroidism: a randomized controlled study comparing parathyroid hormone-(1–34) versus calcitriol and calcium. *J Clin Endocrinol Metab* 2003;88:4214–4220.

40. Olson JA Jr, DeBenedetti MK, Baumann DS, et al. Parathyroid autotransplantation during thyroidectomy. Results of long-term follow-up.[see comment]. *Ann Surg* 1996;223:472–478; discussion 478–480.

41. Rea JL, Khan A. Clinical evoked electromyography for recurrent laryngeal nerve preservation: use of an endotracheal tube electrode and a postcricoid surface electrode. *Laryngoscope* 1998;108: 1418–1420.

42. Otto RA, Cochran CS. Sensitivity and specificity of intraoperative recurrent laryngeal nerve stimulation in predicting postoperative nerve paralysis. *Ann Otol Rhinol Laryngol* 2002;111:1005–1007.

43. Stojadinovic A, Shaha AR, Orlikoff RF, et al. Prospective functional voice assessment in patients undergoing thyroid surgery.[see comment]. *Ann Surg* 2002;236:823–832.

44. Kitamura Y, Shimizu K, Nagahama M, et al. Immediate causes of death in thyroid carcinoma: clinicopathological analysis of 161 fatal cases. *J Clin Endocrinol Metab* 1999;84:4043–4049.

45. Rudow M, Hill AB, Thompson NW, et al. Helium-oxygen mixtures in airway obstruction due to thyroid carcinoma. *Can Anaesth Soc J* 1986;33:498–501.

46. Allo MD, Thompson NW. Rationale for the operative management of substernal goiters. *Surgery* 1983;94:969–977.

47. Sippel RS, Gauger PG, Angelos P, et al. Palliative thyroidectomy for malignant lymphoma of the thyroid. *Ann Surg Oncol* 2002;9:907–911.

48. Mikosch P, Obermayer-Pietsch B, Jost R, et al. Bone metabolism in patients with differentiated thyroid carcinoma receiving suppressive levothyroxine treatment. *Thyroid* 2003;13:347–356.

49. Sawka AM, Gerstein HC, Marriott MJ, et al. Does a combination regimen of thyroxine (T4) and 3,5,3'–triiodothyronine improve depressive symptoms better than T4 alone in patients with hypothyroidism? Results of a double-blind, randomized, controlled trial. *J Clin Endocrinol Metab* 2003;88:4551–4555.

50. Walsh JP, Shiels L, Lim EM, et al. Combined thyroxine/liothyronine treatment does not improve well-being, quality of life, or cognitive function compared to thyroxine alone: a randomized controlled trial in patients with primary hypothyroidism.[see comment]. *J Clin Endocrinol Metab* 2003;88:4543–4550.

51. Walsh JP. Dissatisfaction with thyroxine therapy—could the patients be right? *Curr Opin Pharmacol* 2002;2:717–722.

52. Saravanan P, Chau WF, Roberts N, et al. Psychological well-being in patients on 'adequate' doses of l-thyroxine: results of a large, controlled community-based questionnaire study.[see comment]. *Clin Endocrinol* 2002;57:577–585.

53. Woeber KA. Levothyroxine therapy and serum free thyroxine and free triiodothyronine concentrations. *J Endocrinol Invest* 2002; 25:106–109.

54. Wiersinga WM. Thyroid hormone replacement therapy. *Horm Res* 2001;56:74–81.

55. Fischman J. Reports of thyroid drug's demise were exaggerated. *US News World Rep* 2001;131:57.

56. Anonymous. What is going on with levothyroxine. *Med Lett Drugs Ther* 2001;43:57–58.

57. Bell DS, Ovalle F. Use of soy protein supplement and resultant need for increased dose of levothyroxine. *Endocr Pract* 2001;7: 193–194.

58. Bilezikian JP, Potts JT Jr, Fuleihan Gel H, et al. Summary statement from a workshop on asymptomatic primary hyperparathyroidism:

a perspective for the 21st century [see comment]. *J Bone Miner Res* 2002;17:N2–N11.

59. Potts JT Jr, Ackerman IP, Barker CF, et al. Diagnosis and management of asymptomatic primary hyperparathyroidism: consensus development conference statement. *Ann Intern Med* 1991;114: 593–597.

60. Rothmund M, Wagner P. Reoperations for persistent and recurrent secondary hyperparathyroidism. *Ann Surg* 1988;207:310.

61. Hibi Y, Tominaga Y, Sato T, et al. Re-operation for renal hyperparathyroidism. *World J Surg* 2002;26:1301–1307.

62. Rothmund M, Wagner PK, Schark C. Subtotal parathyroidectomy versus total parathyroidectomy and autotransplantation in secondary hyperparathyroidism: a randomized trial. *World J Surg* 1991;15:745–750.

63. Chen H, Sokoll LJ, Udelsman R. Outpatient minimally invasive parathyroidectomy: a combination of sestamibi-SPECT localization, cervical block anesthesia, and intraoperative parathyroid hormone assay. *Surgery* 1999;126:1016–1022.

64. Johnson LR, Doherty G, Lairmore T, et al. Evaluation of the performance and clinical impact of a rapid intraoperative parathyroid hormone assay in conjunction with preoperative imaging and concise parathyroidectomy. *Clin Chem* 2001;47:919–925.

65. Wells SA Jr, Debenedetti MK, Doherty GM. Recurrent or persistent hyperparathyroidism. *J Bone Miner Res* 2002;17:N158–N162.

66. Kald BA, Mollerup CL. Risk factors for severe postoperative hypocalcaemia after operations for primary hyperparathyroidism. *Eur J Surg* 2002;168:552–556.

67. Hasse C, Sitter H, Brune M, et al. Quality of life and patient satisfaction after re-operation for primary hyperparathyroidism: analysis of long-term results. *World J Surg* 2002;26:1029–1036.

68. Kivlen MH, Bartlett DL, Libutti SK, et al. Re-operation for hyperparathyroidism in multiple endocrine neoplasia type 1. *Surgery* 2001;130:991–998.

69. Mandal AK, Udelsman R. Secondary hyperparathyroidism is an expected consequence of parathyroidectomy for primary hyperparathyroidism: a prospective study. *Surgery* 1998;124:1021–1026; discussion 1026–1027.

70. Fraker DL, Travis WD, Merendino JJ Jr., et al. Locally recurrent parathyroid neoplasms as a cause for recurrent and persistent primary hyperparathyroidism. *Ann Surg* 1991;213:58–65.

Complications in Endocrine Pancreatic Surgery

41

Terry C. Lairmore

■■■ APPROACH TO RESECTION OF ENDOCRINE
PANCREATIC TUMORS 596

■■■ COMPLICATIONS OF ENDOCRINE PANCREATIC
SURGERY 596
Specific Complications 596
General Complications 600

■■■ SUMMARY 601

■■■ REFERENCES 602

The surgical treatment of endocrine pancreatic neoplasms presents unique dilemmas in diagnosis, in the optimal timing and extent of operative intervention, and in the management of postoperative complications that occur with increased frequency in this select group of patients. Neuroendocrine tumors (NETs) of the pancreas and duodenum may occur as sporadic entities or in association with one of several well-defined hereditary endocrine neoplasia syndromes. Sporadic NETs of the pancreas are rare, occurring in only 1 to 2 per million persons. Duodenopancreatic NETs commonly present either with signs and symptoms relating to local growth of the tumor mass or with a specific syndrome of hormone excess, such as profound fasting

Terry C. Lairmore: Texas A & M System Health Sciences Center, College of Medicine, Temple, TX 76508

hypoglycemia, severe peptic ulcer diathesis, vasoactive instability/flushing, or secretory diarrhea. Patients who are members of a known kindred with one of the hereditary endocrine neoplasia syndromes may be diagnosed early as a result of prospective family screening, while sporadic pancreatic endocrine neoplasms tend to present late owing to their rare occurrence and unusual constellation of presenting and clinical findings.

Operative intervention for pancreatic NETs is generally indicated for patients with functional tumors and for tumors with significant malignant potential. Patients with inappropriate hormone oversecretion may develop life-threatening fasting hypoglycemia (insulinoma), severe complications of peptic ulceration, including bleeding, perforation, obstruction, complications from gastroesophageal reflux (gastrinoma), or debilitating secretory diarrhea with associated fluid and electrolyte losses [vasoactive intestinal peptide tumors (VIPomas), or carcinoid tumors]. Rare hormonally active tumors such as glucagonomas and somatostatinomas produce unusual but clinically significant syndromes, including hypoaminoacidemia, diabetes mellitus, deep vein thrombosis (DVT)/pulmonary embolism and cutaneous necrolytic migratory erythema (glucagonomas), or cachexia, steatorrhea, and cholelithiasis (somatostatinomas). Pancreatic NETs that are known to be malignant, or those tumors with significant malignant potential, should also be resected with or without the presence of a specific syndrome of hormone excess. Although pancreatic endocrine neoplasms are generally thought to pursue an indolent clinical course in most patients, regional lymph node metastases and hepatic and distant metastases can occur and be life-limiting due to progression of the tumoral process. In a recent series of patients with NETs in the setting of multiple endocrine neoplasia type 1 (MEN 1) undergoing operation based on traditional indications (hormonally active tumor, tumors >1 cm and perceived to carry significant malignant potential) approximately one-third of patients had lymph node or distant metastases at the time of intervention (1). In one of the largest series (2) of patients undergoing pancreaticoduodenectomy for pancreatic or periampullary NETs (sporadic and familial), the actuarial survival rates at 2, 5, and 7 years were 81%, 73%, and 65%, respectively. Clearly, pancreatic endocrine tumors can be aggressive and result in mortality in a subset of patients.

Pancreatic NETs that are associated with one of the hereditary endocrine neoplasia syndromes present unique diagnostic and therapeutic challenges (1,3). Hereditary cancer syndromes are characterized by a diffuse preneoplastic hyperplasia that precedes the development of discrete tumor foci within the involved tissue, the development of multiple tumors within a target tissue, and the potential for development of tumors in more than one target tissue. Furthermore, in the setting of a familial cancer syndrome, affected patients develop tumors at a much earlier age than patients with corresponding sporadic tumors. For example, in keeping with the two-hit model for a tumor suppressor gene (4), patients with MEN 1 inherit one mutation in the germline and require only one additional genetic event to inactivate the remaining wild-type allele and result in tumor formation. The result is a propensity to develop multiple endocrine tumors at a young age, when patients are otherwise healthy and active. Although group NETs tend to be benign or follow an indolent course, a subset of these tumors may metastasize early to regional lymph nodes, liver, or distant sites with resultant cancer-related mortality. The optimal surgical management of these tumors is complicated by a relative lack of sensitive and specific tumor markers for their early detection, difficulty in accurately localizing small tumors by noninvasive preoperative imaging tests, and uncertainty about the malignant potential or expected natural history of small, apparently benign, tumors (5).

Mention of the controversies surrounding the surgical management of pancreatic NETs is very pertinent to any discussion of the complications of pancreatic endocrine surgery because the potential risks should greatly influence decisions regarding the timing and extent of the operative procedure. Because of the high probability that a small, solitary, grossly encapsulated NET of the pancreas will be benign, enucleation is usually appropriate (1,6,7) (Fig. 41-1). Localized resection preserves pancreatic endocrine and exocrine function and prevents the need for division of the major pancreatic duct or the need for construction of a surgical enteric-pancreatic duct anastomosis. Alternatively, malignant NETs or tumors thought to

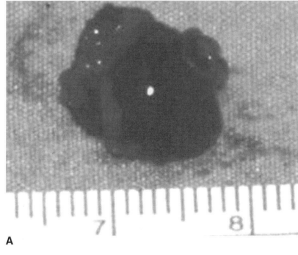

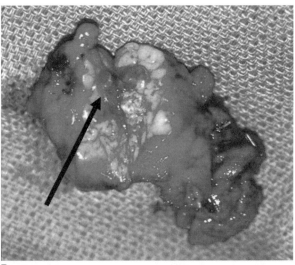

Figure 41-1 Benign insulinoma resections. **A:** A small insulinoma after enucleation from surrounding pancreatic parenchyma. Most insulinomas have no invasion of the surrounding pancreas, and so gross enucleation is curative therapy. **B:** A small insulinoma in the resection distal tail of the pancreas (*arrow*). In some situations there may be less risk of operative complications associated with a limited pancreatic resection than there is with an enucleation. In this situation a low-morbidity resection was preferable.

carry a high risk of malignant progression may require major pancreatic resection. It is obviously desirable to intervene early to prevent malignant spread while preserving pancreatic function and minimizing morbidity and mortality (from either cancer or surgery) (1). The unique aspects of endocrine pancreatic tumors that affect surgical decision-making, outcome, and frequency of postoperative complications include the occurrence of these neoplasms in young patients with normal, soft, nonfibrotic pancreatic parenchyma; the usual absence of dilated pancreatic and biliary ducts; and the significant clinical and financial costs of failing to accurately localize and resect functional tumors or to prevent malignant progression with adequate pancreatic resection.

APPROACH TO RESECTION OF ENDOCRINE PANCREATIC TUMORS

The operative approach to excision of pancreatic and duodenal NETs includes complete exposure of the pancreas by entering the lesser sac, performing an extended Kocher maneuver (mobilization and medial rotation of the duodenum and head of the pancreas off the retroperitoneum), incision of the retroperitoneum at the inferior border of the pancreas, and medial rotation of the spleen and tail of the pancreas. These maneuvers allow thorough inspection and palpation of the entire pancreatic parenchyma. Because 60% to 70% of gastrinomas are located in the submucosa of the duodenal wall, a longitudinal duodenotomy should be performed when hypergastrinemia is present. Somatostatin receptor scintigraphy is very useful to define the extent of disease preoperatively (Fig. 41-2). Intraoperative ultrasonography is critical to the accurate localization of small NETs within the pancreas or duodenum.

COMPLICATIONS OF ENDOCRINE PANCREATIC SURGERY

Specific Complications

Pancreatic or Biliary Fistula

Failure of healing of the enteric-pancreatic or enteric-biliary anastomosis, manifested as a pancreatic or biliary fistula, is a common cause of morbidity following either enucleation or regional pancreatic resection. A postoperative pancreatic fistula may be defined as closed-suction drain output of >50 mL of amylase-rich fluid (>500 IU per L) per day on 3 consecutive days following postop day 7. Typically, the development of a pancreatic fistula is recognized clinically between postoperative days 3 and 7 as increased volume of a milky or particulate drainage that is high in amylase concentration (8). Disruption or failure of healing of the biliary-enteric anastomosis occurs with less frequency and may be difficult to distinguish from a pancreatic-enteric anastomotic leak because of the very close proximity of

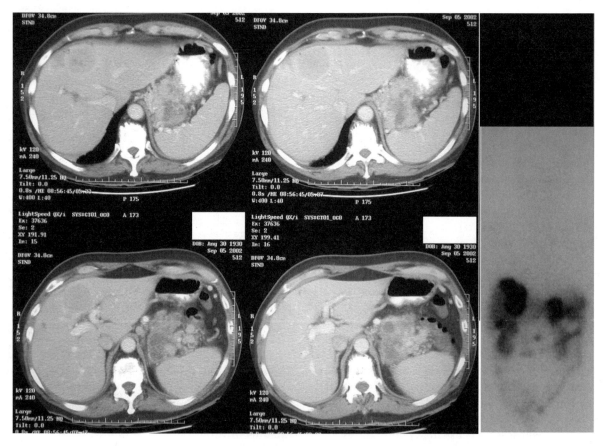

Figure 41-2 Preoperative imaging for malignant tumor resection planning. This patient had a large tumor of the body and tail of the pancreas with liver metastases. The CT scan shown demonstrated the anatomic relationships of the disease, and the somatostatin receptor scintigraphy (*right panel*) showed the extent of the disease and the absence of other distant sites. An operative resection that addressed all of the demonstrated tumor was designed and carried out. The patient has remained a long-term disease-free survivor from this high-grade NET producing VIP.

these two surgically constructed anastomoses. The potential for persistent drainage of enzyme-rich fluid following any disruption of the pancreatic parenchyma, including local enucleation of small NETs, is well recognized. The risk of developing a clinically significant pancreatic fistula may be related to the proximity of the enucleation or resection to the major pancreatic ductal system or to the surgical technique used in dividing the pancreatic parenchyma. Other factors of potential importance include whether simple external drainage of the excision site is employed versus construction of a surgical enteric-pancreatic anastomosis. The presence or absence of proximal pancreatic duct obstruction is also an important factor in healing of the line of pancreatic division or disruption.

The experience from previous large series of patients undergoing pancreaticoduodenectomy for adenocarcinoma in centers of excellence can be cited as a general benchmark of the expected risk of pancreatic fistula following pancreatic resection for endocrine tumors. In studies of patients treated for adenocarcinoma, the incidence of pancreatic fistula ranges from 8% to 25% (8–14). A very similar incidence of pancreatic fistula (10% to 24%) has been reported in patients undergoing resection of pancreatic endocrine tumors (1,2,15,16) (Table 41-1). This complication is a frequent cause of morbidity following pancreatic surgery and is associated with increased costs and prolonged hospital stay. Although nonoperative management often successfully treats this complication, some previous studies have suggested that 20% to 26% of pancreatic fistulas (primarily in patients with adenocarcinoma) were directly related to patient mortality (9,12). A number of operative techniques have been advocated to reduce the frequency of pancreatic fistula, including inversion pancreaticojejunostomy, mucosa to mucosa pancreatic-jejunal

anastomosis, external or internal stent drainage, or a defunctionalized Roux-en-Y jejunal loop to drain the enteric-pancreatic anastomosis.

As a group, patients with endocrine pancreatic tumors have significant anatomic and physiologic differences compared to patients with pancreatic adenocarcinoma. Patients with pancreatic NETs occurring in the setting of one of the hereditary endocrine neoplasia syndromes (multiple endocrine neoplasia type 1, von Hippel-Lindau) are often diagnosed early as a result of prospective screening. Sporadic pancreatic NETs are relatively rare entities that are frequently diagnosed in young patients. These patients are more likely to have soft pancreatic tissue without fibrosis or calcification and nondilated pancreatic and biliary ducts. Importantly, they are also more likely to have fewer medical comorbidities and greater physiologic reserve to overcome potential surgical complications. These clinical features significantly affect operative decision-making, technical concerns, and postoperative outcome.

Small, circumscribed pancreatic NETs may be appropriately enucleated. Transection of the pancreatic parenchyma is usually performed by a combination of electrocautery and ligation of apparent pancreatic ductal or vascular structures. Intraoperative ultrasound is a valuable method to define the proximity of an intrapancreatic neoplasm to the major pancreatic duct or vascular structures. If concern for division of a major pancreatic duct or concern for pancreatic leak exists, some have advocated administration of secretin intravenously and inspection for increased pancreatic secretion from the cut surface of the parenchyma. For enucleations or local pancreatic resections deemed to be at significant risk for development of pancreatic fistula, approximation with a portion of vascularized omentum or construction of enteric-pancreatic drainage should be considered.

TABLE 41-1

COMPLICATION RATES IN SERIES OF PATIENTS UNDERGOING RESECTION OF PANCREATIC AND DUODENAL NEUROENDOCRINE TUMORS

	Phan et al. (2), 1997 (n = 50)[a]	Park et al. (15), 1998 (n = 30)[b]	Lairmore et al. (1), 2000 (n = 21)[c]	Guo et al. (16), 2004 (n = 21)[d]	Total (ave.), (n = 142)
Pancreatic fistula	24%	15%	9.5%	14.6%	15.8%
Biliary fistula	9%		4.8%	2.4%	5.4%
Intra-abdominal abscess	7%	4%	14%		8.3%
Delayed gastric emptying	15%	4%			9.5%
Wound infection	24%	8%	9.5%		13.8%
Transfusion/bleeding		4%	4.8%		4.4%
Pulmonary complication			4.8%		4.8%
Other major complication		12%	9.5%	2.4%	8.0%
Death	2%	0%	4.8%		3.4%

[a]Pancreaticoduodenectomies for periampullary neuroendocrine tumors.
[b]Neuroendocrine tumors of the head of the pancreas.
[c]Enucleation, major pancreatic resection, and pancreaticoduodenectomies in patients with MEN 1.
[d]Nonfunctional neuroendocrine tumors of the pancreas.

The established surgical principles to avoid anastomotic failure of any surgically constructed union of two mucosa-lined structures include preservation of adequate blood supply, avoidance of tension, and meticulous surgical technique. One study of 123 consecutive patients undergoing pancreaticoduodenectomy used critical evaluation of the cut surface of the pancreas for bleeding and revision if deemed necessary and meticulous construction of a tension-free anastomosis under magnification (17). Using this technique, a greatly reduced postoperative pancreatic fistula rate of 1.6% was reported. Although this rate of pancreatic fistula following pancreaticoduodenectomy is exceptionally low compared to previous large published series, the conclusions emphasize attention to the basic tenets of construction of a viable surgical anastomosis.

The use of long-acting somatostatin analogues, such as octreotide acetate or lanreotide, either to decrease the incidence of postoperative pancreatic fistula or to improve healing of established pancreatic fistulas, has been controversial. In conjunction with restriction of oral intake and nasogastric decompression, the rationale for pharmacologic treatment to decrease pancreatic secretion is that fistulas with a lower volume of output should be more likely to heal. Other pharmacologic agents have been employed to decrease gastric and pancreatic secretion, including loperamide, atropine, pirenzepine, H_2-receptor antagonists, and omeprazole or other proton-pump inhibitors, but their effectiveness has yet to be established.

Long-acting somatostatin analogues, such as octreotide acetate, have been evaluated in several randomized controlled trials for efficacy in reducing complications following pancreatic surgery or in promoting healing of enterocutaneous gastrointestinal fistulas. The interpretation of the available data is complicated by differences in the patient characteristics of the study population, the underlying disease processes, the definition of a pancreatic leak or fistula, and variability in the method, timing, and dosage of octreotide administration. In 1992 several studies reported favorable effects of prophylactic octreotide administration, including significantly decreased pancreatic secretion and possible early healing of fistulas. Büchler et al. (18) conducted a large, multicenter double-blind randomized controlled trial in 246 patients undergoing pancreatic surgery. Patients with both pancreatic tumors and chronic pancreatitis were included. Patients were randomized to receive either subcutaneous octreotide 300 micrograms daily in divided doses or placebo for 7 days perioperatively. In the higher risk patients undergoing resection of pancreatic tumors, the complication rate (including pancreatic fistula, abscess, and subsequent sepsis) was 38% of patients receiving octreotide versus 65% of patients given placebo ($p < 0.01$). This study concluded that perioperative treatment with octreotide reduces the occurrence of postoperative complications after pancreatic resection, especially in patients with malignant disease.

Lange et al. from the Surgical Metabolism Section at the NIH reported a randomized prospective trial of postoperative somatostatin analogue in 21 patients undergoing resection of pancreatic NETs (19). Patients were randomized to receive either subcutaneous octreotide 150 μg every 8 hours postoperatively or saline solution. This study showed no significant difference in complications related to pancreatic drainage in the two groups when perioperative octreotide was administered prophylactically.

The combined experience from four early multicenter, randomized controlled trials from Europe (18,20–22) suggested that significant decreases in overall postoperative complications rates are associated with the use of prophylactic octreotide following pancreatic surgery, and some studies reported significant reduction in rates of postoperative pancreatic fistula. However, none of these studies included only those patients undergoing pancreaticoduodenal resections for malignant disease. Two subsequent well-conducted studies from the United States focused on patients undergoing major pancreatic resection for malignancy in which a pancreatic duct-enteric anastomosis is constructed. Lowy et al. (23) from the M.D. Anderson Cancer Center reported the results of a single-institution, randomized trial involving 120 patients undergoing pancreaticoduodenectomy for malignancy. Patients were randomized to receive either octreotide (150 μg subcutaneously every 8 hours through postoperative day 5) or no postoperative treatment. The rate of clinically significant pancreatic leak was 12% in the octreotide group and 6% in the control group ($p = 0.23$), and perioperative morbidity was 30% and 25%, respectively. Therefore, no benefit was seen in the use of prophylactic octreotide to decrease postoperative fistula rate or overall complications. Yeo et al. reported the results of 211 patients undergoing pancreaticoduodenectomy with enteric-pancreatic anastomosis who were randomized to either octreotide 250 μg subcutaneously every 8 hours beginning 1 to 2 hours preoperatively and continuing for 7 days or to saline control (24). The pancreatic fistula rates and overall complication rates were similar in both groups, and the study demonstrated no advantage with prophylactic octreotide administration.

In summary, octreotide has been shown to decrease the volume of pancreatic secretions, and it may have a limited role in the treatment of established enterocutaneous pancreatic secretions (25). Conflicting results exist on the efficacy of perioperative octreotide administration to prevent pancreatic complications, including fistula. Although early trials including pancreatic resections for both benign and malignant disease (18,20–22) suggested decreased pancreatic fistula rates and overall morbidity when octreotide is administered prophylactically, recent randomized studies of the use of octreotide in patients undergoing pancreaticoduodenectomy for malignancy failed to show any benefit (23,24). The one randomized trial specifically focusing on resections of pancreatic NETs (and including both enucleations and major pancreatic resections) also showed no benefit of routine postoperative octreotide to reduce complications (19).

TABLE 41-2

OPERATIVE OUTCOME FOLLOWING RESECTION OF DUODENOPANCREATIC NET IN 21 PATIENTS WITH MEN 1

	Pancr./ Bile Leak	Pancr. Abscess	Other Major Complication	Wound Infection	Transfuse PRBC	Respiratory Failure	Death
Whipple (n = 5)	2	1	0	1	0	1	1[a]
Non-Whipple resection (n = 11)	1	1	0	1	0	0	0
Enucleation (n = 5)	0	1	2	0	1	0	0
Total (%) (n = 21)	3 (14)	3 (14)	2 (9.5)	2 (9.5)	1 (4.8)	1 (4.8)	1 (4.8)

[a]One patient had prohibitive pulmonary disease (FEV$_1$ 700 mL) and a severely symptomatic insulinoma. After an extended ICU stay and successful wean from the ventilator, he suffered a sudden respiratory arrest 6 weeks postop.
Reproduced with permission from Lairmore TC, et al. Duodenopancreatic resections in patients with multiple endocrine neoplasia type 1. *Ann Surg* 2000;231:909–918.

Because octreotide has been shown to reduce the volume of pancreatic secretion, in theory a greater potential benefit might be expected in patients whose treatment involves division of relatively normal, soft pancreatic parenchyma with intact exocrine secretory function. However, multiple large clinical trials suggest a greater potential benefit in patients with chronic pancreatitis, and, when stratified for patients with malignant disease, no benefit can be demonstrated. It is interesting to note that the overall rate of postoperative pancreatic fistula rate is very similar (approximately 10% to 25%) in studies of patients undergoing pancreaticoduodenectomy for malignant disease (8–14) and in patients with NETs (1,2,15,16) undergoing a variety of pancreatic procedures (enucleation, distal pancreatectomy, pancreaticoduodenectomy) with or without construction of a pancreatic-enteric anastomosis. The unique clinical features likely to be present in patients with pancreatic NETs were listed above and include young age, fewer medical comorbidities, nondilated pancreatic/biliary ducts, and the presence of normal, soft, nonfibrosed pancreatic parenchyma. Even though only a subset of patients with NETs requires major pancreatic resection or construction of a pancreatic-enteric anastomosis to adequately excise the tumor, perhaps similar overall fistula rates are seen because of the added small incidence of pancreatic leak from an enucleation site that involves disruption of normal soft pancreatic parenchyma and associated small pancreatic ductules. Patients undergoing major pancreatic resection or enucleation of pancreaticoduodenal NETs develop the expected postoperative complications, including pancreatic or biliary fistulas, peripancreatic abscess, wound complications, bleeding, and cardiopulmonary complications, at rates of approximately 30% to 40% (Table 41-2). However, as a group these patients are more likely to have the attributes of younger age, fewer associated medical conditions, and greater physiologic reserve to overcome these complications. Nonoperative management of pancreas-associated complications is nearly always successful in these patients, and overall outcomes are excellent.

Intra-abdominal Abscess/Peripancreatic Fluid Collection

Approximately 80% of patients with pancreatic fistula following pancreatic resections heal with conservative, nonoperative management requiring no additional percutaneous drainage procedures or operative intervention (8). This nonoperative management may include bowel rest, total parenteral nutrition, pharmacologic intervention (octreotide, H$_2$-receptor antagonists, etc.) where indicated, local wound and skin care, infection control, and continued closed-suction external drainage until the fistula output decreases to a minimal volume. Approximately 10% to 15% of patients require additional invasive intervention, usually image-guided placement of additional percutaneous drainage catheters, to remove undrained or loculated peripancreatic fluid collections. Approximately 5% of patients develop severe sequelae, including sepsis, bleeding, or development of a pancreatic abscess, that require operative intervention.

Pancreatic ductal disruption and anastomotic failure result in leakage of pancreatic exocrine secretions, including pancreatic proteases and lipase, that result in severe inflammatory changes, fistula formation, and tissue necrosis surrounding the pancreas. The result may be a loculated peripancreatic fluid collection or, with the addition of bacterial suprainfection, intra-abdominal abscess, or sepsis. The treatment of intra-abdominal abscess requires appropriate intravenous antibiotics, in combination with adequate percutaneous or operative drainage.

The development of a postoperative intra-abdominal abscess following pancreatic resections is associated with increased mortality and is clearly associated with the occurrence of a leak from the pancreatic or biliary anastomosis. Following pancreaticoduodenectomy for malignant disease, approximately 50% of intra-abdominal abscesses are associated with leakage from the pancreatic anastomosis (8). Less frequently, abscess formation results from anastomotic failure of the hepaticojejunostomy or the gastrojejunostomy. Peripancreatic fluid collections may also occur after enucleation and may develop as an area of loculated fluid that does not communicate effectively with the surgically placed closed-suction drain. Small fluid collections are commonly seen on computed tomography (CT) scans following pancreatic surgery, and most are clinically insignificant in the absence of systemic signs of toxicity or sepsis.

In series of patients undergoing a variety of procedures for resection of neuroendocrine pancreatic or duodenal tumors (1,2,15,16), the incidence of intra-abdominal abscess formation is approximately 7% to 14% and is related to, but somewhat less frequent than, the occurrence of pancreatic or biliary fistula due to anastomotic failure (Table 41-1).

Metabolic Disorders

Operative procedures involving the pancreas carry the potential for adverse sequelae relating to exocrine or endocrine pancreatic function. Postoperative pancreatic function is determined by the extent of organ resection, the underlying disease process, and any preexisting abnormalities of endocrine and exocrine function (26). Few scientific studies available in the literature specifically address preoperative risk factors, the relative risk related to the extent of pancreatic resection, and a rigorous review of surgical outcomes.

In general physiologic terms, the pancreas has digestive functions (exocrine secretion in the postprandial state), endocrine function centered on glucose homeostasis and tight regulatory control of insulin secretion and counter-regulatory hormones, and the interdigestive phase of pancreatic secretion. Both the digestive and interdigestive phases of exocrine and endocrine pancreatic function are affected by major pancreatic resection and are related to the extent of resection as well as the presence of underlying deficiencies.

Exocrine or endocrine pancreatic insufficiency occurs following operative intervention for either chronic pancreatitis or excision of pancreatic malignancies. Varying degrees of pancreatic dysfunction exist in patients with chronic pancreatitis prior to any surgical intervention. Resection of pancreatic tumors may be required in patients with either normal or altered preoperative pancreatic function. Postoperative deficits in exocrine or endocrine secretion are due to a combination of preexisting disease and sequelae that are procedure-related. The specific type of surgical procedure and the magnitude of pancreatic resection have a direct relationship to postoperative impairment of exocrine or endocrine function. The degree of impairment is related to both the extent of pancreatic parenchyma resected and the functional state of the residual pancreas. Enucleations or limited pancreatic resections would be predicted to carry minimal risk for disturbance of digestive or endocrine pancreatic function, although related procedures that affect gastric or biliary secretion may also cause dysfunction due to alterations in the intricate balance of the hormonal and electrolyte physiology of the upper gastrointestinal tract. For instance, the addition of partial gastrectomy to a pancreatic resection results in further impairment in the release of gastrin, pancreatic polypeptide, and cholecystokinin, with resultant effects on overall exocrine digestive function.

The influence of different surgical procedures on pancreatic exocrine function has been investigated in a few clinical studies. In patients undergoing a pylorus-preserving pancreaticoduodenectomy, results following pancreaticojejunostomy versus pancreaticogastrostomy were compared by Jang et al. (27). A significant deterioration of pancreatic exocrine function was seen in patients who were treated with pancreaticogastrostomy compared to patients undergoing pancreaticojejunostomy. The proposed mechanism was early deactivation of pancreatic enzymes by gastric acid. In patients requiring oral supplementation with pancreatic exocrine enzymes following pancreatic surgery, treatment with proton-pump inhibitors is indicated to avoid excess enzyme degradation by increased gastric acid.

Disturbances of endocrine secretion may also occur following operative procedures on the pancreas. Diabetes mellitus may occur after resection of >60% to 75% of the pancreatic parenchyma, especially in patients with preexisting impairment of glucose homeostasis. The most challenging sequela of major pancreatic resection is recurrent hypoglycemia, which may result from increased postoperative insulin sensitivity due to concomitant decrease in glucagon secretion (26).

General Complications

General postoperative complications occur following operation for endocrine pancreatic tumors with a frequency that is expected for similar open, upper-abdominal procedures for either malignant or benign processes. Not surprisingly, these general operative risks are related to the patient's overall health and the existence of associated medical conditions. Because these general surgical risks are not unique to either the decision-making or specific techniques employed for resection of endocrine pancreatic neoplasms, these risks will be acknowledged but not discussed in detail.

Bleeding may occur with either an early or a late time course following pancreatic surgery. Early bleeding may be associated with technical failure of the suture ligation of a small venous or arterial vessel, technical failure of any of several tissue coagulation methods currently used to divide surrounding soft tissues containing an intricate vascular supply, or bleeding related to construction of a surgical anastomosis. Anastomotic bleeding may be manifested as hematobilia, intraluminal gastrointestinal bleeding, or intra-abdominal bleeding. Late bleeding (after postoperative day 5) is more likely to result from complications relating to the development of a pancreatic fistula, such as rupture of an arterial pseudoaneurysm, or erosion of a large vessel. Alternatively, late gastrointestinal bleeding may be associated with marginal ulceration following construction of a gastrojejunostomy. It is reasonable to assume that the risk of postoperative bleeding relating directly to a technical failure should be associated with the magnitude of the required dissection and the need to secure multiple small vessels, the need to perform a major regional pancreatic resection with division of the pancreatic parenchyma, or the requirement for the construction of multiple surgical anastomoses. Because resection of pancreaticoduodenal NETs may frequently be successfully performed without major pancreatic resection, the risk of major postoperative bleeding would be expected to be low. Indeed, in the collected series of 142 patients undergoing resection of NETs reported in Table 41-1, the incidence of significant bleeding requiring transfusion was only 4.4%.

Delayed gastric emptying is a very frequent cause of morbidity following pancreaticoduodenectomy for adenocarcinoma of the pancreas, occurring in up to one-third of patients (8). It may be conservatively defined as the need for gastric decompression for >10 days postoperatively. Patients undergoing resection of endocrine pancreatic tumors develop delayed gastric emptying with reduced frequency (approximately 10%) (Table 41-1). Most patients present with persistent nausea, abdominal fullness, early satiety, or the need for nasogastric tube reinsertion in the first week postoperatively. Poor gastric emptying may occur following any pancreatic procedure but is frequently seen when a gastrojejunostomy has been constructed. Inadequate gastric emptying is multifactorial and may occur even when a water-soluble contrast study demonstrates a patent gastrojejunostomy, with or without associated anastomotic edema. Adequate treatment usually involves continued gastric decompression, judicious use of prokinetic agents, enteral or parenteral feeding as indicated, and patience until oral feeding can be reinitiated.

Other complications, including wound infections, DVT, and significant cardiac or pulmonary events, may also occur following endocrine pancreatic surgery. Wound infections following operation for pancreatic endocrine tumors occur with rates similar to other patients undergoing upper-abdominal operation with or without division of the gastrointestinal tract. Coexistent disorders, including morbid obesity, diabetes, collagen vascular disease, and immunosuppression secondary to underlying medical conditions or steroid use, increase the risk of wound infection. Superficial or deep wound infection occurred in an average of 13.8% of 142 patients undergoing resection of pancreatic endocrine tumors in the collected series summarized in Table 41-1. Wound infection rates ranged from approximately 10% in patients undergoing a variety of procedures, including enucleations and pancreatic resections (1), to approximately 24% in patients undergoing pancreaticoduodenectomy (2). The incidence of DVT was not consistently addressed in the available series of patients undergoing resection of pancreatic endocrine neoplasms; however, these patients appear to be at lower risk than patients with adenocarcinoma of the pancreas. Finally, the frequency of cardiopulmonary or other major complications in the collected series of patients with endocrine pancreatic tumors was approximately 5% to 12%, with an average mortality of 3.4% (Table 41-1). The small mortality rate in the reviewed series was limited to patients undergoing pancreaticoduodenectomy and in almost all cases was associated with patients who had severe preoperative medical limitations.

SUMMARY

NETs of the pancreas are infrequent neoplasms that may occur sporadically or in association with one of several hereditary endocrine neoplasia syndromes. Many patients with NETs, especially in the familial setting, are diagnosed at a young age in the absence of significant medical comorbidities. Furthermore, neuroendocrine pancreatic tumors are more likely to occur in association with soft, nonfibrotic pancreatic parenchyma and without associated dilation of the pancreatic or biliary ducts compared to patients with adenocarcinoma. The unique features of familial endocrine pancreatic tumors, such as those occurring in the MEN 1 syndrome, include multifocal involvement within a target tissue and the development of tumors in multiple target organs. As a general rule, many pancreatic NETs pursue a relatively indolent course, although a subset may metastasize and result in significant morbidity and mortality. Surgical decision-making in these patients should be based on the unique features of these uncommon neoplasms, the tumor's expected natural history, and the most significant operative risks. The most important of these are the risks of postoperative pancreatic fistula formation and the development of peripancreatic abscess and subsequent sepsis. The ideal surgical treatment of pancreatic NETs relieves the patient of significant risk of malignant progression while preserving pancreatic endocrine and exocrine function and minimizing morbidity from either surgery or the underlying disease process.

REFERENCES

1. Lairmore TC, Chen VY, DeBenedetti MK, et al. Duodenopancreatic resections in patients with multiple endocrine neoplasia type 1. *Ann Surg* 2000;231:909–918.
2. Phan GQ, Yeo CJ, Cameron JL, et al. Pancreaticoduodenectomy for selected periampullary neuroendocrine tumors: fifty patients. *Surgery* 1997;122:989–997.
3. Moley JF, Lairmore TC, Phay J. Hereditary endocrinopathies. *Curr Probl Surg* 1999;36:653–764.
4. Knudson AG Jr, Hethcote HW, Brown BW. Mutation and childhood cancer: a probabilistic model for the incidence of retinoblastoma. *Proc Natl Acad Sci U S A* 1975;72:5116–5120.
5. Lairmore TC, Piersall LD, DeBenedetti MK, et al. Clinical genetic testing and early surgical intervention in patients with multiple endocrine neoplasia type 1 (MEN 1). *Ann Surg* 2004;239:637–647.
6. Akerstrom G, Hessman O, Skogseid B. Timing and extent of surgery in symptomatic and asymptomatic neuroendocrine tumors of the pancreas in MEN 1. *Langenbecks Arch Surg* 2002;386(8):558–569.
7. Dralle H, Krohn SL, Karges W, et al. Surgery of resectable nonfunctioning neuroendocrine pancreatic tumors. *World J Surg* 2004;28(12):1248–1260.
8. Yeo CJ. Management of complications following pancreaticoduodenectomy. *Surg Clin North Am* 1995;75(5):913–924.
9. Braasch JW, Gray BN. Considerations that lower pancreatoduodenectomy mortality. *Am J Surg* 1977;133(4):480–484.
10. Edis AJ, Kiernan PD, Taylor WF. Attempted curative resection of ductal carcinoma of the pancreas: review of Mayo Clinic experience, 1951–1975. *Mayo Clin Proc* 1980;55(9):531–536.
11. Grace PA, Pitt HA, Tompkins RK, et al. Decreased morbidity and mortality after pancreatoduodenectomy. *Am J Surg* 1986;151(1):141–149.
12. Trede M, Schwall G. The complications of pancreatectomy. *Ann Surg* 1988;207(1):39–47.
13. Cameron JL, Pitt HA, Yeo CJ, et al. One hundred and forty-five consecutive pancreaticoduodenectomies without mortality. *Ann Surg* 1993;217(5):430–435; discussion 435–438.
14. Cullen JJ, Sarr MG, Ilstrup DM. Pancreatic anastomotic leak after pancreaticoduodenectomy: incidence, significance, and management. *Am J Surg* 1994;168(4):295–298.
15. Park BJ, Alexander HR, Libutti SK, et al. Operative management of islet-cell tumors arising in the head of the pancreas. *Surgery* 1998;124(6):1056–1061; discussion 1061–1062.
16. Guo KJ, Liao HH, Tian YL, et al. Surgical treatment of nonfunctioning islet cell tumor: report of 41 cases. *Hepatobiliary Pancreat Dis Int* 2004;3(3):469–472.
17. Strasberg SM, Drebin JA, Mokadam NA, et al. Prospective trial of a blood supply-based technique of pancreaticojejunostomy: effect on anastomotic failure in the Whipple procedure. *J Am Coll Surg* 2002;194(6):746–758; discussion 759–760.
18. Büchler M, Friess H, Klempa I, et al. Role of octreotide in the prevention of postoperative complications following pancreatic resection. *Am J Surg* 1992;163(1):125–130; discussion 130–131.
19. Lange JR, Steinberg SM, Doherty GM, et al. A randomized, prospective trial of postoperative somatostatin analogue in patients with neuroendocrine tumors of the pancreas. *Surgery* 1992;112(6):1033–1037; discussion 1037-1038.
20. Pederzoli P, Bassi C, Falconi M, et al. Efficacy of octreotide in the prevention of complications of elective pancreatic surgery. *Br J Surg* 1994;81:265–269.
21. Montorsi M, Zago M, Mosca F, et al. Efficacy of octreotide in the prevention of pancreatic fistula after elective pancreatic resections: a prospective, controlled, randomized, clinical trial. *Surgery* 1995;117:26–31.
22. Friess H, Beger HG, Sulkowski U, et al. Randomized controlled multicentre study of the prevention of complications by octreotide in patients undergoing surgery for chronic pancreatitis. *Br J Surg* 1995;82:1270–1273.
23. Lowy AM, Lee JE, Pisters PWT, et al. Prospective, randomized trial of octreotide to prevent pancreatic fistula after pancreaticoduodenectomy for malignant disease. *Ann Surg* 1997;226(5):632–641.
24. Yeo CJ, Cameron JL, Lillemoe KD, et al. Does prophylactic octreotide decrease the rates of pancreatic fistula and other complications after pancreaticoduodenectomy? Results of a prospective randomized placebo-controlled trial. *Ann Surg* 2000;232(3):419–429.
25. Li-Ling J, Irving M. Somatostatin and octreotide in the prevention of postoperative complications and the treatment of enterocutaneous fistulas: a systematic review of randomized controlled trials. *Br J Surg* 2001;88:190–199.
26. Kahl S, Malfertheiner P. Exocrine and endocrine pancreatic insufficiency after pancreatic surgery. *Best Pract Res Clin Gastroenterol* 2004;18(5):947–955.
27. Jang JY, Kim SW, Park SJ, et al. Comparison of the functional outcome after pylorus-preserving pancreaticoduodenectomy: pancreaticogastrostomy and pancreaticojejunostomy. *World J Surg* 2002;26:366–371.

Complications of Breast Surgery

42

Lisa A. Newman

■■■ **INTRODUCTION 603**

■■■ **WOUND COMPLICATIONS 603**
Wound Infections 604
Seroma 606
Hematoma 606
Chronic Pain 607

■■■ **COMPLICATIONS OF MASTECTOMY PROCEDURES 607**
Incisional Dog-ears 607

■■■ **COMPLICATIONS OF LUMPECTOMY 607**
Breast Fibrosis, Breast Lymphedema, and
    Chronic/Recurrent Breast Cellulitis 607
Lumpectomy and Brachytherapy-related
    Complications 608
Angiosarcoma 608

■■■ **COMPLICATIONS OF DIAGNOSTIC OPEN BIOPSY 608**
Sampling Error 608

■■■ **COMPLICATIONS OF AXILLARY STAGING 609**
Complications Associated with ALND 609
Complications Associated with Lymphatic Mapping
    and Sentinel Lymph Node Biopsy 611

■■■ **COMPLICATIONS OF IMMEDIATE BREAST RECONSTRUCTION (IBR) 613**
Skin-sparing Mastectomy 613
IBR and Chest Wall Irradiation 613

■■■ **OTHER ISSUES RELATED TO BREAST SURGERY COMPLICATION RATES 614**
Neoadjuvant Chemotherapy 614

■■■ **REFERENCES 615**

Lisa A. Newman: Breast Cancer Center, University of Michigan Comprehensive Cancer Center, Ann Arbor, MI 48109

INTRODUCTION

The breast is a relatively clean organ, comprised of skin, fatty tissue, and mammary glandular elements that have no direct connection to any major body cavity or visceral structures. In the absence of concurrent major reconstruction, breast surgery is generally not accompanied by large-scale fluid shifts, infectious complications, or hemorrhage. Thus, the breast is largely perceived as being associated with a relatively low risk of surgical morbidity. The breast is, however, the site of the most common cancer afflicting American women, and a myriad of complications can occur in association with the procedures designed to detect and treat breast cancer. Some of these complications are related to the breast itself, and others are associated with axillary staging procedures. This chapter will first address nonspecific complications, followed by discussions of complications that are specific to particular breast-related procedures.

WOUND COMPLICATIONS

As a peripheral, soft tissue organ, wound complications related to breast procedures are relatively minor and frequently managed on an outpatient basis. Studies document that surgical morbidity from breast and/or axillary wound infections, seromas, and hematomas occur in up to 30% of cases. Fewer than half of these will require a prolongation of hospital stay or readmission for inpatient care. Chronic incisional pain can also occur in conjunction with various surgical breast procedures.

Rare complications can also occur in conjunction with various breast procedures. Pneumothorax can be related to either inadvertent pleural puncture during wire localization or to inadvertently deep dissection within an intercostal space. Patients can develop brachial plexopathy related to stretch injury of a malpositioned patient in the operating room (1). The American Society of Anesthesiology recommends upper extremity positioning such that maximal flexion at the shoulder is to 90 degrees, with neutral forearm position, and the use of padded armboards (2).

Thrombosis of the thoracoepigastric vein can occur spontaneously or following breast procedures such as lumpectomy or after percutaneous needle biopsy (3–7). Although thrombosis of the thoracoepigastric vein is not an established breast cancer risk factor, there are case reports of patients who have presented with this condition at the time of breast cancer diagnosis (4). This condition typically presents as a palpable, sometimes tender cord running vertically from the mid-lower hemisphere of the breast toward the abdominal wall. The problem is usually a self-limited condition, and soft-tissue massage can expedite resolution.

Wound Infections

Rates of postoperative infection in breast and axillary incisions have ranged from <1% of cases to nearly 20%, as shown in Table 42-1 (8–21). A meta-analysis by Platt et al. (22) from 1993 analyzed data on 2,587 surgical breast procedures and found an overall wound infection rate of 3.8%. Staphylococcal organisms, introduced via skin flora, are usually implicated in these infections (8,17). Obesity, older age, and diabetes mellitus have been the most consistently identified risk factors for breast wound sepsis. Most investigators (11,14,20,21) have reported that patients undergoing definitive surgery for cancer had a lower risk for wound infection if their diagnosis had been established by prior needle biopsy as opposed to an open surgical biopsy. Nicotine and other components of tobacco cigarettes have well-known adverse effects on small vessels of the skin, resulting in a nearly fourfold increase in risk of wound infection following breast surgery (19). As demonstrated in Table 42-1, there is no consistent correlation between wound infection risk and mastectomy versus lumpectomy as definitive breast cancer surgery.

Perioperative antibiotic coverage to minimize infection rates has been evaluated in both retrospective and prospective randomized controlled trials. Many trials have shown that a single dose of a preoperative antibiotic (usually a cephalosporin) will reduce wound infection rates by 40% (8,13,21,22). A meta-analysis revealed that antibiotic prophylaxis reduced wound infection rates by 38% despite the potential selection bias of antibiotic use, predominantly in higher-risk cases (22). The lowest reported rates of breast wound infections occurred in a phase III study (16) of a long-acting cephalosporin versus a short-acting cephalosporin (0.45% vs. 0.91%). In contrast, Wagman et al. (10) found no effect of perioperative cephalosporin in a placebo-controlled phase III trial involving 118 breast cancer patients (5% vs. 8%); infections in the antibiotic arm were delayed in onset (17.7 days vs. 9.6 days). Gupta et al. (17) reported similar wound infection rates in a phase three study of prophylactic amoxicillin/clavulinic acid (17.7%) versus placebo (18.8%) and concluded that perioperative antibiotics are unnecessary in elective breast surgery. Because of these conflicting results, and in an attempt to minimize cost, many clinicians have adopted the practice of limiting antibiotic prophylaxis to high-risk patients and to cases involving foreign bodies, such as wire localization biopsies. Despite this common practice, wire localization has not been specifically identified as a wound infection risk factor (21).

Incisional cellulitis can be treated with oral antibiotics, but nonresponding cellulitis or extensive soft tissue infection requires intravenous therapy. A minority of breast wound infections progress to a fully developed abscess. The pointing, fluctuant, and exquisitely tender mass of a breast abscess will usually become apparent at a lumpectomy, mastectomy, or axillary incision site 1 to 2 weeks postoperatively. When there is uncertainty regarding the diagnosis, ultrasound imaging may be helpful, but the complex mass that will be visualized can appear identical to a consolidating seroma or hematoma. Aspiration may also confirm the diagnosis, but the possibility of sampling error exists. Definitive management of an abscess requires incision and drainage; curative aspiration of purulent material is rarely successful and the abscess will generally reaccumulate. Incision and drainage can be accomplished by reopening the original surgical wound, and the resulting cavity must be left open to heal by secondary intention. When recurrent cancer is a concern, biopsy of the abscess cavity wall is prudent.

Chronic recurrent periareolar abscess formation does not develop as a consequence of primary breast surgery, but the condition is associated with a high risk of complication following surgical treatment. The condition has been associated with cigarette smoking. Afflicted patients should also be checked for tuberculosis as a factor in recurrent superficial soft tissue infections. Resection of the involved subareolar ductal system(s) is frequently attempted to break the cycle of repeated abscesses, but these procedures are complicated by further wound infection and by the development of chronically draining sinus tracts. The most refractory cases may require complete resection of the nipple-areolar complex, but this strategy should be reserved as a final effort.

TABLE 42-1

SELECTED STUDIES EVALUATING WOUND INFECTION RATES FOLLOWING BREAST SURGERY

Study	No. of Cases	Type of Procedures Analyzed	Type of Study	Wound Infection Rate	Study Findings/Risk Factors for Infection
Platt et al., 1990 (8)	606	Lumpectomy mastectomy ALND reduction mammoplasty	Phase III study of preoperative antibiotics	9.4%	Preoperative antibiotic coverage reduced wound infection rate (6.6% vs. 12.2%)
Hoefer et al., 1990 (9)	101	Mastectomy	Retrospective review	8.9%	*Risk Factor:* • Cautery
Wagman et al., 1990 (10)	118	Mastectomy	Phase III study of preoperative antibiotics	6.8%	Preoperative antibiotics had no effect on wound infection rates (5% vs. 8%)
Chen et al., 1991 (11)		Mastectomy Lumpectomy	Retrospective review	2.6%–11.1%	*Risk Factors:* • Older age • Surgery performed in 1970s vs. 1980s • Prior open diagnostic biopsy vs. single-stage surgery
Vinton et al., 1991 (12)	560	Mastectomy Lumpectomy ALND	Retrospective review	15% (mastectomy) 13% (lumpectomy)	*Risk Factors:* • Older age • Mastectomy vs. lumpectomy • Tobacco smoking • Obesity
Platt et al., 1992 (13)	1981	Mastectomy Lumpectomy ALND Reduction mammoplasty	Retrospective review	3.4%	Preoperative antibiotic coverage reduced wound infection rate (odds ratio 0.59; 95% confidence interval 0.35–0.99)
Lipshy et al., 1996 (14)	289	Mastectomy	Retrospective review	5.3%	*Risk Factor:* Prior open diagnostic biopsy vs. diagnostic needle biopsy (6.9% vs. 1.6%)
Bertin et al., 1998 (15)	18 cases 37 controls	Mastectomy Lumpectomy	Case-control	NA	Preoperative antibiotic coverage reduced wound infection rate *Risk Factors:* • Obesity • Older age
Thomas et al., 1999 (16)	1,766	Mastectomy Lumpectomy ALND	Phase III study of preoperative antibiotics	0.6%	Short-acting vs. long-acting preoperative cephalosporin (0.91% vs. 0.45%)
Gupta et al., 2000 (17)	334	Mastectomy Lumpectomy ALND	Phase III study of preoperative antibiotics	18.3%	Preoperative antibiotics had no effect on wound infection rates (17.7% vs. 18.8%)
Nieto et al., 2002 (18)	107	Mastectomy Lumpectomy ALND	Prospective observational study	7% (mastectomy) 17% (lumpectomy)	*Risk Factors:* • Lumpectomy vs. mastectomy • Older age • Obesity
Sorenson et al., 2002 (19)	425	Mastectomy Lumpectomy ALND	Retrospective review	10.5%	*Risk Factors:* • Tobacco smoking • Diabetes mellitus • Obesity • Heavy ethanol consumption
Witt et al., 2003 (20)	326	Mastectomy Lumpectomy ALND	Prospective observational study	15.3%	*Risk Factors:* • Older age • Obesity • Diabetes mellitus • Prior diagnostic core needle biopsy vs. open diagnostic biopsy
Tran et al., 2003 (21)	320	Mastectomy Lumpectomy	Retrospective review	6.1%	Preoperative antibiotic coverage reduced wound infection rate *Risk Factors:* • Prior open diagnostic biopsy vs. diagnostic needle biopsy (11.1% vs. 9.7%)

ALND, axillary lymph node dissection; NA, not applicable.

Seroma

The rich lymphatic drainage of the breast from intramammary lymphatics to the axillary, supraclavicular, and internal mammary nodal basins establishes a tendency for seroma formation within any closed space that results from breast surgery. Low fibrinogen levels and net fibrinolytic activity within lymphatic fluid may contribute to seroma formation (23,24). The closed spaces of lumpectomy cavities, axillary wounds, and the anterior chest wall cavity left under mastectomy skin flaps will all harbor seroma. After lumpectomy, seroma is advantageous to the patient, as it will usually preserve the normal breast contour even after a large-volume resection, eventually replaced by scar formation as the cavity consolidates. Occasionally the lumpectomy seroma is exuberant, and if the patient experiences discomfort from a bulging fluid collection, simple aspiration of the excess will usually be adequate management.

Seroma formation under the skin flaps of axillary or mastectomy wounds impairs the healing process, and drains are therefore usually left to evacuate postoperative fluid collections. Most breast cancer surgery is performed in the outpatient setting, and patients must be instructed about proper drainage catheter care. After 1 to 3 weeks, skin flaps heal and adhere to the chest wall, as evidenced by diminished drain output. Seroma collections that develop after drain removal can be managed by percutaneous aspiration. Aspiration is usually well-tolerated because the mastectomy and axillary incisions are insensate; these procedures can be repeated as necessary to ensure that skin flaps are densely adherent to the chest wall. Seroma aspiration is necessary in 10% to 80% of axillary lymph node dissection (ALND) and mastectomy cases, according to reported series (23). Axillary surgery limited to the sentinel lymph node biopsy appears to confer a lower risk of seroma formation. This procedure is usually performed without drain insertion, and occasional patients will require subsequent seroma aspiration (25).

Several investigators have studied strategies that might minimize seroma formation in order to decrease the duration that drainage catheters are retained or to obviate drains. Investigators subjected 90 consecutive breast cancer patients undergoing ALND to (a) conventional, prolonged closed suction drainage, (b) 2-day short-term drainage, or (c) no drainage (26). There were no differences in infectious wound complications among the three groups, and at a minimum follow-up of 1 year there were no differences in lymphedema risk. In group 1 the drain was removed at a median of 10 days, with 73% of cases requiring subsequent seroma aspiration. As expected, the short-term and no-drain groups required more frequent seroma aspirations (86% and 97%, respectively). The mean duration of suction drainage or aspiration drainages, or both, was similar for all three groups (25 to 27 days). In all groups fluid accumulation had mostly resolved by 4 weeks, but in each group there were a few patients (approximately 16%) with

prolonged drainage lasting an additional 2 to 3 weeks. Similar findings have been reported in older studies (27,28). The number of drains used and low-vacuum versus high-vacuum suction do not appear to affect the results.

Shoulder immobilization with slings or special wraps to decrease seroma formation has been proposed, but this approach carries the risk of long-term range of motion limitations and may increase the risk of lymphedema (29). Most breast surgeons recommend that patients limit motion at the shoulder to abduction no greater than 90 degrees, and active upper extremity physiotherapy is delayed until drainage catheters are removed. This strategy appears to decrease seroma formation compared to early physiotherapy programs and does not adversely affect long-term range of motion (30,31).

The tissue effects of electrocautery are a well-recognized risk factor for seroma formation (23). Two prospective clinical trials (32,33) have randomized breast cancer patients to surgery with electrocautery versus scalpel only and have demonstrated a lower incidence of seroma formation with the latter technique. Few surgeons are willing to relinquish the convenience and improved hemostasis associated with electrocautery dissection.

Classe et al. (34) reported use of axillary padding in lieu of catheter drains in 207 breast cancer patients undergoing ALND, with seroma formation in 22.2%. In contrast, a second clinical trial that randomized 135 ALND patients to receive a compression dressing for 4 days versus conventional catheter drainage found no benefit from compression dressings (35). Both arms of this study had similar total drainage volumes and drainage catheter durations, and the compression arm had increased seroma aspiration requirements.

Chemical maneuvers to decrease seroma formation have also been investigated. Application of tetracycline as a sclerosing agent has been ineffective (36). Bovine thrombin has been similarly unsuccessful (37). Use of fibrin glues, patches, and/or sealants have appeared promising, but clinical studies in humans have yielded inconsistent results, and it is unclear whether the added expense of these agents is justified (23,38–40).

Hematoma

Widespread use of electrocautery has reduced the incidence of hematoma formation in breast surgery, but this complication occurs in 2% to 10% of cases. Low-volume hematoma cases carry low morbidity, leaving the patient with a more extensive ecchymosis as adjacent soft tissues absorb the hematoma. Large hematomas can be quite painful because of rapid expansion through the closed wound space, and these should be surgically evacuated, with aggressive wound irrigation and reclosure to optimize cosmesis.

An ongoing debate in breast surgery has revolved around the optimal technique for lumpectomy cavity closure. Leaving the cavity open to fill with seroma and closing the overlying skin with deep dermal sutures and a final subcuticular layer has become a conventional wound closure strategy. This method allows for prompt restoration of the breast contour through rapid filling of the lumpectomy cavity, but it requires meticulous hemostasis along the lumpectomy cavity walls prior to skin closure. Absorbable sutures can be used to reapproximate the deeper lumpectomy tissues, and this maneuver has been reported to decrease the risk of hematoma (41). The disadvantage of deep cavity sutures is the potential for compromising the final cosmetic result by altering the underlying breast architecture and causing focal areas of retraction.

The use of a support brassiere in the postoperative period bolsters hemostasis and relieves tension on the skin closure imposed by the weight of the breast. This support is especially important with large, pendulous breasts, where blood vessels running alongside the cavity can be avulsed mechanically if the heavy breast is allowed to suspend unsupported. The patient should be encouraged to wear the support brassiere day and night for several days.

Aspirin-containing products and nonsteroidal anti-inflammatory drugs (NSAIDs) such as ibuprofen have antiplatelet activity, and these medications should be avoided for 1 to 2 weeks prior to surgery. Ketorolac has become a popular intravenous substitute for opiate analgesics during the postoperative period, but this agent is an NSAID and should be used cautiously in order to minimize risk of hematoma (42). Several over-the-counter medications and supplements that are widely used as "herbal supplements" have recently been recognized as contributing to a bleeding diathesis; these include ginseng, ginkgo biloba, and garlic (43,44).

Chronic Pain

A minority of breast cancer patients will experience chronic incisional pain that can be quite debilitating and refractory to standard analgesics, lasting postoperatively for several months to years. This syndrome's etiology remains obscure, although it is commonly assumed to be neuropathic in nature. Frequently described as a "burning," "constricting," or "lancing-type" of ache, chronic pain is reported among mastectomy and lumpectomy patients and is often accompanied by ipsilateral upper extremity symptoms. The incidence of this chronic pain syndrome is uncertain but has been reported to afflict 20% to 30% of patients (45–49). Surprisingly, chronic pain has been reported to occur more commonly following lumpectomy than following mastectomy (45,49). Risk factors include younger age, larger tumors, radiation therapy, chemotherapy, depression, and poor coping mechanisms (46,49,50). This syndrome's intractable quality causes substantial frustration for both patients and surgeons. Successful management has recently been reported with use of serotonin uptake inhibitors, such as amitryptalline and venlafaxine (51).

COMPLICATIONS OF MASTECTOMY PROCEDURES

Incisional Dog-ears

Heavyset patients with thick axillary fat pads are especially prone to being left with triangular or cone-shaped flaps of redundant skin and fatty tissue along the lateral aspect of their mastectomy incisions, commonly known as "dog-ears." Frequently the incisional dog-ear will not be readily apparent while the patient is lying supine on the operating room table, but when she sits or stands upright postoperatively these unsightly protrusions of axillary fat become obvious. They create significant discomfort because they irritate the ipsilateral upper extremity. Similar to the inframammary fold prior to mastectomy, dog-ears can sometimes be the site for recurrent candidal infections.

Numerous surgical approaches have been recommended to either prevent or eliminate the dog-ear problem. One option is to bring the redundant axillary tissue forward and create a "T" or "Y" configuration at the lateral aspect of the transverse mastectomy incision (52). Alternatively, the redundant axillary skin and fatty tissue can be resected either by elongating the standard elliptical mastectomy wound or by using a broad "tear-drop" incision, with the point of the tear-drop oriented medially (53,54).

COMPLICATIONS OF LUMPECTOMY

Breast Fibrosis, Breast Lymphedema, and Chronic/Recurrent Breast Cellulitis

Long-term adverse sequelae related to breast conservation therapy for cancer are being increasingly acknowledged and reported (55,56). These complications are secondary to the combined tissue effects of surgery and radiation therapy. The European Organization for Research and Treatment and the Radiation Therapy Oncology Group have proposed that late effects of breast conservation therapy, including breast edema, fibrosis, and atrophy/retraction, be graded according to the Late Effects of Normal Tissue-Subjective, Objective, Management, and Analytic (LENT-SOMA) scales (57). The LENT-SOMA system stratifies breast symptoms on the basis of pain magnitude as reported by the patient, measurable differences in breast appearance, intervention requirements for control of pain and/or lymphedema, and the presence of image-documented breast sequelae [e.g., photos, mammography, computed tomography (CT)/magnetic resonance imaging (MRI), etc.].

Using the LENT-SOMA four-point grading system, investigators (56) reported grade 3 to 4 toxicity in 4% to 18% of breast cancer patients treated between 1983 and 1984 (XRT fractionation schedule 2.5 Gy 4×/week to 60 Gy, with median follow-up 171 months), with these rates declining to 2% for patients treated in 1994 to 1995 (XRT fractionation schedule 2.0 Gy 5×/week to 55 Gy, with median follow-up 75 months). These findings suggest that the extent of side effects is a function of both follow-up duration and radiation delivery technique. Similarly, investigators (55) reported chronic breast symptoms in 9.9% of breast cancer patients treated by lumpectomy and radiation from 1990 to 1992 and followed for at least 1 year post-treatment.

Recurrent episodes of breast cellulitis occurring several months to years after lumpectomy or breast radiation therapy, or both, are reported to afflict <5% of patients, but this unusual and delayed complication causes significant concern because of the need to rule out an inflammatory breast cancer recurrence (58–62). This condition can present as a myriad of scenarios: acutely inflamed seroma formation, localized mastitis, or diffuse breast pain and swelling. Repeat breast imaging is indicated to detect parenchymal features suggesting recurrence, such as an underlying spiculated mass, and calcifications. If these features are present, an image-guided biopsy should be performed. Benign-appearing cases that are refractory to a standard course of antibiotics should undergo punch biopsy for further evaluation. Occasionally, patients are encountered who ultimately request mastectomy because of intractable pain and inflammation.

The cause of delayed breast edema and cellulitis is incompletely understood but is presumed to be related to lymphatic obstruction affecting intramammary drainage. Risk factors for this condition include history of early postoperative complications such as hematoma and seroma, upper extremity lymphedema, and large-volume lumpectomies (59). Most cases have followed resection of upper outer quadrant tumors. A causative bacterial pathogen is rarely identified, but conventional management includes antibiotic coverage for skin flora. The development of this complication does not appear to carry any cancer-related prognostic significance.

Lumpectomy and Brachytherapy-related Complications

Several breast programs are currently exploring strategies of partial breast irradiation that allow for shortening of the conventional 5 to 6 week external beam program. One such strategy involves insertion of a balloon-type catheter into the lumpectomy cavity for delivery of brachytherapy. This device is typically inserted in the operating room at the time of lumpectomy, with the expectation that margin control will be achieved; if this requirement is not met, additional surgery and a second implantation is required. Although investigations of the long-term efficacy of these accelerated breast irradiation programs are being conducted, experience with catheter-related complications is accumulating. CT imaging is subsequently performed to ensure adequate balloon placement, as defined by a minimum applicator-skin distance of 5 mm, and appropriate

conformance, with uniform contact between the balloon and lumpectomy walls. Optimal positioning can be challenging, but it is essential for delivery of therapy with minimal risk of local complications.

Results from a prospective, multicenter study of the catheter device (63) revealed that of 70 patients enrolled, 21 (30%) could not complete the study because of lumpectomy-related issues (cavity size, skin spacing, or conformance). Of the 54 patients who had a balloon inserted, 57% experienced overlying skin erythema and two patients developed wound infections, including one abscess.

Angiosarcoma

Angiosarcomas of the breast following lumpectomy and x-ray therapy (XRT) for breast cancer are very rare, but they are being reported with increasing frequency (64). These secondary angiosarcomas are distinguished from primary breast angiosarcomas, which occur in relatively younger women and which have no well-defined risk factors. Secondary angiosarcomas occur 4 to 10 years after primary breast cancer treatment (64–66). Lymphedema-related extremity angiosarcoma has a longer latency period from time of breast cancer treatment. The occurrence of breast angiosarcomas in the irradiated field, coupled with the implications for genetic predisposition to radiation-induced tumorigenesis (e.g., ataxia-telangiectasia), has prompted speculation that these lesions have a unique, different etiology. Median survival is poor, averaging 1 to 3 years (64).

COMPLICATIONS OF DIAGNOSTIC OPEN BIOPSY

Sampling Error

The primary potential risk specifically associated with a diagnostic open biopsy is related to missing a cancerous lesion and resecting adjacent fibrocystic tissue, thereby misdiagnosing the patient. This complication exists with palpable masses as well as with screen-detected nonpalpable lesions.

The risk of misdiagnosis with palpable breast masses can be minimized by complete preoperative breast imaging, including mammography and ultrasonography. Palpable lesions that have suspicious imaging should have an initial attempt at percutaneous core needle biopsy to establish a diagnosis. If malignancy is confirmed, cancer-directed management options can be promptly addressed. Neoadjuvant chemotherapy is an option for eligible patients. Although the patient has measureable disease in the breast, the potential benefits of tumor downstaging to improve breast conservation therapy as well as monitoring chemosensitivity responsiveness are available (67). If the percutaneous biopsy is performed and is nondiagnostic, an image-guided needle biopsy can be attempted. Alternatively, percutaneous biopsy may be performed with image guidance as the initial maneuver in order to improve diagnostic accuracy.

If the palpable lesion does not have an imaging correlate, or if needle biopsy strategies are unavailable, a diagnostic open biopsy must be performed. Sampling errors with these procedures are uncommon, but patients with extensive fibrocystic changes can be challenging, especially in cases where the lesion was a self-detected mass that is less dominant on clinical examination. In these cases the breast should be assessed and marked just prior to surgery by the surgeon and patient together, but intraoperative surgical judgment remains critical. Any suspicious masses identified within the open breast wound should be biopsied and oriented appropriately.

The risk of sampling error is greater with nonpalpable breast lesions. Establishing a diagnosis for clinically occult lesions that are identified by mammogram or ultrasound necessarily depends on image guidance. There are advantages to proceeding with an image-guided percutaneous needle biopsy as the initial diagnostic strategy. Cancer patients whose diagnosis has been made via needle biopsy are more likely to have successful breast conservation therapy and require fewer reexcisions for margin control compared to patients who undergo an initial open biopsy for diagnostic purposes (68). A core needle biopsy is preferable to a fine needle aspiration biopsy because of the larger tissue yield, which can distinguish *in situ* from invasive architecture and because the sampling error with a fine needle aspiration biopsy can be as high as 30%, compared to only 5% to 10% with a core needle. If the targeted lesion is small and may be completely resected within the core specimens, a radio-opaque clip should be left in place to facilitate subsequent localization in case surgery is required.

When high-risk lesions such as atypical hyperplasia, radial scar, or lobular carcinoma *in situ* are identified on core needle biopsy, a follow-up open surgical biopsy should be performed. The sampling error rates associated with these findings are substantial, and 10% to 40% will be upstaged to cancer on subsequent open biopsy (69).

Open surgical biopsies of nonpalpable, image-detected breast lesions require image-guided wire localization. The localizing wire can be inserted under either ultrasound or mammographic guidance, depending on which modality best images the abnormal lesion. Magnetic resonance imaging-guided wire localization technology is available in some centers as well. Past strategies for localization have included external skin markings and preoperative injection of dye into the vicinity of the lesion, but these techniques have been largely abandoned because of higher sampling error rates. Insertion of a hooked wire, with two-view confirmatory mammography of the wire position in relation to the abnormal lesion, followed by mammographic or ultrasonographic imaging of the biopsy specimen to document inclusion of the suspicious target, is the routine most widely employed in contemporary breast programs. With this algorithm the likelihood of missing the target should be <5%.

Despite these precautions, risk factors for a sampling error complication include suboptimal wire localization, localizing wire migration between the time of insertion and the time of surgical resection, and migration of a previously inserted clip that was intended to mark the site of a prior core needle biopsy. When a sampling error is recognized intraoperatively, based on specimen imaging, it is quite difficult to reorient the breast anatomy without the localizing wire. In this circumstance it is prudent to resist multiple attempts at "blind" biopsies, as the likelihood of success is low and additional tissue resections will compromise cosmesis. The patient should be informed of the failed procedure, and repeat imaging should be repeated 2 to 4 weeks postoperatively, with plans for another wire localization made accordingly.

COMPLICATIONS OF AXILLARY STAGING

Axillary nodal status remains the most powerful prognostic feature in staging patients with invasive breast cancer. Surgical staging of the axilla is necessary for the majority of newly diagnosed patients, since currently available imaging modalities can easily miss small nodal metastases. The conventional level I/II ALND is the standard means of evaluating the axilla, but lymphatic mapping and sentinel lymph node biopsy has recently emerged as a viable alternative strategy for accurately determining nodal status. Each of these staging procedures is associated with risks for complications.

Complications Associated with ALND

The level I/II ALND is the conventional staging procedure. Random axillary sampling procedures and ALND limited to level I can miss metastases in 20% to 25% of cases. On the other hand, a level III dissection is considered unnecessary unless there is grossly apparent disease present in the axillary apex, because skip metastases to level III occur in only 2% to 3% of cases. The presence of an "axillary arch" has been proposed as an anatomic variant that can increase the risk of sampling error when a standard level I and II ALND is performed (70). The axillary arch is formed by an aberrant segment of latissimus dorsi muscle that extends toward the pectoralis. If the axillary dissection does not encompass lymphatic tissue lateral to these fibers, significant nodal tissue can be missed. Failure to appreciate this anatomic variant has been implicated as a cause of subsequent axillary recurrence (71).

Upper extremity lymphedema is the complication that has generated the most concern following ALND because it is a lifelong risk following the procedure and quite refractory to treatment. Lymphedema has been reported to develop in 13% to 27% of breast cancer patients (25,72–75), but detection rates vary based on how closely patients are followed and the duration of follow-up. Risk of lymphedema is increased in patients after a higher-level axillary dissection compared to less extensive surgery, but lymphedema has been reported to occur even after axillary surgery limited to the sentinel lymph nodes (25). Other risk factors include obesity and regional radiation therapy. Patients can minimize risk of lymphedema by participating in an aggressive and regulated physical therapy program. The problem is aggravated by upper extremity trauma or infection.

The most feared long-term consequence of chronic lymphedema is upper extremity angiosarcoma (76,77). This condition is also known as Stewart-Treves syndrome (78), named for the investigators who first reported the association between postmastectomy lymphedema and the typically bluish-reddish macular lesions or nodules on the skin of the ipsilateral upper extremity. This disease develops approximately 10 years after breast cancer treatment and usually occurs in patients who have received regional irradiation in addition to ALND. Treatment strategies have included wide local excision, amputation, chemotherapy, and radiation, with disappointing results. Most patients succumb to hematogenously disseminated metastases to lung and visceral organs, with a median survival of approximately 2 years.

The axillary dissection exposes the axillary vein, thoracodorsal, long thoracic, and intercostobrachial nerves, as well as the neurovascular bundle to the pectoralis musculature. The intercostobrachial nerves are routinely sacrificed during conventional ALND as they course directly through the nodal tissue en route to the skin of the axilla and upper inner arm, leaving patients with sensory deficits in this distribution. Attempts to preserve these nerves can result in damage that leaves the patient with chronic neuropathic pain of the involved skin. The axillary vein is at risk for hemorrhagic complications as a consequence of direct injury, or thrombosis secondary to traction and compression (Fig. 42-1). The axillary artery and brachial plexus are relatively protected from intraoperative damage because of their deeper and more superior location. The thoracodorsal neurovascular bundle, which courses along the inner aspect of the latissimus dorsi muscle, should be completely exposed and preserved unless there is gross encasement by nodal metastases. Sacrifice of these structures will denervate the latissimus, leaving the patient with weakness of internal rotation and shoulder abduction, and eliminates the thoracodorsal vessels for future use with microvascular anastomoses for free flap reconstructions. Disruption of the long thoracic nerve results in loss of serratus anterior function and a "winged scapula" deformity, an unsightly posterior shoulder bony protrusion. When the medial and lateral pectoral nerves

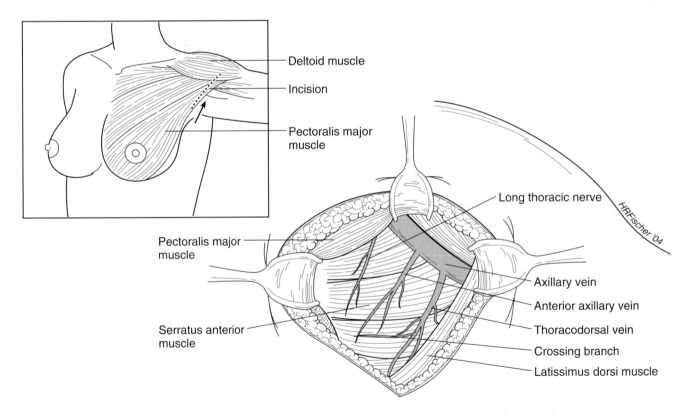

Deltoid muscle

Incision

Pectoralis major muscle

Long thoracic nerve

HRFischer '04

Axillary vein

Anterior axillary vein

Thoracodorsal vein

Crossing branch

Latissimus dorsi muscle

Pectoralis major muscle

Serratus anterior muscle

Figure 42-1 Incision used for axillary dissection (*inset*). Venous structures at risk for injury during axillary dissection include the axillary vein and its branches, including the thoracodorsal vein and its associated thoracodorsal nerve. Injury to the long thoracic nerve may occur more medially.

are transected, denervation atrophy of the pectoral muscles will eventually become apparent and can compromise the cosmetic result substantially.

Axillary webs are bands of scar tissue that develop after ALND in <10% of cases. They are readily apparent as cord-like structures coursing from the surgical bed toward the forearm and occasionally reaching the thumb (79). Axillary webs cause significant tightness and limitation of motion, which in most cases will resolve within a few months. Physical therapy and massage are frequently helpful in alleviating symptoms.

A rare complication of ALND is chyle leak (80), reputed to be secondary to thoracic duct injury. Recently, octreotide has been recommended to control extensive lymphorrhea (81).

Complications Associated with Lymphatic Mapping and Sentinel Lymph Node Biopsy

In 1993 and 1994 the initial reports of lymphatic mapping and sentinel lymph node biopsy for breast cancer patients appeared (82) using radiolabeled isotope and blue dye (83). There was prompt recognition that this technology represented a promising strategy to identify node-negative patients and to spare them the morbidity of a conventional ALND. Since these pioneering studies, dozens of other investigators have reported experiences with lymphatic mapping and sentinel lymph node biopsy in conjunction with a completion ALND. A meta-analysis of these types of studies (84) presented to the American Society of Clinical Oncology in 2002 revealed an overall identification rate of 96% and an overall false-negative rate of 8.4%. This analysis included data from 69 studies involving 10,454 patients. Lower-volume studies, early phase of the learning curve with lymphatic mapping technology, and use of a single mapping agent (blue dye or isotope rather than both) were identified as risk factors for the complications of a failed mapping procedure or obtaining a false-negative sentinel lymph node result.

Table 42-2 summarizes the results of studies that have evaluated specific causes of an inability to identify the sentinel lymph node and features that predict a greater risk of identifying a falsely negative result. Similar to the meta-analysis findings, inexperience with lymphatic mapping and use of a single mapping agent rather than two agents are repeatedly implicated with unsuccessful sentinel lymph node biopsies. The steep learning curve and the benefits of dual versus single mapping agents are explored in recent reviews (85,86).

The original studies of sentinel lymph node biopsy involved intraparenchymal, peritumoral injections of the mapping agent(s), since the goal is to replicate the pathway traversed by tumor cells along intramammary lymphatic channels en route to the sentinel node. If the mapping procedure is performed after an excisional biopsy, there is risk of inadvertent injection into the biopsy cavity. The mapping

agent will not reach the nodal basin. As experience with lymphatic mapping has grown, technical failures have declined and investigators have specifically documented the ability to reliably identify the sentinel lymph node in the setting of prior excisional biopsy (94,95). Injections of skin overlying tumor site further improve sentinel node identification rates because of exuberant uptake by dermal lymphatics (99). With increasing age, lymph nodes can become fatty-replaced and difficult to recognize, contributing to a failed identification. For tumors located in the upper outer quadrant of the breast, extensive background radioactivity (shine-through) impairs the ability to discriminate focal uptake by the sentinel node; the likelihood of missing the true sentinel node and obtaining a false-negative result is increased. In contrast, medially located tumors have been associated with a risk of mapping failure because of the increased likelihood of primary lymphatic drainage to nonaxillary sites. Other reports (100) have found no relationship between tumor location and sentinel node accuracy. An additional factor implicated in mapping inaccuracy is size of the primary tumor; with larger lesions there is risk of tumor embolization causing obstructed lymphatic vessels, thereby altering the pathway that a mapping agent would follow. Although early studies (90) did suggest a correlation between breast tumor size and risk of a false-negative sentinel lymph node biopsy, more recent studies have indicated no association (91,93,101). Investigators (102) have also confirmed the accuracy of sentinel lymph node biopsy for invasive lobular carcinoma.

Many of the potential pitfalls in lymphatic mapping procedures have been obviated by the development of newer mapping techniques, such as subareolar injections of the mapping agent (103–105). This strategy is based on the embryologic development of the breast and its lymphatic drainage system, which begins at the centrally located nipple bud, followed by radial extension peripherally. This pattern leads to the concept that each breast has primary drainage to a discrete cluster of sentinel lymph nodes, as opposed to separate drainage pathways for different areas of the breast. This model permits lymphatic mapping in cases of multicentric breast cancer, which previously had been considered a contraindication to sentinel node biopsy.

Recent studies of lymphatic mapping in patients with multifocal or multicentric disease have demonstrated that sentinel lymph node biopsy is accurate in this setting (106–110). From these studies it appears that the sentinel node can be identified by injection targeting the different breast tumors or by use of the subareolar technique.

Other complications that have been reported following sentinel lymph node biopsy are the same as those that are associated with ALND, including seroma, lymphedema, axillary web formation, and neurosensory disturbances, but the magnitude of risk is lower. Data on long-term follow-up of patients who have undergone sentinel lymph node biopsy alone reveal adverse sequelae in <5% of cases (25,74,111).

TABLE 42-2

SELECTED STUDIES REPORTING RISK FACTORS FOR FAILED LYMPHATIC MAPPING AND/OR FALSE-NEGATIVE SENTINEL LYMPH NODE BIOPSY

Study	Total No. Cases	SLN Identification Rate (%)	SLN False-Negative Rate (%)	Factors Associated with SLN Nonidentification						Factors Associated with SLN FN Risk					
				Learning Curve	Tumor location (Medial Worse)	Older Age Pt	Prior Excisional Biopsy	Single vs. Dual Mapping Agent	Larger Size Tumor	Learning Curve	Tumor Location (Upper/Outer Quadrant Worse)	Older Age Pt	Prior Excisional Biopsy	Single vs. Dual Mapping Agent	Larger Size Tumor
Canavese et al., 2001 (87)	212	97.1	6.5	No	NR										
Albertini et al., 1996 (88)	62	92	0	NR	NR	NR	NA[a]	Yes	NR	No	No	No	No	No	No
McMasters et al., 2000 (89)	806	88	7.2	No	No	Yes	No	Yes	No	No	Yes	No	No	Yes	No
Veronesi et al., 1997 (90)	163	98	4.7	No	No	No	No	NA (Tc only used)	Yes	No	Yes	No	No	NA	Yes
Veronesi et al., 1999 (91)	376	98.7	6.7	No	No	NR	NR	No	No	No	No	No	NR	No	No
Cox et al., 1998 (92)	465	94.4	UK	Yes	NR	NR	No	Yes	NR	Yes	NR	NR	NR	NR	NR
Giuliano et al., 1994 (83)	174	65.5	8.1	Yes	NR	NR	NR	NA (dye only used)	NR	Yes	NR	NR	NR	NR	NR
Bedrosian et al., 2000 (93)	104[b]	99	3.3	NR	NR	NR	NR	NR	No	NR	NR	NR	NR	NR	No
Haigh et al., 2000 (94)	284[c]	81.0	3.2	NR	No	NR	No	NR	No	Yes	No	NR	No	NR	No
Wong et al., 2002 (95)	2206[d]	92.5	8.0	NR	No	NR	No	NR	Yes	NR	No	NR	No	NR	No
Krag et al., 1998 (96)	443	93	12.8	NR	Yes	Yes	Yes	NA (isotope only used)	No	NR	Yes	No	No	NA (isotope only used)	No
O'Hea et al., 1998 (97)	59	93	15	NR	No	NR	No	Yes	No	Yes	No	NR	No	No	Yes
Guenther 1999 (98)	260	81.9	NR[e]	Yes	Yes	NR	No	NA (dye only used)	NA[e]	NA[e]	NA[e]	NA[e]	NA[e]	NA[e]	NA[e]

[a]Patients with prior excisional biopsy excluded from study.
[b]All T2 and T3 tumors.
[c]Including 181 lymphatic mapping cases with prior excisional biopsy.
[d]Medial location worse.
[e]Analyses limited to 47 patients with unsuccessful mapping procedures.
Id, identification; FN, false negative; UOQ, upper outer quadrant; SLN, sentinel lymph node; NR, not reported.

Allergic reactions to the blue dye for mapping procedures must be considered. Table 42-3 demonstrates reported series involving both isosulfan blue and patent blue dye. Within a few minutes to an hour following blue dye injection, up to 2% of patients may experience hemodynamic instability and other sequelae of intraoperative anaphylaxis. Despite the dramatic presentation, these episodes are usually readily responsive to supportive care, which includes discontinuation of the gaseous anesthetics, 100% oxygen, aggressive fluid resuscitation, and pressor support. In most cases the anesthesia and surgical procedure have been resumed and completed uneventfully after the patient has been stabilized. Some surgeons elect to abort the surgical procedure (112) and reschedule the mapping without blue dye, and in one reported case (113) a planned lumpectomy was converted to a mastectomy so that the allergen focus would be completely resected. Many other patients have gone on to undergo successful lumpectomies, but they should be monitored closely for 24 hours because continued uptake of the blue dye from skin and soft tissue can result in protracted or delayed secondary (biphasic) reactions.

"Blue urticaria," a less severe form of blue dye allergy characterized by blue-tinged hives, is another pattern that has been reported (116,122). There is no correlation with past allergy history, and preoperative skin testing is unreliable in identifying highest-risk patients. Individuals may have prior sensitization from exposure to industrial dyes in cosmetics, textiles, detergents, and so on. Routine premedication of all

TABLE 42-3

SELECTED STUDIES OF ALLERGIC REACTIONS TO BLUE DYE IN BREAST CANCER CASES

Study, Year	Blue Dye Type	No. of Cases (Type)	Incidence	No. of 2nd Reactions
Lyew et al., 2000 (114)	Isosulfan blue	1 (anaphylactic)	NR	No
Mullon et al., 2001 (115)	Patent blue			
Cimmino et al., 2001 (116)	Isosulfan blue	5 (3 anaphylactic[a]; 2 blue urticaria)	2%	No
Albo et al., 2001 (117)	Isosulfan blue	7 (all anaphylactic)	1.1%	2/7 (%)
Montgomery et al., 2002 (118)	Isosulfan blue	39 (27 blue hives; 12 anaphylactic)	1.6%	NR
Efron et al., 2002 (113)	Isosulfan blue	1 (anaphylactic)	NR	No
Laurie et al., 2002 (112)	Isosulfan blue	2 (anaphylactic)	NR	No
Stefanutto et al., 2002 (119)	Isosulfan blue	1 (anaphylactic)	NR	No
Crivellaro et al., 2003 (120)	Patent blue	1 (anaphylactic)	NR	No
Sprung et al., 2003 (121)	Isosulfan blue	1 (anaphylactic)	NR	Possibly; protracted hypotension noted

[a]Series includes two cases of lymphatic mapping performed for breast cancer.
NR, not reported.

mapping cases with steroids, antihistamines, and histamine-receptor blockade has been proposed, but justification for the added expense and risks of this approach for a low-incidence allergic reaction has not been documented. Known allergy to triphenylmethane is a contraindication to blue dye use. Methylene blue appears to be less allergenic (123), but caution must be exercised to avoid skin necrosis from dermal injection of this agent.

Blue dyes can also cause a spurious decline in pulse oximetry measurements related to intravascular uptake and interference with spectroscopy; arterial blood gases in these circumstances will reveal normal oxygenation. Blue dyes are contraindicated during pregnancy because the risk of teratogenicity is unknown.

COMPLICATIONS OF IMMEDIATE BREAST RECONSTRUCTION (IBR)

A detailed discussion of breast reconstruction options and complication risks is beyond the scope of this chapter, but a few issues warrant mention. The risks of wound complications associated with any type of reconstruction are increased by smoking, obesity, and chest wall irradiation.

Skin-sparing Mastectomy

The skin-sparing mastectomy technique has become increasingly popular as a means of improving the cosmetic results achieved by immediate breast reconstruction (IBR). The surgeon should take particular care in raising the elongated skin flaps so that risk of retained breast tissue and local recurrence is minimized. When the oncologic principles of the mastectomy are upheld, breast cancer outcome is equivalent for patients undergoing skin-sparing and conventional mastectomy with IBR (124–126).

Localized wound problems such as minor infections, focal epidermolysis, and fat necrosis are usually managed successfully without the need for additional surgery. Fat necrosis associated with a mass may be difficult to distinguish from local recurrence; needle or excisional biopsy may become necessary.

IBR and Chest Wall Irradiation

Chest wall irradiation can compromise reconstruction outcome regardless of whether the mastectomy and IBR are performed before or after the radiation exposure. Mastectomy and IBR performed on a previously irradiated chest wall, as in the setting of patients undergoing surgery for local recurrence or in breast cancer patients with a history of therapeutic chest wall irradiation for Hodgkin disease, is more challenging because of the stiffer, less compliant chest skin. Autogenous tissue reconstructions are usually preferred in this circumstance because of difficulties in expanding the chest wall to accommodate an implant.

Mastectomy and IBR are performed prior to irradiation in cases requiring postmastectomy irradiation—for example, extensive nodal disease, locally advanced breast cancer, or mastectomy flaps with inadequate margin control. In this setting, irradiation of the reconstructed breast increases risk of fat necrosis and wound infection. Implant reconstructions are particularly sensitive to this effect, and up to one half will require explanation because of contractures or recurrent infection (127). Some investigators have reported that transverse rectus abdominus myocutaneous (TRAM) flap reconstructions tolerate irradiation (128), but more recent studies have indicated that in the long term there is increased morbidity, including high rates of fibrosis, shrinkage, and progressive deformity (129). When there is a significant likelihood that postmastectomy irradiation will be required, patients should be informed of the risks associated with IBR and delayed reconstruction should be encouraged. An alternative approach that has been proposed is the insertion of a tissue expander at the time of mastectomy to facilitate skin preservation and expansion, followed by final surgery upon completion of chest wall irradiation as either autogenous tissue reconstruction or exchange to the final implant. Although this strategy may be reasonable in concept, long-term results and rates of attendant infectious morbidity remain to be defined.

OTHER ISSUES RELATED TO BREAST SURGERY COMPLICATION RATES

Neoadjuvant Chemotherapy

The benefits of breast preservation and monitoring of chemosensitivity have led to broadened application for induction chemotherapy regimens. Numerous studies have demonstrated the oncologic and medical safety of this approach. Patients should have surgery timed with the last chemotherapy cycle so that adequate bone marrow recovery has occurred, as evidenced by a platelet count >75,000 and an absolute neutrophil count >1,500. Investigators have reported similar wound complication rates in a retrospective study of nearly 200 patients receiving treatment for locally advanced breast cancer; approximately half of these patients underwent primary mastectomy followed by postoperative chemotherapy, and the other half received treatment in the reverse sequence. Wound infection rates were similar for the two groups, and seroma rates were lower for neoadjuvant chemotherapy patients.

Patients with unifocal breast cancers and no mammographically suspicious calcifications who are receiving induction chemotherapy in order to improve eligibility for breast preservation should have radio-opaque clips inserted into the tumor by the first or second cycle of treatment. If no markers are inserted and the patient has a complete clinical response, she will be committed to a mastectomy because of inability to localize the tumor bed at the time of lumpectomy. Alternatively, patients with diffuse suspicious microcalcifications and patients with multicentric disease should be informed at the time of diagnosis that mastectomy will be required regardless of the magnitude of response to induction chemotherapy because of limited ability to accurately monitor response in these clinical scenarios (130).

The optimal strategy for integrating lymphatic mapping technology into neoadjuvant chemotherapy protocols remains to be defined. As shown in Table 42-4, numerous investigators have reported the accuracy of sentinel lymph node biopsies performed after the delivery of neoadjuvant chemotherapy, and the success rates have been quite varied. Identification rates range from 70% to 100%, and false-negative rates range from 0% to 33%, with averages

TABLE 42-4

SELECTED STUDIES OF LYMPHATIC MAPPING AND SENTINEL LYMPH NODE BIOPSY PERFORMED AFTER NEOADJUVANT CHEMOTHERAPY

Study	T Status	Sample Size	Sentinel Node Identification Rate (%)	False Negative Rate (%)	Metastases Limited to Sentinel Node(s) (%)
Breslin et al., 2000 (131)	2,3	51	85	12	40
Nason et al., 2000 (132)	2,3	15	87	33	≥11
Haid et al., 2001 (133)	1-3	33	88	0	50
Fernandez et al., 2001 (134)	1-4	40	90	20	20
Tafra et al., 2001 (135)	1,2	29	93	0	NR
Stearns et al., 2002 (136)	3,4	T4d (inflammatory) 8	75	40	24
		Noninflammatory 26	88	6	
Julian et al., 2002 (137)	1-3	34	91	0	42
Miller et al., 2002 (138)	1-3	35	86	0	44
Brady, 2002 (139)	1-3	14	93	0	60
Piato et al., 2003 (140)	1,2	42	98	17	0
Balch et al., 2003 (141)	2-4	32	97	5	56
Schwartz et al., 2003 (142)	1-3	21	100	9	64
Reitsamer et al., 2003 (143)	2,3	30	87	7	53
Mamounas et al., 2002 (144) (abstract)	1-3	428	85	11	50

NR, not reported.

approximating 90% and 9%, respectively. Many of these series reveal axillary metastases limited to the sentinel node, comparable to primary surgery cases, supporting the validity of the technology from a biologic perspective. An alternative strategy is to perform the axillary staging via sentinel lymph node biopsy prior to delivery of the neoadjuvant chemotherapy. Unfortunately, this sequence commits many patients to an "unnecessary" completion axillary dissection, as the sentinel node(s) will be the isolated site of metastases in a significant proportion of patients and chemotherapy will sterilize axillary metastases in approximately one-quarter of cases. This issue remains to be further evaluated in prospective clinical trials.

REFERENCES

1. Grunwald Z, Moore JH, Schwartz GF. Bilateral brachial plexus palsy after a right-side modified radical mastectomy with immediate TRAM flap reconstruction. *Breast J* 2003;9:41–43.
2. Warner M, Blitt C, Butterworth J, et al. Practice advisory for the prevention of perioperative peripheral neuropathies. A report by the American Society of Anesthesiologists' Task Force on the prevention of perioperative peripheral neuropathies. *Anesthesiology* 2000;92:1168–1182.
3. Bejanga BI. Mondor's disease: analysis of 30 cases. *J R Coll Surg Edinb* 1992;37:322–324.
4. Catania S, Zurrida S, Veronesi P, et al. Mondor's disease and breast cancer. *Cancer* 1992;69:2267–2270.
5. Harris AT. Mondor's disease of the breast can also occur after a sonography-guided core biopsy. *Am J Roentgenol* 2003;180: 284–285.
6. Hou MF, Huang CJ, Huang YS, et al. Mondor's disease in the breast. *Kaohsiung J Med Sci* 1999;15:632–639.
7. Jaberi M, Willey SC, Brem RF. Stereotactic vacuum-assisted breast biopsy: an unusual cause of Mondor's disease. *Am J Roentgenol* 2002;179:185–186.
8. Platt R, Zaleznik DF, Hopkins CC, et al. Perioperative antibiotic prophylaxis for herniorrhaphy and breast surgery. *N Engl J Med* 1990;322:153–160.
9. Hoefer R, DuBois J, Ostrow L, et al. Wound complications following modified radical mastectomy: an analysis of perioperative factors. *J Am Osteopath Assoc* 1990;90:47–53.
10. Wagman LD, Tegtmeier B, Beatty JD, et al. A prospective, randomized double-blind study of the use of antibiotics at the time of mastectomy. *Surg Gynecol Obstet* 1990;170:12–16.
11. Chen J, Gutkin Z, Bawnik J. Postoperative infections in breast surgery. *J Hosp Infect* 1991;17:61–65.
12. Vinton AL, Traverso LW, Jolly PC. Wound complications after modified radical mastectomy compared with tylectomy with axillary lymph node dissection. *Am J Surg* 1991;161:584–588.
13. Platt R, Zucker JR, Zaleznik DF, et al. Prophylaxis against wound infection following herniorrhaphy or breast surgery. *J Infect Dis* 1992;166:556–560.
14. Lipshy KA, Neifeld JP, Boyle RM, et al. Complications of mastectomy and their relationship to biopsy technique. *Ann Surg Oncol* 1996;3:290–294.
15. Bertin M, Crowe J, Gordon S. Determinants of surgical site infection after breast surgery. *Am J Infect Control* 1998;26:61–65.
16. Thomas R, Alvino P, Cortino GR, et al. Long-acting versus short-acting cephalosporins for preoperative prophylaxis in breast surgery: a randomized double-blind trial involving 1,766 patients. *Chemotherapy* 1999;45:217–223.
17. Gupta R, Sinnett D, Carpenter R, et al. Antibiotic prophylaxis for post-operative wound infection in clean elective breast surgery. *Eur J Surg Oncol* 2000;26:363–366.
18. Nieto A, Lozano M, Moro MT, et al. Determinants of wound infections after surgery for breast cancer. *Zentralbl Gynakol* 2002;124:429–433.
19. Sorensen LT, Horby J, Friis E, et al. Smoking as a risk factor for wound healing and infection in breast cancer surgery. *Eur J Surg Oncol* 2002;28:815–820.
20. Witt A, Yavuz D, Walchetseder C, et al. Preoperative core needle biopsy as an independent risk factor for wound infection after breast surgery. *Obstet Gynecol* 2003;101:745–750.
21. Tran CL, Langer S, Broderick-Villa G, et al. Does reoperation predispose to postoperative wound infection in women undergoing operation for breast cancer?. *Am Surg* 2003;69:852–856.
22. Platt R, Zucker JR, Zaleznik DF, et al. Perioperative antibiotic prophylaxis and wound infection following breast surgery. *J Antimicrob Chemother* 1993;31(Suppl. B):43–48.
23. Pogson CJ, Adwani A, Ebbs SR. Seroma following breast cancer surgery. *Eur J Surg Oncol* 2003;29:711–717.
24. Bonnema J, Ligtensetein D, Wiggers T, et al. The composition of serous fluid after axillary dissection. *Eur J Surg* 1999;165:9–13.
25. Giuliano AE, Haigh PI, Brennan MB, et al. Prospective observational study of sentinel lymphadenectomy without further axillary dissection in patients with sentinel node-negative breast cancer. *J Clin Oncol* 2000;18:2553–2559.
26. Talbot ML, Magarey CJ. Reduced use of drains following axillary lymphadenectomy for breast cancer. *ANZ J Surg* 2002;72: 488–490.
27. Cameron AE, Ebbs SR, Wylie F, et al. Suction drainage of the axilla: a prospective randomized trial. *Br J Surg* 1988;75:1211.
28. Somers R, Jablon L, Kaplan M. The use of closed suction drainage after lumpectomy and axillary dissection for breast cancer: a prospective randomized trial. *Ann Surg* 1992;215: 146–149.
29. Flew J. The effect of restriction of shoulder movement. *Br J Surg* 1979;66:302–305.
30. Lotz M, Duncan M, Gerber L, et al. Early versus delayed shoulder motion following axillary dissection. *Ann Surg* 1981;193: 288–295.
31. Schultz I, Barrholm M, Grondal S. Delayed shoulder exercises in reducing seroma frequency after modified radical mastectomy: a prospective randomized study. *Ann Surg Oncol* 1997;4:293–297.
32. Porter KA, O'Connor S, Rimm E, et al. Electrocautery as a factor in seroma formation following mastectomy. *Am J Surg* 1998; 176:8–11.
33. Keogh G, Doughty J, McArdle C, et al. Seroma formation related to electrocautery in breast surgery—a prospective, randomized trial. *The Breast* 1998;7:39–41.
34. Classe J, Dupre P, Francois T, et al. Axillary padding as an alternative to closed suction drain for ambulatory axillary lymphadenectomy. *Arch Surg* 2002;137:169–173.
35. O'Hea BJ, Ho MN, Petrek JA. External compression dressing versus standard dressing after axillary lymphadenectomy. *Am J Surg* 1999;177:450–453.
36. Rice DC, Morris SM, Sarr MG, et al. Intraoperative topical tetracycline sclerotherapy following mastectomy: a prospective, randomized trial. *J Surg Oncol* 2000;73:224–227.
37. Burak WE Jr, Goodman P, Young D, et al. Seroma formation following axillary dissection for breast cancer: risk factors and lack of influence of bovine thrombin. *J Surg Oncol* 1997;64:27–31.
38. Langer S, Guenther JM, DiFronzo LA. Does fibrin sealant reduce drain output and allow earlier removal of drainage catheters in women undergoing operation for breast cancer? *Am Surg* 2003;69:77–81.
39. Berger A, Tempfer C, Hartmann B, et al. Sealing of postoperative axillary leakage after axillary lymphadenectomy using a fibrin glue coated collagen patch: a prospective randomised study. *Breast Cancer Res Treat* 2001;67:9–14.
40. Moore M, Burak WE Jr, Nelson E, et al. Fibrin sealant reduces the duration and amount of fluid drainage after axillary dissection: a randomized prospective clinical trial. *J Am Coll Surg* 2001;192: 591–599.
41. Paterson ML, Nathanson SD, Havstad S. Hematomas following excisional breast biopsies for invasive breast carcinoma: the influence of deep suture approximation of breast parenchyma. *Am Surg* 1994;60:845–848.

42. Sharma S, Chang DW, Koutz C, et al. Incidence of hematoma associated with ketorolac after TRAM flap breast reconstruction. *Plast Reconstr Surg* 2001;107:352–355.

43. Hodges P, Kam P. The perioperative implications of herbal medicines. *Anaesthesia* 2002;57:889–899.

44. Ang-Lee M, Moss J, Yuan C. Herbal medicines and perioperative care. *JAMA* 2001;286:208–216.

45. Tasmuth T, von Smitten K, Kalso E. Pain and other symptoms during the first year after radical and conservative surgery for breast cancer. *Br J Cancer* 1996;74:2024–2031.

46. Tasmuth T, Blomqvist C, Kalso E. Chronic post-treatment symptoms in patients with breast cancer operated in different surgical units. *Eur J Surg Oncol* 1999;25:38–43.

47. Stevens P, Dibble S, Miastowski C. Prevalence, characteristics, and impact of postmastectomy pain syndrome: an investigation of women's experiences. *Pain* 1995;61:61–68.

48. Carpenter J, Andrylkowski M, Sloan P, et al. Postmastectomy/postlumpectomy pain in breast cancer survivors. *J Clin Epidemiol* 1998;51:1285–1292.

49. Tasmuth T, von Smitten K, Hietanen P, et al. Pain and other symptoms after different treatment modalities of breast cancer. *Ann Oncol* 1995;6:453–459.

50. Bishop SR, Warr D. Coping, catastrophizing and chronic pain in breast cancer. *J Behav Med* 2003;26:265–281.

51. Tasmuth T, Hartel B, Kalso E. Venlafaxine in neuropathic pain following treatment of breast cancer. *Eur J Pain* 2002;6:17–24.

52. Farrar WB, Fanning WJ. Eliminating the dog-ear in modified radical mastectomy. *Am J Surg* 1988;156:401–402.

53. Chretien-Marquet B, Bennaceur S. Dog ear: true and false. A simple surgical management. *Dermatol Surg* 1997;23:547–550; discussion 551.

54. Mirza M, Sinha KS, Fortes-Mayer K. Tear-drop incision for mastectomy to avoid dog-ear deformity. *Ann R Coll Surg Engl* 2003; 85:131.

55. Meric F, Buchholz TA, Mirza NQ, et al. Long-term complications associated with breast-conservation surgery and radiotherapy. *Ann Surg Oncol* 2002;9:543–549.

56. Fehlauer F, Tribius S, Holler U, et al. Long-term radiation sequelae after breast-conserving therapy in women with early-stage breast cancer: an observational study using the LENT-SOMA scoring system. *Int J Radiat Oncol Biol Phys* 2003;55: 651–658.

57. RTOG/EORTC Working Groups. LENT-SOMA scales for all anatomic sites. *Int J Radiat Oncol Biol Phys* 1995;31:1049–1091.

58. Zippel D, Siegelmann-Danieli N, Ayalon S, et al. Delayed breast cellulitis following breast conserving operation. *Eur J Surg Oncol* 2003;29:327–330.

59. Brewer VH, Hahn KA, Rohrbach BW, et al. Risk factor analysis for breast cellulitis complicating breast conservation therapy. *Clin Infect Dis* 2000;31:654–659.

60. Staren ED, Klepac S, Smith AP, et al. The dilemma of delayed cellulitis after breast conservation therapy. *Arch Surg* 1996;131: 651–654.

61. Rescigno J, McCormick B, Brown AE, et al. Breast cellulitis after conservative surgery and radiotherapy. *Int J Radiat Oncol Biol Phys* 1994;29:163–168.

62. Miller SR, Mondry T, Reed JS, et al. Delayed cellulitis associated with conservative therapy for breast cancer. *J Surg Oncol* 1998; 67:242–245.

63. Keisch M, Vicini F, Kuske RR, et al. Initial clinical experience with the MammoSite breast brachytherapy applicator in women with early-stage breast cancer treated with breast-conserving therapy. *Int J Radiat Oncol Biol Phys* 2003;55:289–293.

64. Monroe AT, Feigenberg SJ, Mendenhall NP. Angiosarcoma after breast-conserving therapy. *Cancer* 2003;97:1832–1840.

65. Edeiken S, Russo DP, Knecht J, et al. Angiosarcoma after tylectomy and radiation therapy for carcinoma of the breast. *Cancer* 1992;70:644–647.

66. Feigenberg SJ, Mendenhall NP, Reith JD, et al. Angiosarcoma after breast-conserving therapy: experience with hyperfractionated radiotherapy. *Int J Radiat Oncol Biol Phys* 2002;52: 620–626.

67. Fisher B, Brown A, Mamounas E, et al. Effect of preoperative chemotherapy on local-regional disease in women with operable breast cancer: findings from National Surgical Adjuvant Breast and Bowel Project B-18. *J Clin Oncol* 1997;15:2483–2493.

68. Liberman L, Goodstone S, Dershaw D. One operation after percutaneous diagnosis of nonpalpable breast cancer: frequency and associated factors. *Am J Roentgenol* 2002;178:673–679.

69. Newman L. Surgical management of high-risk breast lesions. *Curr Probl Surg* 2003;20(4):99–112.

70. Petrasek AJ, Semple JL, McCready DR. The surgical and oncologic significance of the axillary arch during axillary lymphadenectomy. *Can J Surg* 1997;40:44–47.

71. Wright FC, Walker J, Law CH, et al. Outcomes after localized axillary node recurrence in breast cancer. *Ann Surg Oncol* 2003;10: 1054–1058.

72. Erickson VS, Pearson ML, Ganz PA, et al. Arm edema in breast cancer patients. *J Natl Cancer Inst* 2001;93:96–111.

73. Beaulac SM, McNair LA, Scott TE, et al. Lymphedema and quality of life in survivors of early-stage breast cancer. *Arch Surg* 2002; 137:1253–1257.

74. Sener SF, Winchester DJ, Martz CH, et al. Lymphedema after sentinel lymphadenectomy for breast carcinoma. *Cancer* 2001;92: 748–752.

75. Roses DF, Brooks AD, Harris MN, et al. Complications of level I and II axillary dissection in the treatment of carcinoma of the breast. *Ann Surg* 1999;230:194–201.

76. Grobmyer SR, Daly JM, Glotzbach RE, et al. Role of surgery in the management of postmastectomy extremity angiosarcoma (Stewart-Treves syndrome). *J Surg Oncol* 2000;73:182–188.

77. Janse AJ, van Coevorden F, Peterse H, et al. Lymphedema-induced lymphangiosarcoma. *Eur J Surg Oncol* 1995;21:155–158.

78. Stewart FW, Treves N. Classics in oncology: lymphangiosarcoma in postmastectomy lymphedema: a report of six cases in elephantiasis chirurgica. *CA Cancer J Clin* 1981;31:284–299.

79. Moskovitz AH, Anderson BO, Yeung RS, et al. Axillary web syndrome after axillary dissection. *Am J Surg* 2001;181:434–439.

80. Caluwe GL, Christiaens MR. Chylous leak: a rare complication after axillary lymph node dissection. *Acta Chir Belg* 2003;103: 217–218.

81. Carcoforo P, Soliani G, Maestroni U, et al. Octreotide in the treatment of lymphorrhea after axillary node dissection: a prospective randomized controlled trial. *J Am Coll Surg* 2003; 196:365–369.

82. Krag DN, Weaver DL, Alex JC, et al. Surgical resection and radiolocalization of the sentinel lymph node in breast cancer using a gamma probe. *Surg Oncol* 1993;2:335–339; discussion 340.

83. Giuliano AE, Kirgan DM, Guenther JM, et al. Lymphatic mapping and sentinel lymphadenectomy for breast cancer. *Ann Surg* 1994;220:391–398; discussion 398–401.

84. Kim T, Agboola O, Lyman G. Lymphatic mapping and sentinel lymph node sampling in breast cancer. *Proceedings of the American Society of Clinical Oncology 2002 annual symposium*, Orlando, FL, 2002.

85. Cox CE, Bass SS, Boulware D, et al. Implementation of new surgical technology: outcome measures for lymphatic mapping of breast carcinoma. *Ann Surg Oncol* 1999;6:553–561.

86. Derossis AM, Fey J, Yeung H, et al. A trend analysis of the relative value of blue dye and isotope localization in 2,000 consecutive cases of sentinel node biopsy for breast cancer. *J Am Coll Surg* 2001;193:473–478.

87. Canavese G, Gipponi M, Catturich A, et al. Technical issues and pathologic implications of sentinel lymph node biopsy in early stage breast cancer patients. *J Surg Oncol* 2001;77:81–87.

88. Albertini JJ, Lyman GH, Cox C, et al. Lymphatic mapping and sentinel node biopsy in the patient with breast cancer. *JAMA* 1996;276:1818–1822.

89. McMasters KM, Tuttle TM, Carlson DJ, et al. Sentinel lymph node biopsy for breast cancer: a suitable alternative to routine axillary dissection in multi-institutional practice when optimal technique is used. *J Clin Oncol* 2000;18:2560–2566.

90. Veronesi U, Paganelli G, Galimberti V, et al. Sentinel-node biopsy to avoid axillary dissection in breast cancer with clinically negative lymph-nodes. *Lancet* 1997;349:1864–1867.

91. Veronesi U, Paganelli G, Viale G, et al. Sentinel lymph node biopsy and axillary dissection in breast cancer: results in a large series. *J Natl Cancer Inst* 1999;91:368–373.

92. Cox CE, Pendas S, Cox JM, et al. Guidelines for sentinel node biopsy and lymphatic mapping of patients with breast cancer. *Ann Surg* 1998;227:645–651; discussion 651–653.

93. Bedrosian I, Reynolds C, Mick R, et al. Accuracy of sentinel lymph node biopsy in patients with large primary tumors. *Cancer* 2000;88:2540–2545.

94. Haigh PI, Hansen NM, Qi K, et al. Biopsy method and excision volume do not affect success rate of subsequent sentinel lymph node dissection in breast cancer. *Ann Surg Oncol* 2000;7:21–27.

95. Wong SL, Edwards MJ, Chao C, et al. The effect of prior breast biopsy method and concurrent definitive breast procedure on success and accuracy of sentinel lymph node biopsy. *Ann Surg Oncol* 2002;9:272–277.

96. Krag D, Weaver D, Ashikaga T, et al. The sentinel node in breast cancer—a multicenter validation study. *N Engl J Med* 1998; 339:941–946.

97. O'Hea BJ, Hill AD, El-Shirbiny AM, et al. Sentinel lymph node biopsy in breast cancer: initial experience at Memorial Sloan-Kettering Cancer Center. *J Am Coll Surg* 1998;186:423–427.

98. Guenther JM. Axillary dissection after unsuccessful sentinel lymphadenectomy for breast cancer. *Am Surg* 1999;65:991–994.

99. Linehan DC, Hill AD, Akhurst T, et al. Intradermal radiocolloid and intraparenchymal blue dye injection optimize sentinel node identification in breast cancer patients. *Ann Surg Oncol* 1999; 6:450–454.

100. Chao C, Wong SL, Woo C, et al. Reliable lymphatic drainage to axillary sentinel lymph nodes regardless of tumor location within the breast. *Am J Surg* 2001;182:307–311.

101. Chung MH, Ye W, Giuliano AE. Role for sentinel lymph node dissection in the management of large (> or = 5 cm) invasive breast cancer. *Ann Surg Oncol* 2001;8:688–692.

102. Grube BJ Hansen NM, Ye X, et al. Tumor characteristics predictive of sentinel node metastases in 105 consecutive patients with invasive lobular carcinoma. *Am J Surg* 2002;184(4):372–376.

103. Klimberg VS, Rubio IT, Henry R, et al. Subareolar versus peritumoral injection for location of the sentinel lymph node. *Ann Surg* 1999;229:860–864; discussion 864–865.

104. Bauer TW, Spitz FR, Callans LS, et al. Subareolar and peritumoral injection identify similar sentinel nodes for breast cancer. *Ann Surg Oncol* 2002;9:169–176.

105. Kern KA. Breast lymphatic mapping using subareolar injections of blue dye and radiocolloid: illustrated technique. *J Am Coll Surg* 2001;192:545–550.

106. Jin Kim H, Heerdt AS, Cody HS, et al. Sentinel lymph node drainage in multicentric breast cancers. *Breast J* 2002;8: 356–361.

107. Kumar R, Jana S, Heiba S, et al. Retrospective analysis of sentinel node localization in multifocal, multicentric, palpable, or non-palpable breast cancer. *J Nucl Med* 2003;2003:7–10.

108. Tousimis E, van Zee K, Fey J, et al. The accuracy of sentinel lymph node biopsy in multicentric and multifocal invasive breast cancers. *J Am Coll Surg* 2003;197:529–535.

109. Zavagno G, Meggiolaro F, Rossi C, et al. Subareolar injection for sentinel lymph node location in breast cancer. *Eur J Surg Oncol* 2002;28:701–704.

110. Schrenk P, Wayand W. Sentinel node biopsy in axillary lymph node staging for patients with multicentric breast cancer. *Lancet* 2001;357:122.

111. Leidenius M, Leppanen E, Krogerus L, et al. Motion restriction and axillary web syndrome after sentinel node biopsy and axillary clearance in breast cancer. *Am J Surg* 2003;185:127–130.

112. Laurie SA, Khan DA, Gruchalla RS, et al. Anaphylaxis to isosulfan blue. *Ann Allergy Asthma Immunol* 2002;88:64–66.

113. Efron P, Knudsen E, Hirshorn S, et al. Anaphylactic reaction to isosulfan blue used for sentinel node biopsy: case report and literature review. *Breast J* 2002;8:396–399.

114. Lyew MA, Gamblin TC, Ayoub M. Systemic anaphylaxis associated with intramammary isosulfan blue injection used for sentinel node detection under general anesthesia. *Anesthesiology* 2000;93:1145–1146.

115. Mostafa A, Carpenter R. Mullon: anaphylaxis to patent blue dye during sentinel lymph node biopsy for breast cancer. *Eur J Surg Oncol* 2001;27:218–219.

116. Cimmino VM, Brown AC, Szocik JF, et al. Allergic reactions to isosulfan blue during sentinel node biopsy—a common event. *Surgery* 2001;130:439–442.

117. Albo D, Wayne JD, Hunt KK, et al. Anaphylactic reactions to iso-sulfan blue dye during sentinel lymph node biopsy for breast cancer. *Am J Surg* 2001;182:393–398.

118. Montgomery LL, Thorne AC, Van Zee KJ, et al. Isosulfan blue dye reactions during sentinel lymph node mapping for breast cancer. *Anesth Analg* 2002;95:385–388, table of contents.

119. Stefanutto TB, Shapiro WA, Wright PM. Anaphylactic reaction to isosulphan blue. *Br J Anaesth* 2002;89:527–528.

120. Crivellaro M, Senna G, Dama A, et al. Anaphylaxis due to patent blue dye during lymphography, with negative skin prick test. *J Investig Allergol Clin Immunol* 2003;13:71–72.

121. Sprung J, Tully MJ, Ziser A. Anaphylactic reactions to isosulfan blue dye during sentinel node lymphadenectomy for breast cancer. *Anesth Analg* 2003;96:1051–1053, table of contents.

122. Sadiq TS, Burns WW III, Taber DJ, et al. Blue urticaria: a previously unreported adverse event associated with isosulfan blue. *Arch Surg* 2001;136:1433–1435.

123. Mostafa A, Carpenter R. Anaphylaxis to patent blue dye during sentinel lymph node biopsy for breast cancer. *Eur J Surg Oncol* 2001;27:610.

124. Newman LA, Kuerer HM, Hunt KK, et al. Presentation, treatment, and outcome of local recurrence after skin-sparing mastectomy and immediate breast reconstruction. *Ann Surg Oncol* 1998;5:620–626.

125. Medina-Franco H, Vasconez LO, Fix RJ, et al. Factors associated with local recurrence after skin-sparing mastectomy and immediate breast reconstruction for invasive breast cancer. *Ann Surg* 2002;235:814–819.

126. Rivadeneira DE, Simmons RM, Fish SK, et al. Skin-sparing mastectomy with immediate breast reconstruction: a critical analysis of local recurrence. *Cancer J* 2000;6:331–335.

127. Newman LA, Kuerer HM, Hunt KK, et al. Feasibility of immediate breast reconstruction for locally advanced breast cancer. *Ann Surg Oncol* 1999;6:671–675.

128. Hunt KK, Baldwin BJ, Strom EA, et al. Feasibility of postmastectomy radiation therapy after TRAM flap breast reconstruction. *Ann Surg Oncol* 1997;4:377–384.

129. Tran NV, Evans GR, Kroll SS, et al. Postoperative adjuvant irradiation: effects on transverse rectus abdominis muscle flap breast reconstruction. *Plast Reconstr Surg* 2000;106:313–317; discussion 318–320.

130. Newman LA, Buzdar AU, Singletary SE, et al. A prospective trial of preoperative chemotherapy in resectable breast cancer: predictors of breast-conservation therapy feasibility. *Ann Surg Oncol* 2002;9:228–234.

131. Breslin TM, Cohen L, Sahin A, et al. Sentinel lymph node biopsy is accurate after neoadjuvant chemotherapy for breast cancer. *J Clin Oncol* 2000;18:3480–3486.

132. Nason KS, Anderson BO, Byrd DR, et al. Increased false negative sentinel node biopsy rates after preoperative chemotherapy for invasive breast carcinoma. *Cancer* 2000;89:2187–2194.

133. Haid A, Tausch C, Lang A, et al. Is sentinel lymph node biopsy reliable and indicated after preoperative chemotherapy in patients with breast carcinoma? *Cancer* 2001;92:1080–1084.

134. Fernandez A, Cortes M, Benito E, et al. Gamma probe sentinel node localization and biopsy in breast cancer patients treated with a neoadjuvant chemotherapy scheme. *Nucl Med Commun* 2001;22:361–366.

135. Tafra L, Verbanac KM, Lannin DR. Preoperative chemotherapy and sentinel lymphadenectomy for breast cancer. *Am J Surg* 2001;182:312–315.

136. Stearns V, Ewing CA, Slack R, et al. Sentinel lymphadenectomy after neoadjuvant chemotherapy for breast cancer may reliably represent the axilla except for inflammatory breast cancer. *Ann Surg Oncol* 2002;9:235–242.

137. Julian TB, Dusi D, Wolmark N. Sentinel node biopsy after neoadjuvant chemotherapy for breast cancer. *Am J Surg* 2002; 184:315–317.

138. Miller AR, Thomason VE, Yeh IT, et al. Analysis of sentinel lymph node mapping with immediate pathologic review in patients

receiving preoperative chemotherapy for breast carcinoma. *Ann Surg Oncol* 2002;9:243–247.

139. Brady EW. Sentinel lymph node mapping following neoadjuvant chemotherapy for breast cancer. *Breast J* 2002;8:97–100.

140. Piato JR, Barros AC, Pincerato KM, et al. Sentinel lymph node biopsy in breast cancer after neoadjuvant chemotherapy. A pilot study. *Eur J Surg Oncol* 2003;29:118–120.

141. Balch GC, Mithani SK, Richards KR, et al. Lymphatic mapping and sentinel lymphadenectomy after preoperative therapy for stage II and III breast cancer. *Ann Surg Oncol* 2003;10:616–621.

142. Schwartz GF, Meltzer AJ. Accuracy of axillary sentinel lymph node biopsy following neoadjuvant (induction) chemotherapy for carcinoma of the breast. *Breast J* 2003;9:374–379.

143. Reitsamer R, Peintinger F, Rettenbacher L, et al. Sentinel lymph node biopsy in breast cancer patients after neoadjuvant chemotherapy. *J Surg Oncol* 2003;84:63–67.

144. Mamounas E, Brown A, Smith R, et al. Accuracy of sentinel lymph node biopsy after neoadjuvant chemotherapy in breast cancer: updated results from NSABP B-27 (abstract #140). *American Society of Clinical Oncology 38th annual meeting*, Orlando, FL, 2002.

Complications of Soft-tissue Tumor Surgery

43

Adam I. Riker   Vernon K. Sondak

■ **MELANOMA 619**
   Excision of the Primary 619
   Complete and Selective Lymph Node Dissection 621
   Blue Dye Reactions 623

■ **SOFT-TISSUE SARCOMAS 624**
   Introduction 624
   Complications of Multimodality Therapy 624
   Complications of Amputation 625
   Complications of Resections for Retroperitoneal
      Sarcomas 625

■ **CONCLUSION 626**

■ **REFERENCES 626**

Soft-tissue tumor surgery includes the management of cutaneous melanoma, soft-tissue sarcoma, and several other types of soft-tissue neoplasms and can be associated with many potential (but rarely life-threatening) complications. Meticulous attention to detail throughout all aspects of soft-tissue surgery will minimize the potential adverse outcomes. A thorough discussion with the patient should include the possible risks of any soft-tissue tumor surgery,

Adam I. Riker: University of South Florida College of Medicine, Tampa, FL 33612
Vernon K. Sondak: University of South Florida, Tampa, FL 33612

such as postoperative bleeding, thromboembolism, infection, hematoma, and/or seroma formation. In particular, large transverse incisions along the trunk with extensive undermining of the surrounding skin flaps are at high risk of seroma/hematoma formation in the postoperative period. Wound infections can occur as soon as 12 to 24 hours after surgery, and special attention should be paid to recognize potentially more lethal and rapid onset infections, such as necrotizing fasciitis or clostridial infections, or both. Cutaneous nerves are necessarily cut during soft-tissue tumor excision, often resulting in transient sensory deficits and numbness surrounding the incision. Depending on the tumor's location, particular discussion should address the possibility of inadvertent damage to, or required sacrifice of, adjacent nerves, arteries, veins, and vital organs or structures. This is especially true for excisions of melanomas on the face, head, and neck, with the possibility of inadvertent damage to many important structures such as the facial, spinal accessory, vagus, and hypoglossal nerves and vascular structures such as the external and internal jugular vein and internal carotid artery.

MELANOMA

Excision of the Primary

The surgical treatment of melanoma begins with the proper management of the primary lesion. When diagnosed early, >90% of all primary melanomas can be successfully excised

TABLE 43-1

LOCAL RECURRENCE AND ASSOCIATED MORTALITY

	Primary Tumor Thickness	Recurrent Rate (%)	5-year Survival Rate (%)	10-year Survival Rate (%)
Ng et al. (2)	<1 to >4 mm	7	61	–
Dong et al. (3)	0.76 to 4.0 mm	–	51	35
Soong et al. (4)	<1 to >4 mm	5	41	37
Urist et al. (5)	0.76 to 4 mm	5	50 (3-yr)	20
Reintgen et al. (6)	0.76 to 4 mm	–	55	–
Kalady et al. (7)	<1 mm	15	60	45

and the patient cured with surgical excision alone. The majority of cutaneous melanomas can be effectively and adequately excised with standard excisions that are elliptically placed with the long axis of the ellipse directed toward the regional nodal basin. The length of the long axis of the ellipse can be estimated to ensure an adequate closure without undue tension or cosmetically displeasing "dog-ears" at the ends. In terms of the wide local excision, efforts should be made to decrease the amount of wound tension along the entire length of the incision. This can be done through careful dissection and undermining of the surrounding skin edges. Transverse incisions that cut across and disrupt the flow of lymphatics may contribute to lymphedema, especially in the lower extremity.

In general, attempts should be made to adequately excise the primary lesion while minimizing scar formation and the need for skin grafts. In some anatomic locations, however, such as the distal extremities, joint lines, face, head and neck, scalp, hands, and feet, a split-thickness skin graft and/or flap closure is the preferred closure, as primary closure is often not possible or increases the risk of undue tension along the incision. Partial-thickness or full-thickness skin grafts are associated with a higher surgical morbidity, cosmetic disfigurement, and overall cost compared to primary closure. The donor site should be examined and chosen pre-operatively and the possibility of skin graft necrosis and poor healing of the graft should be fully explained to the patient prior to surgery. In the era of sentinel lymph node biopsy (SLNB), we have increasingly turned to full-thickness skin grafts harvested from the node biopsy site to close wide excision wounds that would otherwise require split-thickness skin grafting from a third surgical site (1).

It is important to understand that removal of the appropriate surgical margins with the excision of a primary melanoma is instrumental in minimizing the most important potential complication associated with surgical excision: Local tumor recurrence. Local recurrence of disease may be due to the lack of adequate surgical margins or may be a result of microscopic satellites that exist beyond the margins of excision. It is often impossible to differentiate between local persistence and metastasis. The development of a local

recurrence, defined as tumor recurring within 2 cm of the surgical scar, has been associated in many studies with a dismal prognosis, with 40% to 60% of all patients with a local recurrence of melanoma dying of their disease (Table 43-1).

Appropriate surgical margins minimize the chance of local tumor recurrence. A thorough understanding of the past literature and recent recommendations regarding appropriate surgical margins for the excision of a primary melanoma is necessary for optimal patient outcome. For decades, a 3 to 5 cm margin of normal surrounding skin was recommended, with most patients requiring a skin graft in order to cover the large defect created. However, it was recognized that the overall thickness of the primary melanoma influenced the likelihood of a local recurrence, prompting several randomized trials to address this issue (Table 43-2).

TABLE 43-2

PROSPECTIVE CLINICAL TRIALS ADDRESSING MELANOMA SURGICAL MARGINS

WHO Study[a]
- 612 patients with lesions <2 mm
- Randomized between 1-cm and 3-cm margins
- 1 cm margin was safe for melanoma lesions <1 mm thick

Intergroup Melanoma Study[b]
- All patients with primary melanomas from 1–4 mm eligible
- Total of 486 patients randomized to either 2-cm or 4-cm margins
- 2-cm margin adequate with low recurrence rate, less morbidity

United Kingdom Melanoma Study Group[c]
- All patients with melanomas >2.00 mm eligible
- Total of 900 patients randomized to 1-cm vs. 3-cm margins
- 1-cm margin associated with a greater risk of regional recurrence
- No significant difference in overall survival in either group

[a]From Veronesi U, Cascinelli N, Adamus J, et al. Thin stage I primary cutaneous malignant melanoma: comparison of excision with margins of 1 or 3 cm. *N Engl J Med* 1988;322:1159–1162, with permission.
[b]From Balch CM, Urist MM, Karakousis CP, et al. Efficacy of 2-cm surgical margins for intermediate thickness melanomas (1–4 mm). Results of a multi-institutional randomized surgical trial. *Ann Surg* 1993;218(3): 262–267, with permission.
[c]From Thomas JM, Newton-Bishop J, A'Hern R, et al. Excision margins in high-risk malignant melanoma. *N Engl J Med* 2004;350:757–766, with permission.

The first trial to address this issue was the World Health Organization (WHO) Melanoma Group study by Veronesi et al. This trial prospectively randomized patients with primary melanomas ≤ 2.00 mm in Breslow thickness to 1-cm versus 3-cm surgical margins (8). There were no local recurrences at all among patients with primary melanomas of < 1.00 mm, regardless of whether a 1-cm or 3-cm margin was taken. In those patients with primary melanomas between 1 and 2 mm, there were four local recurrences, all occurring within the group that had received 1 cm margins. However, there were no differences noted in either group in terms of disease-free and overall survival. This trial has been recently updated with 15-year follow-up, and there were still no differences noted in disease-free or overall survival (11). This study is important because it provides a clear demonstration that a surgical excision margin of 1 cm is safe and provides excellent local control for melanomas < 1.00 mm in Breslow thickness.

The second prospective trial addressed the efficacy of 2 cm margins compared to 4 cm margins for intermediate thickness melanomas 1 to 4 mm in Breslow thickness (9). The Intergroup Melanoma Committee found a local recurrence rate of 0.8% for patients who had 2 cm margins compared to 1.7% for those who had 4 cm margins taken at the time of surgery. The differences in local recurrence were not statistically significant. There was, however, a significant difference in the number of skin grafts needed, with 46% of the 4-cm group requiring a skin graft but only 11% of the 2-cm group. An update of this trial at a 10-year follow-up reveals no significant differences in local recurrence or disease-free or overall survival (12). This trial clearly demonstrates that a 2-cm margin is safe and effective compared to a 4-cm margin for primary melanomas between 1 and 4 mm, with a marked decrease in the need for skin grafting. Two other trials have examined 2-cm versus 5-cm margins for primary melanomas < 2.00 mm, with both studies showing no difference in local recurrence rates or overall survival (13,14).

The data addressing the recommended surgical margins for thick melanomas (> 4 mm) are not as strong and are mainly based on retrospective analyses. A multi-institutional retrospective review of surgical margins and prognostic factors in patients with thick lesions (> 4 mm) was performed on 278 patients and showed no difference in local recurrence rate, disease-free survival, or overall survival if margins > 2 cm were taken (15). Recently, Thomas et al. prospectively examined the excision margins in high-risk malignant melanoma, considered in this study to be Breslow thickness of 2 mm or greater (10). The median tumor thickness was 3 mm, and patients were randomized to either 1-cm or 3-cm margins of excision. The authors found that a 1-cm margin of excision for melanomas of at least 2 mm in Breslow thickness was associated with a significantly greater risk of combined locoregional recurrence when compared to a 3-cm margin (local recurrence rates examined separately were not different between the two

groups). Although there was no difference between the groups in either melanoma-specific or overall survival, this and other studies suggest that there is a potential increase in the risk of death from melanoma associated with a narrow (1 cm) margin of excision in thick melanomas.

Indeed, this is addressed by Ng et al., who analyzed 1,155 patients who had their primary melanoma excised (2). There were 84 (7%) local recurrences overall, with a total of 33 of those 84 (39%) patients dying of melanoma. The 5-year survival for patients with local recurrence was 59%, compared to 86% for those without a local recurrence ($p < 0.0001$). Other studies examining local tumor recurrence and its impact upon long-term survival have yielded similar results (3–6). Even patients with thin melanomas (≤ 1 mm in thickness) deserve an appropriate surgical margin, as recurrence does occur even in this group and is a harbinger of very poor prognosis and outcome. The current recommendations for excision margins for primary cutaneous melanoma are outlined in Table 43-3 (7).

Complete and Selective Lymph Node Dissection

Historically, the elective lymph node dissection was the main operation performed for the staging of patients presenting with localized melanoma. This involved the removal of clinically nonpalpable lymph nodes, in contrast to palpable adenopathy that would be removed by a therapeutic lymph node dissection. It is still controversial whether a survival advantage is gained after an elective lymph node dissection or if it should be regarded solely as a staging procedure. Regardless, an elective lymph node dissection provides durable local control and accurate staging for most patients with occult lymph node metastases. A therapeutic lymph node dissection, performed for patients with clinically evident regional lymphadenopathy, provides locoregional control of disease and a chance of cure, with 5-year survival rates of 20% to 40% (16–18). Meyer et al. performed 144 therapeutic lymph node dissections in 140

TABLE 43-3

CURRENT RECOMMENDATIONS FOR EXCISION MARGINS FOR CUTANEOUS MELANOMA

Location of Primary Melanoma	Tumor Thickness	Margins
Trunk, proximal extremity	Melanoma *in situ*	5 mm
	≤ 1.00 mm	1 cm
	> 1.00 mm–2.00 mm	1–2 cm
	> 2.00 mm	2 cm
Head/neck, distal extremity	≤ 1.00 mm	1 cm
	> 1.00 mm	At least 1 cm

melanoma patients (14 cervical, 49 axillary, 73 groin) and found a 5-year survival for all patients of 30% (19). In terms of complications associated with each type of nodal dissection, Ingvar et al. compared the morbidity following elective (*n* = 44) versus therapeutic (*n* = 64) lymph node dissections for melanoma patients (20). They found that the total number of complications in the elective group was 39%, compared to 61% in the therapeutic group. Local wound complications dominated, with differences noted in seromas (25% vs. 45%) and skin necrosis, wound infections, and cellulitis (11% vs. 22%). The incidence of lymphedema was higher in the therapeutic group (23%) than in the elective group (10%). This provides a further rationale for surgical management of regional lymph node involvement when occult rather than grossly evident.

Regardless of the approach to patients with clinically localized melanoma, some patients will present with more advanced regional disease. Bulky lymphadenopathy of the axilla is best managed surgically, with a therapeutic complete level I–III axillary lymph node dissection being performed in most cases. Often, bulky adenopathy has grown to the point where large lymph nodes coalesce into a matted mass that may become fixed to the surrounding structures, such as the thoracodorsal neurovascular bundle, long thoracic and intercostal-brachial nerve, axillary vein, and even the brachial plexus. Obvious complications of surgery in such advanced cases include nerve injury to any of the above mentioned nerves, injury to the axillary vein and its branches, thoracic duct injury or other lymphatic injury, and even pneumothorax. Attention to detail and anatomic localization of the thoracodorsal and long thoracic nerves is essential; sacrifice of either of these nerves should be reserved for cases in which the tumor is intimately involving these nerves.

The overall complication rate with regional lymphadenectomy is relatively high, but major and life-threatening problems are rare. Urist et al. describe the surgical morbidity after elective or therapeutic regional lymphadenectomy of the neck (*n* = 48), axilla (*n* = 98), and groin (*n* = 58) in 204 patients with melanoma (21). There was an overall complication rate of 25%, with most patients experiencing wound-related, short-term issues common to all sites of nodal dissection. These included postoperative seroma formation (22%), temporary nerve dysfunction or pain (14%), and wound infections (6%). Wound complications extended the hospital stay an average of 2 to 3 days. Swelling of the leg was measurable in 26% of patients 6 months or longer after undergoing groin dissections, with most of the enlargement confined to the thigh and likely representing prolonged postoperative swelling rather than true "lymphedema." However, 8% of these patients suffered from significant dysfunction from chronic lymphedema involving the entire lower leg. There was a positive correlation between patient obesity and increasing age and the development of at least one postoperative complication. Tonouchi et al. address the

operative morbidity associated with inguinal lymph node dissection (22). They note an overall incidence of moderate to severe complications of 24% for wound infections, 16% for skin flap problems, 12% for seromas, 4% for lymphedema, and 4% for hemorrhage. Interestingly, they found a significantly higher incidence of wound infections and lymphedema after a lazy-S incision compared to a straight incision.

The evaluation and management of the draining lymph node basins in patients with clinically localized melanomas >1.00 mm in Breslow thickness has evolved over the last 10 years. In the past we relied upon the staging information gained from performing a complete (elective) lymph node dissection. We now are able to provide an alternative to a complete node dissection with the SLNB procedure as a viable technique that provides accurate pathological nodal staging. SLNB has become the standard of care at most melanoma centers, providing a surgical technique that is less invasive, with a smaller skin incision that requires a far less extensive dissection of the nodal basin.

Wrightson et al. reviewed the complications associated with SLNB (23). The data are derived from patients enrolled on the Sunbelt Melanoma Trial, which is a randomized prospective trial involving 70 institutions across the United States between 1997 and 2001. Patients between the ages of 18 and 70 with cutaneous melanomas >1.0 mm in Breslow thickness and clinically negative lymph nodes were enrolled. All patients underwent an SLNB with radioactive colloid lymphoscintigraphy to identify all involved lymph node basins followed by isosulfan blue dye. Patients found to have evidence of nodal metastasis with melanoma then underwent a complete lymph node dissection.

Patients were followed with history and physical exams at an initial postoperative visit 2 weeks after surgery, then every 3 months for the first 2 years, every 4 months for the third year, and every 6 months thereafter. An overall assessment of postoperative complications was performed at each visit using a detailed reporting form that included the type of complication, the site and severity of the complication, and the extent of treatment, including whether the patient required reoperation or admission to the hospital. The patient populations were composed of patients who received an SLNB alone (*n* = 2,120) plus patients who had an SLNB followed by a complete lymph node dissection (*n* = 444) because of a tumor-involved sentinel node. The most common complications seen were lymphedema, wound infection, hematoma/seroma formation, and sensory nerve injury. Other complications that were noted included hemorrhage, urinary tract infection, motor nerve injury, deep venous thrombosis, pulmonary complications, and thrombophlebitis. There were no complications associated with the injection of isosulfan blue dye or radioactive colloid in this large series.

The frequency of overall complications was also associated with the site of surgery. After a sentinel node biopsy alone in the axilla or groin, a total of 14 (0.7%) of 2,083 patients developed some degree of lymphedema. It is noteworthy that of these 14 patients, 10 (71%) were patients that had undergone a biopsy of nodes in the inguinal region. There was a significantly higher rate of total number of complications in those patients who underwent a complete inguinal lymph node dissection compared to other node dissections (51.2% inguinal vs. 10% neck, 20% axilla, p <0.0001). Lymphedema was also more common for patients who underwent a complete inguinal lymph node dissection compared to a complete axillary lymph node dissection (31.5% vs. 4.6%, p <0.0001).

This study does not directly compare an SLNB to a complete lymph node dissection but really compares sentinel node biopsy alone to sentinel node biopsy followed by a complete lymph node dissection. It is possible that the performance of two operative procedures compared to a single procedure results in more complications. The reported complication rate of 23.2% in the sentinel node biopsy followed by complete node dissection group is comparable to other published studies examining the complication rate of performing an elective complete lymph node dissection without prior node biopsy. However, although it is fair to say that SLNB causes some complications, the vast majority of these complications are noted to be minor without a lasting impact on the patient. Jansen et al. describe a complication rate of 9% in 200 consecutive sentinel lymph node biopsies for melanoma, all of which were considered minor in nature (24). In terms of lymphedema following a sentinel node biopsy alone for melanoma, Wrone et al. reported five cases for an overall incidence of 1.7% (25), compared to 0.7% as described by Wrightson et al.

Blue Dye Reactions

Isosulfan blue is a rosaniline dye of the triphenylmethane type that is a 2,5-disulfonated isomer of patent blue dye. Isosulfan blue dye (1%) is the only dye approved by the Food and Drug Administration (FDA) in the United States for the visualization of lymphatics. However, other dyes, such as patent blue dye, have been in use outside the United States. Adverse reactions for all such dyes are similar in scope to isosulfan blue and range from mild allergic reactions with hives and erythema to angioneurotic edema with or without laryngospasm and severe cardiovascular collapse. Other symptoms include angioedema, rash, gastrointestinal distress, pulmonary edema, and cardiac arrythmias. The true incidence of reactions to patent blue dye is unknown but is generally reported to be in the range of 0.6% to 1.0%.

Leong et al. describe three cases of adverse reactions to isosulfan blue dye during SLNB for patients with melanoma (26). The three cases, from 406 patients subjected to the procedure (0.74%), varied in severity, but all were associated with a significant and rapid decrease in the systolic blood pressure after the intradermal injection of the isosulfan blue

dye. Most patients will respond to a combination of epinephrine and/or ephedrine infusion with other modes of resuscitative measures such as crystalloid infusion and intravenous infusion of methylprednisolone or hydrocortisone and histamine blockers (diphenhydramine or ranitidine or similar agents). In an attempt to decrease or possibly eliminate the adverse reactions attributed to isosulfan blue dye, Raut et al. instituted a clinical practice protocol that employed preoperative prophylaxis (4 mg of dexamethasone, 50 mg of diphenhydramine, and 20 mg of famotidine) in 654 patients who underwent SLNB for breast cancer (27). They noted no significant difference in the percentage of patients who developed an anaphylactoid reaction compared to a prior series of 639 patients who did not receive prophylaxis (0.7% vs. 1.1%, $p = 0.35$). However, the incidence of wound complications was double (9.2% vs. 4.5%, $p = 0.054$) in the group who received preoperative prophylaxis. Infectious complications were also increased in the prophylaxis group (8.5%) compared to the group without (4.5%), including cellulitis that required intravenous antibiotics and wound abscess requiring incision and drainage. Wound dehiscence was also increased in the prophylaxis group compared to the group receiving no prophylaxis.

Therefore, premedication with steroids is currently not justified and may actually result in an increase in postoperative wound infections and complications. Additionally, the use of preoperative corticosteroids may result in transient immunosuppression of the patient. This is of particular concern in the patient with melanoma, where an intact immune system seems to play a very important role. The additional cost associated with prophylaxis with corticosteroids and other medications is not justified, given the lack of evidence that prophylaxis is beneficial at preventing the rare anaphylactoid reaction to isosulfan blue dye.

Other nonallergic consequences of isosulfan blue dye administration include an acute or more prolonged decline in "apparent" oxygen saturation (SpO_2) as measured by pulse oximetry. This is due to the blue dye's ability to absorb red light, with its peak absorption at 646 nm. The SpO_2 monitor utilizes two wavelengths, 660 and 940 nm, to determine oxyhemoglobin content of blood via a spectrophotometric process. Thus, it is important that the anesthesiologist be aware of such factitious oxygen desaturation readings after the injection of isosulfan blue dye. In one series of patients SpO_2 values decreased by about 5% after the administration of 5 cc of blue dye, with a range of 5% to 10% overall (28). Isosulfan blue injection interfered with SpO_2 readings for as long as 195 minutes with a mean time to the maximal change in SpO_2 reading of 35 minutes (29). Although the changes in SpO_2 readings can be substantial, the time course appears to be predictable, and dual-oximetry analysis (SpO_2 and actual arterial oxygen saturation) is not necessary in an otherwise healthy patient.

It is important to have a clear and open communication with the anesthesiologist prior to the injection of the isosulfan blue dye. The anesthesiologist should establish a preinjection SpO_2 baseline and verify adequate oxygenation and hemodynamic stability prior to blue dye injection. It is important to carefully monitor and evaluate the patient during and after the blue dye injection, as immediate changes in respiratory or cardiac status can then be directly correlated to the injection itself or secondarily to an underlying unknown etiology. Rapid changes in the patient's status should not be falsely attributed to the blue dye injection, and a careful evaluation of the patient should be performed to rule out other possible causative factors that may decrease oxygenation or cause tachycardia and hypotension unrelated to blue dye injection.

Additionally, after blue dye injection, patients may appear to be cyanotic, having a slight ashen and/or pale blue color to their skin. This is due to the dye draining from the lymphatics into the venous system and subsequently into the capillary beds. The patient, as well as the health care personnel who will be involved in the postoperative recovery, should be made aware of this.

SOFT-TISSUE SARCOMAS

Introduction

Like melanoma, sarcomas can occur anywhere in the body and the complications associated with their surgical treatment vary with the anatomic site. Any and all of the complications associated with soft-tissue surgery for other malignancies can occur during and after sarcoma surgery. In addition, multimodality therapy is frequently used in the management of sarcomas. Combining surgery with other treatments—usually radiation and often cytotoxic chemotherapy as well—has the potential to decrease the complications expected from surgery alone but can also lead to increased complications as well. Minimizing the complications associated with sarcoma surgery starts by appropriate selection of candidates for multimodality therapy, but it also depends on the proper performance of the correct surgical procedure.

Complications of Multimodality Therapy

Most soft-tissue sarcomas are treated with the combination of surgery and radiation therapy. Patients with large, intermediate, and high-grade or recurrent sarcomas are all candidates for surgery plus radiation. Although some have maintained that selected small or superficial high-grade sarcomas in favorable locations can be treated successfully with surgery alone (30), most studies demonstrate lower local recurrence rates for all patients with high-grade sarcomas when radiation is added (31,32). Although radiation lowers recurrence rates, it can increase the complications of surgery. Several randomized trials evaluated surgery alone or surgery followed by postoperative radiation as either brachytherapy (31) or external beam radiation (32). Radiation can be administered either before or after surgery, and the complications vary according to the timing of radiation. In a randomized trial, patients who received preoperative radiation were statistically significantly more likely to have wound complications than those receiving radiation after surgery (35% vs. 17%, $p = 0.01$) (Table 43-4). Overall survival was not significantly different between the two groups (33).

TABLE 43-4

WOUND COMPLICATIONS IN A RANDOMIZED TRIAL OF PREOPERATIVE VERSUS POSTOPERATIVE RADIATION FOR PATIENTS WITH RESECTABLE EXTREMITY SARCOMAS

	Preoperative (n = 88)	Postoperative (n = 94)
Wound complications[a]		
Yes	31 (35%)	16 (17%)
Secondary operation for wound repair	14 (45%)	5 (31%)
Invasive procedure for wound management[b]	5 (16%)	4 (25%)
Deep wound packing deep to dermis in area of wound at least 2 cm with or without prolonged dressings >6 weeks from wound breakdown[c]	11 (35%)	7 (44%)
Readmission for wound care[d]	1 (3%)	0
No complications	57 (65%)	78 (83%)

[a] $p = 0.01$ for yes vs. no.
[b] Without secondary operation.
[c] Without secondary operation or invasive procedure.
[d] Without secondary operation, invasive procedure, deep wound packing, or prolonged dressing.
From O'Sullivan B, Davis AM, Turcotte R, et al. Preoperative versus postoperative radiotherapy in soft-tissue sarcoma of the limbs: a randomized trial. *Lancet* 2002;359:2235–2241, with permission.

Complications of surgery and radiation can adversely affect the cosmetic, functional, and quality of life outcomes after sarcoma surgery. One of the most significant long-term complications of surgery plus radiation is pathologic fracture of the underlying bone, since this complication is associated with a very high risk of subsequent amputation. The risk of pathologic fracture increases with the radiation dose delivered to the bone (34). The risk of pathologic fracture is also dramatically increased if extensive stripping of the periosteum of the bone is required as part of the resection of the tumor. To minimize the likelihood of subsequent amputation, patients who are having surgical resections that require extensive resection of the periosteum of weight-bearing long bones combined with radiation should be considered for prophylactic placement of an intramedullary nail (35).

Patients who undergo neoadjuvant (preoperative) chemotherapy may be more likely to have surgical complications. This appears to be particularly true if both chemotherapy and radiation are given together prior to surgery (36). Chemotherapy and radiation present both acute and chronic wound-healing problems that must be considered in the surgical planning. In particular, sarcoma resections typically create large soft-tissue deficits that can take a long time to heal. Preoperative chemotherapy and radiation decrease the chances of successful healing with primary closure, and closure by means of myocutaneous flaps should always be considered when a large surgical defect is created in a patient who received preoperative therapy (37). Irradiated wounds in the trunk and retroperitoneum can present a major challenge to the reconstructive surgeon (38).

Complications of Amputation

With proper selection of patients for preoperative therapy, amputation should rarely be necessary. Although it seems intuitively obvious that amputation is associated with a greater disruption of function and quality of life than limb-sparing surgeries, proving this concept has been surprisingly difficult. Some of this apparent difficulty is due to our relatively crude instruments for assessing these parameters, but much of it reflects the remarkable adaptive capacity of human beings (especially young ones) to adverse circumstances, such that patients compensate for even major amputations remarkably well. Because of this, patients who have a last curative option in amputation should never be denied that option for fear of the procedure's excessive morbidity. Patients may require a great deal of support when faced with a decision regarding amputation; preoperative consultation with a rehabilitation medicine specialist can be extremely helpful in demystifying amputation and correcting misconceptions about amputation's long-term consequences.

On the other hand, one of the reasons that quality of life studies have failed to show limb-sparing surgery to be better

than amputation is because of the complications associated with the more conservative surgery (and the radiation and/or chemotherapy given along with it). Complications like fibrosis or nerve damage, and especially any procedures that result in fixation or marked restriction of major joints, result in significant and long-lasting functional deficits that can dramatically impair quality of life (39).

A particularly problematic complication of amputation is the so-called phantom pain, a series of painful sensations emanating from the extremity's transected nerves and perceived as if the extremity were still in place. Remarkably little is known about how to prevent or treat this complication. Many surgeons suggest infiltrating major nerves with local anesthetic agents prior to transecting them cleanly with a knife; others suggest deepening the general anesthesia at the time of nerve transaction. However, there is little evidence that the technique or the anesthetic circumstances surrounding nerve transaction exert major effects on the subsequent development of phantom pain. Phantom pain is more frequent and severe with more proximal amputations but tends to subside over time. In view of that consideration, most management strategies aim at providing short-term relief through the use of gabapentin, tricyclic antidepressants, and anxiolytics. One randomized trial suggested that dextromethorphan in high doses could minimize the development and intensity of phantom pain (40). Properly fitting prostheses are an essential part of postamputation management, as pressure on the stump can produce symptoms that can be difficult to distinguish from phantom pain but that are much easier to relieve.

Complications of Resections for Retroperitoneal Sarcomas

Approximately 10% to 20% of sarcomas arise in the retroperitoneum, where they can attain great size before becoming symptomatic enough to allow diagnosis. Complete resection is essential in order to have any chance for long-term disease-free survival, but, because of the size and location of the tumors, it often involves concomitant resection of other organs (41). Since resection of one kidney or ureter is not an uncommon requirement, radiographic evidence of bilateral renal function should be sought prior to surgery. To avoid precipitating a hypertensive crisis if a retroperitoneal tumor proves to be a functional extra-adrenal pheochromocytoma (paraganglioma), which may arise in the retroperitoneum, a high index of suspicion needs to be maintained when dealing with upper-retroperitoneal and mid-retroperitoneal tumors just off the midline. If there is any possibility that such a lesion could be a functional endocrine tumor, surgery and even needle biopsy should be deferred until a proper endocrine work-up can be conducted.

Complication rates after resection are high, with concomitant resection of spleen, pancreas, or colon all adding to the likelihood of specific complications. It is important to recognize that partial resection of retroperitoneal sarcomas, leaving gross tumor behind (sometimes referred to as "debulking"), is associated with survival outcomes that are little or no better than with biopsy of the tumor alone (42,43). The complication rates for partial resection, however, are equivalent to those of complete resection (42,44). Thus partial resection conveys all the morbidity without any of the therapeutic benefit and should rarely, if ever, be performed. The goal of any operative procedure for retroperitoneal sarcomas, as with virtually all types of sarcomas, should be complete resection of all gross tumor, ideally with attainment of histologically negative margins.

To avoid situations in which patients are explored only to find that the tumor is unresectable or only incompletely resectable, careful preoperative evaluation is necessary. The tumor's location and size, its relationship to adjacent organs, the presence or absence of local extension and relationship to and/or involvement of major vascular structures, as well as the presence of normal anatomic variants and anomalies of major abdominal arteries and veins, are all crucial pieces of information that need to be provided prior to surgical resection. The most common types of vascular involvement precluding resection are involvement of the proximal superior mesenteric vessels or involvement of bilateral renal vessels. Intraoperative complications may occur due to proximity of the tumor to the inferior vena cava or the iliac veins. Injury to these veins during resection of retroperitoneal sarcomas is more difficult to deal with than injury to the aorta or iliac arteries and can be associated with massive intraoperative blood loss. No one should undertake exploration of a retroperitoneal sarcoma without adequate preparation, including the availability of blood products and, if necessary, vascular surgery backup. In handling a difficult venous injury intraoperatively, it is well to remember several points. The low-pressure bleeding can be temporarily controlled with pressure from laparotomy pads or sponges placed in ring forceps ("sponge sticks"), or both, allowing the anesthesia team to resuscitate the patient and order additional blood products to be delivered and affording the opportunity for additional surgical help to be summoned. The venous injury is often a small hole, not uncommonly from a small, posteriorly located vein branch that has been transected or avulsed. Care should be taken to avoid propagating the tear in the thin-walled vein by injudicious placement of vascular clamps; here again the low-pressure blood flow can often be safely contained by careful placement of sponge sticks above and below the hole, permitting closure with just a few well-placed vascular sutures.

CONCLUSION

Complications of soft-tissue tumor surgery can be minimized by good technique and preoperative preparation but never by skimping on the adequacy of the surgical procedure.

Local recurrence remains the worst, most difficult to treat complication of soft-tissue surgery. Judicious use of multimodality therapy, combined with appropriately but not excessively radical surgery, strikes the proper balance between tumor control and avoidance of complications and highlights the important role the surgical oncologist plays in the management of skin and soft-tissue malignancies.

REFERENCES

1. Dresel A, Kuhn JA, McCarty TM. Sentinel node biopsy site used as a full thickness skin graft donor for cutaneous melanoma. *Am J Surg* 2002;184:176–178.
2. Ng AK, Jones WO, Shaw JH. Analysis of local recurrence and optimizing excision margins for cutaneous melanoma. *Br J Surg* 2001;88:137–142.
3. Dong XD, Tyler D, Johnson JL, et al. Analysis of prognosis and disease progression after local recurrence of melanoma. *Cancer* 2000;88:1063–1071.
4. Soong S, Harrison RA, McCarthy WH, et al. Factors affecting survival following local, regional, or distant recurrence from localized melanoma. *J Surg Oncol* 1998;67:228–233.
5. Urist MM, Balch CM, Soong SJ, et al. The influence of surgical margins and prognostic factors predicting the risk of local recurrence in 3445 patients with primary cutaneous melanoma. *Cancer* 1985;55:1398–1402.
6. Reintgen DS, Cox C, Slingluff CL, et al. Recurrent malignant melanoma: the identification of prognostic factors to predict survival. *Ann Plast Surg* 1992;28:45–49.
7. Kalady MF, White RR, Johnson JL, et al. Thin melanomas: predictive lethal characteristics from a 30-year clinical experience. *Ann Surg* 2003;238:528–537.
8. Veronesi U, Cascinelli N, Adamus J, et al. Thin stage I primary cutaneous malignant melanoma: comparison of excision with margins of 1 or 3 cm. *N Engl J Med* 1988;322:1159–1162.
9. Balch CM, Urist MM, Karakousis CP, et al. Efficacy of 2-cm surgical margins for intermediate thickness melanomas (1-4 mm). Results of a multi-institutional randomized surgical trial. *Ann Surg* 1993;218(3):262–267.
10. Thomas JM, Newton-Bishop J, A'Hern R, et al. Excision margins in high-risk malignant melanoma. *N Engl J Med* 2004;350: 757–766.
11. Santinarni M, Maurici A, Patuzzo R, et al. Impact of clinical trials on the treatment of melanoma. *Surg Oncol Clin N Am* 2001; 10:935–947.
12. Balch CM, Soong SJ, Ross MI, et al. Long term results of a prospective trial comparing 2 cm vs. 4 cm excision margins for 740 patients with 1–4 mm melanomas. *Ann Surg Oncol* 2001;8: 101–108.
13. Khayat D, Rixe O, Martin G, et al. Surgical margins in cutaneous melanoma (2 cm versus 5 cm for lesions measuring less than 2.1 mm thick). *Cancer* 2003;97:1941–1946.
14. Cohn-Cedermark G, Rutqvist LE, Andersson R, et al. Long term results of a randomized study by the Swedish Melanoma Study Group on 2 cm versus 5 cm resection margins for patients with cutaneous melanoma with a thickness of 0.8 to 2.0 mm. *Cancer* 2000;89:1495–1501.
15. Heaton KM, Sussman JJ, Gershenwald JE, et al. Surgical margins and prognostic factors in patients with thick (>4 mm) primary melanoma. *Ann Surg Oncol* 1998;5:322–328.
16. Morton DL, Wanek L, Nizze JA, et al. Improved long-term survival after lymphadenectomy of melanoma metastatic to regional nodes. *Ann Surg* 1991;214:491–501.
17. Warso MA, Das Gupta TK. Melanoma recurrence in a previously dissected lymph node basin. *Arch Surg* 1994;129:252–255.
18. Karakousis CP. Therapeutic lymph node dissection in malignant melanoma. *Ann Surg Oncol* 1998;5:473–478.
19. Meyer T, Merkel S, Gohl J, et al. Lymph node dissection for clinically evident lymph node metastases of malignant melanoma. *Eur J Surg Oncol* 2002;28:424–430.

20. Ingvar C, Erichsen C, Jonsson PE. Morbidity following prophylactic and therapeutic lymph node dissection for melanoma: a comparison. *Tumori* 1984;70:529–533.

21. Urist MM, Maddox WA, Kennedy JE, et al. Patient risk factors and surgical morbidity after regional lymphadenectomy in 204 melanoma patients. *Cancer* 1983;51:2152–2156.

22. Tonouchi H, Ohmori Y, Kobayashi M, et al. Operative morbidity associated with groin dissections. *Surg Today* 2004;34:413–418.

23. Wrightson WR, Wong SL, Edwards MJ, et al. Complications associated with sentinel lymph node biopsy. *Ann Surg Oncol* 2003; 10:676–680.

24. Jansen L, Nieweg OE, Peterse JL, et al. Reliability of sentinel lymph node biopsy for staging melanoma. *Br J Surg* 2000;87: 484–489.

25. Wrone DA, Tanabe KK, Cosimi AB, et al. Lymphedema after sentinel lymph node biopsy for cutaneous melanoma: a report of 5 cases. *Arch Dermatol* 2000;136:511–514.

26. Leong SP, Donegan E, Heffernon W, et al. Adverse reactions to isosulfan blue during selective sentinel lymph node dissection in melanoma. *Ann Surg Oncol* 2000;7:361–366.

27. Raut CP, Daley MD, Hunt KK, et al. Anaphylactoid reactions to isosulfan blue dye during breast cancer lymphatic mapping in patients given preoperative prophylaxis. *J Clin Oncol* 2004;22: 567–568.

28. Heinle E, Burdumy T, Recabaren J. Factitious oxygen desaturation after isosulfan blue injection. *Am Surg* 2003;69:899–901.

29. El-Tamer M, Komenaka IK, Curry S, et al. Pulse oximeter changes with sentinel lymph node biopsy in breast cancer. *Arch Surg* 2003;138:1257–1260.

30. Rydholm A, Gustafson P, Rööser B, et al. Limb-sparing surgery without radiotherapy based on the anatomic location of soft tissue sarcoma. *J Clin Oncol* 1991;9:1757–1765.

31. Pisters PW, Harrison LB, Leung DH, et al. Long-term results of a prospective randomized trial of adjuvant brachytherapy in soft tissue sarcoma. *J Clin Oncol* 1996;14:859–868.

32. Yang JC, Chang AE, Baker AR, et al. Randomized prospective study of the benefit of adjuvant radiation therapy in the treatment of soft tissue sarcomas of the extremity. *J Clin Oncol* 1998;16: 197–203.

33. O'Sullivan B, Davis AM, Turcotte R, et al. Preoperative versus postoperative radiotherapy in soft-tissue sarcoma of the limbs: a randomized trial. *Lancet* 2002;359:2235–2241.

34. Eilber FR, Morton DL, Eckardt JJ, et al. Limb salvage for skeletal and soft tissue sarcomas. Multidisciplinary preoperative therapy. *Cancer* 1984;53:2579–2584.

35. Letson GD, Muro-Cacho CA. Prosthesis in the treatment of sarcomas. *Curr Opin Orthod* 2005 *(in press)*.

36. Delaney TF, Spiro IJ, Suit HD, et al. Neoadjuvant chemotherapy and radiotherapy for large extremity soft-tissue sarcomas. *Int J Radiat Oncol Biol Phys* 2003;56:1117–1127.

37. Peat BG, Bell RS, Davis A, et al. Wound-healing complications after soft-tissue sarcoma surgery. *Plast Reconstr Surg* 1994;93: 980–987.

38. Ladin D, Rees R, Wilkins E, et al. The use of omental transposition in the treatment of recurrent sarcoma of the back. *Ann Plastic Surg* 1993;31:556–559.

39. Gerrand CH, Wunder JS, Kandel RA, et al. The influence of anatomic location on functional outcome in lower-extremity soft-tissue sarcoma. *Ann Surg Oncol* 2004;11:476–4 82.

40. Abraham RB, Marouani N, Weinbroum AA. Dextromethorphan mitigates phantom pain in cancer amputees. *Ann Surg Oncol* 10:268–274.

41. Singer S, Antonescu CR, Riedel E, et al. Histologic subtype and margin of resection predict pattern of recurrence and survival for retroperitoneal liposarcoma. *Ann Surg* 2003;238:358–371.

42. McGrath PC, Neifeld JP, Lawrence W, et al. Improved survival following complete excision of retroperitoneal sarcomas. *Ann Surg* 1984;200:200–204.

43. Heslin MJ, Lewis JJ, Nadler E, et al. Prognostic factors associated with long-term survival for retroperitoneal sarcoma: implications for management. *J Clin Oncol* 1997;15:2832–2839.

44. Pinson CW, ReMine SG, Fletcher WS, et al. Long-term results with primary retroperitoneal tumors. *Arch Surg* 1989;124: 1168–1173.

Complications

of Lymphadenectomy

44

Alliric I. Willis   Jeffrey F. Moley

■ **AXILLARY 628**
Nerve Injury 629
Seroma 629
Major Vascular Injury 630
Lymphedema 630
Treatment of Lymphedema 630
Sentinel Node Biopsy: Comparison with Axillary
    Dissection 630
Allergic Reactions 631

■ **INGUINAL LYMPHADENECTOMY 631**
Treatment of Lower Extremity Lymphedema 632
Saphenous Vein-sparing Inguinal
    Lymphadenectomy 632
Inguinal Sentinel Node Biopsy 632

■ **HEAD AND NECK 633**
Central Neck Dissection Complications (Recurrent
    Laryngeal Nerve, Parathyroids) 633
Radical and Modified Radical Neck Dissection 634
Sentinel Node Biopsy in the Head and Neck 634

■ **ABDOMINAL AND PELVIC 634**

■ **THORACIC 635**

■ **CONCLUSION 635**

■ **REFERENCES 635**

Alliric I. Willis: Fox Chase Cancer Center, Philadelphia, PA 19111
Jeffrey F. Moley: Washington University School of Medicine,
St. Louis, MO 63110

Lymphadenectomy is an integral component of surgical oncology for the diagnosis, staging, and regional control of various cancers. As our understanding of lymphatic metastasis has increased, the benefits of extensive lymphadenectomy for certain cancers have been appreciated. However, with this operation can come significant morbidity from complications related to disruption of the lymphatic system, injury of surrounding structures, wound complications, and functional impairment. In contrast, our appreciation of the benefits of less extensive lymphadenectomy for some cancers has resulted in improvements in frequency and severity of complications. This chapter will focus on complications of lymphadenectomy by region.

AXILLARY

Axillary lymph node dissection is an important component of the surgical staging and treatment of breast cancer as a part of both modified radical mastectomy and breast conserving therapy. Axillary lymph node dissection is also an important part of regional control of melanoma, sarcoma, and other cutaneous cancers that involve the axillary lymph nodes. Indications for axillary dissection include biopsy proven breast cancer; clinically positive lymphadenopathy in the presence of a diagnosis of breast cancer, melanoma, or other cancer; and histologically positive sentinel lymph nodes. The long-term complication rate from axillary dissection is reported to be as high as 25% to 30% and includes lymphedema, numbness, and chronic pain (1).

The anatomical boundaries and structures of importance in an axillary dissection are the lateral border of the pectoralis muscles and the chest wall, along which lies the long thoracic nerve medially, the latissimus dorsi muscle laterally, the axillary vein superiorly, the upper outer breast inferiorly, the thoracodorsal neurovascular bundle posteriorly, and the axillary fascia anteriorly. Careful dissection with attention to identification of structures is essential to minimize the risk of complications. Entering the axillary fascia inferiorly can help avoid injury to the axillary vein. Medial dissection along the pectoralis muscles should avoid injuring the pectoralis neurovascular bundle. Superiorly, care should be taken to avoid skeletonizing the axillary vein to avoid the risk of vessel injury as well as to minimize lymphatic injury.

Nerve Injury

The intercostobrachial nerve can usually be identified coursing across the lower axilla. The axillary contents may be divided to pass over or under the intercostobrachial nerve to preserve it. However, if it is unable to be dissected free of tumor, then it can be sacrificed, which results in the loss of sensation in the upper, inner arm. When no attempt is made to spare the intercostobrachial nerve during axillary dissection, the incidence of arm numbness has been reported to be from 68% to 81% (1,2). The proximal end of the cut nerve should be buried in the pectoralis muscle to avoid painful neuroma formation. Most patients tolerate injury to the thoracodorsal nerve (innervating the latissimus dorsi muscle) well; however, injury to the long thoracic nerve (innervating the serratus anterior muscle) results in winging of the scapula. This injury should be repaired by primary repair or nerve grafting.

Seroma

One of the most common complications of axillary dissection is seroma formation or lymphorrhea, which refers to persistent drainage of axillary lymphatic fluid. This results from transection of lymphatic vessels and may be facilitated by the use of electrocautery, the local inflammatory response, and dead space remaining after removal of the axillary contents (3). It is virtually impossible to prevent lymphatic fluid from accumulating in the wound following axillary dissection. The reported incidence of seroma formation after drain removal following axillary dissection ranges from 35% to as high as 97% in breast cancer patients (3–5). Persistence of lymphorrhea and undrained seromas are associated with wound breakdown and infection.

In a prospective study by Talbot and Magarey published in 2002, three groups of 30 patients each were followed postoperatively after axillary dissection for breast cancer. One group maintained closed suction axillary drainage until the 24-hour drain output was <50 mL. This resulted in an average of 9.6 days of drain placement. The second group had drains removed 2 days after surgery, regardless of the drainage amount. The third group had no drains placed. This study showed that drain placement made no significant difference in the duration of seroma formation after surgery. The duration of seroma accumulation that could be aspirated after surgery was 26.6 days for group one, 25.7 days for group two, and 27.9 days for group three. Additional analysis found that tumor involvement of the nodes, the number of nodes removed, and the type of operation performed (lumpectomy with axillary dissection versus modified radical mastectomy) had no significant effect on seroma formation (5).

Although axillary closed suction drainage remains the standard for controlling lymphorrhea after axillary dissection and preventing seroma formation, some have tried to reduce the amount of lymphorrhea produced. In a study by Carcoforo et al., octreotide, the synthetic somatostatin analog, was investigated in the treatment of lymphorrhea, based on the facts that octreotide has been used in the treatment of abdominal and thoracic lymphatic leaks, somatostatin receptors have been found in lymphatic tissues, and somatostatin analog can reduce local inflammatory responses when given systemically. In this prospective randomized trial involving 261 patients who underwent axillary dissection, 125 patients were treated postoperatively with octreotide (0.1 mg subcutaneously three times daily for 5 days) and compared to a control group of 136 patients for lymphorrhea output and seroma formation. The octreotide group had significantly less lymphorrhea (65.4 mL vs. 94.6 mL) and significantly shorter duration of lymphorrhea (7.1 days vs. 16.7 days) than the control group. There was, however, no significant difference in the length of hospital stay or the length of time that the axillary drains were kept in place. Although the wound complication rate for the control group was three times greater than that of the octreotide group, the overall wound complication rate was only 1.5%. The reported complications associated with octreotide were injection site irritation and gastrointestinal discomfort, although none of these resulted in patients discontinuing treatment (3). Octreotide and new long-acting versions may become more widely used to control lymphorrhea and seroma formation.

Fibrin sealant, a tissue adhesive consisting of fibrinogen and thrombin, has also been reported to reduce the volume of lymphorrhea after lymphatic dissection. Moore et al. reported a phase II, multicenter, prospective, parallel, randomized trial comparing drainage amounts and drain placement duration among 79 patients treated with fibrin sealant and axillary drains to control, standard axillary drainage. Additionally, this trial established a dose response curve for fibrin sealant. In the treatment groups varying doses of fibrin sealant were applied just prior to closing the axilla for lumpectomy with axillary dissection or closing the axilla and skin flaps for modified radical mastectomy. A 4-mL dose of fibrin sealant to the axilla produced a statistically significant reduction in drainage volume and time to drain removal among patients with lumpectomy and axillary dissection. A 16-mL dose to the axilla and an 8-mL dose to the skin flaps resulted in reduction in drainage volume and time to drain removal in modified radical mastectomy patients (6).

Major Vascular Injury

Injury to, or division of, the axillary vein may occur during axillary dissection. The risk of this is increased in patients with bulky axillary nodes, previous operation, or radiation. Although it is debatable whether repair or reconstruction of this vein diminishes long-term complications (7), we recommend repair, vein patch, or autologous vein interposition as indicated, followed by an appropriate period of anticoagulation, if possible.

Lymphedema

One of the most morbid complications of lymphadenectomy is lymphedema, a progressive swelling of the arm characterized by chronic inflammation, fibrosis, and hypertrophy of dermal and subcutaneous tissues. Lymphedema ranges in severity from mild to severe and may be associated with discomfort, increased risk of infections, and development of secondary lymphangiosarcoma (Stewart-Treves syndrome). The overall reported incidence of lymphedema associated with axillary dissection ranges widely from 5% to 80% (8). Causes of lymphedema include injury of lymphatics by surgery, direct effect of tumor on lymphatics (such as metastases that obstruct lymphatic flow), and indirect effects of antitumor treatments such as radiation therapy that can cause fibrosis around lymphatics. Lymphedema can be further defined as acute phase, which is characterized by pitting and is responsive to compression therapy, and chronic phase, which is not pitting, is associated with trophic changes, and is poorly responsive to compression therapy. Tissues affected by lymphedema are more susceptible to infection if injured and are more difficult to heal (8).

Velanovich and Szymanski reported a quality of life study in breast cancer patients with lymphedema. A registry of 827 patients with breast cancer was evaluated defining lymphedema as mid-humerus or mid-radius circumference >1 cm more than the respective circumference of the uninvolved arm. The incidence of lymphedema was 8.3%. A subset of 101 consecutive patients was evaluated using the quality of life assessment instrument SF-36. Comparisons were made within this study group among patients who underwent breast surgery without lymphadenectomy, patients who underwent lymphadenectomy without lymphedema, and patients with lymphadenectomy and lymphedema. In this study patients with lymphedema had significant lower quality of life scores in the domains of role-emotional and bodily pain, while there were no differences in scores between patient groups that did not have lymphedema. Also, there were significantly more patients with lymphedema who had quality of life scores greater than one standard deviation below the national average in the areas of bodily pain, mental health, and general health (9).

Radical lymphadenectomy for melanoma is performed to regionally control the disease in an effort to limit morbidity; however, the procedure itself is associated with significant morbidity. Wrightson et al. reported on the Sunbelt Melanoma Trial, a large scale, multi-institutional, prospective, randomized trial in which complications associated with regional lymph node dissection and sentinel lymph node biopsy (SLNB) were compared. The overall incidence of complications associated with lymphadenectomy was 23%. The complication incidence specifically for axillary dissection was 20%. The incidence of lymphedema with axillary dissection was nearly 5% (10). Serpell et al. reported a prospective study of 64 patients who underwent 73 lymphadenectomies, 34 of which were axillary dissections. The overall incidence of wound complications among axillary dissections was 47% (32% seroma, 6% wound infection, 6% delayed healing, and 3% hematoma). The incidence of lymphedema after axillary dissection was 6% (11).

Treatment of Lymphedema

Strategies for treatment of lymphedema following axillary dissection include meticulous skin care, prevention of infection, massage, compression bandaging, and exercise (12). Drug treatment (benzopyrines) and surgical approaches, including debulking of edematous subcutaneous tissue and lymphaticovenous anastomosis, have been tried, but very limited success has been reported.

Sentinel Node Biopsy: Comparison with Axillary Dissection

Sentinel lymph node biopsy (SLNB) is increasing in popularity and acceptance as an accurate, less invasive technique of assessing axillary lymph node status in patients with clinically negative axillary nodes and isolated or multifocal breast cancer tumors in the same quadrant. The premise for this technique is that the sentinel lymph node, the first lymph node to receive the blue dye marker or technetium-99 sulfur colloid radioactive marker, would be the first lymph node to be involved with axillary nodal metastatic disease. Multiple studies have been reported that validate SLNB as accurate with a low false-negative rate. Patients with sentinel lymph nodes positive for cancer subsequently undergo a complete axillary dissection. The axillary dissection may be performed as a second procedure or during the same operation if the diagnosis is made on frozen section. Burak et al. reported an accuracy of 94% in diagnosing positive sentinel lymph nodes on frozen section (1). Diagnosis on frozen section can prevent the patient from the anxiety associated with a second surgery for axillary dissection. Those who have nodes negative for metastatic disease do not require further surgery and can be spared the risk of complications associated with axillary dissection.

Multiple studies have demonstrated that SLNB significantly reduces the incidence of complications associated with lymphadenectomy. Burak et al. reported a prospective, nonrandomized, controlled study of 96 patients in which they compared 48 patients who underwent SLNB and were found to have negative sentinel nodes to 48 patients who underwent SLNB, were found to have positive nodes, and subsequently underwent axillary dissection. Ninety-four percent of the patients undergoing axillary dissection had that procedure during the same anesthetic as the SLNB, based upon positive frozen section diagnosis. Six percent had a separate procedure performed because the permanent SLNB specimen was read as positive.

The axillary dissection group had significantly more edema as determined by arm circumference at the mid-bicep and antecubital fossa when measured at a minimum of 6 months after surgery. Significantly more axillary dissection patients complained of arm numbness (81%); however, 17% of SLNB patients had complaints of arm numbness. The authors note that no specific attempts were made to spare the intercostobrachial nerve. Significantly fewer SLNB patients had axillary drains placed (16% vs. 100%). The duration of drainage was shorter among SLNB patients (0.5 days vs. 13 days for axillary dissection). Eighty-seven percent of SLNB patients had outpatient procedures, and 70% returned to normal activities <3 days after surgery, compared to 100% of axillary dissection patients who stayed overnight and 73% who returned to normal activities >7 days after surgery (1).

Schrenk et al. reported a prospective study comparing 35 SLNB patients to 35 axillary dissection patients with negative nodes. No SLNB patients had drains placed and none required aspiration after surgery. All the axillary dissection patients had drains placed, and 43% required aspiration after their drains were removed. SLNB patients had no lymphedema based upon arm circumference before and after surgery. Axillary dissection patients had a significantly increased arm circumference in the forearm and upper arm after surgery and a highly significant incidence of postoperative complaints of lymphedema. None of the SLNB patients had complaints of numbness, while 69% of axillary dissection patients had complaints of numbness after surgery. SLNB patients also had significantly fewer complaints of pain and restricted arm mobility (4).

The previously mentioned Sunbelt Melanoma Trial compared complications of regional lymphadenectomy to those of SLNB in melanoma patients. A highly significant difference was found between total complications with axillary SLNB (4%) versus axillary dissection (20%). Lymphedema occurred five times more frequently following axillary dissection. The overall complication incidence with SLNB was nearly 5% (vs. 23% previously mentioned with lymphadenectomy), with hematoma/seroma formation (2%) and wound infection (1%) being more common among SLNB patients (10).

Schijven et al. reported a retrospective study of 213 axillary dissection patients and 180 SLNB patients who were evaluated by their answers on a quality of life questionnaire. Axillary dissection patients had significantly more complaints of postoperative pain, lymphedema, numbness or tingling in the arm and hand, impaired range of motion, and impaired use of the affected arm (2).

Allergic Reactions

Although the incidence of complications is decreased with SLNB, one complication specific to SLNB is reaction to the injected dye. Patent blue dye is the preferred dye in Europe for SLNB. It has been estimated that nearly 3% of the population may be allergic to patent blue dye. Case reports have been published of patients having reactions from rashes and urticaria to anaphylaxis from patent blue dye injections (13,14). In the United States isosulfan blue is the preferred dye marker for SLNB. The incidence of allergic reactions is 1.5%, and as many as 1% may have anaphylaxis. In the Sunbelt Melanoma Trial of over 1,600 SLNBs there were no cases of reactions to isosulfan blue or technetium (10). Radiation safety precautions should be observed when using technetium as a radioactive marker for SLNB. Methylene blue dye has not been as popularly received as a marker for SLNB. In a retrospective study reported by Stradling et al., five of 24 consecutive patients had severe erythematous, ulcerated, or necrotic lesions where methylene blue dye was injected intradermally. No complications were associated with intraparenchymal injection of methylene blue (15). The treatment of patients with allergic reactions to dye includes standard supportive care and the discontinuation of exposure to the inciting agent.

INGUINAL LYMPHADENECTOMY

Inguinal lymphadenectomy is performed for regional control of melanoma, vulvar carcinoma, and anal and penile carcinoma. Other metastasizing cutaneous cancers and sarcoma may also involve inguinal nodes. Anatomically, the boundaries of the superficial inguinal lymph node dissection include several centimeters above the inguinal ligament superiorly, the middle of the adductor longus muscle medially, the apex of the femoral triangle inferiorly, the middle of the sartorius muscle laterally, the subcutaneous fascia anteriorly, and the fascia overlying the quadriceps and sartorious muscles deep. A femoral dissection includes opening the deep fascia, identifying the femoral vein, and removing the deep nodes medial to it. The boundaries of a deep inguinal dissection are from the inguinal ligament inferiorly to the common iliac vessels superiorly with the peritoneum reflected medially and superiorly. Following exposure of the femoral vessels in the upper thigh, soft tissue coverage is best obtained by mobilizing the sartorius muscle from the anterior superior iliac crest and transposing it to cover the femoral vessels by suture to the inguinal ligament.

Complications of inguinal lymphadenectomy are significantly more frequent than other regional lymphadenectomy procedures. Complications from this procedure are the rule rather than the exception, and patients must be prepared accordingly. The main reported complications include prolonged lymphatic drainage and seroma formation, wound infection, necrosis of the inferior flap with prolonged wound healing, and lymphedema. Experience with several recent series addressing different tumor types demonstrates the extremely high prevalence of these problems. The Sunbelt Melanoma Trial experience, reported in 2003, noted an overall complication rate of 51% and an incidence of lymphedema of nearly 32% (10). In 2003, Serpell et al. reported an overall complication incidence of 71% associated with inguinal lymphadenectomy for melanoma (25% infection, 25% delayed wound healing, 46% seroma, and 29% lymphedema) (11).

In a retrospective review from M.D. Anderson from 2002 of 106 inguinal lymphadenectomy procedures in 53 patients with invasive penile cancer, Bevan-Thomas et al. reported an overall complication rate of 57%. Prophylactic and therapeutic dissections had a similar complication rate of approximately 35%. Palliative dissections had a significantly higher incidence of complications at 67% (16).

Gaarenstroom et al. reported a retrospective study of 187 inguinal dissections in 101 patients for diagnosed vulvar carcinoma. The complication rate was 52%. Specific complications were lymphedema (21%), lymphocyst (27%), wound breakdown (11%), wound infection (27%), hematoma (2%), deep venous thrombosis (2%), and pulmonary embolism (2%). A significant association was made between early postoperative complications and late lymphedema. No significant association was found between overall complication rate and postoperative radiation therapy (17). In contrast, Gould et al. reported a retrospective study of 112 inguinal lymphadenectomies in 67 patients with vulvar carcinoma in which they found that early complications (<30 days after surgery) did not predict late complications, and postoperative radiation therapy demonstrated a trend, though not statistically significant, toward association with late lymphedema. Early complications included cellulitis (35%), wound breakdown (19%), lymphedema (5%), and lymphocyst (13%). Late complications included cellulitis (22%), wound breakdown (3%), lymphedema (30%), and lymphocyst (5%) (18).

Rouzier et al. reported a retrospective study of 194 patients who underwent inguinal lymphadenectomy for vulvar carcinoma. Logistic regression analysis showed that lymphedema was associated with radiation therapy, sartorius muscle transposition, and obesity. Wound breakdown was associated with patient age >70 (19).

Treatment of Lower Extremity Lymphedema

For mild cases of lower extremity lymphedema, elevation of the affected limb with appropriate skin care may be adequate. For working patients we recommend twice daily half-hour breaks during which the limb is elevated. This is best achieved by lying flat with the leg up on pillows or propped up against a wall. This may be combined with compression therapy with custom made elastic stockings, multilayer bandaging, or pneumatic pumps. For more severe cases, drug therapy and surgery have been attempted with limited success. Benzopyrones have been shown to reduce edema fluid and increase softness of lyphedematous extremities, but usefulness is limited due to hepatotoxicity. Several surgical procedures have been described for relief of lower extremity lymphedema, including debulking procedures, lymphovenous bypass, and omental autografting. Reports of these procedures are limited by small numbers of patients and variable results, and they are generally not recommended for patients with lymphedema secondary to lymphadenectomy for cancer (20). A recent study from Roswell Park Cancer Institute reported 14 patients with lymphedema following therapeutic groin dissections for melanoma who underwent "complete decongestive physiotherapy" with decrease in lymphedema of 60% (21). This treatment is a combination of manual lymphatic massage, multilayered inelastic bandaging, exercise, and wearing of compression stockings.

Saphenous Vein-sparing Inguinal Lymphadenectomy

The technique of saphenous vein preservation in modified inguinal lymphadenectomy has been associated with a lower incidence of lymphedema, the most debilitating complication of lymphadenectomy. A retrospective review of 139 inguinal dissections in 83 patients compared the incidence of lymphedema in traditional inguinal dissection to saphenous vein-sparing dissection. The incidence of lymphedema in the first 6 months after surgery was reduced from 70% to 32%. Evaluation 6 months to 2 years after surgery found the incidence reduced from 39% to 11% with saphenous vein preservation. Follow-up >2 years after surgery found the incidence to be reduced from 32% in traditional dissections to 2% in saphenous vein-sparing dissections. The likelihood of no complications was significantly higher in the group of patients with the saphenous vein preserved. Wound breakdown and cellulitis were significantly less common in the group of patients with the saphenous vein preserved. There was no significant difference in the rate of disease recurrence between the traditional versus the saphenous vein sparing dissection (22). Saphenous vein preservation was also associated with significantly less lymphedema, wound breakdown, and cellulitis by chi square analysis in the study by Rouzier, but the logistic regression model analysis did not find statistical significance in vein-sparing independently affecting any of those complications (19).

Inguinal Sentinel Node Biopsy

SLNB significantly reduces the rate of complications associated with inguinal lymphadenectomy. The Sunbelt

Melanoma Trial demonstrated a complication rate of 8% among 657 patients undergoing inguinal SLNB and a rate of 1.5% for lymphedema compared to a previously noted total complication rate of 51% for complete inguinal dissection and an incidence of 32% for lymphedema (10). Given the high incidence of complications with inguinal lymphadenectomy, SLNB has great potential to decrease the number of complications by distinguishing those who would most benefit from a complete inguinal dissection.

HEAD AND NECK

Neck dissection is performed for staging and regional control in patients with various cancers of the head and neck, including thyroid. Types of neck dissection include radical neck dissection (removal of nodal levels II–V from the carotid artery to the trapezius muscle en bloc with the internal jugular vein, sternocleidomastoid muscle, and spinal accessory nerve), modified radical neck dissection (same as radical neck dissection, but sparing the internal jugular vein, sternocleidomastoid muscle, and accessory nerve), and central node dissection (level VI paratracheal nodes). Level I neck dissection is frequently performed for cancers of the oral cavity and involves removal of submental and submandibular lymphatic tissue. Variations of these neck dissections are termed functional neck dissections. In those cases the nodal levels removed should be named (e.g., left functional neck dissection—levels II–V). The risk of complications depends on the type of neck dissection performed. Sequelae of radical neck dissection are related to removal of the sternocleidomastoid (cosmetic and weakness), internal jugular vein (possible swelling of the ipsilateral face and neck), and accessory nerve (trapezius paralysis and shoulder weakness). Other potential complications include bleeding, infection, thoracic duct injury, flap necrosis, and other nerve injury (phrenic, hypoglossal, vagus, marginal mandibular). Thoracic duct injury complications can be minimized by identification of the thoracic duct in the inferior aspect of the lateral neck dissection and ligation of the duct if it is injured. Thoracic duct injury leads to chyle leak. This is marked by the accumulation of milky fluid in the drain or incision. Chyle leak is a particularly difficult complication because it rarely stops on its own, even with a low-fat diet, and because over time it results in loss of protein and nutrient-rich fluid that can contribute to malnutrition. If drainage and low-fat diet do not result in cessation of the leak, surgical mass ligation of the duct is necessary. Proper ligation of the thoracic duct entails identification of the structure near its junction with the jugular vein and mass ligation with surrounding soft tissues. The thoracic duct is extremely thin-walled and does not hold a tie or suture well. Mass ligation with surrounding tissues (muscle fascia, fat, lymphatics) ensures stable permanent closure. It is important not to incorporate the phrenic or vagus nerves or vertebral artery into this closure. If neck exploration and closure does not stop the leak, supradiaphragmatic mass ligation by a thoracic approach may be necessary (23). Chyle may also accumulate in the pleural space, causing a chylothorax. This can result from a missed thoracic duct injury or, as in a case report from Kamasaki et al., can rarely occur after the thoracic duct is ligated in the neck, likely secondary to high intraluminal pressures that result in extravasation of chyle through the walls of the duct (24). This type of chyle leak may not present through the neck drain and requires thoracentesis to detect. It has been our experience that surgical correction of this complication is usually necessary (23).

Central Neck Dissection Complications (Recurrent Laryngeal Nerve, Parathyroids)

Complications associated with central neck dissection include recurrent laryngeal nerve (RLN) injury and hypoparathyroidism. RLN injury causes hoarseness and diminishes the effectiveness of cough. Injury to the RLN can be avoided by identification of the nerve throughout its course in the neck and by not using cautery in the vicinity of the nerve (25). If an RLN injury is identified, the results of repair are not always optimal, because the RLN has sensory and mixed adductor and abductor motor fibers. Repair, with careful alignment of fascicles using magnification, is usually appropriate. Nerve grafting may also be performed. Hypocalcemia can be avoided by identification of parathyroids, protection of their blood supply, and autotransplantation of devascularized parathyroids to muscle pockets in the sternocleidomastoid or forearm muscle after mincing into 1 mm by 3 mm fragments (25).

Cheah et al. reported a review of 115 neck dissections performed on 74 patients with thyroid cancer (64% papillary, 32% medullary, and 4% follicular). Postoperatively, 23% had transient hypocalcemia and 0.9% had permanent hypoparathyroidism. One patient had a neck hematoma that required a surgical procedure. There were no nerve palsies and no injuries to the thoracic duct, trachea, or esophagus. Significant factors increasing the risk of hypocalcemia were concurrent neck dissection and thyroidectomy (60% vs. 17% for dissection alone) (26).

Redo central neck dissection is an especially difficult procedure that requires exposure of vital structures through scarred and sometimes radiated tissues. Moley et al. described an effective approach to the central neck in such cases, developing a plane between the sternocleidomastoid muscle and the strap muscles to enter the central neck laterally. In this approach the RLN may be identified early and preserved (27). This approach is also useful in early identification of the carotid artery, jugular vein, vagus, and phrenic nerves. In a report of 52 redo neck dissections for recurrent thyroid cancer, Moley et al. described four thoracic duct injuries and two cases of persistent hypoparathyroidism (25).

Radical and Modified Radical Neck Dissection

Magrin et al. reported a 30-year retrospective study of 193 consecutive bilateral neck dissections. In the last 10 years of the study, the neck dissections were modified to spare the spinal accessory nerves and both internal jugular veins. The spinal accessory nerve was spared in 40% of cases, and the internal jugular vein was spared bilaterally in 6% of cases, with 90% having unilateral ligation. Complications occurred in 61% of the cases. The complications and frequency were: fistulae (30%), local wound infection (26%), wound dehiscence (21%), flap necrosis (20%), chyle fistula (2.5%), pulmonary infection (5%), rupture of vessels (4%), hematoma/seroma (3%), and postoperative mortality (2%). There was no significant survival benefit for elective or therapeutic radical neck dissection when compared to modified radical neck dissection. The authors concluded that bilateral radical neck dissection is a morbid procedure with limited benefit and should not be done as an elective procedure (28).

Modified radical neck dissection is indicated for some patients with melanoma of the head and neck. In the Sunbelt Melanoma Trial, Wrightson et al. reported a postoperative complication incidence of 10% in 50 neck dissection patients with melanoma (10). Serpell et al. also reported a postoperative complication incidence of 10% in ten neck dissection patients with melanoma (11).

Though less morbid than radical neck dissection, modified radical neck dissection still can present significant functional complications. Shoulder dysfunction, frequently a complication of radical neck dissection, is associated with modified radical lymph node dissection as well. In a cross-sectional study from the University of Michigan, Chepeha et al. evaluated 64 patients using the Constant's Shoulder Scale to assess shoulder function postoperatively. Two groups were formed: 32 patients who underwent modified radical neck dissection and 32 patients who underwent selective dissection. The difference between the two procedures is in selectively sparing the level V lymph nodes, which may help prevent scarring and devascularization of the accessory nerve and associated cervical nerve rootlets that can occur with dissection in the posterior triangle. The study found that selective dissection patients had a highly significantly better shoulder function score. The patient's weight, as it likely correlates to better health in this population, was also significantly associated with fewer complications of shoulder function. Radiation therapy was found to be a critical factor, although not independently statistically significant (29).

Another complication associated with neck dissection is fracture of the clavicle postoperatively. The frequency has been reported as approximately 0.5%. It occurs most often as a late complication in association with spinal accessory nerve injury that results in wasting of the trapezius, shoulder drop, and increased torsional forces on the sternoclavicular joint and clavicle (30).

An infrequent but life-threatening complication of neck dissection is postoperative rupture of the internal jugular vein. Cleland-Zamudio et al. evaluated a series of six cases following modified radical and selective neck dissections for primary squamous cell cancer of the head and neck. Factors associated with vein rupture included circumferential dissection of the internal jugular vein low in the neck and fistula in the region of the hypopharynx low in the neck. All patients had a tobacco history and five of the six had poor nutritional status. At emergent re-exploration, each of the involved internal jugular veins was found to be thin-walled and necrotic. They were treated by ligation (31).

A rare complication of neck dissection is vertebral artery injury. A case of bilateral cortical blindness was reported in a patient after right radical neck dissection. Workup revealed a hypoplastic left vertebral artery that possibly embolized a thrombus that developed during the rotation of the neck during the right neck dissection (32).

Sentinel Node Biopsy in the Head and Neck

SLNB using blue dye or radiolabeled marker has demonstrated a potential for minimizing the number of negative neck dissections and reducing complications associated with neck dissection. The Sunbelt Melanoma Trial reported a complication incidence of 2.4% in a total of 370 patients who underwent SLNB in the neck for melanoma (10).

Fukui et al. reported a study of 22 patients with papillary thyroid cancer who had intraoperative SLNB using methylene blue dye injected into the thyroid circumferentially around the tumor. The sentinel nodes were identified by direct vision of the dye passing from the thyroid into the nodes. After removal of the sentinel lymph nodes, subtotal thyroidectomy and modified radical neck dissection were performed. The sentinel lymph node detection rate was 95.5%. Seventy-six percent of the sentinel lymph nodes were identified in the central compartment, while 24% were found in the ipsilateral jugular region. No patients had sentinel nodes found contralaterally, and no patients had sentinel lymph nodes present in both the central and jugular areas. The correlation between the sentinel node status and the final regional node status was 90.5%. Two patients (9.5%) had negative sentinel nodes but positive regional nodes. In the final 11 cases, frozen section of sentinel nodes was performed. There was 100% correlation between the frozen and permanent sentinel node status. There were no complications associated with these procedures (33).

ABDOMINAL AND PELVIC

Extensive abdominal and pelvic lymphadenectomies may be performed for gastric and endometrial cancers. Although not as morbid as those involving the axilla and groin, these lymphadenectomies may result in lymphocyst formation and persistent drain requirements. Franchi et al. reported a study that evaluated the risk factors for postoperative complications of pelvic lymphadenectomy. In this prospective study 133 patients underwent pelvic lymphadenectomy with a complication rate of 34%. The most common complications were lymphocysts and cystitis. Multiple logistic regression analysis found that the only factor significantly associated with postoperative complications was removal of >14 lymph nodes (34). Operative techniques such as omentopexy have been used with some success to reduce the complications of lymphorrhea and lymphocyst formation (35).

Persistent leaking from severed lymphatics due to cauterization is one contributor to lymphadenectomy complications. A prospective, randomized study by Tsimoyiannis et al. evaluated the effectiveness of ultrasonic shears in extended lymphadenectomy for gastric cancer. These shears use ultrasonic waves to denature proteins forming a coagulum that seals vessel walls and thereby would hypothetically prevent lymphorrhea. Forty patients were studied. Twenty underwent resection and lymphadenectomy using traditional monopolar cautery, hemoclips, and ligation. The other 20 underwent resection and lymphadenectomy using ultrasonically activated coagulating shears, reserving hemoclips and ligation only for vessels >3 mm in diameter. The group using the ultrasonic shears had significantly less blood loss intraoperatively and abdominal drainage postoperatively. They also had abdominal drains removed sooner and had a significantly shorter stay. Although there was no difference in the number of patients that were transfused, the patients treated with ultrasonic shears required significantly fewer units of blood (36).

THORACIC

The high frequency of lymphatic metastases from esophageal cancer has made mediastinal lymphadenectomy an important part of the regional treatment of this disease. Complications associated with this include chyle leaks, nerve injury, and pulmonary infections. The standard treatment for chyle leaks includes drainage, total parenteral nutrition, a low-fat diet with medium chain fatty acid supplements, and octreotide to reduce lymphatic production. If this is not effective, supradiaphragmatic mass ligation of the thoracic duct is necessary (23).

The high incidence of nodal metastases to the region of the RLNs increases the risk of RLN injuries in esophageal surgery (37). Griffen et al. reported a prospective series of 228 patients who underwent subtotal esophagectomy and two-field lymphadenectomy. In an effort to reduce nerve injury, the RLN was not dissected out with the removal of nodes in the aortopulmonary window. Cervical lymphadenectomy was not performed. The most common postoperative complication was pulmonary infection at 15%. The incidence of chyle leaks was 0.8%. The incidence of laryngeal nerve palsy was 0.4% (38).

Nishihira et al. reported a prospective randomized trial comparing 32 patients undergoing extended lymphadenectomy, which included superior mediastinal and cervical dissection, to 30 patients undergoing conventional lymphadenectomy for esophageal cancer. There was no significant difference in pulmonary complications. RLN palsy had an incidence of 56% among extended lymphadenectomy patients compared to 30% of conventional lymphadenectomy patients. Extended lymphadenectomy was associated with a significantly higher incidence of phrenic nerve palsy and tracheostomy. However, conventional dissection was associated with a higher incidence of postoperative leakage. The 5-year survival was greater for the extended lymphadenectomy group (66% vs. 48%), but this was not statistically significant (39).

Fujita et al. reported a retrospective study of 302 patients who underwent curative transthoracic esophagectomy with either standard (40), extended (21), total (65), or three-field lymphadenectomy (176). The incidence of RLN palsies was directly related to the extent of lymphadenectomy, with an incidence of 57% overall, 69% three-field, 55% total lymphadenectomy, 20% extended, and 23% standard (37).

CONCLUSION

Lymphadenectomy is an effective means of regional control of cancer, although at the cost of potential morbid complications. Appreciation of these complications and informing the patient beforehand is important. Knowledge of prevention strategies and treatment options is critical for general surgeons performing these operations. SLNB provides a tool for surgeons to better determine which patients will benefit from more extensive lymphadenectomy and which ones can be spared its complications while not compromising cancer treatment.

REFERENCES

1. Burak WE, Hollenbeck ST, Zervos EE, et al. Sentinel lymph node biopsy results in less postoperative morbidity compared with axillary lymph node dissection for breast cancer. *Am J Surg* 2002;183:23–27.
2. Schijven MP, Vingerhoets A, Rutten H, et al. Comparison of morbidity between axillary lymph node dissection and sentinel node biopsy. *Eur J Surg Oncol* 2003;29:341–350.
3. Carcoforo P, Soliani G, Maestroni U, et al. Octreotide in the treatment of lymphorrhea after axillary node dissection: a prospective randomized controlled trial. *J Am Coll Surg* 2003; 196:365–369.
4. Schrenk P, Rieger R, Shamiyeh A, et al. Morbidity following sentinel lymph node biopsy versus axillary node dissection for patients with breast carcinoma. *Cancer* 2000;88:608–614.

5. Talbot M, Magarey C. Reduced use of drains following axillary lymphadenectomy for breast cancer. *ANZ J Surg* 2002;72:488–490.

6. Moore M, Burak WE, Nelson E, et al. Fibrin sealant reduces the duration and amount of fluid drainage after axillary dissection: a randomized prospective clinical trial. *J Am Coll Surg* 2001;192:591–599.

7. Macdonald I. Resection of the axillary vein in radical mastectomy: its relation to the mechanism of lymphedema. *Cancer* 1948;1:618–624.

8. Brennan M, DePompolo R, Garden F. Focused review: postmastectomy lymphedema. *Arch Phys Med Rehabil* 1996;77:S–74–S–80.

9. Velanovich V, Szymanski W. Quality of life of breast cancer patients with lymphedema. *Am J Surg* 1999;177:184–187.

10. Wrightson W, Wong SL, Edwards MJ, et al. Complications associated with sentinel lymph node biopsy for melanoma. *Ann Surg Oncol* 2003;10:676–680.

11. Serpell J, Carne P, Bailey M. Radical lymph node dissection for melanoma. *ANZ J Surg* 2003;73:294–299.

12. Pain S, Purushotham A. Lymphoedema following surgery for breast cancer pain. *Br J Surg* 2000;87(9):1128–1141.

13. Mullan MH, Deacock SJ, Quiney NF, et al. Anaphylaxis to patent blue dye during sentinel lymph node biopsy for breast cancer. *Eur J Surg Oncol* 2001;27:218–219.

14. Woltsche-Kahr I, Komericki P, Kranke B, et al. Anaphylactic shock following peritumoral injection of patent blue in sentinel lymph node biopsy procedure. *Eur J Surg Oncol* 2000;26:313–321.

15. Stradling B, Aranha G, Gabram S. Adverse skin lesions after methylene blue injections for sentinel lymph node localization. *Am J Surg* 2002;184:350–352.

16. Bevan-Thomas R, Slaton J, Pettaway C. Contemporary morbidity from lymphadenectomy for penile squamous cell carcinoma: the M.D. Anderson lymphedema. *Arch Phys Med Rehabil* 2002;167:1638–1642.

17. Gaarenstroom KN, Kenter GG, Trimbos JB, et al. Postoperative complications after vulvectomy and inguinofemoral lymphadenectomy using separate groin incisions. *Int J Gynecol Cancer* 2003;13:522–527.

18. Gould N, Kamelle S, Tillmanns T, et al. Predictors of complication after inguinal lymphadenectomy. *Gynecol Oncol* 2001;82:329–332.

19. Rouzier R, Haddad B, Dubernard G, et al. Inguinofemoral dissection for carcinoma of the vulva: effect of modifications of extent and technique on morbidity and survival. *J Am Coll Surg* 2003;196:442–450.

20. Tiwari A, Cheng KS, Button M, et al. Differential diagnosis, investigation, and current treatment of lower limb lymphedema. *Arch Surg* 2003;138:152–161.

21. Hinrichs C, Gibbs JF, and Driscoll D, et al. The effectiveness of complete decongestive physiotherapy for the treatment of lymphedema following groin dissection for melanoma. *J Surg Oncol* 2004;85:187–192.

22. Zhang S, Sood AK, Sorosky JI, et al. Preservation of the saphenous vein during inguinal lymphadenectomy decreases morbidity in patients with carcinoma of the vulva. *Cancer* 2000;89:1520–1525.

23. Patterson GA, Todd TR, Delarue NC, et al. Supradiaphragmatic ligation of the thoracic duct in intractable chylous fistula. *Ann Thorac Surg* 1981;32(1):44–49.

24. Kamasaki N, Ikeda H, Wang ZL, et al. Bilateral chylothorax following radical neck dissection. *Int J Oral Maxillofac Surg* 2003;32:91–93.

25. Moley JF, Dilley WG, DeBenedetti MK. Improved results of cervical reoperation for medullary thyroid carcinoma. *Ann Surg* 1997;225:734–740.

26. Cheah W, Cumhur A, Ituarte PHG, et al. Complications of neck dissection for thyroid cancer. *World J Surg* 2002;26:1013–1016.

27. Moley JF, Lairmore TC, Doherty GM, et al. Preservation of the recurrent laryngeal nerves in thyroid and parathyroid reoperations. *Surgery* 1999;126(4):673–677; discussion 677–679.

28. Magrin J, Kowalski L. Bilateral radical neck dissection: results in 193 cases. *J Surg Oncol* 2000;75:232–240.

29. Chepeha D, Taylor RJ, Chepeha JC, et al. Functional assessment using Constant's shoulder scale after modified radical and selective neck dissection. *Head Neck* 2002;24:432–436.

30. Halfpenny W, Goodger N. Early fracture of clavicle following neck dissection. *J Laryngol Otol* 2000;114:714–715.

31. Cleland-Zamudio S, Wax MK, Smith JD, et al. Ruptured internal jugular vein: a postoperative complication of modified/selected neck dissection. *Head Neck* 2003;25:357–360.

32. Raj P, Moore PLA, Henderson J, et al. Bilateral cortical blindness: an unusual complication following unilateral neck dissection. *J Laryngol Otol* 2002;116:227–229.

33. Fukui Y, Yamakawa T, Taniki T, et al. Sentinel lymph node biopsy in patients with papillary thyroid carcinoma. *Cancer* 2001;92:2868–2874.

34. Franchi M, Ghezzi F, Riva C, et al. Postoperative complications after pelvic lymphadenectomy for the surgical staging of endometrial cancer. *J Surg Oncol* 2001;78:232–240.

35. Fujiwara K, Kigawa J, Hasegawa K, et al. Effect of simple omentoplasty and omentopexy in the prevention of complications after pelvic lymphadenectomy. *Int J Gynecol Cancer* 2003;13:61–66.

36. Tsimoyiannis E, Jabarin M, Tsimoyiannis JC, et al. Ultrasonically activated shears in extended lymphadenectomy for gastric cancer. *World J Surg* 2002;26:158–161.

37. Fujita H, Sueyoshi S, Tanaka T, et al. Optimal lymphadenectomy for squamous cell carcinoma in the thoracic esophagus: comparing the short- and long-term outcome among the four types of lymphadenectomy. *World J Surg* 2003;27:571–579.

38. Griffen S, Shaw I, Dresner S. Early complications after Ivor Lewis subtotal esophagectomy with two-field lymphadenectomy: risk factors and management. *J Am Coll Surg* 2002;194:285–297.

39. Nishihira T, Hirayama K, Mori S. A prospective randomized trial of extended cervical and superior mediastinal lymphadenectomy for carcinoma of the thoracic esophagus. *Am J Surg* 1998;175:47–51.

Complications of Transplantation

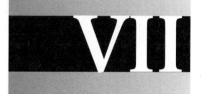

Complications of Renal Transplantation

45

Robert M. Merion

■ OVERVIEW OF RENAL TRANSPLANTATION 639

■ VASCULAR COMPLICATIONS 640
Early Vascular Complications 640
Donor-related Complications 640
Recipient-related Complications 640
Transplant Renal Artery Stenosis 642

■ EARLY POST-TRANSPLANT RENAL
DYSFUNCTION 644
Etiology 644
Diagnosis 645
Treatment 645

■ UROLOGIC COMPLICATIONS 645
Ureteral Obstruction 645
Urinary Extravasation 647
Ureteral Leak 648
Bladder Leak 649
Pelvicalyceal Leak 649

■ LYMPHOCELE 649

■ SUPERFICIAL WOUND INFECTION 650

■ SUBFASCIAL ABSCESS 650

■ ALLOGRAFT FRACTURE 651

■ SPONTANEOUS DECAPSULATION 651

■ HYPERCALCEMIA 651

■ REFERENCES 652

OVERVIEW OF RENAL TRANSPLANTATION

Transplantation of the kidney is usually a straightforward operative procedure not particularly taxing to the surgeon's technical skills. Improved immunosuppressive techniques have resulted in patient survival rates in excess of 95% and graft survival rates in excess of 90% one year following transplantation. As most experienced transplantation surgeons are aware, however, the road to this excellent overall result can have many twists and turns. For example, at least 13% of renal transplant recipients experience a complication related to the urinary system (1). If one also considers nonurologic problems requiring operative intervention, such as local infection, lymphocele, or vascular compromise, it is not an overstatement to suggest that 20% of patients may experience a significant perioperative complication.

Complications after renal transplantation may be related to predisposing recipient factors, issues deriving from characteristics of the kidney donor, donor kidney procurement surgery, preservation-related injury, recipient operative misadventure, or complications of the obligate immunosuppressed state. Effective immunosuppression reduces host resistance to infection and delays wound healing. Transplant recipients themselves are often debilitated as the result of poor nutrition or underlying disease,

Robert M. Merion: University of Michigan, Ann Arbor, MI 48109

especially diabetes mellitus. The transplanted kidney itself may be damaged at the time of organ procurement and may harbor bacterial or viral pathogens. These factors notwithstanding, renal transplantation is safe and effective. Years of previous clinical experience and newer diagnostic techniques to be described in the following paragraphs have allowed for anticipation of problems, with earlier diagnosis and subsequently reduced morbidity and mortality.

VASCULAR COMPLICATIONS

Early Vascular Complications

Most acute vascular complications following renal transplantation are technical in origin and are, therefore, preventable in most cases. In general, early vascular complications can be divided into two categories: those related to organ procurement and those related to the recipient operation.

Donor-related Complications

Deceased Donors

Techniques for the procurement of multiple organs from deceased donors have been standardized for many years (1,2). With the use of *in situ* cold perfusion, the kidneys are protected from warm ischemic injury from the moment of donor aortic cross-clamping, totally avoiding the frantic, hurried removal of organs that may lead to technical misadventure. In the author's experience, the use of *in situ* perfusion combined with en bloc removal of the kidneys for separation on the back bench should very nearly preclude the possibility of injuries to the vascular structures of renal allografts. The latter technique permits easy identification of anomalous vascular structures from within the aorta so that no dissection in the renal hilum is necessary.

Volunteer Living Donors

Injury to a kidney procured from a volunteer living donor is distinctly uncommon. The use of predonation visualization of the renal arterial and venous structures, usually via helical computed tomographic scanning, allows the surgeon to identify potential anomalies such as multiple renal arteries or early renal arterial branching, as well as occult vascular pathology (e.g., aneurysm, fibromuscular dysplasia, and renal artery stenosis). This imaging modality has largely replaced conventional selective renal arteriography (3). Up to 54% of prospective living donors may have anatomical arrangements other than a single artery and vein (4).

Additional factors in the living donor, such as relatively limited operative exposure, shorter lengths of renal artery and vein, the absence of Carrel patches of aorta and vena cava, and the need for direct cannulation of the renal artery for cold perfusion, have on occasion led to a more difficult recipient operation. In the author's experience, however, the incidence of vascular compromise has not been increased.

Laparoscopic donor nephrectomy, introduced in the mid-1990s (5–7), is now used for >50% of living donor renal procurement procedures. A learning curve has been described, as has delayed graft function from the effects of pneumoperitoneum. A brief period of renal rest after dissection and prior to removal, accompanied by administration of mannitol and a modest dose of loop diuretic, is generally recommended to prevent this problem. With experience, excellent renal graft function is routinely obtained. It should be noted that renal vessel and ureter length may be compromised with the use of the laparoscopic technique, but in most cases this does not present an undue challenge for the recipient procedure.

Recipient-related Complications

Arterial Thrombosis

This disastrous complication has a reported incidence of 0.5% to 2% (8,9). In rare instances acute occlusion of the allograft renal artery may be noted at the time of transplantation, when potentially remediable lesions such as intimal tears, native or donor renal artery dissection, improper construction of the arterial anastomosis, or acute angulation of the vessel should be identified and corrected. Multiple renal arteries (particularly if they are not on a common aortic patch), severe atherosclerotic vascular disease in the recipient, and diabetes mellitus may all contribute to an increased risk of arterial compromise. The final death knell of accelerated or hyperacute rejection may be arterial thrombosis. One unusual cause of intraoperative concern about the vascular reconstruction is compression of the proximal iliac artery or vein by a self-retaining retractor. Hypoperfusion or venous engorgement of the transplanted kidney may result, leading to an ill-advised exploration of the anastomotic sites until the offending device is discovered and removed.

Renal dysfunction in the immediate postoperative phase suggests the possibility of arterial thrombosis. Prompt diagnosis is imperative because the transplanted kidney has no collateral circulation to support the renal parenchyma. Although absence or abrupt cessation of urine flow is perhaps the most suggestive sign of arterial thrombosis, the differential diagnosis includes other more common causes. The approach to the patient who develops acute renal failure following transplantation is covered in depth later in this chapter, but the logical steps to follow in a patient with post-transplant anuria start with irrigation of the urinary catheter to rule out obstruction. Once patency of the lower urinary tract is assured, the patient should immediately undergo a bedside ultrasonographic examination of the renal allograft to assess the adequacy of renal perfusion and to measure the renal resistive index.

If renal arteriography can be obtained expeditiously, it may be helpful in planning an operative intervention.

Significant iliac arterial reconstruction may be necessary, with replacement of the artery with prosthetic graft material and reimplantation of the allograft artery into the prosthetic material.

Once the diagnosis of arterial thrombosis is suspected, immediate exploration offers the only hope for salvage. Unfortunately, removal of an infarcted graft is the outcome in virtually all cases, with only a few reports of successful thrombectomy 12 to 48 hours after occlusion (10–12).

Polar Artery Occlusion

Careful attention to the details of organ procurement should prevent missed or inadvertently ligated polar vessels. These circumstances are usually evident at the time of revascularization, with sharp demarcation of the involved segment. Vascular reconstruction should be carried out if at all possible to prevent the sequelae of segmental parenchymal infarction, which include infection, urinary leakage with calyceal cutaneous fistula formation, ureteral infarction, and post-transplant hypertension. If repair is not possible and the parenchyma involved comprises <5% of the renal volume, treatment may be expectant. In most of these cases no problems develop. However, if >5% of the parenchyma is involved, consideration must be given to resection of the infarcted area or complete removal of the transplanted kidney.

Hemorrhage

Secondary hemorrhage from anastomotic leak or mycotic aneurysm is a relatively rare complication of renal transplantation, occurring with an incidence of 0.3% to 2.8% (9,13,14). Although arterial thrombosis and hemorrhage are equally uncommon, the latter is associated with an extremely high mortality, ranging from 33% to 57% (13,15). Hemorrhage that occurs within the first 12 to 24 hours of operation is most likely due to surgical error or incomplete hemostasis, and prompt return to the operating room is indicated.

Later hemorrhage is often related to an infectious complication. Leakage of infected urine, mycotic aneurysm, or necrosis of renal parenchyma secondary to a thrombosed polar artery may be responsible. Attempted repair of an infected, leaking anastomosis can only be described as foolhardy, because bleeding invariably recurs. It is far safer to remove the allograft. Because the arterial anastomosis is usually performed end to side to the external iliac artery, ligation of the ipsilateral native vessel may be necessary. Fortunately, acute limb-threatening lower extremity ischemia is rare in this situation (16).

Because the donor may be the source of contamination that may lead to later life-threatening hemorrhage, administration of prophylactic antibiotics to all recipients of renal allografts is recommended (17).

Vascular Complications of Percutaneous Biopsy

Although percutaneous allograft biopsies are generally safe (18,19), hemorrhage is always a possible complication. Rarely, transplant nephrectomy may be required due to uncontrolled postbiopsy retroperitoneal hemorrhage. Postbiopsy hemorrhage may also occur in the setting of chronic rejection in the late post-transplant period. Fibrosis may prevent contraction around the needle tract, resulting in unabated hemorrhage or massive hematoma necessitating urgent transplant nephrectomy.

Arteriovenous fistulae have also been reported following percutaneous biopsy. Most common are peripheral arteriovenous fistulae, which remain small and asymptomatic and which may spontaneously regress (20). Management is expectant for a small, asymptomatic peripheral arteriovenous fistula. Central hilar fistulae are usually larger, present with a continuous high-pitched bruit, and are associated with evidence of renal dysfunction, hypertension, hemolytic anemia, and, occasionally, heart failure (20–22). Larger, symptomatic fistulae may be treated by ligation, embolization, or nephrectomy (20,23,24).

Renal Vein Thrombosis

The overall incidence of venous thrombosis is about 4% (25). Allograft renal vein thrombosis can occur by means of a number of mechanisms. Improper placement of the graft in the iliac fossa may result in kinking or twisting of the venous anastomosis, especially if the renal vein is left too long. Attention to the orientation of the renal vein and the choice of anastomotic site on the iliac vein are important. The details of expert organ procurement should again be emphasized. Allograft renal vein thrombosis may be encountered in association with severe rejection or concomitantly with arterial thrombosis. In these cases the venous thrombosis is a secondary occurrence.

The usual presentation is heralded by sudden pain at the transplant site, accompanied by swelling and tenderness of the graft. Hematuria, markedly decreased urinary output, and proteinuria may be noted. In many of the reported cases, renal vein thrombosis occurred in the presence of extensive iliofemoral venous thrombosis, often months after transplantation (26–29). Paradoxically, the presentation may include hemorrhage from the transplant incision due to secondary venous rupture of the graft (25). Deep venous thrombosis per se has been reported in 9.3% of cyclosporine-treated renal allograft recipients (30). Somewhat surprisingly, the location of the thrombosis was not influenced by the location of the transplanted kidney.

There are very few successful outcomes when renal vein thrombosis occurs in the early post-transplant period (25). Therefore, prevention is of paramount importance. However, as in arterial thrombosis, prompt recognition and immediate operative intervention are essential for graft salvage.

Transplant Renal Artery Stenosis

Transplant renal artery stenosis is a well-characterized late complication of renal transplantation, generally presenting with hypertension and a variable degree of allograft dysfunction. The long-term effects of uncontrolled hypertension are significant for both allograft and patient. Hence, the differentiation of transplant renal artery stenosis from other causes of post-transplant hypertension is important.

Incidence and Etiology

The etiology of transplant renal artery stenosis is multifactorial. Faulty surgical technique, including injury to the intima of the renal artery during organ procurement, perfusion, or implantation, may lead to anastomotic or postanastomotic stenosis. Kinking, angulation, and torsion of the artery have been proposed as contributing factors. Chronic rejection may generate a so-called immunologic stenosis. Progressive atherosclerotic vascular disease has been noted in recipients of renal allografts and may involve the vessels directly supplying the kidney or result in atheroemboli from the aortoiliac system. Hemodynamic turbulence has been suggested as a possible etiologic factor in end-to-side anastomoses (31,32), but a similar incidence of renal artery stenosis in end-to-end and end-to-side anastomoses (33) refutes this hypothesis. Because many renal transplant patients are hypertensive at baseline and are not studied completely, the true incidence of transplant renal artery stenosis is unknown. The reported incidence ranges from 1.5% to as high as 23% in a study of 100 patients studied with routine post-transplant arteriography (34). Most surgical series report an incidence of 4% to 8% (13,34–40).

Diagnosis

Clinically important hypertension related to transplant renal artery stenosis may become manifest from several weeks to several years after transplant, but most present within 6 to 8 months. New onset of hypertension or exacerbation of preexisting hypertension suggests the diagnosis. Because many patients treated with calcineurin inhibitors experience some degree of hypertension, the pattern of blood pressure elevation in individual patients must be assessed carefully. A bruit may often be heard over the graft. Renal dysfunction may be noted but is often a late sign or an indication that rejection is playing a role. The administration of angiotensin-converting enzyme inhibitors has been associated with severe, usually reversible renal dysfunction in the presence of transplant renal artery stenosis (41,42).

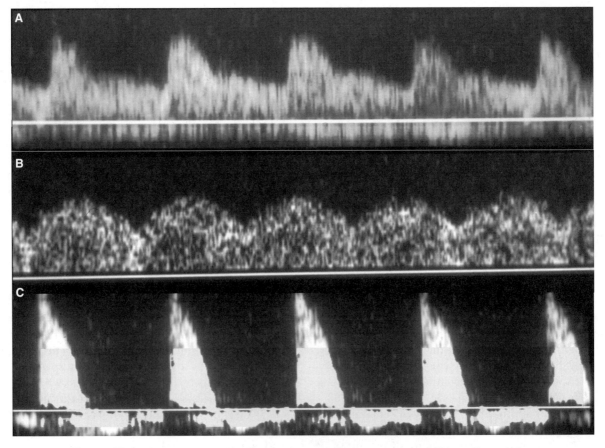

Figure 45-1   A: Normal Doppler ultrasound tracing from a transplanted kidney; **B:** transplant renal artery stenosis showing a tardus waveform; **C:** Doppler ultrasound appearance of reversed diastolic flow associated with allograft rejection or venous obstruction.

Screening of patients suspected of having transplant renal artery stenosis can be accomplished by Doppler ultrasonography (43). In experienced hands this noninvasive modality is highly accurate in determining the presence or absence of transplant renal artery stenosis and can differentiate this entity from other causes of post-transplant allograft dysfunction (Fig. 45-1). Many centers confirm the diagnosis by magnetic resonance angiography (MRA). The MRA is noninvasive and uses a nonnephrotoxic dye load

but is generally lower resolution than a conventional angiogram. The diagnosis of transplant renal artery stenosis should be confirmed by a selective biplane angiographic study to delineate the anatomy and the location, characteristics, and severity of the responsible lesion. Although conventional arteriography using the Seldinger approach has been the standard, recent reports indicate that digital subtraction angiography provides a less invasive alternative in many cases (44). Figure 45-2A is an MRA and Figure 45-2B

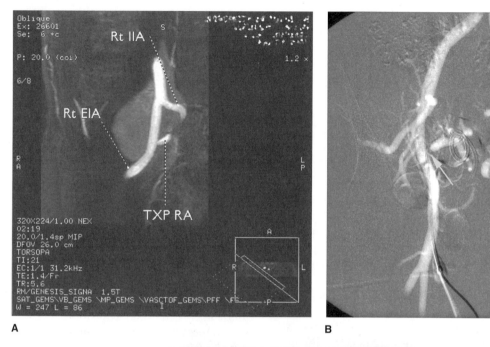

A

B

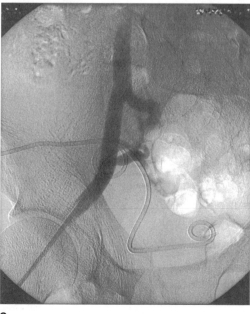

C

Figure 45-2 A: Magnetic resonance angiogram demonstrating a critical stenosis at the anastomosis between the transplant renal artery and the recipient external iliac artery; **B:** conventional digital subtraction angiogram demonstrating the anastomotic stenosis (*arrow*); **C:** the lesion following transluminal balloon angioplasty with resolution of the pressure gradient across the anastomosis (22 mm Hg to 8 mm Hg).

is a conventional angiogram (digital subtraction technique) that shows a tight stenosis at the renal artery anastomosis. The patient had developed increasing hypertension and renal dysfunction 20 months after transplant from a living related donor. The lesion was successfully dilated with percutaneous transluminal angioplasty at the time of angiography (Fig. 45-2C).

There are two basic patterns of stenosis in transplant recipients. The first is an anastomotic lesion that may be associated with poor surgical technique, excessive vessel length, or progression of atherosclerosis. The second pattern is postanastomotic narrowing. A short segment of stenosis suggests technical problems such as injury from the tip of a perfusion cannula or extrinsic compression by fibrous bands, whereas a longer segment may be related to rejection, the so-called immunologic stenosis (35).

Treatment

Before the 1980s the treatment of transplant renal artery stenosis consisted primarily of surgical intervention. The transabdominal approach was thought to be safest because of the relative ease of dissection of the involved blood vessels as compared to the extraperitoneal technique. Identification of the ureter is important during the dissection, as it may lie in close proximity to the renal vasculature. Surgical options include autogenous vein patch angioplasty or bypass, endarterectomy, and excision and reanastomosis. Transplant nephrectomy is only rarely indicated. Among several combined series, the overall success rate for operative treatment was 77% (34,35,39,40). Overall mortality was 3.6%, and up to 15% of grafts were lost as a result of surgical intervention. Results are best in patients who have preserved renal function and who do not have evidence of chronic rejection.

Percutaneous transluminal angioplasty has now largely replaced operative intervention as definitive therapy for transplant renal artery stenosis in most cases. Despite occasional complications (45), the majority of studies show a high rate of success as judged by angiographic and hemodynamic improvement, reduction in systemic blood pressure, improvement in renal function, and lower morbidity and mortality when compared to open surgical techniques (33,46–48). In the largest report so far, 76% of 17 patients had a successful angioplasty by both arteriographic and blood pressure criteria (33). No grafts were lost, and there were no deaths. Anastomotic lesions, which uniformly resisted successful angioplasty by one group (49), were present in 58%. Neither end-to-end nor end-to-side anastomoses were disproportionately represented among patients with transplant renal artery stenosis. Importantly, the study addressed the concern that a high recurrence rate might offset the benefits of balloon dilation. Repeat angiographic studies at an average of 61 weeks after angioplasty showed no instances of recurrence. In two cases absence of blood pressure reduction following angiographically successful

angioplasty was associated with changes of chronic rejection. Normalization of blood pressure occurred after transplant nephrectomy in both patients.

EARLY POST-TRANSPLANT RENAL DYSFUNCTION

Oligoanuric renal failure following transplantation is a common occurrence in most renal transplant programs. Its incidence ranges from <10% up to 60% in reported series (19,50–54). Delayed graft function rates of 20% or less are now common after deceased donor renal transplantation (55).

Etiology

Extrinsic Causes

Many factors may be responsible for post-transplant renal dysfunction. These include vascular thrombosis, lower urinary tract obstruction, and hyperacute or accelerated rejection. Meticulous attention to surgical technique during organ procurement and transplantation prevents most cases of acute vascular compromise and urinary obstruction. Modern immunologic crossmatch testing has nearly eliminated hyperacute rejection. The diagnosis and management of these entities are discussed elsewhere.

Intrinsic Causes

Donor factors that may contribute to an increased incidence of post-transplant oligoanuria after deceased donor transplant include hypovolemia secondary to diabetes insipidus, especially when large doses of vasopressin have been administered; hypotension; hypoxemia; high-dose vasoconstrictor therapy; and prolonged warm ischemia time. Skilled donor maintenance is necessary until the time of nephrectomy to minimize the impact of these factors. As mentioned previously, the use of *in situ* aortic perfusion results in virtually no warm ischemia time. In general, longer periods of cold preservation, whether by simple hypothermia or pulsatile perfusion, result in higher rates of post-transplant acute renal failure (56).

In the recipient, long anastomotic time and multiple renal arteries may contribute to delayed function (57). Adequate hydration and the use of osmotic diuretics have been shown to reduce the incidence of acute tubular necrosis in recipients of kidneys from deceased donors (54). More aggressive strategies of hydration using invasive hemodynamic monitoring techniques have been advocated by some (58,59), but these require the use of a pulmonary artery catheter. The surgeons in the author's group frequently use a central venous catheter and hydrate the patient to an intraoperative central venous pressure between 10 and 12 cm H_2O at the time of revascularization of the kidney. Mannitol is given at a dose of 0.5 to 0.75 gm per kg just prior to release of the vascular clamps, and systolic blood pressure is kept at least 100 mm Hg. Additional intravenous fluid is given postoperatively to keep the central venous pressure around 10 cm H_2O, and urine output is replaced volume for volume for the first 12 to 24 hours. Because of the synergistic nephrotoxic effect of calcineurin inhibitors on ischemically damaged kidneys (60), these agents are withheld until diuresis is established and the serum creatinine has fallen by approximately 25%. Until then, patients receive immunosuppression with an antimetabolite such as mycophenolate mofetil, corticosteroids, and, if delayed graft function will be prolonged, administration of an antilymphocyte antibody.

Diagnosis

The approach to the patient who exhibits intrinsic renal dysfunction immediately following transplantation should focus on rapid identification of correctable underlying causes to reduce the chances of ultimate graft loss. The diagnosis of preservation-associated acute tubular necrosis is one of exclusion.

Urinary Drainage

The first priority should be the assurance of a freely draining urinary catheter. Blood clots in the bladder or in the catheter can frequently be removed by gentle irrigation with sterile saline solution. When doubt exists about the patency of the urinary catheter, there should be no hesitation about replacing it. Ultrasonography should be obtained if there is any suspicion of ureteral obstruction or leak.

Hydration

Inadequate hydration or failure to maintain normovolemia after an initial diuresis may precipitate acute renal failure in the postoperative period. Central venous pressure measured in the recovery room is often lower than that obtained during the operative procedure, and immediate restoration of hydrational status may result in reinstitution of urine flow.

Perfusion

Failure of the previously mentioned strategies to generate urinary output demands investigation of the adequacy of allograft perfusion. The diagnostic modality of choice is ultrasonography with Doppler interrogation of the renal vessels and determination of the resistive index (61). Radionuclide scanning with examination of time-activity curves can demonstrate perfusion abnormalities and identify failure of excretory function compatible with acute tubular necrosis (22,62). In occasional cases such studies may suggest urinary extravasation or obstruction.

Rejection

During the course of post-transplant acute tubular necrosis, it is challenging to identify concomitant allograft rejection. Therefore, percutaneous biopsy is indicated at 7 to 10 day intervals. In this way histologic evidence of tubular regeneration can be seen and occult rejection can be diagnosed and appropriately treated, as previously reported (53).

Treatment

The management of post-transplant acute tubular necrosis is primarily supportive. Dialysis therapy is continued as necessary. If oliguria is established, fluid administration should be restricted to measured losses plus 500 mL per day. Protein and potassium restrictions may be necessary until allograft function improves.

The underlying factors leading to acute tubular necrosis may be more important prognostically than the renal dysfunction itself. Overall, the incidence of acute tubular necrosis appears to be lower among kidneys preserved by pulsatile perfusion than among those preserved with simple hypothermia (53,63). Among kidneys preserved by pulsatile perfusion, however, a higher incidence of acute tubular necrosis was noted if the final pump systolic pressure was >50 mm Hg, and acute tubular necrosis in this setting was associated with poorer graft survival (51). Graft survival rates are significantly lower if early dysfunction occurs (50,51,53,64).

UROLOGIC COMPLICATIONS

In comparison to immunologic barriers, the apparent simplicity of the renal transplant operation may at times lull the operating surgeon into a sense of complacency regarding this procedure. It is particularly frustrating, however, to lose a kidney for technical reasons in the absence of rejection. Fortunately, this is a relatively rare occurrence. Urologic complications account for a large percentage of the technical complications that are encountered in renal transplantation. The reported incidence ranges from 0.9% (65) to 29.6% (66).

Ureteral Obstruction

Incidence

Obstruction of the transplant ureter is a rare complication of renal transplantation. Mundy et al. (67), in a series of 1,000 renal transplants, noted ureteral obstruction to occur in 7.5%. Laughlin et al. (68), in a series of 718 patients, reported an incidence of 3.2%, and Santiago-Delpin et al. (69) reported an incidence of 5.4% in 111 patients. In a series of 808 patients undergoing external ureteroneocystostomy by the Lich technique, ureteral stenosis was noted in 0.7% of patients (70).

Although a rare complication, ureteral obstruction greatly complicates the management of the transplant patient, adds enormously to the expense of the procedure, and may ultimately result in allograft loss or patient death. Mundy et al. (67) reported an overall associated mortality of 19% in patients operated on between 1967 and 1979, with a more recent mortality rate of 12%. The mortality in this context is invariably due to sepsis. A common sequence of events is that poor renal function due to obstruction in the postoperative period is misinterpreted as rejection, with resultant increase in immunosuppression. If urine in the obstructed system is infected, the result is catastrophic. Also, the obstructed ureter often subsequently becomes necrotic; if infected urine is spilled into the peritransplant space, the resultant local infection may be difficult to diagnose and treat. In the past decade the use of ultrasonography to diagnose obstruction and localized fluid collections has markedly improved the management of the transplant patient with a urologic complication (71–73).

Etiology

A wide variety of operative and postoperative conditions may result in obstruction of the renal transplant ureter. The most common problem encountered is stenosis of the distal ureter (Fig. 45-3A) (67). This problem may be due to surgical error in placement of ureteral sutures, ischemia of the distal ureter, improper closure of the submuscular tunnel, hematoma in the submuscular tunnel, or angulation of the ureterovesical anastomosis. Although it is occasionally comforting to think that edema of the distal ureter could result in reversible distal obstruction, in reality this rarely ever happens. Fibrosis of the distal ureter as a cause of obstruction occurs as a sequela of ischemia, which in turn results from damaged or atherosclerotic blood supply of the ureter or in some cases from rejection. Such a complication would typically be seen many months after transplantation. Lymphocele, of which more will be said later, is a frequent cause of renal transplant ureter obstruction (67). The mechanism of obstruction typically involves angulation of the ureterovesical junction. Peritransplant hematoma may have the same effect, and ureteral blood clots secondary to the trauma of harvesting or reimplantation have also been reported as a cause of early post-transplant obstruction (67). Rarely, the operating surgeon may inadvertently position the ureter over the spermatic cord (74), round ligament (67), or inferior epigastric vessels, resulting in obstruction. Finally, stones in the transplanted ureter (67) and a fungus ball, usually secondary to candidal infection of the urine (75,76), have been reported as rare causes of obstruction.

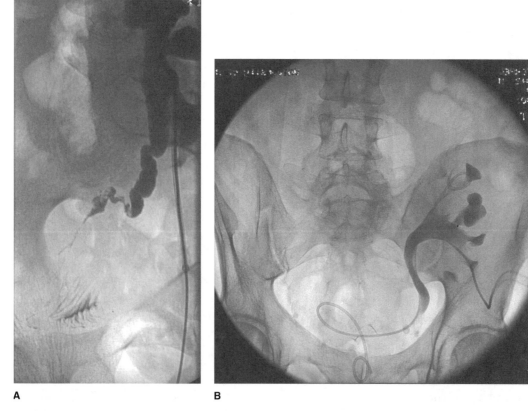

A   B

Figure 45-3   **A:** Percutaneous nephrostogram demonstrating a tight stenosis at the ureteral anastomosis to the bladder; **B:** treatment of the stenosis with a percutaneously placed stent.

Diagnosis

Ultrasonography has completely replaced intravenous pyelography for the initial diagnosis of urologic complications following transplantation because it is accurate, noninvasive, and does not rely on function of the transplant. Routine screening of all transplant patients with ultrasonography has, however, highlighted some pitfalls in interpretation that should be emphasized. First, it is not at all uncommon to diagnose "mild hydronephrosis" in the early post-transplant period in a kidney that is in reality completely unobstructed. The ultrasonographic appearance of dilated calyces and renal pelvis probably results from the profound diuresis occurring after transplantation. Further evaluation is warranted only if this finding persists or worsens in a setting of unsatisfactory renal function. A dynamic renal scan (77) (i.e., radionuclide scan performed before and after furosemide challenge) may be helpful at this point. If not, antegrade pyelography with pressure flow measurements ["Whitaker test" (78)] is a valuable adjunct for the diagnosis of obstruction. Constant intraureteral pressure in the presence of flow of at least 10 mL per minute indicates satisfactory ureteral patency. A second pitfall is that an obstructed ureter occasionally does not produce obvious hydronephrosis by ultrasonographic examination. In these cases the obstruction is high, at the ureteropelvic junction, or prolonged obstruction has resulted in poor function with small volumes of urine. In this difficult situation obstruction usually becomes a diagnosis by exclusion. In the absence of dilated calyces, antegrade pyelography is difficult and operative exploration may be required.

Treatment

Treatment of the obstructed renal transplant ureter may be simple or complex, depending on the cause and timing of the obstruction. However, improvements in interventional genitourinary radiology have made this complication less emergent. Patients most frequently have a percutaneous nephrostomy tube placed at the time of diagnosis and, therefore, are not likely to be septic or uremic if surgery is necessary (Fig. 45-3B). Under these conditions the operating surgeon is more able to evaluate the problem carefully, map out a strategy, and proceed with all available resources.

Under the simplest of circumstances the obstruction is at the level of the distal ureter. A nonoperative technique involves percutaneous antegrade dilatation of the ureteral stricture (79). Under some circumstances, particularly when the stricture occurs late in the transplant course, this technique would seem to hold merit. Standard operative repair involves creation of a new ureterovesical anastomosis, usually with mobilization and resection of the involved ureter. If the operative findings are such that sufficient viable transplant ureter is not available to reach the bladder, the bladder can be extensively mobilized and fixed to the psoas muscle to provide additional length, or a Boari flap of bladder can be advanced to replace the resected ureteral segment. A difficult but common situation may arise when a patient's bladder is found to be contracted, nonpliable, and trabeculated. In this circumstance it may be preferable to mobilize and remove the ipsilateral kidney and anastomose the remaining transplant ureter or renal pelvis to native ureter.

Extensive local drainage, nephrostomy, and urinary catheter drainage are usually indicated after reoperation. Stenting the anastomosis with a soft double-J internal stent is also helpful in many of these circumstances. Despite these measures, further morbidity following treatment of the obstruction is frequent. In one large series (67), 49% of patients developed a further urologic complication (usually urinary fistula) after operative repair of a primary urologic complication. This alarming statistic underscores the importance of meticulous technique in the performance of the procurement and the primary renal transplant operation.

Urinary Extravasation

The first few postoperative weeks after renal transplantation are usually characterized by rapid reduction in the serum creatinine and rapid elevation of the patient's mood. Sometimes, however, the large urine volume of the first few postoperative days falls off dramatically. The patient reports clear drainage from the operative site; fever and systemic sepsis may supervene. This clinical situation, which is suggestive of a urinary leak, requires rapid and accurate diagnosis and effective treatment if loss of the allograft and infectious morbidity are to be avoided. Although it depends greatly on the type of immunosuppressive protocol being used and the historic era from which the report comes, the associated patient mortality for this complication has been as high as 32% (67).

Incidence

Urinary extravasation may occur anywhere from the bladder to the renal transplant calyx. The incidence of extravasation following transplant has varied from 0.1% (69) to 8.5% (68). The most common site is the distal ureter. Predisposing factors relate primarily to the blood supply at this site and thus involve the degree of trauma at the time of procurement, operative handling of the ureter at the time of the transplant procedure, the presence of multiple renal arteries, and possibly the intensity of the rejection process.

Diagnosis

Accurate diagnosis is important because another renal transplant complication, lymphocele, also may be manifested by reduced urine output and a peritransplant fluid collection. A peritransplant fluid collection observed on ultrasonography should be aspirated if it is large (>5 cm in diameter) and accessible (Fig. 45-4). Patients should be placed on broad-spectrum antibiotics prior to this procedure. The fluid specimen is sent for a creatinine determination. If a sufficient concentration gradient exists between fluid and serum creatinine, the diagnosis of urinary leak is established and further diagnostic steps are undertaken to define the extent of the problem. If the fluid creatinine is identical to that of serum, it can be assumed that the fluid is lymph rather than urine. Confirmatory cell counts and differential analysis may be done. An exception may occur if the degree of renal function is such that the kidney makes urine but does not clear creatinine, in which case this differentiation is more difficult. If urinary extravasation is suspected, a cystogram is obtained. This may localize the leak to the bladder or ureterovesical anastomosis, or if there is reflux into the ureter, a higher leak may be identified. If this test is not helpful, antegrade pyelography is required. Flexible fiberoptic cystoscopy with retrograde cannulation of the ureter is usually not an attractive option, because most cases of urinary leak occur in the early post-transplant period, when distension of the bladder with a new suture line would not be advisable. Also, when the ureteroneocytostomy is performed to the dome of the bladder, as in the popular Lich technique, it is technically difficult to cannulate the ureteral orifice even if it can be identified.

One might ask why any further imaging is necessary once the diagnosis of urinary extravasation has been made, because exploration is usually undertaken under these circumstances. Preoperative percutaneous placement of the nephrostomy tube has been found to be easier, more accurate, and less traumatic than intraoperative placement. Also, precise information about the site of the leak may facilitate better preoperative counseling about the risks of the procedure and permits a smaller, more precise operative exposure. In an increasing proportion of cases nonoperative management may be feasible. Further, it occasionally happens that urine appears in the operative site at the time of surgery but no source can be identified. Preoperative imaging prevents this frustrating situation.

Ureteral Leak

The ureter usually leaks because it is ischemic. The relatively tenuous blood supply of the distal ureter is vulnerable to operative trauma at the time of procurement and at reimplantation. Also, the ureter may become ischemic if a lower polar artery has been inadvertently tied off or improperly anastomosed to the recipient blood vessels. Whether or not acute rejection commonly results in ureteral ischemia is not established, but it seems a possibility, because reduction in blood flow to the transplant in general is well documented during acute rejection, and the delicate nature of the ureteral blood supply makes it particularly vulnerable.

Most modest leaks are handled nonoperatively using percutaneous nephrostomy and subsequent advancement across the anastomosis into the bladder. Any significant

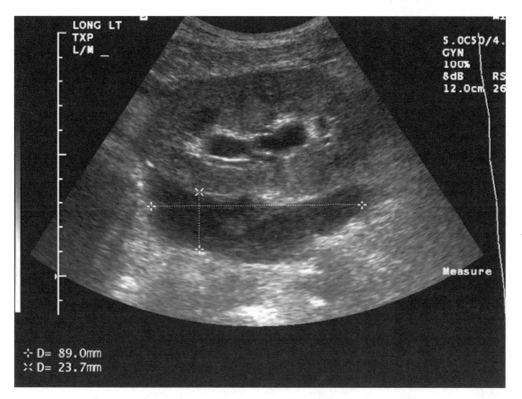

Figure 45-4 Ultrasound image of a urinoma inferior to the renal allograft.

peritransplant urinoma should be separately drained. If ischemia of the ureter has resulted in distal tissue loss and a large leak, operative repair is necessary. Resection of the involved segment with reanastomosis or use of a Boari flap to reestablish urinary continuity is usually performed. Cutaneous ureterostomy might theoretically be used, but in the context of renal transplantation this procedure is not usually a satisfactory long-term solution to the problem of ureteral necrosis. If a generalized ureteral slough has occurred, use of the ipsilateral native ureter is required.

Bladder Leak

The incidence of leakage from the urinary bladder is 0% to 4% (68,69). The opportunity for leakage is higher when the Ledbetter-Politano ureterovesical anastomosis is employed because this procedure involves a large cystotomy not required for the external ureteroneocytostomy. Our group has reported a very low rate of ureterovesical leak in >800 of the latter procedures (70). Another factor of importance is the prior condition of the recipient bladder. If there have been multiple previous operative procedures, the risk of leakage is higher.

Adequate bladder drainage with a urinary catheter is important in preventing postoperative bladder leaks because the profound diuresis that often follows transplantation may put enormous pressure on the new suture line if the bladder cannot empty properly. To avoid this problem, most centers regularly irrigate the catheter with sterile saline solution in the immediate postoperative period. However, prolonged catheter drainage is not necessary and predisposes to bacterial colonization of the bladder and later urethral stricture (80,81). It is necessary in the preoperative evaluation of the transplant recipient to establish that prostatic hypertrophy or urethral stricture does not impair bladder emptying because these factors might also contribute to early postoperative suture line dehiscence.

Most bladder leaks can be repaired primarily or treated conservatively with local drains and prolonged urinary catheterization.

Pelvicalyceal Leak

Urinary extravasation at the calyx is rare and usually the result of trauma to or occlusion of subsegmental arteries. Because there is no effective collateral arterial circulation in the kidney, the result is either loss of renal parenchyma with subsequent fibrosis or necrosis and urinary extravasation. There is a strong association between this complication and the presence of multiple renal arteries in the donor kidney. Calyceal leaks tend to occur later than ureteral or bladder leaks and thus may be harder to diagnose and treat effectively. In one report, seven of eight patients with this complication ultimately lost the transplant and three died (82). Treatment is prolonged nephrostomy tube drainage through the infarct into the involved calyx if possible.

Nephrectomy may be required if infected extravasated urine cannot be adequately drained. Leakage from the renal pelvis is encountered very rarely, probably owing to its rich capillary blood supply. This complication may be associated with operative trauma or, rarely, as a spontaneous complication after transplantation (83). Spontaneous rupture of the renal pelvis presented from 5 to 46 days after transplantation and was not associated with mechanical obstruction. The cause of this complication was not obvious in any case but could have been related to a very brisk diuresis with a functional ureteropelvic obstruction. One case was successfully treated with prolonged nephrostomy drainage, but transplant nephrectomy was required in three cases.

LYMPHOCELE

Incidence

A lymphocele is an extralymphatic collection of lymphatic fluid. Owing to the pelvic location of the renal transplant, an area rich in lymphatics, lymphocele is a common complication of renal transplantation. It is not clear what percentage of peritransplant fluid accumulations develop into clinically significant lymphoceles requiring operative intervention. Most transplant surgeons prefer to follow asymptomatic collections with frequent ultrasonographic examinations until increasing size or deterioration of renal function mandates operative intervention. Clinically oriented series (84–88) have reported this complication to occur in 0% to 22% of patients. A lymphocele typically presents later in the postoperative period than urinary extravasation does. The most common clinical presentation is abdominal mass (72%), ipsilateral leg edema (58%), hypertension (26%), clear drainage from the wound (19%), fever (19%), and decreasing urine output (15%) (89). The patient occasionally presents with rapid progression to anuria (90). The origin of the lymphatic accumulation is primarily from recipient lymphatics severed at the time of surgery, a conclusion drawn by lymphoradiographic studies involving injection of radionuclide into the ipsilateral leg of patients with this condition (91). However, a universal clinical observation is that lymphoceles either present or greatly enlarge during a rejection episode, suggesting that renal hilar lymphatics of the allograft contribute lymph to the lymphocele as well (92).

Diagnosis

The diagnosis of lymphocele has been greatly facilitated by the widespread use of diagnostic ultrasonography. Lymphoceles typically demonstrate fine linear septations not seen with urinoma or abscess (Fig. 45-5). Careful aspiration under sterile conditions with antibiotic coverage is routinely performed to establish the diagnosis.

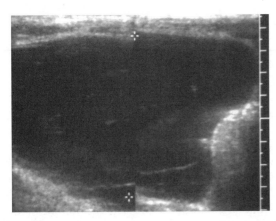

Figure 45-5 High magnification ultrasound image of a lymphocele that demonstrates fine linear septations not typically seen in ultrasound imaging of urinoma or abscess.

Treatment

The treatment of lymphocele may be conservative at first, consisting of complete aspiration under ultrasonographic guidance. Occasionally, this therapy is all that is required. Aspiration should not be repeated as infection may result. External drainage is useless and dangerous because the drained fluid always becomes infected (93). The mean duration from external drainage to complete cessation of drainage was 4.5 weeks. Internal drainage is the treatment of choice. A peritoneal "window" from the lymphocele cavity into the peritoneum is created (laparoscopically in most cases) so that peritransplant lymph has free egress into, and can be reabsorbed by, the peritoneal membrane. Care should be taken to make the window large enough so that bowel cannot become incarcerated in it. Also, the transplant ureter frequently is incorporated into the medial (operated) wall of the lymphocele, and ureteral injury during this procedure has been reported (88).

Certain technical maneuvers at the original transplant procedure seem helpful in preventing lymphoceles. First, most of the large lymphatics coursing from the leg follow the external iliac artery and vein. These can be easily moved out of harm's way. If division is necessary, multiple fine surgical ties are far preferable to electrocautery because lymphatics do not coagulate as do blood vessels. Meticulous ligation of lymphatics near the transplant hilum also may be effective in decreasing lymph leakage from this source.

SUPERFICIAL WOUND INFECTION

Infection of the superficial transplant wound is surprisingly uncommon, given the multitude of predisposing factors in this patient group. When the urine is sterile preoperatively, the transplant wound is considered a clean-contaminated wound. Belzer et al. (94) reported an infection rate of <1%. When infection does occur, *Staphylococcus aureus* is the most common organism on culture.

Prevention of superficial wound infection relies on meticulous operative technique and administration of prophylactic antibiotics. Tissue should be handled gently, and care should be taken to avoid hematoma in the subcutaneous tissue. Copious irrigation of the wound with warm saline before closure of the skin is also beneficial. Drains should be avoided.

Diagnosis of superficial wound infection obligates the surgeon to investigate the possibility that a subfascial infection exists as well.

SUBFASCIAL ABSCESS

Subfascial peritransplant infection is an unusual but potentially grave complication of renal transplantation, with a reported mortality in excess of 20% (65). The clinical presentation with fever and oliguria mimics rejection, and catastrophic results are certain if an underlying abscess is treated with increased immunosuppression. Aggressive and thorough evaluations of patients with a suggestive history are mandatory.

Peritransplant abscess has been reported to be associated with peritransplant hematoma (95–100), post-transplant urinary fistula (97), the presence of infected urine at the time of transplantation (101), and the use of an ileal conduit (102,103) for urinary diversion. Other factors predisposing to abscess formation are more general and include the use of immunosuppressive drugs, poor nutritional status of the transplant recipient, and the location of the transplant incision in the groin area. The diagnosis of this complication is made best by the use of ultrasonography-guided needle aspiration of fluid collections in the appropriate clinical context. The ultrasonographic appearance of the abscess itself is not particularly characteristic, but particulate debris is occasionally noted (73) and multiple linear septations such as would be seen in a lymphocele are not present.

Immediate transplant nephrectomy with wide wound drainage is required if sepsis is extensive, but operative drainage alone is usually satisfactory if the infection is localized, removed from the arterial anastomosis. Immunosuppression can generally be drastically reduced in the setting of sepsis without immediate loss of the allograft. Long-term treatment with broad-spectrum antibiotics is indicated. The offending organisms are Gram-positive in one-half of cases (101). Multiple organisms may be cultured from as many as 30%. The most common organisms encountered were coagulase-positive *S. aureus* and *Escherichia coli.*

Measures to avoid this complication should be undertaken at several levels. Transplant donors with generalized sepsis should be avoided, as well as those donors with active urinary tract infections. However, bacteriuria in the absence of white blood cells is not sufficiently worrisome to discount a donor. Donors and recipients should receive preoperative antibiotics, and serious attempts at eradicating recipient urinary tract infection should be made preoperatively, either with long-term antibiotics or pretransplant native nephrectomy if the source of infection is the kidney or a staghorn calculus. The bladder should be irrigated with povidone-iodine or antibiotic solution just prior to opening the bladder intraoperatively, and the transplant wound should be thoroughly irrigated on completion of all anastomoses. In many cases the organism isolated from the peritransplant infection is identical to the organism cultured preoperatively from the recipient urine (101). The donor artery and vein may be cultured for the presence of infective organisms, and long-term antibiotics should be administered if the results are positive.

An unusual presentation of peritransplant abscess is rupture of the infected fluid into the peritoneal cavity with the development of peritonitis (101,104). This development has an associated mortality of 80% (104).

ALLOGRAFT FRACTURE

Fracture of the renal allograft is rare. The fracture typically occurs late in the course of an episode of acute rejection when the patient has returned to dialysis (105). The patient presents with pain at the site of the transplant and with hypotension. Operative findings vary, but in most reported series the fracture is linear, shallow, and located on the convex surface of the kidney (105,106).

The incidence of allograft fracture ranges from 0.14% (107) to 8.5% (105), with the true figure likely very low. This complication is related to severe swelling of the kidney during acute rejection, but it has been suggested that anticoagulation during hemodialysis may contribute to the bleeding as well (105). It is interesting that fracture of the native kidney has been reported in conditions such as hydronephrosis (108) and pregnancy (109) and in patients receiving anticoagulant therapy (110), indicating that the mechanisms involved are not solely related to immunologic aspects of the rejection process.

Whether or not the transplant can be saved following fracture depends on the clinical circumstances and operative findings. If the fractured area is shallow, there may be some merit in repairing the kidney with pledgeted sutures, as has been reported (111). However, in most circumstances rejection is advanced at the time of rupture and transplant nephrectomy is the wisest alternative, in conjunction with careful and thorough evacuation of the resultant peritransplant hematoma.

SPONTANEOUS DECAPSULATION

A rare but fascinating complication of renal transplantation is spontaneous decapsulation with excessive fluid leakage (112–115). The cause of this complication is not understood. The patient presents with an increasingly large peritransplant fluid collection. At operation the allograft is swollen and decapsulated, with clear fluid leaking from the parenchyma.

A variety of innovative methods has been devised to correct this problem, including painting the capsule with butyl cyanoacrylate, applying lyophilized human dura (115), or diverting the fluid into the peritoneal cavity (113). In five reported cases, four allografts were removed, with the only salvage involving marsupialization of the transplant site into the peritoneal cavity (113). However, intraperitoneal drainage may result in intractable ascites (112,114). Successful treatment of the kidney surface with infrared contact coagulation was recently reported (115).

HYPERCALCEMIA

Virtually all patients with chronic renal failure have secondary hyperparathyroidism as the result of inability to produce 1,25-di-hydroxyvitamin D, renal phosphate retention, and extracellular complexing of circulating calcium. After successful renal transplantation, early postoperative hypercalcemia is common and a significant percentage of patients develop persistent hypercalcemia as well. When the hypercalcemia is resistant to phosphate repletion, this condition has been referred to as tertiary post-transplant hyperparathyroidism, suggesting that the hypertrophic parathyroid glands have become autonomous. Earlier it was assumed that autonomy of parathyroid function was due to the development of an adenoma in the hyperplastic gland. More recent understanding of this situation indicates that true adenomatous degeneration is rare (116) but that hyperplasia may persist for prolonged periods of time even with a well-functioning transplant.

Early post-transplant hypercalcemia occurs in up to 28.6% of renal transplant recipients (117). The most important etiologic factor appears to be slow resolution of hyperactive parathyroid function in combination with increased absorption of calcium as the result of restored 1,25-dihydroxyvitamin D activity (118). In addition, renal transplant recipients are commonly phosphate depleted in the postoperative period, a factor that contributes to hypercalcemia. Finally, aggressive tapering of corticosteroid doses may precipitate hypercalcemia (119). In the past, emergent parathyroidectomy was advocated as treatment for this problem, but current practice is to treat conservatively with aggressive diuresis and elimination of phosphate-binding antacids.

In most cases excess parathyroid function subsides enough in the post-transplant period to avoid long-term hypercalcemia. Some patients do develop long-term hypercalcemia after failure of the hypertrophic glands to involute (117). This condition may persist and, depending on the severity of the hypercalcemia, may adversely influence transplant function (118). Subtotal parathyroidectomy should be reserved for those patients who have serum calcium in excess of 12.5 mg per dL and no other explanation for deterioration in renal allograft function (120).

REFERENCES

1. Garcia-Rinaldi R, Lefrak EA, Defore WW, et al. In situ preservation of cadaver kidneys for transplantation. *Ann Surg* 1975;182:576.
2. Rosenthal JT, Shaw BW Jr, Hardesty RL, et al. Principles of multiple organ procurement from cadaver donors. *Ann Surg* 1983;198:617.
3. Kawamoto S, Montgomery RA, Lawler LP, et al. Multidetector CT angiography for preoperative evaluation of living laparoscopic kidney donors. *Am J Roentgenol* 2003;180:1633–1638.
4. Harrison LH Jr, Flye MW, Seigler HF. Incidence of anatomical variants in renal vasculature in the presence of normal renal function. *Ann Surg* 1978;188:83.
5. Ratner LE, Kavoussi LR, Schulam PG, et al. Comparison of laparoscopic live donor nephrectomy versus the standard open approach. *Transplant Proc* 1997;29:138.
6. Flowers JL, Jacobs S, Cho E, et al. Comparison of open and live donor nephrectomy. *Ann Surg* 1997;226:483.
7. Wolf JS Jr, Marcovich R, Merion RM, et al. Prospective, case-matched comparison of hand-assisted laparoscopic and open surgical live donor nephrectomy. *J Urol* 2000;163:1650–1653.
8. Crosnier J. Extrarenal complications. In: Hamburger J, Crosnier J, Bach J-F, et al, eds. *Renal transplantation theory and practice.* Baltimore, MD: Williams & Wilkins; 1981.
9. Goldman MH, Tilney N, Vineyard GC, et al. A 20-year survey of arterial complications of renal transplantation. *Surg Gynecol Obstet* 1975;141:758.
10. Lee HM, Mendez-Picon G, Pierce JC, et al. Renal artery occlusion in transplant recipients. *Am Surg* 1977;43:186.
11. Nicholson JD, Burleson RL, Bredenberg CE. Survival of a renal allograft after correction of a nearly total acute renal artery occlusion. *Transplantation* 1978;26:131.
12. Swanson DA, Sullivan MJ. Thromboendarterectomy for anuria 4 1/2 years post-renal transplant: a case report. *J Urol* 1976;116:799.
13. Palleschi J, Novick AC, Braun WE, et al. Vascular complications of renal transplantation. *Urology* 1980;16:61.
14. Robson AJ, Evans DB, Calne RY. Secondary hemorrhage from the arterial anastomosis in renal allografts. *Br J Surg* 1972;59:890.
15. Vegeto A, Berardinelli L, Storelli G, et al. Spontaneous rupture of the renal artery in kidney transplantation. *Transplant Proc* 1979;11:1276.
16. Gorey TF, Bulkley GB, Spees EK Jr, et al. Iliac artery ligation. The relative paucity of ischemic sequelae in renal transplant patients. *Ann Surg* 1979;190:753.
17. Pfundstein J, Roghmann MC, Schwalbe RS, et al. A randomized trial of surgical antimicrobial prophylaxis with and without vancomycin in organ transplant patients. *Clin Transplant* 1999;13:245–252.
18. Matas AJ, Sibley R, Mauer M, et al. The value of needle renal allograft biopsy. I. A retrospective study of biopsies performed during putative rejection episodes. *Ann Surg* 1983;197:226.
19. Rohr MS. Renal allograft acute tubular necrosis. II. A light and electron microscopic study of biopsies taken at procurement and after revascularization. *Ann Surg* 1983;197:663.
20. Debruyne FMJ, Koene RAP, Moonen WA, et al. Intrarenal arteriovenous fistula following renal allograft biopsy. *Eur Urol* 1978;4:435.
21. Bennett WM, Strong D, Rosch J. Arteriovenous fistula complicating renal transplantation. *Urology* 1976;8:254.
22. Mandel SR, Mattern WD, Staab E, et al. Use of radionuclide imaging in the early diagnosis and treatment of renal allograft rejection. *Ann Surg* 1975;18(1):596.
23. Baquero A, Morris MC, Cope C, et al. Selective embolization of vascular complications following renal biopsy of the transplant kidney. *Transplant Proc* 1985;17:1751.
24. Navani S, Athanasoulis CA, Monaco AP, et al. Renal homotransplantation: spectrum of angiographic findings of the kidney. *Am J Radiol* 1971;113:433.
25. Merion RM, Calne RY. Allograft renal vein thrombosis. *Transplant Proc* 1985;17:1746.
26. Arruda JA, Gutierrez LF, Jonasson O, et al. Renal-vein thrombosis in kidney allografts. *Lancet* 1973;2:585.
27. Clarke SD, Kennedy JA, Hewitt JC, et al. Successful removal of thrombus from renal vein after renal transplantation. *Br Med J* 1970;1:154.
28. Fletcher EW, Lecky JW, Gonick HC. Selective phlebography of transplanted kidneys. *Clin Radiol* 1970;2(1):144.
29. Smellie WA, Vinik M, Freed TA, et al. Pertrochanteric venography in the study of human renal transplant recipients. *Surg Gynecol Obstet* 1968;126:777.
30. Brunkwall J, Bergqvist D, Bergentz S-E, et al. Postoperative deep venous thrombosis after renal transplantation. Effects of cyclosporine. *Transplantation* 1987;43:647.
31. Morris PJ, Uadav RVS, Kincaid-Smith P, et al. Renal artery stenosis in renal transplantation. *Med J Aust* 1971;29:1255.
32. Oakes DD, Spees EK, McAllister HA, et al. Arterial injury during perfusion preservation: a possible cause of post-transplantation renal artery stenosis. *Surgery* 1981;89:210.
33. Grossman RA, Dafoe DC, Shoenfeld RB, et al. Percutaneous transluminal angioplasty treatment of renal transplant artery stenosis. *Transplantation* 1982;34:339.
34. Lacombe M. Arterial stenosis complicating renal allotransplantation in man: a study of 38 cases. *Ann Surg* 1975;181:283.
35. Dickerman RM, Peters PC, Hull AR, et al. Surgical correction of posttransplant renovascular hypertension. *Ann Surg* 1980;192:639.
36. Kauffman HM, Sampson D, Fos PS, et al. Prevention of transplant renal artery stenosis. *Surgery* 1977;8(1):161.
37. Klarskov P, Brendstrup L, Krarup T, et al. Renovascular hypertension after renal transplantation. *Scand J Urol Nephrol* 1979;13:291.
38. Lacombe M. Correction of renal transplant artery stenosis by transposing iliac arteries. *Urology* 1979;13:21.
39. Lindsey ES, Garbus SB, Golladay ES, et al. Hypertension due to renal artery stenosis in transplanted kidneys. *Ann Surg* 1975;181:604.
40. Tilney NL, Rocha A, Strom TB, et al. Renal artery stenosis in transplant patients. *Ann Surg* 1984;199:454.
41. VanSon WJ, VanderSlikke LB, Hoorntje SJ. Captopril-induced deterioration of graft function in patients with a transplant renal artery stenosis. *Proc Eur Dial Transplant Assoc* 1983;20:325.
42. VanderWoude FJ, VanSon WJ, Tegess AM, et al. Effect of captopril on blood pressure and renal function in patients with transplant renal artery stenosis. *Nephron* 1985;39:184.
43. Rath M, Castro L, Schuler M, et al. Digital subtraction angiography in the diagnosis of arterial complications after renal transplantation. *Eur J Radiol* 1984;4:34.
44. Reinitz ER, Goldman MH, Sais J, et al. Evaluation of transplant renal artery blood flow by Doppler sound-spectrum analysis. *Arch Surg* 1983;118:415.
45. Majeskij A, Munda R. Hazard of percutaneous transluminal dilation in renal transplant arterial stenosis. *Arch Surg* 1981;116:1225.
46. Etheredge SB, Mahony JF, Savdie E. Treatment of renal transplant artery stenosis by percutaneous transluminal dilatation. *Clin Nephrol* 1982;17:217.
47. Gerlock AJ Jr, MacDonell RC Jr, Smith CW, et al. Renal transplant arterial stenosis: percutaneous transluminal angioplasty. *Am J Roentgenol* 1983;140:325.
48. Zajko AB, McLean GK, Grossman RA. Percutaneous transluminal angioplasty and fibrinolytic therapy for renal allograft arterial stenosis and thrombosis. *Transplantation* 1982;33:447.
49. Chandrasoma P, Aberle AM. Anastomotic line renal artery stenosis after transplantation. *J Urol* 1986;135:1159.
50. Anderson GB, Sicard GA, Etheredge EE. Delayed primary renal function and cadaver renal allograft results. *Surg Gynecol Obstet* 1979;149:697.
51. McDonald JC, Vaughn W, Filo RS, et al. Cadaver donor renal transplantation by centers of the Southeastern Organ Procurement Foundation. *Ann Surg* 1981;193:1.
52. Mendez-Picon G, Posner MP, McGeorge MB, et al. The effect of delayed function on long-term survival of renal allografts. *Surg Gynecol Obstet* 1985;161:351.
53. Rocher LL, Landis C, Dafoe DC, et al. The importance of prolonged post-transplant dialysis requirement in cyclosporine-treated renal allograft recipients. *Clin Transplant* 1987;1:29.
54. Tiggeler RGWL, Berden JHM, Hoitsma AJ. Prevention of acute tubular necrosis in cadaveric kidney transplantation by the combined use of mannitol and moderate hydration. *Ann Surg* 1985;201:246.

55. Shoskes DA, Shahed AR, Kim S. Delayed graft function. Influence on outcome and strategies for prevention. *Urol Clin North Am* 2001;28:721–732.

56. Hetzel GR, Klein B, Brause M, et al. Risk factors for delayed graft function after renal transplantation and their significance for long-term clinical outcome. *Transplant Int* 2002;15:10–16.

57. Shimshak RR, Hattner RS, Tucker C, et al. Segmental acute tubular necrosis in kidneys with multiple renal arteries transplanted from living-related donors. *J Nucl Med* 1977;18:1074.

58. Luciani J, Frantz PH, Thibault PH, et al. Early anuria prevention in human kidney transplantation. Advantage of fluid load under pulmonary arterial pressure monitoring during surgical period. *Transplantation* 1979;28:308.

59. Carlier M, Squifflet JP, Pirson Y, et al. Maximal hydration during anesthesia increases pulmonary arterial pressures and improves early function of human renal transplants. *Transplantation* 1982;34:201.

60. Provoost AP, Kaptein L, VanAken M. Nephrotoxicity of cyclosporine A in rats with a diminished renal function. *Clin Nephrol* 1986;25:S162.

61. Baxter GM. Ultrasound of renal transplantation. *Clin Radiol* 2001;56:802–818.

62. Diethelm AG, Dubovsky EV, Whelchel JD. Diagnosis of impaired renal function after kidney transplantation using renal scintigraphy, renal plasma flow and urinary excretion of hippurate. *Ann Surg* 1980;191:604.

63. Wight J, Chilcott J, Holmes M, et al. The clinical and cost-effectiveness of pulsatile machine perfusion versus cold storage of kidneys for transplantation retrieved from heart-beating and non-heart-beating donors. *Health Technol Assess* 2003;7:1–94.

64. Geddes CC, Woo YM, Jardine AG. The impact of delayed graft function on the long-term outcome of renal transplantation. *J Nephrol* 2002;15:17–21.

65. Leary FJ, Woods JE, DeWeerd JH. Urologic problems in renal transplantation. *Arch Surg* 1975;110:1124.

66. MacLean LD, MacKinnon KG, Ingliz FG, et al. When should renal allografts be removed? *Arch Surg* 1969;99:269.

67. Mundy MR, Podesta ML, Bewick M, et al. The urological complications of 1000 renal transplants. *Br J Urol* 1981;53:397.

68. Laughlin KR, Tilney NL, Richie JP. Urologic complications in 718 renal transplant patients. *Surgery* 1984;95:297.

69. Santiago-Delpin EA, Baquero A, Gonzalez Z. Low incidence of urologic complications after renal transplantation. *Am J Surg* 1986;151:374.

70. Ohl DA, Konnak JW, Campbell DA Jr, et al. Extravesical ureteroneocystostomy in renal transplantation. *J Urol* 1988;139:499.

71. Koehler PR, Kanenafo HH, Maxwell JC. Ultrasonic "B"scanning in the diagnosis of complications in renal transplant patients. *Radiology* 1976;119:661.

72. Morley P, Barnett E, Bell PRF, et al. Ultrasound in the diagnosis of fluid collections following renal transplantation. *Clin Radiol* 1975;26:199.

73. Silver TM, Campbell DA Jr, Wicks JD, et al. Peritransplant fluid collections: ultrasonic evaluation and clinical significance. *Radiology* 1981;138:145.

74. Karmi SA, Dagher FJ, Ramos E, et al. Spermatic cord: cause of ureteral obstruction in renal allograft recipients. *Urology* 1978;11:380.

75. Ireton RC, Krieger JN, Rudd TG, et al. Percutaneous endoscopic treatment of fungus ball obstruction in a renal allograft. *Transplantation* 1985;39:453.

76. Walzer Y, Bear RA. Ureteral obstruction of renal transplant due to ureteral candidiasis. *Urology* 1983;21:295.

77. MacGregor RJ, Konnak JW, Thrall JH, et al. Diuretic radionuclide urography in the diagnosis of suspected ureteral obstruction following renal transplantation. *J Urol* 1983;129:708.

78. Whitaker RH. Methods of assessing obstruction in dilated ureters. *Br J Urol* 1973;45:15.

79. Lieberman RP, Glass NR, Crummy AB, et al. Non-operative percutaneous management of urinary fistulas and strictures in renal transplantation. *Surg Gynecol Obstet* 1982;155:667.

80. Loening SA, Banowsky LH, Braun WE, et al. Bladder neck contracture and ureteral stricture as complications of renal transplantation. *J Urol* 1975;114:688.

81. Nerstrom B, Brix E, Clausen E, et al. Late urological complications following human kidney transplantation. *Acta Clin Scand Suppl* 1973;433:113.

82. Goldman MN, Burleson RL, Tilney NL. Calyceal-cutaneous fistulae in renal transplant patients. *Ann Surg* 1976;184:679.

83. Kogan BA, Konnak JW, MacGregor RJ, et al. Spontaneous rupture of renal pelvis after renal transplantation. *Urology* 1981;18:456.

84. Braun WE, Banowsky LH, Straffon RA, et al. Lymphoceles associated with renal transplantation. *Am J Med* 1974;57:714.

85. Griffiths AB, Fletcher EW, Morris PJ. Lymphocele after renal transplantation. *Aust N Z J Surg* 1979;49:626.

86. Howard RJ, Simmons RL, Najarian JS. Prevention of lymphoceles following renal transplantation. *Ann Surg* 1977;186:700.

87. Lindstrom BL, Lindfors O, Eklund B, et al. Surgical complications in 500 kidney transplantations. *Proc Eur Dial Transplant Assoc* 1977;14:353.

88. Schwerzer RT, Cho S, Kountz SL. Lymphoceles following renal transplantation. *Arch Surg* 1972;104:42.

89. Brooks JG, Hulbert JC, Patel AS, et al. The diagnosis and treatment of lymphoceles associated with renal transplantation. A report of six cases and a review of the literature. *Br J Urol* 1978;50:307.

90. Diethelm AG. Anuria secondary to perirenal lymphocele: a complication of renal transplantation. *South Med J* 1972;65:350.

91. Ward K. The origin of lymphoceles following renal transplantation. *Transplantation* 1978;25:346.

92. Cockett ATK, Netto KV. Increased lymphatic drainage from renal transplant. *Urology* 1973;2:571.

93. Olsson CA, Willsche MK, Filoso AM. Treatment of post-transplant lymphoceles: internal versus external drainage. *Transplant Proc* 1976;8:501.

94. Belzer FO, Salvatierra O, Schwerzer RT, et al. Prevention of wound infection by topical antibiotics in high risk patients. *Am J Surg* 1973;126:180.

95. Ehrlich RM, Smith RB. Surgical complications of renal transplantation. *Urology* 1977;10(Suppl. 1):43.

96. Guttman RD. Renal transplantation. II. *N Engl J Med* 1979; 301:1038.

97. Kyriakides GK, Simmons RL, Najarian JS. Wound infections in renal transplant wounds: pathogenetic and prognostic factors. *Ann Surg* 1975;182:770.

98. Lee HM, Madge GE, Mendez-Picon G, et al. Surgical complications in renal transplant recipients. *Surg Clin North Am* 1978;58:285.

99. Schwerzer RT, Kountz SL, Belzer FO. Wound complications in recipients of renal transplants. *Ann Surg* 1973;177:58.

100. Starzl TE, Groth CG, Putnam CW, et al. Urologic complications in 216 human recipients of renal transplants. *Ann Surg* 1970;172:1.

101. Lorber MI, Campbell DA Jr, Konnak JW, et al. Etiology and management of early and late peritransplant infections. *J Urol* 1982; 127:870.

102. Lartro JE, Mustapha N, Mee AD, et al. Ileal urinary diversion in patients with renal transplants. *Br J Urol* 1975;47:603.

103. Markland C, Kelly WD, Buselmeier T, et al. Renal transplantation into iliac urinary conduits. *Transplant Proc* 1972;4:629.

104. Han T, VanHook EJ, Simmons RL, et al. Prognostic factors of peritoneal infections in transplant patients. *Surgery* 1978;84:403.

105. Honan WP, Cheigh JS, Kim SJ. Renal allograft fracture: clinicopathologic study of 21 cases. *Ann Surg* 1977;186:700.

106. Lord RS, Effeney DJ, Hayes JM, et al. Renal allograft rupture: cause, clinical features and management. *Ann Surg* 1973;177:268.

107. Lee HM. Surgical techniques of renal transplantation. In: Morris PJ, ed. *Kidney transplantation, principles and practice.* New York: Grune & Stratton; 1979.

108. Martin KW. Spontaneous circumrenal hematoma: a review and report of two cases. *Br Med J* 1949;2:1118.

109. Bruce AW, Anad SA. Spontaneous rupture of kidney in pregnancy. *J Urol* 1966;95:5.

110. Klinger ME, Tannenbaum B, Elquezabel A. Pseudotumor of the kidney secondary to anticoagulant treatment. *J Urol* 1971;106:507.

111. Dryburgh P, Porter KA, Krom RAF, et al. Should the ruptured renal allograft be removed? *Arch Surg* 1979;114:850.

112. Koene AA, Skotnicki SH, Debruyne FM. Spontaneous renal decapsulation with excessive fluid leakage after transplantation. *N Engl J Med* 1979;300:1030.

113. Nghiem DD, Schulak JA, Corry RJ. Decapsulation of the renal transplant as a mechanism of lymphocele formation. *Transplant Proc* 1982;14:741.

114. Sollinger HW, Starling JR, Oberley T, et al. Severe "weeping" kidney disease after transplantation: a case report. *Transplant Proc* 1983;15:2157.

115. Tiggeler RG, DerSluis RF, Wobbes T, et al. Successful treatment with infrared contact coagulation of excessive fluid leakage after spontaneous decapsulation of a renal allograft. *Transplantation* 1986;41:264.

116. Diethelm AG, Edwards RP, Whelchel JD. The natural history and surgical treatment of hypercalcemia before and after renal transplantation. *Surg Gynecol Obstet* 1982;154:481.

117. Parfitt AM. Hypercalcemic hyperparathyroidism following renal transplantation and complications for population control in the parathyroid gland. *Miner Electrolyte Metab* 1982;8:92.

118. McCarron DA, Bennett WM, Muther RS, et al. Post-transplant hyperparathyroidism demonstration of retained control of parathyroid function by ionized calcium. *Am J Clin Nutr* 1980; 33:1536.

119. Parfitt AM, Kleerkopper M. Clinical disorders of calcium phosphorus and magnesium metabolism. In: Maxwell MH, Kleeman CR, eds. *Clinical disorders of fluid and electrolyte metabolism*, 3rd ed. New York: McGraw-Hill; 1980.

120. David DS, Sakai S, Brennan L. Hypercalcemia after renal transplantation. Long-term follow-up data. *N Engl J Med* 1973;289:398.

Complications of Liver Transplantation

46

Juan D. Arenas   Jeffrey D. Punch

■ COMPLICATIONS DURING DECEASED DONOR ORGAN PROCUREMENT 655

■ PRIMARY NONFUNCTION 656

■ GRAFT REJECTION 656

■ INCISIONAL COMPLICATIONS 656

■ RENAL FAILURE 657

■ RECURRENT DISEASE 657

■ GRAFT VERSUS HOST DISEASE 658

■ INFECTION 658

■ VASCULAR COMPLICATIONS 658

■ HEPATIC ARTERY THROMBOSIS 658

■ PORTAL VEIN THROMBOSIS OR STENOSIS 659

■ COMPLICATIONS OF THE INFERIOR VENA CAVA ANASTAMOSIS 659

■ BILIARY COMPLICATIONS 660

■ COMPLICATIONS OF LIVING DONOR LIVER TRANSPLANTATION 662

■ REFERENCES 663

Liver transplantation is the treatment of choice for patients with end-stage liver disease due to a variety of diseases as well as for patients with severe acute liver failure. This life-saving procedure is primarily limited by the number of available organs. Graft and patient survival rates increased gradually in the 1980s and 1990s but appear to have reached a near plateau over the past 5 years. Currently, the average 1-year graft survival rate in the United States is approximately 80%, while the 1-year patient survival rate is about 85% (1). Patients who survive the first year typically have relatively low mortality rates thereafter (2,3). Early death and graft loss can largely be traced to complications that occur at the time of transplantation or in the perioperative period, while late death is usually due to the cardiovascular disease or the development of immunosuppression-related infection or malignancy (2). Much of the improvement in early mortality can be attributed to improved immunosuppression and advances in the diagnosis and management of complications.

COMPLICATIONS DURING DECEASED DONOR ORGAN PROCUREMENT

The liver transplant procedure truly begins with the donor organ. Despite the recent development of living donor liver transplantation, the vast majority of liver grafts continue to

Juan D. Arenas: Henry Ford Health System, Detroit, MI 48202
Jeffrey D. Punch: University of Michigan, Ann Arbor, MI 48109

derive from deceased donors. Complications that occur during procurement of the liver graft from deceased donors include intraoperative cardiac arrest and injury to the portal vascular structures. Donors who suffer intraoperative cardiac arrest can be considered to be similar to controlled nonheart-beating donors. As such, cardiac arrest of the donor should not be considered a contraindication to donation (4). Similarly, injury to the portal vascular structures should not generally preclude use of a donor graft for transplantation given the multiple options that are available for vascular reconstruction. Laceration of the portal vein can be repaired using a segment of donor iliac vein or vena cava, while injuries to the arterial supply may be salvaged using donor iliac arterial grafts (5). Although embarrassing, the need to reconstruct the hepatic arterial circulation of a donor liver should not cause undue concern, given that reconstruction of a replaced right hepatic artery or other aberrant vessel is frequently necessary despite the finest surgical technique and a satisfactory outcome can be expected (5).

PRIMARY NONFUNCTION

Primary nonfunction of the allograft is the single most disastrous complication following orthotopic liver transplantation. Primary nonfunction is diagnosed by the presence of profound coagulopathy, metabolic acidosis, and hepatic transaminase values that are >3,000 U per mL. The etiology of primary nonfunction is thought to be primarily preservation injury, although recipient factors are important as well (6). Patients rapidly become exceedingly ill with progressive renal, pulmonary, neurologic, and cardiac failure. Survival beyond the fifth postoperative day is uncommon, and the only available therapy is retransplantation. An effective method of temporary hepatic support continues to be elusive despite decades of research (7). Initial reports suggested that prostaglandin E1 may improve immediate liver function (8). Later studies of prostaglandin E1 therapy failed to demonstrate a clinically significant decrease in the rate of primary nonfunction (9). To date, no pharmacologic therapy aimed at preventing primary nonfunction has been shown to be effective in controlled studies.

The primary means of dealing with primary nonfunction in liver transplantation is avoiding its occurrence. Numerous factors have been associated with primary nonfunction, including steatosis of the liver graft, donor age, and prolonged cold ischemia (6,10). Despite intensive scrutiny, objective variables fail to provide strong predictive value about whether a donor liver will function in the recipient. In fact, the factor with the highest predictive value has been the subjective impression of the surgeon who removed the graft from the donor (11).

Currently, patients in the United States with primary nonfunction are eligible to be listed as United Network for Organ Sharing (UNOS) Status 1. This emergency transplant status is reserved for patients who are judged to have <7 days to live without a transplant. Status 1 patients receive regional priority over less ill patients. Despite this advantage, some patients deteriorate during the waiting process. Total hepatectomy with temporary porta-caval shunt has been advocated as a possible means of avoiding the adverse effects associated with the effluent from the nonviable liver graft (12). There is insufficient experience with this technique to evaluate whether it offers a survival benefit.

GRAFT REJECTION

Liver transplantation was revolutionized in the early 1980s by the introduction of cyclosporine and refined in the 1990s by the availability of tacrolimus (13). Despite this success, acute rejection remains relatively common following liver transplantation, with an incidence between 20% and 60% (14,15). Unlike kidney transplantation, the sharing of human leukocyte antigens (HLA) does not appear to decrease rejection rates (16). Also, unlike kidney transplantation, the occurrence of an episode of acute rejection in the first year is not associated with worsened long-term outcome (17). Even late rejection does not carry an adverse prognosis as long as rejection is detected and treated (18). Chronic hepatic graft rejection, a rare phenomenon, manifests as ductopenia, or the "vanishing bile duct syndrome" (19). One group has reported the absence of chronic rejection in a large cohort of children treated with tacrolimus (20). Finally, the availability of newer agents such as mycophenolate mofetil and sirolimus also promise to reduce the problem of chronic liver graft rejection to a negligible level (21,22). Once ductopenic rejection manifests, the only effective treatment to date has been retransplantation.

INCISIONAL COMPLICATIONS

Incisional complications are frequent following liver transplantation, developing in 10% to 15% of patients (23,24). Predisposing factors include poor wound healing due to corticosteroid therapy, a high incidence of wound hematomas secondary to thrombocytopenia and coagulopathy, and attenuated musculature due to ascites and cachexia. Although corticosteroids are currently being greatly reduced, rapidly weaned, or eliminated from immunosuppressive regimens altogether, it is likely that incisional hernias will remain a significant problem following this procedure. Newer immunosuppressive agents, such as everolimus and sirolimus, that profoundly inhibit smooth muscle cellular proliferation are likely to increase the incidence of incisional complications if used perioperatively in liver transplant recipients (25).

Incisional hernia repair should be deferred until the patient has stable graft function and has been withdrawn from corticosteroids or is taking a stable, low dose. Repair of large hernias of the bilateral subcostal incision often entails the use of a large piece of mesh. Investigators report success using laparoscopic technique to repair incisional hernias following liver transplantation (26).

RENAL FAILURE

Renal failure may occur either acutely following the procedure or chronically. Acute renal failure is usually due to acute tubular necrosis. This complication is most often the result of poor renal perfusion during the operation due to intraoperative blood loss or due to insufficient replacement of fluid losses during the procedure. Liver transplant patients are predisposed to the development of acute tubular necrosis because of the physiologic derangements associated with cirrhotic liver disease. These include decreased blood pressure, increased cardiac output, and decreased peripheral vascular resistance. These hemodynamic disturbances are believed to be caused by peripheral shunting of blood due to vasoactive substances that are improperly metabolized in the liver. Together, these factors mean that patients with advanced chronic liver disease are universally prerenal before the operation begins. In addition, many liver transplant patients have preexisting renal insufficiency due to hepato-renal syndrome at the time of transplantation.

It has recently reported that the acute renal failure is associated with excessive increases in intra-abdominal pressure postoperatively (27). This observation suggests that some instances of acute renal failure may be avoided by recognition of intra-abdominal hypertension, defined as >25 mm Hg, and treatment by reexploration and closure of the incision with prosthetic material if necessary (28). This approach has been successful with trauma patients, where the abdominal compartment syndrome has become a widely recognized phenomenon (29).

Chronic renal failure is also a significant problem long term, affecting 10% to 18% of patients within 5 to 10 years (30,31). The use of nephrotoxic immunosuppressive agents such as tacrolimus and cyclosporine that induce progressive loss of renal function is assumed to be the primary cause of most renal insufficiency in this setting. Similar rates of renal failure are also seen in heart and lung transplant recipients (32).

Nephrotoxicity associated with chronic calcineurin inhibitor therapy may be partially abrogated by institution of either mychophenolate mofetil or sirolimus therapy and withdrawing or lowering the dosage of the calcineurin inhibitor without increasing the risk of either acute or chronic graft rejection (33,34). Improvement in renal function appears to be related to the duration of dysfunction. Withdrawal of calcineurin inhibitors after renal insufficiency has reached an advanced stage is not associated with the same degree of improvement in renal function (35). However, attempts at avoiding calcineurin inhibitors altogether have been disappointing due to an increase in early acute rejection (36).

Interestingly, patients who are treated with combined liver/kidney transplantation for chronic liver disease associated with renal failure have fewer episodes of graft rejection compared to recipients of the contralateral grafts from the same donor who received only the kidney grafts or combined kidney/pancreas grafts (37). This phenomenon is believed to be due to the immunological advantage conferred by the liver graft on the kidney graft. The basis for this apparent immunological phenomenon is not understood.

RECURRENT DISEASE

Recurrence of the primary etiology of liver failure has become an increasingly recognized long-term complication of liver transplantation. Hepatitis C viral infection, now the leading cause of cirrhosis in the United States, recurs in the vast majority of cases and leads to cirrhosis within 5 years in 25% of patients (38). The incidence of severe, early recurrence of hepatitis C following liver transplantation appears to be increasing, perhaps due to the increased use of older liver donors (39).

The possibility of recurrent alcoholism has been a concern for liver transplant surgeons since the inception of the procedure. Fortunately, the incidence of recurrent alcohol use in patients receiving liver transplant for alcohol-induced cirrhosis is low, at approximately 15% (40). The incidence of serious liver damage due to recurrent alcohol use is even lower. Given that recidivism rates following conventional alcohol rehabilitation are generally >50%, it appears that liver transplantation is truly the "ultimate eye-opening experience."

For many years it was thought that autoimmune diseases did not recur because of the immunosuppression used to suppress graft rejection. However, careful follow-up of large cohorts of liver recipients has demonstrated that autoimmune diseases do recur in some patients. Primary biliary cirrhosis, primary sclerosing cholangitis, and autoimmune hepatitis each recur in 15% to 20% of patients within 5 years of the transplant (41–43). It is unclear whether maintenance immunosuppression can be manipulated in such a way as to minimize recurrent autoimmune disease. This possibility seems unlikely given that immunosuppression does not play a role in forestalling the development of cirrhosis in these conditions—with the possible exception of autoimmune hepatitis.

It is currently unclear whether cryptogenic cirrhosis, an indication for transplantation in approximately one-sixth of liver transplant candidates, recurs or not. Although chronic inflammation is commonly seen on post-transplant biopsies, the incidence of graft failure is low (44).

GRAFT VERSUS HOST DISEASE

Graft versus host disease (GVHD) occurs when passenger lymphocytes from the donor that are within the graft are transferred to an immunosuppressed host. The transferred cells colonize the recipient and recognize recipient antigens as foreign. Typically the skin, intestines, and bone marrow are involved. Since the liver itself is not foreign relative to the lymphocytes, it is not involved. Despite the large number of donor lymphocytes that are present in a liver graft, GVHD is a very uncommon problem following liver transplantation, with an incidence of <1% (45). This low incidence is probably because donor lymphocytes are usually very immunogenic and are promptly destroyed by the recipient immune system. The incidence of GVHD is higher when the donor is both haplo-identical to the recipient and also homozygous at several HLA alleles. In this situation, the recipient's immune system does not recognize the donor lymphycytes as foreign. Diagnosis is usually made by tissue biopsy of the affected organ and confirmed by the finding of circulating donor lymphocytes using flow cytometry. Treatment of GVHD consists of intensified immunosuppression. Despite therapy, mortality is high (80%), with most patients dying of infection (46).

INFECTION

Since liver transplantation requires suppression of normal immunological responses, infection is an unavoidable complication, affecting as many as 70% of liver transplant recipients (47). In addition to the usual bacterial infections that are associated with postoperative patients, liver transplant recipients are also prone to viral and fungal infections. Acute rejection, obesity, and prolonged hospitalization are clear risk factors for clinically important infections (48,49). Biliary complications also dramatically increase the risk of infection. Approximately 20% of late graft loss (after 1 year) in pediatric liver recipients is attributable to infection (50). Cytomegalovirus (CMV) infection, once a common problem, has become much less common due to the routine use of prophylactic oral ganciclovir and valganciclovir.

Fungal infections may be minimized by prophylaxis with topical mycostatin or oral fluconazol or itraconazol (51). Newer agents such as Amphoterticin B lipid complex may offer improved efficacy against aspergillosis, a rare but deadly opportunistic post-transplant infection (52).

VASCULAR COMPLICATIONS

Vascular complications in general occur at a rate of approximately 10% of all liver transplant recipients. They are a frequent cause of early graft loss. Diagnosis is usually suggested by graft dysfunction and confirmed by Doppler examination of the hepatic vasculature. Extensive ascites, hematoma, body habitus, and bowel gas can make the interpretation of Doppler studies difficult in some patients (53). Many centers advocate contrast computed tomography (CT), and it can be an alternative noninvasive technique. Magnetic resonance evaluation is the choice if patients have allergic reactions to contrast or impaired renal function due to the use of iodinated contrast material (54). Magnetic resonance scanning may also be useful for confirmation of ultrasound studies and for evaluation of hepatic outflow problems. Selective angiography remains the gold standard for diagnosing vascular complications.

HEPATIC ARTERY THROMBOSIS

Hepatic artery thrombosis (HAT), the most common vascular complication of orthoptic liver transplantation (OLT), has an incidence of 4% to 12% in adult patients and up to 40% in children, with a mortality rate of as high as 50% to 60% (55). The clinical presentation of HAT varies from mild transaminase elevation due to ischemic changes in the liver parenchyma to delayed bile leak, bile duct strictures, and relapsing bacteremia and sepsis. Acute thrombosis in the first week after a liver transplant is associated with biliary necrosis and graft failure and invariably requires retransplantation if thrombectomy cannot be performed (56). In contrast, late HAT has a variable clinical course with one-third of patients not requiring intervention (57).

Multiple risk factors for HAT have been identified. Technical factors include a difference in the caliber of donor and recipient arteries, preexisting lesions such as hepatic artery dissection in the donor, or recipient or celiac stenosis in the donor. A recipient:donor weight ratio of >1.25 is a clear risk factor. The need for reconstructive arterioplasty in the presence of nonstandard donor anatomy, present in as many as 50% of donor livers, is known to predispose to HAT. Nontechnical factors also predispose to hepatic artery problems, most likely because they are associated with graft edema and poor flow. Nontechnical factors include prolonged cold ischemia time, ABO type incompatibility, biopsy proven rejection within the first week post-transplant, donor positive/recipient negative CMV status, and the G20210A prothrombin polymorphism (55,58). Recently, a strong association between cigarette smoking and increased incidence of arterial thrombosis has been found in OLT recipients. Smoking cessation at least 2 years before OLT decreased the risk (59).

In some instances, hepatic artery stenosis is diagnosed because of an elevation of hepatic enzymes, because of a new onset biliary complication, or on the basis of a Doppler study obtained for some other, unrelated reason. Although Doppler ultrasonography may suggest this

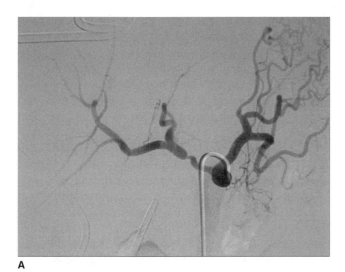

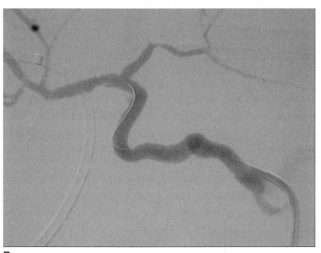

Figure 46-1 **A:** Selective hepatic arteriogram demonstrating anastomotic narrowing of the hepatic artery. **B:** Arteriogram following balloon angioplasty showing resolution of the narrowing.

problem, confirmation with angiography is usually required (Fig. 46-1A). Most stenoses occur at either the anastomotic site or because of clamp injury on the native vessel. When detected early in the postoperative period, abdominal exploration with takedown and thrombectomy may be an effective therapeutic option (60). In some instances when recipient inflow is the problem, the use of additional donor arterial graft is necessary to reestablish arterial flow. In cases of late arterial stenosis, selective angiography and balloon angioplasty may be successful (Fig. 46-1B). When the donor arterial system is damaged and after a revision there is absence of flow, retransplantation is necessary.

Hepatic artery pseudoaneurysm is an uncommon but life-threatening complication after OLT. It occurs more commonly in the presence of infected biloma or after using arterial graft reconstruction. Hepatic artery pseudoaneurysms can rupture intraperitoneally and lead to massive hemorrhage. Treatment options include surgical resection

and reconstruction using homograft, embolization, or exclusion with stent placement (61).

PORTAL VEIN THROMBOSIS OR STENOSIS

Portal vein complications following OLT are relatively uncommon, occurring at a rate of only 1% to 3% (62). Venous complications are usually the result of a technical surgical problem, such as size discrepancy, misalignment, or purse-stringing causing turbulent flow. A higher incidence of portal vein problems is seen in patients who have had previous portal vein operations or prior thrombosis of the portal system. Patients typically present with complications of portal hypertension, including variceal bleeding and ascites.

Doppler ultrasound examination is usually the first diagnostic tool, but it is inadequate to assess portal pressure gradients across a stricture or focal narrowing. Percutaneous transhepatic direct portography allows the measurement of pressures across a stenotic area, with values of >5 mm Hg being considered significant. Percutaneous transluminal angioplasty with or without stent placement may also be a good choice for this particular problem (Fig. 46-2) (63–65). In cases where there is a recalcitrant stricture, surgical intervention, including thrombectomy, placement of a venous jump graft, or creation of a porto-systemic shunt, may be necessary. In very severe cases in which frank hepatic decompensation occurs, retransplantation may be the only option.

COMPLICATIONS OF THE INFERIOR VENA CAVA ANASTAMOSIS

Complications arising from the vena cava anastamosis, either stenosis or occlusion, account for a small percentage of all complications. Vena cava problems that take place intraoperatively relate to venous tears in the recipient's cava, which may lead to catastrophic hemorrhage or air embolism. Rapid sternotomy and control of the intrapericardial portion of the inferior vena cava may be life-saving in this situation. Posttransplant complications can relate to size discrepancy between the donor and recipient, allowing for rotation of the graft and kinking at the level of the suprahepatic vena cava anastomosis. This circumstance is particularly problematic when the donor is small relative to the recipient. Inferior vena cava (IVC) thrombosis can be caused by a hypercoagulable state or by technical errors, such as including the back wall of the anastamosis when suturing the front wall. Hepatic outflow problems usually present with lower extremity edema or severe ascites, or both.

The incidence of outflow problems appears to be related to surgical technique. The traditional bicaval anastomotic technique involves resection of the intrahepatic portion of

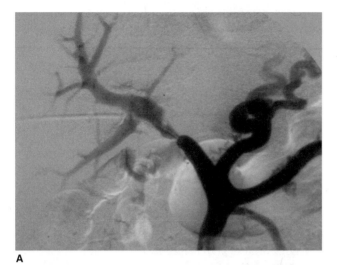

A

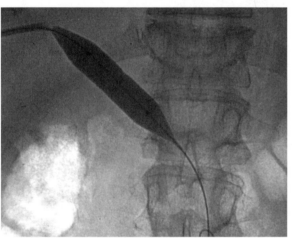

B

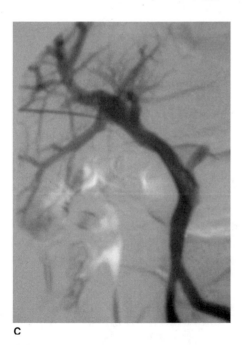

C

Figure 46-2 **A:** Transhepatic portal venogram showing narrowing of the portal vein anastamosis. **B:** Balloon angioplasty of the portal vein at the area of narrowing. **C:** Portal venogram following angioplasty showing resolution of the anastamotic narrowing.

the recipient vena cava and separate suprahepatic and infrahepatic anastamosis of the donor vena cava to the recipient (Fig. 46-3A). The incidence of caval obstruction using this technique is 1% to 2% (66). More recently, the "piggyback technique," involving preservation of the recipient cava, oversewing of the donor infrahepatic cava, and end-to-side anastamosis between the donor and recipient suprahepatic cava, has been advocated as a means of obviating veno-venous bypass (Fig. 46-3B) (67,68). The incidence of caval complications using the piggyback technique appears to be higher, at approximately 4% (69). Outflow stenosis appears to be more common if the combined orifice of two, rather than three, hepatic veins is used for the anastamotic site on the recipient (69). In many cases hepatic vein or suprahepatic cava stenosis can be successfully treated noninvasively with the use of balloon angioplasty or stenting, or both (70,71).

BILIARY COMPLICATIONS

Biliary complications after liver transplantation continue to cause substantial morbidity in both the early and late perioperative periods. In spite of better understanding of the biliary tree blood supply, improved surgical technique, and the use of absorbable suture material, the reported biliary complication rate varies from 10% to 30% (72). The pathogenesis of biliary complications is multifactorial. The single most important factor appears to be poor or absent arterial flow. The transected donor bile duct is totally dependent on arterial flow from the liver graft. Factors that have been associated with biliary problems include prolonged cold and warm ischemia time, sphincter of Oddi dysfunction, CMV infection, vascular rejection, and ABO incompatibility. Recipients with a diagnosis of primary sclerosing cholangitis have a higher rate of biliary complications.

Early diagnosis and treatment of biliary complications is paramount. Diagnostic procedures should take place urgently when bilirubin or alkaline phosphatase levels remain abnormally elevated in the perioperative period or when these values rise after a period of decline. Biliary leak or stricture is suggested by the development of abdominal pain, nausea, or persistent fever and by the development of ascites with a bilirubin level greater than serum. Whenever a biliary complication is identified, it is important to rule out hepatic arterial thrombosis with a Doppler ultrasound examination.

Two general techniques are used for biliary anastomosis in liver transplantation—duct to duct and Roux-en-Y hepatico-jejunostomy. In addition, a T-tube or other type of biliary stent may be used, allowing for monitoring of bile production and for contrast injection for diagnostic purposes (73). When a biliary stent is in place and a biliary complication is suspected, a cholangiogram through the stent is the first diagnostic test that should be performed. In the absence of a stent, an ultrasound examination followed

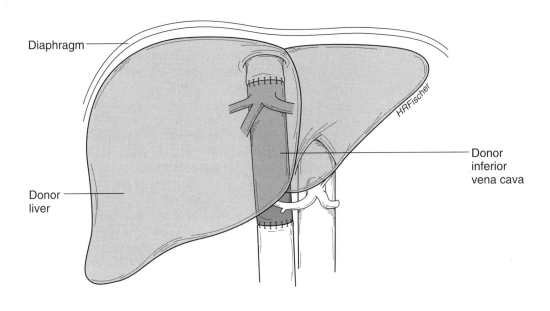

A

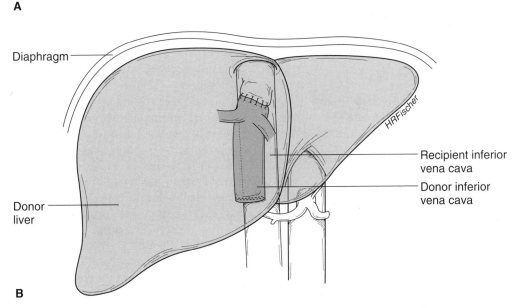

B

Figure 46-3 A: Liver transplant using bicaval technique showing the relationship between the donor liver, the donor cava, and the recipient cava. **B:** Liver transplant using the piggyback technique showing the relationship between the donor liver, the donor cava, and the recipient cava.

by either HIDA scan or endoscopic retrograde cholangiopancreatography (ERCP) is appropriate. ERCP has the advantage of being potentially both diagnostic and therapeutic when combined with sphincterotomy and the insertion of an internal stent. Percutaneous transhepatic cholangiography is a more invasive alternative that is usually reserved for cases where ERCP is not possible, such as patients with Roux-en-Y bile duct reconstruction.

The initial management of biliary complications can generally be nonoperative. Management should include intraluminal and external drainage, antibiotic administration as indicated, and reevaluation at 4 to 6 weeks. In cases where initial studies show a large defect and in cases where the leak is not controlled through percutaneous measures, operative

repair using a Roux-en-Y hepatico-jejunostomy is indicated. Similarly, anastomotic strictures can generally be managed nonoperatively using percutaneous cholangioplasty. When anastomotic strictures persist beyond two attempts at balloon dilatation and stent replacement, operative repair should be performed (Fig. 46-4) (74,75).

Late leaks, after 1 month post-transplant, are associated with T-tube removal. The incidence of this problem is about 35%, but episodes are usually short-lived and resolve after a period of observation with antibiotic therapy. In some instances, it may be advisable to insert a small feeding tube or other drain through the previously formed tract to serve as a drain until symptoms resolve. ERCP or percutaneous transhepatic cholangiogram (PTC) injection and ultrasound

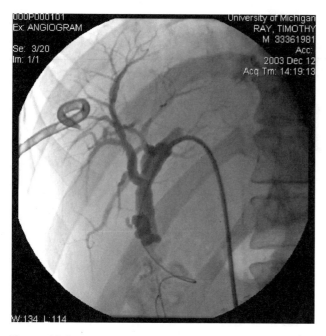

Figure 46-4 Transhepatic cholangiogram showing severe stenosis of the bile duct at the anastomosis that did not respond to balloon dilatation. This stenosis was successfully treated with Roux-en-Y hepatico-jejunostomy.

or CT guided placement of drains is necessary in cases where abdominal pain and/or fluid collections persist. Surgical intervention is only rarely necessary when a large defect is identified that cannot be controlled noninvasively (75).

COMPLICATIONS OF LIVING DONOR LIVER TRANSPLANTATION

Since its inception in 1989, living donor liver transplantation has gradually become a standard treatment for patients with liver failure. Originally developed to overcome the inadequate number of organ donors for children, the technique has more recently been applied to adult liver transplantation for the same reason (76). Several complications are relatively unique to living donor transplantation. It has been said that living donor transplantation is the only surgical procedure that has a potential mortality of 200%, causing the death of both the donor and the recipient. It is interesting to compare living donor liver transplantation, which has only recently been developed, to living donor kidney transplantation. In the 1950s, the first successful kidney transplants used living donors (identical twins) (77). Since that time, living donor kidney transplantation has become increasingly accepted to the point that living kidney donors now outnumber deceased kidney donors. The mortality of donating a kidney is approximately 0.03% (78). The long-term consequences of donating a kidney appear to be minimal (79). In contrast, the risk of donating the right hepatic lobe is not yet known, but it may be as high as 0.5% to 1%, leading some experts to question the development of the practice of adult to adult donation (80).

In addition to ethical issues related to donor mortality, the morbidity of the procedure is significant, with more than 12% to 20% of donors experiencing major complications (81,82). The risk of donor morbidity appears to be higher for right lobe donors than for left lateral segment donors. In right lobe donors, biliary complications occur in approximately 15% of cases (83). Although most biliary problems can be treated nonoperatively with ERCP or percutaneous drainage, some require operative repair. Although the donor liver regenerates, the long-term consequences of the donor operation are unknown (84).

Biliary complications are particularly common after living donor liver transplantation, with an incidence of between 16% and 38% (85). Biliary reconstruction is usually performed in living donor liver transplantation using a Roux-en-Y hepatico-jejunostomy, although duct-to-duct anastamosis has been reported. Depending on the plane of transection, a single or double anastomosis may be necessary. The use of intrabiliary stenting is common practice. Most programs evaluate the duct anatomy at the time of abdominal exploration with either intraoperative cholangiography or probe exploration through the cystic duct after cholecystectomy. When the two ducts are in close proximity, a ductoplasty can be performed, allowing the creation of a single orifice and a larger anastomotic opening (86).

One of the major difficulties during the development of the living donor technique has been the choice of graft. For pediatric recipients the left lateral segment comprising segments 2 and 3 has usually been selected. However, when the recipient is large (<30 kg), it may be necessary to use an extended left graft that includes segment 1 (the caudate lobe) or segment 4, or both. Adult recipients generally require a right lobe graft in order to supply sufficient hepatic mass for the recipient. The mass of the donor graft should be at least 1% of the recipient's body mass in order to support the recipient until a normal hepatic mass can regenerate, a process that takes several weeks. Grafts that are <1% of recipient body weight exhibit risk of post-transplant graft dysfunction (87). Graft dysfunction is manifested by prolongation of prothrombin time, necessitating continued infusions of fresh frozen plasma and persistent elevation of total bilirubin that may require retransplantation in some cases. Morbidity and mortality due to septic complications are also more common. Recipient factors are also known to play a role, as the small-for-size syndrome is observed more commonly when the recipient is extremely ill (88). One theory regarding the etiology of the graft dysfunction in small-for-size syndrome is that the hepatic dysfunction relates to "hyperperfusion" of the graft with portal blood, which causes a compensatory decrease in hepatic arterial flow. Methods to attenuate graft dysfunction with small-for-size grafts by temporarily shunting portal blood away from the graft have been suggested and are currently being evaluated (89).

REFERENCES

1. Roberts JP, Brown RS Jr, Edwards EB, et al. Liver and intestine transplantation. *Am J Transplant* 2003;3(Suppl. 4):78–90.
2. Rabkin JM, De la Melena V, Orloff SL, et al. Late mortality after orthotopic liver transplantation. *Am J Surg* 2001;181:475–479.
3. Pruthi J, Medkiff KA, Esrason KT, et al. Analysis of causes of death in liver transplant recipients who survived more than 3 years. *Liver Transpl* 2001;7:805–811.
4. Moon JI, Nishida S, Butt F, et al. Multi-organ procurement and successful multi-center allocation using rapid en bloc technique from a controlled non-heart-beating donor. *Transplantation* 2004;77(9):1476–1477.
5. Goldstein RM, Secrest CL, Klintmalm GB, et al. Problematic vascular reconstruction in liver transplantation. Part I. Arterial. *Surgery* 1990;107(5):540–543.
6. Strasberg SM, Howard TK, Molmenti EP, et al. Selecting the donor liver: risk factors for poor function after orthotopic liver transplantation. *Hepatology* 1994;20(4 Pt 1):829–838.
7. Adham M. Extracorporeal liver support: waiting for the deciding vote. *ASAIO J* 2003;49(6):621–632.
8. Takaya S, Doyle H, Todo S, et al. Reduction of primary nonfunction with prostaglandin E1 after clinical liver transplantation. *Transplant Proc* 1995;27(2):1862–1867.
9. Henley KS, Lucey MR, Normolle DP, et al. A double-blind, randomized, placebo-controlled trial of prostaglandin E1 in liver transplantation. *Hepatology* 1995;21(2):366–372.
10. Marsman WA, Wiesner RH, Rodriguez L, et al. Use of fatty donor liver is associated with diminished early patient and graft survival. *Transplantation* 1996;62(9):1246–1251.
11. Zamir GA, Markmann JF, Abrams J, et al. The fate of liver grafts declined for subjective reasons and transplanted out of a local organ procurement organization. *Transplantation* 2000;70(8):1149–1154.
12. Oldhafer KJ, Bornscheuer A, Fruhauf NR, et al. Rescue hepatectomy for initial graft non-function after liver transplantation. *Transplantation* 1999;67(7):1024–1028.
13. Calne RY. Immunosuppression in liver transplantation. *N Engl J Med* 1994;331(17):1154–1155.
14. Jain A, Kashyap R, Dodson F, et al. A prospective randomized trial of tacrolimus and prednisone versus tacrolimus, prednisone and mycophenolate mofetil in primary adult liver transplantation: a single center report. *Transplantation* 2001;72(6):1091–1097.
15. Demetris AJ, Ruppert K, Dvorchik I, et al. Real-time monitoring of acute liver-allograft rejection using the Banff schema. *Transplantation* 2002;74(9):1290–1296.
16. Toyoki Y, Renz JF, Mudge C, et al. Allograft rejection in pediatric liver transplantation: comparison between cadaveric and living related donors. *Pediatr Transplant* 2002;6(4):301–307.
17. Wiesner RH, Rakela J, Ishitani MB, et al. Recent advances in liver transplantation. *Mayo Clin Proc* 2003;78(2):197–210.
18. Ramji A, Yoshida EM, Bain VG, et al. Late acute rejection after liver transplantation: the Western Canada experience. *Liver Transpl* 2002;8(10):945–951.
19. Ludwig J, Wiesner RH, Batts KP, et al. The acute vanishing bile duct syndrome (acute irreversible rejection) after orthotopic liver transplantation. *Hepatology* 1987;7(3):476–483.
20. Jain A, Mazariegos G, Pokharna R, et al. The absence of chronic rejection in pediatric primary liver transplant patients who are maintained on tacrolimus-based immunosuppression: a long-term analysis. *Transplantation* 2003;75(7):1020–1025.
21. Pfitzmann R, Klupp J, Langrehr JM, et al. Mycophenolate mofetil for treatment of ongoing or chronic rejections after liver transplantation. *Transplant Proc* 2002;34(7):2938–2939.
22. Neff GW, Montalbano M, Slapak-Green G, et al. A retrospective review of sirolimus (Rapamune) therapy in orthotopic liver transplant recipients diagnosed with chronic rejection. *Liver Transpl* 2003;9(5):477–483.
23. Janssen H, Lange R, Erhard J, et al. Causative factors, surgical treatment and outcome of incisional hernia after liver transplantation. *Br J Surg* 2002;89(8):1049–1054.
24. Gomez R, Hidalgo M, Marques E, et al. Incidence and predisposing factors for incisional hernia in patients with liver transplantation. *Hernia* 2001;5(4):172–176.
25. Guilbeau JM. Delayed wound healing with sirolimus after liver transplant. *Ann Pharmacother* 2002;36(9):1391–1395.
26. Andreoni KA, Lightfoot H Jr, Gerber DA, et al. Laparoscopic incisional hernia repair in liver transplant and other immunosuppressed patients. *Am J Transpl* 2002;2(4):349–354.
27. Biancofiore G, Bindi ML, Romanelli AM, et al. Postoperative intra-abdominal pressure and renal function after liver transplantation. *Arch Surg* 2003;138(7):703–706.
28. Biancofiore G, Bindi ML, Romanelli AM, et al. Renal failure and abdominal hypertension after liver transplantation: determination of critical intra-abdominal pressure. *Liver Transpl* 2002;8(12):1175–1181.
29. Ivatury RR, Sugerman HJ, Peitzman AB. Abdominal compartment syndrome: recognition and management. *Adv Surg* 2001;35:251–269.
30. Cohen AJ, Stegall MD, Rosen CB, et al. Chronic renal dysfunction late after liver transplantation. *Liver Transpl* 2002;8(10):916–921.
31. Gonwa TA, Mai ML, Melton LB, et al. End-stage renal disease (ESRD) after orthotopic liver transplantation (OLTX) using calcineurin-based immunotherapy: risk of development and treatment. *Transplantation* 2001;72(12):1934–1939.
32. Ojo AO, Held PJ, Port FK, et al. Chronic renal failure after transplantation of a nonrenal organ. *N Engl J Med* 2003;349(10):931–940.
33. Raimondo ML, Dagher L, Papatheodoridis GV, et al. Long-term mycophenolate mofetil monotherapy in combination with calcineurin inhibitors for chronic renal dysfunction after liver transplantation. *Transplantation* 2003;75(2):186–190.
34. Nair S, Eason J, Loss G. Sirolimus monotherapy in nephrotoxicity due to calcineurin inhibitors in liver transplant recipients. *Liver Transpl* 2003;9(2):126–129.
35. Neau-Cransac M, Morel D, Bernard PH, et al. Renal failure after liver transplantation: outcome after calcineurin inhibitor withdrawal. *Clin Transplant* 2002;16(5):368–373.
36. Hirose R, Roberts JP, Quan D, et al. Experience with daclizumab in liver transplantation: renal transplant dosing without calcineurin inhibitors is insufficient to prevent acute rejection in liver transplantation. *Transplantation* 2000;69(2):307–311.
37. Fong TL, Bunnapradist S, Jordan SC, et al. Analysis of the United Network for Organ Sharing database comparing renal allografts and patient survival in combined liver-kidney transplantation with the contralateral allografts in kidney alone or kidney-pancreas transplantation. *Transplantation* 2003;76(2):348–353.
38. Ghobrial RM. Retransplantation for recurrent hepatitis C. *Liver Transpl* 2002;8(10 Suppl. 1):S38–S43.
39. Charlton M. The impact of advancing donor age on histologic recurrence of hepatitis C infection: the perils of ignored maternal advice. *Liver Transpl* 2003;9(5):535–537.
40. Jauhar S, Talwalkar JA, Schneekloth T, et al. Analysis of factors that predict alcohol relapse following liver transplantation. *Liver Transpl* 2004;10(3):408–411.
41. Sylvestre PB, Batts KP, Burgart LJ, et al. Recurrence of primary biliary cirrhosis after liver transplantation: histologic estimate of incidence and natural history. *Liver Transpl* 2003;9:1086–1093.
42. Kugelmas M, Spiegelman P, Osgood MJ, et al. Different immunosuppressive regimens and recurrence of primary sclerosing cholangitis after liver transplantation. *Liver Transpl* 2003;9(7):727–732.
43. Molmenti EP, Netto GJ, Murray NG, et al. Incidence and recurrence of autoimmune/alloimmune hepatitis in liver transplant recipients. *Liver Transpl* 2002;8(6):519–526.
44. Heneghan MA, Zolfino T, Muiesan P, et al. An evaluation of long-term outcomes after liver transplantation for cryptogenic cirrhosis. *Liver Transpl* 2003;9(9):921–928.
45. Burdick JF, Vogelsang GB, Smith WJ, et al. Severe graft-versus-host disease in a liver-transplant recipient. *N Engl J Med* 1988;318(11):689–691.
46. Sanchez-Izquierdo JA, Lumbreras C, Colina F, et al. Severe graft versus host disease following liver transplantation confirmed by PCR-HLA-B sequencing: report of a case and literature review. *Hepatogastroenterology* 1996;43(10):1057–1061.
47. Kibbler CC. Infections in liver transplantation: risk factors and strategies for prevention. *J Hosp Infect* 1995;30(Suppl.):209–217.

48. Wade JJ, Rolando N, Hayllar K, et al. Bacterial and fungal infections after liver transplantation: an analysis of 284 patients. *Hepatology* 1995;21(5):1328–1336.

49. Nair S, Cohen DB, Cohen MP, et al. Postoperative morbidity, mortality, costs, and long-term survival in severely obese patients undergoing orthotopic liver transplantation. *Am J Gastroenterol* 2001;96(3):842–845.

50. Wallot MA, Mathot M, Janssen M, et al. Long-term survival and late graft loss in pediatric liver transplant recipients—a 15-year single-center experience. *Liver Transpl* 2002;8(7):615–622.

51. Sharpe MD, Ghent C, Grant D, et al. Efficacy and safety of itraconazole prophylaxis for fungal infections after orthotopic liver transplantation: a prospective, randomized, double-blind study. *Transplantation* 2003;76(6):977–983.

52. Linden PK, Coley K, Fontes P, et al. Invasive aspergillosis in liver transplant recipients: outcome comparison of therapy with amphotericin B lipid complex and a historical cohort treated with conventional amphotericin B. *Clin Infect Dis* 2003;37(1):17–25.

53. Huang DZ, Le GR, Zhang QP, et al. The value of color Doppler ultrasonography in monitoring normal orthotopic liver transplantation and postoperative complications. *Hepatobiliary Pancreat Dis Int* 2003;2(1):54–58.

54. Glockner JF, Forauer AR, Solomon H, et al. Three-dimensional gadolinium-enhanced MR angiography of vascular complications after liver transplantation. *Am J Roentgenol* 2000;174(5):1447–1453.

55. Oh CK, Pelletier SJ, Sawyer RG, et al. Uni-and multi-variate analysis of risk factors for early and late hepatic artery thrombosis after liver transplantation. *Transplantation* 2001;71(6):767–772.

56. Sheiner PA, Varma CV, Guarrera JV, et al. Selective revascularization of hepatic artery thromboses after liver transplantation improves patient and graft survival. *Transplantation* 1997;64(9):1295–1299.

57. Bhattacharjya S, Gunson BK, Mirza DF, et al. Delayed hepatic artery thrombosis in adult orthotopic liver transplantation—a 12-year experience. *Transplantation* 2001;71(11):1592–1596.

58. Mas VR, Fisher RA, Maluf DG, et al. Hepatic artery thrombosis after liver transplantation and genetic factors: prothrombin G20210A polymorphism. *Transplantation* 2003;76(1):247–249.

59. Pungpapong S, Manzarbeitia C, Ortiz J, et al. Cigarette smoking is associated with an increased incidence of vascular complications after liver transplantation. *Liver Transpl* 2002;8(7):582–571.

60. Abbasoglu O, Levy MF, Vodapally MS, et al. Hepatic artery stenosis after liver transplantation—incidence, presentation, treatment, and long term outcome. *Transplantation* 1997;63(2):250–255.

61. Bonham CA, Kapur S, Geller D, et al. Excision and immediate revascularization for hepatic artery pseudoaneurysm following liver transplantation. *Transplant Proc* 1999;31(1-2):443.

62. Sieders E, Peeters PM, TenVergert EM, et al. Early vascular complications after pediatric liver transplantation. *Liver Transpl* 2000;6(3):326–332.

63. Cherukuri R, Haskal ZJ, Naji A, et al. Percutaneous thrombolysis and stent placement for the treatment of portal vein thrombosis after liver transplantation: long-term follow-up. *Transplantation* 1998;65(8):1124–1126.

64. Gonzalez-Tutor A, Abascal F, Cerezai L, et al. Transjugular approach to treat portal vein stenosis after liver transplantation—a case report. *Angiology* 2000;51(6):511–514.

65. Bhattacharjya T, Olliff SP, Bhattacharjya S, et al. Percutaneous portal vein thrombolysis and endovascular stent for management of posttransplant portal venous conduit thrombosis. *Transplantation* 2000;69(10):2195–2198.

66. Glanemann M, Settmacher U, Langrehr JM, et al. Results of end-to-end cavocavostomy during adult liver transplantation. *World J Surg* 2002;26(3):342–347.

67. Navarro F, Le Moine MC, Fabre JM, et al. Specific vascular complications of orthotopic liver transplantation with preservation of the retrohepatic vena cava: review of 1361 cases. *Transplantation* 1999;68(5):646–650.

68. Nemec P, Cerny J, Hokl J, et al. Hemodynamic measurement in liver transplantation. Piggyback versus conventional techniques. *Ann Transplant* 2000;5(1):35–37.

69. Parrilla P, Sanchez-Bueno F, Figueras J, et al. Analysis of the complications of the piggy-back technique in 1,112 liver transplants. *Transplantation* 1999;67(9):1214–1217.

70. Borsa JJ, Daly CP, Fontaine AB, et al. Treatment of inferior vena cava anastomotic stenoses with the Wallstent endoprosthesis after orthotopic liver transplantation. *J Vasc Interv Radiol* 1999;10(1):17–22.

71. Frazer CK, Gupta A. Stenosis of the hepatic vein anastomosis after liver transplantation: treatment with a heparin-coated metal stent. *Australas Radiol* 2002;46(4):422–425.

72. Feller RB, Waugh RC, Selby WS, et al. Biliary strictures after liver transplantation: clinical picture, correlates and outcomes. *J Gastroenterol Hepatol* 1996;11(1):21–25.

73. Sawyer RG, Punch JD. Incidence and management of biliary complications after 291 liver transplants following the introduction of transcystic stenting. *Transplantation* 1998;66(9):1201–1207.

74. Sung RS, Campbell DA, Rudich SM, et al. Long-term follow-up of percutaneous transhepatic balloon cholangioplasty in the management of biliary strictures after liver transplantation. *Transplantation* 2004;77(1):110–115.

75. Roumilhac D, Poyet G, Sergent G, et al. Long-term results of percutaneous management for anastomotic biliary stricture after orthotopic liver transplantation. *Liver Transpl* 2003;9(4):394–400.

76. Marcos A, Fisher RA, Ham JM, et al. Right lobe living donor liver transplantation. *Transplantation* 1999;68(6):798–803.

77. Murray J, Merril J, Harrison J. Kidney transplantation between seven pairs of identical twins. *Ann Surg* 1958;148:343.

78. Starzl TE. Living donors. *Transpl Proc* 1987;19:174–175.

79. Johnson EM, Anderson JK, Jacobs C, et al. Long-term follow-up of living kidney donors: quality of life after donation. *Transplantation* 1999;67(5):717–721.

80. Cronin DC II, Millis JM, Siegler M. Transplantation of liver grafts from living donors into adults—too much, too soon. *N Engl J Med* 2001;344(21):1633–1637.

81. Umeshita K, Fujiwara K, Kiyosawa K, et al. Japanese liver transplantation society. Operative morbidity of living liver donors in Japan. *Lancet* 2003;362(9385):687–690.

82. Brown RS Jr, Russo MW, Lai M, et al. A survey of liver transplantation from living adult donors in the United States. *N Engl J Med* 2003;348(9):818–825.

83. Ito T, Kiuchi T, Egawa H, et al. Surgery-related morbidity in living donors of right-lobe liver graft: lessons from the first 200 cases. *Transplantation* 2003;76(1):158–163.

84. Shiffman ML, Brown RS Jr, Olthoff KM, et al. Living donor liver transplantation: summary of a conference at The National Institutes of Health. *Liver Transpl* 2002;8(2):174–188.

85. Lo CM. Complications and long-term outcome of living liver donors: a survey of 1,508 cases in five Asian centers. *Transplantation* 2003;75(Suppl. 3):S12–S15.

86. Egawa H, Inomata Y, Uemoto S, et al. Biliary anastomotic complications in 400 living related liver transplantations. *World J Surg* 2001;25(10):1300–1307.

87. Inomata Y, Uemoto S, Asonuma K, et al. Right lobe graft in living donor liver transplantation. *Transplantation* 2000;69(2):258–264.

88. Kiuchi T, Tanaka K, Ito T, et al. Small-for-size graft in living donor liver transplantation: how far should we go? *Liver Transpl* 2003;9(9):S29–S35.

89. Boillot O, Mechet I, Le Derf Y, et al. Portomesenteric disconnection for small-for-size grafts in liver transplantation: preclinical studies in pigs. *Liver Transpl* 2003;9(9):S42–S46.

Complications
of Pancreatic
Transplantation

47

Dixon B. Kaufman

■ RATIONALE OF PANCREATIC
TRANSPLANTATION FOR PATIENTS
WITH TYPE 1 DIABETES MELLITUS 665

■ OUTCOME MEASURES OF PANCREATIC
TRANSPLANTATION 666
General Causes and Incidence of Pancreas Graft
Loss 668

■ COMPLICATIONS OF PANCREATIC
TRANSPLANTATION 669
Pancreas Transplant Recipient Selection 669
Cadaveric Pancreas Donor Selection and
Procurement 670
Pancreas Transplantation Surgery 671
Complications in the Postoperative Setting 673

■ TECHNICAL AND IMMUNOLOGICAL PROGRESS
IN PANCREATIC TRANSPLANTATION 680

■ REFERENCES 681

Dixon B. Kaufman: Northwestern University, Feinberg School of
Medicine, Chicago, IL 60611

Illustrations for Figures 47-3 to 47-5 and 47-8 to 47-11 by
Simon Kim.

RATIONALE OF PANCREATIC
TRANSPLANTATION FOR PATIENTS
WITH TYPE 1 DIABETES MELLITUS

The prevalence of type 1 diabetes in the United States is estimated to be 1,000,000 individuals, and 35,000 new cases are
diagnosed each year. The discovery of insulin as a therapeutic
agent in 1927 revolutionized the treatment of diabetes mellitus by changing it from a rapidly fatal disease into a chronic
illness. Unfortunately, this increased longevity brought
to the fore serious secondary complications, including
nephropathy, neuropathy, retinopathy and macrovascular
and microvascular complications in survivors 10 to 20
years after disease onset. The metabolic, microvascular, and
macrovascular complications of diabetes are responsible for
increased mortality in patients with type 1 diabetes compared to the general US population (1). In 2002, the national
direct and indirect costs of type 1 and type 2 diabetes, including hospital and physician care, laboratory tests, pharmaceu-
tical products, and patient workdays lost because of disability
and premature death, exceeded $130 billion (2).

Hyperglycemia is the most important factor in the
development and progression of secondary complications
of diabetes. The Diabetes Control and Complication Trial
demonstrated that the microvascular and, possibly,
macrovascular complications of diabetes may be prevented
by maintaining euglycemia (3,4). This realization has lead

to a search for alternative methods of treatment designed to achieve better glycemic control so that the progression of long-term complications can be altered.

Currently there is no practical artificial endocrine pancreas, a mechanical insulin-delivery device coupled with an automated glucose-sensory apparatus, that could administer insulin with the degree of control necessary to produce a near-constant euglycemic state without risk of hypoglycemia. Since severe hypoglycemia is life-threatening, persons with type 1 diabetes are resigned to manually regulating blood glucose levels by various forms of insulin administration. As a consequence, patients with type 1 diabetes typically exhibit wide deviations of plasma glucose levels from hour to hour and from day to day. Because hypoglycemia is intolerable, glucose control must err on the high side. Therefore, patients must live with relative chronic hyperglycemia.

The only treatments that influence the progression of secondary complications include β cell replacement therapy with pancreas or islet transplantation and intensive insulin therapy. Since diabetes is not a rapidly fatal disease, and because transplant procedures require the patient to receive life-long immunosuppression, the results of islet or pancreas transplantation must be sufficiently efficacious and safe to warrant application in place of standard medical management of the primary disease. Currently, islet transplantation is an experimental procedure for highly selective cases. Pancreas transplantation is a proven therapeutic treatment option for diabetes and is superior to manual intensive insulin therapy with regard to the efficacy of achieving glycemic control and beneficial effects on diabetic secondary complications.

A successful pancreas transplant produces an immediate normoglycemic and insulin-independent state that normalizes hemoglobin A1C levels for as long as the graft functions. Transplantation also has the added physiological properties of pro-insulin and C-peptide release not possible with intensive insulin therapy (5). Through improved metabolic control, many secondary complications of diabetes, including diabetic neuropathy (6), autonomic neuropathy-associated sudden death (7), and diabetic nephropathy in both uremic and nonuremic patients (8,9) may be markedly improved. A successful pancreas transplant significantly improves quality of life (10) and life expectancy (11,12).

Approximately 1,300 pancreas transplants are performed annually in the United States. Of these, 85% to 90% involve a simultaneous pancreas and kidney (SPK) transplant for patients with type 1 diabetes and chronic renal failure. These individuals are excellent candidates for an SPK transplant from the same donor because the immunosuppressive medications that are needed are similar to those for a kidney transplant alone and the surgical risk of adding the pancreas is low. The benefits of adding a pancreas transplant to ameliorate diabetes are profound—transplantation saves lives (11,12). The second category for pancreas transplantation consists of patients with type 1 diabetes who have received a previous kidney transplant from either a living or deceased donor. This group accounts for approximately 10% of patients receiving pancreas transplants. The important consideration is that of surgical risk, since the risk of immunosuppression has already been assumed.

The third category for pancreas transplantation is composed of nonuremic, non-kidney transplant patients with type 1 diabetes. In this situation one assesses the risk of immunosuppression to be less than the risk of diabetes treated with conventional exogenous insulin. Some of these patients with diabetes have extremely labile disease, such that there is difficulty with day-to-day living associated with frequent emergency room visits and inpatient hospitalizations for hypoglycemia or diabetic ketoacidosis. Other patients have significant difficulty with hypoglycemic unawareness that results in unconsciousness without warning. For select patients this state can be a devastating problem that affects their employment and their ability to keep a driver's license and creates concern about lethal hypoglycemia while asleep.

The indications for a pancreas transplant alone are essentially identical to indications for patients being considered for an islet transplant. However, in the former situation there are fewer contraindications with respect to body mass index and insulin requirements.

OUTCOME MEASURES OF PANCREATIC TRANSPLANTATION

The most important outcome measures of pancreas transplantation are defined in terms of patient and graft survival and rejection. The definition of patient survival is obvious. Pancreas graft losses are defined as: (i) patient death with a functioning graft or (ii) loss of insulin independence irrespective of whether the pancreas allograft is in place or removed. Rejection is an immunologic host response to the foreign graft that will destroy it unless antirejection medications are effectively administered. The definition of a rejection episode usually requires tissue biopsy confirmation. Patients are treated with a short course of anti–T-cell antibody, often in conjunction with corticosteroids.

The most valuable and complete information on the results of pancreas transplantation comes from the International Pancreas Transplant Registry (IPTR) and the Scientific Registry of Transplant Recipients (SRTR) of the Organ Procurement and Transplant Network (OPTN). The IPTR is supported primarily by the National Institute of Diabetes & Digestive & Kidney Diseases (NIDDK) at the National Institutes of Health (NIH) and by the United Network for Organ Sharing (UNOS). The IPTR is located at the University of Minnesota.

The SRTR is the scientific arm of the OPTN, where data on all transplants in the United States have been collected since 1987. The SRTR supports ongoing evaluation of the scientific and clinical status of solid-organ transplantation, including pancreas transplants. Funding comes from the

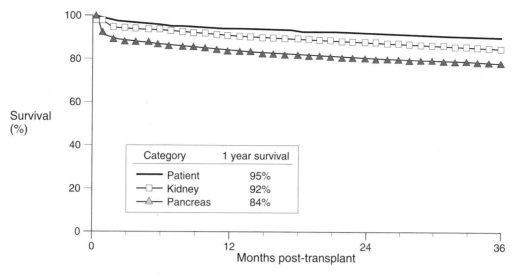

Figure 47-1 Patient, kidney, and pancreas survival rates of simultaneous pancreas-kidney transplant recipients (n = 3885, 1/1/98–1/1/02). (From International Pancreas Transplant Registry, 2003, with permission.)

Health Resources and Services Administration (HRSA), a division of the U.S. Department of Health and Human Services (HHS). The SRTR is administered by University Renal Research and Education Association (URREA), a nonprofit health research organization, in collaboration with the University of Michigan.

In addition to the national databases, multicenter studies and single center experiences with pancreas transplantation have also been valuable in reporting results of specific technical and immunosuppressive protocols.

Figure 47-1 shows patient, kidney, and pancreas graft survival rates in SPK transplant recipients in the most recent era analyzed (1998 to 2002) by the IPTR. These are the best outcomes reported to date, with 1-year patient, kidney, and pancreas graft survival rates of 95%, 92%, and 84%, respectively. Single center reports from the most active SPK transplant programs show wide variability of kidney and pancreas graft survival rates (Table 47-1) (13). The phenomenon is often referred to as "the center effect."

TABLE 47-1

ONE-YEAR PANCREAS AND KIDNEY ALLOGRAFT SURVIVAL RATES IN SIMULTANEOUS PANCREAS-KIDNEY TRANSPLANT RECIPIENTS AT THE TOP FIVE MOST ACTIVE CENTERS IN THE UNITED STATES[a]

Center	No. Transplants	Actual Graft Survival (%)	Expected Graft Survival (%)[b]	p Value
PANCREAS ALLOGRAFT				
United States	2,240	86.3		
University of Wisconsin Hosp. (Madison)	135	91.69	84.63	0.017
Fairview University Medical Center (Minneapolis)	77	75.06	83.29	0.073
Northwestern University (Chicago)	74	95.95	86.64	0.021
Ohio State University Hospital (Columbus)	73	87.39	86.54	0.999
Jackson Memorial Hospital (Miami)	70	92.86	87.27	0.230
KIDNEY ALLOGRAFT				
United States	2,240	91.98		
University of Wisconsin Hosp. (Madison)	1,305	92.26	92.11	0.999
Fairview University Medical Center (Minneapolis)	77	82.44	90.46	0.037
Northwestern University (Chicago)	74	98.65	92.32	0.049
Ohio State University Hospital (Columbus)	73	94.37	91.88	0.666
Jackson Memorial Hospital (Miami)	70	97.14	91.86	0.172

[a]Adult (age >18 years) recipients transplanted between 7/1/99–12/31/01.

[b]Based on SRTR data on US graft failure rates adjusted for donor and recipient characteristics (see http//www.ustransplant.org).

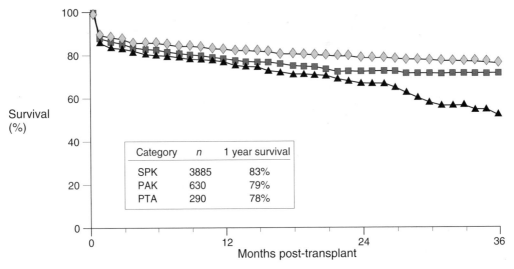

Figure 47-2 Pancreas transplant survival rates according to transplant category (1/1/97–10/10/01). SPK, simultaneous pancreas/kidney; PAK, pancreas after kidney; PTA, pancreas transplant alone. (From International Pancreas Transplant Registry, 2003, with permission.)

Figure 47-2 shows the comparative survival rates of the pancreas graft among the three transplant groups (SPK, PAK, and PTA) for the current era analyzed. These results demonstrate that pancreas allograft loss commonly occurs.

General Causes and Incidence of Pancreas Graft Loss

The IPTR database has information on the general causes and incidence of pancreas graft loss for each of the three recipient categories (SPK, PAK, and PTA). Tables 47-2, 47-3, and 47-4 show the rates of graft loss by etiology according to time post-transplant. The two most important general categories of graft loss are technical and immunological. The most common cause of pancreas graft failure within the first 6 months post-transplant in all three recipient categories is technical. The absolute rate of pancreas graft loss within the first 6 months post-transplant is approximately 10% in SPK transplant recipients and 20% in PAK and PTA recipients. Technical failures account for >60% of the cases

of pancreas graft loss within this early time period. Immunologic causes of graft loss, acute and chronic rejection, become more important after the 6-month period. The absolute rate of pancreas graft loss from rejection within the first year post-transplant is actually very low. The current rate of immunologic loss in SPK transplant recipients is only 2% at 1 year. The immunologic risk for graft loss for the technically successful cases of PAK and PTA transplants has been reduced to only 3% to 5% at 1 year. Patient death at a time when the transplanted organs are functional is another important cause of graft loss, especially in the SPK and PAK transplant category.

The specific causes and rates of technical failures are described in Table 47-5. The most important cause of technical failure is pancreas graft thrombosis. It occurs in approximately 4% to 9% of cases. Recipients of an SPK transplant are at the lowest risk, and patients receiving a PTA are at the highest risk. Graft losses due to infection, pancreatitis, bleeding, or a duodenal leak are relatively rare. Knowledge of the technical aspects of the surgical

TABLE 47-2

CAUSES AND RATES OF PANCREATIC GRAFT LOSS IN SPK TRANSPLANT RECIPIENTS (1/98–5/03)

	0–6 Months (%)	7–12 Months (%)	1–2 Years (%)	2–4 Years (%)
Technical failure	63.1	11.2	15.8	4.6
Acute rejection	4.3	11.2	12.3	8.0
Chronic rejection	2.7	22.5	24.5	33.1
Death with function	19.9	39.3	34.5	31.1

TABLE 47-3

CAUSES AND RATES OF PANCREATIC GRAFT LOSS IN PAK TRANSPLANT RECIPIENTS (1/98–5/03)

	0–6 Months (%)	7–12 Months (%)	1–2 Years (%)	2–4 Years (%)
Technical failure	61.9	22.5	20.0	18.8
Acute rejection	6.9	12.2	12.5	15.6
Chronic rejection	7.5	22.5	25.0	18.8
Death with function	12.7	26.5	22.5	34.4

procedures pertaining to pretransplant organ procurement and pancreas graft implantation shed light on the potential complications of pancreas transplantation.

COMPLICATIONS OF PANCREATIC TRANSPLANTATION

Pancreas transplant recipients may fall victim to several common and potentially life-threatening complications. Awareness, meticulous postoperative care, and surveillance are paramount in preventing or promptly diagnosing a complication before it becomes severe. Anticipation of potential complications within the context of the various stages of the transplant procedure is also an important discipline. Complications may be anticipated and averted in the settings of recipient selection, donor selection and procurement, and pancreas transplantation surgery and in the postoperative management setting.

Pancreas Transplant Recipient Selection

In the evaluation phase of a pancreas transplant candidate, the history of disease, the review of systems, and the physical examination are conducted in a manner that focuses on specific comorbid conditions that may compromise transplant outcome. Contraindications to solitary pancreas transplantation include patients with type 1 diabetes who have normal renal function and do not exhibit a brittle course, hypoglycemic unawareness, or evidence of nephropathy. For patients who have an indication for pancreas transplantation, it is important to exclude significant medical contraindications, including recent malignancy, active or chronic untreated infection, advanced forms of major extrarenal disease (i.e., coronary artery disease), life expectancy of <1 year, sensitization to donor tissue, noncompliance, active substance abuse, and uncontrolled psychiatric disorder (Table 47-6).

Pre-existing morbidities have direct implications for predicting and, therefore, avoiding postoperative complications. Premature cardiovascular disease and advanced coronary artery disease are the most important comorbidities in patients with type 1 diabetes, especially those with diabetic nephropathy (14–16). There is a fourfold elevation in cardiovascular mortality in type 1 diabetics without proteinuria compared to the general population. In type 1 diabetics with proteinuria, cardiovascular mortality is 37 times higher than it is in the general population (15). The diabetic, uremic patient has several risk factors in addition to diabetes for development of coronary artery disease, including hypertension, hyperlipidemia, and smoking. Because of the neuropathy associated with diabetes, patients are often asymptomatic because ischemia-induced angina is not perceived. The prevalence of significant (>50% stenosis) coronary artery disease in patients with diabetes starting treatment for end-stage renal disease is estimated to be 45% to 55%.

TABLE 47-4

CAUSES AND RATES OF PANCREATIC GRAFT LOSS IN PTA TRANSPLANT RECIPIENTS (1/98–5/03)

	0–6 Months (%)	7–12 Months (%)	1–2 Years (%)	2–4 Years (%)
Technical failure	65.8	4.76	17.9	25.0
Acute rejection	10.1	4.8	10.7	20.0
Chronic rejection	5.1	42.9	28.6	30.0
Death with function	6.3	9.5	25.0	15.0

TABLE 47-5

CAUSES OF TECHNICALLY FAILED PANCREAS TRANSPLANTS ACCORDING TO RECIPIENT CATEGORY (1/99–5/03)

	SPK (%)	PAK (%)	PTA (%)
Thrombosis	4.3–6.4	5.4–8.7	7.0–9.0
Infection	1.1	0.5–2.2	1.0–1.1
Pancreatitis	0.3–0.8	0.3–0.7	0.0–2.5
Bleeding	0.3–0.5	0.0–0.2	0.0–0.5
Anastomotic leak	0.3–0.7	0.5–0.7	0.5

The interventional screening studies to detect significant, treatable coronary artery disease require a uniform methodology. Noninvasive screening that has high sensitivity and specificity for significant coronary artery disease can be used in low-risk patients. Patients considered at moderate or high risk for significant coronary artery disease should undergo coronary arteriography to determine the severity and location of the lesions. A liberal policy of coronary angiography is reasonable because the current noninvasive tests are relatively insensitive. Also, the techniques of coronary angiography have changed in the last few years, allowing for selected arteriography with very low-dose, less toxic contrast agents using biplanar imaging techniques. The nephrotoxic risk of angiography has been reduced considerably, if a left ventriculogram is omitted, in a preuremic patient with creatinine clearance >20 mL per minute.

Patients with coronary lesions amenable to angioplasty with stenting or bypass grafting should be treated, re-evaluated, and then reconsidered for transplantation. The goal of revascularization is to diminish the perioperative risk of the transplant procedure and to prolong the duration of life post-transplant. Patients who have experienced long waiting periods prior to pancreas transplantation should have their cardiac status assessed at regular intervals.

TABLE 47-6

CONTRAINDICATIONS TO PANCREAS TRANSPLANTATION

1. Omission of consent for organ donation from family
2. Incompatible blood group
3. Donor HLA class I antigen generating a positive immunological crossmatch
4. History of type 1 or type 2 diabetes mellitus in donor
5. Donor viral infectious disease of HIV, hepatitis B and/or C
6. Significant bacterial and/or fungal infection of the donor
7. Significant and prolonged donor hemodynamic instability
8. History of previous donor pancreatic surgery
9. Intra-abdominal trauma to the donor pancreas

Autonomic neuropathy is prevalent and may manifest as neurogenic bladder dysfunction, gastropathy, and orthostatic hypotension. Neurogenic bladder dysfunction is an important consideration in patients receiving a bladder-drained, pancreas-alone transplant or an SPK transplant (17). Inability to sense bladder fullness and to empty the bladder predisposes to urine reflux and high postvoid residuals. These problems may adversely affect renal allograft function, increase the incidence of bladder infections and pyelonephritis, and predispose to graft pancreatitis.

Impaired gastric emptying, gastroparesis, is an important consideration with significant implications in the post-transplant period. Patients with severe gastroparesis may have difficulty tolerating the oral immunosuppressive medications that are essential to prevent rejection of the transplants.

The combination of orthostatic hypotension and recumbent hypertension results from dysregulation of vascular tone. This condition has implications for blood pressure control post-transplant, especially in patients with bladder-drained pancreas transplants that are predisposed to volume depletion. Careful reassessment of post-transplant antihypertensive medication requirement is important.

Diabetic retinopathy is a nearly ubiquitous finding in patients with diabetes and end-stage renal disease. Blindness is not an absolute contraindication to transplantation since many blind patients lead very independent life styles. Although rarely a problem, it should be confirmed that a patient with significant vision loss has an adequate support system to ensure help with travel and immunosuppressive medications.

Lower extremity peripheral vascular disease is significant in patients with diabetes. Uremic diabetic patients are at risk for amputation of a lower extremity. These problems typically begin with a foot ulcer associated with advanced somatosensory neuropathy. The risk is further complicated by sensory and motor neuropathies in patients with long-standing diabetes. Vascular disease may have implications for the rehabilitation post-transplant and is an indicator for potential risk for injury to the feet and subsequent diabetic foot ulcers.

Mental or emotional illnesses, including neuroses and depression, are common. Diagnosis and appropriate treatment of these illnesses is an important pretransplant consideration with important implications for ensuring a high degree of medical compliance.

Cadaveric Pancreas Donor Selection and Procurement

Identification of suitable cadaveric organ donors for pancreas transplantation is an important and often underappreciated determinant of outcome. Misjudgment regarding the quality of the transplantable organs may have significant downstream adverse consequences post-transplant. In a sense, the transplant operation begins with organ procurement.

In general, the criteria that determine an appropriate donor for pancreas transplantation are more stringent than for kidney or liver donors. Cadaveric pancreas organ donors are typically between the ages of 10 and 55. The lower age limit does not relate to the metabolic efficiency of the pediatric endocrine pancreas to regulate blood sugar control in an adult. Rather, the lower age limit of a pediatric donor pancreas reflects the anticipated small size of the splenic artery, which may preclude successful construction of the arterial Y-graft needed for pancreas allograft revascularization. With respect to upper age limits, the use of pancreata from older donors has been associated with increased technical failure due to pancreas graft thrombosis, a higher incidence of post-transplant pancreatitis, and decreased pancreas graft survival rates.

The body weight of the cadaveric organ donor is an important consideration. Obese donors >100 kg are frequently found not to be suitable pancreas donors. Obese patients may have a history of type 2 diabetes, or the pancreas may be found to be unsuitable for transplantation because of a high degree of adipose infiltration of the pancreas.

Importantly, pancreata from relatively older donors (age 55 to 65) and obese organ donors are associated with very successful islet isolation recovery required for islet transplantation. Therefore, application of β cell replacement therapy should be considered for nearly all cadaveric organ donors.

Donor hemodynamic stability and need for inotropic support is an important consideration. Hemodynamic stability has more influence on the anticipated function of the kidney allograft than it does on initial endocrine function of the pancreas allograft in the case of an SPK transplant. Deceased donors who have experienced a significant period of cardiac arrest or who require high doses of prolonged inotropic support frequently exhibit slow deterioration of renal function that may result in delayed renal allograft function in the SPK transplant recipient.

The most important determinant of suitability of the pancreas for transplantation is direct examination of the organ during surgical procurement. The experience of the procurement team is important. During procurement that judgment regarding the degree of fibrosis, adipose tissue infiltration into the parenchyma, trauma, and specific vascular anomalies can be made. Pancreata with heavy infiltration of adipose tissue are believed to be relatively intolerant of cold preservation and the potential of a high degree of saponification due to reperfusion pancreatitis following revascularization. These organs may be more suitable for islet isolation.

The important vascular anomaly that must be evaluated during procurement is the occurrence of a replaced or accessory right hepatic artery originating from the superior mesenteric artery (SMA). The presence of a replaced right hepatic artery is no longer an absolute contraindication for the use of the pancreas for transplantation. Experienced procurement teams will be able to successfully separate the liver and the pancreas either *in situ* or on the backbench, without sacrificing quality of either organ for transplantation.

A few important caveats determine if this maneuver is possible. The replaced right hepatic artery must be dissected to the junction with the SMA. If the replaced right hepatic artery traverses deep into the parenchyma of the head of the pancreas, requiring extensive dissection, this circumstance may preclude the pancreas for transplantation. The SMA is divided distal to the origin of the replaced right hepatic artery, preserving intact a short length of SMA with a carrel patch for the liver graft. Occasionally, there is a large inferior pancreaticoduodenal arterial branch vascularizing the head of the pancreas that originates proximal to the origin of the replaced right hepatic artery. The inferior pancreaticoduodenal vessels are critical to vascularization of the head of the pancreas because the gastroduodenal artery is routinely ligated during the process of hepatic artery mobilization for the liver transplant. In the case of a very proximal origin of the inferior pancreaticoduodenal artery, dividing the SMA at the appropriate location for proper liver procurement would significantly impair vascularization of the head of the pancreas and preclude its use for transplantation. Evaluation of the arterial vascularity of the pancreaticoduodenal allograft can be tested on the backbench by several methods: (i) injection of Renografin into the SMA or Y-graft and obtaining an x-ray; (ii) intra-arterial injection of fluorescein, with visualization using a Wood lamp; and (iii) performing a methylene blue angiogram.

The use of marginal and nonheartbeating donors for pancreas transplantation has been reported. If the pancreas is deemed suitable, there is the added consideration of the effect of delayed kidney graft function in a uremic SPK transplant candidate. The use of marginal and nonheartbeating donors for pancreas alone transplantation is a selective decision made on a case-by-case basis.

The use of living related and unrelated pancreas donors has also been described. A distal pancreatectomy is performed for a segmental pancreas transplant. Anecdotal cases of combined live donor partial pancreatectomy and nephrectomy have also been reported. These procedures are not widely performed and are confined to one or two pancreas transplant programs.

Pancreas Transplantation Surgery

The surgical techniques for pancreas transplantation are diverse (Figs. 47-3, 47-4, 47-5). The principles are consistent, however, and include providing adequate arterial blood flow to the pancreas and duodenal segment, adequate venous outflow from the pancreas, and management of the pancreatic exocrine secretions. The native pancreas is not removed.

Pancreas graft arterial revascularization is typically accomplished using the recipient right common or external iliac

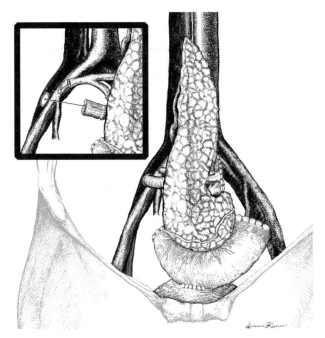

Figure 47-3 Pancreaticoduodenal allograft with exocrine bladder-drainage and systemic venous drainage. (Reprinted from Stuart FP, Abecassis MM, Kaufman DB. *Organ Transplantation*, 2nd ed. Georgetown: Landes Bioscience, 2003:166, with permission.)

artery. The Y-graft of the pancreas is anastomosed end-to-side. Positioning of the head of the pancreas graft cephalad or caudad is not relevant with respect to successful arterial revascularization. There are two choices for venous revascularization—systemic and portal. Systemic venous revascularization commonly involves the right common iliac vein, or right external iliac vein. If portal venous drainage is used, it is necessary to dissect the superior mesenteric vein at the root of the mesentery. The pancreas portal vein is anastomosed end-to-side to a branch of the superior mesenteric vein. This anastomosis may influence the methodology of arterial revascularization using a long Y-graft placed through a window in the mesentery to reach the right common iliac artery. Portal venous drainage of the pancreas is more physiologic with respect to immediate delivery of insulin to the recipient liver. Portal drainage results in diminished circulating insulin levels relative to those in systemic venous-drained pancreas grafts. The route of venous drainage has no documented clinically relevant differences in glycemic control.

There are several methods of managing the exocrine drainage of the pancreas. Pancreatic exocrine drainage may be handled via anastomosis of the duodenal segment to the bladder or by anastomosis to the small intestine. The bladder-drained pancreas transplant is a very important modification that was introduced about 1985. This technique significantly improved the procedure's safety by minimizing the occurrence of intra-abdominal abscess from leakage of enteric-drained pancreas grafts. With the successful application of the new immunosuppressant

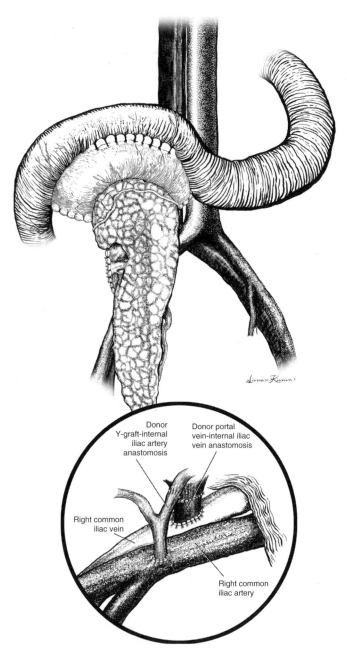

Figure 47-4 Pancreaticoduodenal allograft with exocrine enteric-drainage and venous systemic drainage. (Reprinted from Stuart FP, Abecassis MM, Kaufman DB. *Organ transplantation*, 2nd ed. Georgetown: Landes Bioscience, 2003:167, with permission.)

agents and reduction in the incidence of rejection, enteric drainage of pancreas transplants has enjoyed a rebirth.

Enteric drainage of the pancreas allograft is physiologic with respect to the delivery of pancreatic enzymes and bicarbonate into the intestines for reabsorption. Enterically drained pancreases can be constructed with or without a Roux-en-Y intestinal limb. The enteric anastomosis can be made side-to-side or end-to-side with the duodenal segment of the pancreas. The anastomosis may be hand sewn or accomplished with the stapler. The risk of intra-abdominal abscesses is extremely low (18), and the avoidance of the

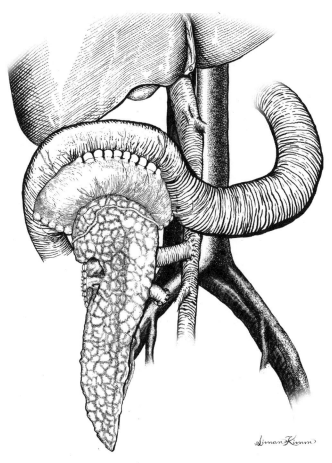

Figure 47-5   Pancreaticoduodenal allograft with exocrine enteric-drainage and portal venous drainage. (Reprinted from Stuart FP, Abecassis MM, Kaufman DB. *Organ transplantation*, 2nd ed. Georgetown: Landes Bioscience, 2003:168, with permission.)

bladder-drained pancreas has significant implications with respect to potential complications that include bladder infection, cystitis, urethritis, urethral injury, balanitis, hematuria, metabolic acidosis, and the requirement for enteric conversion. Currently, approximately 75% of pancreas transplants are performed with enteric drainage, and the remainder are performed with bladder drainage.

The options of enteric versus bladder drainage depend on the choice of venous drainage and the clinical scenario of the pancreas transplant. For portally drained pancreas transplants, bladder drainage is not an option. For recipients of an SPK transplant, enteric drainage is the technique of choice because there is no urinary monitoring benefit and the morbidities as described above are significant. In the cases of PAK and PTA, bladder drainage has two important advantages: (i) urinary monitoring for rejection and (ii) placement of the graft, allowing access for percutaneous biopsy for diagnosis of rejection. In the latter situation the advantages of monitoring outweigh the morbidities associated with bladder drainage, at least in the short term, when the risk of immunologic graft loss is significant.

The pancreas is typically drained into the bladder if a pancreas transplant alone or pancreas-after-kidney transplant is performed in order to use measurement of urinary amylase as a method of detecting rejection. However, some programs have had good experience with enteric drainage of the pancreas transplant alone, using other markers for rejections, such as clinical signs and symptoms of pancreas graft pancreatitis and serum amylase or lipase levels coupled with biopsy.

Complications in the Postoperative Setting

Table 47-7 outlines the most common complications in the early postoperative period.

Thrombosis

Vascular thrombosis is the most important early complication of pancreatic transplantation (19). Thrombosis can occur at any time post-transplant but typically occurs within 48 hours and usually within 24 hours of the transplant. Thrombosis is generally due to venous thrombosis of the transplant pancreas portal vein. The incidence is approximately 5% to 8%. Arterial thrombosis is less common and is usually associated with atherosclerotic vessels. The etiology of thrombosis is not entirely defined but is believed to be associated with reperfusion pancreatitis, the

---

TABLE 47-7

POTENTIAL EARLY COMPLICATIONS OF PANCREATIC TRANSPLANTATION

Thrombosis
    Arterial
    Venous

Hemorrhage
    Pancreatic graft
    Vascular anastomosis

Infection
    Bacterial or fungal
        Peripancreatic fluid
        Superficial wound
        Urinary tract

Metabolic
    Acidosis
    Hyperkalemia, hypokalemia, hypocalcemia,
       hypomagnesemia
    Dehydration

Gastrointestinal
    Anastomotic leak (enteric drained graft)
    Mechanical obstruction

Urologic
    Hematuria
    Bladder anastomotic leak (bladder-drained
      graft)
    Urethral injury/stenosis

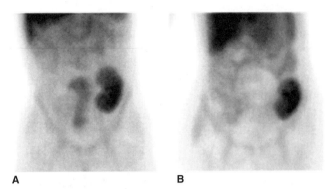

A   **B**

Figure 47-6 Technetium-99m hexamethyl propylene amine oxime (^{99}mTc-HMPAO) radionucleotide scintigraphic scan of a well-perfused simultaneous pancreas-kidney (SPK) transplant **(A)** and of an SPK transplant recipient with acute thrombosis of the pancreaticoduodenal allograft **(B)**. Images were recorded 0 to 5 minutes after labeled contrast injection.

relatively low-flow state of the pancreas graft, and unrecognized concomitant prothromotic disorders (20). The quality of the pancreas graft, the age of the donor, and the cold ischemia time also influence graft thrombosis rates.

Acute venous thrombosis is heralded by a sudden rise in serum glucose, pain directly over the pancreatic graft, and, occasionally, ipsilateral lower extremity swelling from extension of the thrombus into the common iliac vein.

Confirmatory noninvasive diagnostics may be helpful when the clinical picture is not consistent with loss of pancreas graft viability. Perfusion imaging of the graft using technetium-99m hexamethyl propylene amine oxime (HMPAO) may reveal loss of pancreas graft perfusion and a photopenic region (21). Figure 47-6 illustrates a normal perfusion scan of the pancreas and kidney grafts of an SPK transplant recipient and an abnormal scan wherein the pancreas allograft is not perfused. Ultrasonography is often used to determine the quality of vascular flow to and from the pancreaticoduodenal allograft. Ultrasonography

advantages include the portable nature of the scanning device, but the quality of results is highly dependent on the skills of the technician and radiologist. Completed tomography is usually not the diagnostic test of choice but may reveal findings consistent with pancreas allograft thrombosis that include an enlarged and inhomogeneous pancreas graft (Fig. 47-7).

Management of pancreatic graft thrombosis requires urgent operative intervention—either thrombectomy and vascular revision or graft excision. The findings at surgery usually reveal an ischemic, dusky, and nonviable pancreas and duodenal segment, with fresh clot in the graft portal vein (Fig. 47-8). Salvage of the thrombosed graft is not to be expected, but anecdotal salvage has been described (22). Fortunately, as a result of advances in cold preservation, technical modifications, and widespread use of postoperative anticoagulation, this is a complication of decreasing incidence.

Anticoagulation therapy is routinely used to reduce the incidence of pancreatic graft thrombosis. Although there is no standard protocol for optimal anticoagulation regimen early post-transplant, most centers employ a combination approach involving a heparin agent and an antiplatelet agent such as aspirin. The concern with instituting anticoagulation therapy is the increased risk of postoperative hemorrhage. Although the thrombosis/hemorrhage dichotomy complicates postoperative patient care, the management of mild postoperative bleeding is more acceptable than the irreversible consequences of allograft thrombosis.

Hemorrhage

This complication is common whenever any major vascular procedure is performed. The use of postoperative anticoagulation to diminish the frequency of allograft thrombosis increases the risk of this complication. Bleeding from the vascular anastomotic site and ligatures or cut surfaces of the

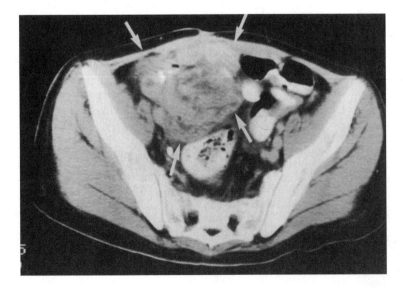

Figure 47-7 CT image of pancreas graft thrombosis showing an enlarged and inhomogeneous graft. (Reprinted from Letourneau JG, Day DL, Ascher NL. *Radiology of organ transplantation.* St. Louis: Mosby, 1991:269, with permission.)

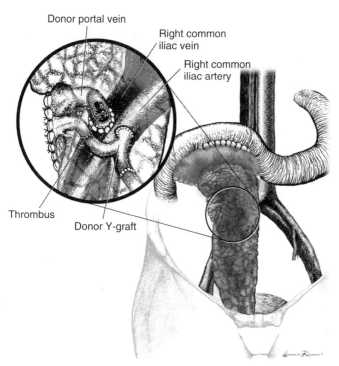

Figure 47-8 Intraoperative vignette of the surgical findings of acute pancreatic graft thrombosis.

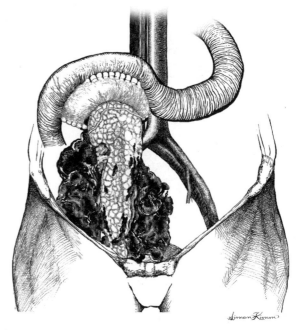

Figure 47-9 Intraoperative vignette of the surgical findings of acute intra-abdominal hemorrhage in a pancreatic graft recipient.

pancreatic graft will result in an intra-abdominal accumulation of hematoma. Clinical suspicion, physical examination, serial blood counts, and attention to abdominal drain effluents often reveal postoperative hemorrhage. Frequently, discontinuation of anticoagulants/antiplatelet agents, correction of coagulation abnormalities by administration of platelets, vasopressin, vitamin K, fresh-frozen plasma, cryoprecipitate, and so on, and medical support is all the therapy that is required. Aggressive resuscitative efforts and operative intervention consisting of celiotomy with evacuation of hematoma and control of hemorrhage are essential if hemodynamic instability develops. The intraoperative findings reveal fresh and clotted hematoma, often without a definitive bleeding source (Fig. 47-9). The hematoma is washed out, exploration for a source of bleeding is conducted, coagulopathy is corrected, and the viability of the pancreas (and kidney) is confirmed. Gastrointestinal (GI) bleeding may occur after the enteric-drained pancreas from a combination of perioperative anticoagulation and bleeding from the suture line of the duodenoenteric anastomosis (23). Suture line bleeding is self-limited and will manifest as diminished hemoglobin level associated with heme-positive or melanotic stool. Conservative management is appropriate; reoperative exploration is unusual.

Transplant Pancreatitis

Pancreatitis of the allograft occurs to some degree in all patients postoperatively. A temporary elevation in serum amylase levels is common for 48 to 96 hours post-transplant.

Most episodes are transient and mild without significant clinical consequence. It is common for patients receiving an SPK transplant to have a greater degree of fluid retention for several days post-transplant, compared to kidney transplant alone recipients. Though not proven, fluid retention may be related to graft pancreatitis that ensues in the perioperative period. The retained fluid is mobilized early postoperatively. It is important to minimize the risk of delayed kidney graft function by shortening cold ischemia time so that the retained third-space fluid may be rapidly eliminated to avoid an episode of heart failure or pulmonary edema.

Complications Associated with Bladder Drainage

Many mild to moderately severe complications arise because of the unusual physiologic consequences of draining pancreatic exocrine secretions into the bladder (24) (Fig. 47-10). The pancreas transplant eliminates approximately 500 cc of richly bicarbonate fluid with pancreatic enzymes into the bladder each day. Change in pH of the bladder accounts, in part, for an increase in urinary tract infections. In some cases a foreign body, such as an exposed suture from the duodenocystotomy, acts as a nidus for urinary tract infections or stone formation. Acute postoperative hematuria of the bladder-drained pancreas is usually due to ischemia/reperfusion injury to the duodenal mucosa or to a bleeding vessel on the suture line that is aggravated by antiplatelet or anticoagulation protocols to minimize vascular thrombosis. Small amounts of hematuria require only close observation, but larger clots may

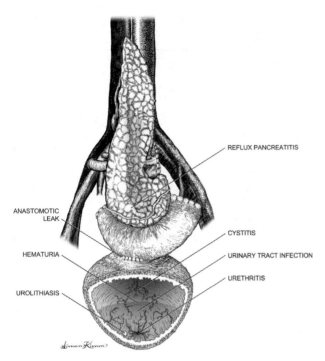

REFLUX PANCREATITIS

ANASTOMOTIC
LEAK

HEMATURIA

UROLITHIASIS

CYSTITIS

URINARY TRACT INFECTION

URETHRITIS

Figure 47-10 Postoperative complications associated with the bladder-drained pancreas transplant.

need continuous bladder irrigation or direct cytoscopic evaluation and cautery. Occasionally it is necessary to perform a formal open cystotomy with suture ligation of the bleeding vessel intraoperatively.

Sterile cystitis, urethritis, and balanitis may occur after bladder-drained pancreas transplantation due to the effect of the pancreatic enzymes on urinary tract mucosa. Cystitis is more common in male recipients. Urethritis can progress to urethral perforation and perineal pain. Conservative treatment with catheterization and operative enteric conversion are the extremes of the continuum of treatment.

Metabolic/fluid/electrolyte complications may be exacerbated by the procedure of pancreatic exocrine bladder drainage. Metabolic acidosis routinely develops as a consequence of bladder excretion of large quantities of the alkaline pancreatic secretions. Patients must receive oral bicarbonate supplementation to minimize the degree of acidosis. Bladder drained pancreas recipients may have difficulty compensating for the added fluid losses. Some immunosuppressive agents (e.g., mycophenolate mofetil) induce lower gastrointestinal dysfunction, resulting in increased bowel activity of a watery nature that may exacerbate the propensity for dehydration in the patient with a bladder-drained pancreas allograft. Careful monitoring of serum electrolytes and acid-base balance is necessary. Electrolyte and fluid repletion may be necessary to avoid dehydration. Patients should be started on fluid and bicarbonate supplementation early and educated about this entity prior to discharge in order to prevent severe dehydration and possible graft loss.

Reflux pancreatitis can result in acute inflammation of the pancreas graft, mimicking acute rejection. Reflux pancreatitis is associated with pain and hyperamylasemia and is believed to be secondary to reflux of urine through the ampulla and into the pancreatic ducts. Often the urine is contaminated with bacteria. Bacterial contamination occurs in patients with neurogenic bladder dysfunction. This complication is managed acutely by Foley catheterization. The patient may require a complete workup of the cause of bladder dysfunction, including a pressure flow study and voiding cystourethrogram. In older male patients, even mild hypertrophy of the prostate has been described as a cause of reflux pancreatitis. If recurrent graft pancreatitis occurs, enteric conversion may be indicated.

Urine leak from breakdown of the duodenal segment can occur and is usually encountered within the first 2 to 3 months post-transplant, but it can occur years postoperatively. Leak is the most serious postoperative complication of the bladder-drained pancreas. The onset of abdominal pain with elevated serum amylase, which can mimic reflux pancreatitis or acute rejection, is a typical presentation. Supporting imaging studies utilizing a cystogram or computed tomography (CT) scanning are necessary to confirm the diagnosis. Operative repair is usually required. The degree of leakage can be best determined intraoperatively and proper judgment made about whether direct repair is possible or more aggressive surgery involving enteric diversion (25) (Fig. 47-11) or graft pancreatectomy is indicated.

Infection

The most serious complication of the pancreas transplantation is leak and intra-abdominal abscess. Patients present with fever, abdominal discomfort, and leukocytosis. Computed tomographic study of the abdomen is helpful to confirm clinical suspicion and to localize infected peripancreatic fluid collections (Fig. 47-12). Duodenoenteric anastomotic leak occurs as a result of an ischemic duodenal stump, technical error, or duodenal stump blowout. Percutaneous access of intra-abdominal fluid collections for Gram stain and culture is essential. The flora is typically mixed with bacteria and possibly fungus (26), particularly *Candida*. Broad-spectrum antibiosis is essential. Surgical exploration is required if conservative methods of percutaneous drainage do not adequately control established infection.

Intraoperative findings usually reveal fibrinous adhesive disease with interloop abscess. Exploration repair of a duodenal graft leak is necessary. A decision must be made on whether the infection can be eradicated without removing the pancreas allograft. Incomplete eradication of the infection will result in progression to sepsis and multiple organ system failure. Peripancreatic infections can result in development of a mycotic aneurysm at the arterial anastomosis that could cause arterial rupture. Transplant pancreatectomy is indicated if mycotic aneurysm is diagnosed.

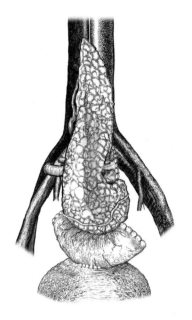

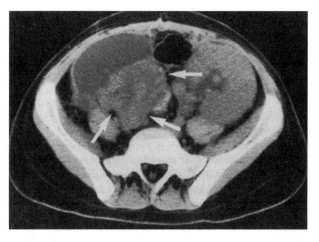

Figure 47-12 Computed tomographic study of a well-marginated, low-density fluid collection anterior to the pancreas transplant (*arrows*). (Reprinted from Letourneau JG, Day DL, Ascher NL. *Radiology of organ transplantation*. St. Louis: Mosby, 1991:278, with permission.)

Immunologic Complications

The most important threat to loss of a functioning pancreas allograft is acute rejection. The graft's fate is intimately linked to the efficacy and safety of immunosuppressive agents and the recipient's medical compliance. Through judicious application of immunosuppression, both rejection and infectious complications may be avoided. Pancreatic allograft monitoring to diagnose acute rejection in a timely manner is essential to achieve long-term survival. Overtreatment of a suspected rejection episode can be a serious cause of infectious morbidity and mortality in pancreas transplant recipients.

Pancreas allograft rejection can be characterized as hyperacute, acute, and chronic. Hyperacute rejection occurs minutes to hours following revascularization of the pancreas graft. Hyperacute rejection occurs when preformed anti-HLA antibodies bind to graft endothelium, activate the compliment cascade, and produce capillary microthombi. Hyperacute rejection is rare if the pretransplant screening crossmatch is nonreactive. This form of rejection can be a difficult diagnosis because of the relatively high incidence of early organ failure due to vascular thrombosis. The few cases published describe negative crossmatches in recipients with high panel-reactive antibody levels (27).

Acute pancreatic graft rejection typically occurs 3 to 12 months post-transplant but can happen later if medical noncompliance occurs. Acute rejection is primarily a function of cell-mediated cytotoxicity. The initial cellular targets of rejection are endothelial cells, acinar, and ductal epithelial cells. Islets and β cells are not primary targets of allo-immune rejection (27). Islets may be involved late in rejection and may also stop functioning before becoming involved with inflammatory cells (28,29).

Chronic rejection is a more indolent process that occurs relatively late in the course of transplantation. The most notable contributing factor includes multiple acute

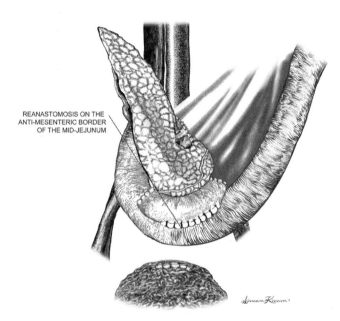

REANASTOMOSIS ON THE
ANTI-MESENTERIC BORDER
OF THE MID-JEJUNUM

Figure 47-11 Surgical procedure of enteric conversion of the bladder-drained pancreaticoduodenal transplant.

The occurrence of intra-abdominal abscess has been greatly reduced with greater recognition of the suitability of cadaveric pancreas grafts for transplantation. Improved perioperative antibiosis, including antifungal agents, has contributed to the decreased incidence of intra-abdominal infection as well. There is no convincing evidence that a Roux-en-Y intestinal reconstruction decreases incidence. Perhaps the most significant contribution to reducing intra-abdominal abscesses is the efficacy of the immunosuppressive agents in reducing acute rejection and thereby minimizing the need for intensive antirejection immunotherapy.

rejection episodes (30). Chronic rejection in the pancreas is characterized by arterial narrowing and interstitial fibrosis with variable loss of acinar and islet tissue (29,31). Arteriopathy causes progressive ischemic damage to the acinar and islet tissues, resulting in extensive pancreatic fibrosis.

Diagnosis

The clinical presentation of pancreas allograft rejection can be subtle. Only 5% to 20% of patients with pancreatic graft rejection present with obvious clinical symptoms. The pancreatic graft undergoing acute rejection becomes inflamed. Patients experience pain and discomfort due to surrounding peritoneal irritation, but rejection is difficult to distinguish clinically from benign graft pancreatitis. Fever as a clinical symptom of rejection is uncommon, partly due to maintenance immunosuppressive therapy with prednisone. If the workup for infection is negative, fever is highly suspicious for rejection. A paralytic ileus or acute abdomen rarely occurs but can be caused by rejection-induced pancreatitis. Inflammation of the surrounding organs, such as the small and large intestine, may result in a dynamic ileus or diarrhea, respectively.

Laboratory markers are commonly relied on to guide subsequent imaging studies or biopsy. Profound destruction of exocrine pancreatic tissue occurs prior to significant deterioration in endocrine pancreatic function (32). Hyperglycemia is a late parameter of rejection and is usually apparent only after extensive destruction of the islets has taken place. Hyperglycemia is not useful to diagnose acute rejection that is likely to be reversed. Hyperglycemia is also a sign of development of peripheral insulin resistance (type 2 diabetes). Differentiation of loss of β cell insulin production (rejection) is accomplished by measurement of C-peptide levels. Using pancreas-specific serum markers to detect rejection is problematic due to the pathophysiology of the exocrine pancreas. Rejection, as well as pancreatitis, infection, or preservation injury, leads to damage of acinar tissue, with subsequent enzyme and cytokine release. The causes of destruction of pancreas acinar tissue are multiple and, with pancreas-specific serum parameters only, difficult to differentiate.

An increase in serum amylase usually occurs with rejection and precedes a decline in urinary amylase (in recipients with bladder-drained pancreas) (33,34). Post-transplant hyperamylasemia can be caused by any process inducing pancreatic inflammation. In addition, serum amylase is also derived in large part from other tissues, including salivary glands and intestine. Several studies of SPK transplant recipients showed elevated human anodal trypsinogen (HAT) levels during clinically diagnosed rejection episodes (35). HAT levels are frequently elevated in the early post-transplant period, which may reflect preservation or procurement injury rather than rejection. Renal dysfunction, pancreatitis, trauma, and bladder outlet obstruction may also influence HAT levels. One study included both renal biopsies and HAT levels performed on SPK and PAK recipients, finding HAT a reliable marker of pancreas rejection in all cases (36).

In the context of SPK transplantation, the kidney allograft is the best indicator of a rejection episode. Rejection of the kidney allograft will manifest as a rise in serum creatinine. Increased serum creatinine will prompt ultrasound and biopsy of the kidney allograft, and if rejection is diagnosed, antirejection therapy is instituted. If there is a concurrent pancreas graft rejection process, the antirejection therapy will reverse the process in both organs.

Bladder drainage is a widely used technique for management of exocrine secretion in pancreatic transplantation because it also allows graft exocrine function to be monitored by measuring pancreatic enzymes secreted directly into the urine (37). Bladder drainage is mostly used in recipients of PAK and PTA. The technique is becoming less frequently used in SPK transplant recipients because monitoring renal allograft function serves as a better indication of rejection (and a surrogate marker of pancreas graft rejection) and there is less morbidity of enteric drainage. Serial urine amylase measurement has emerged as a very common surveillance and diagnostic laboratory test. A reduction in urinary amylase activity, relative hypoamylasuria, is the most commonly used biochemical marker of acute rejection in the PAK and PTA recipient categories. By monitoring urinary amylase levels, antirejection treatment can begin before hyperglycemia occurs. Urinary amylase measurements are simple, without morbidity, and relatively inexpensive, and most laboratories can perform them. One of the limitations of urinary amylase monitoring is that a decrease in activity does not necessarily mean rejection. Reduced urinary amylase levels may be caused by other factors, such as preservation injury in the early post-transplant period, pancreatitis, fibrosis, thrombosis, ductal obstruction, prolonged fasting, hydration status, and diuresis (38).

Needle core biopsy is the standard for the diagnosis of pancreas allograft rejection in the context of PAK and PTA. For most solid organ transplants histologic evaluation of graft biopsies became the standard assessment for rejection early on. For pancreas transplantation the development was different for two reasons. It is rare that isolated pancreatic rejection occurs in SPK transplant recipients without simultaneous renal allograft rejection. In these patients most rejection episodes involve either the kidney alone or the kidney and the pancreas simultaneously (39). This observation has promoted the perception that pancreatic graft rejection can be monitored indirectly by relying on serum creatinine changes or kidney graft biopsies. For SPK transplants the kidney serves as an excellent surrogate marker for rejection. In recipients of solitary pancreas transplants (PTA, PAK), serum creatinine levels or kidney biopsies cannot be used as markers of rejection, and, given the inadequacies of laboratory parameters, biopsies are therefore essential for monitoring solitary pancreas transplants. In SPK transplant recipients, isolated pancreatic graft rejection can occur and pancreatic graft biopsies may become necessary if a change in exocrine or endocrine laboratory parameters occurs without an elevation in serum creatinine.

Currently, the vast majority of pancreatic graft biopsies are obtained either percutaneously or cystoscopically and only rarely by laparotomy or laparoscopy. Most centers prefer ultrasound-guided, percutaneous biopsy, performed under local anesthesia. If it is impossible to obtain tissue for histology or if overlying bowel prohibits sampling, the cystoscopic approach is employed for bladder-drained grafts. Laparotomy or laparoscopy and biopsy is reserved for grafts inaccessible by the aforementioned approaches when the risks of empiric antirejection therapy outweigh those of surgery.

Immunosuppression

Over the past decade pancreas transplantation results have improved significantly due to advances in immunosuppression. The principles of immunosuppressive therapy for pancreas recipients are similar to those applied to recipients of other solid-organ allografts. The advent of more effective immunomodulating agents has reduced the frequency and severity of pancreatic allograft rejection episodes. However, acute rejection continues to be the most challenging event in the course of pancreatic graft recipients.

The use of induction therapy has been shown to significantly improve pancreas graft survival rates in several subgroups. According to data from the IPTR, the use of induction therapy in SPK transplant recipients with systemic venous-enteric exocrine drainage significantly improves pancreas graft survival rates (40,41). Interestingly, pancreas graft survival is not improved with induction therapy in the subgroups with portal venous-enteric or bladder drainage. Furthermore, SPK transplant recipients who receive induction therapy benefit from a reduced incidence and severity of biopsy-confirmed, treated, acute kidney rejection episodes. For solitary pancreas recipients (PAK and PTA), the addition of induction therapy is associated with a clinically significant improvement in pancreas graft survival rates.

Maintenance immunosuppressive agents used for pancreas transplantation fall into the following categories: (a) corticosteroids, (b) calcineurin inhibitors (cyclosporine and tacrolimus), (c) antimetabolites (azathioprine and mycophenolate mofetil), and (d) cell cycle inhibitors (sirolimus). In 2002 solitary pancreas recipients received corticosteroids in approximately 90% of cases, tacrolimus in 91% (cyclosporine 8%), mycophenolate mofetil in 70% (azathioprine 1%), and sirolimus in 18%. Therefore, in 2002 the most frequently used combination of maintenance therapy at discharge was tacrolimus, mycophenolate mofetil, and corticosteroids.

Trends in the uses of maintenance therapies over the past 10 years for solitary (PAK and PTA) transplant recipients are depicted in Figure 47-13. The dominant use of tacrolimus today represents a marked shift from earlier eras. The U.S. Food and Drug Administration (FDA) approved

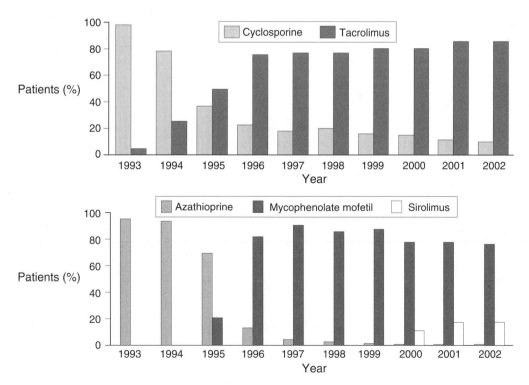

Figure 47-13 Trends in maintenance immunosuppression in recipients of solitary pancreas transplants. (From 2003 OPTN/SRTR Annual Report, with permission.)

tacrolimus for marketing for kidney transplantation in 1994. In 1993 cyclosporine accounted for virtually 100% of the calcineurin inhibitor use in pancreas transplantation. Since that time, tacrolimus use has increased yearly and reached 91% in 2002. The FDA approved mycophenolate mofetil for marketing for kidney transplantation in 1995, and it was used in only 14% of solitary pancreas transplant cases that year (azathioprine was used in 72% of cases). However, within 1 year, nearly 80% of solitary pancreas transplant recipients received mycophenolate mofetil, with only 12% receiving azathioprine. The use of azathioprine has diminished yearly and dropped to 1% usage in 2002. In 1999 the FDA approved the use of sirolimus for marketing for kidney transplantation. For pancreas transplantation this agent is usually used in combination with a calcineurin inhibitor and as a substitute for an antimetabolite. The use of sirolimus has been relatively slow to penetrate the market, compared to the rapid spread of tacrolimus and mycophenolate mofetil. In 2002 sirolimus was used for 18% of solitary pancreas cases.

Similar trends in maintenance immunosuppression were also observed for recipients of SPK transplants. In 2002, 86% of SPK transplant recipients received corticosteroids, 88% tacrolimus (9% cyclosporine), 79% mycophenolate mofetil, and 18% sirolimus. On the basis of these data, one can extrapolate that the most common maintenance immunosuppressive regimen used in SPK transplant recipients included tacrolimus, mycophenolate mofetil, and corticosteroids.

Trends in the uses of maintenance therapies over the past 10 years for SPK transplant recipients are depicted in Figure 47-14. The use of tacrolimus rose from 17% in 1994 to 88% in 2002. Because tacrolimus is used as a replacement for cyclosporine, cyclosporine usage has dropped from nearly 100% of cases in 1993 to only 9% of cases in 2002. Similar trends in the use of antimetabolites are seen with respect to azathioprine and mycophenolate mofetil. In 1993 azathioprine was used in nearly 100% of cases, dropping to 1% in 2002; mycophenolate mofetil usage grew from 25% in 1995 to 79% in 2002. From 2000 to 2002 sirolimus usage rose from 12% to 18% of cases.

TECHNICAL AND IMMUNOLOGICAL PROGRESS IN PANCREATIC TRANSPLANTATION

Table 47-8 shows that the overall rate of technical failure has progressively diminished since 1987. In the early period (1987 to 1992) the technical failure rate was 15% to 24%. In the most current era (2001 to 2003) the rate has decreased to 7% to 8%. Pancreas transplant results have steadily improved. According to the SRTR and the IPTR, over the past 10 years pancreas graft survival in SPK recipients has increased from 74% to 84% (42). For PAK transplantation, pancreas graft survival has shown steady improvement over the 10-year interval 1993 through 2002 from a 1-year patient survival rate of 65% to 82%. For patients receiving a PTA, the pancreas graft functional survival rates over the past 10 years has improved from 55% to 80%.

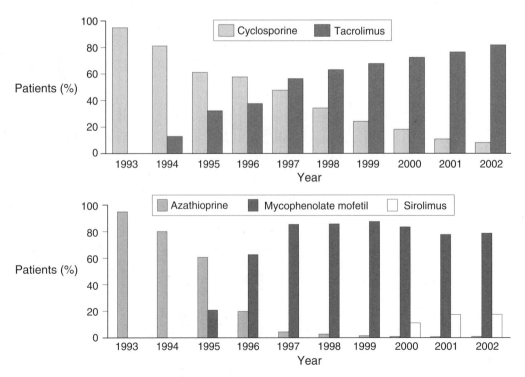

Figure 47-14 Trends in maintenance immunosuppression in recipients of simultaneous pancreas-kidney transplants. (From 2003 OPTN/SRTR Annual Report, with permission.)

TABLE 47-8				
TECHNICAL FAILURE RATE OF PANCREAS TRANSPLANTATION (10/87–12/03)				
	1987–1992 (%)	1993–1995 (%)	1996–1998 (%)	1999–2000 (%)	2001–2003 (%)
SPK	15	12	10	10	7
PAK	21	17	19	13	7
PTA	24	20	18	14	8

Changes in clinical practice patterns regarding the use of the maintenance immunosuppressive agents have had a significant beneficial effect on outcomes of pancreas transplantation (40). To illustrate the point, three eras have been identified over the last decade (1993 to 2002) in which OPTN pancreas transplant data are available that depicts the progressive improvement in outcome. The period of 1993 to 1995 reflects use of today's "second line" immunosuppressants (cyclosporine and azathioprine), 1996 to 1998 is the period in which new agents (tacrolimus, mycophenolate, and sirolimus) were introduced, and 1999 to 2002 reflects the period of mature integration of the new "first line" immunosuppressive agents into mainstream use. Figure 47-15 shows pancreas allograft 1-year survival rates according to transplant era. Pancreas graft survival rates increased from 80% to 84% in SPK transplant recipients and increased from 60% to 77% in solitary pancreas transplant recipients. Figure 47-16 shows 1-year rejection rates according to transplant era. Rejection rates decreased from 59% to 20% in SPK transplant recipients and decreased from 56% to 23% in solitary pancreas transplant recipients.

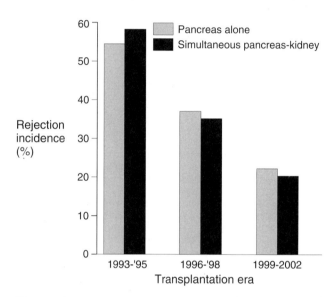

Figure 47-16 Pancreas allograft 1-year rejection rates according to transplant era. Outcomes based on data from the Organ Procurement And Transplant Network (OPTN) as of January 2, 2004. Outcomes represent all US cases of simultaneous pancreas-kidney (SKP) and pancreas-alone transplants performed from January 1993 to December 2002.

Aggregate outcome information from national databases and single center reports (43) demonstrate that improvements in the technical and immunologic approaches to pancreatic transplantation have moved the field forward. However, further refinements are needed to decrease complication rates. Continued advances in immunotherapy combined with technical refinements will make pancreatic transplantation a safer and more widely applied treatment option for patients with diabetes.

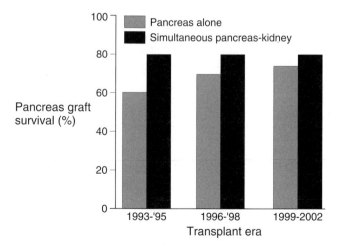

Figure 47-15 Pancreas allograft 1-year survival rates according to transplant era. Outcomes based on data from the Organ Procurement and Transplant Network (OPTN) as of January 2, 2004. Outcomes represent all US cases of simultaneous pancreas-kidney and pancreas-alone transplants performed from January 1993 to June 2002.

REFERENCES

1. Portuese E, Orchard T. Mortality in insulin-dependent diabetes. In: Harris MI, Cowie CC, Stern MP, Boyko EJ, Reiber GE, Bennett PH, eds. *Diabetes in America*, Washington, DC: US Government Printing Office; 1995:221–232.
2. National Diabetes Data Group, National Institutes of Health. *Diabetes in America*, 2nd ed. Bethesda, MD: National Institutes of Health, 1995. NIH Publication No. 95-1468.
3. Epidemiology of Diabetes Interventions and Complications (EDIC) Research Group. Effect of intensive diabetes treatment

on carotid artery wall thickness in the epidemiology of diabetes interventions and complications. Epidemiology of Diabetes Interventions and Complications (EDIC) Research Group. *Diabetes* 1999;48:383–390.

4. DCCT/EDIC Research Group. Effect of intensive therapy on the microvascular complications of type 1 diabetes mellitus. *JAMA* 2002;287:2563–2569.

5. Morel P, Goetz F, Moudry-Munns KC, et al. Long term metabolic control in patients with pancreatic transplants. *Ann Intern Med* 1991;115:694–699.

6. Navarro X, Kennedy WR, Loewenson RB, et al. Influence of pancreas transplantation on cardiorespiratory reflexes, nerve conduction, and mortality in diabetes mellitus. *Diabetes* 1990;39:802–806.

7. Kennedy WR, Navarro X, Goetz FC, et al. Effects of pancreatic transplantation on diabetic neuropathy. *N Engl J Med* 1990;322:1031–1037.

8. Fioretto P, Mauer SM, Bilous RW, et al. Effects of pancreas transplantation on glomerular structure in insulin-dependent diabetic patients with their own kidneys. *Lancet* 1993;342:1193–1196.

9. Bilous RW, Mauer SM, Sutherland DE, et al. The effects of pancreas transplantation on the glomerular structure of renal allografts in patients with insulin-dependent diabetes. *N Engl J Med* 1989;321:80–85.

10. Zehr PS, Milde FK, Hart LK, et al. Pancreas transplantation: assessing secondary complications and life quality. *Diabetologia* 1991;34(Suppl. 1):S138–S140.

11. Ojo AO, Meier-Kriesche HU, Hanson JA, et al. Impact of simultaneous pancreas-kidney transplantation on long-term patient survival. *Transplantation* 2001;71:82–90.

12. Mohan P, Safi K, Little DM, et al. Improved patient survival in recipients of simultaneous pancreas-kidney transplant compared with kidney transplant alone in patients with type 1 diabetes mellitus and end-stage renal disease. *Br J Surg* 2003;90:1137–1141.

13. http://ustransplant.org/csr_0104/center.php 2/1/2004.

14. Kroslewski AS, Kosinski EJ, Warram JH, et al. Magnitude and determinants of coronary artery disease in juvenile-onset, insulin-dependent diabetes mellitus. *Am J Cardiol* 1987;59:750–755.

15. Borch-Johnsen K, Kreiner S. Proteinuria: value as predictor of cardiovascular mortality in insulin dependent diabetes mellitus. *Br Med J* 1987;294:1651–1654.

16. Grundy SM, Benjamin IJ, Burke GL, et al. Diabetes and cardiovascular disease: a statement for healthcare professionals from the American Heart Association. *Circulation* 1999;100:1134–1146.

17. Blanchet P, Droupy S, Eschwege P, et al. Urodynamic testing predicts long-term urological complications following simultaneous pancreas-kidney transplantation. *Clin Transplant* 2003;17:26–31.

18. Pirsch JD, Odorico JS, D'Alessandro AM, et al. Intra-abdominal infection in enteric versus bladder-drained simultaneous pancreas-kidney transplant recipients. *Transplantation* 1998;66:1746–1750.

19. Troppmann C, Gruessner AC, Benedetti E, et al. Vascular graft thrombosis after pancreatic transplantation: univariate and multivariate operative and nonoperative risk factor analysis. *J Am Coll Surg* 1996;182:285–316.

20. Wullstein C, Woeste G, Zapletal C, et al. Prothromotic disorders in uremic type-1 diabetics undergoing simultaneous pancreas and kidney transplantation. *Transplantation* 2003;76:1691–1695.

21. Booster MH, Schoenmakers EA, Rijnders AJ, et al. Perfusion imaging of pancreas allografts using technetium-99m hexamethyl propylene amine oxime. *Transplant Int* 1992;5(Suppl.1):S265–S267.

22. Gilabert R, Fernandez-Cruz L, Real MI, et al. Treatment and outcome of pancreatic venous graft thrombosis after kidney—pancreas transplantation. *Br J Surg* 2002;89:355–360.

23. Barone GW, Webb JW, Hudec WA. The enteric drained pancreas transplant: another potential source of gastrointestinal bleeding. *Am J Gastroenterol* 1998;93:1369–1371.

24. Sollinger HW, Messing EM, Eckhoff DE, et al. Urologic complications in 210 consecutive simultaneous pancreas-kidney transplants with bladder drainage. *Ann Surg* 1993;218:561–568.

25. West M, Gruessner AC, Metrakos P, et al. Conversion from bladder to enteric drainage after pancreaticoduodenal transplantations. *Surgery* 1998;124:883–893.

26. Benedetti E, Gruessner AC, Troppmann C, et al. Intra-abdominal fungal infections after pancreatic transplantation: incidence, treatment, and outcome. *J Am Coll Surg* 1996;183:307–316.

27. Sibley RK. Pancreas transplantation. In: Sale GE, ed. *The Pathology of Organ Transplantation*, Boston, MA: Butterworth-Heineman; 1990:179–215.

28. Nakhleh RE, Gruessner RWG, Swanson PE, et al. Pancreas transplant pathology: a morphologic immunohistochemical, and electron microscopic comparison of allogeneic grafts with rejection, syngeneic grafts, and chronic pancreatitis. *Am J Surg Pathol* 1991;15:246–256.

29. Nakhleh RE, Sutherland DER. Pancreas rejection: Significance of histopathologic findings with implication of classification for rejection. *Am J Surg Pathol* 1992;16:1098–1107.

30. Humar A, Khwaja K, Ramcharan T, et al. Chronic rejection: the next major challenge for pancreas transplant recipients. *Transplantation* 2003;76:918–923.

31. Papadimitriou JC, Drachenberg CB, Klassen DK, et al. Histological grading of chronic pancreas allograft rejection/graft sclerosis. *Am J Transplant* 2003;3:599–605.

32. Dragstedt LR. Some physiologic problems in surgery of the pancreas. *Ann Surg* 1943;118:576–593.

33. Tyden G, Gunnarsson R, Ostman J, et al. Laboratory findings during rejection of segmental pancreatic allografts. *Transplant Proc* 1984;16:715–717.

34. Cheng SS, Munn SR. Posttransplant hyperamylasemia is associated with decreased patient and graft survival in pancreas allograft recipients. *Transplant Proc* 1994;26:428–429.

35. Marks WH, Borgstrom A, Sollinger H, et al. Serum immunoreactive anodal trypsinogen and urinary amylase as biochemical markers for rejection of clinical whole-organ pancreas allografts having exocrine drainage into the urinary bladder. *Transplantation* 1990;49:112–115.

36. Perkal M, Marks C, Lorber MI, et al. A three-year experience with serum anodal trypsinogen as a biochemical marker for rejection in pancreatic allografts. False positives, tissue biopsy, comparison with other markers, and diagnostic strategies. *Transplantation* 1992;53:415–419.

37. Prieto M, Sutherland DE, Fernandez-Cruz L, et al. Experimental and clinical experience with urine amylase monitoring for early diagnosis of rejection in pancreas transplantation. *Transplantation* 1987;43:73–79.

38. Munn SR, Engen DE, Barr D, et al. Differential diagnosis of hypoamylasuria in pancreas allograft recipients with urinary exocrine drainage. *Transplantation* 1990;49:359–362.

39. Gruessner RWG, Dunn DL, Tzardis PJ, et al. Simultaneous pancreas and kidney transplants versus single kidney transplants and previous kidney transplants in uremic patients and single pancreas transplants in nonuremic diabetic patients: comparison of rejection, morbidity, and long-term outcome. *Transplant Proc* 1990;22:622–623.

40. Gruessner AC and Sutherland DE. Pancreas transplant outcomes for United States (US) and Non-US cases as reported to the United Network for Organ Sharing (UNOS) and the International Pancreas Transplant Registry (IPTR) as of October, 2002. In: Cecka JM, Terasaki PI, eds. *Clinical Transplants 2002*. Los Angeles, CA: UCLA Tissue Typing Laboratory, 2002:41–77.

41. Kaufman DB. Induction therapy. In: Gruessner RWG, Sutherland DE, eds. *Transplantation of the Pancreas*. New York: Springer-Verlag, 2004:267–300.

42. Gruessner AC, Sutherland DE. Analysis of United States (US) and Non-US pancreas transplants reported to the United Network for Organ Sharing (UNOS) and the International Pancreas Transplant Registry (IPTR) as of October, 2001. In: Cecka JM, Terasaki PI, eds. *Clinical transplants 2001*. Los Angeles, CA: UCLA Tissue Typing Laboratory, 2001:41–72.

43. Kaufman DB, Leventhal JR, Gallon LG, et al. Technical and immunological progress in simultaneous pancreas-kidney transplantation. *Surgery* 2002;132:545–555.

Complications of Pulmonary Transplantation

Christine L. Lau   *Bryan F. Meyers*

48

■ **TECHNICAL COMPLICATIONS 683**
Suboptimal Donor Procurements 684
Complications During Recipient Operation 684

■ **POSTOPERATIVE COMPLICATIONS 686**
Ischemia-reperfusion Injury 686
Airway Complications 688
Infections 690

■ **PLEURAL SPACE COMPLICATIONS 693**
Hyperinflation 693
Pneumothorax 693
Pleural Effusion 693
Empyema 693

■ **REJECTION 694**
Acute Rejection 694
Chronic Allograft Rejection/Bronchiolitis Obliterans
    Syndrome 694

■ **NONPULMONARY COMPLICATIONS 695**
Gastrointestinal Complications 695
Post-transplant Lymphoproliferative Disease 695
Atrial Dysrhythmias 696
Renal Failure 696

Hyperammonemia 696
Thrombotic Thrombocytopenic Purpura
    (TTP)–Hemolytic Uremic Syndrome (HUS) 697

■ **CONCLUSION 697**

■ **REFERENCES 697**

Christine L. Lau: University of Michigan, Ann Arbor, MI 48109
Bryan F. Meyers: Washington University School of Medicine, St.
Louis, MO 63110

Over the past three decades, lung transplantation has become an accepted treatment option for a variety of end-stage pulmonary diseases. Improvements in organ preservation, surgical techniques, infection prophylaxis, and immunosuppression medications have resulted in durable and steady improvements in lung transplant outcomes and have allowed for expanded uses of lung transplantation. As a result of these evolutionary changes, recipients are surviving longer after transplant and some late complications arising from the procedure and years of immunosuppression are becoming increasingly evident. It is thus important to have a working knowledge of the common complications, when these complications are most likely to occur, and how best to treat them.

TECHNICAL COMPLICATIONS

It is important to identify and correct technical complications that arise during the lung transplant operation.

Transplant operations of all types are unique in that they have two components: the retrieval of the organ from the donor and the implantation of the organ into the recipient. Technical complications can occur during either phase of the operation, but the main burden of either type of complication will fall upon the recipient. A unique exception to that statement occurs in the instance of living-related lobar transplantation, a phenomenon in which two living donors each donate a lower lobe of one lung to allow the recipient to receive bilateral lobes as lung replacements. In this extraordinary situation, three persons are susceptible to perioperative complications. This chapter will focus on complications borne by the recipients, but interested readers can learn about potential pitfalls for lobar donors by reviewing the report by Battafarano et al. (1).

Suboptimal Donor Procurements

Atrial Cuff and Pulmonary Vein Injuries

Despite the best efforts of both the heart and lung procurement teams to equitably share the left atrial cuff, the donor lungs will occasionally arrive at the recipient operating room with insufficient atrial cuff or injuries to the pulmonary vein orifices. When injuries do occur, they most frequently involve the right inferior pulmonary vein. Such injuries usually occur as a result of poor visibility or undue haste during the division of the left atrial cuff. When a pulmonary vein orifice has been lacerated, repair begins by dividing the pericardium overlying the vein, exposing the vessel until it disappears into the lung parenchyma. Small branches of the vein may have been divided if the vein orifice has been entered. These are identified and oversewn to prevent troublesome bleeding after reperfusion.

Casula et al. (2) have described a technique of augmenting the pulmonary veins using donor pericardium when the left atrium cuff is inadequate. This method can be used to create a cuff even when the superior and inferior pulmonary veins have been completely separated. A running 5-0 polypropylene suture is used around each vein orifice, tacking the intima to the pericardium and creating a "neoatrial cuff." Scissors are then used to trim the newly created pericardial cuff and separate it from the other hilar structures. This pericardial cuff substitutes for donor atrium in the atrial anastomosis. Alternatively, donor superior vena cava or redundant donor pulmonary artery can be used for the reconstruction if there is inadequate tissue.

Pulmonary Artery Injuries

The bifurcation of the pulmonary artery should always be left attached to the lung graft at the time of procurement. Even when a heart transplant is planned from the same donor, division of the pulmonary artery at the distal extent of the main trunk, proximal to the bifurcation, leaves sufficient length of artery for the safe implantation of the heart.

Common locations for pulmonary artery injuries during the donor procurement include the right pulmonary artery as it travels behind the aorta or, even more problematic, posterior to the superior vena cava. Since the right pulmonary artery is substantially longer than the left, injury to this vessel behind the aorta rarely requires repair and the artery can be simply trimmed distal to the laceration. More serious injuries to the right pulmonary artery can occur deep to the superior vena cava. At this location the first branch of the right pulmonary artery can be lacerated, and repair, rather than trimming, is required. The laceration can simply be repaired in most cases, but if a more complex reconstruction of the truncus anterior is required, a patch or complete reimplantation may be used to prevent loss of diameter in the repaired vessel. The repair can be performed with a segment of donor vena cava, azygous vein, or redundant donor pulmonary artery.

Bronchial and Parenchymal Injuries

It is unusual for any significant injury to occur to the lung parenchyma or main bronchi during procurement. Most parenchymal injuries would simply result in a prolonged air leak after implantation. Special care should be taken to avoid injury to the lung parenchyma when the implantation is to be performed with cardiopulmonary bypass, as even small parenchymal injuries may lead to endobronchial bleeding under circumstances of profound anticoagulation for bypass.

Parenchymal injury in a different sense can occur in an atraumatic manner due to technical problems with delivery of the flush solution used to cool and preserve the lungs during the period of extracorporeal ischemia. Inadequate flushing of the lungs may lead to profound ischemia reperfusion injury and poor initial graft function. One extreme example occurred in a bilateral lung transplant performed by the authors for cystic fibrosis. On the routine postoperative perfusion scan, no flow was seen perfusing the left lung. A pulmonary arteriogram demonstrated a patent anastomosis without evidence of technical flaws to account for the absent blood flow in the lung. Re-exploration revealed an edematous ischemic lung with severe reperfusion injury requiring removal of the graft. The conclusion was that the flush of the preservative solution had somehow been directed down the right pulmonary artery preferentially and exclusively, thus exposing the left lung to the "no-reflow phenomenon" due to severe ischemic injury.

Complications During Recipient Operation

Phrenic Nerve Injuries

Dense adhesions present at the time of explantation can increase the risk of bleeding and of injuries to the phrenic nerve and left recurrent laryngeal nerve. These adhesions are most likely to be present in patients with septic lung diseases (cystic fibrosis and bronchiectasis) and in patients who have had previous thoracic surgery. Particularly dense adhesions have been seen in emphysema patients who have undergone previous lung volume reduction surgery. In a multicenter experience of 35 lung transplant patients who had previously undergone lung volume reduction surgery, phrenic nerve injury was recorded in two patients (5.7%) (3). Frequently the phrenic nerve is adherent to the lung volume reduction staple line and makes its dissection tedious and dangerous. To avoid injury to the phrenic nerve, we have opted to leave the staple line and a small amount of residual lung tissue attached to the phrenic nerve using a lung stapler to divide the densely attached tissue. The use of electrocautery to dissect mediastinal adhesions will greatly increase the risk of phrenic nerve injury.

If a phrenic nerve is injured, little can be done to remedy the situation acutely. In the setting of bilateral transplant, the fact that both lungs are being replaced will mitigate the impact of a unilateral phrenic injury. In these circumstances the overall outcome will be satisfactory and there is a risk for under-reporting of complications. If a phrenic nerve injury occurs during a unilateral transplant, the transplant's benefit to the patient will be greatly diminished. It has been exceedingly rare in our experience or in the reported literature for a patient to require diaphragmatic plication after lung transplantation.

Hemorrhage

Hemorrhage was once a frequent complication after lung transplantation. Indeed, in the early experience of some programs undertaking heart-lung and en bloc double-lung transplants, approximately 25% of patients required reoperation for postoperative hemorrhage. However, with current surgical techniques, such as posterolateral thoracotomy for single-lung transplantation and the "clamshell" or "sternal-sparing clamshell" incisions for bilateral lung replacement, surgical exposure is superb (4). In addition to improved surgical exposure, it has been observed that aprotinin administration has reduced intraoperative and postoperative bleeding, especially in patients with extensive pleural adhesions requiring cardiopulmonary bypass.

Pulmonary Hypertension and Hypoxemia

Persistent pulmonary hypertension and unexplained hypoxemia can occur as a result of stenosis at the pulmonary artery anastomosis. A nuclear perfusion scan that demonstrates less than anticipated flow to a single-lung graft or unequal distribution of flow in a bilateral lung recipient can suggest this problem. Occasionally, transesophageal echocardiography can visualize a stenotic vascular anastomosis. Contrast angiography should be performed in any patient for whom there is such a concern. At the time of angiography the pressure gradient across the pulmonary artery anastomosis

should be determined. A gradient of 15 to 20 mm Hg is commonly encountered, especially in single-lung recipients in whom most cardiac output may be directed to the transplanted lung or in bilateral recipients with a high cardiac output. The clinical situation dictates the need for anastomotic revision. Dramatic reduction in flow should not be accepted, as the donor bronchus is totally dependent on pulmonary arterial collateral flow.

Compromised flow across the atrial anastomosis can also occur as a result of unsatisfactory anastomotic technique. Impaired venous outflow results in elevated venous pressure and ipsilateral pulmonary edema. Pulmonary artery pressures remain unexpectedly high in this situation, and flow through the graft is less than expected. Transesophageal echocardiography is often useful in visualizing the patency and flow through the atrial anastomoses. Contrast studies may be helpful in demonstrating a reduced level of flow through the anastomosis. Open exploration is occasionally necessary to confirm the diagnosis and conduct appropriate repair.

Sternal Complications

The bilateral trans-sternal thoracotomy provides excellent exposure to the hila and pleural spaces, but problems have been reported with poor sternal healing with the use of this incision. Brown et al. (5) report a prevalence of 36% for sternal disruption in transverse bilateral thoracosternotomy for lung transplantation in their institution, and they cite disruption rates of 20% to 60% at institutions worldwide. Lung transplant recipients may be particularly prone to poor sternal healing because of their debilitated state and the routine use of postoperative corticosteroids (6). A common sternal healing complication is "sternal override," which results because of the tendency toward angulation and anterior displacement of the distal sternum, a translational movement that is not prevented by sternal wires. The solution to sternal override has been the addition of coaxial stabilization—either long, thin Kirschner wires or short, stout Steinmann pins—placed within the cancellous bone of the sternum to eliminate sternal override and translational movement at the bony closure. The problem with such wires is their tendency to migrate. We have removed numerous wires from many patients after the discovery of their migration from the sternum to various locations in the body. Such retrievals have required interventions ranging from a local anesthetic to liberate a wire eroding through the anterior chest wall to a general anesthetic and a laparoscopic procedure to remove a Kirschner wire from the pouch of Douglas. An additional serious problem is deep sternal wound infection after transverse sternotomy. We have encountered this problem in several patients, and it has required operative and bedside wound debridement with additional antibiotics and a prolonged hospital stay. The estimated prevalence for all sternal closure complications in one historical control group is 34%. We routinely avoid sternal division and have found that bilateral anterior thoracotomies alone can provide adequate exposure in most circumstances. Additionally, in rare selected cases we also advocate modified approaches such as a combined left posterolateral and right anterior thoracotomy to optimize the left hilar exposure without the need for either sternal division or for a separate positioning, preparing, and draping.

POSTOPERATIVE COMPLICATIONS

The numerous complications that can occur after transplantation often occur along a predictable time course. Detailed discussion of the most important complications follows.

Ischemia-reperfusion Injury

Ischemia-reperfusion injury represents the most frequent cause of early mortality and prolonged ICU stay. A variety of factors, such as poor preservation techniques, prolonged ischemic time, or unsuspected donor lung pathology such as contusion, pulmonary thromboembolism, or aspiration, all play a role in the development of primary graft dysfunction. Hyperacute rejection is exceedingly rare, but it must be a consideration in cases of early severe lung dysfunction. The condition is characterized by noncardiogenic pulmonary edema and progressive lung injury over the first few hours following implantation. In its most severe form ischemia reperfusion injury is described as primary graft failure that pathologically appears as diffuse alveolar damage (Fig. 48-1). Irrespective of the cause, it is important to establish a diagnosis of early graft dysfunction and rule out other treatable conditions. One may perform open lung biopsy at the time of implantation if graft dysfunction is immediately apparent in the operating room. Additionally, serologic evaluation for anti-HLA antibodies may reveal evidence for hyperacute rejection in some of these patients.

Fortunately, severe reperfusion injury has not commonly been encountered in recent years. Superior strategies of

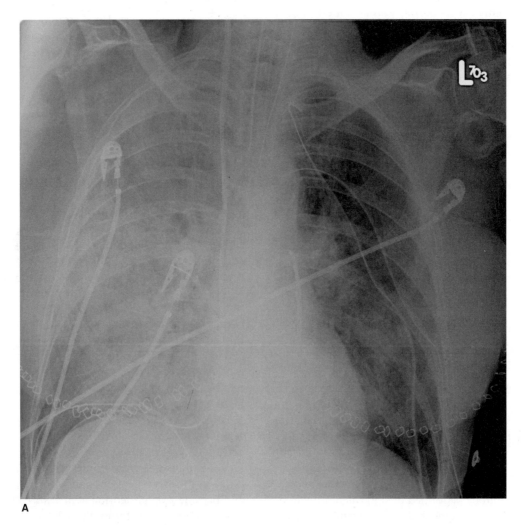

A

Figure 48-1   A: Chest radiograph showing severe right-sided ischemia-reperfusion injury following bilateral lung transplantation. Right lung was implanted first.

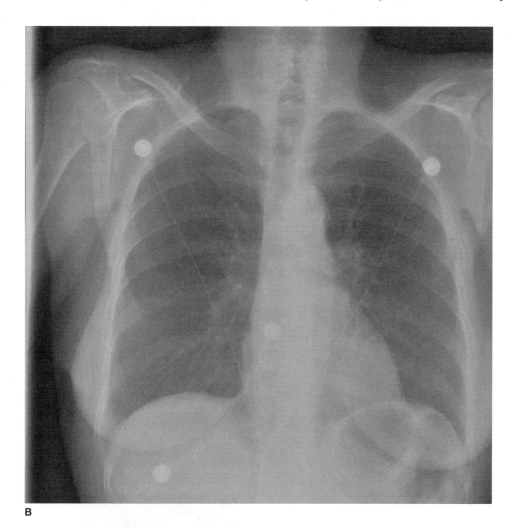

B

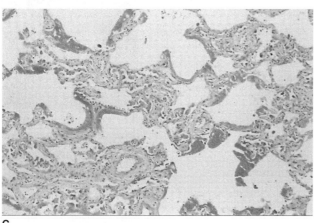

C

Figure 48-1 (*continued*) **B:** Chest radiograph of the same patient after resolution of ischemia-reperfusion injury. **C:** Transbronchial biopsy showing diffuse alveolar damage characteristic of ischemia-reperfusion injury.

lung preservation have evolved (7). It is clear from experimental (8) and clinical work (9) that low potassium dextran solution provides superior preservation than the high potassium preservation solutions previously in use. In addition, experimental work suggests that nitric oxide added to the flush solution at the time of harvest provides a preservation advantage (10). On the other hand, lung hyperinflation is an excellent model of postreperfusion pulmonary edema. One must therefore be particularly careful to avoid lung hyperinflation during harvest and storage of the donor lungs. Each of these factors has contributed to a reduction in the frequency of ischemia-reperfusion injury.

The notion of "controlled reperfusion" originally described efforts to reduce cardiac dysfunction after reperfusion of acutely ischemic myocardium at the time of coronary artery revascularization. Recently, the use of controlled reperfusion, in combination with leukocyte depletion (11–17), has shown promise as a preventive strategy for ischemia-reperfusion injury. Lick et al. (18) reported a small, nonrandomized series in humans using this technique and reported no reperfusion injury in the treated cohort of patients. At the time of reperfusion, leukocyte-filtered, pharmacologically modified perfusate is pumped into the newly implanted pulmonary artery at a controlled rate (200 mL per minute) and pressure (<20 mm Hg) for 10 minutes. The lung is ventilated with 50% inspired oxygen concentration during the period to further reduce the opportunity for oxygen radical mediated reperfusion injury.

In cases of established ischemia-reperfusion injury, proper treatment includes diuresis and maximal ventilatory support with simultaneous avoidance of additional ventilator induced injury. In most cases the reperfusion injury will resolve over 24 to 48 hours. Inhaled nitric oxide is of benefit in severe reperfusion injury as it decreases pulmonary artery pressure and improves the Pao_2/Fio_2 ratio (19). Recently, inhaled prostacyclin has shown promise as an economical alternative to nitric oxide (20).

Although standard intensive ventilatory and pharmacologic interventions generally suffice, severe graft dysfunction or coexisting cardiac failure may require extracorporeal membrane oxygenation (ECMO) support. Investigators have reported results of the use of ECMO after lung transplantation (21) and have found the technique to be satisfactory when the lung failure occurs immediately (<24 hours post-transplant). The etiology of graft failure in these cases was reperfusion lung injury. The frequency of reperfusion injury severe enough to warrant this therapy was <3% of all transplant operations. When deterioration occurs after 24 hours, it is often multifactorial and will be associated with lasting pathologic changes in the pulmonary parenchyma that are less likely solved by temporary ECMO support. An alternative approach to severe, reversible allograft dysfunction is reported by Eriksson and Steen (22), who have successfully used core cooling to reduce oxygen requirements and avoid ECMO while the lung injury heals.

Airway Complications

Airway complications were formerly a major cause of morbidity and mortality after pulmonary transplantation. Using standard methods of implantation, the donor bronchus is rendered ischemic, without reconstitution of its systemic bronchial artery circulation. The donor bronchus relies on collateral pulmonary artery blood flow during the first few days after transplantation. It has been demonstrated that pulmonary collateral flow makes a substantial contribution to bronchial viability at the level of the distal bronchus and lobar origin. A shortened donor bronchial length (two rings proximal to the upper lobe takeoff) reduces the length of donor bronchus dependent on collateral flow. Superior preservation, improved sepsis prophylaxis, and better immunosuppression have reduced the incidence of airway

complications. In a review of one experience, Date et al. (23) reported a reduction of the prevalence of anastomotic complications from 14% to 4%.

Airway complications are identified in a number of ways. Routine postoperative bronchoscopic surveillance generally provides early evidence that an anastomotic complication has occurred. On occasion, computed tomography (CT), performed for some other indication, demonstrates an unexpected airway stenosis or dehiscence. In fact, we learned that CT scanning is a useful diagnostic tool in the evaluation of documented or suspected donor airway complications (Fig. 48-2). Late airway stenoses generally manifest with symptoms of dyspnea, wheeze, or decreased FEV_1. Bronchoscopic assessment confirms the diagnosis. A normal bronchial anastomotic suture line will demonstrate a narrow rim of epithelial slough that ultimately heals.

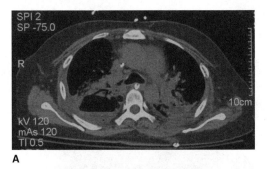

A

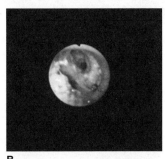

B

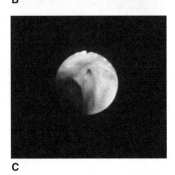

C

Figure 48-2 **A:** CT scan suggestive of right bronchial anastomotic dehiscence with a small amount of mediastinal air tracking from the right bronchial anastomosis and multiple loculated pneumothoraces. **B:** Bronchoscopy findings of right anastomotic dehiscence with a defect in the membranous wall. **C:** Follow-up bronchoscopy showing closing of the defect with a residual "pinhole," which ultimately healed.

Occasionally one can observe patchy areas of superficial necrosis of donor bronchial epithelium. These areas are also of no concern and ultimately heal without causing problems. Minor degrees of bronchial dehiscence are also of little long-term consequence. Membranous wall defects generally heal without any airway compromise, whereas cartilaginous defects usually result in some degree of late stricture. Significant dehiscence (>50% of the bronchial circumference) may result in compromise of the airway. This problem should be managed expectantly by mechanical debridement of the area to maintain satisfactory airway patency. A stent can be placed only if the distal main airway remains intact. Occasionally, a significant dehiscence results in direct communication with the pleural space, resulting in pneumothorax and a significant air leak following chest tube insertion. If the lung remains completely expanded and the pleural space is evacuated, the leak will ultimately seal and the airway may heal without significant stenosis. Similarly, a dehiscence may communicate directly with the mediastinum, resulting in significant mediastinal emphysema. If the lung remains completely expanded and the pleural space is filled, adequate drainage of the mediastinum can be achieved by placing a drain in close proximity to the anastomotic line by way of mediastinoscopy. This step will also result in satisfactory healing of the anastomosis, often without stricture.

A high incidence of postoperative airway dehiscence has been recently reported with the early use of sirolimus in lung transplant recipients (24). In a series of 15 patients treated in the early postoperative period with sirolimus, four patients experienced anastomotic dehiscences, and three of these four died. The use of sirolimus in the early post-transplant period should be discouraged.

Anastomotic Stenosis

Chronic airway stenoses can present significant management problems. A right main bronchial anastomotic stricture is generally managed easily by repeated dilatation and ultimate placement of an endobronchial stent. There is usually sufficient length for placement of a right main bronchial orifice stent without impingement of the right upper lobe bronchus. On the left side, however, strictures can be somewhat more difficult to manage. Dilatation of the distal left main bronchus is technically more difficult because of the angulation of that bronchus. In addition, the lobar bifurcation immediately distal to the usual site of anastomosis does not provide a suitable length of bronchus distal to the stricture for placement of large-caliber dilating bronchoscopes. Finally, Silastic stents placed across a distal left main bronchial anastomotic stricture may occlude the upper or lower lobe orifice as they bridge the stricture.

Silastic stents are tolerated exceptionally well. Patients may, however, require daily inhalation of N-acetylcystine

to keep the stents patent. De Hoyos et al. (25) reported that the stents have resulted in dramatic improvement in pulmonary function. Fortunately, most of these stents have proven to be required only temporarily. After several months, most stented anastomotic strictures maintain satisfactory patency without the stent in place.

Self-expanding metal stents have benefited from impressive technological improvement in recent years. These stents come in a wide variety of lengths and diameters, and they have been exceptionally easy to insert. In rare situations in which the airways distal to an anastomotic stricture are too small to accept a Silastic stent or when a Silastic stent will obstruct one bronchus while stenting another, the use of a self-expanding metal stent may suit the purpose. A caveat is that granulation tissue will rapidly overgrow an uncovered metal mesh stent, sometimes making it impossible to remove.

Finally, a recent addition to the armamentarium is a self-expanding plastic stent without interstices that allow granulation tissue ingrowth. This stent appears to incorporate the best aspects of the two predecessor stents and combine them in a useful device. Long-term data concerning stability and function of these stents are lacking.

Anastomotic Infections

Because of the inherent ischemia occurring at the bronchial anastomosis after lung transplantation, fungal infections may develop at this site. *Aspergillus* and *Candida* have been identified as potential pathogens that can cause life-threatening bronchial anastomotic infection (26). Nunley et al. (27) identified 15 (24.6%) saprophytic fungal infections involving the bronchial anastomoses in 61 recipients, with the majority of these infections due to *Aspergillus* species. Stenotic airway complications were more frequently seen in recipients with anastomotic infections (46.7%) compared to those without fungal infections (8.7%). Specific complications from fungal infections arising at the bronchial anastomoses included bronchial stenosis, bronchomalacia, and fatal hemorrhage. A variety of interventions, including bronchial stenting, balloon dilatation, electrocauterization, laser debridement, and radiation brachytherapy, have been used to treat these complications. Additionally, in this series three fatalities were associated (4.9%) with saprophytic bronchial anastomotic infections.

If bronchoscopic inspection reveals extensive anastomotic pseudomembranes, a biopsy of the site should be performed to rule out an invasive fungal infection. The optimal treatment of bronchial anastomotic fungal infection is unknown. Success has been reported with a combination of systemic and inhaled antifungal agents. The addition of the inhaled antifungal therapy seems appropriate because aerosolization allows direct drug delivery to the poorly vascularized anastomosis. Debridement of the site may also be necessary (28,29).

Infections

Lung transplant recipients are at increased risk for a variety of infectious complications due to the chronic immunosuppression and abnormal physiology of the post-transplant lung. Infections with typical bacterial pathogens and opportunistic infections are both common. Collectively, infections represent the leading cause of death in the early postoperative interval and remain an important cause of morbidity and mortality throughout the post-transplant period. Evidence suggests that many early infections may induce immune and nonimmune inflammatory responses that predispose the recipient to acute or chronic allograft rejection, or both.

Bacterial

Bacterial infections are most common in the early post-transplant period and remain the primary cause of mortality during this time (30). The most common organisms involved are those colonizing the donor or the recipient or iatrogenic bacteria that populate individual institutional ICUs. Gram-negative pathogens such as *Pseudomonas ssp.*, *Klebsiella*, and *Haemophilus influenzae* are responsible for most early post-transplant bacterial pneumonias, but Gram-positive organisms such as *Staphylococcus aureus* are also causes. Less commonly *Actinomyces* (Fig. 48-3), *Mycobacterium tuberculosis*, and atypical *Mycobacterium* have been seen in lung transplant recipients (30,31). Analysis of trends in individual hospital bacterial susceptibilities should guide selection of empiric therapy with adjustments as necessary when sensitivities are available. At one institution all lung transplant patients receive a 7 to 10 day course of postoperative broad-spectrum antimicrobial prophylaxis (e.g., vancomycin and cefipime). This antibiotic regimen is modified depending on the results of cultures

obtained from the donor and recipient prior to transplantation (especially in patients with cystic fibrosis who have preoperative pathogens with known sensitivities). Antibiotics may be continued depending on the recipient's bronchial cultures after transplantation.

Blood stream infections have been identified as an important cause of early postoperative morbidity and mortality. In one report, bloodstream infection was documented in 25% of lung transplant recipients, with *S. aureus* and *Pseudomonas aeruginosa* singled out as the most common pathogens. Pneumonia and catheter-related infection represented the most common etiology for post-transplant blood stream infection and infection was associated with a significantly increased risk for postoperative death. These results highlight the importance of appropriate antibiotic selection and the need to minimize the duration of central lines (32).

Viral

Cytomegalovirus

Cytomegalovirus (CMV) disease is the most common infectious postoperative complication after lung transplantation. This virus causes infection in 13% to 75% of transplant patients depending on the specific definitions of infection and on the type and duration of pharmacologic CMV prophylaxis (33,34). Lung transplant recipients who are serologically CMV-negative preoperatively and who receive serologically CMV-positive donor lungs are at the highest risk of developing severe, life-threatening disease from primary infection. On the other hand, such infection is not usually seen in donor negative/recipient negative transplants (33). The optimal approach to the prevention of post-transplant CMV infection remains controversial. Most centers employ a regimen of 12 weeks of IV ganciclovir (5 mg per kg qd) post-transplantation in the high-risk (donor positive/recipient negative) mismatch patients. Some centers employ a shorter course of IV ganciclovir (e.g., 4 weeks) in all "at-risk" lung recipients. In a randomized prospective trial, Kruger et al. have recently demonstrated that hyperimmune globulin against CMV alone is ineffective in the prevention of CMV viremia or pneumonitis after lung transplant (35). As an additional preventive measure, one may use CMV-negative or leukocyte-reduced blood products in all instances, except major bleeding requiring large volume rapid transfusion (33).

"CMV infection" refers to detection of the virus in the serum or bronchial alveolar lavage using conventional culture, shell vial assay, or qualitative serum assay (e.g., polymerase chain reaction or CMV DNA by hybrid capture). "CMV disease," on the other hand, is defined by the presence of "cytomegalic" cells (CMV inclusion bodies or cells positive on immunoperoxidase stain) on tissue biopsies (Fig. 48-4) or the isolation of CMV from a tissue specimen in the presence of clinical findings consistent with CMV infection. Most CMV infections respond to 14 to 21 days of

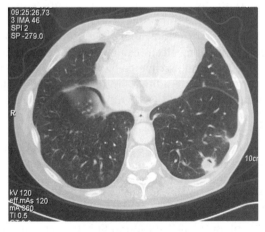

Figure 48-3   CT scan showing a lung abscess that was aspirated and found to be *Actinomyces*. Patient initially presented with fevers and chills. The patient was subsequently treated with ampicillin with resolution of the abscess.

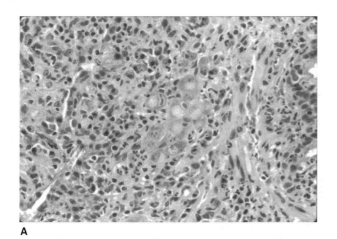

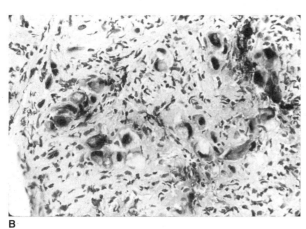

Figure 48-4 A: Transbronchial lung biopsy showing Cytomegalovirus (CMV) pneumonitis with demonstration of CMV inclusion bodies (hematoxylin and eosin). **B:** Demonstration of CMV inclusion bodies by immunoperoxidase staining.

IV ganciclovir (5 mg per kg b.i.d.). The dose should be adjusted for leukopenia and renal dysfunction. When patients fail to respond to IV ganciclovir therapy, drug resistance should be considered and Foscarnet or Cidofovir therapy may be instituted (36). However, because of the significant nephrotoxicity of these second line agents, formal testing for ganciclovir resistance should be performed when suspected. Acute renal failure has been reported in a lung transplant recipient treated with Cidofovir (37). Valganciclovir, an oral ganciclovir derivative with bioavailability comparable to intravenous formulations of ganciclovir, has recently been introduced for use in transplantation. Currently ongoing prospective studies will define the indications, efficacy, and cost effectiveness of oral valganciclovir in the lung transplant population.

Community Acquired Respiratory Viral Infections

Community acquired respiratory viral infections, including respiratory syncytial virus (RSV) adenovirus, parainfluenza, and influenza, cause significant morbidity and mortality in lung transplant recipients (38–42). These viral respiratory infections occur over a broad time range after

transplantation, and different mechanisms may account for early and late post-transplant infection. Early viral infection may result from nosocomial transmission or reactivation of latent virus. In contrast, late post-transplant respiratory viral infection is more likely to be community acquired. A seasonal variation is seen with RSV (January to April), while infection with adenovirus and parainfluenza occur throughout the year.

The majority of viral infections produce acute symptoms, including cough, wheeze, dyspnea, and fever. Presentation of influenza may be atypical with gastrointestinal (GI) symptoms predominating. New radiographic findings in lung transplant recipients with viral respiratory infections indicate severe infection and are a marker for poor prognosis (40). Symptomatic adenoviral infection, in particular, is typically associated with new radiologic abnormalities and is frequently fatal (40).

Treatment options for respiratory viral infections are limited. Aerosolized ribavirin has shown benefit in the treatment of RSV and parainfluenza infection in children (43). Intravenous immunoglobulin to RSV has been used in prevention and treatment of RSV infections in infants (44). Although the efficacy of these agents in lung transplant recipients remains unclear, it has been recommend that all patients with severe symptomatic RSV or parainfluenza infection receive aerosolized ribavirin. Ribavirin is also recommended in patients with radiographic abnormalities in the setting of RSV or parainfluenza infection, given the increased potential to progress to respiratory failure. Care for adenovirus is currently supportive as no definitive therapies are currently available. A trial of reduced immunosuppression appears worthwhile, although the risk for rejection must be considered. Reports of the use of intravenous ribavirin or immunoglobulin have suggested potential value in adenoviral infections in pediatric, bone marrow recipient, and AIDS patients (45–48). Intravenous ribavirin has also been used with some success in a pediatric patient with adenoviral infection after liver transplantation (49). Treatment for influenza in nonimmunocompromised patients consists of several potential drugs, including amantadine, rimantadine, and the newer neuraminidase inhibitors such as zanamivir and oseltamivir (50,51). The use of these agents in lung transplant recipients requires further study.

Because treatment options for community acquired viral infections in lung transplant recipients are limited, the main goal in this population is prevention. It is routine for all lung transplant recipients to receive yearly influenza vaccines. Unfortunately, the response to influenza vaccine in solid-organ transplant recipients is impaired and revaccination does not seem to improve the vaccine response (43). In a series of heart transplant patients, the efficacy of the influenza vaccine was significantly impaired. Although vaccination was less effective compared to nonimmunosuppressed individuals, 50% of patients still reached protective serum antibody titers against two of the three virus strains (52). Therefore, routine influenza immunization is still recommended but serologic testing may be indicated (41). Importantly, all close contacts should receive influenza vaccination with the intended goal of decreasing the risk of infection to the transplant patient. Lung transplant recipients should avoid contact with family and friends with respiratory symptoms, especially children, to minimize risks of acquiring community viral infection. Frequent hand washing should be encouraged after contact with infected patients.

Fungal Infections

Fungal infections are a major problem after lung transplantation and occur early and late after transplant. *Aspergillus* and *Candida* account for the majority of these fungal infections (53) (Fig. 48-5). *Candida albicans* is commonly isolated from bronchial washings after transplant and its presence usually represents colonization (30), but it may also be invasive (54). *Aspergillus* can also represent colonization, but because of the potential for invasive life-threatening infections, strong consideration needs to be given for treatment. More than

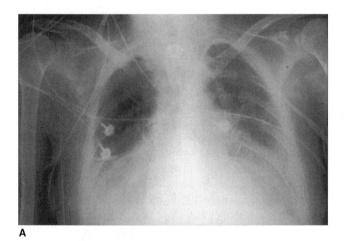

A

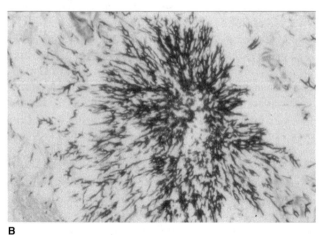

B

Figure 48-5 **A:** Chest radiograph of patient with invasive pulmonary *Aspergillus*. **B:** Histopathologic examination of patient with *Aspergillus* (hematoxylin and eosin, ×20).

50% of cases of *Aspergillus* colonization and infection occur within 6 months after transplantation. Mortality rates associated with invasive *Aspergillus* pneumonia or disseminated infection approached 60% in one series of lung transplant recipients (55).

Although risk factors for post-transplant fungal infection are not well defined, pretransplant colonization or prior treated infection may identify patients at higher risk for post-transplant infection. In patients with a single-lung transplant, one obvious potential reservoir of persistent *Aspergillus* is the native lung (30,56). Aspergilloma lesions found in the recipient explanted lungs have been associated with reduced post-transplant survival (57). Patients with cystic fibrosis and positive preoperative sputum cultures for *Aspergillus* are at higher risk for postoperative infections (58).

Nocardia infections are increasingly recognized as complications of lung transplantation (59). Although *Nocardia asteroides* accounts for the most transplant-related nocardiosis, a case of disseminated infection with *Nocardia brasiliensis* (60) in a single-lung transplant recipient has been reported. Although the mortality is high for immunocompromised patients with *N. brasiliensis,* prompt diagnosis and early initiation of appropriate therapy may improve outcome.

Reports of other fungal infections such as *Histoplasma, Coccidiomycosis, Mucormycosis, Zygomycetes,* and *Cryptococcus* are also documented (30). *Scedosporium apiospermum* is an uncommon cause of disseminated infection, but, importantly, it is resistant to amphotericin B (61). *Pneumocystis carinii,* now classified as a fungus, remains a rare cause of infection because of the routine use of effective prophylaxis in all lung transplant recipients. Dematiaceous fungi, such as *Mucormycosis,* are also infrequent causes of postoperative infection.

Treatment for fungal infection is based on the specific organism causing the infection; amphotericin B has been the drug of choice for *Aspergillus* and *Fusarium.* Newer options that may be as effective with less toxicity include liposomal formulations of amphotericin, voriconazole, and caspofungin. Voriconazole must be used with caution in lung transplant recipients because of its extensive list of known drug interactions. High-dose azole therapy (itraconazole, voriconazole) may be used for *Scedosporium. Nocardia* infections are treated with trimethoprim-sulfamethoxazole. Most candidal infections can be treated with fluconazole. Nonalbicans *Candida* species, however, are increasingly resistant to Diflucan but can be effectively treated by new drugs such as voriconazole. Single-lung transplant should probably not be performed in patients with mycetomas as adequate removal of fungal organisms cannot be achieved and the newly transplanted lung will be at increased risk of colonization and infection (57). Prolonged therapy is required for all fungal infections.

Because of the potential morbidity and mortality associated with fungal infections, several antifungal prophylactic strategies have been used in lung transplant recipients, often employing either systemic or inhaled antifungal agents, or both (62). However, enthusiasm for the use of systemic antifungal therapies is limited by the lack of *in vitro* activity against some infections, drug interactions, and significant treatment-limiting toxicities. Furthermore, the use of inhaled amphotericin B has been associated with significant subjective intolerance leading to treatment discontinuation in up to 50% of patients (63).

One lung transplant group has recently demonstrated the safety and tolerability of inhaled amphotericin B lipid complex (ABLC) in >50 lung transplant recipients. Because of the lipid properties, it was hypothesized that ABLC would be more effectively nebulized with greater pulmonary deposition than conventional amphotericin B. Consistent with this hypothesis, very low rates of intolerance and very low rates of fungal infection were seen in patients who received nebulized ABLC (64). Although further study is needed, nebulized ABLC seems a promising approach to prevent fungal infections without systemic toxicities after lung transplantation.

PLEURAL SPACE COMPLICATIONS

Hyperinflation

When undersized lungs are used in recipients, one may observe increased airway pressures when suction is applied to the chest tubes (65). Presumably the negative pleural pressure inhibits the lungs, elastic recoil and leads to detrimental hyperinflation. With hyperinflation, alveoli do not completely decompress during exhalation, resulting in an increase in functional residual capacity. As more mechanical breaths are delivered, a stacking of the breaths occurs and the lungs function on a flatter portion of the volume-pressure curve. In extreme cases, this can lead to detrimental alveolar hyper-expansion and hemodynamic instability. Awareness of the potential for acute hyperinflation can lead to preventive measures such as avoidance of chest tube suction or water seal while the patient is on positive pressure ventilation.

Pneumothorax

Pneumothorax is encountered primarily in two circumstances. The most common circumstance is the development of insignificant pneumothoraces in patients with obstructive lung disease, either emphysema or cystic fibrosis, who have undergone bilateral replacement and have received lungs smaller than the pleural space into which they are implanted. Often a minimal degree of bilateral pneumothorax occurs subsequent to chest tube removal. In general, these pneumothoraces can be ignored and the pleural air will eventually resorb and any remaining space will fill with fluid. Pneumothorax can occur infrequently

as a result of airway dehiscence with communication into the pleural space. This is a rare occurrence and is usually readily managed by intercostal tube drainage with appropriate re-expansion of the underlying lung.

Pleural Effusion

Pleural effusions are common, particularly in recipients whose lung volume is somewhat smaller than the pleural space. A sympathetic effusion will occur in association with underlying pulmonary infection or rejection. These effusions, as with others, generally clear with appropriate therapy of the underlying parenchymal condition.

Empyema

Pleural empyema is an uncommon complication following lung transplantation, but its occurrence is associated with a significant mortality (Fig. 48-6). Spontaneous development of an empyema is rare. More commonly, an empyema develops after a prolonged air leak or as a result of open lung biopsy performed on a patient receiving high-dose corticosteroids. Persistent air leak and failure to achieve re-expansion of the lung and subsequent pleurodesis result in a chronic pleural space that eventually will become infected. Nunley et al. performed a retrospective review of 392 transplant recipients and found empyema documented in 14 patients (3.6%) (66). In this series empyemas tended to occur early in the post-transplant period, and 28.6% (four patients) with empyemas died secondary to related infectious complications. No predominant organism was isolated in empyemic fluid with Gram-positive, Gram-negative, and saprophytic organisms seen. There was no relationship between the development of an empyema and the type of transplant performed or whether the transplant was done for a septic or nonseptic lung diagnosis. Surgeons

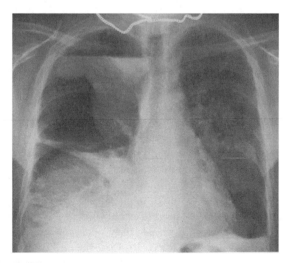

Figure 48-6 Chest radiograph showing empyema of the native lung following single-lung transplantation.

have treated a number of patients who developed empyemas by open drainage by rib resection or by creation of a Clagett window or Eloesser flap. Interestingly, an empyema rarely occurs as a result of bronchial dehiscence in communication with the pleural space.

REJECTION

Both acute and chronic lung allograft rejection contribute substantially to morbidity in lung transplant recipients. Chronic lung rejection remains the major limitation to long-term success in lung transplantation today. Hyperacute rejection has only anecdotally been reported in the literature (67–69). Saint Martin et al. (70) performed immunofluorescence with C3, immunoglobin M, and immunoglobin G and found no evidence of humoral rejection in 106 biopsies. In this report, only one patient had a high reactivity pretransplant panel of reactive antibodies (PRA), suggesting a low risk for hyperacute rejection. Conversely, others have reported immunohistochemical findings of humoral injury in some recipients with high PRA (71). Interestingly, investigators have recently reported evidence suggesting that a frequently occurring septal capillary injury syndrome may represent humoral injury in lung allografts (72).

Acute Rejection

Acute allograft rejection is one of the most common complications following lung transplantation. Most recipients experience at least one episode of acute rejection within the first year following transplant (73,74). In 1990, the Lung Rejection Study Group developed a system to characterize lung allograft rejection based on histologic criteria detected in lung biopsy specimens, with emphasis on perivascular and intersitial infiltration of mononuclear cells. Note is also made of the coexistence of airway inflammation (75). Modest revisions in this system were described in 1995 (76). In recent years, airway-centered inflammation (lymphocytic bronchitis/bronchiolitis) has been associated with subsequent development of chronic lung allograft dysfunction characterized by the pathologic lesion of bronchiolitis obliterans (77). In addition, it is clear that there is an association between frequency and severity of acute rejection episodes and the subsequent development of bronchiolitis obliterans (77). Thus early detection of acute rejection and alteration of immunosuppression to deal with this problem may have a significant impact in the subsequent reduction of chronic lung allograft dysfunction.

In the early years of lung transplant experience, clinical parameters were often used to establish a clinical diagnosis of acute rejection. Unfortunately, dyspnea, low-grade fever, perihilar infiltrates, leukocytosis, hypoxia, and the clinical response to intravenous bolus doses of corticosteroid are nonspecific findings. Pathologic assessment of multiple transbronchial biopsy specimens has proven to be the "gold" standard for the diagnosis of acute lung allograft rejection (75,78,79). Indeed, many programs have adopted a program of prophylactic surveillance transbronchial biopsy (74,78,80–83). However, this strategy is controversial and a number of active lung transplant programs have abandoned it (84,85).

Since acute rejection is a predictor of bronchiolitis obliterans syndrome (BOS), induction and maintenance immunosuppression regimens, as well as treatment strategies for documented acute rejection, are subjects of intense interest. Induction therapy with either a cytolytic agent or an interleukin-2 receptor (IL-2R) blocker has been shown to reduce early rejection rates (86). Due to ease of administration, a low rate of side effects, similar efficacy, and fewer secondary infections, the IL-2R blockers are becoming the induction agents of choice for centers adhering to such a protocol.

Treatment of acute rejection has two goals: to treat the acute problem and to reduce the likelihood of further acute rejection episodes. Conventional therapy has been intravenous methylprednisolone in a dose of 10 to 15 mg per kg for 3 to 5 days (87). Although this strategy often accomplishes resolution of perivascular infiltrates, airway-centered inflammation has been more refractory to therapy. Depending on the maintenance steroid dose, 2 to 3 weeks of an oral steroid taper is usually prescribed. As acute therapy is initiated, the maintenance immunosuppression regimen should be scrutinized. A frequent first adjustment is a switch from maintenance cyclosporine to tacrolimus in the event of cyclosporine toxicity or acute rejection episodes despite adequate cyclosporine dosage (88,89). The roles of newer agents such as sirolimus or leflunomide, a pyrimidine synthesis inhibitor, are evolving in lung transplantation based on success in other solid-organ transplants (90–93). Low calcineurin inhibitor drug levels warrant investigation, especially for new medications activating the cytochrome P450 enzyme pathway and enhancing calcineurin inhibitor metabolism (e.g., dilantin, rifampin, nafcillin) (94).

Chronic Allograft Rejection/Bronchiolitis Obliterans Syndrome

The descriptive term "bronchiolitis obliterans syndrome" (BOS) has been used to describe a late decline from a postoperative baseline first second expired volume (FEV_1) that is not attributable to acute rejection, infection, or mechanical obstruction due to a bronchial anastomotic complication. The pathologic lesion associated with this decline is bronchiolitis obliterans (Fig. 48-7). A working formulation was created to characterize and grade BOS (95) and has been recently revised (96).

BOS is a very common condition following lung transplantation (97). Most observers believe that every recipient will develop some degree of BOS with long-term follow-up.

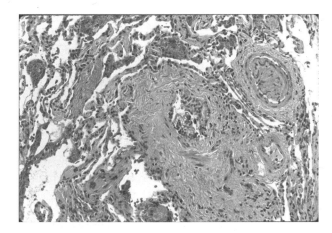

Figure 48-7 Transbronchial lung biopsy showing bronchiolitis obliterans with scarring and fibrosis of the small airways (hematoxylin and eosin).

Actuarial freedom from BOS at 1, 3, and 5 years posttransplant is 82%, 42%, and 25%, respectively (98).

The specific causes of BOS are not clear. Evidence suggests that both alloimmune and nonalloimmune mechanisms are important (99). Recipients who have more frequent and severe episodes of acute allograft rejection are more likely to develop subsequent BOS (77). Nonimmune mechanisms may also be important. Lung transplant recipients appear to have a high incidence of gastroesophageal reflux disease (GERD). Patients without GERD have a much lower incidence of BOS than those with uncorrected GERD. Improvement of BOS has been noted in recipients with GERD who underwent corrective fundoplication (100).

Until we have a better understanding of the molecular and cellular mechanisms of BOS, we are not likely to make much progress in its treatment. This goal is hampered by the lack of a suitable experimental model of the bronchiolitis obliterans lesion. A definitive solution for chronic allograft rejection may come through the development of strategies to promote immune tolerance or permanent acceptance of the graft by the recipient without the need for immunosuppression.

NONPULMONARY COMPLICATIONS

Gastrointestinal Complications

GI complications are frequent in lung transplant recipients, occurring in as many as 50% of patients in some series (101). Frequently reported nonsurgical GI complications include esophagitis, pancreatitis, gastric atony, adynamic colonic ileus, gastroesophageal reflux, peptic ulcer disease, gastritis, gastrointestinal bleeding, CMV hepatitis, CMV colitis, diverticulitis, cholecystitis, and clostridium difficile colitis/diarrhea. The majority of these nonsurgical GI complications occur in the first month postoperatively and most respond to conservative therapy (101). Acute

abdominal processes requiring surgical intervention have a reported incidence of 4% to 17% in lung transplant recipients and include, in decreasing occurrence, bowel perforation, appendicitis, cholecystitis, colitis, and pneumatosis intestinalis (102). Post-transplant lymphoproliferative disease (PTLD) may present as an acute abdominal process, secondary to intussusception or bowel perforation. Surgical GI complications can occur at any time after transplantation, and immunosuppression may initially mask their severity. When emergent operative exploration is required, such an intervention has significant associated morbidity and mortality. Elective abdominal surgical procedures can be performed safely in this population with acceptable morbidity (103).

Post-transplant Lymphoproliferative Disease

PTLD is a well-recognized complication after solid-organ and bone marrow transplantation with an incidence between 4% to 10% after lung transplantation (104–107). Investigators have reported a 6.1% incidence of PTLD after lung transplantation in the adult population (106). PTLD includes a spectrum of disease entities ranging from atypical lymphoid proliferation to malignant non-Hodgkin lymphoma (108,109). Most commonly, the neoplastic cells are of B-cell origin and there are often associations between PTLD and the presence of Epstein-Barr virus (EBV) (110). Cytotoxic T cells are involved in destroying cells presenting EBV in the context of MHC I. It has been proposed that an immunocompromised recipient experiencing a primary EBV infection may not be capable of destroying the virus infected B cells, resulting in EBV-driven B-cell proliferation. In lung transplant recipients, a strong correlation has been reported between negative EBV serology prior to transplantation and the subsequent development of PTLD. Studies have reported a 6.8- to 20- fold increased risk of development of PTLD in recipients who were EBV-negative pretransplantation (105,111). Some have proposed that EBV carried in the donor lung lymphocytes results in a primary infection in the recipient. However, some reports have shown the recipient to be the origin of the lymphocytes in PTLD (112). The use of induction therapy (113) and the presence of CMV infection (114) have both been suggested as contributing factors to the development of PTLD.

PTLD often occurs in the first year after transplantation and shows a predilection for the thorax, most commonly the lung allograft (104–107). Cases of PTLD that present after the first year, in contrast, are usually extrathoracic, commonly arising in the abdomen and pelvis (106). In one series, of the 16 reported cases of PTLD that occurred after the first year, 14 of 16 (88%) were extrathoracic. Late cases of PTLD in the abdomen and pelvis occur at a median time of 5.8 years after transplantation (115). Interestingly, in all late cases occurring in the abdomen and pelvis, the recipients were EBV-positive prior to transplant. Late occurring abdominal and pelvic PTLD cases were most commonly malignant non-Hodgkin lymphomas, and despite aggressive therapy the prognosis was poor. In contrast, the patients who presented with early PTLD, unless disseminated at diagnosis, had a favorable prognosis and often responded to simply decreasing the level of immunosuppression (115).

Treatment of PTLD is based on the stage and progression of disease. Initially, a trial of reduction of immunosuppression is attempted, particularly with disease limited to the allograft. Many investigators have recommended the simultaneous use of antiviral therapy (111). Although chemotherapy has been used in patients with widespread disease or who have progression of disease, treatment related mortality is considerable. In one reported study, 75% of PTLD patients treated with chemotherapy died as a result of sepsis (111). Recently, Rituximab, a humanized anti-CD20 monoclonal antibody, has shown promise as a treatment option (116). Only a few cases of its use in the lung transplant population have been reported. Verschuuren et al. (116) reported complete remission in three lung transplant patients treated with Rituximab. Complications occurred in two, one relapsed with a partial CD20 negative PTLD, and the other developed hypogammaglobulinemia with subsequent sepsis and death.

Preventative strategies have been contemplated. In adult lung transplantation, it does not appear prudent to match recipient and donor EBV status, because >90% of the population is EBV-positive by the time they are 35 years old. This strategy may have more value in children who have a higher percentage of EBV-negative recipients. Malouf et al. (117) reported that prophylactic use of antiviral therapy might reduce the incidence of PTLD.

Atrial Dysrhythmias

Atrial dysrhythmias frequently occur after lung transplantation. In one series, 68 of 209 patients (33%) developed arterial dysrhythmias (118). The median time to onset was 4 days. Atrial fibrillation was the most common atrial dysrhythmia (53%), followed by supraventricular tachycardia (23%), atrial flutter (18%), and multifocal atrial tachycardia (6%). Eighty-eight percent of atrial dysrhythmias were treated with medical therapy alone, while 12% underwent an additional intervention (cardioversion or ablation). Patients with atrial dysrhythmias had higher rates of reintubation, additional operative intervention, and longer ICU and hospital stays. Use of cardiopulmonary bypass, age of recipient, and time on the waiting list were identified as significant risk factors for atrial dysrhythmias.

Renal Failure

Renal failure is a common complication following lung transplantation because of the necessary use of calcineurin inhibitors. Ishani et al. (119) reviewed the course of 219 lung and heart-lung transplant recipients surviving at least 6 months post-transplant and found that by 6 months 200 patients (91.3%) had a decrease in renal function. Doubling of creatinine from pretransplant baseline occurred in 34%, 43%, and 53% at 1, 2, and 5 years, respectively. End-stage renal disease occurred in 16 lung transplant recipients (7.3%) at a median duration of 28 months. The majority of recipients who developed ESRD had received cyclosporine (13/16), compared to only three who had received tacrolimus. Of the patients who developed ESRD, 44% (7) received hemodialysis alone and 56% (9) received kidney transplants. Risk factors associated with time to doubling of creatinine by multivariate analysis were serum creatinine at 1 month post-transplant and the number of cumulative follow-up periods with the diastolic blood pressure >90 mm Hg. Compared to cyclosporine, the use of tacrolimus in the first 6 months following transplantation was associated with a decreased risk for time to doubling of serum creatinine. It is apparent that prevention of subsequent renal failure in lung transplant recipients requires preserving renal function early in the course of transplantation. Early identification of high-risk recipients for renal dysfunction should prompt aggressive blood pressure control in these recipients and consideration of change in immunosuppressive protocol (120). Other studies have found the underlying pulmonary diagnosis to be a risk factor for the subsequent development of renal insufficiency. Recipients with cystic fibrosis had the greatest impairment in renal function and recipients with pulmonary hypertension had the least impairment (121).

Hyperammonemia

Hyperammonemia following lung transplantation has been reported as a potentially fatal complication (122–124). The development of hyperammonemia appears to occur early in the post-transplant period. In one recent study, 6 (4.1%) of 145 lung transplant recipients developed hyperammonemia, all within the first 26 days after transplantation (123). A high mortality rate was seen in the population that developed hyperammonemia (67% vs. 17%). The majority of patients with hyperammonemia develop neurologic symptoms, including encephalopathy, lethargy, agitation, seizure, tremors, and coma. Risk factors for the development of hyperammonemia include major gastrointestinal complications, use of total parenteral nutrition, and lung transplantation for primary pulmonary hypertension. Treatment includes discontinuation of exogenous nitrogen, high caloric intake to depress catabolism, lactulose, neomycin, agents used to treat hyperammonemia in congenital urea cycle defects (sodium phenylacetate, sodium benzoate, and arginine hydrochloride), and the use of hemodialysis (125).

Thrombotic Thrombocytopenic Purpura (TTP)–Hemolytic Uremic Syndrome (HUS)

An infrequent but potentially serious complication following lung transplantation is thrombotic thrombocytopenic purpura (TTP)-hemolytic uremic syndrome (HUS). More common in other solid-organ transplants, especially kidney transplants, these syndromes are characterized by microangiopathic hemolysis, thrombocytopenia, and renal failure (126). Disease is most common within the first 3 months post-transplantation, and 96% of cases occur within the first year. This complication is associated with the use of calcineurin inhibitor therapy. The critical component of treatment is prompt initiation of plasma exchange. In addition to plasma exchange, aspirin, dipyridamole, or glucocorticoids can be used (127). Hemodialysis or renal transplantation is required in lung transplantation patients who develop renal failure from this syndrome. Mortality is in the range of 13% (126).

CONCLUSION

Complications occur commonly in lung transplant recipients because of their general debilitation and the requirement for lifelong immunosuppression. Prevention and early recognition of these complications is important to prevent morbidity and mortality in this high-risk population.

REFERENCES

1. Battafarano RJ, Anderson RC, Meyers BF, et al. Perioperative complications after living donor lobectomy. *J Thorac Cardiovasc Surg* 2000;120:909–915.
2. Casula RP, Stoica SC, Wallwork J, et al. Pulmonary vein augmentation for single lung transplantation. *Ann Thorac Surg* 2001;71: 1373–1374.
3. Lau CL, Guthrie TJ, Chaparro C, et al. Lung transplantation in recipients with previous lung volume reduction surgery. *J Heart Lung Transplant* 2003;22:S183.
4. Pasque MK, Cooper JD, Kaiser LR, et al. An improved technique for bilateral lung transplantation: rationale and initial clinical experience. *Ann Thorac Surg* 1990;49:785–791.
5. Brown RP, Esmore DS, Lawson C. Improved sternal fixation in the transsternal bilateral thoracotomy incision. *J Thorac Cardiovasc Surg* 1996;112:137–141.
6. Meyers BF, Sundaresan RS, Guthrie T, et al. Bilateral sequential lung transplantation without sternal division eliminates post-transplantation sternal complications. *J Thorac Cardiovasc Surg* 1998;117:358–364.
7. Matsuzaki Y, Waddell TK, Puskas JD, et al. Amelioration of post-ischemic lung reperfusion injury by PGE1. *Am Rev Respir Dis* 1993;148:882 889.
8. Maccherini M, Keshavjee SH, Slutsky AS, et al. The effect of low-potassium-dextran versus Euro-Collins solution for preservation of isolated type II pneumocytes. *Transplantation* 1991;52:621–626.
9. Fischer S, Matte-Martyn A, De Perrot M, et al. Low-potassium dextran preservation solution improves lung function after human lung transplantation. *J Thorac Cardiovasc Surg* 2001;121:594–596.
10. Yamashita M, Schmid RA, Ando K, et al. Nitroprusside ameliorates lung allograft reperfusion injury. *Ann Thorac Surg* 1996;62: 791–797.
11. Halldorsson A, Kronon M, Allen BS, et al. Controlled reperfusion after lung ischemia: implications for improved function after lung transplantation. *J Thorac Cardiovasc Surg* 1998;115:415–425.
12. Halldorsson A, Kronon M, Allen BS, et al. Controlled reperfusion prevents pulmonary injury after 24-hours of lung preservation. *Ann Thorac Surg* 1998;66(2):174–180.
13. Clark SC, Sudarshan C, Khanna R, et al. Controlled reperfusion and pentoxifylline modulates reperfusion injury after single lung transplantation. *J Thorac Cardiovasc Surg* 1998;115:1335–1341.
14. Bhabra MS, Hopkinson DN, Shaw TE, et al. Controlled reperfusion protects lung grafts during a transient early increase in permeability. *Ann Thorac Surg* 1998;65:187–192.
15. Halldorsson AO, Kronon MT, Allen BS, et al. Lowering reperfusion pressure reduces the injury after pulmonary ischemia. *Ann Thorac Surg* 2000;69:198–203.
16. Clark SC, Sudarshan CD, Dark JH. Controlled perfusion of the transplanted lung [comment]. *Ann Thorac Surg* 2001;71: 1755–1756.
17. Fiser SM, Kron IL, Long SM, et al. Controlled perfusion decreases reperfusion injury after high-flow reperfusion. *J Heart Lung Transplant* 2002;21:687–691.
18. Lick SD, Brown PS, Kurusz M, et al. Technique of controlled reperfusion of the transplanted lung in humans. *Ann Thorac Surg* 2000;69:910–912.
19. Date H, Triantafillou A, Trulock E, et al. Inhaled nitric oxide reduces human lung allograft dysfunction. *J Thorac Cardiovasc Surg* 1996;111:913–919.
20. Fiser SM, Cope JT, Kron IL, et al. Aerosolized prostacyclin (epoprostenol) as an alternative to inhaled nitric oxide for patients with reperfusion injury after lung transplantation. [Erratum appears in *J Thorac Cardiovasc Surg* 2001 Jun;121(6):1136.] *J Thorac Cardiovasc Surg* 2001;121:981–982.
21. Meyers BF, Sundt TM, Henry S, et al. Selective use of extracorporeal membrane oxygenation is warranted after lung transplantation. *J Thorac Cardiovasc Surg* 2000;120:20–28.
22. Eriksson LT, Steen S. Induced hypothermia in critical respiratory failure after lung transplantation. *Ann Thorac Surg* 1998;65: 827–829.
23. Date H, Trulock EP, Arcidi JM, et al. Improved airway healing after lung transplantation: an analysis of 348 bronchial anastomoses. *J Thorac Cardiovasc Surg* 1995;110:1424–1433.
24. King-Biggs MB, Dunitz JM, Park SJ, et al. Airway anastomotic dehiscence associated with use of sirolimus immediately after lung transplantation. *Transplantation* 2003;75:1437–1443.
25. de Hoyos A, Patterson GA, Maurer J. Pulmonary transplantation: early and late results. *J Thorac Cardiovasc Surg* 1992;103:295–306.
26. Kramer MR, Denning DW, Marshall SE, et al. Ulcerative tracheobronchitis after lung transplantation. A new form of invasive aspergillosis. *Am Rev Respir Dis* 1991;144:552–556.
27. Nunley DR, Gal AA, Vega JD, et al. Saprophytic fungal infections and complications involving the bronchial anastomosis following human lung transplantation. *Chest* 2002;122:1185–1191.
28. Palmer SM, Perfect JR, Howell DN, et al. Candidal anastomotic infection in lung transplant recipients: successful treatment with a combination of systemic and inhaled antifungal agents. *J Heart Lung Transplant* 1998;17:1029–1033.
29. Hadjiliadis D, Howell DN, Davis RD, et al. Anastomotic infections in lung transplant recipients. *Ann Transplant* 2000;5:13–19.
30. Chaparro C, Kesten S. Infections in lung transplant recipients. *Clin Chest Med* 1997;18:339–351.
31. Bassiri AG, Girgis RE, Theodore S. Actinomyces odontolyticus thoracopulmonary infections. Two cases in lung and heart-lung transplant recipients and review of the literature. *Am J Respir Crit Care Med* 1995,152:374–376.
32. Palmer SM, Alexander BD, Sanders LL, et al. Significance of blood stream infection after lung transplantation: analysis in 176 consecutive patients. *Transplantation* 2000;69:2360–2366.
33. Ettinger NA, Bailey TC, Trulock EP, et al. Cytomegalovirus infection and pneumonitis. Impact after isolation lung transplantation. *Am Rev Respir Dis* 1993;147:1017–1023.
34. Gutierrez CA, Chaparro C, Drajden M, et al. Cytomegalovirus viremia in lung transplant recipients receiving ganciclovir and immune globulin. *Chest* 1998;113:924–932.

35. Kruger RM, Paranjothi S, Storch GA, et al. Impact of prophylaxis with cytogam alone on the incidence of CMV viremia in CMV-seropositive lung transplant recipients. *J Heart Lung Transplant* 2003;22:754–763.

36. Zamora MR. Controversies in lung transplantation: management of cytomegalovirus infections. *J Heart Lung Transplant* 2002;21:841–849.

37. Zedtwitz-Liebenstein K, Presterl E, Deviatko E, et al. Acute renal failure in a lung transplant patient after therapy with cidofovir. *Transpl Int* 2001;14:445–446.

38. Palmer SM Jr, Henshaw NG, Howell DN, et al. Community respiratory viral infection in adult lung transplant recipients [comment]. *Chest* 1998;113:944–950.

39. Holt ND, Gould FK, Taylor CE, et al. Incidence and significance of noncytomegalovirus viral respiratory infection after adult lung transplantation. *J Heart Lung Transplant* 1997;16:416–419.

40. Matar LD, McAdams HP, Palmer SM, et al. Respiratory viral infections in lung transplant recipients: radiologic findings with clinical correlation. *Radiology* 1999;213:735–742.

41. Garantziotis S, Howell DN, McAdams HP, et al. Influenza pneumonia in lung transplant recipients: clinical features and association with bronchiolitis obliterans syndrome [comment]. *Chest* 2001;119:1277–1280.

42. McCurdy LH, Milstone A, Dummer S. Clinical features and outcomes of paramyxoviral infection in lung transplant recipients treated with ribavirin. *J Heart Lung Transplant* 2003;22:745–753.

43. Blumberg EA, Albano C, Pruett T, et al. The immunogenicity of influenza virus vaccine in solid organ transplant recipients. *Clin Infect Dis* 1996;22:295–302.

44. Wandstrat TL. Respiratory syncytial virus immune globulin intravenous. *Ann Pharmacother* 1997;31:83–88.

45. Zahradnik JM. Adenovirus pneumonia. *Semin Respir Infect* 1987;2:104–111.

46. Jurado M, Navarro JM, Hernandez J, et al. Adenovirus-associated haemorrhagic cystitis after bone marrow transplantation successfully treated with intravenous ribavirin. *Bone Marrow Transplant* 1995;15:651–652.

47. McCarthy AJ, Bergin M, De Silva LM, et al. Intravenous ribavirin therapy for disseminated adenovirus infection. *Pediatr Infect Dis J* 1995;14:1003–1004.

48. Maslo C, Girard PM, Urban T, et al. Ribavirin therapy for adenovirus pneumonia in an AIDS patient. *Am J Respir Crit Care Med* 1997;156:1263–1264.

49. Shetty AK, Gans HA, So S, et al. Intravenous ribavirin therapy for adenovirus pneumonia. *Pediatr Pulmonol* 2000;29:69–73.

50. Cox NJ, Subbarao K. Influenza. *Lancet* 1999;354:1277–1282.

51. The MIST (Management of Influenza in the Southern Hemisphere Trialists) Study Group. Randomised trial of efficacy and safety of inhaled zanamivir in treatment of influenza A and B virus infections [comment]. [Erratum appears in *Lancet* 1999 Feb 6;353(9151):504.] *Lancet* 1998;352:1877–1881.

52. Dengler TJ, Strnad N, Buhring I, et al. Differential immune response to influenza and pneumococcal vaccination in immunosuppressed patients after heart transplantation. *Transplantation* 1998;66:1340–1347.

53. Grossi P, Farina C, Fiocchi R et al, Italian Study Group of Fungal Infections in Thoracic Organ Transplant Recipients. Prevalence and outcome of invasive fungal infections in 1,963 thoracic organ transplant recipients: a multicenter retrospective study. *Transplantation* 2000;70:112–116.

54. Kanj SS, Welty-Wolf K, Madden J, et al. Fungal infections in lung and heart-lung transplant recipients. Report of 9 cases and review of the literature. *Medicine* 1996;75:142–156.

55. Mehrad B, Paciocco G, Martinez FJ, et al. Spectrum of *Aspergillus* infection in lung transplant recipients: case series and review of the literature. *Chest* 2001;119:169–175.

56. Westney GE, Kesten S, DeHoyos A, et al. *Aspergillus* infection in single and double lung transplant recipients. *Transplantation* 1996;61:915–919.

57. Hadjiliadis D, Sporn TA, Perfect JR, et al. Outcome of lung transplantation in patients with mycetomas [comment]. *Chest* 2002;121:128–134.

58. Nunley DR, Ohori P, Grgurich WF, et al. Pulmonary aspergillosis in cystic fibrosis lung transplant recipients. *Chest* 1998;114:1321–1329.

59. Husain S, McCurry K, Dauber J, et al. Nocardia infection in lung transplant recipients. *J Heart Lung Transplant* 2002;21:354–359.

60. Palmer SM, Kanj SS, Davis RD, et al. A case of disseminated infection with nocardia brasiliensis in a lung transplant recipient. *Transplantation* 1997;63:1189–1190.

61. Raj R, Frost AE. Scedosporium apiospermum fungemia in a lung transplant recipient. *Chest* 2002;121:1714–1716.

62. Calvo V, Borro JM, Morales P et al, Valencia Lung Transplant Group. Antifungal prophylaxis during the early postoperative period of lung transplantation. *Chest* 1999;115:1301–1304.

63. Erjavec Z, Woolthuis GM, de Vries-Hospers HG, et al. Tolerance and efficacy of amphotericin B inhalations for prevention of invasive pulmonary aspergillosis in haematological patients. *Eur J Clin Microbiol Infect Dis* 1997;16:364–368.

64. Palmer SM, Drew RH, Whitehouse JD, et al. Safety of aerosolized amphotericin B lipid complex in lung transplant recipients. *Transplantation* 2001;72:545–548.

65. Kozower BD, Meyers BF, Ciccone AM, et al. Potential for detrimental hyperinflation after lung transplantation with application of negative pleural pressure to undersized lung grafts. *J Thorac Cardiovasc Surg* 2003;125:430–432.

66. Nunley DR, Grgurich WF, Keenan RJ, et al. Empyema complicating successful lung transplantation. *Chest* 1999;115:1312–1315.

67. Frost AE, Jammal CT, Cagle PT. Hyperacute rejection following lung transplantation. *Chest* 1996;110:559–562.

68. Bittner HB, Dunitz J, Hertz M, et al. Hyperacute rejection in single lung transplantation—case report of successful management by means of plasmapheresis and antithymocyte globulin treatment. *Transplantation* 2001;71:649–651.

69. Choi JK, Kearns J, Palevsky HI, et al. Hyperacute rejection of a pulmonary allograft. Immediate clinical and pathologic findings. *Am J Respir Crit Care Med* 1999;160:1015–1018.

70. Saint Martin GA, Reddy VB, Garrity DR, et al. Humoral (antibody-mediated) rejection in lung transplantation. *J Heart Lung Transplant* 1996;15:1217–1222.

71. Lau CL, Palmer SM, Posther KE, et al. Influence of panel-reactive antibodies on posttransplant outcomes in lung transplant recipients. *Ann Thorac Surg* 2000;69:1520–1524.

72. Magro CM, Deng A, Pope-Harman A, et al. Humorally mediated posttransplantation septal capillary injury syndrome as a common form of pulmonary allograft rejection: a hypothesis. *Transplantation* 2002;74:1273–1280.

73. Husain AN, Siddiqui MT, Holmes EW, et al. Analysis of risk factors for the development of bronchiolitis obliterans syndrome. *Am J Respir Crit Care Med* 1999;159:829–833.

74. Hopkins PM, Aboyoun CL, Chhajed PN, et al. Prospective analysis of 1,235 transbronchial lung biopsies in lung transplant recipients. *J Heart Lung Transplant* 2002;21:1062–1067.

75. Yousem SA, Berry GJ, Brunt EM, et al. A working formulation for the standardization of nomenclature in the diagnosis of heart and lung rejection: lung rejection study group. *J Heart Lung Transplant* 1990;9:593–601.

76. Yousem SA, Berry GJ, Cagle PT, et al. Revision of the 1990 working formulation for the classification of pulmonary allograft rejection: lung rejection study group. *J Heart Lung Transplant* 1996;15:1–15.

77. Sharples LD, McNeil K, Stewart S, et al. Risk factors for bronchiolitis obliterans: a systematic review of recent publications. *J Heart Lung Transplant* 2002;21:271–281.

78. Trulock EP, Ettinger NA, Brunt EM, et al. The role of transbronchial lung biopsy in the treatment of lung transplant recipients: an analysis of 200 consecutive procedures. *Chest* 1992;102:1049–1054.

79. Higenbottam T, Stewart S, Penketh A, et al. Transbronchial lung biopsy for the diagnosis of rejection in heart-lung transplant patients. *Transplantation* 1988;46:532–539.

80. Sibley RK. The role of transbronchial biopsies in the management of lung transplant recipients. *J Heart Lung Transplant* 1993;12:308–324.

81. Boehler A, Vogt P, Zollinger A, et al. Prospective study of the value of transbronchial lung biopsy after lung transplantation. *Eur Respir J* 1996;9:658–662.

82. Guilinger RA, Paradis IL, Dauber JH, et al. The importance of bronchoscopy with transbronchial biopsy and bronchoalveolar lavage in the management of lung transplant recipients. *Am J Respir Crit Care Med* 1995;152:2037–2043.

83. Baz MA, Layish DT, Govert JA, et al. Diagnostic yield of bronchoscopies after isolated lung transplantation [comment]. *Chest* 1996;110:84–88.

84. Tamm M, Sharples LD, Higenbottam TW, et al. Bronchiolitis obliterans syndrome in heart-lung transplantation: surveillance biopsies. *Am J Respir Crit Care Med* 1997;155:1705–1710.

85. Valentine VG, Taylor DE, Dhillon GS, et al. Success of lung transplantation without surveillance bronchoscopy. *J Heart Lung Transplant* 2002;21:319–326.

86. Brock MV, Borja MC, Ferber L, et al. Induction therapy in lung transplantation: a prospective, controlled clinical trial comparing OKT3, anti-thymocyte globulin, and daclizumab. *J Heart Lung Transplant* 2001;20:1282–1290.

87. Trulock EP. Lung transplantation. *Am J Respir Crit Care Med* 1997;155:789–818.

88. Vitulo P, Oggionni T, Cascina A, et al. Efficacy of tacrolimus rescue therapy in refractory acute rejection after lung transplantation. *J Heart Lung Transplant* 2002;21:435–439.

89. Horning NR, Lynch JP, Sundaresan SR, et al. Tacrolimus therapy for persistent or recurrent acute rejection after lung transplantation. *J Heart Lung Transplant* 1998;17:761–767.

90. Kahan BD, The Rapamune US Study Group. Efficacy of sirolimus compared with azathioprine for reduction of acute renal allograft rejection: a randomised multicentre study [comment]. *Lancet* 2000;356:194–202.

91. Hong JC, Kahan BD. Sirolimus rescue therapy for refractory rejection in renal transplantation. *Transplantation* 2001;71:1579–1584.

92. Snell GI, Levvey BJ, Chin W, et al. Rescue therapy: a role for sirolimus in lung and heart transplant recipients. *Transplant Proc* 2001;33:1084–1085.

93. Williams JW, Mital D, Chong A, et al. Experiences with leflunomide in solid organ transplantation. *Transplantation* 2002;73:358–366.

94. Chakinala MM, Trulock EP. Acute allograft rejection after lung transplantation: diagnosis and therapy. *Chest Surg Clin N Am* 2003;13:525–542.

95. Cooper JD, Billingham M, Egan T, et al., International Society for Heart and Lung Transplantation. A working formulation for the standardization of nomenclature and for clinical staging of chronic dysfunction in lung allografts. *J Heart Lung Transplant* 1993;12:713–716.

96. Estenne M, Maurer JR, Boehler A, et al. Bronchiolitis obliterans syndrome 2001: an update of the diagnostic criteria. *J Heart Lung Transplant* 2002;21:297–310.

97. Hertz MI, Taylor DO, Trulock EP, et al. The registry of the international society for heart and lung transplantation: nineteenth official report-2002. *J Heart Lung Transplant* 2002;21:950–970.

98. Meyers BF, Lynch J, Trulock EP, et al. Lung transplantation: a decade of experience. *Ann Surg* 1999;230:362–370; discussion 370–361.

99. Estenne M, Hertz MI. Bronchiolitis obliterans after human lung transplantation. *Am J Respir Crit Care Med* 2002;166:440–444.

100. Davis RD, Lau CL, Eubanks S, et al. Improved lung allograft function following fundoplication in lung transplant patients with GERD. *J Thorac Cardiovasc Surg* 2003;125:533–542.

101. Lubetkin EI, Lipson DA, Palevsky HI, et al. GI complications after orthotopic lung transplantation. *Am J Gastroenterol* 1996;91:2382–2390.

102. Hoekstra HJ, Hawkins K, de Boer WJ, et al. Gastrointestinal complications in lung transplant survivors that require surgical intervention. *Br J Surg* 2001;88:433–438.

103. Pollard TR, Schwesinger WH, Sako EY, et al. Abdominal operations after lung transplantation. *Arch Surg* 1997;12:714–718.

104. Armitage JM, Kormos RL, Stuart RS, et al. Posttransplant lymphoproliferative disease in thoracic organ transplant patients: ten years of cyclosporine-based immunosuppression. *J Heart Lung Transplant* 1991;10:877–887.

105. Aris RM, Maia DM, Neuriner IP, et al. Post-transplantation lymphoproliferative disorder in the Epstein-Barr virus-naive lung transplant recipient. *Am J Respir Crit Care Med* 1996;154:1712–1717.

106. Paranjothi S, Yusen RD, Kraus MD, et al. Lymphoproliferative disease after lung transplantation: comparison of presentation and outcome of early and late cases. *J Heart Lung Transplant* 2001;20:1054–1063.

107. Levine SM, Angel L, Anzueto A, et al. A low incidence of posttransplant lymphoproliferative disorder in 109 lung transplant recipients [comment]. *Chest* 1999;116:1273–1277.

108. Swerdlow SH. Classification of the posttransplant lymphoproliferative disorders: from the past to the present. *Semin Diag Pathol* 1997;14:2–7.

109. Schaar CG, Van Der Pijl JW, Van Hoek B, et al. Successful outcome with a "quintuple approach" of posttransplant lymphoproliferative disorder. *Transplantation* 2001;71:47–52.

110. Montone KT, Litzky LA, Wurster A, et al. Analysis of Epstein-Barr virus associated posttransplantation lymphoproliferative disorder after lung transplantation. *Surgery* 1996;119:544–551.

111. Wigle DA, Chaparro C, Humar A, et al. Epstein-Barr virus serology and posttransplant lymphoproliferative disease in lung transplantation. *Transplantation* 2001;72:1783–1786.

112. Wood BL, Sabath D, Broudy VC, et al. The recipient origin of posttransplant lymphoproliferative disorders in pulmonary transplant patients. *Cancer* 1996;78:2223–2228.

113. Swinnen LJ, Costanzo-Nordin MR, Fisher SG, et al. Increased incidence of lymphoproliferative disorder after immunosuppression with the monoclonal antibody OKT3 in cardiac transplant recipients. *N Engl J Med* 1990;323:1723–1728.

114. Walker RC, Marshall WF, Strickler JG, et al. Pretransplantation assessment of the risk of lymphoproliferative disorder. *Clin Infect Dis* 1995;20:1346–1353.

115. Hachem R, Patterson G-A, Trulock EP. Abdominal-pelvic lymphoproliferative disease after lung transplantation. *J Heart Lung Transplant* 2003;22:S194.

116. Verschuuren EA, Stevens SJ, van Imhoff GW, et al. Treatment of posttransplant lymphoproliferative disease with Rituximab: the remission, the relapse, and the complication. *Transplantation* 2002;73:100–104.

117. Malouf MA, Chhajed PN, Hopkins P, et al. Anti-viral prophylaxis reduces the incidence of lymphoproliferative disease in lung transplant recipients. *J Heart Lung Transplant* 2002;21:547–554.

118. Lau C, Trulock E, Guthrie T, et al. Post-operative atrial dysrhythmias after lung transplantation. *J Heart Lung Transplant* 2004;23:150A.

119. Ishani A, Erturk S, Hertz MI, et al. Predictors of renal function following lung or heart-lung transplantation. *Kidney Int* 2002;61:2228–2234.

120. Soccal PM, Gasche Y, Favre H, et al. Improvement of drug-induced chronic renal failure in lung transplantation [comment]. *Transplantation* 1999;68:164–165.

121. Broekroelofs J, Navis GJ, Stegeman CA, et al. Long-term renal outcome after lung transplantation is predicted by the 1-month postoperative renal function loss. *Transplantation* 2000;69:1624–1628.

122. Lichtenstein GR, Kaiser LR, Tuchman M, et al. Fatal hyperammonemia following orthotopic lung transplantation [comment]. *Gastroenterology* 1997;112:236–240.

123. Lichtenstein GR, Yang YX, Nunes FA, et al. Fatal hyperammonemia after orthotopic lung transplantation. *Ann Intern Med* 2000;132:283–287.

124. Tuchman M, Lichtenstein GR, Rajagopal BS, et al. Hepatic glutamine synthetase deficiency in fatal hyperammonemia after lung transplantation [comment]. *Ann Intern Med* 1997;127:446–449.

125. Berry GT, Bridges ND, Nathanson KL, et al. Successful use of alternate waste nitrogen agents and hemodialysis in a patient with hyperammonemic coma after heart-lung transplantation [comment]. *Arch Neurol* 1999;56:481–484.

126. Singh N, Gayowski T, Marino IR. Hemolytic uremic syndrome in solid-organ transplant recipients [comment]. *Transpl Int* 1996;9:68–75.

127. George JN. How I treat patients with thrombotic thrombocytopenic purpura-hemolytic uremic syndrome. *Blood* 2000;96:1223–1229.

Complications of Heart Transplantation

49

Francis D. Pagani

■ **INTRODUCTION 700**

■ **COMPLICATIONS IN THE EARLY PERIOPERATIVE PERIOD 700**
Acute Allograft Failure 700
Arrhythmias 702
Technical Factors 703

■ **COMPLICATIONS IN THE FIRST YEAR 703**
Cardiac Allograft Rejection 703
Infection 706

■ **COMPLICATIONS AFTER THE FIRST YEAR 711**
Transplant Coronary Artery Disease 711
Malignancies 714

■ **OTHER MAJOR COMPLICATIONS 715**
Chronic Renal Insufficiency 715
Hypertension 716
Hyperlipidemia 716
Hyperglycemia 717
Osteoporosis 717
Abdominal and Gastrointestinal Complications 717

■ **REFERENCES 719**

INTRODUCTION

Heart transplantation represents the most successful long-term treatment option available for patients with end-stage

Francis D. Pagani: University of Michigan, Ann Arbor, MI 48109

heart disease. Despite its success in improving both survival and quality of life for patients with refractory congestive heart failure, heart transplantation is associated with significant early and long-term morbidity and mortality. The overall expected 1-year survival for all patients following heart transplantation is approximately 80% to 85%, with a linear attrition rate of 4% per year (Fig. 49-1) (1,2). Fifty percent of heart transplant recipients survive approximately 10 years. For those patients who survive the first year following heart transplantation, median survival is 12 years (1).

A temporal pattern for the development of specific complications following heart transplantation is well documented (Fig. 49-2) (3). Complications contributing directly to early mortality and morbidity within the first 30 days following heart transplantation are generally due to primary allograft failure and, to a lesser extent, infection and allograft rejection. Within the first year, infectious complications and complications of acute allograft rejection dominate causes of mortality and morbidity. After the first year, the development of cardiac-allograft vasculopathy and post-transplant lymphoproliferative disease increases, with infectious causes contributing to a lesser extent. The development of renal insufficiency, hypertension, and endocrine abnormalities (i.e., diabetes mellitus and osteoporosis) also significantly contributes to late morbidity and decrement in quality of life.

COMPLICATIONS IN THE EARLY PERIOPERATIVE PERIOD

Acute Allograft Failure

The incidence of acute allograft failure following cardiac transplantation approximates 2% to 5% in most large

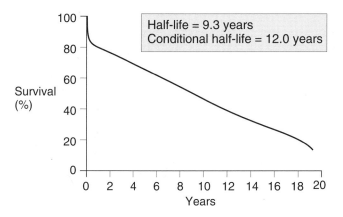

Figure 49-1 Heart transplant survival. (Reprinted from Taylor DO, Edwards LB, Mohacsi PJ, et al. The registry of the international society for heart and lung transplantation: twentieth official adult heart transplant report—2003. *J Heart Lung Transplant* 2003;22:616–624.)

TABLE 49-1

RISK FACTORS FOR EARLY ACUTE ALLOGRAFT FAILURE

Recipient Factors
Congenital etiology
Higher serum creatinine at transplant
Pas-PCWP
Mean RAP
PRA >10%
Previous sternotomy
>1 Previous sternotomy
Ventilator dependence
Days on ventricular assist device
Donor Factors
Older donor age
Abnormal echo
Diabetes
Longer ischemic time

Adapted from Young JB, Naftel DC, Ewald G, et al. Determinants of early graft failure following cardiac transplantation: a ten year multi-institutional, multi-variable analysis. *J Heart Lung Transplant* 2001;20:212 [abstract]; Naftel DC, Brown RN. Survival after heart transplantation. In: Kirklin JK, Young JB, McGiffin DC, eds. *Heart transplantation: medicine, surgery, immunology, and research.* New York: Churchill Livingstone, 2002:587–614.

series and is the most common cause of death within the first 30 days (approximately 40% to 45% of early deaths) (Fig. 49-3) (2 – 6). The incidence of acute allograft failure has remained relatively constant over the past 10 years (5). Multiple recipient and donor characteristics that adversely influence the incidence of early acute allograft failure have been reported (Table 49-1) (5,7).

Early allograft failure following heart transplantation is predominantly due to right-sided circulatory failure as a consequence of elevated recipient pulmonary vascular resistance or donor right ventricular contractile dysfunction secondary to brain death, myocardial contusion (i.e., cardiopulmonary resuscitation or blunt thoracic trauma), or ischemic injury (8 – 10). Elevated preoperative recipient pulmonary vascular resistance has been identified as an independent predictor for early post-transplant mortality and correlates in a linear fashion

with mortality following heart transplantation (Fig. 49-4) (1,2,11 – 13). Acute allograft failure may also manifest as biventricular dysfunction as a result of ischemia-reperfusion injury to the donor organ secondary to inadequate myocardial protection or prolonged allograft ischemic time. For allograft ischemic times greater than approximately 2 hours, there is an increasing risk of death from allograft failure (Fig. 49-5) (1). Acute allograft failure secondary to accelerated or hyperacute rejection is more unusual. In some instances, the cause of allograft failure remains unexplained.

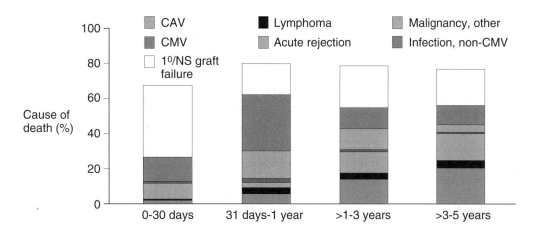

Figure 49-2 Causes of death by time following heart transplantation. CAV, cardiac allograft vasculopathy; CMV, cytomegalovirus; NS, nonspecific. (Reprinted from Hosenpud JD, Bennett L, Keck BM, et al. The registry of the international society for heart and lung transplantation: eighteenth official report—2001. *J Heart Lung Transplant* 2001;20:805–815.)

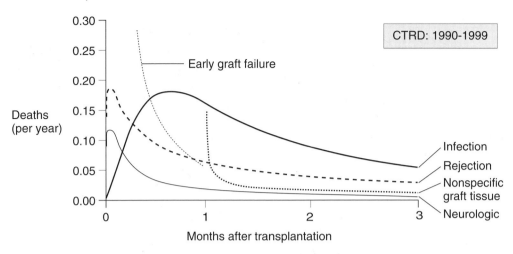

Figure 49-3 Hazard functions for the specific causes of death during the first 4 months following heart transplantation. (Reprinted from Kirklin JK, Naftel DC, Bourge RC, et al. Evolving trends in risk profiles and causes of death after heart transplantation: a ten-year multi-institutional study. *J Thorac Cardiovasc Surg* 2003;125:881–890.)

Arrhythmias

Bradycardia secondary to sinus node dysfunction occurs frequently following heart transplantation but is generally asymptomatic and resolves early within the first few days to weeks (14,15). Atrioventricular block is less common and more likely to remain permanent. Late bradycardias are rare and represent an adverse prognostic sign. Early treatment of symptomatic bradycardia due to sinus node dysfunction may include temporary external pacing or administration of intravenous (e.g., isoproterenol) or oral (e.g., terbutaline) β-adrenergic agents. Permanent pacemaker implantation is required for bradycardia that remains persistent and symptomatic. The reported incidence of permanent pacemaker implantation following heart transplantation is

strongly influenced by surgical technique and is significantly less when bicaval anastomosis rather then biatrial technique is used (16−18). Since the introduction of the bicaval anastomosis, early sinus node dysfunction has been significantly reduced, and permanent pacing is now required in only 1% to 2% of patients.

Any type of supraventricular tachyarrhythmia may occur following heart transplantation. The overall incidence of atrial arrhythmias is high, with atrial flutter being the most common arrhythmia reported (19−21). An association between atrial arrhythmias, early allograft rejection, and subsequent late allograft vasculopathy has been reported (19,22). The occurrence of ventricular arrhythmias early following heart transplantation is very unusual and may represent ischemic allograft injury or significant allograft

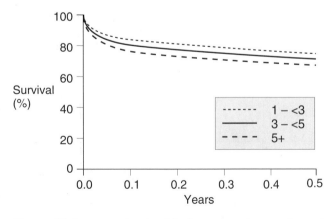

Figure 49-4 Actuarial survival for heart transplants performed between April 1994 and June 2001 categorized by pulmonary vascular resistance (Wood units). (Reprinted from Taylor DO, Edwards LB, Mohacsi PJ, et al. The registry of the international society for heart and lung transplantation: twentieth official adult heart transplant report—2003. *J Heart Lung Transplant* 2003;22:616–624.)

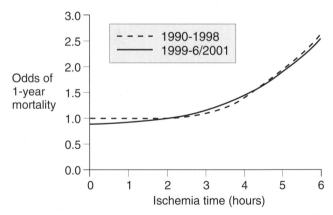

Figure 49-5 Actuarial survival for heart transplants performed between April 1994 and June 2001 categorized by allograft ischemic time. (Reprinted from Taylor DO, Edwards LB, Mohacsi PJ, et al. The registry of the international society for heart and lung transplantation: twentieth official adult heart transplant report—2003. *J Heart Lung Transplant* 2003;22:616–624.)

rejection. Late ventricular arrhythmias may occur in association with allograft ischemia secondary to coronary artery vasculopathy.

Technical Factors

Although technical complications directly related to the operative procedure are unusual, they still have a significant impact on early postoperative morbidity and mortality. Complications related to operative technique include atrial thrombosis at the suture line (23,24), atrial distortion with subsequent atrioventricular valvular incompetence (25,26), acquired cor-triatiatum with mitral inflow obstruction (27,28), pulmonary artery anastomotic distortion (29), chronotropic insufficiency or heart block (30), and aneurysm of the ascending aorta (31). Minimizing the amount of residual recipient left atrium, proper alignment of the aortic and pulmonic anastomoses, use of the bicaval technique, and ensuring apposition of recipient endothelium to donor endothelium during creation of the atrial anastomosis significantly reduce these technical pitfalls.

COMPLICATIONS IN THE FIRST YEAR

Cardiac Allograft Rejection

Acute allograft rejection remains a significant cause of mortality and morbidity following heart transplantation within the first year (Fig. 49-2). Approximately 60% of adult transplant recipients will experience one or more episodes of acute allograft rejection within 6 months following heart transplantation, while approximately one-third of patients remain free of allograft rejection at 1 year (Fig. 49-6) (32). Approximately 25% of patients will experience another

rejection episode within 1 month of the previous episode. The greatest risk for recurrence of allograft rejection is within 1 month of the previous rejection episode (32). Beyond 1 year, there is a significant decrease in number of episodes of acute allograft rejection (33). Patients experiencing late episodes of acute allograft rejection are typically those who have experienced recurrent episodes of rejection during the first year following heart transplantation (34).

Multiple recipient and donor characteristics that adversely influence the occurrence of acute allograft rejection have been reported (Table 49-2) (32,35). The most significant risk factor for the development of hyperacute or early acute allograft rejection is the presence of preformed recipient anti–human leukocyte antigens (HLA) antibodies directed against the donor allograft. A panel-reactive antibody value >10% is indicative of significant sensitization in cardiac-allograft recipients and is a risk factor for the development of acute rejection during the early posttransplant period. High reactivity is also a risk for early death from acute or chronic rejection, particularly if directed against class I HLA antigens (36–39). This finding also applies to heart transplant recipients who have developed anti-HLA class II antibodies against the donor organ, although the degree of risk is less clearly defined. (36,40).

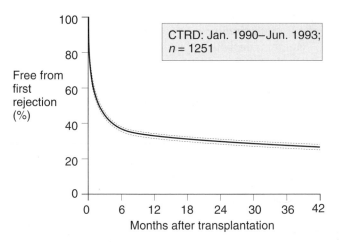

Figure 49-6 Actuarial and parametric freedom from initial rejection following heart transplantation. (Reprinted from Kubo SH, Naftel DC, Mills RM, et al. Risks factors for late recurrent rejection after heart transplantation: a multi-institutional, multi-variable analysis. *J Heart Lung Transplant* 1995;14:409–418.)

TABLE 49-2

RISK FACTORS FOR CARDIAC ALLOGRAFT REJECTION

Factors Influencing Earlier Initial Rejection Following Heart Transplantation
Younger age (among adult recipients)
Female gender (donor and recipient)
If white recipient: higher number of HLA mismatches
Black recipient race
Risk Factors for Increased Cumulative Rejection Episodes during First Year Following Heart Transplantation
Younger age or recipient
Female gender (donor and recipient)
HLA-DR mismatches
Induction therapy
Risk Factors for Recurrent Rejection during the First Year Following Heart Transplantation
Female gender (donor and recipient)
Younger recipient age (except infant)
Positive CMV serology before transplant
Induction therapy (use of OKT3)
Fewer months since transplant
Fewer months since last rejection
Greater number of previous infections
Increased donor ischemic time

Adapted from Jarcho J, Naftel DC, Shroyer TW, et al. The Cardiac Transplant Research Database Group. Influence of HLA mismatch on rejection after heart transplantation: a multi-institutional study. *J Heart Lung Transplant* 1994;13:583–596 and Kubo SH, Naftel DC, Mills RM, et al. Risks factors for late recurrent rejection after heart transplantation: a multi-institutional, multi-variable analysis. *J Heart Lung Transplant* 1995;14:409–418.

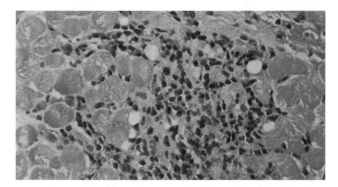

Figure 49-7 Endomyocardial biopsy representative of grade 2 cellular rejection. Interstitial inflammatory infiltrate consisting mostly of lymphocytes and some macrophages. The infiltrate covers an area of about 300 to 500 μm, thus representing a large area of myocyte dropout. Vacuoles are present mostly within myocytes, but others are difficult to assign to a specific cell type (H&E, ×40). (Reprinted from Rodriguez R. The pathology of heart transplant biopsy specimens: revisiting the 1990 ISHLT working formulation. *J Heart Lung Transplant* 2003;22:3–15.)

Acute allograft rejection is a cellular process characterized by a mononuclear inflammatory response composed predominantly of a lymphocytic cell type that is directed against the donor allograft (Fig. 49-7). The rejection phenomenon is a diffuse process and typically involves both the left and right ventricles, thus permitting diagnosis of rejection by representative endomyocardial biopsies of the right ventricular septum. Cellular-mediated allograft rejection is graded on histologic analysis of endomyocardial biopsies according to established criteria (Table 49-3) (41). Additional research has characterized the lymphocytic infiltrate and immune response.

TABLE 49-3

DEFINITIONS FOR GRADING OF CELLULAR-MEDIATED ALLOGRAFT REJECTION: INTERNATIONAL SOCIETY FOR HEART AND LUNG CLASSIFICATION

Grade 0	No evidence of cellular rejection
Grade 1A	Focal perivascular or interstititial infiltrate without myocyte injury
Grade 1B	Multifocal or diffuse sparse infiltrate without myocyte injury
Grade 2	Single focus of dense infiltrate with myocyte injury
Grade 3A	Multifocal dense infiltrates with myocyte injury
Grade 3B	Diffuse, dense infiltrates with myocyte injury
Grade 4	Diffuse and extensive polymorphous infiltrate with myocyte injury; may have hemorrhage, edema, and microvascular injury

Use the term injury to include one or more of the following: myocyte encroachment, architectural distortion, and dropout, as well as reversible and irreversible cell injury. Substituting the term aggressive infiltrates with dense infiltrates may be more appropriate.
Adapted from Rodriguez R. The pathology of heart transplant biopsy specimens: revisiting the 1990 ISHLT working formulation. *J Heart Lung Transplant* 2003;22:3–15.

The inflammatory response within the allograft during acute cellular rejection is promoted by a number proinflammatory molecules, such as interleukin-2 (IL-2), that correlate with episodes of rejection (42–45). In addition to cytokines, increased expression of a number of adhesion molecules have been reported that correlate with upcoming rejection (intercellular adhesion molecule 1 and E-selectin) or correlate with the response to therapy of the rejection process (vascular adhesion molecule 1) (42,46–52). The induction of chemokine gene and protein expression within the allograft, detected with serial endomyocardial biopsies, also coincides with leukocyte graft infiltration (53–55). These chemokines include the T-cell chemoattractants inducible protein 10 (IP)-10, monokine induced by IFN-[gamma] (Mig), interferon inducible-T cell α chemoattractant (I-TAC), regulated on activation normal T-cell expressed and secreted (RANTES), and their receptors CXCR3 and CCR5.

In addition to a cellular-mediated allograft rejection process, humoral-mediated allograft rejection may contribute to the pathogenesis of acute allograft rejection (42,56). The main histologic features of humoral rejection include intravascular polymorphonuclear leukocytes and macrophages with associated endothelial swelling; vasculocentric, lymphocyte-poor inflammatory infiltrate; and myocyte injury, including myocyte necrosis in areas adjacent to affected vessels with infiltrates (42). Evaluation of endomyocardial biopsies from the allograft with immunohistochemical techniques identifies deposition near capillaries, arterioles, and small arteries of pathologic markers of humoral rejection, including IgG, IgM, IgA, C1q, C3d, C4d, fibrinogen, and fibrin. The presence of swollen macrophages within capillaries can be demonstrated by staining with CD68/KP1 (monocytes/macrophages) and CD34 (endothelium) antibodies (Fig. 49-8) (42,56). The finding of donor-specific anti-HLA antibodies in the serum of the recipient further supports the diagnosis of humoral-mediated rejection. More pronounced humoral-mediated allograft rejection may be associated with a lymphocytic or mixed cellular infiltrate.

Humoral-mediated allograft rejection typically presents within the first 3 weeks postoperatively but can be observed up to 6 months or later following heart transplantation (57). When compared to cellular-mediated allograft rejection, humoral-mediated allograft rejection typically occurs earlier following heart transplantation, is more highly associated with hemodynamic abnormalities or left ventricular dysfunction, is more resistant to augmented immunosuppression, is associated with a higher frequency of allograft loss and mortality, and is more highly associated with the subsequent development of coronary allograft vasculopathy (56). Risk factors for the development of humoral-mediated allograft rejection include recipient female gender, a history of repeat transplantation, elevated recipient panel-reactive antibody screen, recipient cytomegalovirus (CMV) seropositivity, positive perioperative T-cell flow cytometry crossmatch, and possibly prior sensitization to OKT3 (56).

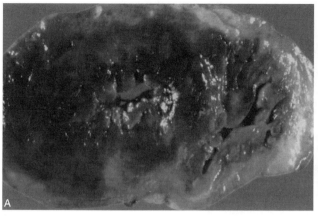
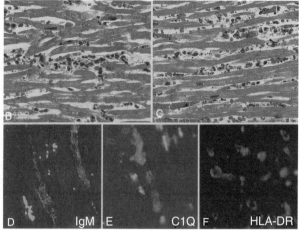

Figure 49-8 Representative gross anatomical and histologic analysis of humoral-mediated cardiac allograft rejection. **A:** Cross-section of a heart from a patient who died of humoral rejection (HR). There is diffuse myocardial hemorrhage within both the left and right ventricular walls. **(B, C)** Microscopic sections show intravascular macrophages and neutrophils. There is congestion of capillaries with focal interstitial hemorrhage (original magnification ×33). Immunofluorescence studies show capillary positivity (green fluorescence) for IgM **(D)**, C1q **(E)**, and HLA-DR **(F)**. Yellow fluorescence represents lipofucsin granules in myocytes (original magnification ×120). (Reprinted from Michaels PJ, Espejo ML, Kobashigawa J, et al. Humoral rejection in cardiac transplantation: risk factors, hemodynamic consequences and relationship to transplant coronary artery disease. *J Heart Lung Transplant* 2003;22:58–69.)

Right ventricular endomyocardial biopsy is the most reliable method of assessing allograft rejection in heart transplant recipients. Endomyocardial biopsy is performed under fluoroscopic or echocardiographic guidance along with right heart catheterization to assess filling pressures and to calculate cardiac index. Endomyocardial biopsies are initially performed weekly in adults for the first month and then every 2 to 4 weeks over the next 2 months (58). The frequency of endomyocardial biopsy is generally decreased to every 3 to 4 months for the remainder of the first year and less frequently during the second year in recipients who demonstrate no episodes of allograft rejection (59). Endomyocardial biopsies are indicated for significant changes in clinical status such as unexplained tachycardia, arrhythmia, hypotension, fever, abnormal hemodynamics, or new echocardiographic abnormalities. The ability of endomyocardial biopsy to detect allograft rejection has limitations due to sampling error as a result of small biopsy size, the heterogeneous nature of acute cellular rejection, and interobserver variability and skill (60,61). A failure rate as high as 14% has been reported in the detection of moderate to severe rejection when at least three fragments show mild rejection (60). Biopsies obtained within the first 4 to 6 weeks following transplantation frequently demonstrate changes consistent with ischemic myocardial necrosis.

The primary method of management of allograft rejection is prevention with maintenance immunosuppressive therapy. The most common management strategy involves triple drug therapy, based on a calcineurin inhibitor (cyclosporine or tacrolimus), accompanied by an antiproliferative agent (mycophenolate or, less commonly, azathioprine or cyclophosphamide), and corticosteroids. Recent evidence suggests benefit with use of a calcineurin inhibitor and corticosteroids, along with sirolimus or everolimus (62,63). Attempts to wean corticosteroid therapy are made after 3 to 6 months. Female gender, degree of HLA mismatch, and prior rejection history are adverse factors influencing steroid withdrawal. Treatment of an acute episode of cellular-mediated allograft rejection is complex, based on factors that include clinical features such as presence of abnormal myocardial function, histologic severity of the rejection episode, and time course following heart transplantation during which the rejection episode occurs (Tables 49-4–49-6).

The infrequent occurrence of humoral rejection and problems in diagnosis have made it difficult to evaluate the most effective form of treatment. Anecdotal reports have documented resolution with pulsed high-dose corticosteroids, cytolytic therapy with OKT-3 or ATG, cyclophsophamide, IVIg, and plasmapheresis (64). Cyclophosphamide is effective in inhibiting B-cell activity and may improve outcome. Intermittent therapeutic plasmapharesis removes circulating antibodies against HLA and endothelial antigens. Heparin administration has been proposed to inhibit vascular smooth muscle cell proliferation. Heparin binding to the endothelium may inhibit allogenic recognition of receptors on the endothelial surface and improve coronary flow. Photopheresis with ultraviolet A light following treatment with 8-methoxypsoralen has been effective in treating cellular rejection in highly sensitized transplant recipients and may also be useful in the treatment of humoral rejection.

TABLE 49-4

TREATMENT OF ISOLATED ACUTE CELLULAR REJECTION WITHOUT HEMODYNAMIC COMPROMISE

Biopsy Grade	Therapy	Follow-up
IA	None	Routine follow-up
IB	Prednisone (3 mg/kg PO) × 3 d ± taper	Rebiopsy in 2–4 wk
II	Prednisone (3 mg/kg PO) × 3 d ± taper	Same as above
IIIA	Methylprednisolone (IV) or prednisone (same dose as above)	Rebiopsy in 1–2 wk
IIIB	Same protocol as for recurrent or persistent rejection	Rebiopsy in 1 wk
IV	Same protocol as for rejection with hemodynamic compromise	Rebiopsy in 1 wk

Adapted from Bourge RC, Rodriguez ER, Tan CD. Cardiac allograft rejection. In: Kirklin JK, Young JB, McGiffin DC, eds. *Heart transplantation: medicine, surgery, immunology, and research.* New York: Churchill Livingstone, 2002:464–520.

Humoral-mediated allograft rejection frequently recurs, and overall allograft loss exceeds 20%.

Infection

Infection is a leading cause of mortality during the first year following heart transplantation (Fig. 49-3) (65–67). Approximately 40% of transplant recipients have one or more major infectious episodes, with the cumulative incidence of infections per patient averaging 0.4 at 3 months, 0.55 at 6 months, and 0.62 at 12 months (65). The risk of infection depends on the net state of immunosuppression of the patient and exposure to potential pathogens (Table 49-7) (68). The majority of infections occur with a predictable time course following transplantation, largely

due to the consistency of treatment regimens with immunosuppressive drugs (Fig. 49-9).

The risk of first infection following heart transplantation is highest during the first month. Risk factors for infection early following heart transplantation include older recipient age, ventilator support at the time of transplantation, ventricular assist device at the time of transplantation, the use of OKT3 induction therapy, and positive donor CMV serology (69). Infection in the early period is dominated by bacterial nosocomial infections with gram-negative bacilli and *Staphylococcus* species. (65). *Pseudomonas aeruginosa*, *Proteus* species, and *Klebsiella* are more commonly observed in transplant recipients than in routine postoperative cardiac surgical patients. The more debilitated the patient or the more invasive the degree of preoperative support, the higher the likelihood of infectious morbidity. The lung is consistently the most common

TABLE 49-5

STRATEGIES FOR TREATMENT OF RECURRENT OR PERSISTENT REJECTION WITHOUT HEMODYNAMIC COMPROMISE

Initial treatment with intravenous methylprednisolone plus cytolytic therapy (OKT3 or ATGAM)
Consider one or more of the following:
 Convert from azathioprine to mycophenolate or cyclophosphamide (if evidence of humoral rejection)
 Convert from cyclosporine to tacrolimus
 Raise maintenance prednisone to 0.2 mg/kg/d
 Initiate photophoresis
 Add methotrexate (rarely needed)
 Total lymphoid radiation (only as last resort because of potential for late megakaryocytic leukemia)

Adapted from Bourge RC, Rodriguez ER, Tan CD. Cardiac allograft rejection. In: Kirklin JK, Young JB, McGiffin DC, eds. *Heart transplantation: medicine, surgery, immunology, and research.* New York: Churchill Livingstone, 2002:464–520.

TABLE 49-6

THERAPEUTIC STRATEGY FOR REJECTION WITH HEMODYNAMIC COMPROMISE

Always consider this a life-threatening event
Methylprednisolone 1 g IV daily for 3 d
Prompt inotropic support
Swan-Ganz catheter for hemodynamic monitoring
Prompt plasmapharesis daily for 3 d
Cytolytic therapy with ATGAM or OKT3
Heparin therapy
Continue maintenance immunosuppression
Schedule photophoresis

Adapted from Bourge RC, Rodriguez ER, Tan CD. Cardiac allograft rejection. In: Kirklin JK, Young JB, McGiffin DC, eds. *Heart transplantation: medicine, surgery, immunology, and research.* New York: Churchill Livingstone, 2002:464–520.

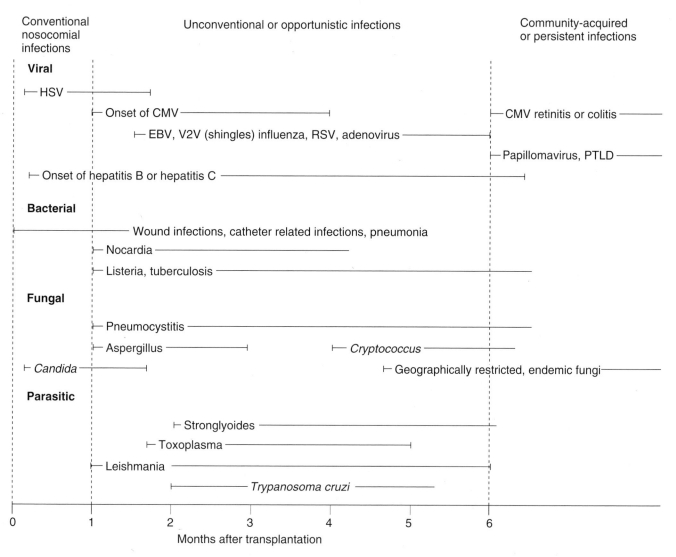

| Conventional nosocomial infections | Unconventional or opportunistic infections | Community-acquired or persistent infections |

Viral

├─ HSV ───────┤

├─ Onset of CMV ───────────────┤   ├─ CMV retinitis or colitis ───────

├─ EBV, V2V (shingles) influenza, RSV, adenovirus ───────┤

├─ Papillomavirus, PTLD ───────

├─ Onset of hepatitis B or hepatitis C ──────────────────────────────────

Bacterial

├───────── Wound infections, catheter related infections, pneumonia

├─ Nocardia ─────────────────────────

├─ Listeria, tuberculosis ───────────────────────────────

Fungal

├─ Pneumocystitis ───────────────────────────────

├─ Aspergillus ───────────────┤   ├─ *Cryptococcus* ───────────

├─ *Candida* ───────┤   ├─ Geographically restricted, endemic fungi ───────

Parasitic

├─ Stronglyoides ─────────────────────

├─ Toxoplasma ───────────────────────

├─ Leishmania ───────────────────────

├──────── *Trypanosoma cruzi* ────────

0   1   2   3   4   5   6

Months after transplantation

Figure 49-9   Time course of infections following organ transplantation. Exceptions to the usual sequence of infections after transplantation suggest the presence of unusual epidemiologic exposure or excessive immunosuppression. Zero indicates the time of transplantation. Solid lines indicate the most common period for the onset of infection; dotted lines and arrows indicate periods of continued risk at reduced levels. HSV, herpes simplex virus; CMV, cytomegalovirus; EBV, Epstein–Barr virus; VZV, varicella–zoster virus; RSV, respiratory syncytial virus; PTLD, post-transplantation lymphoproliferative disease. (Reprinted from Fishman JA, Rubin RH. Medical progress: infection in organ-transplant recipients. *N Engl J Med* 1998; 338:1741–51.)

site of infection (28%), followed by bloodstream (26%), gastrointestinal tract (17%), urinary tract (12%), skin (8%), and wound (7%) (65).

Infectious risk for viral and opportunistic organisms remains high from postoperative months 1 through 6 as a result of the cumulative effects of immunosuppression. Although pulmonary infections remain common, central nervous system and gastrointestinal infections may occur. The clinical effects of viruses such as CMV, Epstein–Barr virus, and other human herpes-viruses and opportunistic infections due to *Pneumocystis carinii*, *Aspergillus*, and *Listeria monocytogenes* become important. Routine prophylaxis is required to prevent a number of viral and opportunistic

infections (Table 49-8). After 6 months the risk of serious opportunistic infections and viral illnesses becomes less. Those at particular risk for infectious complications, particularly opportunistic infections with *P. carinii*, *L. monocytogenes*, *Nocardia asteroides*, *Cryptococcus neoformans*, and *Aspergillus*, include patients with recurrent rejection episodes who have heightened intensity of immunosuppression regimens late in the transplant period.

CMV is the most important infectious pathogen in cardiac transplant recipients (65,68,70). Two critical steps in the pathogenesis of CMV infection include reactivation from latency and systemic dissemination. Following heart transplantation, approximately 20% of recipients will

TABLE 49-7

FACTORS AFFECTING THE IMMUNOSUPPRESSIVE STATE OF THE TRANSPLANT RECIPIENT

Immunosuppressive therapy: dose, duration, and temporal sequence
Underlying immune deficiency: autoimmune disease, functional immune deficits
Integrity of the mucocutaneous barrier: catheters, epithelial surfaces
Devitalized tissue, fluid collections
Neutropenia, lymphopenia
Metabolic conditions
Uremia
Malnutrition
Diabetes
Alcoholism with cirrhosis
Infection with immunomodulating viruses
Cytomegalovirus
Epstein–Barr virus
Hepatitis B and C viruses
Human immunodeficiency virus

Adapted from Fishman JA, Rubin RH. Medical progress: infection in organ-transplant recipients. *N Engl J Med* 1998; 338:1741–1751.

have experienced one or more infections with CMV by 2 years. The peak incidence of infection with CMV occurs between the first and second month following heart transplantation, but the period of time to onset of CMV disease

has been steadily increasing (71). Risk factors for the development of CMV infection include the serologic status of the donor and recipient. A seronegative recipient with seropositive donor has the greatest risk (Fig. 49-10). The use of induction therapy or treatment of rejection episodes with OKT-3 or antilymphocyte globulin significantly increases the risk of symptomatic CMV disease and activation from latency (Table 49-9). Additional factors include allogeneic reactions and systemic infection or inflammation.

The effects of acute CMV infection include fever with constitutional symptoms, laboratory abnormalities including leucopenia, thrombocytopenia, atypical lymphocytosis, and elevation of liver transaminases. The sites of CMV infection include the bloodstream (43% of infections), lungs (CMV pneumonitis, 30%), and gastrointestinal tract (8%). Less common features include hepatitis, CMV myocarditis, chorioretinitis, and central nervous system involvement. Long-term sequelae of CMV infection include cardiac-allograft vasculopathy, post-transplant lymphoproliferative disorder, and increased risk of developing opportunistic infections (Fig. 49-11).

The diagnosis of disease due to CMV is accomplished by demonstrating viremia or tissue invasion. CMV antigenemia assay is commonly used for detection of CMV in peripheral blood. Quantitative PCR or hybrid capture assay for CMV DNA provides the most sensitive technology

TABLE 49-8

INFECTION PROPHYLAXIS AFTER HEART TRANSPLANTATION

Infectious Complication	Prophylaxis
Pneumocystis carinii	Trimethoprim/sulfamethoxazole 1 gd (1 yr); for patients allergic to sulfonamides, dapsone 50 mg gd (1 yr) or pentamidine 300 mg via nebulizer every month (1 yr)
Mucocutaneous candidiasis	Topical, nonabsorbable antifungal (nystatin) 500,000 units t.i.d (6 mo)
Toxoplasmosis recipient (–)/donor (+)	Pyrimethamine 25 mg gd and leucovorin 10 mg gd (6 mo)-serology is checked at 3 mo, 6 mo, and 1 y
Cytomegalovirus recipient (–)/donor (+)	Ganciclovir IV (6 wk), then ganciclovir 1 g t.i.d PO (6 wk) Cytogam 150 mg/kg IV within 72 hours after transplant, then every 2 wk × 4 doses; then 100 mg/kg IV every 4 wk × 2 doses
Recipient (+) or any course of OKT3 or antithymocyte globulin	Ganciclovir IV during hospitalization, then ganciclovir 1 g t.i.d PO (6 wk), then acyclovir 200 mg PO t.i.d for 6 mo
Recipient (–)/donor (–)	Acyclovir 200 mg t.i.d PO (6 mo)
Epstein-Barr virus recipient (–)/donor (+)	EBV IgM IgG serologies are checked at 6 wk, 3 mo, and every 3 mo for the first year and then every 6 mo until seroconversion; at seroconversion patient is treated with ganciclovir IV (6 wk), then ganciclovir PO 1 g t.i.d for 6 mo, then acyclovir 200 mg t.i.d for 6 mo
Herpes simplex 1 and 2	Acyclovir 200 mg t.i.d PO (6 mo)

Adapted from Bourge RC, Rodriguez ER, Tan CD. Cardiac allograft rejection. In: Kirklin JK, Young JB, McGiffin DC, eds. *Heart transplantation: medicine, surgery, immunology, and research.* New York: Churchill Livingstone, 2002:464–520.

TABLE 49-9

RISK OF CLINICAL DISEASE DUE TO CMV INFECTION IN DIFFERENT POPULATIONS OF HEART TRANSPLANT RECIPIENTS

Donor CMV Serotype Status	Recipient CMV Serotype Status	Antilymphocyte Antibody Therapy	Incidence of Clinical Disease (%)
Positive	Negative	—	50–75
Positive or negative	Positive	No	10–15
Positive or negative	Positive	Induction antirejection	25, 50–75
Negative	Negative	—	0^a

[a]In donor negative/recipient negative transplants, CMV disease is uncommonly seen under two circumstances: transfusion of viable leukocyte containing blood products from a seropositive donor or acquisition of virus in the community through intimate person-to-person contact.

Adapted from Rubin RH. Prevention and treatment of cytomegalovirus disease in heart transplant patients. *J Heart Lung Transplant* 2000;19:731–735.

for detection of CMV in tissue or fluid. Demonstration of virus on biopsy of infected tissue is used in some cases.

Antiviral agents are used in three modes to treat the sequelae of CMV infection (72). Antiviral therapy may be used for the prophylaxis. The prevention of CMV infection through prophylaxis is an important strategy for heart transplant recipients (Table 49-8). Due to the limited data available, however, there is currently no consensus on the optimal prophylactic regimen. The intensity of prophylaxis must be proportional to the intensity of immunosuppression and to the risk of viral reactivation; prophylaxis must be initiated before reactivation of the virus; and effective antiviral prophylaxis must be maintained for at least 3 months to prevent relapses after premature termination of

prophylaxis. Antiviral therapy with ganciclovir reduces the incidence of CMV disease in CMV-positive recipients (73). Recent data suggest that valganciclovir, an orally administered prodrug of ganciclovir that achieves serum levels similar to ganciclovir, may be effective for prevention of CMV disease in transplant recipients (74).

Antiviral therapy is used in a therapeutic mode to treat established infection with the aim of eradicating active infection, limiting lasting pathologic effect, and preventing recurrence. The generally accepted standard for treatment of CMV disease is 2 to 3 weeks of intravenous ganciclovir (adjusted for renal function). Prior to the availability of ganciclovir, the mortality associated with CMV pnuemonitis was as high as 75%. With ganciclovir, contemporary

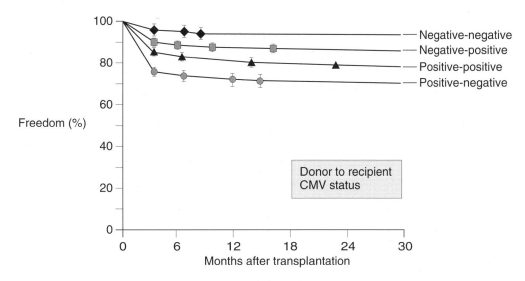

Figure 49-10 Actuarial freedom from initial cytomegalovirus (CMV) infection according to CMV serologic status of donor and recipient before transplantation. Dashed lines indicate duration of follow-up. Error bars indicate ± standard error. (Reprinted from Kirklin JK, Naftel DC, Levine TB, et al. Cytomegalovirus after heart transplantation. Risk factors for infection and death: a multiinstitutional study. *J Heart Lung Transplant* 1994;13:394–404.)

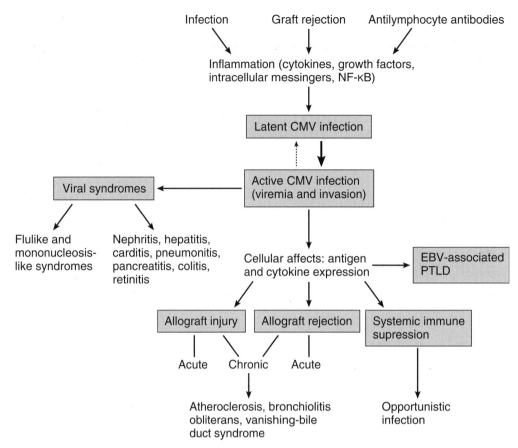

Figure 49-11 Role of cytomegalovirus (CMV) infection in transplant recipients. Mediators of systemic inflammation link the activation of CMV infection to allograft injury and rejection, to infection with opportunistic pathogens, and to the development of cancer in organ-transplant recipients. EBV, Epstein–Barr virus; PTLD, post-transplantation lymphoproliferative disease. (Reprinted from Fishman JA, Rubin RH. Medical progress: infection in organ-transplant recipients. *N Engl J Med* 1998;338:1741–1751.)

mortality of CMV pneumonitis is <15%. Duration of therapy has not been clearly established, but 2 to 3 weeks is usually recommended. Many clinicians believe that tissue-invasive disease should be treated for longer periods (up to 6 weeks). With the current availability of quantitative measures of CMV viral load, it may be advisable to continue treatment until at least one viral load measure is zero, with all symptoms resolved. In patients with severe disease, particularly pneumonitis, CMV hyperimmune globulin may be used in combination with ganciclovir, although this combination has not been clearly substantiated outside of bone marrow transplant recipients. CMV infection relapse rate can be as high as 20% in seropositive individuals and even higher among patients with primary infection.

Antiviral therapy can be used in a pre-emptive mode in patients at very high risk of developing clinical infection and disease. This population of patients is defined as having received cytolytic therapy for induction or treatment of rejection or having a high likelihood of developing clinical infection by demonstrating laboratory evidence of CMV infection by CMV antegenemia or quantitative PCR testing but lacking clinically apparent disease. Antiviral therapy is initiated on the basis of viremia.

Transmission of infection from donor to recipient remains a significant concern following heart transplantation. Routine screening of the donor for a number of infectious agents minimizes this risk (Table 49-10). The consequences of seroconversion for hepatitis B (HVB) in recipients suggest significant long-term sequelae. In heart

TABLE 49-10

ROUTINE SEROLOGY SCREENING OF THE DONOR ORGAN

HIV antibody
HTLV-1 antibody
Hepatitis B virus surface antigen (HBsAg)
Hepatitis B virus surface antibody (anti-HBs)
Hepatitis B virus core antibody (anti-HBc)
Hepatitis C virus antibody (HCV)
Cytomegalovirus (CMV)
Treponemal antigen (syphilis)
Toxoplasma antibody
Epstein-Barr antibody
West Nile virus

transplant recipients who acquired HBsAg positivity after transplantation, 56% developed severe fibrosis and cirrhosis within a mean of 7.4 years after infection. Eighteen percent of deaths in HBsAg-positive patients were due to HBV-related liver failure, with the adverse effect of HBV infection on survival apparent beyond 10 years (75). The use of organs from donors who are IgG HBcAb-positive, IgM HBcAb-negative, and HBsAg-negative has been reported and suggests a low risk of HBV transmission (76). The use of organs from donors who are HBsAb-positive probably carries a very significant risk of HBV transmission.

The sequelae of transmission of hepatitis C (HCV) infection from donor to the recipient has been difficult to assess due to limited data. Lake et al. have reported on the long-term outcome of HCV-positive recipients and found no difference in survival compared to a UNOS control group (77). There was a 50% incidence of liver dysfunction and greater proportion of deaths due to liver disease in the HCV-positive recipients. Ong et al. reviewed the outcomes of HCV antibody-negative cardiac recipients receiving HCV antibody-positive donor hearts. Twenty-three of 28 patients developed detectable viremia, of whom seven developed HCV-related liver disease. Four of the seven patients developed severe cholestatic hepatitis, which contributed to a significantly poorer survival compared to patients receiving hearts from HCV antibody-negative donors (78). On the basis of the limited data available it is reasonable to avoid the transplantation of HCV-positive donor hearts into HCV-negative recipients.

Transmission of protozoal infection with *Toxoplasma gondii* is an important consideration for heart transplant recipients. Pneumonitis, myocarditis, and encephalitis are the most common clinical syndromes that usually first present with undifferentiated fever. In heart transplant recipients, the risk of toxoplasmosis due to reactivation of latent infection is low (79). The highest risk of developing disease is in the setting of primary infection (seronegative

recipient who acquires the parasite from a seropositive donor) via the graft (80). In one study, a higher incidence of previous *T. gondii* infection was observed among recipients (16%) compared to donors (6%) reflecting the increasing seroprevalence of infection with increasing age (71). Only 5.6% of patients were donor seropositive/recipient seronegative. Of the 32 donor positive/recipient negative patients for serology testing, 16 were receiving trimethoprimsulfamethoxazole or pyrimethamine prophylaxis or both, and none of those 16 patients developed toxoplasmosis. However, four (25%) of the 16 donor positive/recipient negative patients who were not taking either trimethoprimsulfamethoxazole or pyrimethamine developed toxoplasmosis, and all died of the infection. None of the 98 patients who were seropositive for *T. gondii* preoperatively developed clinical evidence of reactivation of the infection. Whether a single tablet (double-strength) taken twice daily, 3 times each week, is sufficient to prevent toxoplasmosis in the donor positive/recipient negative group is unclear at this time, and it seems prudent that for those patients a 6-week course of pyrimethamine be added (81).

COMPLICATIONS AFTER THE FIRST YEAR

Transplant Coronary Artery Disease

Cardiac allograft vasculopathy is an accelerated and diffuse form of obliterative coronary arteriosclerosis that is a major cause of late death for patients who survive the first year following heart transplantation (Fig. 49-12) (82–85). In a multicenter study of 2,609 heart transplantation recipients, 42% of patients demonstrated evidence of cardiac-allograft vasculopathy on coronary angiography by 5 years following transplantation (86). The average incidence of angiographically demonstrable cardiac-allograft

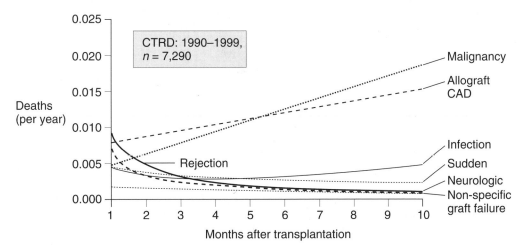

Figure 49-12 Hazard functions for specific causes of death after the first year following heart transplantation. (Reprinted from Kirklin JK, Naftel DC, Bourge RC, et al. Evolving trends in risk profiles and causes of death after heart transplantation: a ten-year multi-institutional study. *J Thorac Cardiovasc Surg* 2003;125:881–890.)

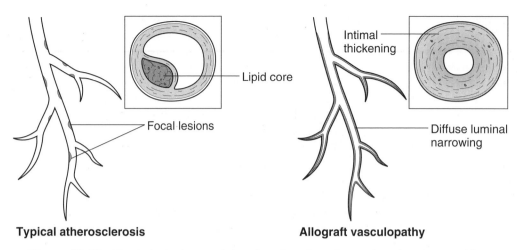

Figure 49-13 Morphologic characteristics of cardiac allograft vasculopathy. (Reprinted from Avery RK. Cardiac-allograft vasculopathy. *NEJM* 2003;349:829–830.)

vasculopathy is approximately 10% to 12% per patient year (84,85).

Cardiac allograft vasculopathy involves diffuse narrowing and occlusion of the coronary arteries and differs pathologically from typical coronary artery atherosclerosis characterized by a more focal distribution (Fig. 49-13). Endothelial dysfunction is an early feature of cardiac-allograft vasculopathy and progresses over time. Immulogic and nonimmunologic factors are believed to result in a repetitive endothelial cell injury that elicits a sustained inflammatory response within the arterial wall, followed by intimal hyperplasia, proliferation of vascular smooth muscle cells, and mononuclear cell infiltration. Concentric, circumferential, and longitudinal intimal thickening affect the epicardial arteries with pruning of extramural and intramyocardial branches. Events occurring during the first year after transplantation appear to

be important in pathogenesis. Transplantation vasculopathy is characterized by intense intimal proliferation in large-caliber and small-caliber vessels. Severe intimal thickening is associated with an increased rate of cardiac events, such as sudden death, myocardial infarction, allograft dysfunction, and failure and need for retransplantation (86).

Multiple risk factors for the development of cardiac-allograft vasculopathy have been identified that suggest a complicated interrelationship between immunologic and nonimmunologic mechanisms that combine to create an environment that facilitates endothelial injury and pathologic remodeling (87–90) (Figs. 49-14 and 49-15; Table 49-11). Data supporting the role of early recurrent rejection episodes in the development of cardiac-allograft vasculopathy have not been consistent (90–92). Other data suggest that the development of cardiac-allograft vasculopathy

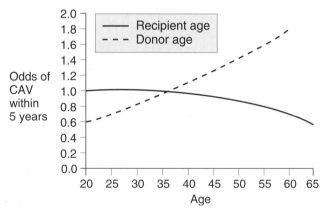

Figure 49-14 Effect of recipient and donor age on the odds of developing cardiac allograft vasculopathy (CAV) within 5 years post-transplant for heart transplants performed between April 1994 and June 1997 (*n* = 4,797). (Reprinted from Taylor DO, Edwards LB, Mohacsi PJ, et al. The registry of the international society for heart and lung transplantation: twentieth official adult heart transplant report—2003. *J Heart Lung Transplant* 2003;22: 616–624.)

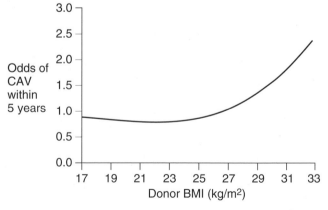

Figure 49-15 Effect of donor body mass index (BMI) on the odds of developing cardiac allograft vasculopathy (CAV) between 5 and 7 years post-transplant for heart transplants performed between April 1994 and June 1997 (*n* = 839). (Reprinted from Taylor DO, Edwards LB, Mohacsi PJ, et al. The registry of the international society for heart and lung transplantation: twentieth official adult heart transplant report—2003. *J Heart Lung Transplant* 2003;22: 616–624.)

TABLE 49-11
RISK FACTORS FOR THE DEVELOPMENT OF CARDIAC ALLOGRAFT VASCULOPATHY

Risk Factor
Diagnosis: coronary artery disease
Panel-reactive antibodies >20%
Donor history of hypertension
Female donor
Hospitalized for rejection within 5 years of transplant

Adapted from Taylor DO, Edwards LB, Mohacsi PJ, et al. The registry of the international society for heart and lung transplantation: twentieth official adult heart transplant report—2003. *J Heart Lung Transplant* 2003;22:616–624.

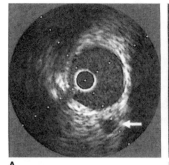 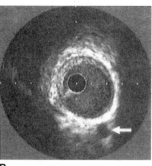

A   **B**

Figure 49-16 Intravascular ultrasound for the evaluation of cardiac allograft vasculopathy. Identical site in the left circumflex artery (*arrow*) from a baseline (**A**) and 1-year follow-up (**B**) study. There is no intimal thickening at baseline. However, when the same site is identified using pericardium and a branch vessel as a landmark, significant intimal thickening (0.6 mm) is identified at the same site. This is an example of *de novo* lesion of transplant vasculopathy. (Reprinted from Kapadia SR, Nissen SE, Ziada KM, et al. Development of transplant vasculopathy and progression of donor transplant atherosclerosis: a comparison by serial intravascular ultrasound imaging. *Circulation* 1998; 98:2672–2678.)

is associated with chronic allograft rejection through allorecognition that results in CD4 T-cell activation and expansion of T-cell clones with specificity for multiple HLA-DR allopeptides (93–96). Activation of T cells can elicit B-cell activation with *de novo* development of anti-HLA IgG antibodies to the allograft. The development of anti-HLA antibodies, as well as antibodies to antigens expressed by endothelial cells, has been shown to be predictive of the development of graft atherosclerosis (97–99). Anti-HLA antibody production in the recipient may thus correlate with a high risk for transplantation-related vasculopathy by both reflecting an activated T-cell recognition pathway and an efficient alloantigen-presentation arm of the immune response. Evidence implicating the degree of major histocompatibility complex (MHC) mismatch with subsequent development of cardiac-allograft vasculopathy has not been uniformly observed (100).

Nonimmunologic factors such as hyperlipidemia, obesity, oxidant stress, allograft ischemia/reperfusion injury, older donor age, mechanism of donor death, viral infections, and CMV disease are also thought to influence the development of cardiac-allograft vasculopathy (86–89). Infection with CMV has been associated with the development of cardiac-allograft vasculopathy, more severe angiographic disease, and a 5-year graft loss twice that of CMV-negative patients (101). Depletion of vascular tissue phasminogen-activator (t-PA) occurring within 3 months following transplantation has been associated with a 8.3-fold increase in risk for the development of angiographically evident coronary disease and a greater likelihood of death or repeat transplantation.

Early identification of cardiac-allograft vasculopathy is important to permit early intervention that may alter the long-term prognosis. Annual coronary angiography is performed for diagnostic and surveillance purposes. Intravascular ultrasound, when added to conventional coronary angiography, provides a more sensitive diagnostic tool for early disease stages and reveals progressive and concentric luminal narrowing of the vessel (Fig. 49-16).

Dobutamine echocardiography is also helpful in identifying myocardial ischemia in patients with coronary allogaft vasculopathy but is limited by its sensitivity. Recent data have demonstrated a correlation between circulating chemokine levels and the development of coronary artery vasculopathy in humans (102). ITAC/CXCL11, a CXCR3 ligand, may have a causative role in the pathogenesis of this disease and may provide a way to prospectively identify patients at risk for the development of coronary artery vasculopathy.

Therapy for allograft vasculopathy has been disappointing, and strategies are usually directed toward its prevention. The use of calcium antagonists, angiotension converting enzyme (ACE) inhibitors, hydroxymethylglutaryl Co-A reductase inhibitors, antioxidants, and intensified immunosuppression provide modest benefit (103–107). Due to the diffuse nature of cardiac-allograft vasculopathy, percutaneous and surgical revascularization procedures have a limited role. Transmyocardial revascularization has been performed, but little success has been reported. Repeat transplantation for significant coronary allograft vasculopathy is the only method of cure. Outcomes following repeat transplantation for cardiac-allograft vasculopathy approach that of primary transplantation.

Cellular proliferation has been identified as a central process in the pathogenesis of allograft vasculopathy. Sirolimus and everolimus, drugs of a new class of macrocyclic immunosuppressive agents with unique antiproliferative activity, have recently been shown to reduce the incidence and progression of cardiac-allograft vasculopathy (108–113). Unlike calcineurin inhibitors, sirolimus does not inhibit interleukin production from antigen-induced T-cell activation but rather inhibits cellular proliferation and migration in response to alloantigens.

Sirolimus binds to FK506-binding protein 12 (FKBP12). The sirolimus-FKBP12 dimeric molecule inhibits the mammalian target of rapamycin and upregulates the cyclin-dependent kinase inhibitor p27kip1, leading to inhibition of cell cycle progression at the G1 to S phase (114,115). Use of sirolimus in kidney allograft recipients has been shown to be effective in reducing allograft rejection (116,117). Use of sirolimus in heart transplantation recipients is more limited. In a recent, randomized study of 46 patients, sirolimus appeared to slow the progression of established cardiac-allograft vasculopathy (62).

Investigators recently reported a large, multicenter, randomized trial comparing everolimus and azathioprine, each in combination with prednisone and cyclosporine, for the prevention of vasculopathy after heart transplantation (63). Statin lipid-lowering agents were administered to all patients. Intravascular ultrasonography was performed at base line and at 12 months. In the groups receiving everolimus, significantly fewer patients reached the composite primary end point of death, graft loss or repeat transplantation, loss to follow-up, rejection of grade 3A or higher, or rejection involving hemodynamic compromise. Rates of graft loss and death did not differ significantly among the study groups, but the group receiving azathioprine had a higher incidence of rejection of at least grade 3A than did the everolimus groups. Intravascular ultrasonography showed that change in intimal variables, including maximal intimal thickness, was significantly smaller in both everolimus groups. The incidence of vasculopathy was lower in the everolimus groups, particularly the higher-dose group. This is the first study to demonstrate the effect of a particular immunosuppressive regimen on the development of allograft vasculopathy. If these differences persist in subsequent years, this effect of everolimus could translate into a substantial long-term benefit for patients who received the drug.

The differential incidence of infections is also of interest. With approximately 75% of patients receiving prophylaxis against CMV infection, the incidence of CMV disease was considerably lower in the everolimus groups than in the azathioprine group. It is possible that this difference contributed to the lower incidence of allograft vasculopathy in the groups given everolimus, but a causal effect is not yet clear.

Malignancies

Heart transplant recipients have a markedly increased incidence of lymphoproliferative malignancies and carcinomas of the skin (118). Malignancies are a major cause of late mortality following heart transplantation (Fig. 49-12). Lymphomas occur in approximately 6% of heart transplant recipients and constitute 22% of all malignancies, compared to 5% of the general population (119,120). Cancers of the prostate, colon and rectum, female breast, and uterine cervix occur at a similar prevalence compared

to the general population. The combination of immunosuppression and a history of smoking may account for an increased risk of developing lung cancer in heart transplant recipients (121). No relationship has been demonstrated between the type of maintenance immunosuppression and the risk of malignancy (122).

Over 90% of post-transplant lymphomas are non-Hodgkin type and consist mostly of abnormal proliferations of B lymphocytes. These tumors display a variety of morphologies ranging from simple B-cell hyperplasia to aggressive monoclonal immunoblastic varieties and are more correctly characterized as a post-transplant lymphoproliferative disease (PTLD). PTLD is more common in heart and heart-lung recipients than in kidney recipients, and is more common in pediatric patients compared to adults (119). Extranodal involvement is seen in >70% of cases; central nervous system and intra-abdominal involvement are particularly common (119,123).

Epstein-Barr virus (EBV) is believed to have a relationship to PTLD through induction of B-cell proliferation. EBV-seronegative recipients are at greater risk, but PTLD may also occur during EBV reactivation (118). Induction therapy or treatment of rejection episodes with cytolytic agents such as antilymphcyte globulin or OKT3 increases the risk of PTLD. Swinnen et al. reported a markedly increased incidence when the cumulative OKT-3 dose exceeded 75 mg; however, this observation has not been consistently demonstrated (124). There is general consensus that cytotoxic immunosuppressive drugs may permanently eliminate T-cell clones that are necessary for controlling malignant cells or latent oncogenic viruses.

The clinical presentation of PTLD is very heterogeneous (118,125). Early disease generally occurs within the first 12 months and is frequently localized or nodal disease. Focal lymphadenopathy is a common initial presentation. Early PTLD is generally polyclonal by DNA analysis and often regresses following reduction in immunosuppression. In contrast, late PTLD presents with disseminated disease, demonstrates monoclonal B-cell proliferation, fails to respond to reduced immunosuppression, and carries a 1-year mortality rate in excess of 75%. CNS involvement may occur in up to 27% of patients (118,125). Aggressive monoclonal B-cell types of PTLD may occur within the first year.

The association between PTLD and viral infections has promoted the use of antiviral prophylaxis during the early post-transplant period and during periods of augmented immunosuppression. Reduction in immunosuppression may be effective in approximately 60% of cases (118,125). Additional treatments include excision of the lesion if localized, localized radiation therapy for discrete masses or central nervous system lesions, or modified non-Hodgkin chemotherapy for widespread disease.

In addition to lymphoproliferative disorders, there is a significantly increased risk of developing nonmelanoma skin cancers following heart transplantation. Squamous cell carcinoma of the skin is more prevalent than basal cell carcinoma. This trend is opposite of that observed in the general population (118). Therapy for treatment of skin cancers following heart transplantation follows traditional dermatologic approaches based on histology and clinical stage of the disease.

OTHER MAJOR COMPLICATIONS

Chronic Renal Insufficiency

Heart transplant recipients are at an increased risk of developing chronic renal dysfunction (Fig. 49-17). Up to 20% of patients may develop severe renal dysfunction, with 4% to 8% of patients requiring renal replacement therapy within 5 to 10 years (126−129). In a significant number there is a decrease in the glomerular filtration rate by 30% to 50% during the first 6 months after transplantation that is followed by stabilization or a slower rate of loss of renal function (127). This decline is almost 10 times as great as expected in a healthy population (130). Subsequent initiation of dialysis has a significantly adverse influence on survival, with only 60% of patients surviving 1 year following the start of dialysis (128).

Calcineurin inhibitors (e.g., cyclosporine and tacrolimus) are associated with both the acute and chronic nephrotoxicity that occurs following transplantation (131−133). Calcineurin inhibitors contribute to acute nephrotoxicity by causing constriction of afferent renal arterioles that results in a decrease in glomerular filtration rate (133). Cyclosporine has also been shown to induce elevation of endothelin-1 (134) and to stimulate the renin-angiotensin-aldosterone system (135). Acute nephrotoxicity is dose dependent and reversible. The chronic effects of cyclosporine nephrotoxicity

are characterized by progressive afferent arteriolopathy and interstitial fibrosis (132,136). These chronic pathologic abnormalities of the kidney are also observed in patients receiving chronic calcineurin inhibitors in settings other than organ transplantation (e.g., treatment of psoriasis) (137).

The chronic nephrotoxic effects of calcineurin inhibitors are thought to be irreversible and dose independent (132,138). Risk factors for the development of renal insufficiency have not been clearly defined but may include recipient age at the time of heart transplantation and glomerular filtration rate at 1 year following heart transplantation. In one 5-year retrospective analysis of adult patients who survived for >1 year following heart transplantation, patients were divided into three groups based on perioperative renal function: (1) preoperative creatinine concentration <1.5 mg per dL and a postoperative creatinine <2.0 mg per dL; (2) preoperative creatinine of <1.5 mg per dL but a postoperative creatinine of >2.0 mg per dL; and (3) preoperative creatinine of >1.5 mg per dL (139). Nearly 30% of patients experienced chronic renal insufficiency defined as serial serum creatinine >2.0 mg per dL on two or more monthly examinations. The mean preoperative serum creatinine was 1.6 mg per dL in patients who experienced chronic renal insufficiency, whereas it was 1.3 mg per dL in patients who did not. The fraction of patients in whom chronic renal insufficiency developed was highest in Group 3 (55.3%), lower in Group 2 (25.5%), and lowest in Group 1 (18.7%). After adjusting for multiple potentially confounding variables, including cyclosporine dosage, the risk of chronic renal insufficiency linearly decreased in the three groups, stratified by perioperative renal function.

Although pretransplant serum creatinine was the best predictor of the development of chronic renal insufficiency in this study (139), the pathophysiology of chronic renal

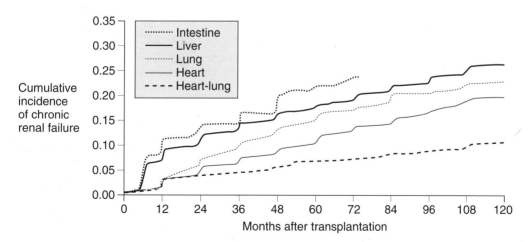

Figure 49-17 Cumulative incidence of chronic renal failure among 69,321 persons who received nonrenal organ transplants in the United States between January 1, 1990 and December 31, 2000. The risk of chronic renal failure was estimated with a noncompeting-risk model. Measurements of renal function were obtained at 6-month intervals during the first year and annually thereafter. (Reprinted from Ojo AO, Held PJ, Port FK, et al. Chronic renal failure after transplantation of a nonrenal organ. *N Engl J Med* 2003;349:931–940.)

insufficiency appears more complex and probably results from multiple interacting factors. These factors include the acute and chronic nephrotoxic effects of calcineurin inhibitors, abnormal renal function in patients with advanced heart failure, transplant operation with associated cardiopulmonary bypass, recipient age, immunologic factors, and risk factors for chronic renal insufficiency such as hypertension, diabetes mellitus, and hypercholesterolemia. Histologic evidence of progressive glomerulosclerosis and loss of functioning glomeruli is present in patients treated with calcineurin inhibitors despite maintaining a stable serum creatinine (140). Thus, all patients treated with calcineurin inhibitors are likely to have some renal damage, but the degree of functional impairment is highly dependent on the degree of pretransplant renal disease.

There is no effective treatment to reverse progressive renal dysfunction following heart transplantation. Alterations in cyclosporine dosing regimens have been proposed but have not been consistently demonstrated to have a significant impact (141). There is no consistent data to suggest that treatment with calcium channel blockers, statins, or ACE-inhibitors has a significant benefit on long-term renal function (127,142). Calcineurin-sparing immunosuppressive protocols have been proposed as one alternative to reduce the risk of chronic renal insufficiency secondary to calcineurin inhibitors. Although protocols using mycophenolate and sirolimus without calcineurin inhibitors have been proposed, there are only anecdotal data regarding safety and efficacy in the setting of heart transplantation. Alternative strategies involve reduction of doses of calcineurin inhibitors with introduction of non-nephrotoxic immunosuppressants such as mycophenolate mofetil and sirolimus. This strategy is currently being investigated extensively in renal transplantation and has been shown to improve renal function, at least in the short term (143,144). Similar approaches might be effective in recipients of non-renal transplants as well. The substitution of mycophenolate mofetil for azathioprine, with a concomitant reduction in the dose of calcineurin inhibitors, has been reported to improve renal function without increasing the rate of allograft rejection (145,146). In addition to changes in immunosuppressive therapy, continued long-term management of nonimmunologic factors (i.e., hypertension, diabetes mellitus) is important.

Hypertension

The development of systemic hypertension is a significant complication following heart transplantation. The incidence of hypertension has been reported to range from 40% to 90% in the era of calineurin inhibitors (147). The overwhelming factor responsible for the development of hypertension following heart transplantation is the use of calcineurin inhibitors. Additional risk factors include male gender, a family history of hypertension, and recipient age >20 years (148). The additional influence of these factors

in the setting of calcineurin use is relatively minor (148,149). Calcineurin inhibitors contribute to the development of hypertension by a direct effect on sympathetic stimulation (150), neurohormonal activation (151), and peripheral vasoconstriction through release of endothelin-1 (152). Although corticosteriods may contribute to the development of hypertension secondary to mineralocorticoid effect, heart transplant recipients on steroid-free immunosuppressive regimens have a similar degree of postoperative hypertension.

The treatment of post-transplant hypertension is similar to that of essential hypertension. Calcium channel blocking agents are usually the first line of therapy for hypertension in patients treated with cyclosporine. Diltiazem has the advantage of decreasing cyclosporine dose and therefore decreasing immunosuppression costs. ACE inhibitors are also used for treatment of hypertension in transplant recipients. A randomized trial comparing diltiazem and lisinopril in the treatment of post-tranplant hypertension demonstrated equal efficacy (153). Monotherapy is effective in <50% of patients. Therapy with both agents is generally required to obtain adequate blood pressure regulation, and peripheral α-adrenergic blocking agents such as doxazosin, peripheral arterial dilators such as hydralazine and minoxidil, and centrally acting sympathetic inhibitors such as clonidine may be useful adjuvants in therapy to calcium channel blockers and ACE-inhibitors if first line therapy is not sufficient in controlling blood pressure.

Hyperlipidemia

The incidence of hyperlipidemia following heart transplantation is as high as 60% to 80% and is manifested by elevated serum levels of total cholesterol, low-density lipoprotein (LDL) cholesterol, apolipoprotein B, and triglyceride levels (154). Hyperlipidemia in the post-transplant setting is related to the use of cyclosporine (155,156). Cyclosporine blood levels have been shown to correlate directly with total plasma cholesterol, LDL cholesterol, and apoB and inversely with HDL cholesterol and apoA-I (the antiatherogenic protein component of HDL). In addition, significant correlation with the total cholesterol/HDL ratio and cyclosporine levels has been reported (156).

The benefits of cholesterol reduction in patients with coronary artery disease and in high-risk patients without established coronary artery disease are well established. All cause mortality is markedly and significantly reduced owing to a dramatic reduction in coronary end points. The benefit of treatment of hyperlipidemia in heart transplant recipients has been recently demonstrated in a study of 97 heart transplant recipients randomized to therapy with or without pravastatin (157). Pravastatin at doses of 20 to 40 mg daily produced a 22% lowering of total plasma cholesterol. There was no change in the number of episodes of rejection, but there was a dramatic reduction in episodes of rejection associated with hemodynamic compromise and marked improvement in survival. There was also a lower incidence of coronary vasculopathy, as determined by angiography or intravascular ultrasound. The mechanism of this effect was most likely related to cholesterol reduction. A significant decrease was noted in the cytotoxicity of natural killer cells, suggesting that an immunologic mechanism may also contribute to the effectiveness of this intervention. Despite the potential for rhabdomyolysis in patients receiving pravastatin together with cyclosporine, no elevation of creatine kinase, transaminases, myositis, or rhabdomyolysis were documented over the 12-month study.

Hyperglycemia

The reported incidence of diabetes mellitus following transplantation has varied widely (from 2% to 46%) due to variations in the criteria used to define diabetes mellitus after transplantation. The onset of diabetes mellitus after organ transplantation is related to immunosuppressive therapy. Exogenous glucococorticoid administration causes diabetes mellitus in predisposed individuals by exacerbating insulin resistance. Glucocorticoids impair hepatic and extrahepatic actions of insulin, probably at the postreceptor level, as glucocorticoid administration affects neither binding of insulin to its receptor nor the number of insulin receptors. Glucocorticoids stimulate hepatic synthesis of glucose from amino acids and glycerol, stimulate the deposition of glucose in the liver as glycogen, diminish glucose utilization, increase protein breakdown, and activate lipolysis. The net effect of these alterations is to increase blood glucose levels.

Several animal studies have demonstrated that cyclosporine interferes with glucose metabolism. Cyclosporine accumulates in pancreatic islet cells, causing decreased B-cell volume, diminished insulin secretion, and hyperglycemia (158). These effects are reversible with discontinuation of the drug. In addition, cyclosporine may potentiate the diabetogenic effects of glucocorticoids by decreasing steroid clearance, as the cytochrome P450 system metabolizes both drugs. Tacrolimus has been shown to have a direct toxic effect on pancreatic islet cells similar to that of cyclosporine. However, with more conservative dosing, this agent can be effectively used without an excessive risk of diabetes.

Osteoporosis

Osteoporosis is a disease characterized by low bone mass that results in a significantly increased risk of fracture. Osteoporosis is diagnosed by bone mineral density criteria developed by the World Health Organization that are generally obtained from evaluation with dual-energy x-ray absorptiometry. Heart transplant recipients are at particular risk for developing osteoporosis due to prolonged periods of immobilization, poor nutrition, and corticosteroid therapy associated with postoperative immunosuppression. Corticosteroids suppress osteoblast function, inhibit bone formation, inhibit intestinal calcium absorption, and stimulate renal calcium excretion. These effects may lead to secondary hyperparathyroidism with increased osteoclastic bone resorption, decreased production of skeletal growth factors, and alteration of the hypothalamic-pituitary-gonadal axis, resulting in hypogonadism. Postmenopausal women, children, and patients >50 are at greatest risk of osteoporosis following heart transplantation; however, almost all heart transplant recipients have some degree of bone mineral density loss (159).

The most rapid demineralization occurs during the first 6 to 12 months following transplantation, with less or no subsequent bone loss thereafter (160–162). Some studies have demonstrated recovery of bone mineral density during the second and third post-transplant years (163). The overall incidence of severe osteoporosis at 2 years following heart transplantation was 28% as measured in the lumbar spine and 20% by measurements from the femoral neck (161).

Fracture prevalence approximates 5% to 30% (164). Fractures most commonly involve the spine and occur during the first 6 months after transplantation. Women are at increased risk of fracture, perhaps because their pretransplant bone mineral density is lower than men. No pretransplant biochemical or densitometric measurement reliably predicts fracture in individual patients. The amount of bone loss is directly related to dose and duration of corticosteroid exposure. The process of bone loss in heart transplant recipients is believed to be mulitfactorial and includes the effects of corticosteroids in addition to the adverse effects of cyclosporine on bone remodeling and the high prevalence of post-transplant renal insufficiency (159,165).

Early therapeutic measures to reduce the degree of bone loss following heart transplantation are essential. Therapy focuses on (a) supplementation of elemental calcium (15,000 mg per day); (b) administration of vitamin D preparations (i.e., calcitriol); (c) use of bisphosphonates to inhibit bone resorption; and (d) institution of a physical exercise training program. In selected patients, measurement of gonadal hormones with appropriate replacement therapy and utilization of calcitonin for patients who do not tolerate bisphosphonates may be indicated. Patients in whom osteoporosis is diagnosed by pretransplant bone mineral density measurements should be treated with antiresorptive therapy prior to transplantation.

Abdominal and Gastrointestinal Complications

Minor and major life-threatening gastrointestestinal complications occur at a relatively high frequency following heart transplantation (Table 49-12). The reported incidence

TABLE 49-12

GASTROINTESTINAL COMPLICATIONS FOLLOWING HEART TRANSPLANTATION

Risk Factor	Complications
Immunosupression	
Corticosteroids	Peptic ulceration, bleeding, perforation, toxic megacolon, intestinal perforation, pancreatitis
Cyclosporine	Hepatocellular injury, cholelithiasis
Azathioprine	Cholestatic/hepatocellular injury, pancreatitis
Mycophenolate mofetil	Diarrhea, nausea, vomiting, abdominal pain
Infection	
CMV	Esophagitis, gastritis with gastric bleeding or ulceration, colitis, hepatitis
HSV	Oral ulceration, esophagitis, colitis
Adenovirus	Colitis
Clostridium difficile	Pseudomembranous colitis
Salmonella	Diarrhea
Candida albicans	Pharyngitis, esophagitis
Post-transplant lymphoproliferative disease	Bowel obstruction, perforation

CMV, cytomegalovirus; HSV, herpes simplex virus.
Adapted from Rayburn BK. Other long-term complications. In: Kirklin JK, Young JB, McGiffin DC, eds. *Heart transplantation.* New York: Churchill Livingstone; 2002.

of gastrointestinal complications in several series has varied from 9% to 34% (166–169). Variability in the reported incidence of gastrointestinal complications is partly attributable to the definitions authors use to identify patients in retrospective reviews. If one considers presentation of gastrointestinal symptoms requiring investigation with endoscopy or barium enema, as opposed to identifying patients by operative events, the incidence of gastrointestinal abnormalities or complications following heart transplantation may be as high as 42% (168). The majority of complications occur within the first 3 to 5 years following heart transplantation, with the greatest risk occurring within the first 30 days (166,167). The majority of complications appear to require operative intervention (167).

In a retrospective review of 240 patients undergoing heart transplantation from December 1985 to June 1994, investigators reported gastrointestinal complications in 21 patients (9.3%), with hepatobiliary (29%), peptic ulcer disease (14%), and pancreatic (14%) complications being the most prevalent (167). Twelve procedures (63%) were either emergently or urgently performed, and seven procedures (37%) were carried out electively. Operative mortality was 33% in patients requiring an emergent or urgent intervention, while there was no operative mortality among patients who had an elective procedure.

In a report of 131 patients undergoing heart or heart-lung transplantation between July 1983 and December 1989 (166), 28 patients (21%) had 38 gastrointestinal complications that included visceral perforations, gastrocutaneous fistula, retroperitoneal abscess, cholecystitis, gastric atony,

perianal abscess, gastrointestinal bleeding, esophagitis, pancreatitis, pancreatic abscess, hepatitis, CMV infection, and diarrhea. Thirteen (46%) of 28 patients required 17 operative procedures. Age, gender, race, and number of rejection episodes did not correlate with the occurrence of a gastrointestinal complication.

The frequency and nature of gastrointestinal complications has been examined by reviewing the indications and findings of endoscopic and surgical procedures involving the gastrointestinal tract in 159 patients undergoing heart transplantation (168). Sixty-seven patients (42%) had gastrointestinal symptoms significant enough to warrant either endoscopic, radiologic, or surgical procedures. Forty-seven patients (30%) underwent esophagogastroduodenoscopy or upper gastrointestinal roentgenography with a high frequency of esophagitis, gastritis, duodenitis, and gastroduodenal ulcers. Thirty-two patients (20%) underwent barium enema or endoscopic procedures of the lower gastrointestinal tract, with the most frequent findings being benign polyps and colitis. Opportunistic infections, especially with CMV, were frequent and were diagnosed only by endoscopic procedures, indicating an advantage of endoscopy over barium studies in these patients. Twenty-three patients (15%) underwent surgical procedures for gastrointestinal complications with a 2.5% mortality.

Gastrointestinal disease following heart transplantation is thought to occur as a consequence of: (a) operation in debilitated patients with sequelae of long-standing heart failure; (b) utilization of cardiopulmonary bypass with potential for low flow states; and (c) the effects of postoperative immunosuppression. Corticosteroids have been associated with an increased risk of peptic ulceration, bowel perforation, gastrointestinal bleeding, and pancreatitis. Investigators have observed a higher maintenance dose of prednisone in patients with gastrointestinal complications compared to patients without gastrointestinal complications (167). However, the relationship between pulse corticosteroid therapy and the onset of abdominal complications has not been consistent. In addition to corticosteroids, other factors that may increase risk for gastrointestinal complications requiring a surgical procedure include a pretransplant diagnosis of ischemic cardiomyopathy and history of previous abdominal operation (169).

Gastrointestinal complications following heart transplantation require prompt and aggressive therapy to limit morbidity and mortality. The presence of immunosuppression with higher doses of steroids in the early perioperative period may mask the manifestations of gastrointestinal complications, thus delaying institution of therapy. The mortality of gastrointestinal complications is greatest in the first 30 days following heart transplantation (169–171).

REFERENCES

1. Taylor DO, Edwards LB, Mohacsi PJ, et al. The registry of the international society for heart and lung transplantation: twentieth official adult heart transplant report—2003. *J Heart Lung Transplant* 2003;22:616–624.
2. Marelli D, Laks H, Kobashigawa JA, et al. Seventeen-year experience with 1,083 heart transplants at a single institution. *Ann Thoracic Surg* 2002;74:1558–1566.
3. Hosenpud JD, Bennett L, Keck BM, et al. The registry of the international society for heart and lung transplantation: eighteenth official report—2001. *J Heart Lung Transplant* 2001;20:805–815.
4. Kirklin JK, Naftel DC, Bourge RC, et al. Evolving trends in risk profiles and causes of death after heart transplantation: a ten-year multi-institutional study. *J Thorac Cardiovasc Surg* 2003;125: 881–890.
5. Young JB, Naftel DC, Ewald G, et al. Determinants of early graft failure following cardiac transplantation: a ten year multi-institutional, multi-variable analysis. *J Heart Lung Transplant* 2001; 20:212. [abstract].
6. Jahania MS, Mullett TW, Sanchez JA, et al. Acute allograft failure in thoracic organ transplantation. *J Cardiac Surg* 2000;15:122–128.
7. Naftel DC, Brown RN. Survival after heart transplantation. In: Kirklin JK, Young JB, McGiffin DC, eds. *Heart transplantation: medicine, surgery, immunology, and research*, New York: Churchill Livingstone, 2002:587–614.
8. Bittner HB, Chen EP, Biswas SS, et al. Right ventricular dysfunction after cardiac transplantation: primarily related to status of donor heart. *Ann Thorac Surg* 1999;68:1605–1611.
9. Bittner HB, Chen EP, Kendall SW, et al. Brain death alters cardiopulmonary hemodynamics and impairs right ventricular power reserve against an elevation of pulmonary vascular resistance. *Chest* 1997;111:706–711.
10. Bittner HB, Chen EP, Craig D, et al. Preload-recruitable stroke work relationships and diastolic dysfunction in the brain-dead organ donor. *Circulation* 1996;94(Suppl. 9):II320–II325.
11. Murali S, Kormos RL, Uretsky BF, et al. Preoperative pulmonary hemodynamics and early mortality after orthotopic cardiac transplantation: the Pittsburgh experience. *Am Heart J* 1993; 126:896–904.
12. Chen JM, Levin HR, Michler RE, et al. Reevaluating the significance of pulmonary hypertension before cardiac transplantation: determination of optimal thresholds and quantification of the effect of reversibility on perioperative mortality. *J Thorac Cardiovasc Surg* 1997;114:627–634.
13. Chen EP, Bittner HB, Davis RD Jr, et al. Effects of nitric oxide after cardiac transplantation in the setting of recipient pulmonary hypertension. *Ann Thorac Surg* 1997;63:1546–1555.
14. Holt ND, McComb JM. Cardiac transplantation and pacemakers: when and what to implant. *Card Electrophysiol Rev* 2002; 6:140–151.
15. Miyamoto Y, Curtiss E, Kormos R, et al. Bradyarrhythmias after heart transplantation. *Circulation* 1990;82(Suppl. IV):313–317.
16. Blanche C, Nessim S, Quartel A, et al. Heart transplantation with bicaval and pulmonary venous anastomoses. A hemodynamic analysis of the first 117 patients. *J Cardiovasc Surg* 1997;38: 561–566.
17. Brandt M, Harringer W, Hirt S, et al. Influence of bicaval anastomosis on late occurrence of atrial arrhythmia after heart transplantation. *Ann Thorac Surg* 1997;64:70–72.
18. Milano C, Shah A, Van Tright P, et al. Evaluation of early postoperative results after bicaval versus standard cardiac transplantation and review of the literature. *Am Heart J* 2000; 140:717–721.
19. Cui G, Tung T, Kobashigawa J, et al. Increased incidence of atrial flutter associated with the rejection of heart transplantation. *Am J Cardiol* 2001;88:280–284.
20. Scott CD, Dark JH, McComb JM. Arrhythmias after cardiac transplantation. *Am J Cardiol* 1992;70:1061–1063.
21. Jacquet L, Ziady G, Stein K, et al. Cardiac rhythm disturbances early after orthotopic heart transplantation: prevalence and clinical importance of the observed abnormalities. *J Am Coll Cardiol* 1990;16:832–837.
22. Tahara K, Ninomiya I, Kajihara H, et al. The significance of atrial monophasic action potentials for monitoring rat cardiac allograft rejection. *J Heart Lung Transplant* 1998;17:954–958.
23. Castedo E, Burgos R, Canas A, et al. Left atrial thrombosis after heart transplantation. *Cardiovasc Surg* 2003;11:247–249.
24. Derumeaux G, Habib G, Schleifer DM, et al. Standard orthotopic heart transplantation versus total orthotopic heart transplantation. A transesophageal echocardiography study of the incidence of left atrial thrombosis. *Circulation* 1995;92(Suppl. 9):H196–H201.
25. Sahar G, Stamler A, Erez E, et al. Etiological factors influencing the development of atrioventricular valve incompetence after heart transplantation. *Transplant Proc* 1997;29:2675–2676.
26. De Simone R, Lange R, Sack F-U, et al. Atrioventricular valve insufficiency and atrial geometry after orthotopic heart transplantation. *Ann Thorac Surg* 1995;60:1686–1693.
27. Law Y, Belassario A, West L, et al. Supramitral valve obstruction from hypertrophied native atrial tissue as a complication of orthotopic heart transplantation. *J Heart Lung Transplant* 1997; 16:922–925.
28. Oaks TE, Rayburn BK, Brown ME, et al. Acquired cor triatriatum after orthotopic cardiac transplantation. *Ann Thorac Surg* 1995; 59:751–753.
29. Dreyfus G, Jebara VA, Couetil JP, et al. Kinking of the pulmonary artery: a treatable cause of acute right ventricular failure after heart transplantation. *J Heart Transplant* 1990;9:575–576.
30. Laske A, Carrel T, Niederhauser U, et al. Modified operation technique for orthotopic heart transplantation. *Eur J Cardiothorac Surg* 1995;9:120–126.
31. Defraigne JO, Vadhat O, Lavigne JP, et al. Aneurysm of the ascending aorta after cardiac transplantation. *Ann Thorac Surg* 1992;54:983–984.
32. Kubo SH, Naftel DC, Mills RM, et al. Risks factors for late recurrent rejection after heart transplantation: a multi-institutional, multi-variable analysis. *J Heart Lung Transplant* 1995; 14:409–418.
33. Miller L. Long-term complications of cardiac transplantation. *Prog Cardiovasc Dis* 1991;33:229–282.
34. Winters G, Costanzo-Nordin M, O'Sullivan E, et al. Predictors of late acute orthotopic heart transplant rejection. *Circulation* 1989;80(Suppl. III):106–110.

35. Jarcho J, Naftel DC, Shroyer TW et al, The Cardiac Transplant Research Database Group. Influence of HLA mismatch on rejection after heart transplantation: a multi-institutional study. *J Heart Lung Transplant* 1994;13:583–596.

36. Kobashigawa J, Sbad A, Drinkwater D, et al. Pretransplant panel reactive-antibody screens: are they truly a marker for poor outcome after cardiac transplantation? *Circulation* 1996;94(Suppl. II):II-294–II-297.

37. George JF, Kirklin JK, Shroyer MT, et al. Utility of posttransplantation panel-reactive antibody measurements for the prediction of rejection frequency and survival of heart transplant recipients. *J Heart Lung Transplant* 1995;14:856–864.

38. Lavee J, Kormos RL, Duqesnoy RJ, et al. Influence of panel reactive antibody and lymphocytotoxic crossmatch on survival after heart transplantation. *J Heart Lung Transplant* 1991;10:921–930.

39. Loh E, Bergin JD, Couper GS, et al. Role of panel reactive antibody cross reactivity in predicting survival after orthotopic heart transplantation. *J Heart Lung Transplant* 1994;13:194–201.

40. Itescu S, Tung TC, Burke EM, et al. Preformed IgG antibodies against major histocompatibility complex class II antigens are major risk factors for high-grade cellular rejection in recipients of heart transplantation. *Circulation* 1998;98:786–793.

41. Billingham ME, Cary NR, Hammond ME, et al. A working formulation for the standardization of nomenclature in the diagnosis of heart and lung rejection: Heart Rejection Study Group. The International Society for Heart and Lung Transplantation. *J Heart Transplant* 1990;9:587–593.

42. Rodriguez R. The pathology of heart transplant biopsy specimens: revisiting the 1990 ISHLT working formulation. *J Heart Lung Transplant* 2003;22:3–15.

43. Ruan XM, Qiao JH, Trento A, et al. Cytokine expression and endothelial cell and lymphocyte activation in human cardiac allograft rejection: an immunohistochemical study of endomyocardial biopsy samples. *J Heart Lung Transplant* 1992;11:1110–1115.

44. Torry RJ, Labarrere CA, Torry DS, et al. Vascular endothelial growth factor expression in transplanted human hearts. *Transplantation* 1995;60:1451–1457.

45. Van Hoffen E, van Wichen D, Stuij I, et al. In situ expression of cytokines in human heart allografts. *Am J Pathol* 1996;149:1991–2003.

46. Deng MC, Bell S, Huie P, et al. Cardiac allograft vascular disease. Relationship to microvascular cell surface markers and inflammatory cell phenotypes on endomyocardial biopsy. *Circulation* 1995;91:1647–1654.

47. Ohtani H, Strauss HW, Southern JF, et al. Intercellular adhesion molecule-1 induction: a sensitive and quantitative marker for cardiac allograft rejection. *J Am Coll Cardiol* 1995;26:793–799.

48. Herskowitz A, Mayne AE, Willoughby SB, et al. Patterns of myocardial cell adhesion molecule expression in human endomyocardial biopsies after cardiac transplantation. Induced ICAM-1 and VCAM-1 related to implantation and rejection. *Am J Pathol* 1994;145:1082–1094.

49. Briscoe DM, Yeung AC, Schoen FJ, et al. Predictive value of inducible endothelial cell adhesion molecule expression for acute rejection of human cardiac allografts. *Transplantation* 1995;59:204–211.

50. Qiao JH, Ruan XM, Trento A, et al. Expression of cell adhesion molecules in human cardiac allograft rejection. *J Heart Lung Transplant* 1992;11:920–925.

51. Ferran C, Peuchmaur M, Desruennes M, et al. Implications of de novo ELAM-1 and VCAM-1 expression in human cardiac allograft rejection. *Transplantation* 1993;55:605–609.

52. Tanio JW, Basu CB, Albelda SM, et al. Differential expression of the cell adhesion molecules ICAM-1, VCAM-1, and E-selectin in normal and posttransplantation myocardium. Cell adhesion molecule expression in human cardiac allografts. *Circulation* 1994;89:1760–1768.

53. Melter M, Exeni A, Reinders ME, et al. Expression of the chemokine receptor CXCR3 and its ligand IP-10 during human cardiac allograft rejection. *Circulation* 2001;104:2558.

54. Zhao DX, Hu Y, Miller GG, et al. Differential expression of the IFN-gamma-inducible CXCR3-binding chemokines, IFN-inducible protein 10, monokine induced by IFN, and IFN-inducible T cell alpha chemoattractant in human cardiac allografts: association with cardiac allograft vasculopathy and acute rejection. *J Immunol* 2002;169:1556.

55. Fahmy NM, Yamani MH, Starling RC, et al. Chemokine and chemokine receptor gene expression indicates acute rejection of human cardiac transplants. *Transplantation* 2003;75:72.

56. Michaels PJ, Espejo ML, Kobashigawa J, et al. Humoral rejection in cardiac transplantation: risk factors, hemodynamic consequences and relationship to transplant coronary artery disease. *J Heart Lung Transplant* 2003;22:58–69.

57. Lones M, Czer L, Trento A, et al. Clinical-pathological features of humoral rejection in cardiac allografts: a study in 81 consecutive patients. *J Heart Lung Transplant* 1995;14:151–162.

58. Sethi G, Kosaraju S, Arabia F, et al. Is it necessary to perform surveillance endomyocardial biopsies in heart transplant recipients? *J Heart Lung Transplant* 1995;14:1047–1051.

59. White J, Guiraudon C, Pflugfelder P, et al. Routine surveillance myocardial biopsies are unnecessary beyond one year after heart transplantation. *J Heart Lung Transplant* 1995;14:1052–1056.

60. Sharpes L, Cary N, Large S, et al. Error rates with which endomyocardial biopsy specimens are graded for rejection after cardiac transplantation. *Am J Cardiol* 1992;70:527–530.

61. Nielson H, Sorensen F, Nielsen B, et al. Reproducibility of the acute rejection diagnosis in human cardiac allografts. The Stanford classification and the international grading system. *J Heart Lung Transplant* 1993;12:239–243.

62. Mancini D, Pinney S, Burkhoff D, et al. Use of rapamycin slows progression of cardiac transplantation vasculopathy. *Circulation* 2003;108:48–53.

63. Eisen HJ, Tuzcu EM, Dorent R, et al. Everolimus for the prevention of allograft rejection and vasculopathy in cardiac-transplant recipients. *N Engl J Med* 2003;349:847–858.

64. De Marco T, Damon LE, Colombe B, et al. Successful immunomodulation with intravenous gamma globulin and cyclophosphamide in an alloimmunized heart transplant recipient. *J Heart Lung Transplant* 1997;16:360–365.

65. Miller L, Naftel D, Bourge R, et al. Infection after heart transplantation: a multiinstitutional study. *J Heart Lung Transplant* 1994;13:381–393.

66. Hunt SA. Current status of cardiac transplantation. *JAMA* 1998;280:1692–1698.

67. Robbins RC, Barlow CW, Oyer PE, et al. Thirty years of cardiac transplantation at Stanford University. *J Thorac Cardiovasc Surg* 1999;117:939–951.

68. Fishman JA, Rubin RH. Medical progress: infection in organ-transplant recipients. *N Engl J Med* 1998;338:1741–1751.

69. Smart FW, Naftel DC, Costanzo MR, et al. Risk factors for early, cumulative, and fatal infections after heart transplantation: a multiinstitutional study. *J Heart Lung Transplant* 1996;15:329–341.

70. Macdonald P, Keogh A, Marshman D, et al. A double-blind placebo-controlled trial of low-dose ganciclovir to prevent cytomegalovirus disease after heart transplantation. *J Heart Lung Transplant* 1995;14:32–38.

71. Montoya JG, Giraldo LF, Efron B, et al. Infectious complications among 620 consecutive heart transplant patients at Stanford University Medical Center. *Clin Infect Dis* 2001;33:629–640.

72. Rubin RH. Prevention and treatment of cytomegalovirus disease in heart transplant patients. *J Heart Lung Transplant* 2000;19:731–735.

73. Merigan TC, Renlund DG, Keay S, et al. A controlled trial of ganciclovir to prevent cytomegalovirus disease after heart transplantation. *N Eng J Med* 1992;326:1182.

74. Pescovitz MD, Rabkin J, Merion RM, et al. Valganciclovir results in improved oral absorption of ganciclovir in liver transplant recipients. *Antimicrob Agents Chemother* 2000;44:2811–2815.

75. Wedemeyer H, Pethig K, Wagner D, et al. Long-term outcome of chronic hepatitis B in heart transplant recipients. *Transplantation* 1998;66:1347–1353.

76. Wachs ME, Amend WJ, Ascher NL, et al. The risk of transmission of hepatitis B from HBsAg(-), HBcAb(+), HBIgM(-) organ donors. *Transplantation* 1995;59:230–234.

77. Lake KD, Smith CI, LaFrost SKM, et al. Outcomes of hepatitis C positive (HCV+) heart transplant recipients. *Transplant Proc* 1997;29:581–582.

78. Ong JP, Barnes DS, Younossi ZM, et al. Outcome of de novo hepatitis C virus infection in heart transplant recipients. *Hepatology* 1999;30:1293–1298.

79. Israelski DM, Remington JS. Toxoplasmosis in the non-AIDS immunocompromised host. *Curr Clin Topics Infect Dis* 1993;13:322–356.

80. Luft BJ, Billingham M, Remington JS. Endomyocardial biopsy in the diagnosis of toxoplasmic myocarditis. *Transplant Proc* 1986;18:1871–1873.

81. Wreghitt TG, Gray JJ, Pavel P, et al. Efficacy of pyrimethamine for the prevention of donor-acquired *Toxoplasma gondii* infection in heart and heart-lung transplant patients. *Transplant Int* 1992;5:197–200.

82. Julius BK, Attenhofer JCH, Sutsch G, et al. Incidence, progression and functional significance of cardiac allograft vasculopathy after heart transplantation. *Transplantation* 2000;69:847–854.

83. Constanzo M, Naftel D, Pritzker M, et al. Heart transplant coronary artery disease detected by coronary angiography: a multi-institutional study of preoperative donor and recipient risk factors. *J Heart Lung Transplant* 1998;17:744–753.

84. Uretsky B, Murali S, Reedy S, et al. Development of coronary artery disease in cardiac transplant patients receiving immunosuppressive therapy with cyclosporine and prednisone. *Circulation* 1987;76:827–834.

85. Gao S, Schroeder J, Alderman E, et al. Clinical and laboratory correlates of accelerated coronary artery disease in the cardiac transplant patient. *Circulation* 1987;76(Suppl. 5):56–61.

86. Kapadia SR, Nissen SE, Ziada KM, et al. Development of transplant vasculopathy and progression of donor transplant atherosclerosis: a comparison by serial intravascular ultrasound imaging. *Circulation* 1998;98:2672–2678.

87. Gould DS, Auchincloss HJ. Direct and indirect recognition: the role of MHC antigens in graft rejection. *Immunol Today* 1999;20:77–82.

88. Avery RK. Viral triggers of cardiac allograft dysfunction. *N Engl J Med* 2001;344:1545–1547.

89. Young J. Allograft vasculopathy. *Circulation* 1999;100:458–460.

90. Mehra MR, Ventura HO, Chambers RB, et al. The prognostic impact of immunosuppression and cellular rejection on cardiac allograft vasculopathy: time for a reappraisal. *J Heart Lung Transplant* 1997;16:743–751.

91. Kobashigawa JA, Miller L, Yeung A, et al. Does acute rejection correlate with the development of transplant coronary artery disease? A multi-center study using intravascular ultrasound. Sandoz/CVIS Investigators. *J Heart Lung Transplant* 1995;14(6 Pt 2):S221–S226.

92. Stovin PG, Sharples LD, Schofield PM, et al. Lack of association between endomyocardial evidence of rejection in the first six months and the later development of transplant-related coronary artery disease. *J Heart Lung Transplant* 1993;12(1 Pt 1):110–116.

93. Liu Z, Sun YK, Xi YP, et al. Contribution of direct and indirect recognition pathway to T cell alloreactivity. *J Exp Med* 1993;177:1643–1650.

94. Liu Z, Colovai AI, Tugulea S, et al. Indirect recognition of donor HLA-DR peptides in organ allograft rejection. *J Clin Invest* 1996;98:1150–1157.

95. Tugulea S, Ciubotariu R, Colovai AI, et al. New strategies for early diagnosis of heart allograft rejection. *Transplantation* 1997;64:842–847.

96. Vanderlugt CJ, Miller SD. Epitope spreading. *Curr Opin Immunol* 1996;8:831–836.

97. Rose EA, Pepino P, Barr M, et al. Relation of HLA antibodies and graft atherosclerosis in human cardiac allograft recipients. *J Heart Lung Transplant* 1992;3:S120–S123.

98. Reed EF, Hong B, Ho E, et al. Monitoring of soluble HLA alloantigens and anti-HLA antibodies identifies heart allograft recipients at risk of transplant associated coronary artery disease. *Transplantation* 1996;61:556.

99. Dunn MJ, Crisp S, Rose ML, et al. Anti-endothelial antibodies and coronary artery disease after cardiac transplantation. *Lancet* 1992;339:1566.

100. Richenbacher PR, Kemna MS, Pinto FJ, et al. Coronary artery intimal thickening in the transplanted heart. An in vivo intracoronary ultrasound study of immunologic and metabolic risk factors. *Transplantation* 1996;61:46–85.

101. Lowry R, Allen E, Hu C, et al. What are the implications of cardiac infection with cytomegalovirus before heart transplantation? *J Heart Lung Transplant* 1994;13:122–128.

102. Kao J, Kobashigawa J, Fishbein MC, et al. Elevated serum levels of the CXCR3 chemokine ITAC are associated with the development of transplant coronary artery disease. *Circulation* 2003;107:1958–1961.

103. Mehra M, Ventura H, Smart F, et al. An intravascular ultrasound study of the influence of angiotensin converting enzyme inhibitors and calcium entry blockers on the development of cardiac allograft vasculopathy. *Am J Cardiol* 1995;75:853–854.

104. Launch R, Ballester M, Marti V, et al. Efficacy of augmented immunosuppressive therapy for early vasculopathy in heart transplantation. *J Am Coll Cardiol* 1998;32:413–419.

105. Schroeder J, Gao S, Alderman E, et al. A preliminary study of diltiazem in the prevention of coronary artery disease in heart transplant recipients. *N Engl J Med* 1993;328:164–170.

106. Kobashigawa JA, Katznelson S, Laks H, et al. Effect of pravastatin on outcomes after cardiac transplantation. *N Engl J Med* 1995;333:621–627.

107. Wenke K, Meiser B, Thiery J, et al. Simvastatin reduces graft vessel disease and mortality after heart transplantation: a 4 year randomized trial. *Circulation* 1997;96:1398–1402.

108. Marx S, Jayaraman T, Go L, et al. Rapamycin-FKBP inhibits phosphorylation of retinoblastoma protein and blocks vascular smooth muscle cell proliferation. *Circ Res* 1995;76:412–417.

109. Poon M, Marx SO, Gallo R, et al. Rapamycin inhibits vascular smooth muscle cell migration. *J Clin Invest* 1996;98:2277–2283.

110. Sehgal S. Rapamune (RAPA, rapamycin, sirolimus): mechanism of action immunosuppressive effect results from blockade of signal transduction and inhibition of cell cycle progression. *Clin Biochem* 1998;31:335–340.

111. Poston R, Billingham M, Hoyt E, et al. Rapamycin reverses chronic vascular disease in a novel cardiac allograft model. *Circulation* 1999;100:67–74.

112. Gallo R, Padurean A, Jayaraman T, et al. Inhibition of intimal thickening after balloon angioplasty in porcine coronary arteries by targeting regulators of the cell cycle. *Circulation* 1999;99:2164–2170.

113. Sousa J, Costa M, Abizaid A, et al. Lack of neointimal proliferation after implantation of sirolimus-coated stents in human arteries. *Circulation* 2001;103:192–194.

114. Luo Y, Marx S, Koff A, et al. Rapamycin resistance tied to defective regulation of p27kip1. *Mol Cell Biol* 1996;16:6744–6751.

115. Marx S, Marks A. Bench to bedside: the development of rapamycin and its application to stent restenosis. *Circulation* 2001;104:852–855.

116. Kahan B, Podbielski J, Napoli K, et al. Immunosuppressive effects and safety of a sirolimus/cyclosporine combination regimen for renal transplantation. *Transplantation* 1998;66:1040–1046.

117. Groth C, Backman L, Morales J, et al. Sirolimus (rapamycin) based therapy in human renal transplantation. *Transplantation* 1999;67:1036–1042.

118. Hunt S. Malignancy in organ transplantation: heart. *Transplant Proc* 2002;34:1874–1876.

119. Penn I. Incidence and treatment of neoplasia after transplantation. *J Heart Lung Transplant* 1993;12:S328–S336.

120. Haldas J, Wang W, Lazarchick J. Post-transplant lymphoproliferative disorders: T-cell lymphoma following cardiac transplant. *Leuk Lymphoma* 2002;43:447–450.

121. Johnson WM, Baldrusson O, Gros TJ. Double jeopardy: lung cancer after cardiac transplantation. *Chest* 1998,113.1720–1723.

122. Couetil J, McGoldrick J, Wallwork J, et al. Malignant tumors after heart transplantation. *J Heart Lung Transplant* 1991;9:622–626.

123. Penn I, Porat G. Central nervous system lymphomas in organ allograft recipients. *Transplantation* 1995;59:240–244.

124. Swinnen L, Costanzo-Nordin M, Fisher SG, et al. Increased incidence of lymphoproliferative disorder after immunosuppression with the monoclonal antibody OKT-3 in cardiac-transplant recipients. *N Eng J Med* 1990;323:1723–1728.

125. Armitage J, Kormos R, Stuart R, et al. Posttransplant lymphoproliferative disease in thoracic organ transplant patients: ten years

of cyclosporine-based immunosuppression. *J Heart Lung Transplant* 1991;10:877–887.

126. van Gelder T, Balk AH, Zietse R, et al. Renal insufficiency after heart transplantation: a case-control study. *Nephrol Dial Transplant* 1998;13:2322–2326.

127. Lindelow B, Bergh CH, Herlitz H, et al. Predictors and evolution of renal function during 9 years following renal transplantation. *J Am Soc Nephrol* 2000;11:951–957.

128. Goldstein DJ, Zuech N, Sehgal V, et al. Cyclosporine-associated end-stage nephropathy after cardiac transplantation: incidence and progression. *Transplantation* 1997;63:664–668.

129. Ojo AO, Held PJ, Port FK, et al. Chronic renal failure after transplantation of a nonrenal organ. *N Engl J Med* 2003;349: 931–940.

130. Granerus G, Aurell M. Reference values for 51Cr-EDTA clearance as a measure of glomerular filtration rate. *Scand J Clin Lab Invest* 1982;41:611–616.

131. Meyers BD, Ross J, Newton L, et al. Cyclosporine-associated chronic nephropathy. *N Engl J Med* 1984;311:699–705.

132. Bennett WM. Insights into chronic cyclosporine nephrotoxicity. *Int J Clin Pharm Ther* 1996;34:515–519.

133. Andoh TF, Burdmann EA, Bennett WM. Nephrotoxicity of immunosuppressive drugs: experimental and clinical observations. *Semin Nephrol* 1997;17:34–45.

134. Grieff M, Loertscher R, Shohaib SA, et al. Cyclosporine-induced elevation in circulating endothelin-1 in patients with solid-organ transplants. *Transplantation* 1993;56:880–884.

135. Julien J, Farge D, Kreft-Jais C, et al. Cyclosporine-induced stimulation of the renin-angiotensin system after liver and heart transplantation. *Transplantation* 1993;56:885–891.

136. Feutren G, Mihatsch MJ. Risk factors for cyclosporine induced nephropathy in patients with autoimmune diseases. *N Engl J Med* 1992;326:1654–1660.

137. Young EW, Ellis CN, Messana JM, et al. A prospective study of renal structure and function in psoriasis patients treated with cyclosporine. *Kidney Int* 1994;46:1216–1222.

138. Waser M, Maggiorini M, Binswanger U, et al. Irreversibility of cyclosporine-induced renal function impairment in heart transplant recipients. *J Heart Lung Transplant* 1993;12:846–850.

139. Vossler MR, Ni H, Toy W, et al. Pre-operative renal function predicts development of chronic renal insufficiency after orthotopic heart transplantation. *J Heart Lung Transplant* 2002;21:874–881.

140. Falkenhain ME, Cosio FG, Sedmak DD. Progressive histologic injury in kidneys from heart and liver transplant recipients receiving cyclosporine. *Transplantation* 1996;62:364–370.

141. Furlanut M, Baraldo M, Pea F, et al. Effect of fluctuations of blood cyclosporine concentrations on renal function. *Transplant Proc* 1994;26:2574–2575.

142. Chan C, Maurer J, Cardella C, et al. A randomized controlled trial of verapamil on cyclosporine nephrotoxicity in heart and lung transplant recipients. *Transplantation* 1997;63:1435–1440.

143. Pascual M, Theruvath T, Kawai T, et al. Strategies to improve long-term outcomes after renal transplantation. *N Engl J Med* 2002;346:580–590.

144. Pascual M, Curtis J, Delmonico F, et al. A prospective, randomized clinical trial of cyclosporine reduction in stable patients greater than 12 months after renal transplantation. *Transplantation* 2003;75:1501–1505.

145. Tedoriya T, Keogh AM, Kusano K, et al. Reversal of chronic cyclosporine nephrotoxicity after heart transplantation—potential role of mycophenolate mofetil. *J Heart Lung Transplant* 2002;21:976–982.

146. Soccal PM, Gasche Y, Favre H, et al. Improvement of drug-induced chronic renal failure in lung transplantation. *Transplantation* 1999;68:164–165.

147. Starling RC, Cody RJ. Cardiac transplant hypertension. *J Heart Lung Transplant* 1990;65:106–111.

148. Ozdogan E, Banner N, Fitzgerald M, et al. Factors influencing the development of hypertension after heart transplantation. *J Heart Lung Transplant* 1990;9:548–553.

149. Thompson ME, Shapiro AP, Johnsen AM, et al. The contrasting effects of cyclosporine A and asathioprine on arterial blood pressure and renal function following cardiac transplantation. *Int J Cardiol* 1986;11:219–229.

150. Scherrer U, Vissing SF, Morgan BJ, et al. Cyclosporine induced sympathetic activation and hypertension after heart transplantation. *N Eng J Med* 1990;323:693–699.

151. Julien J. Cyclosporin induced stimulation of the rennin-angiotensin system after liver and heart transplantation. *Transplantation* 1993;56:885–891.

152. Ong AC. Effect of cyclosporine A on endothelin synthesis by cultured human renal cortical epithelial cells. *Transplantation* 1993;8:748–753.

153. Brozena SC, Johnson MR, Ventura HO, et al. Effectiveness and safety of diltiazem or lisinopril in treatment of hypertension after heart transplantation. *J Am Coll Cardiol* 1996;27:1707–1712.

154. Ballantyne CM, Radovancevic B, Farmer JA, et al. Hyperlipidemia after heart transplantation: report of a 6 year experience with treatment recommendations. *J Am Coll Cardiol* 1992;19:1315.

155. Hilbrands LB, Demacker PN, Hoitsma AJ, et al. The effects of cyclosporine and prednisone on serum lipid and (apo) lipoprotein levels in renal transplant recipients. *J Am Soc Nephrol* 1995;5:2073–2081.

156. Kuster GM, Drexel H, Bleisch JA, et al. Relation of cyclosporine blood levels to adverse effects on lipoproteins. *Transplantation* 1994;57:1479–1483.

157. Kobashigawa JA, Katznelson S, Laks H, et al. Effect of provastatin on outcomes after cardiac transplantation. *N Eng J Med* 1995;333:621–627.

158. Hahn HJ, Dunger A, Laube F, et al. Toxic effects of cyclosporine on the endocrine pancreas of Wistar rats. *Transplantation* 1986; 41:44–47.

159. Negri AL, Perrone S, Gallo R, et al. Osteoporosis following heart transplantation. *Transplant Proc* 1996;28:3321–3324.

160. Berguer DG, Krieg MA, Thiebaud D. Osteoporosis in heart transplant recipients: a longitudinal study. *Transplant Proc* 1994;26: 2649–2651.

161. Shane E, Rivas MC, Siverberg SJ, et al. Osteoporosis and bone morbidity in cardiac transplant recipients. *Am J Med* 1993;94: 257–264.

162. Shane E, Rivas M, McMahon DJ, et al. Bone loss and turnover after cardiac transplantation. *J Clin Endocrinol Metab* 1997;82: 1497–1506.

163. Henderson NK, Sambrook PN, Kelly PJ, et al. Bone mineral loss and recovery after cardiac transplantation. *Lancet* 1995;2:905.

164. Shane E, Rivas M, Staron R, et al. Fracture after cardiac transplantation: a prospective longitudinal study. *J Clin Endocrinol Metab* 1996;81:1740–1746.

165. Klaushofer K, Hoffmann O, Stewart PJ, et al. Cyclosporine A inhibits bone resorption in cultured neonatal mouse calvaria. *J Pharmacol Exp Ther* 1987;243:584–590.

166. Augustine SM, Yeo CJ, Buchman TG, et al. Gastrointestinal complications in heart and heart-lung transplant patients. *J Heart Lung Transplant* 1991;10:547–556.

167. Sharma S, Reddy V, Ott G, et al. Gastrointestinal complications after orthotopic cardiac transplantation. *Eur J Cardiothorac Surg* 1996;10:616–620.

168. Steck TB, Durkin MG, Costanzo-Nordin MR, et al. Gastrointestinal complication and endoscopic findings in heart transplant patients. *J Heart Lung Transplant* 1993;12:244–251.

169. Fazel S, Everson EA, Stitt LW, et al. Predictors of general surgical complications after heart transplantation. *J Am Coll Surg* 2001; 193:52–59.

170. Watson CJE, Jamieson NV, Johnston PS, et al. Early abdominal complications following heart and heart-lung transplantation. *Br J Surg* 1991;78:699–704.

171. Kirklin JK, Holm A, Aldrete JS, et al. Gastrointestinal complications after cardiac transplantation. Potential benefit of early diagnoses and prompt surgical intervention. *Ann Surg* 1990; 211(5):538–541.

Complications of
Pediatric Surgery

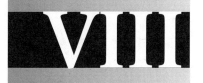

Surgical Complications in Newborns

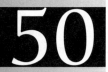

Ronald B. Hirschl

■ OVERVIEW 725

■ INTESTINAL OBSTRUCTION IN THE
   NEWBORN 725
   Congenital Duodenal Obstruction 726
   Malrotation 728
   Jejunoileal Obstruction 730
   Meconium Ileus 733
   Hirschsprung Disease 735
   Imperforate Anus 738

■ THORACIC ANOMALIES 742
   Congenital Pulmonary Airway
      Malformation (CPAM) 742
   Pulmonary Sequestration 743
   Foregut Duplication Cyst 744
   Esophageal Atresia and Tracheoesophageal Fistula 744
   Congenital Diaphragmatic Hernia (CDH) 749

■ ABDOMINAL WALL DEFECTS 751
   Gastroschisis 751
   Omphalocele 753

■ ACQUIRED NEWBORN SURGICAL
   PROBLEMS 754
   Pyloric Stenosis 754
   Necrotizing Enterocolitis 756

■ REFERENCES 758

Ronald B. Hirschl: University of Michigan, Ann Arbor, MI 48109

OVERVIEW

Disease processes manifested by newborns are almost always related to an underlying birth anomaly. The complications associated with such anomalies are related to the effects that the birth defect has upon cardiopulmonary physiology or organ system function. For example, depending on the associated cardiopulmonary compromise, a congenital pulmonary airway malformation (CPAM) or congenital diaphragmatic hernia (CDH) may prove to be lethal at birth or manifest itself only in the ensuing months or years.

In most cases, the outcome of newborns and infants following operative intervention is determined by the associated direct cardiopulmonary effects, such as with CDH, or related to the presence of other anomalies, especially neurologic or cardiac defects. Although there are a few exceptions, correction of a gastrointestinal, pulmonary, abdominal wall, or diaphragmatic anomaly is straightforward, with little morbidity and mortality associated with the procedure itself. Rather it is the other associated anomalies and the effect of the birth defect upon the heart, lungs, or nervous system that adversely affect outcome.

INTESTINAL OBSTRUCTION IN THE NEWBORN

Bilious vomiting is the hallmark of bowel obstruction that requires operative intervention in the newborn. Newborns with bowel obstruction should have an orogastric or naso-gastric tube placed to continuous suction to prevent vomiting and pulmonary aspiration and to decompress the gastrointestinal (GI) tract. Fluid resuscitation should be performed until appropriate urine output is noted (1 to 2 mL/kg/h). The electrolyte status should be evaluated and any aberrancies corrected prior to administration of anesthetics. The newborn should be placed in a warm environment since the surface-to-mass ratio of the newborn is high and the ability to maintain normothermia is limited. Radiographic evaluation typically begins with an abdominal flat plate and either a cross-table lateral or left lateral decubitus assessment. Further radiographic evaluation varies depending on the specific clinical picture and abnormalities observed. Typically, an upper GI contrast series allows assessment of the presence, etiology, and location of a proximal obstruction, whereas a contrast enema is frequently performed to rule out obstruction in the colon or terminal ileum. A contrast enema may also be performed to rule out a second colonic obstruction downstream from the primary anomaly that the surgeon otherwise might miss. In order to minimize the risk of ischemia and bowel necrosis, the workup of bowel obstruction in the newborn should be performed emergently until the diagnosis of malrotation with volvulus has been excluded.

Congenital Duodenal Obstruction

Congenital duodenal obstruction with duodenal dilation is due to atresia in 76% of cases and stenosis in 23% of cases. Causes include the presence of a duodenal web (18%), annular pancreas (36%), absence of a portion of the duodenum (10%), or a malrotation with either volvulus or the presence of Ladd bands (36%) (1). The presence of this anomaly may be appreciated on prenatal ultrasound usually due to identification of polyhydramnios (41%) or a dilated stomach and duodenum (double bubble, 87%) (2). Nearly half of patients with duodenal obstruction are premature (<37 weeks gestation) (3). Typical presenting symptoms in the first 1 to 2 days of life include feeding intolerance and emesis. The latter is usually bilious unless the obstruction is distal to the ampulla of Vater, which it is in 5% to 10% of cases. Plain abdominal radiographs demonstrate the classic "double-bubble" of an air-filled, dilated stomach and proximal duodenum in 77% of patients (Fig. 50-1) (3). Air can be used as a contrast agent by injecting 20 mL through the nasogastric tube during performance of the radiograph. The distal small intestine and colon remain gasless with a duodenal atresia. In contrast, in the setting of a duodenal web with an opening or a malrotation with Ladd bands or volvulus, gas is often present in the downstream GI tract. The importance of the distinction is that the urgency with which operation is performed is reduced if malrotation with volvulus is excluded as a likely diagnosis. However, in most cases prompt surgical intervention is appropriate. If a classic

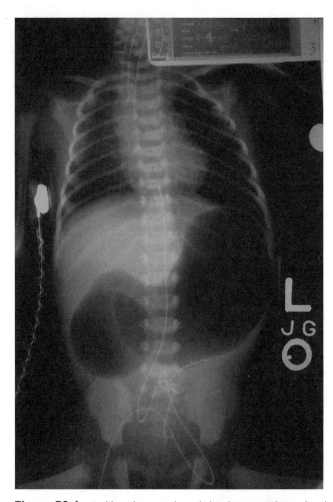

Figure 50-1 A dilated stomach and duodenum without distal gas is noted in a newborn. This is the classic "double-bubble" finding in a patient with duodenal atresia.

double-bubble is observed, further radiographic study usually is unnecessary.

A right supraumbilical incision with mobilization of the duodenum is typically used for the exploration, although some surgeons have recommended a transumbilical or laparoscopic approach (4,5). After a Kocher maneuver, the markedly dilated proximal duodenum and the decompressed distal duodenum are identified. If malrotation is present, a Ladd procedure is the best approach (see below). Otherwise, mobilization of the right colon and ligament of Treitz with derotation of the small bowel is often helpful to expose the entire duodenum. The most difficult maneuver involves determining the site of the obstruction because a "windsock" deformity may be present such that the origin of the atresia or stenosis may be proximal to the change in caliber of the duodenum. One must be certain that a corrective procedure is not performed distal to the actual obstruction. To avoid this complication, a small longitudinal incision may first be made along the anterolateral, distal aspect of the dilated portion of the duodenum. The anterolateral aspect is used in order to avoid the ampulla of

Vater during subsequent anastomosis. A catheter is passed proximally and distally to identify the location of the obstruction. Alternatively, a small gastrotomy may be performed and a catheter passed distally into the duodenum. Gentle pressure applied to the catheter at the site of obstruction may demonstrate the site of attachment of a windsock by the presence of an indentation on the surface of the dilated duodenum (Fig. 50-2). If a simple web is present, the longitudinal incision can be extended across the anterolateral aspect of the web and the web incised after identification of the ampulla of Vater. Identification of the ampulla is best performed by compressing the gallbladder and observing the site of bile drainage into the duodenum. The ostium of the ampulla of Vater is often located at the

base of or even within the web. In this case excision of the web is ill-advised and incision is carefully performed after identification of the ampulla of Vater in order to avoid injury to, or obstruction of, the biliary tract. Transverse closure of the longitudinal incision, as in a Heinike-Mikulicz pyloroplasty, effectively bypasses the obstruction once the web is partially incised.

Alternatively, bypass of the obstructing lesion with a duodenoduodenostomy is performed in 81% of cases (6). This consists of a "diamond" anastomosis between a transverse incision in the proximal dilated duodenum and a longitudinal incision in the distal duodenum. The initial exploratory duodenal incision allows correct placement of the second incision for this anastomosis either distal or

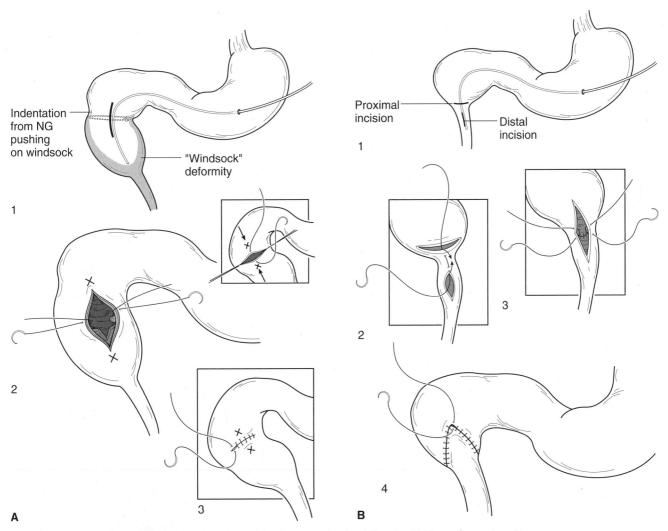

Figure 50-2   A: A web that is forming a "windsock" deformity. (*1*) The catheter placed into a gastrotomy demonstrates the proximal attachment of the membrane. Traction sutures are applied at this point. (*2*) A longitudinal incision is made and the anterior aspect of the membrane incised/resected. The ampulla of Vater is usually at the base of the web in the medial aspect (*arrow*) (*3*) The incision is closed transversely. **B:** Alternatively, a duodenoduodenostomy (diamond anastomosis) may be performed around the obstruction. (*1*) A transverse incision is made proximally and a longitudinal incision distally. (*2*) The middle of the proximal incision is approximated to the proximal aspect of the distal incision. (*3*) A diamond shape is formed by the anastomosis, thus giving the procedure the name. (*4*) The completed anastomosis is demonstrated.

proximal depending on where the obstruction is located (Fig. 50-2). The proximal incision is extended horizontally just above the obstruction and the distal in a longitudinal direction starting just downstream from the obstruction. The proximal duodenal incision is approximately 1 cm in length and maintained on the anterolateral aspect of the duodenum to avoid injury to the biliary tract or the pancreas during suture placement. The distal incision is also approximately 1 cm in length and placed on the antimesenteric border. In the rare circumstance (10%) where a wide gap exists between the ends of the duodenum, a loop of proximal jejunum may be brought to the duodenum through the mesocolon for a duodenojejunostomy.

Although rare, distal atresia is present in up to 3% of cases. Thus it is imperative that the small bowel be explored for findings of a distal atresia. One approach is to inject saline through the entire bowel via a catheter placed through the duodenal incision prior to anastomosis (3).

Morbidity and mortality for these infants are frequently due to complications from prematurity, trisomy 21, congenital heart disease, and other associated anomalies. Feeding is often delayed for days to weeks (mean of 13 days) due to duodenal dysfunction in the proximal dilated duodenum (7). Clinicians may need to increase feeds slowly and to tolerate higher volumes of feeding residuals in the newborn after operation. Some surgeons suggest that placement of a transanastomotic feeding tube at the time of correction of the duodenal atresia allows earlier initiation of feeding, while others suggest that this may not be the case (8,9). Still others perform a plication or resection of the redundant duodenum at the time of the initial operation (10). Rarely is reoperation required in the newborn period. Upper GI contrast studies should be performed only if feeding intolerance persists for a number of weeks. Chromosomes should be assessed for trisomy 21, which is present in 21% of patients with duodenal obstruction (7).

Postoperative complications include anastomotic obstruction (3%), congestive heart failure (9%), prolonged ileus (4%), pneumonia (5%), and superficial wound infection (3%) (3). Late complications include reoperation for adhesive obstruction in 15%, blind loop syndrome or bile reflux gastritis in 22%, gastroesophageal reflux (GER) disease unresponsive to medical management that requires antireflux surgery (Nissen fundoplication) in 5%, duodenal dilation in 22%, diminished peristalsis in 20%, delayed emptying in 12%, and luminal narrowing in 7% (7,11). Late duodenal dysmotility resulting in megaduodenum will require tapering duodenoplasty in 4% of patients (3).

The operative mortality rate (4%) is due to complex congenital heart anomalies, as is the late mortality (10%) (3). The overall long-term survival is 86%.

Malrotation

At approximately 8 to 10 weeks of development, the midgut, which consists of the intestines oriented on the blood supply of the superior mesenteric artery, rotates 270 degrees counterclockwise (from the perspective of the surgeon looking toward the base of the mesentery), which leads to fixation of the proximal small bowel at the ligament of Treitz, attachment of the cecum and right colon in the right lower quadrant, and broad fixation of the base of the small bowel mesentery to the retroperitoneum. If this rotation fails to occur, the small intestine remains on the right side of the abdomen, the cecum is typically at a location other than the right lower quadrant, and the bowel overall remains unfixed. The entire midgut is thus mobile and prone to a twist, or volvulus, which is the form of presentation in 31% of patients but 85% of newborns (12,13). Volvulus may compromise superior mesenteric artery inflow and venous blood outflow, leading to ischemia or necrosis of the entire small intestine and transverse colon (Fig. 50-3). In addition, peritoneal bands that cross over the distal portions of the duodenum and the proximal jejunum are residue of the failed rotation. These bands, known as Ladd bands, may partially obstruct the duodenum and small bowel.

Ninety-one percent of patients with symptomatic malrotation present in the first year of life, with 51% in the first week and 65% in the first month of life (14). Thus only 15% present after the first year. An occasional older patient presents with intermittent midgut volvulus and recurrent abdominal pain.

One of the most common complications of treatment for malrotation and acute midgut volvulus is the failure to recognize this entity promptly, with ensuing loss of the entire midgut. The primary symptom of acute midgut volvulus is sudden onset of bilious vomiting (15). It is incumbent upon clinicians to pursue the diagnosis of malrotation in infants with bilious vomiting. With midgut volvulus, as the distal bowel empties, the abdomen is often scaphoid rather than distended. Physical examination is surprisingly unremarkable until later in the process when

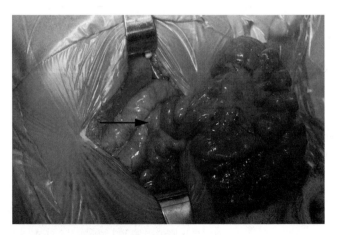

Figure 50-3 Malrotation with volvulus. The arrow demonstrates the site of the volvulus. Note that the volvulus is in a clockwise direction and that the small bowel is ischemic.

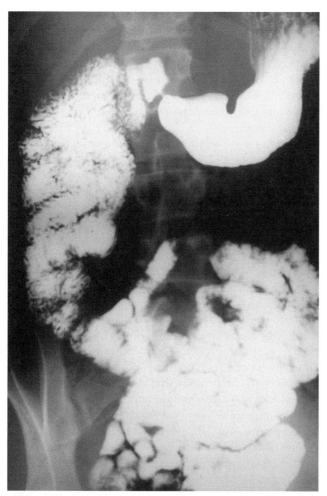

Figure 50-4 Classic upper GI with small bowel follow-through in a patient with malrotation. Note that the duodenojejunal junction never passes to the left of the midline (spine) and the jejunum is on the right side of the abdomen.

intestinal ischemia and necrosis develop. At that point, abdominal distension, tenderness, and hematochezia are often present. As the course progresses, hypovolemia, shock, and acidosis ensue. Contrast radiography evaluation of the course of the duodenum demonstrates that the duodenojejunal junction remains to the right of the midline and the normal posterior and cephalad fixation of the duodenum at the ligament of Treitz is absent (Fig. 50-4) (16). If volvulus is present, a corkscrew appearance of the duodenojejunal junction is noted.

Midgut volvulus is one of the most serious emergencies in the neonate. Once the diagnosis of malrotation is made in the symptomatic patient, immediate laparotomy is indicated even if radiologic and clinical signs of volvulus are absent. The child should be rapidly resuscitated either in the operating room or while the operating room is being readied. Ladd procedure consists of the following: (i) Exploration of the midgut; (ii) Counterclockwise derotation of a midgut volvulus (if present) since the volvulus is almost always clockwise from the surgeon's perspective. Two or more rotations of the bowel may be required and

the process of derotation can be very confusing. One must continue to derotate until the entire mesentery can be broadly followed to the base; (iii) Performance of a Kocher maneuver with division of Ladd bands (which may be causing the obstruction). Failure to lyse all of Ladd bands may result in persistent obstruction or recurrence of volvulus; (iv) Broadening of the mesentery of the proximal jejunum and the transverse colon, which, along with subsequent adhesion formation, will prevent recurrent volvulus; (v) Return of the intestine to the abdomen without any twists in the mesentery and placement of the cecum in the left lower quadrant to further broaden the mesentery; and (vi) Appendectomy because of the potential of a difficult diagnosis of appendicitis in the future with the inappropriate location of the appendix (17). There is no value in fixing—or need to fix—the intestines to the retroperitoneum. If compromised bowel is noted, a second look at 24 hours is an option. Another approach may entail resection of clearly necrotic bowel with either reanastamosis if the status of the remaining bowel is certain or staple closure of the ends in areas of compromise with reexploration at 24 hours. If possible, sufficient length of intestine is maintained to avoid the short gut syndrome. Performance of an ileostomy is usually necessary only if there is continued question of intestinal viability at reexploration. Necrosis of the entire midgut makes survival unlikely and excessive morbidity a likely outcome with requirement for life-long parenteral nutrition or small bowel transplantation (18).

Postoperative complications are relatively few. Recurrence of midgut volvulus occurs in <2% of patients and is thought to be related to a failure to lyse all of the Ladd bands. Adhesive bowel obstruction occurs in 1% to 10% of patients and can be treated with nasogastric decompression, although lysis of adhesions, sometimes via a laparoscopic approach, may be required. Malrotation is associated with a duodenal atresia or a partially obstructing web in 11% of patients (14). To exclude this, one option is to pass a Foley catheter through the duodenum via a small gastrotomy and withdraw it with the balloon gently inflated in order to ensure that a duodenal web or other obstruction does not exist.

In those with short bowel syndrome, complications are associated with long-term parenteral nutrition, fluid and electrolyte abnormalities, and liver failure. The length of bowel sufficient for enteral nutrition traditionally has been considered to be 15 cm with an intact ileocecal valve and 40 cm without, although recent data suggest that it is not just the length, but also the character of the bowel that determines successful provision of enteral feeding (19).

Perioperative mortality is 4% and is primarily associated with sepsis from massive intestinal necrosis (13). Mortality is at least 50% in those with extensive (>75%) small bowel infarction (20). Mortality may be increased in those with congenital heart disease. The incidence of malrotation is increased in those with congenital heart disease, especially in those with the heterotaxia or polysplenia syndrome. However, approximately 15% of such patients will develop acute midgut volvulus. In conjunction with the cardiologist, the surgeon must consider the risk-benefit of a Ladd procedure in these patients with asymptomatic malrotation and congenital heart disease.

Jejunoileal Obstruction

Among cases of jejunoileal obstruction, atresia occurs in 95% while stenosis occurs in 5% (6). The diagnosis of bowel obstruction is made on the basis of fetal ultrasound in 29% of cases via identification of enlarged loops of bowel in conjunction with maternal polyhydramnios, although about 50% of positive scans are false-positive studies (3,21). Associated *in utero* causes of jejunoileal atresia include volvulus in 27%, malrotation in 19%, gastroschisis in 17%, and intussusception in 2%. Other anomalies are unusual with jejunoileal atresia (7%) (3).

The diagnosis can be made by plain radiography when a large loop of dilated, air-filled bowel is noted. The enlarged loops are usually thumb-sized or greater on the newborn radiograph (rule of thumb). If such large, dilated loops are noted, further preoperative diagnostic studies are not required except for a contrast enema, which often demonstrates a diminutive and unused colon and rules out colonic pathology, which can be missed during exploration. Peritoneal calcification is noted in 12% of patients, indicating prior *in utero* perforation and saponification of fat from pancreatic enzymes in the extruded meconium.

Different types of jejunoileal atresia are observed (Fig. 50-5). Type I (membranous) occurs in 23%, type II (fibrous cord) in 27%, and type IIIa (mesenteric gap) in 18%. Multiple atresias (type IV) are observed in 24% of cases (3). The "apple-peel" or "Christmas-tree" deformity occurs in approximately 10% of cases and is associated with atresia near the ligament of Treitz and precarious, retrograde blood supply from the ileocolic, middle colic, or right colic arterial distribution to the distal bowel (22).

As long as radiologic findings exclude malrotation with volvulus, intravenous fluids may be administered, a nasogastric tube placed, and a timely, but not emergent, operation performed. The bowel is eviscerated and any twists reduced via a supraumbilical transverse incision. Examination for malrotation must be deliberate so that this anomaly is not missed. A seromuscular biopsy of the rectum can be performed just proximal to the peritoneal reflection to evaluate for Hirschsprung disease. Because between 6% and 20% of newborns may have more than one atresia, a 10 French catheter is placed into the small bowel distal to the atresia and saline gently infused until it reaches the terminal ileum. If no contrast enema was performed, saline is infused to the rectum to rule out the presence of another atretic segment of bowel. The dilated proximal segment should be resected to a reasonable caliber of bowel (≈1 cm) to prevent subsequent anastomotic dysfunction since the massively dilated proximal bowel has smooth muscle hyperplasia and ineffective peristalsis.

If resection would compromise bowel length, an antimesenteric tapering enteroplasty of the proximal bowel can reduce the lumen size. This entails resection of the most bulbous end of the proximal bowel, placement of a 20 French catheter into the proximal end, and resection of the excess caliber of bowel using a stapling device (6,23). The staple line should be reinforced with 5-0 Vicryl sutures to prevent a leak.

A discrepancy in caliber between the proximal and distal bowel will still be present and, therefore, a proximal end to distal oblique anastomosis is performed by resecting the proximal bowel at a 90-degree angle and the distal bowel at a 45-degree angle (Fig. 50-6). An antimesenteric incision on the distal bowel can equalize the caliber. The bowel anastomosis is very similar to a vascular anastomosis and is performed with one layer of interrupted 5-0 Vicryl suture starting at the mesenteric border, with the knots on the inside of the bowel to evert the bowel edges. Any discrepancy in size between the bowel ends can be adjusted as the anastomosis proceeds around the antimesenteric border. The closure is continued three-fourths of the way around, at which point the closure is started in the other direction. The final few sutures placed are of the Lembert type. It is critical that these final sutures are not placed near the antimesenteric area of the bowel as this might compromise the distal lumen.

In patients with compromised blood supply or in the setting of meconium ileus or meconium peritonitis, a primary anastomosis may be inadvisable because of the risk of leak. In this case a double barrel enterostomy should be performed. If an apple-peel deformity is noted with tenuous blood supply to the distal bowel, an anastomosis may be performed while being careful to avoid a twist in the distal bowel mesentery. Alternatively, forming a proximal enterostomy while leaving the distal bowel intact may be the best option. In patients with gastroschisis, the thickened bowel often precludes resection and anastomosis. In this case the bowel is reduced and the atresia addressed approximately 3 weeks later, when the bowel inflammation and thickening have resolved. Over 50% of patients with jejunoileal atresia require parenteral nutrition (6). Central venous access should be established before or at the time of operation.

Patients with meconium ileus and all others with volvulus and atresia should have a workup for cystic fibrosis. Suction rectal biopsy to evaluate for Hirschsprung disease should be performed in the 9% of patients with colonic atresia and those with volvulus and atresia in the terminal ileum (24). Anastomotic leak is associated with jejunoileal atresia when it is accompanied by Hirschsprung disease.

Postoperative complications include adhesive bowel obstruction (24%), functional obstruction at the site of the anastomosis (9%), and the occasional anastomotic leak or stricture (4%) (3). Prolonged dysfunction of the proximal dilated intestine is quite common, and days to weeks may pass before enteral feeds are established. Evaluation for

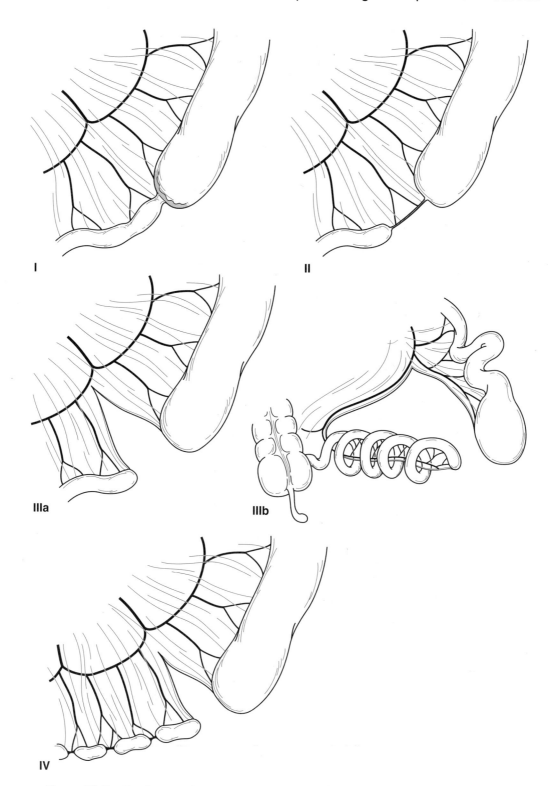

Figure 50-5 Classification of jejunoileal atresia describes the pathology as type I (mucosal web), type II (fibrous cord), type IIIa (mesenteric gap defect), type IIIb ("apple peel"), or type IV (multiple atresias).

bowel obstruction by contrast enema or upper GI contrast study should be performed after a few weeks if feedings are not tolerated. Typically, a contrast study demonstrates a widely patent anastomosis. If the anastomosis is patent and feeding intolerance persists, a revision of the anastomosis with resection of additional bowel and/or enteroplasty to reduce the proximal bowel caliber may be required. Anastomotic complications, such as a leak, may be indicated by persistent pneumoperitoneum or, more commonly, by development of a fistula. If sepsis is present,

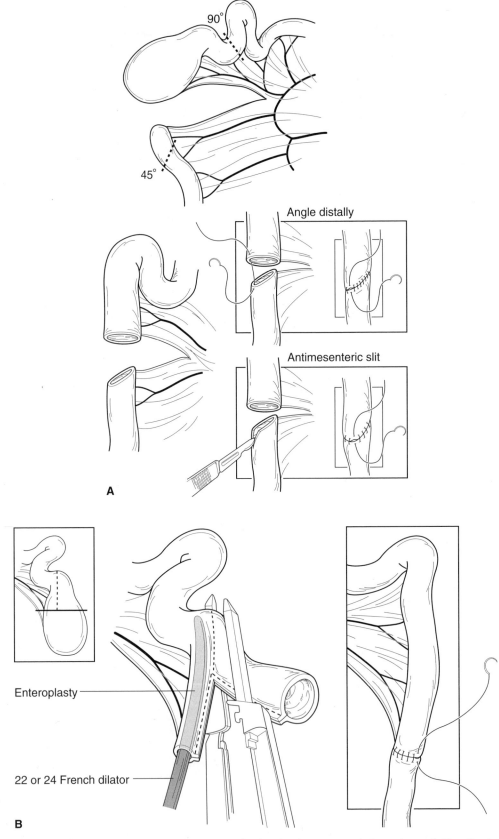

Figure 50-6   A: For jejunoileal atresia, an end-to-back anastomosis is performed. The distal bowel, which has the smaller caliber even after resection of the bulbous proximal end, is divided on an angle to equalize the proximal and distal bowel caliber. Often an additional antimesenteric slit is required. The anastomosis is accomplished with 5-0 Vicryl. **B:** An enteroplasty using a 22 or 24 French catheter stent and staples is used for high jejunal atresia.

operative intervention is required. If not, antibiotic treatment and parenteral nutrition allow resolution of the leak and fistula. If a leak is present without fistula or sepsis, drain placement, most commonly through the incision or a small separate right lower quadrant incision, may be necessary.

Bacterial overgrowth is a long-term complication that manifests as vomiting, diarrhea, and abdominal distension. Bacterial overgrowth is treated with metronidazole and, if acute and severe, a short course of broad-spectrum intravenous antibiotics. Occasionally, resection of a dilated segment or enteroplasty will be required to resolve recurrent bacterial overgrowth. Chronic blood loss from the anastomosis or an adjacent ulcer can occur many years after the initial operation. Although the exact etiology is unclear, this is thought to be due to ischemia at the anastomosis. Resection and revision of the anastomosis is curative, although the ulcer may be near but not at the anastomosis and can, therefore, be easily missed.

Short-term survival has increased in recent years to approximately 85% to 90% (6,25). Even those with an apple-peel deformity are expected to survive and, despite early morbidity, will likely have an excellent long-term outcome (26). The perioperative mortality of approximately 1% is mainly related to associated anomalies such as congenital heart disease and sepsis. The long-term causes of death are mainly related to the short bowel syndrome observed in 25% of patients with jejunoileal atresia (3). Parenteral nutrition has markedly enhanced outcome in patients with atresia. However, those patients with short bowel syndrome and long-term dependency on parenteral nutrition may endure numerous episodes of catheter sepsis, probably related to translocation of enteric organisms. In addition, cholestasis from parenteral nutrition with associated liver failure is a potentially lethal complication in infants that is not as prevalent in adults. Liver and small bowel transplantation have not yet had a consistent impact upon outcome in those with this complication. Vitamin deficiencies can also occur.

Meconium Ileus

Meconium ileus is present in approximately 20% of newborns with cystic fibrosis (27). With meconium ileus, secretion of viscous intestinal mucus, an abnormal concentrating process in the proximal bowel, and impaired pancreatic enzyme secretion together result in bowel obstruction because of the presence of thick, tenacious meconium in the midileum and pellets of gray, inspissated meconium in the distal ileum (Fig. 50-7). The hallmark of the newborn with meconium ileus is abdominal distention at birth, with multiple doughy loops of dilated bowel noted on palpation. Bilious emesis occurs and the newborn fails to pass meconium in the first 24 to 48 hours of life. Meconium ileus is divided into uncomplicated and complicated. The uncomplicated meconium ileus is simple obstruction of the terminal ileum and occurs in 55% of cases (28,29). In contrast, meconium-filled bowel may twist and produce a volvulus, resulting in ischemic necrosis with associated perforation (19%) and/or atresia (48%) (30). Perforation, with intraperitoneal dissemination of sterile meconium, may lead to isolated regions of calcification (meconium peritonitis) or even the development of a large meconium-containing

Pathology of meconium ileus: character of contents in various parts of the bowel

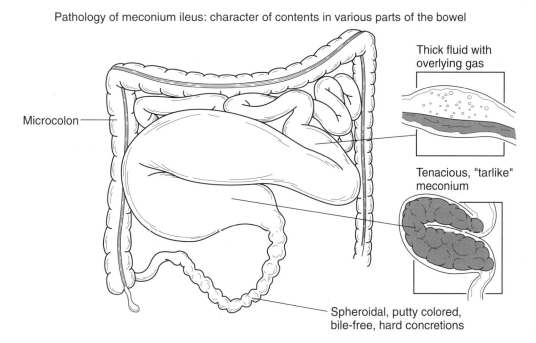

Figure 50-7 Typical intestinal findings in the setting of meconium ileus.

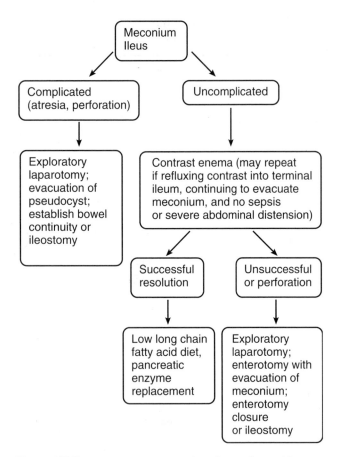

Figure 50-8 Management approach to the newborn with meconium ileus.

pseudocyst (19%). Extra intestinal anomalies are uncommon with meconium ileus.

For uncomplicated meconium ileus, a contrast enema can be both diagnostic and therapeutic (Fig. 50-8). Gastrograffin, hypaque, or Conray may be used to perform the study; the osmolarity of the contrast agent does not appear to be of significance. A small, unused microcolon is noted with thick, inspissated meconium in the terminal ileum. The distal small bowel must be filled or the therapeutic aspect of the study will not be successful. The hypertonicity of the gastrograffin likely draws fluid into the bowel lumen, which aids in mobilizing the meconium. The newborn undergoing such studies must be kept warm and well hydrated: typical fluid requirements are 150 mL/kg/d, and monitoring of urine output and vital signs in an ICU is required. Adding an emulsifying agent, such as Tween 80 or N-acetylcysteine (Mucomyst), may enhance the treatment's effectiveness (31). Contrast studies are effective at relieving the obstruction in 40% to 60% of patients with simple meconium ileus (30). Additional enemas may be performed over the ensuing days as long as progress is made refluxing contrast into the ileum, meconium is being mobilized and evacuated, and complications, such as perforation, worsening abdominal distension, or sepsis, are not encountered. Perforation will

occur in 3% and requires operative intervention with bowel resection and evacuation of the meconium (see below).

If contrast enemas are unsuccessful, operative intervention is evacuation of the obstructing meconium from the terminal ileum. An enterotomy in the dilated ileum just proximal to the change in lumen caliber provides access to milk meconium out by external massage and by irrigation of the bowel via an 8 to 10 French catheter with warm saline, 2% to 4% N-acetylcysteine, or gastrograffin. Thick meconium is evacuated through the enterotomy or flushed into the colon. The appendix can be removed and a catheter placed into the base of the appendix to flush the terminal ileum and colon. If the meconium cannot be successfully evacuated, the bowel has been compromised, or an atretic or stenotic segment is identified, the involved segment of ileum should be resected. In general, a simple end-to-end anastomosis is preferred because the long-term surgical morbidity is lower than with an enterostomy (32,33). If peritonitis, bowel compromise, concern for bowel dysfunction, or concurrent medical problems make an anastomosis risky, formation of an ileostomy with an adjacent mucous fistula is an alternative, with plans for establishing bowel continuity 4 to 6 weeks later (29).

Atresia should be treated by resection with adequate bowel preservation as outlined in the section on jejunoileal atresia. Before the anastomosis is performed, the distal meconium should be evacuated as described above. Meconium ascites or a meconium pseudocyst is often the result if an *in utero* perforation has occurred. The goal of operations in the setting of meconium ascites or a pseudocyst is to identify the site of perforation and to ensure bowel continuity. In many cases, an ileostomy is required. The rind that forms the pseudocyst is left on the bowel, thus avoiding injury. In general, careful blunt dissection allows separation of the loops of bowel until the entire small bowel is mobilized.

Recent improvements in perioperative care and management of patients with cystic fibrosis have resulted in an increase in survival rates to between 90% to 100% (29,30,33). Dilute 10% N-acetylcysteine is administered through the nasogastric tube after resolution of the obstruction to prevent recurrent inspissated secretions. Anastomotic leak is unusual. Postoperative care is specifically aimed at treatment of pulmonary problems with excellent pulmonary hygiene and administration of antibiotics. Parenteral nutrition is administered until enteral feeding of a predigested, low long chain fatty acid formula, such as Pregestamil, is tolerated. Oral pancreatic enzyme administration is necessary with the initiation of feeding. A sweat chloride test cannot be performed in the first 3 weeks of life because of inadequate sweat production in newborns. Either a sweat chloride test after the first 3 weeks of life or cytogenetics for the ΔF508 and other common mutations is useful since 21% of patients with meconium ileus will not have laboratory or clinical evidence of cystic fibrosis (34). Closure of the ileostomy is often accompanied by bowel dysfunction. One option to determine if the patient is ready for ostomy closure is refeeding of the ileostomy output down the mucus fistula.

Long-term complications are related to the cystic fibrosis and its treatment. The distal intestinal obstruction syndrome (DIOS) or meconium ileus equivalent occurs in 9% of patients with cystic fibrosis and is more frequently observed among patients with cystic fibrosis who previously had meconium ileus (32). This syndrome may be associated with inadequate enzyme replacement or fluid intake and is usually successfully managed with administration of gastrograffin as an enema or orally. Colonic strictures can occur in association with high-dose enzyme administration and require operative colonic resection (35). Rectal prolapse can occur between 1 to 3 years of age and in general resolves with oral enzyme therapy or rectal cautery and sclerotherapy. Intussusception and gall bladder disease can also occur in patients with cystic fibrosis.

Hirschsprung Disease

During the first 12 weeks of fetal development neuroenteric cells migrate from the neural crest to the upper GI tract, from which they advance to the distal large intestine. Failure of this results in Hirschsprung disease, with absence of ganglion cells in the submucosal as well as the intermuscular planes of the distal intestine. Submucosal noncholinergic, nonadrenergic nerve hypertrophy is also observed. Perhaps as a result of absence of nitric oxide synthase, the distal aganglionic area is in spasm and presents as an obstruction to the proximal intestine that dilates and develops a hypertrophic muscularis (36). The aganglionic segment is almost always continuous and limited to the descending or rectosigmoid region in 75% to 80% of patients; long segment or total colonic disease occurs in 15% to 20% (37,38).

The diagnosis of Hirschsprung disease may be difficult to make. The infant with constipation, failure to pass meconium in the first 24 hours of life, failure to thrive, vomiting, and/or abdominal distension should be evaluated for Hirschsprung disease (39). Likewise, the surgeon should consider Hirschsprung disease in the setting of any unexplained perforation of the distal intestinal tract in the neonate so that the diagnosis is not missed. Older patients may present with enterocolitis, in which diarrhea, abdominal distension, vomiting, fever, and lethargy are the result of stasis and intestinal epithelial infection. Frequently used diagnostic tests include a contrast enema and a rectal biopsy. The contrast enema is used to examine for a "transition zone" between the dilated proximal bowel and the narrowed distal colon/rectum. The transition zone, especially if it is distal, may be missed if the enema catheter balloon is inflated during the study or a bowel preparation is used. For the same reason, rectal exams and enemas should not be performed in proximity to the exam. Failure to pass the contrast on a repeat

abdominal radiograph 24 hours later suggests the diagnosis of Hirschsprung disease.

Either a full-thickness or a suction rectal biopsy is the definitive method for establishing the diagnosis. A suction rectal biopsy is performed approximately 2 cm above the anus and must be of sufficient depth and contain enough tissue (approximately three times as much submucosa as mucosa) to allow the pathologist to conclude that no ganglion cells are present. Both the aganglionosis and the nerve hypertrophy must be identified to avoid a mistaken diagnosis of Hirschsprung disease: An area of hypoganglionosis exists for approximately 1 cm in the anal canal. Thus, an absence of ganglion cells may be noted if the biopsy is performed too close to the anus, but the absence of hypertrophic nerves will prevent one from mistakenly concluding that Hirschsprung disease is the diagnosis. The full-thickness rectal biopsy may be performed by excising a piece of rectum under direct vision, which allows one to ensure that the biopsy was taken from the correct location and provides a thorough pathologic evaluation of both the submucosal and the myenteric plexus. However, the full-thickness biopsy must be performed in the operating room under anesthesia and the resulting inflammation and scarring may complicate the submucosal dissection required for correction of Hirschsprung disease. Complications of rectal biopsy are exceedingly rare and include perforation and bleeding. Whichever approach to biopsy is used, one should not rely only on frozen sections to make the diagnosis of Hirschsprung disease since the reliability of the frozen section is limited (40). The diagnosis of Hirschsprung disease may be especially difficult to make when the aganglionic segment is "ultrashort" because the rectal biopsy and the contrast enema may appear normal. Anorectal manometry will, however, demonstrate failure of rectal relaxation with distension. Ultrashort segment Hirschsprung disease may be treated with a posterior myotomy/myectomy (POMM), as described below.

Three operations comprise the majority of those performed in the setting of Hirschsprung disease: the Soave, the Swenson, and the Duhamel procedures (Fig. 50-9) (41,42). The intent of each is to bring the bowel with ganglion cells in proximity to the anus. For the Soave procedure, the portion with aganglionosis is resected to the peritoneal reflection, at which point a mucosectomy is performed to within 1 cm of the dentate line. The aganglionated and ganglionated portion of bowel are then identified by frozen section of seromuscular biopsies performed at the peritoneal reflection and just above an obvious transition zone. Although frozen section may be inadequate to document the absence of ganglion cells and the diagnosis of Hirschsprung disease, it is reasonable for identifying the presence of ganglion cells and the status of the pulled-through segment (40). However, inappropriate use of either a nonganglionated portion of the bowel or a segment from the transition zone may be used in the pull-through if an inexperienced pathologist is mistaken in assessing whether

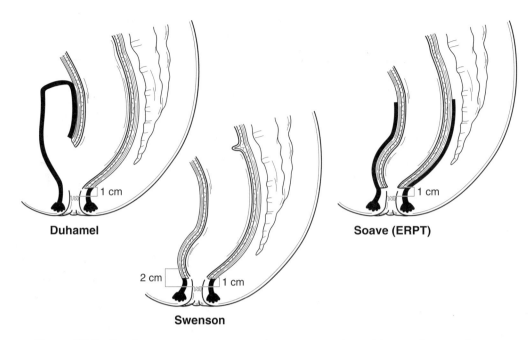

Figure 50-9 The three most common types of operations performed for Hirschsprung disease. The dark black lines indicate remnant portions of aganglionated bowel. In the Soave procedure, the aganglionated bowel proximal to the anastomosis has the mucosa removed.

ganglion cells and hypertrophic nerves are present. Once a ganglionated portion above the transition zone is identified, it is then pulled through the cuff and approximated to the mucosa just proximal to the dentate line. The pulled-through segment must not be twisted. Postoperative enterocolitis and anastomotic stricture formation may be higher with the Soave procedure than with the other Hirschsprung disease procedures (43).

The Swenson operation involves dissection of the rectum to approximately 1.5 to 2 cm from the dentate line. The full thickness of the rectum is then everted and excised to that point as the ganglionated bowel is pulled through and an anastomosis performed. Care must be taken during this procedure to dissect exactly on the surface of the rectum and to minimize anterior dissection in order to avoid injury to the vas deferens and the pelvic innervation involved with bladder and penile/ejaculatory function. These complications are rare, although they are more common with this technique (44,45). Finally, for the Duhamel procedure the aganglionic sigmoid/rectum is resected down to the peritoneal reflection. The ganglionated bowel is brought anterior to the sacrum and anastomosed to a transverse posterior rectal incision performed 1 to 2 cm proximal to the dentate line. A GIA stapler is then placed into the anus with one limb in the native rectum and one into the pulled-through segment. The GIA stapler is then used to form a common pouch in which the anterior portion is the aganglionated rectum and the posterior is the ganglionated pulled-through bowel. One must ascertain that the GIA stapler has fired correctly and that the staple line is intact without evidence of bleeding. This is a fairly simple operation to perform. However, failure to eliminate

the septum completely may leave a diverticulum that can accumulate feces, dilate, and result in rectal dysfunction and formation of a fecaloma. To prevent this complication, the proximal portion of the rectum can be approximated to the pulled-through segment, thus eliminating the diverticulum (46). Constipation may be more common with the Duhamel procedure (45).

Over the last few decades pull-through operations for Hirschsprung disease have typically been done in two stages, with a primary colostomy formed followed by the pull-through at 9 to 12 months of age. Most recently, primary pull-through operations have been performed without colostomy formation. This approach has not been associated with a greater complication rate, although the incidence of postoperative enterocolitis may be increased (47). In fact, problems with the stoma when a two-stage approach is used may contribute to a higher rate of complications among those managed with two stages (48). Even pull-through operations can be safely performed in one stage in the neonatal period (42).

Minimally invasive approaches to the Soave operation have become favored recently. A laparoscopic approach to mobilization of the sigmoid colon followed by a perineal approach to the mucosectomy allows transanal removal of the aganglionic segment in continuity with the remainder of the bowel followed by anastomosis of the normal sigmoid colon to the mucosa just proximal to the dentate line (49). It is now clear that laparoscopy is not required for a transanal approach in the setting of rectosigmoid disease (50). Thus the mucosectomy is initiated transanally at approximately 1 cm above the dentate line and continued until the muscularis of the rectum can be intussuscepted from the anus. At that point, the rectosigmoid muscularis is incised circumferentially and the full-thickness rectosigmoid colon mobilized by dividing the blood supply as it is exposed at the anus. A transition zone is usually visible and frozen section biopsies are used to confirm that the aganglionated bowel is completely excised. A coloanal anastomosis is then performed. Before doing so it is critical both to divide the posterior aspect of the rectal cuff and to ensure that the remainder of the cuff is not prolapsed. Failure to do so may result in telescoping of the cuff over the distal aspect of the pulled-through bowel with associated compression. One must also be careful to avoid a twist in the sigmoid colon as it is pulled down toward the anus. A preoperative contrast enema allows identification of the transition zone, which determines the feasibility of the transanal approach. In addition, the contrast enema allows identification of bowel that is dilated to the point where it is unreasonable to pull the bowel through the muscular cuff. Such dilated bowel must be identified before the mucosectomy has been performed. Laparoscopy can be used to identify bowel with a caliber that would prevent performance of a pull-through. In that case, a colostomy should be performed at a level within the ganglionated bowel as defined by seromuscular biopsy and frozen section. Laparoscopic mobilization of the colon can also be used to augment a transanal operation in long segment Hirschsprung disease in which the aganglionic segment extends out of the rectosigmoid area.

Total colonic Hirschsprung disease occurs in approximately 10% of patients. The diagnosis is difficult to ascertain because a transition zone is often not evident on contrast enema. Rectal biopsy provides evidence for Hirschsprung disease. If initial intraoperative biopsies fail to show ganglion cells, an appendectomy should be performed with examination for ganglion cells within the appendix in order to discern if total colonic Hirschsprung disease is present. Most often an ileostomy is performed, although a primary pull-through can be considered. Nutritional deficiencies, failure to thrive, and fluid and electrolyte disturbances are common in patients with total colonic Hirschsprung disease. Sodium repletion should be documented via measurement of urine sodium. Serum bicarbonate levels should be assessed and replaced if necessary. Parenteral nutrition is frequently required and associated catheter sepsis is frequent. A Martin modification of the Duhamel procedure, in which a long beveled ileorectal anastomosis is performed, may enhance absorption, but the incidence of enterocolitis is high (51). Occasionally extensive small bowel aganglionosis is also encountered. With extensive small bowel aganglionosis, long-term parenteral nutrition is required (70%) and mortality is high (40%) (52).

The complications associated with operations performed for Hirschsprung disease are, except as noted previously, independent of the type of operation performed. Rarely, complications such as twisting or necrosis of the pulled-through segment, anastomotic disruption, cuff abscess, and enterocutaneous fistulas may occur and are best managed with formation of a colostomy (53). Reoperative procedures are often required in those with twisting of the pulled-through segment and enterocutaneous fistulas (50,54). The most common complication is enterocolitis, which occurs in 20% to 50% of patients (55,56). The etiology of enterocolitis is unclear, but it is thought to result from stasis and associated bacterial overgrowth. Interestingly, the incidence of enterocolitis decreases with advancing age and is rarely observed past childhood. As mentioned previously, children typically present with diarrhea, vomiting, abdominal distension, fever, and lethargy (56). Rectal examination demonstrates explosive diarrhea, and abdominal radiograph often reveals a dilated sigmoid colon with a cutoff sign. The treatment may be outpatient with oral metronidazole if the enterocolitis is mild or inpatient with broad-spectrum intravenous antibiotics if it is more severe. Rectal irrigation with metronidazole (10 mL per kg) with colonic decompression via advancement of a rectal tube often helps to resolve this process. Enterocolitis usually resolves with treatment using rectal washouts and intravenous antibiotics for 2 to 3 days. The patient is then discharged on oral metronidazole for 2 to 4 weeks. For recurrent enterocolitis, rectal washouts or dilatations, or both, can be performed at home and ciprofloxacin can be used instead of metronidazole. A contrast enema should be performed to evaluate for a twist in the pull-through or evidence of obstruction (Fig. 50-10). Any obstruction related to the anastomosis or cuff should be dilated (57). Although a rare cause of enterocolitis, aganglionosis of the pulled-through segment should be evaluated by rectal biopsy (58). Persistent enterocolitis may be addressed by injection of botulinum toxin (Botox) into the internal sphincter (59). In some cases the advantages of Botox injection will be long-lasting, while in others it will demonstrate benefit for 3 to 6 months. Reinjection of Botox is an option. If enterocolitis persists, a POMM is performed, which is successful at completely resolving symptoms in 75% of patients. A posterior myotomy is best performed by incising the full thickness of the pulled-through segment and the rectum for a distance proximally of approximately 8 cm starting at the dentate line followed by closure of the mucosa. Alternatively, a posterior myectomy may be initiated with a transverse incision of the mucosa at the posterior aspect of the dentate line and development of a submucosal plane for 5 to 8 cm. The strip of full-thickness muscle extending proximally is then excised and the mucosa reapproximated. Antibiotics are administered. Complications from this procedure are rare.

One of the most common postoperative problems in patients with Hirschsprung disease is perianal excoriation (55%) (60). This is more commonly a problem in the newborn and may lead to severe perianal skin breakdown. It is best to start prophylactic treatment with perianal barrier creams after operation. Administration of H_2 blockers may be of benefit. Postoperative strictures occur in 5% to 22% of patients and are more often observed in

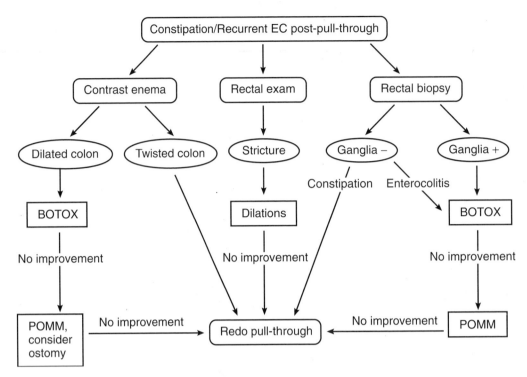

Figure 50-10   Flow chart for workup and treatment of patients with chronic constipation or recurrent enterocolitis after a pull-through operation for Hirschsprung disease. Note: Botox injection may be used as a test for proceeding on to posterior myotomy/myectomy (POMM). Should the patient derive long-term benefit from Botox, no further treatment is needed. If the patient develops transient improvement with Botox, a POMM should be considered.

the newborn (60,61). Rectal examination in the first 2 to 3 weeks will determine if a stricture is developing. The stricture will often resolve over the ensuing weeks. If not, daily rectal dilatation by the parents may be necessary.

Most children do well postoperatively and have regular bowel movements without difficulty. Constipation is managed with stool softeners and enemas. POMM is beneficial in 90% of those with severe refractory constipation (Fig. 50-10) (62). However, POMM is rarely beneficial in the setting of a retained aganglionic segment, which is relatively common among those with persistent, severe constipation (58). Aganglionosis may be acquired due to ischemia because the intraoperative evaluation of the histology was incorrect or the pull-through was performed in a transition zone in which ganglion cells were variably present along with hypertrophic nerves. Performance of a pull-through of the bowel in the transition zone is associated with an increased incidence of enterocolitis and constipation and may require reoperative pull-through (63). Interestingly, the distribution of ganglion cells may extend for 2 to 2.5 cm further in one area than another (64). Thus, identification of ganglion cells in one portion of the circumference of the bowel does not mean that ganglion cells are present in all areas. Contrast enema should also be performed in the setting of severe constipation to assess for a dilated proximal colon or other evidence of obstruction or a twisted pull-through segment. Intestinal neuronal dysplasia (IND), in which giant ganglia, ectopic ganglia, hyperplasia of the submucosal plexus, and

increased acetylcholinesterase activity in the lamina propria are observed on biopsy, is associated with Hirschsprung disease and postoperative constipation (65). IND may require additional bowel resection and redo pull-through. Reoperations for complications after procedures for Hirschsprung disease are necessary in a few patients, usually due to refractory stricture, recurrent enterocolitis, fistula formation, twist in the pull-through segment, rectal prolapse, or retention of an aganglionic segment (54,66,67). Any of the common operations for Hirschsprung disease can be performed secondarily. A mucosectomy of the previously relocated segment can be performed as a redo Soave pull-through (67). A Duhamel often allows operation in a fresh plane if a Soave was previously performed. Most patients (75% to 94%) are continent following a redo pull-through for Hirschsprung disease (68).

Continence is good to normal in 75% to 85% of patients after pull-through, although soiling may be observed in up to 50% (45,69–71).

Imperforate Anus

Imperforate anus occurs because of an arrest of the normal descent of the rectum to the perineum. The diagnosis should be apparent at the initial newborn examination, although a large perineal fistula or ectopic anus can easily be missed. Patients are divided into those in whom the end of the rectum is above the sphincter muscles (high), partially through the sphincter mechanism (intermediate), or fully through the sphincter mechanism (low). From a clinical point of view, however, it is only necessary to distinguish low anomalies from intermediate/high anomalies. Two-thirds of males have high/intermediate lesions, whereas two-thirds of females have low malformations. The distinction between the high/intermediate form and the low type is complicated, needs to be made in the first 24 hours of life, and affects treatment, since the operations and approaches are very different. Examination of the perineum often provides important clues. The following are all suggestive of a low anomaly: a well-developed perineum with an anal dimple; extra skin in the midline (bucket handle); presence of an anocutaneous fistula along the perineum, at the posterior vagina in a female or the scrotal raphe in a male; or meconium seen through a membrane (Fig. 50-11). Therefore, in both males and females, the absence of a fistula or anal membrane suggests the presence of an intermediate/high lesion, although it may take 24 hours before signs of meconium on the perineum appear. In contrast, a flat perineum (rocker bottom) with a poorly developed sacrum is indicative of a high/intermediate lesion. The majority of those patients with an intermediate/high anomaly have an associated fistula to the genitourinary tract: a rectoprostatic or rectobulbar urethral fistula in the male and a rectovaginal or rectovestibular fistula in the female. Thus, meconium may be noted in the urine of the male or

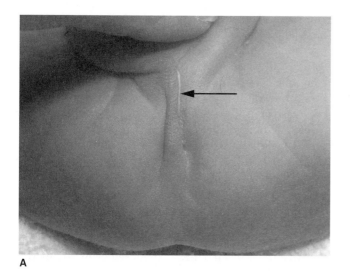

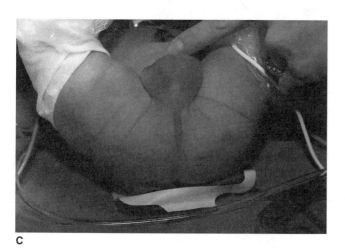

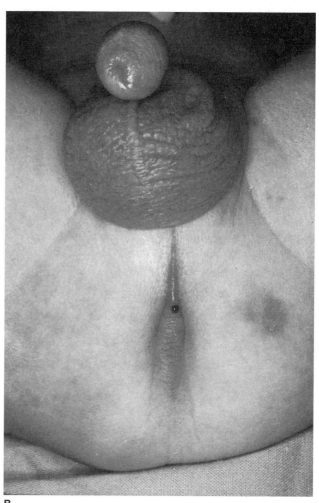

Figure 50-11 **A:** A low imperforate anus in a male. Note the well-formed anal dimple and "bucket handle" deformity. There is a fistula with a streak of white meconium extending anteriorly along the scrotal raphe (*arrow*). This indicates the presence of a low anomaly. **B:** Another low anomaly with a well-developed anal dimple and meconium on the perineum extending anteriorly along the raphe. **C:** A high imperforate anus. Note that there is no fistula and the anal dimple is not as well developed. Additional studies were required to establish whether this was an intermediate/high or low anomaly. Distinguishing whether the patient has a low or intermediate/high imperforate anus is important since the management is distinctly different.

coming from the vagina of the female with an intermediate/high anomaly. Additional techniques for ascertaining the type of lesion include (a) needle aspiration of the perineum to assess whether return of meconium is within 1 cm of the perineum, (b) lateral pelvic radiography after 24 hours of life with the newborn in the prone position to assess the distance between the rectal pouch and the anal skin, or (c) ultrasound evaluation of the perineum, allowing visualization of a distal rectal pouch and documentation of the distance between the anal dimple and the rectum. These techniques can be inaccurate if meconium is impacted in the rectal pouch during pelvic radiography or if the needle or ultrasound probe indents the anal skin during aspiration or ultrasound evaluation. Magnetic resonance imaging (MRI) probably provides the most accurate information (72). Most important, if the diagnosis of a low lesion cannot be established, the newborn should be considered to have an intermediate/high anomaly.

Over half of newborns with imperforate anus have additional anomalies (73). Specifically, the VATERS or VACTERL associations [having two or three of the following: V (vertebral anomalies), A (anal atresia), C (congenital heart disease), TE (tracheoesophageal fistula [TEF]) or esophageal atresia (EA), R (reno-urinary anomalies), and L (radial limb defect)] occur in 44% of patients (74,75). The most significant of these associated anomalies are cardiac lesions that affect 21% (74). One-third have bony sacral abnormalities that affect bladder and rectal innervation and function. Occult spinal dysraphism, consisting of tethered cord with or without associated lipoma of the cord, occurs in 14% and may lead to bowel or bladder dysfunction if not corrected (76). Other important associated problems that should be identified to avoid long-term complications include cryptorchidism (19%), vesicoureteral reflux, and vaginal abnormalities (74,77). Workup of the patient with imperforate anus should include spine radiographs, a spinal and renal ultrasound, an echocardiogram, and a voiding cystourethrogram to evaluate for vesicoureteral reflux.

Treatment of imperforate anus depends on the level and type of lesion. If an obstructive anomaly is present, orogastric or nasogastric suction should be used to prevent aspiration and intravenous antibiotics should be administered. In general, intermediate/high lesions are managed with a colostomy, although some surgeons are proponents of correction in the newborn period either via standard posterior sagittal anorectoplasty (PSARP) in girls or via laparoscopic repair (78,79). The colostomy is usually performed in the descending/sigmoid colon. The colostomy is preferably divided to prevent fecal contamination of the distal loop and the urinary tract or vagina. The colostomy is sewn to the fascia in two layers to prevent prolapse and evisceration, often with a skin bridge between the proximal and distal end of the colon. A distal colostogram is performed after colostomy formation to ascertain the specific lesion and to document the presence and location of a fistula. The presence of a urinary-rectal fistula in the male may

lead to urinary tract infection. All such patients should be placed on prophylactic antibiotics.

Corrective operation by performance of a PSARP is accomplished at 2 to 12 months of life (Fig. 50-12). First a urethral catheter is placed, which may go into the rectum instead of the bladder. If this occurs, it can be rectified later during the operation. The PSARP procedure first involves electrostimulation and identification of the external sphincter, division of the perineum from the anterior border of the external sphincter muscle to the coccyx, and division of all muscles of continence, including the levator ani, in the midline. It is important that one stay exactly in the midline or the rectum may be brought down off to one side of the muscle complex or levator ani. The rectum is identified and opened. The rectourethral, rectovaginal, or rectovestibular fistula is divided from within the rectum and closed with care taken to avoid compromising the urethral lumen, which would lead to urethral stricture formation. Identification of the rectum can be difficult, especially in the case of a bladder fistula, which requires a combined abdominoperineal approach; injury to the urethra can result if it is not done appropriately. Placement of a gastroscope with a light or a dilator through the colostomy may assist with identification of the distal rectum visually or via palpation. Once the fistula is ligated, the rectum is mobilized by developing a submucosal plane where the rectum abuts the urethra and bladder in order to avoid injury to the urogenital structures, including the vas deferens and the seminal vesicles. Once dissection has extended for approximately 1 cm, the full-thickness rectum can be dissected and freed. The rectum is then approximated to the anus as the levator ani and associated muscles of continence are reconstructed in the midline around the rectum. Specifically, the rectum should sit in front of/above the levator ani and inside the external sphincter. The length of rectum should be such that moderate tension is placed on the neoanus so that the anus cosmetically appears normal and mucosal prolapse does not occur. The blood vessels to the distal aspect of the rectum are divided during mobilization; only those required should be divided in order to avoid ischemia to the distal rectum.

Most low malformations can be definitively repaired in the newborn period. In both males and females, an anal membrane may be punctured and dilated or managed with an anoplasty in which the membrane is incised for the distance of the external sphincter, as identified by electrostimulation, and the mucosa sutured to the skin. A perineal fistula is addressed by incision of the skin and rectum back to the posterior margin of the external sphincter, with suture approximation of the rectal mucosa to the skin (cutback anoplasty). If meconium (often white) is present along the scrotal raphe, the pearls of meconium should be unroofed lest they increase in size and become infected. In the female, mobilization of an anterior fourchette or vestibular fistula requires posterior transposition of the fistula to the proper

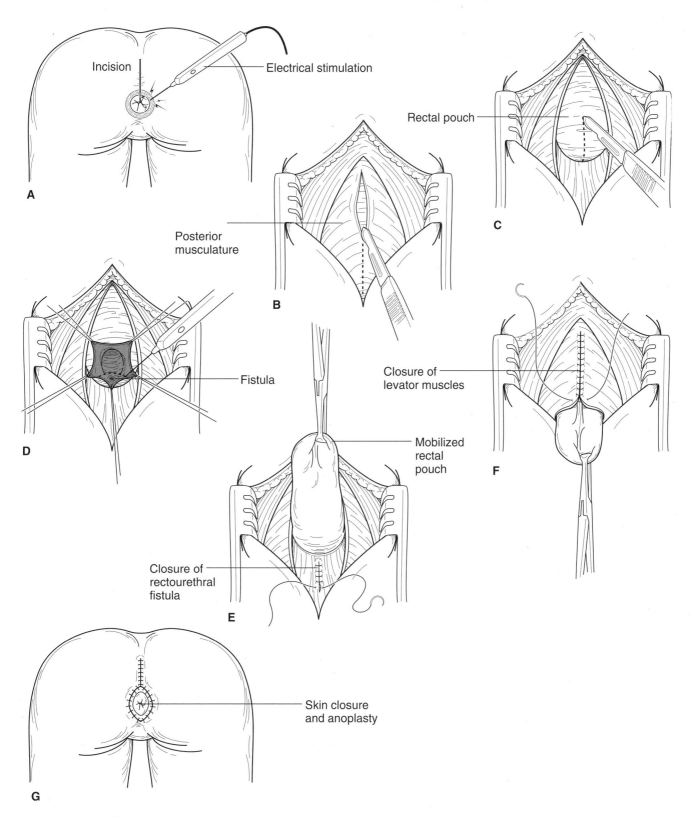

Figure 50-12 The essential features of the posterior sagittal anorectoplasty used for intermediate and high malformations, which are usually associated with rectourinary or rectovaginal fistulas. **A:** Electrical stimulation to identify the external sphincter location. **B:** Midline incision through all posterior musculature. **C:** Identification of the rectal pouch and incision into the posterior, inferior wall of the rectum. **D:** Identification and dissection of the rectourethral fistula from the rectum. **E:** Closure of the rectourethral fistula and anterior muscle complex and mobilization of the rectal pouch. **F:** Closure of the posterior musculature over the rectal pouch. **G:** Skin closure and anoplasty.

site of the anus. This procedure can be performed by making a circumferential incision around the fistula accompanied by a midline perineal incision (tennis racquet) extending back to the posterior margin of the external sphincter as defined by electrostimulation. The most difficult part of this operation is dissection of the rectum from the vagina since the two have a common wall. Entry into the vagina is preferred to entry into the rectum. Careful cautery dissection usually allows separation of the two. Complete separation must be performed or the rectum will be tethered anteriorly during attempts to transpose it posteriorly. The anoplasty is performed after the rectum is brought through the external sphincter and the perineum reconstructed. Alternatively, the perineum may be left intact and separate incisions made around the fistula and at the site of the anoplasty (Pott anoplasty). The rectum is mobilized as described above and then pulled through the anoplasty incision. The procedure for correcting an anterior fistula in a female is somewhat more complex and, therefore, is usually performed beyond 8 weeks of age.

Immediate postoperative complications include ischemia of the distal rectum and wound infection. Both these complications resolve without intervention if a colostomy is present. Femoral nerve palsy can occur due to compression of the femoral nerves with the patient in the prone position and can be prevented by appropriate padding. Postoperative urinary retention is usually due to preoperative dysfunction, which is present in a majority of patients with imperforate anus, even with a normal sacrum, and can be treated with intermittent catheterization or with cystostomy tube placement (80). Bladder function typically improves with time. Antibiotic prophylaxis should be administered if vesicoureteral reflux is identified or if intermittent bladder catheterization is being performed. A rectal dilatation program is initiated at 2 to 3 weeks after operation to prevent stricture formation. It is initially performed by the family once or twice per day until a no. 12 to 14 dilator can be advanced through the neoanus of the newborn/infant. The frequency of dilatations is sequentially decreased over the ensuing 6 months. Colostomy closure is performed only after the neoanus has been dilated to the size indicated above. Occasionally an anal stricture forms despite a dilatation program. An anoplasty with posterior division of the stricture and approximation of the mucosa to the skin can then be performed if necessary. Alternatively, skin flaps can be placed into the sites of stricture incision in order to prevent recurrence (81). Rectal mucosal prolapse is managed by excision of the redundant mucosa. An atonic megarectum can result after PSARP and require resection by endorectal pull-through (82,83). If the rectum is large at the time of initial PSARP, tapering may be indicated to attempt to prevent this complication. Recurrent rectourethral fistulas occur, though rarely, and can require redo PSARP, which is successful at enhancing continence in most cases (84,85). Likewise, a redo PSARP may be of benefit in patients in whom MRI evaluation of placement of the rectum within

the levator and sphincter muscles demonstrates an inappropriately placed anus and rectum (86).

The postoperative mortality should be <5% for low imperforate anus and 15% for the high/intermediate variety and is usually the result of associated anomalies (87,88). Patients should be followed carefully for evidence of genitourinary problems. Evaluation for sacral anomalies and presence of a tethered spinal cord should be performed. Newborns with low malformations have an excellent outlook, with fecal continence documented in 50% to 75% of patients and normal anorectal function in 52% (83,89,90). The remainder of the patients have occasional accidents or soiling and fair to normal continence. Constipation may, however, be a problem in 25% and vaginal abnormalities and scarring may be an issue that often requires operative intervention in a substantial number of patients (91).

Approximately 80% of patients with high/intermediate anomalies have reasonable results, with occasional soiling noted in some of these patients (83,92). The remaining patients have fair to poor results, with varying degrees of continence. The functional results are mostly related to the presence of sphincter muscle hypoplasia and the abnormal sacral innervation that may be observed in patients with intermediate or high anomalies. Bladder continence is affected as well. Those with sacral incontinence accompanied by constipation are managed with enemas. A Malone antegrade continent enema procedure may be an option to provide social acceptability to patients with persistent incontinence (93). This technique uses the appendix for access to deliver enemas to the colon and may be effective in the constipated or incontinent patient. The artificial bowel sphincter and electrically stimulated gracilis neosphincter are two techniques that have been used for the treatment of patients with refractory fecal incontinence with reasonable success (94). If severe incontinence persists, a permanent colostomy may be a reasonable solution.

THORACIC ANOMALIES

Congenital Pulmonary Airway Malformation (CPAM)

CPAM consists of an arrest of airway development such that large cysts (macrocystic) or small cysts (microcystic) are formed (95,96). The anomalies are often identified *in utero* and may spontaneously decrease in size or even disappear prior to delivery (97,98). In a minority of patients, the CPAM compresses the adjacent lung and esophagus, resulting in polyhydramnios and physiologic compromise both *in utero* and after birth—*in utero* this may manifest itself through development of nonimmune hydrops, which is associated with a high mortality rate (99). Identification of *in utero* hydrops in a patient with CPAM is an indication for delivery or, if lung maturity will not allow delivery, fetal intervention, which may entail aspiration of a major cyst, cyst-amniotic fluid shunt placement, or lung lobe resection

(100–102). Following birth, resection of the involved lung is indicated in newborns who are symptomatic (97). Intubation and ventilation should be undertaken with care and only when necessary since overexpansion of the involved lobe(s) may occur. Extracorporeal life support or extracorporeal membrane oxygenation (ECLS or ECMO) may be necessary if gas exchange is compromised either preoperatively or postoperatively due to lung compression or the development of pulmonary hypertension (103).

No intervention is recommended at birth in asymptomatic newborns, which form the majority (104). CPAMs do not regress after birth. Because of the potential for infection and the development of rhabdomyosarcoma and other malignancies during childhood, most surgeons recommend excision at 3 to 12 months of age (105,106). Doppler ultrasound or CT imaging with contrast optimally is performed preoperatively to evaluate for an aberrant systemic artery, which is seen in a pulmonary sequestration. CPAMs are often similar in presentation to a sequestered lobe, although the latter is almost always in the lower lobe. Operative resection of the involved lobe is undertaken with care to identify an aberrant arterial vessel in case one is present, which usually is observed entering the thorax through the inferior pulmonary ligament. Incidental division of this vessel without control and ligation may lead to retraction of the vessel below the diaphragm and massive bleeding. Standard lobe resection via thoracotomy is otherwise undertaken, although a number of surgeons are proponents of a thoracoscopic approach (107,108). If the lesion is in more than one lobe (14%), segmental resection or nonanatomical resection with a stapling device is performed. Pneumonectomy is specifically avoided because of the risk of mediastinal shift and compromise of ventilation in newborns and infants (109). Persistent air leak is usually limited to those undergoing segmental resection and will most often resolve with chest tube suction over a period of days to weeks. Alternatively, placement of a thoracoscope through the chest tube site with injection of fibrin glue at the site of the air leak may lead to resolution. Placement of fibrin glue over the raw surface of the lung at the time of segmental resection can primarily prevent air leak.

Associated anomalies, including renal agenesis or dysgenesis, diaphragmatic hernia, imperforate anus, intestinal atresia, or congenital heart disease, occur in 20% of cases. In the absence of hydrops, mortality should be minimal (101).

Pulmonary Sequestration

Pulmonary sequestrations derive their arterial blood supply from the systemic arterial circulation, usually via one or more large arteries that extend from below the diaphragm and enter the thorax through the inferior pulmonary ligament (Fig. 50-13). The sequestered lobe can be either intralobar (73%) or extralobar (27%). Sequestrations of the intralobar variety are incorporated into the surrounding lung and often have a normal venous drainage (110). In contrast,

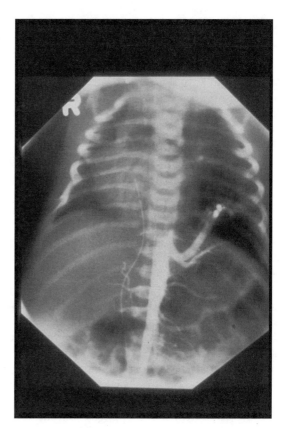

Figure 50-13 Angiogram demonstrating a left pulmonary sequestration with a large aortic systemic arterial blood supply extending from below the diaphragm. Failure to control this vessel during resection of the sequestration may result in potentially exsanguinating hemorrhage as the vessel retracts below the diaphragm.

extralobar sequestrations are separate from the normal lung, have a separate pleural covering, and drain blood to the azygous veins (111). Sequestrations are more commonly found in or adjacent to the lower lobe (110). Arteriovenous fistulas with hemoptysis or high output heart failure may occur. Neither variety typically has communication with the airway, although the intralobar sequestrations may be aerated from the surrounding lung. Intralobar sequestrations are frequently associated with recurrent infections in the lobe and require excision, usually via lobectomy. Extralobar sequestrations are excised for diagnosis without lung resection. It is critical to identify the large arteries in the inferior pulmonary ligament or extending directly from the aorta, which uniformly accompany these lesions, in order to ligate them (112). Failure to recognize such vessels may result in disruption and exsanguination as the vessel(s) retract beneath the diaphragm. Rarely, the sequestration can cause compression of the adjacent lung with development of respiratory insufficiency (88). Operative complications are rare and include persistent air leak and hemothorax (110). The persistent air leak will usually resolve with thoracostomy suction. If the leak does not resolve, then thoracoscopy with application of fibrin glue to the site of the air leak should be performed.

Foregut Duplication Cyst

The lungs and the esophagus develop from the foregut. It is sometimes difficult to distinguish between developmental cysts that are pulmonary (bronchogenic cysts) and esophageal (esophageal duplication cysts) in origin. In fact, 71% of intramural esophageal cysts contain respiratory epithelium (113). Foregut duplication cysts are lined by respiratory or gastrointestinal epithelium, and both have been noted in a single cyst (114). Approximately 25% of patients present due to incidental cysts detected on chest radiograph in asymptomatic individuals (115). Otherwise, cysts are identified if they produce cough, dyspnea, recurrent pneumonia, hemoptysis, or dysphagia or if the cyst becomes infected (116). Such cysts can compress the tracheobronchial tree and create life-threatening airway obstruction, especially in newborns and infants and if they are subcarinal in location (115,117–119). Thus they should be addressed operatively in the symptomatic newborn. Intrapulmonary cysts may be mistaken for a lung abscess if air-fluid levels are present from an airway communication. Intrapulmonary cysts are excised via lobectomy (115). Mediastinal cysts can be large and daunting to the surgeon, but a plane of dissection is usually found that allows relatively easy resection. Foregut duplication cysts may be intimately involved with the esophagus, but they rarely communicate with the esophageal lumen. Instead, they typically can be dissected from the muscularis of the esophagus leaving the mucosa intact. Thus esophageal resection should rarely be required. Occasionally they may communicate with the trachea or tracheobronchial tree. Short-term complications include air leak if there is communication with the tracheobronchial tree and recurrence if the cyst is not completely resected (113,120). Long-term complications are rare.

Esophageal Atresia and Tracheoesophageal Fistula

Patients with esophageal atresia (EA) frequently have an *in utero* history of polyhydramnios and a small or absent stomach on ultrasound (121). After birth, difficulty with handling secretions is often accompanied by choking and coughing with feeding. Usually an unsuccessful attempt is made at passing a nasogastric or orogastric tube. Curling of the tube in the dilated proximal esophageal pouch is pathognomonic for EA. If not recognized and controlled by proximal pouch placement of a Repogle tube, which has perforations only near the end of the tube, aspiration of oral secretions may occur. In addition, gastric secretions may reflux up through a TEF, if present, and lead to further lung contamination and the development of pneumonia. Placing the newborn on antibiotics and maintaining the newborn in a 30-degree to 45-degree upright position will inhibit reflux of gastrointestinal contents into the tracheobronchial

tree. Intravenous antibiotics should be administered prophylactically because of the risk of pneumonia. Mechanical ventilation should be performed only if necessary because of the risk of gastric perforation when a TEF is present (122). Gastric perforation is often associated with the sudden development of abdominal distension and respiratory compromise. This should be managed with needle paracentesis of the abdomen en route to surgery, where the lower esophagus is occluded with a catheter introduced through the perforation. Thoracotomy with division of the fistula, creation of an esophageal anastomosis if appropriate, and repair of the gastric perforation are then in order.

Air in the abdomen on radiograph suggests the presence of a distal TEF (85%), and, conversely, its absence indicates a pure EA (7%) (Fig. 50-14). Radiologic evaluation, performed with careful administration of contrast medium into the upper pouch with the patient sitting upright to avoid aspiration, will verify the diagnosis of EA and prevent a proximal TEF from being missed. A proximal fistula is present in approximately 1% of patients and may be missed at the time of operation because the fistula may be proximal and high up in the thorax at a level above routine dissection (Fig. 50-15). Proximal fistulas are often associated with smaller caliber and shorter proximal pouches (extending at most down to the T1 vertebra) because of the *in utero* decompression of the proximal pouch that the fistula provides. The presence of a small proximal pouch suggests that the anastomosis will be under considerable tension. Bronchoscopy may be performed to identify a proximal fistula in the operating room prior to repair of the EA/TEF. However, bronchoscopy may miss small proximal fistulas, and contrast study of the proximal pouch appears to be the best approach.

Since 64% of patients have associated anomalies, a search for congenital defects should be undertaken (123). Approximately 15% of patients with EA and TEF have a constellation of findings compatible with the VATER or VACTERL association (vertebral defects, anal atresia, cardiac anomalies, TEF and EA, renal defects, and limb abnormalities). The most common anomalies are cardiac (38%) and are responsible for many of the deaths associated with EA and TEF. Renal anomalies should be identified so that renal damage is not incurred.

In general, patients with EA and a distal TEF have adequate esophageal length to allow primary reconstruction. Thus, a repair is undertaken within the first 24 to 48 hours unless contraindicated by prematurity, the presence of congenital heart disease, or another physiologically compromising situation. In that case, temporizing with proximal pouch Repogle suction and a gastrostomy tube with plans for delayed repair may be the best strategy. Otherwise, an approach through the right chest using a muscle-sparing incision is performed with access via the fourth intercostal space. However, the presence of a right aortic arch should be identified on echocardiography in 2% of patients with

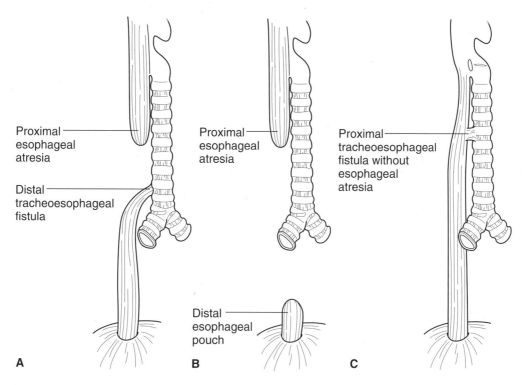

Figure 50-14 The three most common forms of esophageal atresia and tracheoesophageal fistula. **(A)** constitutes 85% of the total, while **(B)** and **(C)** together make up another 10%. The rarer types are not depicted.

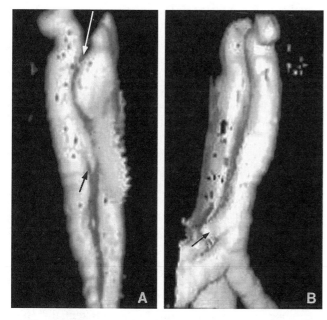

Figure 50-15 **A:** Three-dimensional CT reconstruction of the trachea and esophagus. White arrow on proximal tracheoesophageal fistula, which was missed at the initial operation, black arrow on remnant pouch. **B:** Similar reconstruction from different rotational angle depicts accessory bronchus (*arrow*). (From Islam S, Cavanaugh E, Honeke R, et al. Diagnosis of a proximal tracheoesophageal fistula using three-dimensional CT scan: a case report. *J Pediatr Surg* 2004;39(1):100–102, with permission).

the EA/TEF anomaly so that a left thoracic approach can be used (124). Anastomosis via a right thoracotomy in the presence of a right aortic arch is associated with a high anastomotic leak rate (42%) and often requires a left thoracotomy for completion of the operation (125). A double aortic arch makes division of the TEF and esophagoesophagostomy difficult via either approach. The distal TEF is identified in the region of the carina and is divided (Fig. 50-16). Prior to division of the fistula, maintenance of oxygenation may be tenuous and requires that the surgeon intermittently allow expansion of the right lung. This problem with oxygenation usually resolves once the fistula is ligated. A few millimeters of esophageal tissue are left on the trachea during division of the TEF in order to avoid compromise of the tracheal lumen. In contrast, leaving too much esophagus on the trachea can compromise the length of the distal esophageal segment and result in an airway diverticulum, which can serve as a source of ongoing airway contamination. The tracheal closure is checked for an air leak while under saline with application of sustained airway pressure. The distal esophagus can be mobilized without fear of it being devascularized. The proximal esophageal pouch is best identified by having the anesthesiologist advance a catheter placed through the mouth into the pouch. A suture is placed in the apex of the proximal pouch for manipulation in order to avoid trauma due to

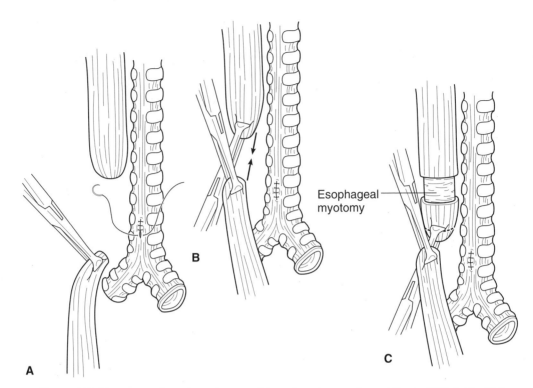

Figure 50-16   Repair of esophageal atresia (EA) and tracheoesophageal fistula (TEF) **A:** The TEF has been divided and the tracheal opening closed with 5–0 or 6–0 PDS suture. **B:** The feasibility of primary anastomosis between the two esophageal segments is being assessed. **C:** A circumferential proximal esophagomyotomy is being used to gain additional length.

repeated grasping of the tissue. The pouch is mobilized in the upper mediastinum; care is taken while mobilizing the anterior esophagus because of the risk of entry into the membranous trachea. Use of cautery should be limited, especially in the apex of the thorax, because of the risk of thermal injury to the recurrent laryngeal nerve. An esophagoesophagostomy is performed in most cases under mild to moderate levels of tension. Care must be used to ensure that sutures include the full thickness of the esophagus since the mucosa can easily retract. A nasogastric tube is passed through the anastomosis into the stomach to ensure patency of the distal esophagus. Gastrostomy tubes are done only if the presence of other anomalies suggests that tube feeding will be required. Most surgeons use a retropleural approach and place a drainage tube near, but not on, the anastomosis at the end of the operation to contain a postoperative anastomotic leak, which occurs in 16% of cases (123). Small openings in the pleura are unimportant and should not be closed when a retropleural approach is used. Silk sutures are associated with a two- to three fold increase in the incidence of anastomotic leak (126). Oropharyngeal suctioning is limited to <6 cm from the lips in order to avoid trauma to the anastomosis. An esophageal contrast study is performed approximately 7 days after operation. If the anastomosis appears intact, feedings are initiated, antibiotics are discontinued, and the retropleural chest tube is removed.

In patients with isolated EA without a TEF, the distal esophagus is typically short, which precludes immediate repair. Some patients with EA and a distal TEF will still have a long gap between the proximal and distal esophagus (>3 cm). Both of these situations present a challenge to the surgeon. In both situations, a decision must be made on whether to attempt to salvage the native esophagus. One option for management is to ligate the fistula, if present, to place a gastrostomy tube, and to allow growth of the proximal and distal pouch over the ensuing 3 months prior to an attempt at a primary repair (127). Daily dilation of the proximal pouch may enhance lengthening. Another option is to mobilize the entire distal and proximal esophagus, to perform the anastomosis under considerable tension, and to maintain the patient sedated with the head in the flexed position to decrease postoperative anastomotic tension (128). Alternatively, a proximal or distal pouch circular myotomy of Livaditis may be performed, which increases the length by 1 to 2 cm (Fig. 50-16) (129,130). With this technique the muscularis is divided circumferentially while the mucosa is carefully maintained intact. Two or three proximal myotomies may be used to enhance length. Unfortunately, complications such as leaks, stricture, outpouching of the esophagus at the site of the myotomy, and esophageal dysfunction are associated with this technique (131). A spiral myotomy may be used to decrease the outpouching associated with myotomy.

Other innovative techniques for lengthening the esophagus when the proximal and distal segments cannot be brought together include a multistaged approach in which an esophagostomy is formed on the chest and sequentially lengthened every 2 to 3 weeks by advancing the esophagostomy inferiorly along the chest wall (132). This technique allows sham feedings, which are important for normal feeding development, to take place. Another approach promoted by Scharli involves transverse division of the lesser curvature of the stomach along with ligation of the left gastric artery (133). This technique is similar to a Collis procedure, except that it is performed along the lesser curvature and is effective at lengthening the distal esophagus (134). Foker, et al. have suggested placing externalized sutures on the ends of the esophagus to apply tension with eventual approximation of the ends (135). An intriguing approach developed by Gough suggests formation of a flap from the dilated proximal fistula, which is then tubularized in order to enhance proximal esophageal length (136). Whatever approach is used, a long gap adversely affects the outcome with regard to death (18%), anastomotic leak (31%), stricture (44%), and GER (56%) (137).

In general, all attempts are made at salvaging the native esophagus (138). However, when the esophagus cannot be approximated or if complications of stricture, recurrent GER, or esophageal dysfunction persist, esophageal replacement is an alternative. Right or left colon, jejunum, or the stomach, either as a reversed-gastric tube or a gastric transposition, can be used (139–143). Although an effective solution to establishing esophageal continuity, the complication rate with esophageal replacement is substantial and includes an anastomotic leak rate of approximately 30%, stricture formation in 20% to 60%, and a mortality of 5% (139–141,144,145). Anastomotic leaks almost always resolve spontaneously. When a colon conduit is used, it can be placed behind the hilum of the lung on either side or in a substernal position, although the latter is associated with a higher stenosis rate (139). A vagotomy is effective in preventing the development of ulcers when a colon conduit is used. The colon may become redundant in the chest, leading to dysfunction and stasis (16%). Reoperation is necessary in approximately 50% of patients and is most often performed to redo the esophagocolic or cologastric anastomoses due to strictures (144,146). Gastrocolic reflux may also occur, and approximately 20% will ultimately require replacement of the colon graft, which is best managed by performance of a gastric transposition or a free jejunal graft (144,146).

Another option for esophageal replacement is the reverse gastric tube, which is formed by creating a tube from the greater curvature of the stomach. This is most often brought up to the neck through what would have been the esophageal bed. Complications are similar to those of the colonic substitutes with the addition of leak from the long suture line. In addition, compromise of the stomach size in newborns may be a problem. Finally, gastric transposition is a successful option since the blood supply to the stomach is excellent and the operation is technically easier than other alternatives. This option can be used even when previous operations have been performed on the stomach (143). The right and left gastroepliploic arteries are maintained intact while the stomach is otherwise mobilized. The distal esophageal segment is excised and the fundus preferably brought through the posterior mediatinum, which limits the potential complication of gastric distension. The posterior aspect of the stomach must be anchored to the sternocleidomastoid muscles in the infant and to the prevertebral fascia in the older patient to prevent retraction of the stomach into the thorax. A pyloromyotomy should be performed to enhance gastric emptying. The dumping syndrome occurs in a minority of patients in the postoperative period but typically resolves over the first year. Care must be taken to avoid a twist in any of the conduits performed, which may result in ischemia or obstruction (147). Dissection must be maintained on the proximal esophagus to avoid injury to the recurrent laryngeal nerves.

The simultaneous presentation of EA/TEF and duodenal atresia is a difficult clinical situation. Duodenal atresia occurs in 10% of patients with isolated EA and the lack of air in the GI tract can delay diagnosis of the duodenal atresia until a gastrostomy tube is placed. An intraoperative contrast study at the time of gastrostomy tube placement helps to identify this combined anomaly (127). Imperforate anus should be addressed by performing a colostomy unless a primary, laparoscopic repair of the imperforate anus is to be performed.

Patients with a TEF but no EA (4%) often have episodes of gastric distention during crying and choking, recurrent pneumonia, and cyanotic spells during feeding. The diagnosis is best made by a contrast swallow, bronchoscopy, or esophagoscopy which may demonstrate the H-type fistula between the trachea and esophagus. A Fogarty catheter may be placed through the fistula at the time of bronchoscopy to help with identification of the fistula at operation. Ligation of the fistula is usually performed via a right cervical approach. The recurrent laryngeal nerve must be identified to prevent the most common complication of this procedure, which is injury to this nerve. Recurrence of the fistula is rare.

Overall survival rate is 95% (123). Mortality is usually secondary to associated anomalies and is associated with the presence of major cardiac disease and birth weight <1,500 g (Table 50-1) (148). Immediate postoperative complications include small anastomotic leaks on postoperative contrast study in 15% of EA/TEF patients with primary repair. Almost all small leaks will resolve spontaneously with continuation of IV antibiotics and chest tube drainage. A repeat study is performed 1 week later, and oral feedings are held until the leak resolves. Disruption of the anastomosis occurs in approximately 5% due to excess tension, ischemia, or poor surgical technique and presents with persistent pneumothorax, respiratory distress, pleural

TABLE 50-1

PREDICTORS OF SURVIVAL FROM ESOPHAGEAL ANOMALY

Group	Total, *n*	Dead, *n*	Survival Rate (%)
I Birth weight >1,500 g without major congenital heart disease	293	10	97
II Birth weight <1,500 g or major congenital heart disease	70	29	59
III Birth weight <1,500 g and major congenital heart disease	9	7	22

fluid, and/or sepsis. The disruption should be managed with either direct repair of the anastomosis, preferably with reinforcement with an intercostal muscle flap or a pleural or pericardial patch, or with formation of a cervical esophagostomy and placement of a gastrostomy tube with subsequent esophageal replacement (149). Stricture formation occurs in approximately 15% of cases and is often associated with a prior anastomotic leak. Most strictures are responsive to repeated antegrade dilatation initially at a frequency of approximately every 2 to 3 weeks. Esophagoscopy should be performed before dilatation to assess the anastomotic caliber and after to ensure that full-thickness perforation has not occurred. In narrow strictures a wire passed under endoscopic and/or fluoroscopic guidance will allow safe passage of sequentially larger Savory dilators under fluoroscopic guidance to safely enlarge the anastomosis. Contrast injection at the end of the dilatation can be performed to identify a leak at the site of the stricture. Rarely, strictures that are refractory to routine dilatation require placement of a gastrostomy tube with maintenance of a silicone "string" from the nares internally to the gastrostomy tube. The ends of the string can be tied externally and taped on the infant's back. Vigorous dilations with Tucker dilators can then be performed on a recurring basis. Occasionally, refractory strictures may require resection or even esophageal replacement. However, refractory strictures are most often due to the presence of reflux and respond to dilatation once a fundoplication has been performed. Thus GER should be investigated if a stricture does not respond after two or three dilatations.

Leak from the trachea or compromise of the tracheal lumen is unusual but requires operation in the former and bronchoscopic evaluation in the latter. Recurrent TEF occurs in 3% of cases and is usually associated with a postoperative leak. This complication requires reoperation, with division and ligation of the fistula (123). Recurrent pneumonia, coughing, and choking are frequently noted. Esophagoscopy with the patient prone, or balloon catheter obstruction of the distal esophagus during esophageal contrast administration can enhance identification of the fistula. High resolution CT may help to identify a recurrent fistula or a missed proximal fistula (150). Thoracotomy with fistula ligation is required. A 2 French balloon catheter should first be passed through the fistula under bronchoscopic guidance to allow intraoperative identification of the fistula. Once the fistula is ligated, a pleural or pericardial flap should be interposed between the trachea and esophagus to help prevent recurrence. Injection of fibrin glue into the fistula may result in closure of the communication without thoracotomy (151).

The most common long-term problems associated with EA include GER (40% to 60%), tracheomalacia (16%), and esophageal dysfunction (123,152). GER is likely due to the tension placed on the distal esophagus with compromise of the native antireflux mechanisms and shortening of the intra-abdominal esophagus. Recurrent pneumonia, reactive airway disease, cyanotic spells, and persistent anastomotic stricture can be symptoms/signs of GER in the EA/TEF patient. GER symptoms are present in at least 20% to 40% of adult patients with previous EA/TEF (153,154). Evaluation with upper GI contrast study and/or 24-hour pH probe may document the diagnosis (155). GER is typically first managed with prokinetic agents and proton pump inhibitors, although approximately 30% to 40% of patients require a fundoplication (123,152). A 360-degree Nissen fundoplication is most frequently performed, although a Nissen fundoplication may exacerbate the esophageal dysfunction associated with EA/TEF (156). Under those circumstances, recurrent reflux, esophageal dilation and dysfunction, and dysphagia may result in an adverse outcome (157). A Thal fundoplication is a reasonable alternative because of the partial nature of the wrap, but the Thal's failure rate has proven to be too high. As a result, the optimal approach is to perform a floppy Nissen fundoplication. Since studies have demonstrated a relatively high incidence of Barrett esophagitis among patients with repaired EA/TEF (5% to 7%), long-term endoscopic surveillance of these patients is important (154,158).

Tracheomalacia results in stridor and a barking cough in newborns, although some patients may present with apnea. This is the result of a weakness in the tracheal wall such that the anterior and posterior tracheal walls coapt during expiration. Bronchoscopy during spontaneous breathing demonstrates the collapse in the distal third of the trachea. Mild symptoms in most patients can be followed with expected resolution as the patient grows. Life-threatening symptoms require operation in 6% (123). An aortopexy, in which the anterior aspect of the aortic arch is approximated to the posterior sternum, is effective in almost all patients at resolving the symptoms of tracheomalacia (159). A Palmaz airway stent or tracheostomy may be of benefit should the aortopexy fail (160). It is frequently difficult to determine if the symptoms observed are due to tracheomalacia, stricture, or GER (161).

Esophageal dysmotility is present in the majority of EA/TEF children, and 40% to 75% of adult EA/TEF patients have mild-to-severe dysphagia and esophageal dysmotility (153,154,162,163). In most cases, the dysphagia is tolerable and in infants can be managed by feeding while the patient is sitting up. An occasional patient develops a diverticulum proximal to the anastomosis that requires resection. Scoliosis develops in 8% of patients, probably due to fusion of the ribs at the site of the thoracotomy, which prevents ipsilateral spine growth and results in anterior chest wall deformities in 20%. A number of surgeons are now performing EA/TEF repair via a thoracoscopic approach that may prevent these complications (164). Foreign body impaction occurs in 13% of patients with corrected EA/TEF (165).

Congenital Diaphragmatic Hernia (CDH)

CDH occurs due to failure of the pleuroperitoneal canal to close at 6 to 8 weeks of development. The diaphragmatic defect is in the posterolateral aspect and is referred to as Bochdalak hernia. The CDH is left-sided in 78% and typically contains the small and large intestine and the spleen and may contain the stomach and the left lobe of the liver (166). With a right CDH, the liver and the abdominal viscera are typically in the hemithorax. This anomaly remains one of the most frustrating and challenging for pediatric surgeons because of the high associated postnatal mortality (37%) in otherwise mostly robust, healthy newborns. This high mortality rate is related to the effect of the herniated abdominal viscera on the developing heart and lungs, although developmental studies in animals suggest that the lung hypoplasia may precede the diaphragmatic defect and serve as the primary insult (167,168). By whatever mechanism, both the ipsilateral and contralateral lungs are hypoplastic, with the alveolar number on the ipsilateral side decreased by at least 90% and the contralateral lung decreased by 60% (Fig. 50-17) (169). There is a marked reduction in the number of alveoli and pulmonary arterial branches. In addition, pulmonary arteries in newborns

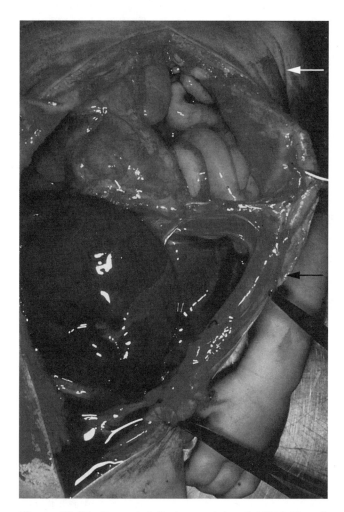

Figure 50-17 Congenital diaphragmatic hernia (CDH). Note the lip of the diaphragmatic defect (*black arrow*) and the left lobe of the liver that is at the opening of the defect. In some cases the left lobe of the liver may actually reside in the left chest. The small bowel is seen in the left hemithorax. The heart is shifted to the right. The major complications in patients with CDH are pulmonary hypertension and lung hypoplasia. The latter is demonstrated in this image by the small lung to the right of the heart and a diminutive lung on the left (*white arrow*).

with CDH demonstrate a thickened media with the presence of abnormal smooth muscle in small arterioles (170). As a result of a decrease in the total cross-sectional area of the pulmonary arterial vessels, along with increased muscularization of small arteries, which promotes vasospasm, pulmonary hypertension persists in the perinatal period when it is necessary for pulmonary pressures to drop in order to transition from fetal to newborn circulation. As a result, postnatal fetal circulation persists with right-to-left shunting of blood across the foramen ovale and patent ductus arteriosus. This, in conjunction with the presence of pulmonary hypoplasia, which inhibits gas exchange, results in further increase in $PaCO_2$ and reduction in PaO_2 and pH, all of which augment pulmonary arterial vasospasm. This increases the right-to-left shunt and reduces pulmonary blood flow. A vicious cycle persists, which, if not interrupted, can result in severe respiratory failure and death. Outcome in CDH appears to depend on the degree of pulmonary hypoplasia and reactive pulmonary hypertension (171,172).

Most patients with CDH present in the first 24 hours, although approximately 10% to 20% present later (173). The diagnosis of CDH is typically made on chest radiograph where bowel in the chest, along with mediastinal shift to the side opposite the hernia, is noted. An upper GI contrast study can be confirmatory if there is question of a hiatal hernia, a congenital cystic lesion of the lung, or an eventration. Survival is related to the size of the diaphragmatic defect, and the stomach's location may act as a surrogate for defect size. Thus the presence of the stomach in the chest is associated with 30% survival, but survival is nearly 100% if it is in the abdomen (174,175). The ability to reduce $Paco_2$ <40 mm Hg with reasonable levels of ventilation also predicts survival (176).

Unfortunately, the anomaly is identified on fetal ultrasound in only 45% of fetuses with CDH (177). Those infants who are identified *in utero* should be delivered at a center that has capabilities of performing state-of-the art care for the newborn with CDH, including extracorporeal life support (ECLS, ECMO). Amniocentesis should be performed to establish the karyotype since trisomy 13, 18, and 21 may be associated with CDH. At the time of birth a nasogastric tube should be inserted to avoid GI distension. An endotracheal tube should be placed for ventilation. Bag mask ventilation should be avoided because of the risk of gaseous distension of the viscera both in the abdomen and the chest. An umbilical arterial line is placed and intravenous access established. An umbilical venous catheter may result in vessel disruption due to the angulation of the vessels in the rotated liver if the left lobe is in the chest (178). After stabilization a right radial artery blood gas should be evaluated. Inability to produce an arterial oxygen saturation of 100% and a $Paco_2$ <50 mm Hg suggests severe lung hypoplasia incompatible with life. Conventional mechanical ventilation techniques should be applied while avoiding ventilator-induced lung injury, which can result in acute lung deterioration and chronic lung disease. An arterial oxygen saturation >85% and a $Paco_2$ <60 mm Hg are acceptable. High frequency oscillatory ventilation can be applied, although it is questionable whether this enhances survival (179,180). Application of inhaled nitric oxide in newborns with CDH may actually increase the need for ECLS (181). Echocardiography should be performed to evaluate for congenital heart disease.

If gas exchange cannot be enhanced, ECLS is instituted, preferably prior to marked cardiopulmonary deterioration (182). An oxygenation index [O.I. = (mean airway pressure * Fio_2/Pao_2) * 100] of >25 is an indication for ECLS. ECLS allows for lung rest, resolution of pulmonary hypertension, and avoidance of ventilator-induced lung injury while providing adequate gas exchange. Venoarterial access via the right carotid artery and the right internal jugular vein is often used because this configuration provides cardiac support. Patients with CDH who require ECLS have lower left ventricular mass and associated hemodynamic compromise and, therefore, may require cardiac support (183). However, a double lumen venovenous configuration provides adequate support in most CDH patients and has the advantages of avoiding carotid artery ligation, providing well-oxygenated blood to the lungs and the heart, and minimizing the risk for arterial embolization (184). Hemorrhagic complications are the most common clinical complications, due to anticoagulation, occurring in 43% of patients overall. The most common locations for bleeding are a surgical repair site (24%), head (11.5%), cannulation site (7.5%), and gastrointestinal (5%) (185). Bleeding complications are most common in those undergoing diaphragmatic hernia repair while on ECLS (58%). For this reason it is preferable that diaphragmatic hernia repair be delayed until the patient has weaned from ECLS or is just about to be removed from extracorporeal support. When operation on ECLS is required, administration of aminocaproic acid (AMICAR) may reduce bleeding complications (186). Current overall survival of CDH patients who require ECLS is 53% (187).

The operation for CDH is no longer an emergency. In fact, survival may be increased and the need for ECLS decreased if a very delayed approach to the repair of the diaphragmatic defect is taken, although some studies dispute this (188–190). Either way, a delay in repair does not appear to be detrimental, and thus in most centers the diaphragm is repaired once the physiologic issues have resolved. Typically the defect is approached via a subcostal incision, although a thoracic approach can be used. In approximately 20% of patients, a sac consisting of peritoneum and pleura that contains the herniated viscera is present and must be excised to allow full lung expansion. The viscera are carefully reduced. If the patient has been on ECLS, the spleen and liver are enlarged and prone to injury. Extralobar sequestration is observed in some patients with CDH and should be resected with care to control the systemic arteries extending through the inferior pulmonary ligament from the aorta to the sequestered lobe. The posterior leaf of the diaphragm typically has to be freed from the peritoneum, after which an assessment is made of whether sufficient diaphragm is present for primary repair. If so, 3-0 prolene mattress sutures are used for the repair. In approximately 50% of patients a patch is required to complete the diaphragmatic closure (166). Typically, inadequate muscle is present posterolaterally. Use of prosthetics such as Goretex or SIS allows a loose repair but may be associated with high rates (40% to 80%) of diaphragmatic hernia recurrence, especially when little or no diaphragmatic muscle is present (191–193). In addition, with use of a prosthetic the risk of infection is low but present. Posterior sutures of 3-0 prolene are all placed and then tied to approximate the prosthesis to the muscle. The patch is approximated to the ribs where the native diaphragm is absent. The needle is passed around individual ribs to provide a strong closure. One must be careful to ensure that bowel does not get entrapped between the sutures or the patch and the rib. An alternative is to use an internal oblique and transversalis muscle flap to close the diaphragmatic defect, which may reduce the risk of recurrence (194). To do this, the muscle is separated from the external oblique at the upper aspect of the subcostal incision and folded downward. Division of the posterior lower ribs aids in creating the flap. However, the extensive dissection should be undertaken only if the risk for imminent initiation of ECLS and associated anticoagulation is low. Likewise, correction of the typical malrotation with a Ladd procedure is performed only if it appears unlikely that ECLS will be required. An appendectomy is specifically not performed if a prosthesis has been placed because of the risk of infection. A chest tube may be placed, although one must be careful to avoid application of excess negative pressure. This can induce a shift in the mediastinum with associated hemodynamic compromise (109). In general, the abdomen is closed primarily. Alternatively, abdominal wall closure may not be possible because the peritoneal cavity is poorly developed. Mesh closure of the abdominal wall or even placement of a silo may be necessary to avoid the complications associated with increased intra-abdominal pressure (see section on abdominal wall defects) and compromise of diaphragmatic excursion in a patient with concomitant CDH and respiratory insufficiency.

Postoperative complications are predominantly associated with the cardiorespiratory sequelae associated with CDH. Chylothorax occurs in 10% of patients after repair and is increased among those patients requiring ECLS (195). Recurrent hernias are managed with transabdominal reoperation and generous use of a patch to decrease tension on the repair. The survival rate for patients with CDH is 63% (166). Associated anomalies are present in 40% of newborns with CDH and most commonly involve heart defects (63%) (196). The combination of CDH and congenital heart disease confers a worse prognosis (41%), especially in those with univentricular disease (5%).

The long-term morbidity in patients with CDH is substantial. Chronic lung disease is present in 50% of survivors at 1 year of age (197). In most patients, pulmonary function normalizes over time, although pulmonary blood flow to the ipsilateral side remains reduced, especially in those patients who required ECLS (198,199). GER is evident in up to 81% of patients at the time of discharge and in 50% at 1 year (200). The esophagus is ectatic in 70% of patients with CDH, likely related to kinking of the gastroesophageal junction when the stomach is in the hemithorax (201). Tube feedings are required in over half of the patients at the time of discharge, but most are tolerating oral feeds within the first few years. Malrotation is present in most patients with CDH. The incidence of subsequent volvulus is 3% to 9% (202,203). Bowel obstruction occurs in approximately 10%.

Spinal and chest wall abnormalities are potential long-term problems in children with CDH and include pectus deformities in 33% and thoracic spine scoliosis in 12% (203). A thoracoscopic approach to the repair may ameliorate problems with scoliosis, which appears to be related to the thoracotomy incision (204).

Developmental delay classified as mild or moderate is evident in 45% of patients, but these findings tend to improve over time. Those managed with ECLS demonstrate severe neurologic abnormalities in 20% to 40% of patients. Hearing deficits are observed in 21%.

ABDOMINAL WALL DEFECTS

Gastroschisis

The newborn with gastroschisis has a smooth 2-cm to 5-cm opening almost always to the right of an intact umbilical cord through which the stomach, small intestine, and colon are typically herniated. The liver is almost never eviscerated and associated anomalies are mostly limited to those of the GI tract where the bowel is often short and atresia occurs in 10% to 15% (205).

Prenatal diagnosis via ultrasound occurs in most infants (206). Controversy exists as to whether newborns diagnosed *in utero* should be delivered early and by Cesarean section to prevent injury to and swelling of the bowel (207). However, there is now substantial data to suggest that there is minimal, if any, advantage to preterm or Cesarean section delivery (208–210). At the time of delivery, a nasogastric tube should be placed to prevent vomiting and aspiration. The bowel should be examined and any twists in the mesentery or constriction of the viscera from a small opening relieved immediately to avoid vascular compromise. Dehydration and hypothermia from insensible fluid and heat losses are prevented by administration of intravenous fluids, wrapping of the viscera with a gauze dressing, and placement of the lower portion of the newborn's body in a bowel bag. The viscera should be supported by the gauze so that they remain on top of the abdomen, rather than falling over to the side, to avoid vascular obstruction, especially venous outflow obstruction, which can lead to increased bowel edema. Broad-spectrum antibiotics should be administered to prevent infection.

After resuscitation the newborn is taken to the operating room. The size of the peritoneal cavity is often limited and can make safe reduction of the viscera challenging. Rectal irrigation is performed, along with manual massage of the intestines, to evacuate as much meconium as possible, thus reducing the volume of the intra-abdominal contents. Likewise, a Foley catheter is inserted to decompress the bladder. After cleansing of the bowel with betadine and establishing a sterile field, the fingers are used to stretch the anterior abdominal fascia in an attempt to enlarge the peritoneal cavity. The small and large bowels are typically matted together with a peel on the surface, edematous, thickened, foreshortened, and, at times, ischemic-appearing. The bowel should be handled gently and operations on the bowel avoided. Any attempt to remove peel risks bowel injury, including perforation, and development of an enterocutaneous fistula. When jejunoileal atresia is identified, a primary anastomosis should be performed only if the edema and peel are minimal. Otherwise, there is a reasonable risk of anastomotic leak and stricture. In most cases (80%) the atresia should be left intact at the initial operation (205). The bowel should be re-explored at 3 to 4 weeks with repair of the atresia. If a silo was placed initially, the bowel should be evaluated at the time of fascial closure and a primary resection of the atresia with anastomosis performed if the thickening has resolved. In some circumstances an enterostomy is required, especially in the setting of colonic atresia.

Primary closure of the abdominal wall is successful in approximately 80% of newborns (206,211). The viscera are gently reduced while avoiding twists in the mesentery. The edge of the opening is incised and the fascia identified circumferentially. Vicryl sutures are then placed to close the fascia; this is often done in a horizontal fashion because the tension is less than with a vertical fascial closure. Communication between the surgeon and the anesthesiologist allows recognition of adverse effects of the closure: significant increase in airway pressures, compromise of hemodynamics, or development of acidosis due to excess intra-abdominal pressure. Examination of the newborn's thighs may demonstrate cyanosis due to venous congestion. Intra-abdominal pressure may be measured via the nasogastric or bladder catheter. If signs of increased abdominal pressure are observed, the bowel should be removed to decompress the abdomen and a silo placed (see below). At times the viscera may be successfully reduced, but fascial closure leads to physiologic compromise. In that case a Vicryl or small intestinal submucosa mesh (Surgisis ES; Cook Tissue Engineering Products, Bloomington, IN) may be used to augment the fascia, although a ventral hernia may result. Failure to recognize the signs of increased intra-abdominal pressure may lead to reduced visceral and renal blood flow and associated bowel necrosis and renal failure.

If the bowel cannot be safely reduced, a staged closure using a prosthesis is useful. Spring-loaded preformed silos are now available in different sizes and are easy to place, which precludes the need to manually construct the silo and to sew the silo to the relatively tenuous fascia (Fig. 50-18) (212). In some cases, the abdominal wall defect is enlarged to avoid a funnel type configuration of the silo, which could lead to compression of the bowel at the base of the silo with ischemia and necrosis. As much of the intestine as is safe is reduced. The silo is wrapped in betadine-moistened gauze to prevent infection and suspended from the over bed warmer in order to encourage gravity-assisted reduction of the remaining viscera. Over the ensuing days the viscera are

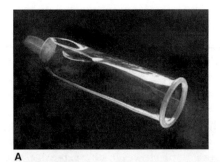

A

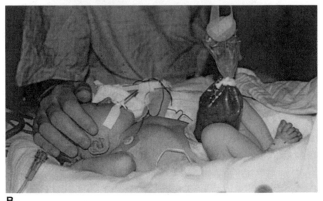

B

Figure 50-18   A: A preformed, spring-loaded silo (Specialty Surgical Products, Victor, MT) used to contain the bowel in patients with gastroschisis. **B:** The silo is in place with the round, spring-loaded base inside the peritoneal cavity. The umbilical tapes are tied sequentially lower to reduce the bowel into the abdomen over a period of days.

gradually reduced by compressing or twisting the silo and tying an umbilical tape sequentially lower on the silo every 12 to 24 hours. One must be careful to avoid injury to the bowel during these maneuvers; the silo is constructed of a transparent material specifically to allow monitoring of the bowel's status. The viscera are usually reduced within a week such that the base of the silo is flat. The patient is then taken back to the operating room and the fascia closed as described above.

Postoperative mechanical ventilation is required in most newborns, and care should be taken to avoid ventilator-induced lung injury as a result of high intra-abdominal pressure. Oliguria unresponsive to fluid administration, cyanosis and edema of the legs and lower abdomen, and compromised ventilation are all indications for silo placement or release of the umbilical tape on the silo. Patients with gastroschisis have an approximately 50% increase in fluid requirements when compared to other newborns (213).

There is a growing trend toward placement of a silo rather than attempting to close the abdomen primarily (214). It has been suggested that primary closure may be traumatic to the bowel and place the newborn at risk for physiologic compromise and pulmonary barotrauma (215). Spring-loaded silo placement can be performed at the bedside in the newborn intensive care unit (ICU). Closure of the gastroschisis defect can then occur once the viscera are reduced. This approach may be associated with a decrease in time on the mechanical ventilator, time to initial and full feedings, and complication rate (214).

Postoperative complications, in addition to those mentioned above, include delay in return of GI function (median time to initiation of feedings is 15 days with full enteral intake achieved by 22 days) (216). Support with parenteral nutrition is required in most patients. As such, central access should be achieved early in the course, although catheter-related sepsis is a potential complication. Postoperative bowel obstruction is relatively uncommon and an upper GI contrast study is performed only after approximately 3 weeks without return of GI function. Patients with gastroschisis are also at risk for infection as long as the silo is in place; as a result, broad-spectrum antibiotics are administered while the silo is in place. The complication of silo separation from the fascia, which often occurred after 7 to 10 days, has diminished with application of the spring-loaded silo. If this complication occurs, a pseudomembrane has usually formed beneath the silo, which can be allowed to granulate. Skin graft closure of the abdominal wall is possible once infection has been resolved using topical silver sulfadiazine. Short bowel syndrome may occur as a result of bowel compromise from elevated intra-abdominal pressure in 60% of patients. An enterocutaneous fistula may develop from an anastomotic leak or a suture-induced intestinal injury. Malrotation, if not corrected at the time of the initial operation, may result in jejunal obstruction due to Ladd bands or volvulus.

Survival is over 90% (206,217). By 6 months of age, intestinal function has returned to normal. GER is observed in 16% of patients with gastroschisis, likely related to the presence of increased intra-abdominal pressure (218).

Omphalocele

In contrast to gastroschisis, an omphalocele consists of an abdominal wall defect at the umbilicus, a peritoneal and amnion covering or sac, a normal umbilical cord that attaches to the sac, and umbilical vessels that radiate over the defect. These characteristics of an omphalocele allow it to be differentiated from a gastroschisis even when the sac ruptures, as it does in approximately 10% of cases (219). The liver is present in approximately half of the defects.

Associated anomalies are present in approximately 30% to 60% of newborns with omphalocele and are a source of major morbidity and mortality for such patients (220). Congenital heart disease occurs in 20% and may increase operative risk (221). Abnormal karyotypes are observed in 29% and the Beckwith-Wiedemann Syndrome in 10% (222). The latter patients have macroglossia, which can obstruct the airway, and may have hypoglycemia, which requires preoperative recognition and treatment.

The initial management of omphalocele is similar to that previously described for gastroschisis. Prevention of hypothermia and dehydration is paramount. Treatment with broad-spectrum antibiotics is initiated. Endotracheal intubation and mechanical ventilation is frequently required. The sac is left intact and is covered with a moist gauze to prevent dessication and to decrease heat and fluid losses. Evaluation for other chromosomal and developmental anomalies, especially those that are cardiac, is undertaken.

If the defect is <4 cm in size, it is considered a hernia of the umbilical cord. Closure of a defect of this size is fairly straightforward and primary closure should be performed. The management of omphaloceles >4 cm is more challenging and complicated and is associated with a poorly developed peritoneal cavity. Coverage of the omphalocele defect is the primary goal. The skin-amnion junction is incised circumferentially and the fascia mobilized; caution should be exercised when dissecting over the superior aspect of the liver since the hepatic veins are often superficial in this location because of the downward position of the liver in the omphalocele. Injury to and bleeding from the hepatic veins can result. Examination of the diaphragm should be performed in case an associated defect is present. With a large omphalocele, primary closure is rarely possible. Thus, staged reductions are typically employed. A silo is created from Dacron-reinforced silastic or Goretex (W.L. Gore and Assoc., Inc.; Newark, DE) and is sewn to the fascial edges. The mesh is sequentially gathered in the midline every 12 to 24 hours until the fascial edges are nearly approximated. During this process one must balance aggressively tightening the mesh with avoiding undue tension on the mesh; excess tension could lead to premature separation of the mesh from the fascia. The patient should also be monitored for evidence of high intra-abdominal pressure resulting in hypercarbia, oliguria, hemodynamic compromise, and acidosis. Such high pressures could compromise ventilation, renal blood flow, cardiac output, intestinal perfusion, and venous drainage from the lower extremities. The intra-abdominal pressure can be assessed using a nasogastric tube or a bladder catheter and should be maintained <20 cm H_2O. Once it is nearly approximated, the fascia can then be closed with removal of the mesh, although a reasonable option is to close the skin while leaving part of the mesh in place. If the mesh remnant is substantial, subsequent staged operations may be performed to remove the mesh and to approximate the fascia in the midline. If fascia or skin closure is not achieved within 7 to 10 days, the mesh is at risk for becoming infected and may separate, leaving granulation tissue underneath. This presents a challenging wound care problem that may be complicated by the development of enterocutaneous fistulas and sepsis. Application of homograft and other artificial wound coverings should be considered. One option is to allow the wound to epithelialize (223). An alternative is split-thickness skin graft placement, which is often effective once wound infection is controlled.

Traditionally, the omphalocele sac is excised during staged reduction except for where it is adherent to the liver. To excise the sac in that location could result in liver injury and bleeding. Should bleeding occur, pressure and clot enhancing agents should be applied. Unfortunately, once the sac is excised, reduction must be achieved within the following 7 to 14 days. Some surgeons have recommended leaving the sac intact and sequentially gathering the sac to achieve reduction (224). Alternatively, mesh can be sutured to the skin-amnion junction and progressively tightened to reduce the bowel and liver within the abdomen (225). Once reduction is accomplished, the linea alba is approximated, leaving the amnion intact. This technique allows staged reduction without a commitment to rapid closure. If the mesh separates, the sac is still in place. Another approach is to enhance the rate of successful closure of the defect using external compression by wrapping of the omphalocele (Fig. 50-19) (226,227).

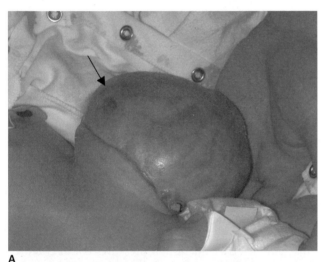

A

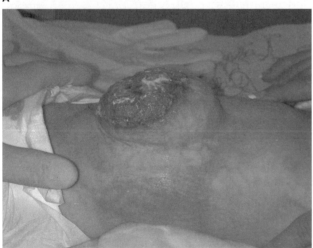

B

Figure 50-19 **A:** An omphalocele at birth. Note the dark area on the superior aspect (*arrow*), which denotes the liver in the omphalocele. This omphalocele was treated expectantly with compression wrapping and Silvadene. **B:** Note the reduction in the size of the omphalocele over the ensuing months.

Some have recommended simply allowing the sac to epithelialize over a number of months (228). Application of Silvadene, rather than mercurochrome, which can cause mercury poisoning, results in eschar formation of the sac. Contraction and flattening of the omphalocele is often the result, although a massive ventral hernia usually remains. One may be trading complications associated with current attempts at fascial closure with those in the future.

Return of GI function is often delayed in patients with a large omphalocele. Parenteral nutrition support will uniformly be required. Mechanical obstruction can occur but is unusual. Lung and chest wall hypoplasia and chronic respiratory insufficiency is reasonably common among patients with giant omphaloceles, and tracheostomy tube placement may be required. Staged reduction, with its associated effect upon the diaphragm, is frequently complicated by the lung dysfunction.

Survival is 80% to 90% and is mostly related to the impact of associated anomalies (220,229). Most patients do well in the long term and have a good quality of life (222,230). In children with omphalocele the incidence of GER is high (43%), likely due to the effects of elevated intra-abdominal pressure (218). Ventral hernias frequently need to be addressed, especially in those in whom a nonoperative approach was undertaken. A staged approach to closure of the ventral hernia is required in those with massive ventral hernias. The incidence of cryptorchidism is increased in patients with omphalocele (16%), presumably because of the decreased intra-abdominal pressure present during the usual *in utero* testicular descent (231).

ACQUIRED NEWBORN SURGICAL PROBLEMS

Pyloric Stenosis

Hypertrophic pyloric stenosis typically presents with projectile nonbilious vomiting in the newborn at 2 to 8 weeks of age. Palpation of the upper abdomen reveals the classic "olive" rolling under the examining hand in 72% of patients and in and of itself is an indication for operation (232). The olive can be easily missed unless a nasogastric tube is placed to decompress the stomach and the infant is quieted with feeding of 5% dextrose water. An ultrasound demonstrating a pylorus longer than 15 to 19 mm or with a wall thickness >3 mm is considered diagnostic, although the patient's age and prematurity should be taken into account to avoid misdiagnosis (233,234). The ultrasound is operator-dependent and may not be accurate if the radiologist is inexperienced (235). An upper GI contrast study should demonstrate an elongated, narrowed pyloric channel and "shouldering" of the pyloric mass upon the antrum. The barium should be evacuated from the stomach after the study via a nasogastric tube to prevent aspiration.

Patients with pyloric stenosis have been vomiting and must be sufficiently resuscitated before operation. Many patients will have a degree of hypochloremic, hypokalemic, metabolic alkalosis (236). Bicarbonate levels >30 mEq per L are of concern and >35 mEq per L are even more so. Preoperative resuscitation is advised in most patients unless the bicarbonate is <30 mEq per L, the chloride normal, and urine output excellent by history.

The stomach should be aspirated before induction of anesthesia to prevent aspiration even if a nasogastric tube was in place prior to operation (237). The pyloric musculature is divided via a Ramstedt pyloromyotomy while the mucosa is maintained intact. The operation is typically performed using a right upper quadrant transverse incision, although supraumbilical and laparoscopic approaches have been used with success (238,239). The laparoscopic approach uses a 5-mm umbilical port for the scope and both a right and left upper quadrant stab wound for placement of 3-mm instruments. With the open technique the antrum is first delivered, followed by "rocking" the pylorus out through the incision. Failure to make an incision of adequate size will make delivery of the pylorus difficult and potentially result in trauma to the serosa of the antrum or even perforation. From this point the open and laparoscopic techniques are similar. Vessels on the surface of the pylorus are scored with the electrocautery since deeper use of cautery may lead to potential injury to the mucosa. An incision with a knife is then performed from a point just proximal to the duodenum up onto the antrum. With the laparoscopic technique, it is important to make the incision long enough and deep enough to facilitate subsequent spreading of the pyloric muscle. The back of a knife blade (open) or the sheathed arthrotomy knife (laparoscopic) is then insinuated into the incision and twisted to further spread the edges of the pyloric muscle. The Ramstedt pyloromyotomy spreader is then used to engage the edges and complete the pyloromyotomy. The first spread should be generous in order to crack the pylorus and expose the underlying mucosa. It is important to engage the spreader equally between the edges of the pylorus so that the edges are perpendicular rather than oblique, which makes completion of the pyloromyotomy difficult. In order to avoid perforation, the pyloromyotomy should not extend onto the duodenum. There is a color change at the pyloroduodenal junction, which, along with palpation with a finger or instrument, allows identification of the distal end of the pylorus. The pyloromyotomy should extend proximally onto the antrum for approximately 1 cm until the circular muscles of the antrum are identified. Failure to extend the pyloromyotomy proximally to this point risks an incomplete pyloromyotomy and postoperative feeding intolerance. The mucosa should be visible for the entire length of the pyloromyotomy, and the two halves of the pylorus should be tested to see that they easily move longitudinally separately from each other. A volume of 30 to 60 mL of air is injected through an NG tube, the duodenum occluded

just distal to the pylorus, and the stomach compressed while observing for leak of air or bile from the pyloromyotomy site. Perforation of the mucosa occurs in 2% of patients and is usually at the duodenal end of the pyloromyotomy (240). The mucosa can be closed directly with a 5-0 Vicryl suture. A better alternative is to approximate the gastric side of the opening to the pyloric muscle at the duodenal end with interrupted 5-0 Vicryl sutures (Fig. 50-20). Consideration should be given to suturing the omentum to the pyloromyotomy site to reinforce the closure. Alternatively, the serosa of the pyloromotomy site can be closed with 4-0 Vicryl sutures and the pylorus turned 90 or 180 degrees, where another pyloromyotomy is performed. The results of either approach appear to be equivalent (240). Nasogastric suction should be maintained for 48 hours after such a repair. Small amounts of bleeding from the surface or edges of the pyloromyotomy may be seen and will uniformly stop without cautery. Cauterizing the mucosa should never be attempted because of the risk of perforation.

Feedings are often initiated 4 to 6 hours after the procedure and can be given ad libitum (241). Emesis in the first day or two after the operation occurs in 44% of patients and is thought to be secondary to gastritis (242). The laparoscopic approach is associated with a similar operative time and length of stay when compared to the open technique (239). The perforation rate appears to be higher with the open technique, while the incidence of incomplete pyloromyotomy may be higher with the laparoscopic approach (243). As mentioned previously, at the end of the operation one must carefully check the pyloromyotomy site for leaks. Persistent vomiting occurs in approximately 5% and usually resolves, although vomiting that persists beyond 3 to 5 days should raise concern for an incomplete pyloromyotomy (242). An upper GI study will not be helpful in distinguishing an incomplete

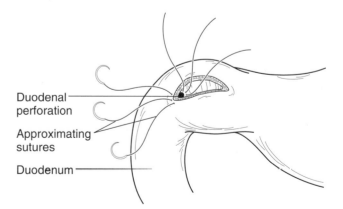

Figure 50-20 Repair of a duodenal perforation following pyloromyotomy. The opening in the mucosa is almost always adjacent to the duodenum. Three or four sutures are placed approximating the mucosa to the seromuscular layer of the duodenum. Note that the pyloromyotomy is carried proximally onto the antrum until the gastric circular fibers are encountered in order to ensure that the pyloromyotomy is adequate.

pyloromyotomy because changes in the pylorus are not observed for many weeks after adequate pyloromyotomy. In the case of prolonged feeding intolerance, parenteral nutrition should be initiated. If gastric outlet obstruction persists over the next 1 to 2 weeks, reoperation should be considered. Administration of intravenous or oral atropine may treat the symptoms of pyloric stenosis and serve as an alternative to reoperation in this setting (244). Unrecognized perforation can be devastating; the incidence should be <1%. Any infant manifesting fever, lethargy, and/or physiologic instability should undergo upper GI contrast study to evaluate for a leak. The incidence of wound infections may be higher than expected for a clean case (4%), and for that reason it is recommended that antibiotics such as Cephazolin be administered in the perioperative period (245). Postoperative wound fascial dehiscence, which used to be a concern when operations were performed in malnourished infants, is now an unusual complication.

Necrotizing Enterocolitis

The etiology of necrotizing enterocolitis (NEC) is unclear, but the result is hypoperfusion of the mesenteric blood supply with intestinal ischemia leading to bacterial invasion and necrosis. Although it can occur in full-term newborns, the risk of NEC increases with gestational age >35 to 36 weeks (246). Administering enteral feeds, especially with hyperosmolar solutions, appears to augment the risk of NEC. However, neonates who have never been fed are susceptible. NEC may be associated with either a single site of perforation in 50% of cases or multiple, discontinuous segments with bowel thinning, pneumatosis, and even frank necrosis. This is in contrast to idiopathic spontaneous intestinal perforation (SIP), in which a perforation without associated necrosis is noted on the antimesenteric border of the terminal ileum (247).

The most difficult aspect of the surgical treatment of NEC is the decision on when to intervene operatively. In the absence of pneumoperitoneum or evidence for bowel necrosis, the patient is managed with nasogastric suction, broad-spectrum antibiotics, fluid resuscitation, and frequent monitoring of hemodynamics, urine output, platelet count, white blood cell count, blood gas values, electrolytes, and abdominal radiographs. Clinical signs and symptoms consistent with ongoing sepsis (lethargy, temperature instability, apnea, bradycardia, shock) despite antibiotic therapy, an erythematous or discolored abdomen, palpable loops of bowel, a falling platelet count or one that remains <150,000 cells per mm³, oliguria, neutropenia, and metabolic acidosis are all relative indications for operation (248). Portal vein gas, which occurs in 9% to 20% of patients with NEC, and a gasless, distended abdomen are harbingers of advanced disease likely to require operative intervention. Pneumoperitoneum is a firm indication for operative intervention in the setting of NEC. Up to 56% of patients will require operation at some point during their course (249).

Operation is undertaken following resuscitation, usually in the newborn ICU to avoid the hypothermia and deterioration in hemodynamics, oxygenation, and ventilation parameters observed during transport of the critically ill premature newborn (250). A tense abdomen may require drainage prior to laparotomy if it is physiologically embarrassing. Venous access for parenteral nutrition is required postoperatively; as such, central access is obtained at the time of the exploratory laparotomy. It is critical to keep the newborn warm. A supraumbilical, transverse incision is created and a finger used to eviscerate the bowel, which may be matted with adhesions. The entire GI tract is examined and areas of necrosis identified and resected. Cases in which an isolated area of perforation is identified in the terminal ileum may be treated with a primary anastomosis. Otherwise an ileostomy is created during operation in almost all cases of NEC (89%) (251). This is performed by bringing the bowel out through either the supraumbilical incision or through a separate 1-cm incision in the right lower quadrant while carefully maintaining the mesenteric blood supply. The former facilitates subsequent ostomy closure, while the latter is of advantage should a dehiscence of the supraumbilical incision occur. The bowel is sutured to the external oblique fascia at four points around the circumference of the enterostomy in order to prevent the frequent complication of peristomal hernia. Typically, a mucous fistula is created along with the enterostomy, which allows a local operation at the time of takedown of the enterostomy. Stoma and wound complications occur in 39% of patients operated upon for NEC and include wound infection, dehiscence, and stomal prolapse, retraction, necrosis, or stricture (252).

In cases in which the extent of disease is patchy but involves a minority of the small bowel, all ischemic and necrotic regions are excised. In contrast, if the majority of the bowel is compromised, then only frankly necrotic, but not ischemic, areas should be resected because of the risk of short bowel syndrome. The ends of the bowel may be ligated with re-exploration in 24 to 48 hours. Alternatively, if an enterostomy is created that is proximal to all ischemic regions such that all distal areas are defunctionalized, then reexploration may be required only if refractory sepsis develops. Multiple enterostomies or anastomoses distal to the most proximal enterostomy may be required. Alternatively, multiple segments distal to the enterostomy may be placed over a feeding tube "stent" in hopes of preserving bowel length and preventing the short bowel syndrome (253). These segments may even autoanastomose. A proximal jejunostomy may be associated with fluid management challenges and electrolyte imbalance.

Pan-involvement with necrosis of the majority of the small bowel occurs in 12% of patients and occurs equally in both premature and full-term newborns (254). Resection would be uniformly associated with the development of short bowel syndrome. Mortality in patients with pan-involvement is nearly 100%, especially in premature newborns. As such, most surgeons do not perform resection but instead choose to withdraw support.

An alternative strategy to operation in the newborn with NEC is peritoneal drainage (255). This involves placement of a Penrose drain under local anesthesia via a 1-cm incision placed in the right lower quadrant, which is the most likely site of perforated NEC. During drain placement the bowel is examined locally for viability and a catheter is passed to the left upper and lower quadrants in order to irrigate the abdomen. A drain is then placed through the right lower quadrant incision toward the left side of the abdomen. Interestingly, studies suggest that using this approach, 32% of patients with perforated NEC survive and require no further operations while 24% succumb soon after drainage. Laparotomy is required within 24 hours in 24%, and operation for delayed strictures becomes necessary in an additional 19%. The survival among those with perforated NEC appears to be equivalent among those undergoing laparotomy when compared to those managed with peritoneal drainage and may depend more on the underlying comorbidities than on the operative approach (256,257). Others have suggested that peritoneal drainage is most effective in patients with isolated SIP, while most patients with NEC require subsequent laparotomy (258). As such, most practitioners apply peritoneal drainage to the premature newborn with perforated NEC and perform laparotomy if physiologic parameters do not improve in the ensuing 24 hours, although the salvage rate for laparotomy following peritoneal drainage is low (256).

An extraordinary and potentially devastating complication of operation for NEC is spontaneous liver hemorrhage (259). The liver in premature newborns has less stromal components and is prone to laceration and bleeding. As such, extreme care should be taken to avoid liver injury to patients with NEC. If bleeding does occur, packing with application of hemostatic agents and correction of coagulopathy should be undertaken rather than attempts at suture ligation (260).

It is rare for newborns with enterostomies to tolerate full feedings unless the stoma is in the terminal ileum and the amount of bowel resected was minimal. Administration of immodium may decrease gut motility, enhance the success of feeding, and limit fluid and electrolyte losses. The urine sodium and serum bicarbonate should be followed and repleted when deficient. In general, the enterostomy is closed at 4 to 6 weeks after the operation but preferably not until the premature newborn reaches approximately 2 kg in weight. Closure of an enterostomy may be challenging for the surgeon and physiologically disruptive for the premature newborn because of the presence of dense adhesions. Anastomotic leaks are rare but do occur, although they often close spontaneously given conservative management for a number of weeks. If the newborn is thriving with enteral feedings despite the presence of an ostomy, closure can be postponed. Factors such as the onset of cholestatic jaundice, the presence of excessive stoma output, failure to

thrive, and development of a stricture at the site of the stoma may indicate early stoma closure. Stoma strictures may be prevented by intermittent dilation of the stoma opening with a small blunt-tipped catheter.

Recurrent NEC occurs in approximately 5% of patients and can frequently be treated nonoperatively (261). Abscess development is rare in newborns, although it can occur and may be diagnosed and drained readily by abdominal ultrasound. Multiple operations are required in 55% of patients with NEC (252). Strictures occur in 29% of patients with NEC, most commonly in those treated without laparotomy, and are most often seen in the large intestine (70%) and the terminal ileum, with the splenic flexure being most common (Fig. 50-21). Most patients with strictures demonstrate feeding intolerance, bowel obstruction, or hemoccult positive stools. A contrast enema is usually diagnostic for the most common large intestinal strictures. Because of the risk of distal stricture a contrast enema is performed before enterostomy closure in all patients.

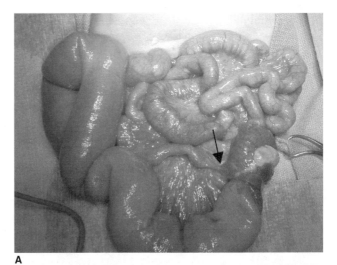

A

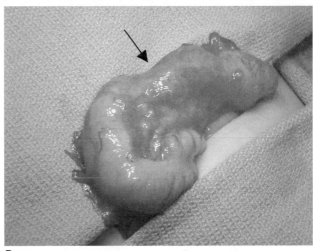

B

Figure 50-21 Strictures following necrotizing enterocolitis in the newborn in the **(A)** terminal ileum (*arrow*) and the **(B)** distal transverse colon (*arrow*).

The mortality associated with NEC is related to the prematurity and associated comorbidities as well as complications of the short bowel syndrome (262). Overall survival among patients with NEC is 87% and is decreased (68%) among those patients whose weight is >1,000 g, in those who have diffuse intestinal involvement, and in premature newborns with four or more comorbidities (30%) (251,254,257). Those patients with SIP have a higher survival rate (88%) even though they have lower gestational age and increased incidence of respiratory distress syndrome (263). Limited ileal resection for NEC is associated with a subsequent increased prevalence of cholelithiasis and a risk of vitamin B_{12} deficiency (264). Otherwise, limited ileocecal resection is not associated with increased morbidity or mortality (265). Intestinal problems occur in 25% of patients over the long term and are mostly associated with development of the short bowel syndrome, which was covered earlier in this chapter (254).

Neurodevelopment is significantly delayed in infants with NEC, such that 55% have severe neurologic deficit when compared to 23% of non-NEC controls (266). Long-term growth does not differ between infants with and without NEC.

REFERENCES

1. Grosfeld JL, Rescorla FJ. Duodenal atresia and stenosis: reassessment of treatment and outcome based on antenatal diagnosis, pathologic variance, and long-term follow-up. *World J Surg* 1993;17:301–309.
2. Lawrence MJ, Ford WD, Furness ME, et al. Congenital duodenal obstruction: early antenatal ultrasound diagnosis. *Pediatr Surg Int* 2000;16:342–345.
3. Dalla Vecchia LK, Grosfeld JL, West KW, et al. Intestinal atresia and stenosis: a 25-year experience with 277 cases. *Arch Surg* 1998;133:490–496; discussion 496–497.
4. Rothenberg SS. Laparoscopic duodenoduodenostomy for duodenal obstruction in infants and children. *J Pediatr Surg* 2002;37:1088–1089.
5. Soutter AD, Askew AA. Transumbilical laparotomy in infants: a novel approach for a wide variety of surgical disease. *J Pediatr Surg* 2003;38:950–952.
6. Rescorla FJ, Grosfeld JL. Intestinal atresia and stenosis: analysis of survival in 120 cases. *Surgery* 1985;98:668–676.
7. Spigland N, Yazbeck S. Complications associated with surgical treatment of congenital intrinsic duodenal obstruction. *J Pediatr Surg* 1990;25:1127–1130.
8. Arnbjornsson E, Larsson M, Finkel Y, et al. Transanastomotic feeding tube after an operation for duodenal atresia. *Eur J Pediatr Surg* 2002;12:159–162.
9. Upadhyay V, Sakalkale R, Parashar K, et al. Duodenal atresia: a comparison of three modes of treatment. [see comment]. *Eur J Pediatr Surg* 1996;6:75–77.
10. Adzick NS, Harrison MR, deLorimier AA, et al. Tapering duodenoplasty for megaduodenum associated with duodenal atresia. *J Pediatr Surg* 1986;21:311–312.
11. Kokkonen ML, Kalima T, Jaaskelainen J, et al. Duodenal atresia: late follow-up. *J Pediatr Surg* 1988;23:216–220.
12. Seashore JH, Touloukian RJ. Midgut volvulus. An ever-present threat. *Arch Pediatr Adolesc Med* 1994;148:43–46.
13. Prasil P, Flageole H, Shaw KS, et al. Should malrotation in children be treated differently according to age? *J Pediatr Surg* 2000;35:756–758.
14. Ford EG, Senac MO, Srikanth MS, Jr., et al. Malrotation of the intestine in children. *Ann Surg* 1992;215:172–178.
15. Millar AJ, Rode H, Cywes S, et al. Malrotation and volvulus in infancy and childhood. *Semin Pediatr Surg* 2003;12:229–236.
16. Long FR, Kramer SS, Markowitz RI, et al. Radiographic patterns of intestinal malrotation in children. *Radiographics* 1996;16:547–556; discussion 556–560.
17. Torres AM, Ziegler MM. Malrotation of the intestine. *World J Surg* 1993;17:326–331.
18. Severijnen R, Hulstijn-Dirkmaat I, Gordijn B, et al. Acute loss of the small bowel in a school-age boy. Difficult choices: to sustain life or to stop treatment? *Eur J Pediatr* 2003;162:794–798.
19. Wilmore DW. Factors correlating with a successful outcome following extensive intestinal resection in newborn infants. *J Pediatr* 1972;80:88–95.
20. Messineo A, MacMillan JH, Palder SB, et al. Clinical factors affecting mortality in children with malrotation of the intestine. *J Pediatr Surg* 1992;27:1343–1345.
21. Phelps S, Fisher R, Partington A, et al. Prenatal ultrasound diagnosis of gastrointestinal malformations. *J Pediatr Surg* 1997;32:438–440.
22. Zerella JT, Martin LW. Jejunal atresia with absent mesentery and a helical ileum. *Surgery* 1976;80:550–553.
23. Thomas CG, Jr. Jejunoplasty for the correction of jejunal atresia. *Surg Gynecol Obstet* 1969;129:545–546.
24. Lally KP, Chwals WJ, Weitzman JJ, et al. Hirschsprung's disease: a possible cause of anastomotic failure following repair of intestinal atresia. *J Pediatr Surg* 1992;27:469–470.
25. Touloukian RJ. Diagnosis and treatment of jejunoileal atresia. *World J Surg* 1993;17:310–317.
26. Waldhausen JH, Sawin RS. Improved long-term outcome for patients with jejunoileal apple peel atresia. *J Pediatr Surg* 1997;32:1307–1309.
27. Lai HJ, Cheng Y, Cho H, et al. Association between initial disease presentation, lung disease outcomes, and survival in patients with cystic fibrosis. *Am J Epidemiol* 2004;159:537–546.
28. Murshed R, Spitz L, Kiely E, et al. Meconium ileus: a ten-year review of thirty-six patients. *Eur J Pediatr Surg* 1997;7:275–277.
29. Mushtaq I, Wright VM, Drake DP, et al. Meconium ileus secondary to cystic fibrosis. The East London experience. *Pediatr Surg Int* 1998;13:365–369.
30. Rescorla FJ, Grosfeld JL, West KJ, et al. Changing patterns of treatment and survival in neonates with meconium ileus. *Arch Surg* 1989;124:837–840.
31. Kao SC, Franken EA, Jr. Nonoperative treatment of simple meconium ileus: a survey of the society for pediatric radiology. *Pediatr Radiol* 1995;25:97–100.
32. Fuchs JR, Langer JC. Long-term outcome after neonatal meconium obstruction. *Pediatrics* 1998;101:E7.
33. Del Pin CA, Czyrko C, Ziegler MM, et al. Management and survival of meconium ileus. A 30-year review. *Ann Surg* 1992;215:179–185.
34. Fakhoury K, Durie PR, Levison H, et al. Meconium ileus in the absence of cystic fibrosis. *Arch Dis Child* 1992;67:1204–1206.
35. Lloyd-Still JD, Beno DW, Kimura RM, et al. Cystic fibrosis colonopathy. *Curr Gastroenterol Rep* 1999;1:231–237.
36. O'Kelly TJ, Davies JR, Tam PK, et al. Abnormalities of nitric-oxide-producing neurons in Hirschsprung's disease: morphology and implications. *J Pediatr Surg* 1994;29:294–299; discussion 299–300.
37. Reding R, de Ville de Goyet J, Gosseye S, et al. Hirschsprung's disease: a 20-year experience. *J Pediatr Surg* 1997;32:1221–1225.
38. Polley TZ, Coran AG, Wesley JR, et al. Jr. A ten-year experience with ninety-two cases of Hirschsprung's disease. Including sixty-seven consecutive endorectal pull-through procedures. *Ann Surg* 1985;202:349–355.
39. Lewis NA, Levitt MA, Zallen GS, et al. Diagnosing Hirschsprung's disease: increasing the odds of a positive rectal biopsy result. *J Pediatr Surg* 2003;38:412–416; discussion 412–416.
40. Maia DM. The reliability of frozen-section diagnosis in the pathologic evaluation of Hirschsprung's disease. *Am J Surg Pathol* 2000;24:1675–1677.

41. Pierro A, Fasoli L, Kiely EM, et al. Staged pull-through for rectosigmoid Hirschsprung's disease is not safer than primary pull-through. *J Pediatr Surg* 1997;32:505–509.

42. Wilcox DT, Bruce J, Bowen J, et al. One-stage neonatal pull-through to treat Hirschsprung's disease. *J Pediatr Surg* 1997;32:243–245; discussion 245–247.

43. Minford JL, Ram A, Turnock RR, et al. Comparison of functional outcomes of Duhamel and transanal endorectal coloanal anastomosis for Hirschsprung's disease. *J Pediatr Surg* 2004;39:161–165; discussion 161–165.

44. Sherman JO, Snyder ME, Weitzman JJ, et al. A 40-year multinational retrospective study of 880 Swenson procedures. *J Pediatr Surg* 1989;24:833–838.

45. Moore SW, Albertyn R, Cywes S, et al. Clinical outcome and long-term quality of life after surgical correction of Hirschsprung's disease. *J Pediatr Surg* 1996;31:1496–1502.

46. Soper RT, Miller FE. Modification of Duhamel procedure: elimination of rectal pouch and colorectal septum. *J Pediatr Surg* 1968;3:376.

47. Teitelbaum DH, Cilley RE, Sherman NJ, et al. A decade of experience with the primary pull-through for Hirschsprung disease in the newborn period: a multicenter analysis of outcomes. *Ann Surg* 2000;232:372–380.

48. Langer JC, Fitzgerald PG, Winthrop AL, et al. One-stage versus two-stage Soave pull-through for Hirschsprung's disease in the first year of life. *J Pediatr Surg* 1996;31:33–36; discussion 36–37.

49. Georgeson KE, Cohen RD, Hebra A, et al. Primary laparoscopic-assisted endorectal colon pull-through for Hirschsprung's disease: a new gold standard. *Ann Surg* 1999;229:678–682; discussion 682–673.

50. Langer JC, Durrant AC, de la Torre L, et al. One-stage transanal Soave pullthrough for Hirschsprung disease: a multicenter experience with 141 children. *Ann Surg* 2003;238:569–583; discussion 583–565.

51. Davies MR, Cywes S. Inadequate pouch emptying following Martin's pull-through procedure for intestinal aganglionosis. *J Pediatr Surg* 1983;18:14–20.

52. Ziegler MM, Royal RE, Brandt J, et al. Extended myectomy-myotomy. A therapeutic alternative for total intestinal aganglionosis. *Ann Surg* 1993;218:504–509; discussion 509–511.

53. Elhalaby EA, Hashish A, Elbarbary MM, et al. Transanal one-stage endorectal pull-through for Hirschsprung's disease: a multicenter study. *J Pediatr Surg* 2004;39:345–351; discussion 345–351.

54. Weber TR, Fortuna RS, Silen ML, et al. Reoperation for Hirschsprung's disease. *J Pediatr Surg* 1999;34:153–156; discussion 156–157.

55. Van Leeuwen K, Geiger JD, Barnett JL, et al. Stooling and manometric findings after primary pull-throughs in Hirschsprung's disease: perineal versus abdominal approaches. *J Pediatr Surg* 2002;37:1321–1325.

56. Elhalaby EA, Coran AG, Blane CE, et al. Enterocolitis associated with Hirschsprung's disease: a clinical-radiological characterization based on 168 patients. *J Pediatr Surg* 1995;30:76–83.

57. Hackam DJ, Filler RM, Pearl RH, et al. Enterocolitis after the surgical treatment of Hirschsprung's disease: risk factors and financial impact. [see comment]. *J Pediatr Surg* 1998;33:830–833.

58. Wildhaber BE, Pakarinen M, Rintala RJ, et al. Posterior myotomy/myectomy for persistent stooling problems in Hirschsprung's disease. *J Pediatr Surg* 2004;39:920–926; discussion 920–926.

59. Langer JC, Birnbaum E. Preliminary experience with intrasphincteric botulinum toxin for persistent constipation after pull-through for Hirschsprung's disease. *J Pediatr Surg* 1997;32:1059–1061; discussion 1061–1052.

60. Wester T, Rintala RJ. Early outcome of transanal endorectal pull-through with a short muscle cuff during the neonatal period. *J Pediatr Surg* 2004;39:157–160; discussion 157–160.

61. Hadidi A. Transanal endorectal pull-through for Hirschsprung's disease: experience with 68 patients. *J Pediatr Surg* 2003;38:1337–1340.

62. Blair GK, Murphy JJ, Fraser GC, et al. Internal sphincterotomy in post-pull-through Hirschsprung's disease. *J Pediatr Surg* 1996;31:843–845.

63. Farrugia MK, Alexander N, Clarke S, et al. Does transitional zone pull-through in Hirschsprung's disease imply a poor prognosis? *J Pediatr Surg* 2003;38:1766–1769.

64. White FV, Langer JC. Circumferential distribution of ganglion cells in the transition zone of children with Hirschsprung disease. *Pediatr Dev Pathol* 2000;3:216–222.

65. Schmittenbecher PP, Sacher P, Cholewa D, et al. Hirschsprung's disease and intestinal neuronal dysplasia—a frequent association with implications for the postoperative course. *Pediatr Surg Int* 1999;15:553–558.

66. Langer JC. Repeat pull-through surgery for complicated Hirschsprung's disease: indications, techniques, and results. *J Pediatr Surg* 1999;34:1136–1141.

67. van Leeuwen K, Teitelbaum DH, Elhalaby EA, et al. Long-term follow-up of redo pull-through procedures for Hirschsprung's disease: efficacy of the endorectal pull-through. *J Pediatr Surg* 2000;35:829–833; discussion 833–824.

68. Wilcox DT, Kiely EM. Repeat pull-through for Hirschsprung's disease. *J Pediatr Surg* 1998;33:1507–1509.

69. Ludman L, Spitz L, Tsuji H, et al. Hirschsprung's disease: functional and psychological follow up comparing total colonic and rectosigmoid aganglionosis. *Arch Dis Child* 2002;86:348–351.

70. Teitelbaum DH, Drongowski RA, Chamberlain JN, et al. Long-term stooling patterns in infants undergoing primary endorectal pull-through for Hirschsprung's disease. *J Pediatr Surg* 1997;32:1049–1052; discussion 1052–1043.

71. Bai Y, Chen H, Hao J, et al. Long-term outcome and quality of life after the Swenson procedure for Hirschsprung's disease. *J Pediatr Surg* 2002;37:639–642.

72. McHugh K, Dudley NE, Tam P, et al. Pre-operative MRI of anorectal anomalies in the newborn period. *Pediatr Radiol* 1995;25(Suppl. 1):S33–S36.

73. Boocock GR, Donnai D. Anorectal malformation: familial aspects and associated anomalies. *Arch Dis Child* 1987;62:576–579.

74. Hassink EA, Rieu PN, Hamel BC, et al. Additional congenital defects in anorectal malformations. *Eur J Pediatr* 1996;155:477–482.

75. Rittler M, Paz JE, Castilla EE, et al. VACTERL association, epidemiologic definition and delineation. *Am J Med Genet* 1996;63:529–536.

76. Tsakayannis DE, Shamberger RC. Association of imperforate anus with occult spinal dysraphism. *J Pediatr Surg* 1995;30:1010–1012.

77. Cortes D, Thorup JM, Nielsen OH, et al. Cryptorchidism in boys with imperforate anus. *J Pediatr Surg* 1995;30:631–635.

78. Adeniran JO. One-stage correction of imperforate anus and rectovestibular fistula in girls: preliminary results. *J Pediatr Surg* 2002;37:E16.

79. Georgeson KE, Inge TH, Albanese CT. Laparoscopically assisted anorectal pull-through for high imperforate anus—a new technique. *J Pediatr Surg* 2000;35:927–930; discussion 930–921.

80. De Filippo RE, Shaul DB, Harrison EA, et al. Neurogenic bladder in infants born with anorectal malformations: comparison with spinal and urologic status. [see comment]. *J Pediatr Surg* 1999;34:825–827; discussion 828.

81. Anderson KD, Newman KD, Bond SJ, et al. Diamond flap anoplasty in infants and children with an intractable anal stricture. *J Pediatr Surg* 1994;29:1253–1257.

82. Powell RW, Sherman JO, Raffensperger JG, et al. Megarectum: a rare complication of imperforate anus repair and its surgical correction by endorectal pullthrough. *J Pediatr Surg* 1982;17:786–795.

83. Nixon HH, Puri P. The results of treatment of anorectal anomalies: a thirteen to twenty year follow up. *J Pediatr Surg* 1977;12:27–37.

84. Nakayama DK, Templeton JM, Ziegler MM, Jr., et al. Complications of posterior sagittal anorectoplasty. *J Pediatr Surg* 1986;21:488–492.

85. Kulshrestha S, Kulshrestha M, Yadav A, et al. Posterior sagittal approach for repair of rectourethral fistula occurring after perineal surgery for imperforated anus at birth. *J Pediatr Surg* 2000;35:1155–1160.

86. Tsugawa C, Hisano K, Nishijima E, et al. Posterior sagittal anorectoplasty for failed imperforate anus surgery: lessons learned from secondary repairs. *J Pediatr Surg* 2000;35:1626–1629.

87. Chowdhary SK, Chalapathi G, Narasimhan KL, et al. An audit of neonatal colostomy for high anorectal malformation: the developing world perspective. *Pediatr Surg Int* 2004;20:111–113.

88. Bratu I, Flageole H, Chen MF, et al. The multiple facets of pulmonary sequestration. *J Pediatr Surg* 2001;36:784–790.

89. Heikkinen M, Rintala R, Luukkonen P, et al. Long-term anal sphincter performance after surgery for Hirschsprung's disease. *J Pediatr Surg* 1997;32:1443–1446.

90. Javid PJ, Barnhart DC, Hirschl RB, et al. Immediate and long-term results of surgical management of low imperforate anus in girls. *J Pediatr Surg* 1998;33:198–203.

91. Fleming SE, Hall R, Gysler M, et al. Imperforate anus in females: frequency of genital tract involvement, incidence of associated anomalies, and functional outcome. *J Pediatr Surg* 1986;21:146–150.

92. Bliss DP Jr, Tapper D, Anderson JM, et al. Does posterior sagittal anorectoplasty in patients with high imperforate anus provide superior fecal continence? *J Pediatr Surg* 1996;31:26–30; discussion 30–22.

93. Ellsworth PI, Webb HW, Crump JM, et al. The Malone antegrade colonic enema enhances the quality of life in children undergoing urological incontinence procedures. *J Urol* 1996;155:1416–1418.

94. da Silva GM, Jorge JM, Belin B, et al. New surgical options for fecal incontinence in patients with imperforate anus. *Dis Colon Rectum* 2004;47:204–209.

95. Morotti RA, Cangiarella J, Gutierrez MC, et al. Congenital cystic adenomatoid malformation of the lung (CCAM): evaluation of the cellular components. *Hum Pathol* 1999;30:618–625.

96. Kim WS, Lee KS, Kim IO, et al. Congenital cystic adenomatoid malformation of the lung: CT-pathologic correlation. *AJR Am J Roentgenol* 1997;168:47–53.

97. Sauvat F, Michel JL, Benachi A, et al. Management of asymptomatic neonatal cystic adenomatoid malformations. *J Pediatr Surg* 2003;38:548–552.

98. Roggin KK, Breuer CK, Carr SR, et al. The unpredictable character of congenital cystic lung lesions. *J Pediatr Surg* 2000;35:801–805.

99. Taguchi T, Suita S, Yamanouchi T, et al. Antenatal diagnosis and surgical management of congenital cystic adenomatoid malformation of the lung. *Fetal Diagn Ther* 1995;10:400–407.

100. Morin L, Crombleholme TM, D'Alton ME, et al. Prenatal diagnosis and management of fetal thoracic lesions. *Semin Perinatol* 1994;18:228–253.

101. Miller JA, Corteville JE, Langer JC, et al. Congenital cystic adenomatoid malformation in the fetus: natural history and predictors of outcome. *J Pediatr Surg* 1996;31:805–808.

102. Adzick NS, Harrison MR, Flake AW, et al. Fetal surgery for cystic adenomatoid malformation of the lung. *J Pediatr Surg* 1993; 28:806–812.

103. Atkinson JB, Ford EG, Kitagawa H, et al. Persistent pulmonary hypertension complicating cystic adenomatoid malformation in neonates. *J Pediatr Surg* 1992;27:54–56.

104. van Leeuwen K, Teitelbaum DH, Hirschl RB, et al. Prenatal diagnosis of congenital cystic adenomatoid malformation and its postnatal presentation, surgical indications, and natural history. *J Pediatr Surg* 1999;34:794–798; discussion 798–799.

105. Murphy JJ, Blair GK, Fraser GC, et al. Rhabdomyosarcoma arising within congenital pulmonary cysts: report of three cases. *J Pediatr Surg* 1992;27:1364–1367.

106. Hasiotou M, Polyviou P, Strantzia CM, et al. Pleuropulmonary blastoma in the area of a previously diagnosed congenital lung cyst: report of two cases. *Acta Radiol* 2004;45:289–292.

107. Coran AG, Drongowski R. Congenital cystic disease of the tracheobronchial tree in infants and children. Experience with 44 consecutive cases. *Arch Surg* 1994;129:521–527.

108. Gluer S, Scharf A, Ure BM, et al. Thoracoscopic resection of extralobar sequestration in a neonate. *J Pediatr Surg* 2002;37: 1629–1631.

109. Becmeur F, Horta P, Christmann D, et al. Mediastinal stabilization by an expansion prosthesis in postoperative congenital diaphragmatic hernia with severe pulmonary hypoplasia. *Eur J Pediatr Surg* 1995;5:295–298.

110. Halkic N, Cuenoud PF, Corthesy ME, et al. Pulmonary sequestration: a review of 26 cases. *Eur J Cardiothorac Surg* 1998;14: 127–133.

111. Tsolakis CC, Kollias VD, Panayotopoulos PP, et al. Pulmonary sequestration. Experience with eight consecutive cases. *Scand Cardiovasc J* 1997;31:229–232.

112. Conran RM, Stocker JT. Extralobar sequestration with frequently associated congenital cystic adenomatoid malformation, type 2: report of 50 cases. *Pediatr Dev Pathol* 1999;2: 454–463.

113. Nobuhara KK, Gorski YC, La Quaglia MP, et al. Bronchogenic cysts and esophageal duplications: common origins and treatment. *J Pediatr Surg* 1997;32:1408–1413.

114. Kim KW, Kim WS, Cheon JE, et al. Complex bronchopulmonary foregut malformation: extralobar pulmonary sequestration associated with a duplication cyst of mixed bronchogenic and oesophageal type. *Pediatr Radiol* 2001;31:265–268.

115. Di Lorenzo M, Collin PP, Vaillancourt R, et al. Bronchogenic cysts. *J Pediatr Surg* 1989;24:988–991.

116. Ribet ME, Copin MC, Gosselin BH, et al. Bronchogenic cysts of the lung. *Ann Thorac Surg* 1996;61:1636–1640.

117. Cohen SR, Geller KA, Birns JW, et al. Foregut cysts in infants and children. Diagnosis and management. *Ann Otol Rhinol Laryngol* 1982;91:622–627.

118. Yerman HM, Holinger LD. Bronchogenic cyst with tracheal involvement. *Ann Otol Rhinol Laryngol* 1990;99:89–93.

119. Harle CC, Dearlove O, Walker RW, et al. A bronchogenic cyst in an infant causing tracheal occlusion and cardiac arrest. *Anaesthesia* 1999;54:262–265.

120. Merry C, Spurbeck W, Lobe TE, et al. Resection of foregut-derived duplications by minimal-access surgery. *Pediatr Surg Int* 1999;15:224–226.

121. Langer JC, Hussain H, Khan A, et al. Prenatal diagnosis of esophageal atresia using sonography and magnetic resonance imaging. *J Pediatr Surg* 2001;36:804–807.

122. Maoate K, Myers NA, Beasley SW, et al. Gastric perforation in infants with oesophageal atresia and distal tracheo-oesophageal fistula. *Pediatr Surg Int* 1999;15:24–27.

123. Engum SA, Grosfeld JL, West, KW, et al. Analysis of morbidity and mortality in 227 cases of esophageal atresia and/or tracheoesophageal fistula over two decades. *Arch Surg* 1995;130:502–508; discussion 508–509.

124. Bowkett B, Beasley SW, Myers NA, et al. The frequency, significance, and management of a right aortic arch in association with esophageal atresia. *Pediatr Surg Int* 1999;15:28–31.

125. Babu R, Pierro A, Spitz L, et al. The management of oesophageal atresia in neonates with right-sided aortic arch. [see comment]. *J Pediatr Surg* 2000;35:56–58.

126. Chittmittrapap S, Spitz L, Kiely EM, et al. Anastomotic leakage following surgery for esophageal atresia. *J Pediatr Surg* 1992; 27:29–32.

127. Ein SH, Shandling B. Pure esophageal atresia: a 50-year review. *J Pediatr Surg* 1994;29:1208–1211.

128. Boyle EM, Irwin ED, Foker JE, Jr., et al. Primary repair of ultra-long-gap esophageal atresia: results without a lengthening procedure. *Ann Thorac Surg* 1994;57:576–579.

129. Giacomoni MA, Tresoldi M, Zamana C, et al. Circular myotomy of the distal esophageal stump for long gap esophageal atresia. *J Pediatr Surg* 2001;36:855–857.

130. Sharma AK, Wakhlu A. Simple technique for proximal pouch mobilization and circular myotomy in cases of esophageal atresia with tracheoesophageal fistula. *J Pediatr Surg* 1994;29: 1402–1403.

131. Lai JY, Sheu JC, Chang PY, et al. Experience with distal circular myotomy for long-gap esophageal atresia. *J Pediatr Surg* 1996;31: 1503–1508.

132. Kimura K, Nishijima E, Tsugawa C, et al. Multistaged extrathoracic esophageal elongation procedure for long gap esophageal atresia: experience with 12 patients. *J Pediatr Surg* 2001;36: 1725–1727.

133. Fernandez MS, Gutierrez C, Ibanez V, et al. Long-gap esophageal atresia: reconstruction preserving all portions of the esophagus by Scharli's technique. *Pediatr Surg Int* 1998;14:17–20.

134. Evans M. Application of Collis gastroplasty to the management of esophageal atresia. *J Pediatr Surg* 1995;30:1232–1235.

135. Foker JE, Linden BC, Boyle EM Jr, et al. Development of a true primary repair for the full spectrum of esophageal atresia. *Ann Surg* 1997;226:533–541; discussion 541–533.

136. Gough MH. Esophageal atresia—use of an anterior flap in the difficult anastomosis. *J Pediatr Surg* 1980;15:310–311.

137. Brown AK, Tam PK. Measurement of gap length in esophageal atresia: a simple predictor of outcome. *J Am Coll Surg* 1996;182:41–45.

138. Rescorla FJ, West KW, Scherer LR, et al. III. The complex nature of type A (long-gap) esophageal atresia. *Surgery* 1994;116:658–664.

139. Pompeo E, Coosemans W, De Leyn P, et al. Esophageal replacement with colon in children using either the intrathoracic or retrosternal route: an analysis of both surgical and long-term results. *Surg Today* 1997;27:729–734.

140. McCollum MO, Rangel SJ, Blair GK, et al. Primary reversed gastric tube reconstruction in long gap esophageal atresia. *J Pediatr Surg* 2003;38:957–962.

141. Spitz L, Kiely E, Pierro, A. Gastric transposition in children—a 21-year experience. *J Pediatr Surg* 2004;39:276–281; discussion 276–281.

142. Khan AR, Stiff G, Mohammed AR, et al. Esophageal replacement with colon in children. *Pediatr Surg Int* 1998;13:79–83.

143. Hirschl RB, Yardeni D, Oldham K, et al. Gastric transposition for esophageal replacement in children: experience with 41 consecutive cases with special emphasis on esophageal atresia. *Ann Surg* 2002;236:531–539; discussion 539–541.

144. Ahmad SA, Sylvester KG, Hebra A, et al. Esophageal replacement using the colon: is it a good choice? *J Pediatr Surg* 1996;31:1026–1030; discussion 1030–1021.

145. Ruangtrakool R, Spitz L. Early complications of gastric transposition operation. *J Med Assoc Thai* 2000;83:352–357.

146. Dunn JC, Fonkalsrud EW, Applebaum H, et al. Reoperation after esophageal replacement in childhood. *J Pediatr Surg* 1999;34:1630–1632.

147. Chan KL, Saing H. Iatrogenic gastric volvulus during transposition for esophageal atresia: diagnosis and treatment. *J Pediatr Surg* 1996;31:229–232.

148. Spitz L, Kiely EM, Morecroft JA, et al. Oesophageal atresia: at-risk groups for the 1990s. *J Pediatr Surg* 1994;29:723–725.

149. Chavin K, Field G, Chandler J, et al. Save the child's esophagus: management of major disruption after repair of esophageal atresia. *J Pediatr Surg* 1996;31:48–51; discussion 52.

150. Islam S, Cavanaugh E, Honeke R, et al. Diagnosis of a proximal tracheoesophageal fistula using three-dimensional CT scan: a case report. *J Pediatr Surg* 2004;39:100–102.

151. Gutierrez C, Barrios JE, Lluna J, et al. Recurrent tracheoesophageal fistula treated with fibrin glue. *J Pediatr Surg* 1994;29:1567–1569.

152. Wheatley MJ, Coran AG, Wesley JR, et al. Efficacy of the Nissen fundoplication in the management of gastroesophageal reflux following esophageal atresia repair. *J Pediatr Surg* 1993;28:53–55.

153. Deurloo JA, Ekkelkamp S, Bartelsman JF, et al. Gastroesophageal reflux: prevalence in adults older than 28 years after correction of esophageal atresia. *Ann Surg* 2003;238:686–689.

154. Krug E, Bergmeijer JH, Dees J, et al. Gastroesophageal reflux and Barrett's esophagus in adults born with esophageal atresia. *Am J Gastroenterol* 1999;94:2825–2828.

155. Bergmeijer JH, Bouquet J, Hazebroek FW, et al. Normal ranges of 24 hour pH metry established in corrected esophageal atresia. *J Pediatr Gastroenterol Nutr* 1999;28:162–163.

156. Bergmeijer JH, Tibboel D, Hazebroek FW, et al. Nissen fundoplication in the management of gastroesophageal reflux occurring after repair of esophageal atresia. *J Pediatr Surg* 2000;35:573–576.

157. Lindahl H, Rintala R. Long-term complications in cases of isolated esophageal atresia treated with esophageal anastomosis. *J Pediatr Surg* 1995;30:1222–1223.

158. Schier F, Korn S, Michel E, et al. Experiences of a parent support group with the long-term consequences of esophageal atresia. *J Pediatr Surg* 2001;36:605–610.

159. Vazquez-Jimenez JF, Sachweh JS, Liakopoulos OJ, et al. Aortopexy in severe tracheal instability: short-term and long-term outcome in 29 infants and children. *Ann Thorac Surg* 2001;72:1898–1901.

160. Tazuke Y, Kawahara H, Yagi M, et al. Use of a Palmaz stent for tracheomalacia: case report of an infant with esophageal atresia. *J Pediatr Surg* 1999;34:1291–1293.

161. Delius RE, Wheatley MJ, Coran AG, et al. Etiology and management of respiratory complications after repair of esophageal atresia with tracheoesophageal fistula. *Surgery* 1992;112:527–532.

162. Tomaselli V, Volpi ML, Dell'Agnola CA, et al. Long-term evaluation of esophageal function in patients treated at birth for esophageal atresia. *Pediatr Surg Int* 2003;19:40–43.

163. Dutta HK, Grover VP, Dwivedi SN, et al. Manometric evaluation of postoperative patients of esophageal atresia and tracheoesophageal fistula. *Eur J Pediatr Surg* 2001;11:371–376.

164. Bax KM, van Der Zee DC. Feasibility of thoracoscopic repair of esophageal atresia with distal fistula. *J Pediatr Surg* 2002;37:192–196.

165. Zigman A, Yazbeck S. Esophageal foreign body obstruction after esophageal atresia repair. *J Pediatr Surg* 2002;37:776–778.

166. Clark RH, Hardin WD, Hirschl RB, Jr., et al. Current surgical management of congenital diaphragmatic hernia: a report from the Congenital Diaphragmatic Hernia Study Group. *J Pediatr Surg* 1998;33:1004–1009.

167. Iritani I. Experimental study on embryogenesis of congenital diaphragmatic hernia. *Anat Embryol* 1984;169:133–139.

168. Harrison MR, Jester JA, Ross NA, et al. Correction of congenital diaphragmatic hernia in utero. I. The model: intrathoracic balloon produces fatal pulmonary hypoplasia. *Surgery* 1980;88:174–182.

169. Bohn D, Tamura M, Perrin D, et al. Ventilatory predictors of pulmonary hypoplasia in congenital diaphragmatic hernia, confirmed by morphologic assessment. *J Pediatr* 1987;111:423–431.

170. Yamataka T, Puri P. Pulmonary artery structural changes in pulmonary hypertension complicating congenital diaphragmatic hernia. *J Pediatr Surg* 1997;32:387–390.

171. Price MR, Galantowicz ME, Stolar CJ, et al. Congenital diaphragmatic hernia, extracorporeal membrane oxygenation, and death: a spectrum of etiologies. *J Pediatr Surg* 1991;26:1023–1026; discussion 1026–1027.

172. Dillon PW, Cilley RE, Mauger D, et al. The relationship of pulmonary artery pressure and survival in congenital diaphragmatic hernia. *J Pediatr Surg* 2004;39:307–312; discussion 307–312.

173. Manning PB, Murphy JP, Raynor SC, et al. Congenital diaphragmatic hernia presenting due to gastrointestinal complications. *J Pediatr Surg* 1992;27:1225–1228.

174. Burge DM, Atwell JD, Freeman NV, et al. Could the stomach site help predict outcome in babies with left sided congenital diaphragmatic hernia diagnosed antenatally? *J Pediatr Surg* 1989;24:567–569.

175. Hatch EI, Kendall J, Blumhagen J Jr., et al. Stomach position as an in utero predictor of neonatal outcome in left-sided diaphragmatic hernia. *J Pediatr Surg* 1992;27:778–779.

176. Bohn DJ, James I, Filler RM, et al. The relationship between PaCO2 and ventilation parameters in predicting survival in congenital diaphragmatic hernia. *J Pediatr Surg* 1984;19:666–671.

177. Lewis DA, Reickert C, Bowerman R, et al. Prenatal ultrasonography frequently fails to diagnose congenital diaphragmatic hernia. *J Pediatr Surg* 1997;32:352–356.

178. Nakstad B, Naess PA, de Lange C, et al. Complications of umbilical vein catheterization: neonatal total parenteral nutrition ascites after surgical repair of congenital diaphragmatic hernia. *J Pediatr Surg* 2002;37:E21.

179. Cacciari A, Ruggeri G, Mordenti M, et al. High-frequency oscillatory ventilation versus conventional mechanical ventilation in congenital diaphragmatic hernia. *Eur J Pediatr Surg* 2001; 11:3–7.

180. Azarow K, Messineo A, Pearl R, et al. Congenital diaphragmatic hernia—a tale of two cities: the Toronto experience. *J Pediatr Surg* 1997;32:395–400.

181. The Neonatal Inhaled Nitric Oxide Study Group (NINOS). Anonymous inhaled nitric oxide and hypoxic respiratory failure in infants with congenital diaphragmatic hernia. *Pediatrics* 1997;99:838–845.

182. Shanley CJ, Hirschl RB, Schumacher RE, et al. Extracorporeal life support for neonatal respiratory failure. A 20-year experience. *Ann Surg* 1994;220:269–280; discussion 281–262.

183. Schwartz SM, Vermilion RP, Hirschl RB, et al. Evaluation of left ventricular mass in children with left-sided congenital diaphragmatic hernia. *J Pediatr* 1994;125:447–451.

184. Heiss KF, Clark RH, Cornish JD, et al. Preferential use of venovenous extracorporeal membrane oxygenation for congenital diaphragmatic hernia. *Pediatr Surg* 1995;30:416–419.

185. Vazquez WD, Cheu HW. Hemorrhagic complications and repair of congenital diaphragmatic hernias: does timing of the repair make a difference? Data from the Extracorporeal Life Support Organization. *J Pediatr Surg* 1994;29:1002–1005; discussion 1005–1006.

186. Wilson JM, Bower LK, Lund DP, et al. Evolution of the technique of congenital diaphragmatic hernia repair on ECMO. *J Pediatr Surg* 1994;29:1109–1112.

187. Registry ELSO. The ELSO Registry Report. Ann Arbor, Michigan; 2004.

188. Reickert CA, Hirschl RB, Schumacher R, et al. Effect of very delayed repair of congenital diaphragmatic hernia on survival and extracorporeal life support use. *Surgery* 1996;120:766–772; discussion 772–763.

189. Nio M, Haase G, Kennaugh J, et al. A prospective randomized trial of delayed versus immediate repair of congenital diaphragmatic hernia. *J Pediatr Surg* 1994;29:618–621.

190. de la Hunt MN, Madden N, Scott JE, et al. Is delayed surgery really better for congenital diaphragmatic hernia?: a prospective randomized clinical trial. [see comment]. *J Pediatr Surg* 1996;31: 1554–1556.

191. Atkinson JB, Poon MW. ECMO and the management of congenital diaphragmatic hernia with large diaphragmatic defects requiring a prosthetic patch. *J Pediatr Surg* 1992;27:754–756.

192. Hajer GF, vd Staak FH, de Haan AF, et al. Recurrent congenital diaphragmatic hernia; which factors are involved? *Eur J Pediatr Surg* 1998;8:329–333.

193. Tsang TM, Tam PK, Dudley NE, et al. Diaphragmatic agenesis as a distinct clinical entity. *J Pediatr Surg* 1995;30:16–18.

194. Scaife ER, Johnson DG, Meyers RL, et al. The split abdominal wall muscle flap—a simple, mesh-free approach to repair large diaphragmatic hernia. *J Pediatr Surg* 2003;38:1748–1751.

195. Hanekamp MN, Tjin ADGC, van Hoek-Ottenkamp WG, et al. Does V-A ECMO increase the likelihood of chylothorax after congenital diaphragmatic hernia repair? *J Pediatr Surg* 2003; 38:971–974.

196. Fauza DO, Wilson JM. Congenital diaphragmatic hernia and associated anomalies: their incidence, identification, and impact on prognosis. *J Pediatr Surg* 1994;29:1113–1117.

197. Bernbaum J, Schwartz IP, Gerdes M, et al. Survivors of extracorporeal membrane oxygenation at 1 year of age: the relationship of primary diagnosis with health and neurodevelopmental sequelae. *Pediatrics* 1995;96:907–913.

198. Nagaya M, Akatsuka H, Kato J, et al. Development in lung function of the affected side after repair of congenital diaphragmatic hernia. *J Pediatr Surg* 1996;31:349–356.

199. Wohl ME, Griscom NT, Strieder DJ, et al. The lung following repair of congenital diaphragmatic hernia. *J Pediatr* 1977;90:405–414.

200. D'Agostino JA, Bernbaum JC, Gerdes M, et al. Outcome for infants with congenital diaphragmatic hernia requiring extracorporeal membrane oxygenation: the first year. *J Pediatr Surg* 1995;30:10–15.

201. Stolar CJ, Levy JP, Dillon PW, et al. Anatomic and functional abnormalities of the esophagus in infants surviving congenital diaphragmatic hernia. *Am J Surg* 1990;159:204–207.

202. Rescorla FJ, Shedd FJ, Grosfeld JL, et al. Anomalies of intestinal rotation in childhood: analysis of 447 cases. *Surgery* 1990;108:710–715; discussion 715–716.

203. Lund DP, Mitchell J, Kharasch V, et al. Congenital diaphragmatic hernia: the hidden morbidity. *J Pediatr Surg* 1994;29:258–262; discussion 262–254.

204. Arca MJ, Barnhart DC, Lelli JL, Jr., et al. Early experience with minimally invasive repair of congenital diaphragmatic hernias: results and lessons learned. *J Pediatr Surg* 2003;38:1563–1568.

205. Snyder CL, Miller KA, Sharp RJ, et al. Management of intestinal atresia in patients with gastroschisis. *J Pediatr Surg* 2001;36: 1542–1545.

206. Driver CP, Bruce J, Bianchi A, et al. The contemporary outcome of gastroschisis. *J Pediatr Surg* 2000;35:1719–1723.

207. Lenke RR, Hatch EI, Jr. Fetal gastroschisis: a preliminary report advocating the use of cesarean section. *Obstet Gynecol* 1986;67:395–398.

208. Dunn JC, Fonkalsrud EW, Atkinson JB, et al. The influence of gestational age and mode of delivery on infants with gastroschisis. *J Pediatr Surg* 1999;34:1393–1395.

209. Bethel CA, Seashore JH, Touloukian RJ, et al. Cesarean section does not improve outcome in gastroschisis. *J Pediatr Surg* 1989;24: 1–3; discussion 3–4.

210. Huang J, Kurkchubasche AG, Carr SR, et al. Benefits of term delivery in infants with antenatally diagnosed gastroschisis. [see comment]. *Obstet Gynecol* 2002;100:695–699.

211. Singh SJ, Fraser A, Leditschke JF, et al. Gastroschisis: determinants of neonatal outcome. *Pediatr Surg Int* 2003;19:260–265.

212. Minkes RK, Langer JC, Mazziotti MV, et al. Routine insertion of a silastic spring-loaded silo for infants with gastroschisis. [see comment]. *J Pediatr Surg* 2000;35:843–846.

213. Mollitt DL, Ballantine TV, Grosfeld JL, et al. A critical assessment of fluid requirements in gastroschisis. *J Pediatr Surg* 1978;13: 217–219.

214. Schlatter M, Norris K, Uitvlugt N, et al. Improved outcomes in the treatment of gastroschisis using a preformed silo and delayed repair approach. *J Pediatr Surg* 2003;38:459–464; discussion 459–464.

215. Schwartz MZ, Tyson KR, Milliorn K, et al. Staged reduction using a Silastic sac is the treatment of choice for large congenital abdominal wall defects. *J Pediatr Surg* 1983;18:713–719.

216. Molik KA, Gingalewski CA, West KW, et al. Gastroschisis: a plea for risk categorization. *J Pediatr Surg* 2001;36:51–55.

217. Saxena AK, Hulskamp G, Schleef J, et al. Gastroschisis: a 15-year, single-center experience. *Pediatr Surg Int* 2002;18:420–424.

218. Koivusalo A, Rintala R, Lindahl H, et al. Gastroesophageal reflux in children with a congenital abdominal wall defect. *J Pediatr Surg* 1999;34:1127–1129.

219. Mahour GH, Weitzman JJ, Rosenkrantz JG, et al. Omphalocele and gastroschisis. *Ann Surg* 1973;177:478–482.

220. Heider AL, Strauss RA, Kuller JA, et al. Omphalocele: clinical outcomes in cases with normal karyotypes. *Am J Obstet Gynecol* 2004;190:135–141.

221. Greenwood RD, Rosenthal A, Nadas AS, et al. Cardiovascular malformations associated with omphalocele. *J Pediatr* 1974;85: 818–821.

222. Boyd PA, Bhattacharjee A, Gould S, et al. Outcome of prenatally diagnosed anterior abdominal wall defects. *Arch Dis Child Fetal Neonatal Ed* 1998;78:F209–F213.

223. Krasna IH. Is early fascial closure necessary for omphalocele and gastroschisis? *J Pediatr Surg* 1995;30:23–28.

224. Hong AR, Sigalet DL, Guttman FM, et al. Sequential sac ligation for giant omphalocele. *J Pediatr Surg* 1994;29:413–415.

225. de Lorimier AA, Adzick NS, Harrison MR, et al. Amnion inversion in the treatment of giant omphalocele. *J Pediatr Surg* 1991;26:804–807.

226. Brown MF, Wright L. Delayed External Compression Reduction of an Omphalocele (DECRO): an alternative method of treatment for moderate and large omphaloceles. *J Pediatr Surg* 1998;33:1113–1115; discussion 1115–1116.

227. Barlow B, Cooper A, Gandhi R, et al. External silo reduction of the unruptured giant omphalocele. *J Pediatr Surg* 1987;22:75.

228. Hatch EI, Baxter R. Surgical options in the management of large omphaloceles. *Am J Surg* 1987;153:449–452.

229. Dunn JC, Fonkalsrud EW. Improved survival of infants with omphalocele. *Am J Surg* 1997;173:284–287.

230. Koivusalo A, Lindahl H, Rintala RJ, et al. Morbidity and quality of life in adult patients with a congenital abdominal wall defect: a questionnaire survey. *J Pediatr Surg* 2002;37:1594–1601.

231. Koivusalo A, Taskinen S, Rintala RJ, et al. Cryptorchidism in boys with congenital abdominal wall defects. *Pediatr Surg Int* 1998;13:143–145.

232. Godbole P, Sprigg A, Dickson JA, et al. Ultrasound compared with clinical examination in infantile hypertrophic pyloric stenosis. [see comment]. *Arch Dis Child* 1996;75:335–337.
233. Kovalivker M, Erez I, Shneider N, et al. The value of ultrasound in the diagnosis of congenital hypertrophic pyloric stenosis. *Clin Pediatr* 1993;32:281–283.
234. Haider N, Spicer R, Grier D, et al. Ultrasound diagnosis of infantile hypertrophic pyloric stenosis: determinants of pyloric length and the effect of prematurity. *Clin Radiol* 2002;57:136–139.
235. Neilson D, Hollman AS. The ultrasonic diagnosis of infantile hypertrophic pyloric stenosis: technique and accuracy. *Clin Radiol* 1994;49:246–247.
236. Miozzari HH, Tonz M, von Vigier RO, et al. Fluid resuscitation in infantile hypertrophic pyloric stenosis. *Acta Paediatr* 2001;90:511–514.
237. Cook-Sather SD, Tulloch HV, Liacouras CA, et al. Gastric fluid volume in infants for pyloromyotomy. *Can J Anaesth* 1997;44:278–283.
238. Karri V, Bouhadiba N, Mathur AB, et al. Pyloromyotomy through circumumbilical incision with fascial extension. *Pediatr Surg Int* 2003;19:695–696.
239. Campbell BT, McLean K, Barnhart DC, et al. A comparison of laparoscopic and open pyloromyotomy at a teaching hospital. *J Pediatr Surg* 37:1068–1071; discussion 1068–1071.
240. Royal RE, Linz DN, Gruppo DL, et al. Repair of mucosal perforation during pyloromyotomy: surgeon's choice. *J Pediatr Surg* 1995;30:1430–1432.
241. Puapong D, Kahng D, Ko A, et al. Ad libitum feeding: safely improving the cost-effectiveness of pyloromyotomy. *J Pediatr Surg* 2002;37:1667–1668.
242. Luciani JL, Allal H, Polliotto S, et al. Prognostic factors of the postoperative vomiting in case of hypertrophic pyloric stenosis. *Eur J Pediatr Surg* 1997;7:93–96.
243. Yagmurlu A, Barnhart DC, Vernon A, et al. Comparison of the incidence of complications in open and laparoscopic pyloromyotomy: a concurrent single institution series. *J Pediatr Surg* 2004;39:292–296; discussion 292–296.
244. Yamataka A, Tsukada K, Yokoyama-Laws Y, et al. Pyloromyotomy versus atropine sulfate for infantile hypertrophic pyloric stenosis. *J Pediatr Surg* 2000;35:338–341; discussion 342.
245. Poon TS, Zhang AL, Cartmill T, et al. Changing patterns of diagnosis and treatment of infantile hypertrophic pyloric stenosis: a clinical audit of 303 patients. *J Pediatr Surg* 1996;31:1611–1615.
246. Wilson R, Kanto WP, McCarthy BJ, Jr., et al. Age at onset of necrotizing enterocolitis: an epidemiologic analysis. *Pediatr Res* 1982;16:82–85.
247. Pumberger W, Mayr M, Kohlhauser C, et al. Spontaneous localized intestinal perforation in very-low-birth-weight infants: a distinct clinical entity different from necrotizing enterocolitis. *J Am Coll Surg* 2002;195:796–803.
248. Hutter JJ, Hathaway WE, Wayne ER, et al. Jr. Hematologic abnormalities in severe neonatal necrotizing enterocolitis. *J Pediatr* 1976;88:1026–1031.
249. Butter A, Flageole H, Laberge JM, et al. The changing face of surgical indications for necrotizing enterocolitis. *J Pediatr Surg* 2002;37:496–499.
250. Frawley G, Bayley G, Chondros P, et al. Laparotomy for necrotizing enterocolitis: intensive care nursery compared with operating theatre. *J Paediatr Child Health* 1999;35:291–295.
251. de Souza JC, da Motta UI, Ketzer CR, et al. Prognostic factors of mortality in newborns with necrotizing enterocolitis submitted to exploratory laparotomy. *J Pediatr Surg* 2001;36:482–486.
252. Chwals WJ, Blakely ML, Cheng A, et al. Surgery-associated complications in necrotizing enterocolitis: a multiinstitutional study. *J Pediatr Surg* 2001;36:1722–1724.
253. Lessin MS, Schwartz DL, Wesselhoeft CW, Jr., et al. Multiple spontaneous small bowel anastomosis in premature infants with multisegmental necrotizing enterocolitis. *J Pediatr Surg* 2000;35:170–172.
254. Chardot C, Rochet JS, Lezeau H, et al. Surgical necrotizing enterocolitis: are intestinal lesions more severe in infants with low birth weight? *J Pediatr Surg* 2003;38:167–172.
255. Ein SH, Shandling B, Wesson D, et al. A 13-year experience with peritoneal drainage under local anesthesia for necrotizing enterocolitis perforation. *J Pediatr Surg* 1990;25:1034–1036; discussion 1036–1037.
256. Dimmitt RA, Meier AH, Skarsgard ED, et al. Salvage laparotomy for failure of peritoneal drainage in necrotizing enterocolitis in infants with extremely low birth weight. *J Pediatr Surg* 2000;35:856–859.
257. Ehrlich PF, Sato TT, Short BL, et al. Outcome of perforated necrotizing enterocolitis in the very low-birth weight neonate may be independent of the type of surgical treatment. *Am Surg* 2001;67:752–756.
258. Cass DL, Brandt ML, Patel DL, et al. Peritoneal drainage as definitive treatment for neonates with isolated intestinal perforation. *J Pediatr Surg* 2000;35:1531–1536.
259. VanderKolk WE, Kurz P, Daniels J, et al. Liver hemorrhage during laparotomy in patients with necrotizing enterocolitis. *J Pediatr Surg* 1996;31:1063–1066; discussion 1066–1067.
260. Pumberger W, Kohlhauser C, Mayr M, et al. Severe liver haemorrhage during laparotomy in very low birthweight infants. [see comment]. *Acta Paediatr* 2002;91:1260–1262.
261. Stringer MD, Brereton RJ, Drake DP, et al. Recurrent necrotizing enterocolitis. *J Pediatr Surg* 1993;28:979.
262. Stevenson DK, Kerner JA, Malachowski N, et al. Late morbidity among survivors of necrotizing enterocolitis. *Pediatrics* 1980;66:925–927.
263. Okuyama H, Kubota A, Oue T, et al. A comparison of the clinical presentation and outcome of focal intestinal perforation and necrotizing enterocolitis in very-low-birth-weight neonates. *Pediatr Surg Int* 2002;18:704–706.
264. Davies BW, Abel G, Puntis JW, et al. Limited ileal resection in infancy: the long-term consequences. *J Pediatr Surg* 1999;34:583–587.
265. Fasoli L, Turi RA, Spitz L, et al. Necrotizing enterocolitis: extent of disease and surgical treatment. *J Pediatr Surg* 1999;34:1096–1099.
266. Sonntag J, Grimmer I, Scholz T, et al. Growth and neurodevelopmental outcome of very low birthweight infants with necrotizing enterocolitis. *Acta Paediatr* 2000;89:528–532.

Surgical Complications in Children

James D. Geiger

THORACIC SURGERY 764
Chest Infections 764
Respiratory Foreign Bodies 767
Pectus Excavatum 768

GASTRIC SURGERY 768
Gastrostomy 768
Gastrocutaneous Fistula 769
Fundoplication 770

SMALL-BOWEL SURGERY 771
Meckel Diverticulum 771
Intussusception 772

COLON SURGERY 774
Appendicitis 774

SURGERY FOR DEFECTS OF THE ABDOMINAL WALL 774
Umbilical Hernia 774
Inguinal Hernia 775

LIVER SURGERY 776
Biliary Atresia 776
Choledochal Cyst 778
Liver Tumors 779

PANCREAS SURGERY 780
Acute Pancreatitis 780
Hyperinsulinism 780

SPLEEN SURGERY 781
Splenectomy 781
Postsplenectomy Sepsis 781
Splenosis 781

REFERENCES 781

James D. Geiger: University of Michigan, Ann Arbor, MI 48109

THORACIC SURGERY

Chest Infections

Although most serious pediatric chest infections are treated medically, several suppurative conditions can lead to surgical complications both in diagnosis and management.

Mediastinitis

Acute mediastinitis follows bacterial and chemical soiling of the mediastinum by perforation of the pharynx, trachea, or esophagus. Perforation usually results from external trauma, surgery, foreign bodies, or instrumentation (1–4). Because the mediastinum offers no anatomic barriers to the spread of infection within it, early diagnosis and treatment is critical to reducing morbidity and mortality.

Acute mediastinitis is usually heralded by a high fever, chest pain, dyspnea, cyanosis, and marked tachycardia and leukocytosis. In neonates, acute mediastinitis may present with more subtle signs of sepsis, such as lethargy, temperature instability, and leukopenia. Radiographs show medistinal emphysema, and crepitation will sometimes be apparent on palpation of the neck or chest wall. If the diagnosis is delayed and sepsis develops, the mortality can be significant, but it is less significant than seen in adults (5).

The management of mediastinitis depends on the etiology and whether there is ongoing contamination or leak into the mediastinum or pleural space. Drainage is essential for an abscess or a continued contamination from an esophageal perforation. The mediastinum can be drained by a cervical, transthoracic, retropleural, or anterior route, depending on the site of ongoing contamination.

Esophageal Perforation

Perforations generally occur in low birth weight premature infants. Typically, a nasogastric tube perforates the hypopharynx and courses along the esophagus until it perforates the mediastinal parietal pleura into a pleural space (6). Tubes terminating in the pericardium and retroperitoneum have been reported. Less commonly, endotracheal tubes or suction catheters can lead to perforation of the pharynx or cervical esophagus.

The diagnosis of perforation is suspected if intubation is difficult or if excessive blood-tinged oropharyngeal secretions are noted. An abnormal course of the nasogastric tube on radiographic examination indicates the presence of the perforation. Pneumomediastinum occurs variably. Esophagram confirms the diagnosis. Delayed diagnosis can lead to systemic sepsis. Diagnostic errors can lead to unnecessary thoracic exploration. Esophageal perforation may be mistaken for esophageal atresia, or the injury may be misinterpreted to be intrathoracic when, in fact, a cervical injury is present (7). Perforation into the pleural space may produce a large tension pneumothorax. When the diagnosis of pharyngoesophageal perforation is made quickly, evacuation of pneumothoraces, antibiotics, gastric decompression, and hyperalimentation are usually adequate therapy with a high rate of survival (8,9). Surgical drainage is rarely necessary for these injuries and is usually reserved for extensive extravasation or an abscess.

Thoracic Esophageal Perforations

Perforations of the thoracic esophagus may follow trauma, endoscopic or dilation procedures, or disruption of an esophageal anastomosis. Most of these perforations are small contained leaks occurring after dilation of an esophageal stricture. Nonoperative treatment is usually effective. If a contrast esophagram demonstrates a contained perforation in the mediastinum with free drainage back into the esophagus, intravenous antibiotics and hyperalimentation with close observation should be adequate therapy (1,5,10). Major perforation of the thoracic esophagus not contained within the mediastinum requires thoracotomy, closure of the perforation site, pleural drainage, and intravenous antibiotics. In some cases esophageal diversion is also required.

Lung Abscess

Lung abscess is primarily a medical disease with surgical implications. There are many causes of lung abscess in children, including bacterial and fungal pneumonias, cystic fibrosis (CF), foreign body aspiration, lung cysts, bronchiectasis, immune deficiencies, sequestration, and chronic granulomatous disease. Aspiration of gastric contents, in children with neurologic deficits or in patients with abnormal esophageal motility such as achalasia or esophageal atresia, is a significant risk factor for the development of aspiration pneumonia and lung abscess.

The initial, and often only, treatment is specific antibiotics with postural drainage and chest physiotherapy (11,12). Whenever possible, a specific bacteriologic diagnosis should be made before treatment. In some cases needle aspiration guided by computed tomography (CT), ultrasound, or bronchoscopy is helpful in the identification of the pathogen and can also provide drainage of the abscess (13,14). Bronchoscopy with removal of an obstructing foreign body can be curative for a distal abscess. The antibiotics of choice depend on the results of Gram stain and culture findings. Empiric antimicrobial therapy should include a penicillinase-resistant agent active against *Staphylococcus aureus* and an agent active against anaerobes. A course of at least 3 weeks is usually indicated. Surgical resection is reserved for the rare patient who does not respond to prolonged antibiotic therapy. This is more likely in a patient with centrally located fungal abscess or multiple abscess, as well as those with an abscess within a congenital lung lesion. In general, anatomic lobectomy is the best approach with the lowest rate of complications (15). In some cases, a segmentectomy or wedge resection may be effective. Endobronchial spill with contralateral lung contamination is a possible and potentially significant complication of thoracotomy for lung abscess or severe pneumonia. Use of a selective bronchial blocker, minimal manipulation of the abscess, and needle aspiration of the abscess once the chest is opened may minimize the morbidity associated with thoracotomy in these circumstances.

Empyema

Pleural effusions and empyemas can complicate up to 20% of bacterial pneumonias. Despite advances in antimicrobial therapy and the use of the pneumococcus conjugate vaccine, several studies have noted an increase in the incidence of empyema as well as an increase in resistant organisms (16). In some studies methicillin-resistant staphylococcus is a frequent pathogen (17).

In addition to antibiotics, multiple treatment modalities exist for pleural effusions and empyemas, including thoracentesis, chest tube drainage, instillation of fibrinolytic therapy into the pleural cavity, and decortication (18,19). In the last 10 years the use of video-assisted thoracic surgery (VATS) has dramatically changed the management of complicated pneumonia (20). The less invasive nature of VATS, as well as the excellent published results, has led to the recommendation of an early surgical approach to drain the pleural space effectively (Fig. 51-1) (21,22). Early thoracoscopic intervention, when compared to a stepwise approach of thoracentesis followed by chest tube placement, appears to lead to excellent outcomes with significantly shorter length of stay (17,23,24). Chest CT is useful for identifying patients with loculated effusions who are more likely to fail a nonsurgical approach. Rarely is open thoracotomy with decortication required.

Bronchiectasis

Bronchiectasis is abnormal dilation of the bronchi and bronchioles associated with chronic suppurative disease of the airways (25). The disease usually develops as a result of bronchial obstruction or of an antecedent infection such as pneumonia. Bronchiectasis is rarer than it was in the 1940s and 1950s, when it ranked as one of the most frequent indications for pulmonary resection in children (26,27). Today most children with bronchiectasis have an underlying congenital pulmonary anomaly, CF, or an immunologic deficiency.

The preferred treatment for bronchiectasis is nonoperative, consisting of antibiotics, postural drainage, and avoidance of inhaled toxins. Pulmonary resection is rarely required except when the disease is discretely localized chronic infection causing contamination of the other lung fields (28,29). The decision to proceed with operation especially in CF patients must be made very carefully as it can be difficult to predict the benefit that lobectomy or segmental resection will provide (28,29).

Cystic Fibrosis

CF is hereditary and transmitted by a mendellian recessive gene, which was cloned and characterized in 1989 (30). There has been dramatic improvement in the medical management of the complications of CF. The median survival is now well over 30 years of age compared to less than a year when the disorder was first described in 1938 (31). Progressive infection and inflammation in the lower airways continue to limit the length and quality of life for most patients with CF and often leads to a number of pulmonary complications. Infection with an active host inflammatory response is present in CF airways from early in life. Infection is commonly caused by *S. aureus, Hemophilus influenzae, Pseudomonas aeruginosa,* and *Burkholderia cepacia*. Airway obstruction with viscous secretions is characteristic of CF and is the primary factor in perpetuating infection and inflammation. The course of the lung disease is inexorably progressive, although the rate of progression is variable depending on a number of factors, including genotype, nutritional status, exposure to environmental toxins, exposure to secondhand smoke, and aerobic activity (32,33). The earliest chest radiographic

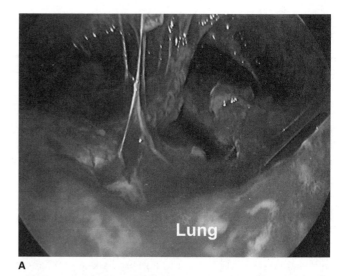

A

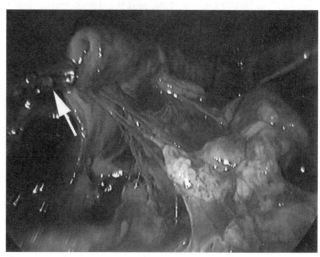

B

Figure 51-1 A: Thoracoscopic view of fibronous empyema. **B:** Atraumatic grasper (*arrow*) removing the fibronous peel and breaking down adhesions.

abnormality is hyperinflation, often with right upper lobe mucous retention (34). This progresses to widespread bronchial dilation, cyst, linear shadows, and infiltrates. The clinical course is marked by episodic exacerbations of the pulmonary infection and inflammation treated with antibiotic therapy, postural drainage, and physiotherapy. With intense oral and often intravenous antibiotic therapy, as well as the intense airway clearance therapy, the length and frequency of these pulmonary exacerbations can be decreased. This in turn should delay scarring and loss of pulmonary function (35,36).

Pneumothorax occurs in 5% to 8% of patients with CF (37). It is one of the two acutely life-threatening complications of CF lung disease (hemoptysis is the other). Pneumothorax is more common in older patients with more severe lung disease. Patients present with sudden onset of chest pain and dyspnea; however, both the exam and initial x-ray may not be very impressive as the stiff CF lung may resist collapse. Simple tube thoracostomy is adequate treatment for most pneumothoraces, but the rate of recurrence is high. The definitive treatment, both for prompt resolution and prevention, involves ablating the pleural space with chemical pleurodesis or surgical pleurectomy and manual pleural abrasion (37). Unfortunately, these ablative procedures may make future lung transplantation more difficult. Thoracoscopy is a very reasonable approach for this group of patients. In some cases oversewing or resection of surgical blebs is required to control a persistent air leak. Less commonly, a pulmonary resection may be needed. Minor hemoptysis with streaks of blood mixed in with expectorated mucous is common, especially in adults. Massive hemoptysis (300 to 500 mL in 24 hours) is less common [5% in one large series (38)]. Minor hemoptysis needs little attention beyond reassurance and treatment as for pulmonary exacerbation. Some patients benefit from additional vitamin K and stopping drugs that might interfere with clotting. Major hemoptysis may be self-limited, but careful monitoring in the hospital is essential and transfusion may be required. If massive hemoptysis is persistent, bronchial artery embolization may be required (39).

Despite the advances in management, CF patients ultimately develop progressive respiratory failure. Lung transplantation is an acceptable approach to irreversible respiratory failure, with either cadaveric or living lobar transplants. The outcome for lung transplantation is improving, with 5-year survival rates approaching 70% in a number of series (40,41).

Respiratory Foreign Bodies

Foreign body aspiration is a common and serious problem among children, accounting for 7% of lethal accidents in children aged 1 to 3 years (42). Foreign body aspiration may result in either airway compromise and death or serious sequelae such as recurrent pulmonary infection, atelectasis, and bronchiectasis (43). Early diagnosis and removal of the foreign body is critical to preventing complications (44). However, diagnosis can be delayed due to poor history and nonspecific findings on physical exam and chest x-ray. Lateral decubitus chest radiographs can at times be helpful in showing hyperinflation associated with a radiolucent foreign body. However, because of the risks of overlooked foreign body aspiration there should be a low threshold to proceeding with bronchoscopy for both diagnosis and treatment (Fig. 51-2) (45).

Patients with chronic respiratory tract foreign bodies may present with a recent diagnosis of asthma, fever, hemoptysis, pneumonia, or pulmonary abscess. This group of patients should be considered for diagnostic bronchoscopy (46). When there is a relatively low suspicion for aspirated foreign body, flexible bronchoscopy can be completed. When there is a high suspicion, rigid bronchoscopy is useful due to the

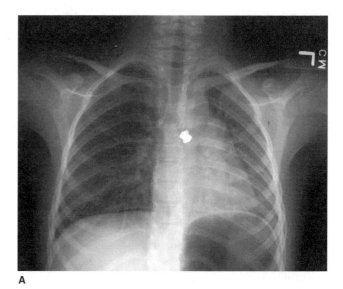

A

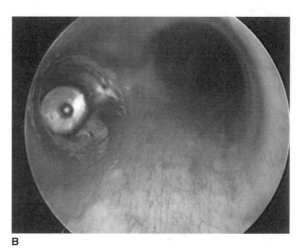

B

Figure 51-2 A: Chest x-ray showing aspirated metallic foreign body in left mainstem bronchus. **B:** Rigid bronchoscopic view of the foreign body obstructing the left mainstem bronchus.

broader array of instruments available for the removal of even difficult foreign bodies.

Complications of bronchoscopy are more common in patients with chronic foreign bodies due to the development of granulation tissue, stenosis, pneumonia, and bronchiectasis. Some patients who have bronchoscopies without identifying a foreign body may have a worsening of their symptoms following the procedure due to exacerbation of an underlying infectious process. It is important that these patients are watched closely in the recovery room and admission considered if there are any persistent postprocedure respiratory symptoms. The rigid bronchoscope provides a protective sheath for the removal of many sharp foreign bodies. Pneumothorax and airway laceration are relatively uncommon complications (47).

When aspiration of peanuts is suspected, early bronchoscopy is critical for a good outcome. Peanuts that have been in the airway for some time become softer and an inflammatory reaction is initiated, making removal quite difficult (48). Fogarty catheters and ureteral stone baskets may facilitate removal of difficult foreign bodies.

Pectus Excavatum

Pectus chest deformities are among the most common major congenital anomalies, occurring in approximately 1 in every 400 births (49). Pectus excavatum is commonly recognized during the first year of life. It is frequently asymptomatic until adolescent skeletal growth occurs and the deformity becomes much more severe (50). There is some evidence to indicate that pectus excavatum deformities cause physiologic impairment and limitations, and there is little controversy that the defects can lead to adverse cosmetic and psychological affects (51–53).

Until recently most surgeons performed a small number of pectus operations for pectus excavatum each year, primarily using modifications of the operation popularized by Ravitch (54), Welch (55), Haller (56), and others. With the advent of the Nuss procedure first reported in 1998 (57), the number of pectus operations has significantly increased because of the reported lower morbidity, an easier-to-complete operation, and excellent outcomes of the Nuss procedure. These two approaches accomplish the pectus excavatum repair in quite a different manner and therefore have a different pattern of complications.

Complications of the Ravitch Procedure

Although a number of variations of the operative technique have been reported, the major concepts are: (i) resection of deformed costal cartilages with preservation of the perichondral sheaths, (ii) wedge anterior sternal osteotomy with elevation of the lower sternum to the desired level, and (iii) some type of internal or external fixation to support the sternum. Early complications following the Ravitch procedure are limited and generally include wound infection, pneumothorax, and pleural effusion (58,59). Most pneumothoraces can be observed unless there is associated pulmonary compromise. Recurrence of the pectus deformity has been reported in up to 5% of patients and appears to be more common in those who do not have at least temporary internal fixation of the sternum (60). Delaying repair until at least 10 years of age should minimize the extent of remodeling of the chest that occurs with growth. Marfan patients have a higher risk of recurrence and long-term internal fixation should be considered.

Acquired Jeune disease (acquired thoracic chondrodystrophy syndrome) occurs when too extensive resection of the costal cartilages leads to failure of subsequent chest wall growth (60). Although this can occur at any age, children who undergo pectus repair at younger ages seem to be at greater risk. Hypertrophic scar formation in the anterior chest incision can compromise an otherwise excellent cosmetic result. Minimizing trauma to the skin flaps and

antiscar measures in the postoperative period can prevent this complication. In some instances excision of the hypertrophic scar is needed. Other complications, including a floating sternum and migration of the substernal fixation device, can occur (61,62).

Complications of the Nuss Procedure

Many pediatric surgeons now repair most pectus excavatum defects with the Nuss procedure. This procedure, which is less invasive, avoids an anterior chest incision, cartilage resection, and sternal osteotomy by placing a carefully preformed, convex steel bar under the sternum through bilateral thoracic incisions (57). Early respiratory complications, such as pneumothorax and pleural effusion, appear to occur at a similar rate as in the Ravitch procedure (63,64). Modification of the Nuss procedure with use of thoracoscopy to guide dissection of the anterior mediastinum and placement of the bar should significantly reduce the risk of cardiac perforation seen very early in the experience with this procedure when the dissection of the mediastinum was completed blindly (65). Pericarditis and pericardial fusion has been reported but in general do not require intervention. Wound infection occurs in 2% to 3% of patients and may necessitate bar removal (66). Bar displacement occurs in 5% to 10% of patients, and a number of techniques to reduce this complication have now been described (67,68). Our preference is to use heavy-gauge sternal wire placed around a rib to secure the bar (Fig. 51-3). Although postoperative pain is significant with both approaches, necessitating epidural pain management, patients undergoing the Nuss procedure require longer courses of oral narcotics, and in some cases the severe pain leads to early bar removal. The recurrence rate appears to be under 10% and can be decreased by keeping the bar in place for a total of 3 years (65). The outcome of patients with severe asymmetric defects has been less satisfactory with the Nuss procedure, requiring either significant modifications or completion of a later Ravitch-type procedure. Other less common complications include allergic reactions to the bar (69), scoliosis, secondary rib deformities due to the bar (70), and extraosseous bone formation (71), which may make bar removal more difficult.

GASTRIC SURGERY

Gastrostomy

Gastrostomy is a procedure used frequently in the care of pediatric surgical patients. Depending on the clinical variables, gastrostomy tube placement can be accomplished with an open laparotomy, a percutaneous endoscopic approach, or a laparoscopic approach. As the indications for placement of gastrostomy tubes have broadened, the procedure is being completed on patients with significant

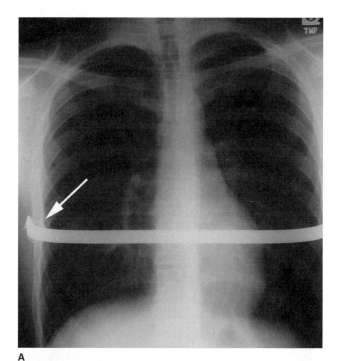

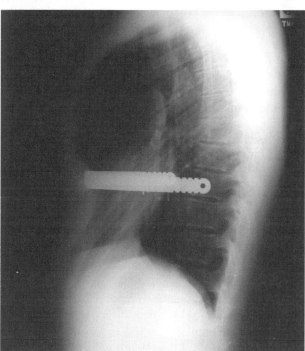

Figure 51-3 Anterior-posterior (**A**) and lateral (**B**) chest x-rays demonstrate Nuss bar position and use of heavy-gauge sternal wires around a rib for fixation (*arrow*).

comorbidities. Despite this, the complication rate overall is fairly low, but when complications do occur they can lead to significant morbidity and even mortality (72). Minor complications such as gastrostomy site infections, granulation tissue, and leakage occur in a significant percentage of patients and postoperative care is important in preventing these problems (73).

Location of the gastrostomy tube on the abdominal wall is important and requires planning. During percutaneous endoscopic gastrostomy (PEG) or laparoscopic gastrostomy placement, it is important to mark the costal margin with a marking pen before insufflation of the stomach or abdomen is initiated. If this step is not completed, especially in small children, the gastrostomy tube may end up right on the costal margin, leading to significant gastrostomy site complications and the need to be repositioned.

Accurate placement of the gastrostomy tube into the stomach is not always straightforward, even in open surgery, and especially in neonates with pure esophageal atresia who have microgastria. In addition, PEG tube placement can lead to a development of gastroenteric, most commonly gastrocolic, fistulas in up to 3% of patients (74). Abnormal anatomy or previous surgery may contribute to this complication, and in this group of patients a laparoscopic or laparoscopic-assisted approach is warranted. The diagnosis of a gastroenteric fistula following a PEG can be difficult and is often delayed (75). This problem often becomes apparent at the time of the first gastrostomy tube change.

A common complication of gastrostomy is inadvertent removal by either the patient or the treating medical personnel. If the tube was placed with an open or laparoscopic approach that included tacking sutures of the stomach to the posterior fascia, then replacement of the tube by an appropriately trained person may be possible, but correct tube placement should be confirmed with a contrast study. In PEG placement, early dislodgement will require a redo PEG if recognized promptly or potentially a laparoscopic or open procedure if significant abdominal contamination has occurred. In chronically placed gastrostomy tubes, family members and caregivers can be trained in tube replacement. This should be done rapidly because the gastrostomy stoma can close quickly. A smaller tube, such as a Foley catheter, can be placed until a new gastrostomy tube can be inserted.

In some patients significant leakage from the gastrostomy site leading to enlargement of the gastrostomy wound and prolapse of gastric mucosa occurs. Delayed gastric emptying and increased intra-abdominal pressure, as in cerebral palsy patients with severe spasticity, increases the risk of this complication (73). In many patients this can be managed by discontinuation of the gastrostomy tube for at least 24 hours to allow the stoma to close partially. A larger balloon catheter may also be of help in sealing the leak and allowing the site to heal. A number of topical agents may assist in protecting the skin and stimulating healing of the site. In difficult cases the gastrostomy tube can be converted to a gastrojejunal feeding tube. If this is unsuccessful, this site can be surgically revised (76).

Gastrocutaneous Fistula

When a patient no longer requires a gastrostomy, the tube is discontinued. Closure of the gastrostomy site occurs spontaneously in the majority of patients. In 20% to 40% a persistent gastrocutaneous fistula develops (77–79). The most important factor predisposing to the persistence of a gastrocutaneous fistula appears to be the length of time the tube was in place before removal. Local measures, such as cautery of the epithelialized track, occlusive wound dressings, and installation of fibrin glue, may facilitate closure of a gastrocutaneous fistula in some patients (80). A significant percentage of patients with a persistent gastrocutaneous fistula requires surgical closure. The gastrocutaneous fistula is mobilized and the stomach is closed separately from the facial closure.

Fundoplication

Gastroesophageal reflux disease (GERD) is a relatively benign condition in the younger infant. Most patients improve, at least symptomatically, during the first 18 months of life. In older children and adults, GERD is often a chronic disease, unlikely to resolve spontaneously. Some children, such as those with neurologic disorders or chronic pulmonary disease, are at particular risk for complications of poorly controlled GERD. In fact, in some patients GERD may be the primary agent inducing respiratory disease such as asthma (81). In some infants it may be a cause of sudden death (82). Medical treatment of GERD has traditionally involved administration of antisecretory and prokinetic agents (83). Proton pump inhibitors, widely used in children for the past few years, are effective in treating esophagitis. The loss of the use of cisapride has significantly depleted the armamentarium of prokinetic agents. Therefore the management of other complications of reflux, including pulmonary aspiration of gastric contents (with subsequent pneumonia and reactive airway disease), apparent life-threatening events, and failure to thrive, may necessitate antireflux surgery.

The development of minimally invasive (laparoscopic) fundoplication has recently increased the number of referrals for antireflux surgeries (84). Fundoplication remains one of the three most common major surgical procedures performed in infants and children by pediatric surgeons in the United States. In many studies fundoplication has been shown to be highly effective in preventing reflux, emesis, and many of the complications associated with GERD. However, due to the alteration of the gastroesophageal anatomy and function antireflux surgery may lead to a variety of side effects or complications. The Nissen fundoplication, either laparoscopic or open, is the most common procedure, but some surgeons prefer partial fundoplication such as the Thal fundoplication. In all procedures fundoplication is designed to prevent GERD by correcting hiatal herniation, lengthening the intra-abdominal portion of the esophagus, tightening the crura, and increasing the pressure at the level of the lower esophageal sphincter (LES). Fundoplication is successful in abolishing GERD symptoms in 80% to 90% of patients

in long-term follow-up studies (85). However, both short and long-term complications occur and can at times be very difficult to manage.

Immediate complications of a primary laparoscopic fundoplication should be very rare events. In general, patients undergoing Nissen fundoplication have a short length of stay, often <48 hours.

Erroneous diagnosis of GERD may cause failure of fundoplication to improve preoperative symptoms. Conditions commonly mimicking GERD and associated with a high incidence of problems after surgery include cyclic vomiting, rumination, gastroparesis, and eosinophilic esophagitis. It is critical that these conditions are considered before surgery (86).

Side effects directly related to antireflux surgery include dysphagia due to a tight fundoplication, herniation of the wrap through the hiatus, development of a periesophageal hernia, or a small-bowel obstruction from adhesions (87).

Dysphagia

Dysphagia is a common problem in the early postoperative period (88). This is especially true in toddlers, who often take longer to adjust to the fundoplication. This early dysphagia, which is most likely made worse by the edema and inflammation associated with the normal healing process, resolves over the first few months in the vast majority of patients. In <15% of patients dysphagia is persistent due to a tight fundoplication or overzealous closure of the hiatus. In this group esophageal dilation may improve symptoms dramatically without compromising the fundoplication. The dilation should not be performed before 8 weeks postoperatively. In some patients persistent dysphagia necessitates revision of the fundoplication.

Gas-bloat Syndrome

Dyspeptic symptoms such as fullness, early satiety, abdominal pain, and bloating occur in a significant number of patients after antireflux surgery. The "gas-bloat syndrome" may impair the symptomatic success of antireflux surgery. Patients with severe gas-bloat syndrome suffer episodes of retching and abdominal pain. The use of a venting gastrostomy is often helpful but may not relieve the symptoms completely. Patients with abnormal motility leading to delayed gastric emptying, impaired gastric accommodation, or gastric hypersensitivity are at increased risk for development of gas-bloat syndrome (89). Many pediatric surgeons use preoperative emptying studies to determine if a patient is at risk for gas-bloat syndrome, adding a pyloromyotomy or pyloroplasty to the antireflux procedure in children with delayed gastric emptying. Although some studies have demonstrated a benefit of this approach (90,91), other series have reached different conclusions (92). It is well established that fundoplication improves the emptying of liquids. Gastric emptying scintiscans showing delay in emptying of a liquid meal are probably not the best indication for a drainage procedure, and use of solid phase emptying maybe more helpful. The treatment of gas-bloat symptoms is challenging, and there are no controlled studies evaluating the different pharmacological interventions available to treat these symptoms. Prokinetic agents such as metoclopramide, erythromycin, and octreotide have been used to treat gas-bloat symptoms. Metoclopramide is often the first prokinetic agent used, but the high prevalence of central nervous system side effects limits its use. New prokinetic agents are needed. Anticholinergics, tricyclic antidepressants, and antagonist to $5HT_3$ receptors, such as ondansetron, may have some efficacy due to their effect on gastric hypersensitivity. Patients with severe gas-bloat syndrome and a gastrostomy tube in place may benefit from conversion of the gastrostomy to a gastrojejunal feeding tube. In patients who have failed multiple fundoplications and still have chronic problems, esophagogastric dissociation with a Roux-en-Y esophagojejunostomy may be an option (93,94). Dumping syndrome, characterized by postprandial nausea, retching, diaphoresis, diarrhea, and wide swings in serum glucose have been reported to occur in up to 30% of children who undergo fundoplication (95). When suspected, dumping syndrome should be evaluated with a glucose tolerance test and treated with small feedings of complex carbohydrates.

Anatomic Failure

Anatomic or physiologic failure of Nissen fundoplication occurs in 2% to 25% of patients and is more frequent in those with neurologic conditions. Herniation of the fundoplication into the hiatus is the most common cause of anatomic failure and occurs at a higher frequency after laparoscopic approaches (96,97) (Fig. 51-4). Meticulous closure of the esophageal hiatus by crural approximation and securing the fundoplication by suturing the wrap to the crus or securing the intra-abdominal esophagus to the crura may help prevent a wrap migration. If only a small portion of the fundoplication is herniated, the wrap may still be functional and revision may not be needed. Loosening or complete breakdown of a fundoplication can occur and is more common in patients with repeated retching and delayed gastric emptying. When a fundoplication still appears anatomically intact on upper gastrointestinal (GI) study, the decision to complete a redo fundoplication is much more complex and definitive evidence of recurrent reflux by pH monitoring is required (87).

SMALL-BOWEL SURGERY

Meckel Diverticulum

Meckel diverticulum is the most common congenital anomaly of the GI tract, with an incidence of approximately 2%

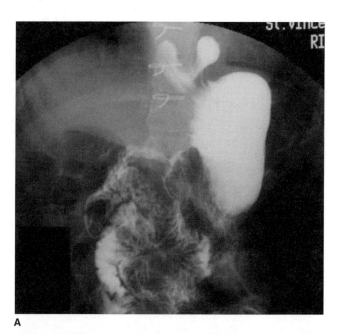

A

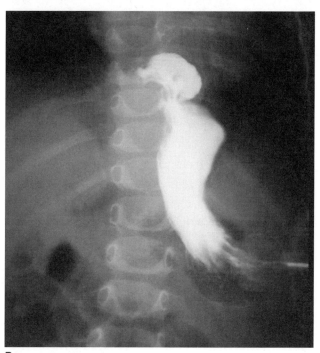

B

Figure 51-4 A and **B:** Upper gastrointestinal contrast studies showing transdiaphragmatic herniation after laparoscopic Nissen fundoplication.

(98). Although the incidence in asymptomatic patients is nearly equal in men and women, the symptomatic form occurs more frequently in men. Meckel diverticulum is a remnant of the omphalomesenteric duct, which normally should regress between the fifth and seventh weeks of fetal life. Complications of a Meckel diverticulum are obstruction, inflammation, perforation, or hemorrhage (99). The "rule of two" is often quoted in regard to Meckel diverticulum: 2% incidence, two types of heterotopic mucosa (gastric

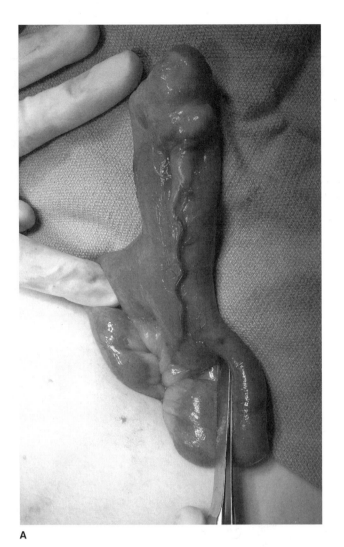

A

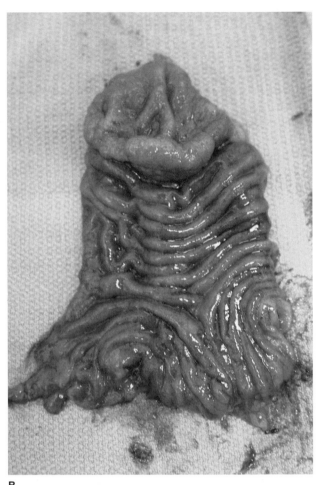

B

Figure 51-5   **A:** Operative photos of bleeding Meckel diverticulum. **B:** Opened Meckel demonstrates gastric mucosa in tip of diverticulum.

and pancreatic) (Fig. 51-5), located within 2 feet of the ileocecal value, about 2 inches in length (and 2 cm in diameter), and usually symptomatic before 2 years of age. However, one detailed population study demonstrated a lifetime risk of developing complications from a Meckel diverticulum at 6.4% and found that the risks were similar throughout all age groups (100).

The most common clinical presentations of Meckel diverticulum are lower GI bleeding, intestinal obstruction (usually due to intussusception or volvulus) (101), and inflammatory complications (99). In the case of lower GI hemorrhage, a technetium-pertechnetate or Meckel scan is often used to demonstrate ectopic gastric mucosa in the Meckel. However, in a significant percentage of cases diagnostic laparoscopy may ultimately be needed to evaluate for a bleeding Meckel diverticulum (102,103).

Laparoscopy or a combination of laparoscopy and minilaparotomy can be used to manage most of the complications of Meckel diverticulum (102,104). Whether an

open resection with transverse suture closure or a mechanical stapling device is used, resection should be accomplished with a very low rate of complications. Anastomotic leak, partial obstruction due to narrowing of the ileum, bowel obstruction, or persistent GI bleeding are the major complications (105,106).

In general, when an asymptomatic Meckel diverticulum is identified, resection should be performed, especially in younger patients who have a greater chance of developing complications (100,105,107). Resection in asymptomatic patients can be accomplished with very low morbidity, however. If the patient has abnormal bowel or distal obstruction, resection may not be prudent.

Intussusception

Ileocolic intussusception is the most common form of intussusception of the intestine, classically occurring at 4 to 12 months of age (108,109). The diagnosis is often unsuspected and confused with other entities. Frequently, the infant may present with severe lethargy, obtundation, and nonspecific complaints, and a workup for sepsis or meningitis is undertaken without considering the possibility of intussusception (110,111). The classic history includes awakening from sleep with severe spasms of pain during which the knees are drawn up onto the abdomen. The child recovers between spasm episodes, but then the pain recurs, eventually followed by vomiting and the passage of bloody mucous per rectum. Infants with unrecognized intussusception may go on to develop severe hypovolemic shock and intestinal ischemia. Before diagnostic evaluation begins, patients must be adequately rehydrated with intravenous fluids. Intravenous antibiotics are important prior to attempts at hydrostatic or air reduction of the intussusception (111).

Contrast enema or ultrasound is often used in the diagnosis of intussusception (112). Once intussusception is identified, nonoperative treatment using controlled hydrostatic reduction or air enema has a success rate of 85% to 90% (113) (Fig. 51-6). Contraindications to attempted enema reduction include clinical evidence of hypovolemia, shock, peritonitis, or radiographic evidence of perforation with free air. Patients with severe hypovolemia may be rehydrated and then undergo an attempt at reduction by enema. There are factors such as younger age, rectal bleeding, radiographic signs of intestinal obstruction, or longer duration of signs and symptoms that decrease the success rate of reduction. However, successful reduction can be achieved in the presence of any of these factors, and none of them preclude an attempted enema reduction if the patient is well hydrated and clinically stable (113).

The success rates of either hydrostatic reduction or pneumatic reduction using fluoroscopy are comparable. The perforation rate is <2% in nearly all the series reported, and many large series have perforation rates less than a half percent (113). Recurrence rates after radiologic reduction average approximately 10% (114,115). Patients who have a lead point such as a Meckel diverticulum have a much lower rate of successful reduction.

Surgery for intussusception has evolved due to the advances in laparoscopic surgery. The conventional approach consists of a right transverse incision positioned just above the umbilicus. The intussusception is reduced by gentle finger pressure on the apex of the intussuscepted intestine in the descending or transverse colon. The intussusceptum should be gently pushed back from the distal end and usually not pulled. If a pathologic lead point is recognized, resection is performed. A number of series indicate that laparoscopy may be a very appropriate initial approach for surgical reduction of classic ileocolic intussusception (116–118). In addition, some authors have reported a combined approach using laparoscopy and pneumatic enema (119). If a pathologic lead point is recognized, resection can be performed.

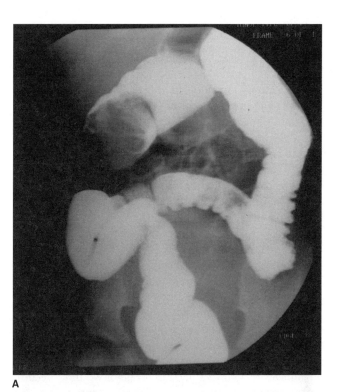

A

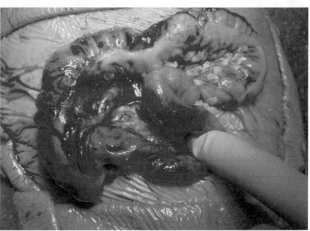

B

Figure 51-6 **A:** Barium enema demonstrates ileocolic intussusception that would not reduce further. **B:** Intraoperative photo shows now reduced ileocolic segment, but a section of bowel was necrotic, requiring resection.

If the intussusception cannot be reduced, the involved segment is resected and a primary end-to-end anastomosis is completed. A decision on whether to remove the appendix at the time of laparotomy or laparoscopy is an arbitrary one, although most surgeons remove it. Feedings are usually started the day after surgery, and patients are discharged from the hospital within 48 hours unless there is a persistent ileus. Immediate postoperative complications are rare, though long-term morbidity related to adhesions has been reported. The current mortality rate in children with intussusception in developed countries is <1% (111).

COLON SURGERY

Appendicitis

Appendectomy is one of the most common surgical procedures performed in children. Due to advances in the therapy of appendicitis, including improved antibiotics, improved imaging both for diagnosis and treatment of complications, and improvement in the surgical techniques, the mortality of appendicitis in the United States is nearly zero. However, perforation rates over the last 70 years remain essentially unchanged (120) and appendicitis continues to lead to significant morbidity. A number of controversies regarding the management of acute appendicitis remain unresolved.

Since the introduction of laparoscopic appendectomy in 1983 by Semm (121), numerous prospective randomized trials have compared laparoscopic and open appendectomies in adult patients (122–124). There have been no true randomized studies of laparoscopic versus open appendectomy in children. Clearly, laparoscopic appendectomy is technically feasible and safe and may offer some advantages related to a decreased rate of wound infection and shorter hospital stays. The complication rate between the two approaches seems to be similar in the retrospective series that have been reported (125–128). In cases where the diagnosis is uncertain, especially in teenage girls, laparoscopy offers the advantage of a complete view of the abdomen, especially the pelvic structures. One somewhat unique complication of the laparoscopic approach is the possibility of completing only a partial appendectomy and leaving an appendiceal stump (129). Care must be given to ensure that the base of the appendix at the cecum is clearly identified before removal of the appendix.

There is a wide range of clinical presentation in children with acute appendicitis, from mild inflammation of the appendix to ruptured appendicitis with diffuse peritonitis or localized abscess formation. The perforation rate varies significantly among different series but is often >50% for children <8 years old (120). There is no consensus on the optimum timing of appendectomy in patients undergoing treatment for a perforated appendix. The complication rate between either early appendectomy or delayed appendectomy does not appear to be dramatically different in the retrospective series that have been reported (120,130–132). The major complications, which are all higher in perforated appendicitis, include intra-abdominal abscess, prolonged ileus, small-bowel obstruction, wound infection, pneumonia, and urinary retention. Intra-abdominal abscess rates range from roughly 1.3% to 7% in pediatric series. Although some surgeons use closed suction drainage following appendectomy for perforated appendix, the utility remains unproven (133–136). Other variations in surgical technique, including the use of an endoscopic bag for removal of the appendix, may help to decrease rates of intra-abdominal abscess and wound infections.

There has been concern that perforated appendix may lead to a higher rate of tubal infertility and ectopic pregnancy in women. This rate has been reported to be from 1.6% to 4.8% (137). However, due to confounding variables and other methodologic weaknesses of these studies, a causal relationship cannot definitively be supported (138). One potential advantage of interval laparoscopic appendectomy is the ability to assess the tubes and complete a tubal lysis if significant scarring is present.

Appendicitis continues to be a major challenge for surgeons in both diagnosis and treatment. Further studies will hopefully resolve some of the controversies and lead to even further lowering of the significant morbidity associated with appendicitis.

SURGERY FOR DEFECTS OF THE ABDOMINAL WALL

Umbilical Hernia

Umbilical hernias are common in infants and young children. The natural history of umbilical hernia is spontaneous closure, usually in the first three years of life (139). African American infants appear to have a high incidence of umbilical hernias and, in particular, large umbilical hernias (140,141). Expectant or nonoperative management is reasonable for the majority with umbilical hernias. Umbilical hernia defects with a small diameter (<1 cm) are more likely to close spontaneously than those with large diameters (>1.5 cm) (142). The incidence of umbilical hernia has been reported to be 18% to 20% in term babies weighing 2,500 g and as high as 84% in premature infants weighing 1,000 to 1,500 g (143). In general, it is common practice to wait until at least approximately 4 to 5 years of age before repairing umbilical hernia, and some defects may even close after 5 years of age (139). Defects >2 cm in diameter or those umbilical hernias that become symptomatic are indications for earlier operative intervention. It is important to distinguish an umbilical hernia from supraumbilical or epigastric hernias, which are caused by defects along the linea alba between the umbilicus and the xiphoid process.

Although the complications of umbilical hernia are believed to be rare (144), the frequency of incarceration and strangulation reported in the literature ranges from 6% to 37% (145–148). The frequency of incarceration appears to be increased for defects measuring 0.5 to 1.5 cm and does not appear to be dramatically different in infants >1 year of age compared to those <1 year of age.

Repair of an umbilical hernia is performed as an outpatient procedure with the patient under general anesthesia. Removal of the hernia sac down to a strong fascial edge and precise placement of interrupted sutures, usually in a transverse orientation, are important principals to reduce postoperative complications. The umbilical skin is tacked to the fascia to create a cosmetically acceptable umbilicus. In some instances, when there is significant redundant skin, this must be excised and a formal umbilicoplasty completed (149,150).

The most common postoperative complications include wound hematoma, which can be reduced with precise hemostasis and a pressure dressing (140). Wound infections are rare but should be treated with early wound drainage to avoid breakdown of the repair. Repair of very large umbilical defects or in patients <1 year of age increase the rate of recurrence. Visceral injuries are extremely rare, especially with an interrupted closure in which all the sutures are tied after placement.

Inguinal Hernia

Inguinal hernia repair is one of the most common general surgery operations performed by pediatric surgeons. The incidence of inguinal hernia in children ranges from 0.8% to 4.4% and is higher in infants, with approximately one-third of hernias occurring in children >6 months of age (151). The incidence is highest in premature infants, with reports ranging from 16% to 25% (152–154). An inguinal hernia does not resolve spontaneously and must be repaired due to the risk of incarceration, particularly during the first few months of life (Fig. 51-7). Sixty-nine percent of incarcerated hernias occur before the age of 1 year, and in these younger patients the hernia is often irreducible (155,156). In most patients elective inguinal hernia repair is done as an outpatient with an extremely low risk of anesthetic complications. Premature infants and older children with cardiac, respiratory, or other disorders that increase the risk of anesthesia often require overnight hospitalization for monitoring (157).

Contralateral Exploration

Among children undergoing hernia repair, there is up to a 30% chance that a hernia will develop on the contralateral side, requiring subsequent repair (158). Routine contralateral exploration, done frequently in the past, is less common today, with surgeons choosing either observation alone or selective exploration based on the use of laparoscopy at the time of the repair of the symptomatic hernia. Those who advocate observation and repair of a metachronous hernia only if it becomes clinically apparent believe the approach leads to lower cost and complications (159,160). The alternative is to use laparoscopy through the symptomatic side hernia sac. The technique has been modified to allow an accurate determination of an open processus vaginalis, which is then repaired (161,162). This approach will identify a patent processus vaginalis in about 20% to 30% of children and can be accomplished rapidly and without complication (163).

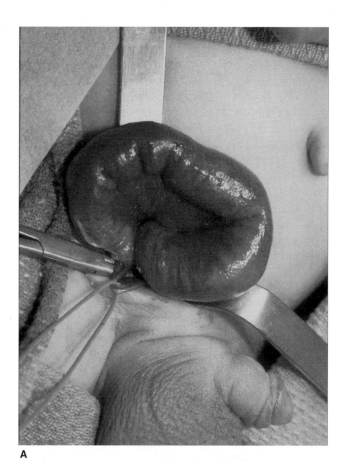

A

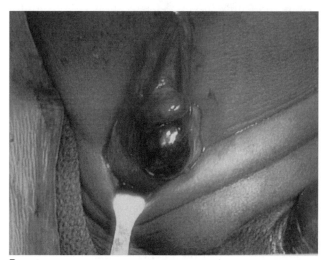

B

Figure 51-7 A: Strangulated bowel due to an incarcerated inguinal hernia in a 4-week-old infant that necessitated resection. **B:** Ischemic testicle in the same patient, which at 3-month follow-up was no longer palpable due to atrophy.

Premature Infants

There is strong evidence of an increased risk of postoperative life-threatening apnea in premature infants after repair of an inguinal hernia (164,165). Our current practice is to admit for overnight observation all premature infants who are <50 weeks postconception age. The timing of repair of inguinal hernia in premature infants when the hernia is recognized before discharge from the hospital is more controversial. Some advocate early repair when the baby is otherwise ready for discharge related to the issues surrounding the prematurity (166). These children are still at risk for significant respiratory complications and may require time on the ventilator postoperatively (167). Others advocate delayed herniorrhaphy when infants are older and have been out of the hospital for some time (168). Delayed surgery must be balanced against the risk of incarceration and development of testicular atrophy (169). Patients with Hunter, Hurler, Ehlers-Danlos, or and Marfan syndromes frequently have inguinal hernias and are prone to recurrence unless the floor of the inguinal canal is repaired in addition to the usual high ligation of the sac. Use of prosthetic material at the initial repair may decrease the rate of recurrence in these high-risk populations.

Cystic Fibrosis

The incidence of inguinal hernia in children with CF is also increased to between 6% and 15% (170). Based on vasectomy studies, the incidence of absent vas deferens in the general population is 0.5% to 1%; however, in CF patients abnormalities of the vas deferens are very common (171). These abnormalities range from obstruction to complete absence of the vas deferens and are usually symmetrical. Failure to identify the vas deferens at operation should, therefore, lead to investigation for CF.

Complications

A number of complications occur following inguinal herniorrhaphy, and nearly all these complications appear to occur at an increased rate in premature infants.

It is difficult to determine the precise incidence of recurrence after repair of an indirect inguinal hernia, but, in general, the reported recurrence rate for uncomplicated hernias is 0% to 0.8% (172–174). The recurrence rate is increased in patients undergoing operations for incarcerated hernia and in premature infants. Most recurrent hernias are indirect and result from not identifying the process vaginalis during the initial operative procedure or due to improper ligation of the sac (174). Some patients will recur with a direct hernia that results from failure to recognize a direct hernia at the initial operation or due to new pathology as a result of damage to the posterior wall during the initial dissection. Injury to the vas deferens can occur by either transection (approximately 25% of vasal injuries) or compression (175). The exact incidence of vas deferens injury is difficult to quantify because this injury is unlikely to be recognized until adulthood and possibly then only if the injury is bilateral. From a number of studies, however, the incidence appears to be approximately 0.8% to 2% (175). Studies of male fertility and hernia sac pathology studies have helped to estimate the incidence of

vas injury (176,177). To reduce the incidence of injury to the vas, it must be identified and protected throughout resection and division of the hernia sac. Crushing of the vas deferens with a clamp or forceps may also lead to permanent injury (178). Minimizing traction on the vas during dissection of the processus vaginalis and careful ligation of the sac also helps to avoid injury. At the completion of inguinal herniorrhaphy, it is routine to palpate the testicles in the scrotum. Oversight of this maneuver can lead to an iatrogenic undescended testicle, which may ultimately require orchiopexy. Some premature infants have a very poorly developed gubernaculum, and, if the testicle does not sit in the scrotum securely, a simple orchiopexy should be considered.

Scrotal swelling is most commonly related to fluid accumulation or postoperative hydrocele and less commonly due to hematoma. In general, postoperative hydrocele can be managed expectantly and resolves spontaneously (179). In some cases aspiration or reoperation is needed.

Testicular atrophy can occur due to operative injury to the testicular vesicles or may occur preoperatively with incarcerated hernias in which the testicular blood supply is compromised by the incarcerated viscus (179–182).

Injury to the bladder can occur during mobilization of the cord structures when dissection is carried medially through the rectus muscle (172,183). The abdominal wall is extremely thin in infants, and the bladder, being mistaken for a hernia sac, can be mobilized in error. If the bladder is entered, the defect should be repaired in layers and decompression of the bladder considered.

Inadvertent trauma to bowel, ovary, or the fallopian tube can occur in the lumen of the hernia sac. This is avoided by opening the sac and inspecting the contents before transecting it if it is not absolutely clear that the hernia sac is empty. Wound infection of inguinal hernias is uncommon and may be minimized by the use of collodion or other tissue adhesive to seal the wound.

LIVER SURGERY

Biliary Atresia

Biliary atresia is the most common neonatal cholestatic disorder, occurring in approximately 1 of 8,000 (Asian countries) to 1 of 15,000 (Western countries) live births, and is characterized by complete fibrotic obliteration of the lumen of all or part of the extrahepatic biliary tree within 3 months of life (184). The etiologic factors and pathogenesis of the obliteration of the biliary tree remain poorly understood (185). In approximately 20% of patients with biliary atresia, the presence of at least one other congenital anomaly suggests that defective development of the bile ducts plays a role in these cases (185,186). The more common form (found in 80% of patients) of biliary atresia is not associated with other congenital anomalies and has been termed the perinatal or acquired form. It is believed that various perinatal or postnatal events trigger progressive injury and fibrosis of a normally developed biliary tree (185,187). Despite these potential disparate etiologies, the clinical phenotype of these two forms of biliary atresia may be identical. The diagnosis of biliary atresia should be considered in any newborn whose jaundice persists after 14 days of age. Conjugated hyperbilirubinemia is present, and the majority of infants develop acholic stools and hepatomegaly. A number of diagnostic tests, including ultrasound, hepatic scintigraphy, and, more recently, magnetic resonance cholangiography, have been used to diagnosis biliary atresia. However, intraoperative cholangiography and liver biopsy definitively establish the diagnose of biliary atresia (188). This can often be accomplished with a laparoscopic-assisted or minilaparotomy approach. Intraoperative cholangiography that fails to demonstrate a lumen in some portion of the extrahepatic biliary tree, surgical findings of a fibrotic, nonpatent bile duct, and characteristic findings on liver and bile duct histology confirm the diagnosis.

Kasai Portoenterostomy

Optimal therapy for patients with biliary atresia is the Kasai procedure, in which a Roux-en-Y loop of jejunum is connected to the portal plate identified during careful dissection of the fibrotic bile duct remnants (189). If performed by an experienced pediatric surgeon, the portoenterostomy yields bile drainage from the liver into the intestinal tract in approximately 70% to 80% of patients, resulting in resolution of the acholic stools and resolution of jaundice (190–192). Although some patients may have excellent bile drainage when undergoing the operation after 120 days of life (193), in general the results both in terms of bile flow and longer term survival are improved if the operation is completed before 90 days of age (190).

Recently there has been an interest in adjuvant medical therapy to enhance liver function and potentially decrease further fibrosis. Immunosuppression with corticosteroids or use of ursodeoxycholic acid to stimulate bile flow and as a cytoprotective agent has been used (194,195). Randomized studies will be needed to definitively prove the benefit of these agents. Antibiotic prophylaxis against cholangitis, as well as supplementation with fat-soluble vitamins, are indicated (196,197). The long-term outcome after the Kasai operation depends on several factors, such as the time of the operation and the extent of liver fibrosis, as well as recurrent bouts of cholangitis (185,190,191,198). If a portoenterostomy is not performed in patients with biliary atresia, 50% to 80% of children will die (without liver transplantation) from biliary atresia by age 1 year and 90% to 100% will die by age 3 years (199,200). Successful portoenterostomy, when performed at 60 to 90 days of age, is associated with a 10-year survival rate ranging from 40% to 60% (190,200). If the portoenterostomy is not successful in establishing bile

flow, survival without liver transplantation is similar to, or worse than, that of patients not undergoing surgery.

Liver transplantation has improved survival in patients with biliary atresia significantly and is indicated for patients with biliary atresia who do not undergo an attempt at portoenterostomy because of delayed diagnosis, those in whom portoenterostomy has failed to reestablish bile flow, and those with decompensated cirrhosis and end-stage liver disease despite initial success of portoenterostomy. Long-term survival after liver transplantation for biliary atresia approaches 80% to 90% (201,202).

Complications

Failure to Achieve Bile Flow. If performed by an experienced pediatric surgeon, the portoenterostomy should yield bile drainage from the liver into the intestinal tract in approximately 70% to 80% of patients (190–192). Whether the operation was technically completed correctly is always a concern in those patients who do not develop good bile flow. However, reoperation in this group of patients has not led to significantly improved outcome, and further adhesions may complicate the later transplant procedure. In general, the only group of patients who may benefit from revision of a hepatic portoenterostomy are those who initially had good bile excretion but in whom the good bile flow suddenly ceases (186,203,204).

Cholangitis. In addition to the common postoperative complications associated with abdominal surgery in infancy, cholangitis is the most frequent and serious complication after portoenterostomy. The reported incidences range from 40% to 60% (196,203,205). The cause of postoperative cholangitis is not entirely clear but is thought to be due to reflux of intestinal contents toward the porta hepatis. Predisposing factors to infection are intrahepatic biliary statis in patients with lower rates of bile flow. Attacks of cholangitis are manifested by fever, decreased quantity of bile, and a progressive increase in serum bilirubin levels. Early postoperative cholangitis may lead to a cessation of bile flow, and repeated attacks may cause a progressive deterioration of hepatic function. Prophylactic antibiotics are helpful in reducing the incidence of cholangitis. For recurrent cholangitis, Neomycin or Ciprofloxacin is beneficial (206,207). A number of modifications to the Roux-en-Y biliary construction have been reported to help prevent cholangitis. In a long-term study recently reported from the Japanese Biliary Atresia Registry (JBAR), complex modifications such as the Roux-en-Y with an intestinal valve and the Suruga-II, in which a total biliary conduit is created and then later restored at a second operation, did not lower the rate of cholangitis compared to the conventional Roux-en-Y procedure (190,208). Ascending cholangitis can develop during or after viral actions related to decreased bile flow and bile stasis. During the first 6 to 12 months after portoenterostomy, most fevers with any evidence of increased liver dysfunction or reduction in stool pigmentation should be treated as if cholangitis is present. In general, broad-spectrum intravenous antibiotics, including anaerobic coverage, are best. If there are no signs of sepsis, intravenous corticosteroid pulse therapy for 5 to 7 days using intravenous methylprednisolone may increase drainage. Patients with persistent or recurring cholangitis can be evaluated with hepatic scintigraphy and ultrasonography to rule out a rare afferent limb obstruction.

Portal Hypertension. A variable degree of hepatic fibrosis is usually present in patients with biliary atresia at the time of initial surgery. In addition, many patients may continue to have some degree of bile stasis and progressive fibrosis ultimately leading to the development of portal hypertension. Portal hypertension may become clinically manifest by the finding of progressive hepatosplenomegaly. Patients can also develop complications of portal hypertension, including GI hemorrhage from esophageal or gastric varices, thrombocytopenia and/or pancytopenia related to hypersplenism, ascites, spontaneous bacterial peritonitis, portosystemic encephalopathy, or portopulmonary syndrome. Significant variceal hemorrhage has been reported in 20% to 60% of patients with biliary atresia (200,205). Patients with variceal hemorrhage are treated with both pharmacologic and endoscopic methods. In some patients splenectomy and portosystemic shunts may be temporizing measures while the patient is being evaluated for liver transplantation (209).

Outcome. The JBAR, a nationwide registry of children with biliary atresia in Japan, recently reported overall 5-year and 10-year survival rates of 75.3% (553 of 734) and 66.7% (72 of 108) (190). A large multicenter review of the outcome of all children diagnosed with biliary atresia in France between 1986 and 1996 evaluated the combined results of portoenterostomy with liver transplantation and found the 10-year survival for 472 patients with biliary atresia was 68%. The 10-year actuarial survival with the native liver after portoenterostomy was 29%, and 5-year survival after liver transplantation was 71%. Prognostic factors predictive of overall 10-year survival were the performance of the portoenterostomy, age at portoenterostomy (survival of 80.4% with surgery at age >45 days vs. 68.5% at <45 days), anatomic pattern of atresia (100% for atresia of the common bile duct vs. only 65.4% for complete extrahepatic atresia), the presence of polysplenia syndrome (48.3% for yes vs. 69.9% for no), and the experience of the center performing the portoenterostomy (54% for ≤2 new patients per year, 59.8% for 3 to 5 per year, and 77.8% for >20 per year). The same factors predicted 5-year and 10-year survival with the native liver after portoenterostomy. In the context of current therapeutic options, 70% to 80% of patients with biliary atresia in North America require liver transplantation during the first two decades of life, despite initial success with portoenterostomy. Consequently, biliary atresia accounts for 40% to 50% of all liver transplants performed in children. The National Institutes of Health has recently funded a

Biliary Atresia Clinical Research Consortium. It is only through such multicentered collaborative approaches that major advances in our understanding of biliary atresia leading to improved outcomes will occur.

Choledochal Cyst

Choledochal cyst is a rare congenital dilation of the bile ducts. The estimated incidence in western countries varies between 1 in 100,000 and 1 in 150,000. The incidence is significantly higher in Asia and occurs more commonly in girls (210). The most widely used subdivision of choledochal cyst is Todani classification (211). Type 1 cysts are the most frequently encountered and maybe caused by an abnormal arrangement of the pancreatic and biliary ducts, also known as "common channel," which occurs in up to 92% of patients with choledochal cyst (212–214) (Fig. 51-8).

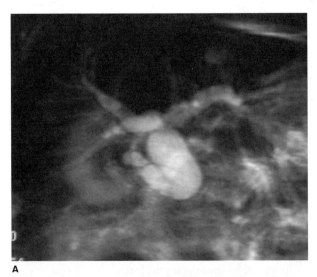

A

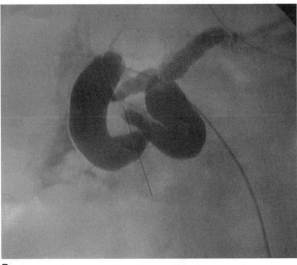

B

Figure 51-8 **A:** Magnetic resonance cholangiopancreatography (MRCP) demonstrates a type I choledochal cyst with excellent correlation with the intraoperative cholangiogram (**B**) in the same patient.

If a choledochal cyst is not resected, a high incidence (20% to 30%) of cholangiocarcinoma has been reported, mainly after the second decade of life (215,216). The incidence of asymptomatic choledochal cyst identified both prenatally and in neonates has increased due to advances in diagnostic imaging (217,218). Choledochal cyst can present at any age; abdominal pain, jaundice, cholangitis, and pancreatitis are frequent presenting symptoms. Early diagnosis followed by cyst excision, and Roux-en-Y reconstruction of the biliary tract is the treatment of choice, even in asymptomatic children. Early complications of complete cyst excision and Roux-en-Y hepatic reconstruction occur at a quite low rate. Biliary leak, Roux-en-Y anastomotic leak, afferent limb obstruction, pancreatitis and/or pancreatic duct injury, and early cholangitis have all been reported (211,219–221).

Long-term complications include cholangitis, and these patients should be evaluated for the possible development of intrahepatic bile duct stones or anastomotic stricture (220–222). Patients who have undergone complete cyst excision may still have an increased risk of development of cholangiocarcinoma at sites distant from the anastomosis, and long-term follow up is necessary (223). Investigators have made recommendations for preventing complications related to Roux-en-Y hepatic-jejunostomy (224). These include completing an end-to-end anastomosis if possible or, if not, minimizing the length of the end of the blind pouch in an end-to-side anastomosis. They recommend that the length of the Roux-en-Y limb be individualized based on the patient's size, as this may lengthen with age, and they recommend a long side-to-side jejunostomy.

Liver Tumors

The most common indication for hepatic resection in children is hepatoblastoma (HB), followed by hepatocellular carcinoma (HCC) and then a number of other malignant and benign conditions, as listed in Table 51-1 (225). There is general agreement that complete surgical resection is the cornerstone of treatment for patients with HB and HCC and the only opportunity for cure (226–228).

Hepatoblastoma

HB occurs most frequently in the first few years of life, whereas HCC usually occurs in older children and adolescents. Historically, only 30% of patients with HB were amenable to primary surgical resection. Currently, with the help of more sophisticated imaging and surgical techniques, the rate is probably closer to 50%. Approximately 50% of the tumors that are unresectable at the time of diagnosis can be made resectable with systemic chemotherapy (227). Cisplatin (CDDP)-based chemotherapy is capable of reducing tumor volume and treating pulmonary metastasis. Thus, roughly 75% of all tumors can be resected completely (229). Orthotopic liver transplantation can augment the percentage of patients who can undergo complete resection of their disease and should be considered early in patients with central tumors involving the portal structures or the hepatic veins or with multifocal disease in both lobes (230). Transplant has not been a formal part of the major cooperative group studies but does appear to significantly improve survival in children with advanced HB (230,231).

Complications of Hepatic Resection

Most of the morbidity and mortality after hepatectomy is related to intraoperative blood loss and transfusion requirements (232). Therefore, control of intraoperative bleeding should be the cornerstone of any strategy for major liver resections—and even in minor resections of centrally located tumors. Improved preoperative imaging with the use of CT 3D-reconstructions of the tumor and vascular anatomy facilitates better preoperative planning (233,234). The use of intraoperative ultrasound is also beneficial for real-time identification of the tumor and hepatic vasculature (235). A number of surgical techniques for vascular control during hepatectomy have been advocated and have led to reduced intraoperative blood loss. The Pringle maneuver, controlling only blood inflow, is effective and offers the advantage of simplicity, but patients are still exposed to the danger of retrograde bleeding from the hepatic veins and inferior vena cava, as well as air embolism. Total hepatic venous exclusion (THVE), consisting of both liver inflow and outflow occlusion, provides a bloodless surgical field during hepatic transaction. However, due to the interruption of inferior vena caval blood flow, it is complicated by hemodynamic instability in 20% to 30% of patients (233,236). Selective hepatic venous exclusion appears to be as effective as THVE for controlling both inflow and outflow, with the advantage of not disturbing IVC patency. This technique involves disconnecting the liver from the retrohepatic IVC and meticulous dissection of the hepatic veins (237). This procedure

TABLE 51-1

INCIDENCE OF PRIMARY HEPATIC TUMORS IN CHILDHOOD

Tumor	Number of Patients	Percent
Hepatoblastoma	532	43
Hepatocellular carcinoma	284	23
Sarcoma	79	6
Benign vascular tumor	166	13
Mesenchymal hamartoma	75	6
Adenoma	22	2
Focal nodular hyperplasia	22	2
Miscellaneous	57	5

Adapted from Weinberg AG, Finegold MJ. Primary hepatic tumors of childhood. *Hum Pathol* 1983;14:512.

is technically demanding and potentially hazardous, especially in children in whom the hepatic veins are short and intraparenchymal.

A number of other technical advances, including new devices for division of the liver parenchyma, local and systemic hemostatic agents, and understanding the effects of liver ischemia, should facilitate further reductions in liver resection morbidity and mortality (233,238). Normal liver parenchyma can safely tolerate continuous normothermic ischemia for as long as 90 minutes and intermittent ischemia for as long as 120 minutes (237). In addition to the major complications of hemorrhage and air embolism, a number of postoperative complications, including bile leak, abscess, pleural effusion, ascites, wound infection, and respiratory complications, have been reported (232). Most of these complications are directly related to the degree of intraoperative blood loss and the difficulty of the hepatic resection. Careful dissection of the bile ducts prior to parenchymal transection may reduce injury to the remaining hepatic duct.

PANCREAS SURGERY

Acute Pancreatitis

Most cases of acute pancreatitis in children result from systemic infection, trauma, choledocholithiasis, anomalies of the pancreatobiliary duct system, and drugs (239). Other causes include idiopathic disease, metabolic disorders, familial pancreatitis, and Crohn disease. Traumatic injury to the pancreas is often related to a direct impact to the epigastrium, such as bicycle handlebar injuries (240). Diagnosis is confirmed by CT or ultrasound, but it is sometimes delayed because of subtle clinical signs. Over 50% of patients develop pseudocysts; however, more than three-fourths resolve without surgery (239–241). Pancreatic transection can occur due to abdominal trauma. Although somewhat controversial, the majority of these patients can be managed without operation (242,243). In patients with pseudocysts that do not resolve with nonoperative management, cystgastrostomy is the most common drainage option (244,245). In some patients, this can be accomplished endoscopically or even with a transgastric laparoscopic approach (246). Roux-en-Y cystojejunostomy may be appropriate for a pancreatic pseudocyst that cannot be approached through the stomach.

The current medical management of pancreatitis is principally supportive, including aggressive hydration, management of metabolic complications and pain, and minimization of pancreatic stimulation by fasting, with nutritional support by parenteral or jejunoenteral feedings. The efficacy of pharmacologic interventions remains largely anecdotal and unproved (239).

Severe pancreatitis progressing to pancreatic necrosis is uncommon. When patients show signs of severe clinical pancreatitis, imaging studies should be obtained to evaluate for areas on pancreatic necrosis that can lead to infection in 30% to 70% of patients. A fine needle aspiration can be used to diagnose infected necrotic pancreatic tissue. If this group of patients does not respond to supportive measures and broad-spectrum antibiotic coverage, then drainage of the infected material may be indicated (247). Surgery for chronic pancreatitis is indicated in a small percentage of patients (248).

Hyperinsulinism

Congenital hyperinsulinism (CHI) is characterized by profound hyperglycemia related to inappropriate insulin secretion. The disease includes focal and diffuse forms, which share a similar presentation but appear to result from different molecular mechanisms (249,250).

The overall incidence of persistent hyperinsulinemia and hyperglycemia of infancy (PHHI) is 1 in 50,000 births; and autosomal recessive inheritance with a risk of 1 in 2,500 has been recognized in Saudi Arabian and Ashkenazi Jewish people (with mutations in SUR gene) (249,251). Untreated or undertreated PHHI leads to almost certain neurologic impairment and often death. Historically, half of the infants surviving treatment for PHHI had neurologic impairment, with increased age at the time of surgery being associated with an increased incidence of neurologic damage. Even those who appear intact have been shown to have impaired head growth (249). It is now well recognized that neonates with CHI may have either diffuse involvement of the pancreatic B cells or focal adenomatous islet cell hyperplasia (252,253). Clinically, these two forms of CHI are indistinguishable. Patients with diffuse disease often require near total pancreatectomy, which has the long-term risk of diabetes mellitus (254). Conversely, babies with focal disease can potentially be cured with a selective partial pancreatectomy with little risk of subsequent diabetes (250,252). A number of diagnostic tests has been evaluated for discriminating between these two forms of CHI, including transhepatic portal venous sampling, selection arterial stimulation with calcium with hepatic venous sampling, and 18-fluoro-dopa positron-emission tomography (PET) scan (250). Patients who are identified to have focal lesions should undergo a surgery without significant delay. Diffuse disease is initially treated medically, but >50% of patients ultimately require surgical resection (250). The current recommendation for diffuse disease is a 95% resection, leaving only a rim of tissue on the duodenum and bile duct. Although a 95% pancreatectomy successfully controls hyperinsulinism in the majority of the infants, it can be associated with major intraoperative and postoperative morbidity (255). This can include hemorrhage, injury to the splenic vein and/or spleen, and bile duct injuries. Inadvertent splenic injuries should be treated by splenorrhaphy if technically feasible to avoid the risk of postsplenectomy sepsis in this young group of patients.

SPLEEN SURGERY

Splenectomy

Splenectomy is a surgical procedure that is indicated for a variety of hematologic disorders, severe hypersplenism, occasionally trauma, and other causes, as indicated in Table 51-2. The laparoscopic approach has been adopted for many of the hematologic indications for splenectomy. Overall, in the retrospective studies reported, the complications of the two approaches seem equivalent. Laparoscopic splenectomy offers improved cosmesis and possibly shorter hospital stays (256–258). Excellent results with a lateral open approach have also been reported, and it is unlikely the two procedures will ever be compared directly (259). Careful dissection of the splenic hilum after complete mobilization of the spleen is required to avoid injury to the pancreas, leading to postoperative pancreatitis and, potentially, pseudocyst formation. Injury to the greater curve of the stomach must be avoided during ligation or coagulation of the short gastric vessels. With preoperative antibiotics and careful attention to hemostasis, the risk of subphrenic abscess is low. When this does occur, it can usually be treated by percutaneous drainage. Accessory spleens are identified in 20% to 30% of patients and should be removed (260,261).

TABLE 51-2

POTENTIAL INDICATIONS FOR SPLENECTOMY IN CHILDREN

Chronic Hemolytic Anemias
Hereditary spherocytosis
Autoimmune hemolytic anemia
Thalassemia intermedia
β-Thalassemia

Chronic Thrombocytopenias
Idiopathic thrombocytopenic purpura
Thrombotic thrombocytopenic purpura

Severe Hypersplenism
Severe cytopenia, pain, splenic infarction
Myeloproliferative disorders
Myeloid metaplasia
Chronic myelogenous leukemia
Congestive splenomegaly (portal hypertension)
Storage diseases (Gaucher)
Parasitic diseases

Primary Malignant Conditions
Splenic lymphoma
Angiosarcoma

Splenic Lesions
Cysts: Post-traumatic, congenital, echnococcal
Hodgkin disease (rarely for staging)

Trauma
Irreparable ruptured spleen
Ruptured spleen with other abdominal trauma requiring operation

---

Postsplenectomy Sepsis

The most lethal complication of splenectomy is postsplenectomy sepsis caused by encapsulated organisms such as *pneumococci*, *Haemophilus influenza*, or *meningococci* (262). In elective hematologic cases, patients should be immunized with *pneumococci*, *haemophilus type B*, and *meningococci* vaccines before splenectomy (263). The duration of postsplenectomy antibiotic prophylaxis using penicillin or an equivalent antibiotic is controversial but should be at least until 5 years of age and for a minimum of 1 year postsplenectomy (263). Many authorities have maintained antibiotic prophylaxis until the age of 18 and then left further prophylaxis at the discretion of the patient and the patient's primary care physician. The incidence of sepsis among postsplenectomy patients is approximately 3% to 4% in large population studies and carries a mortality of approximately 1.5% (262). The incidence of infection is highest among patients with thalassemia major and sickle-cell anemia (262). Critical to the prevention of postsplenectomy infection is the education of parents on the significance of early diagnosis and aggressive treatment of any febrile illnesses (263).

Splenosis

During splenectomy, especially for hematologic diseases, careful attention is needed to avoid parenchymal disruption or spill of splenic tissue. This is especially true in laparoscopic splenectomy when the spleen is placed into a bag intracorporeally before being fragmented and removed. Splenosis, the autotransplantation of splenic tissue, can occur at splenectomy and may lead to recurrent disease (260,264).

REFERENCES

1. Martinez L, Rivas S, Hernandez F, et al. Aggressive conservative treatment of esophageal perforations in children. *J Pediatr Surg* 2003;38(5):685–689.
2. Morzaria S, Walton JM, MacMillan A. Inflicted esophageal perforation. *J Pediatr Surg* 1998;33(6):871–873.
3. Kerschner JE, Beste DJ, Conley SF, et al. Mediastinitis associated with foreign body erosion of the esophagus in children. *Int J Pediatr Otorhinolaryngol* 2001;59(2):89–97.
4. Samad L, Ali M, Ramzi H. Button battery ingestion: hazards of esophageal impaction. *J Pediatr Surg* 1999;34(10):1527–1531.
5. Engum SA, Grosfeld JL, West KW, et al. Improved survival in children with esophageal perforation. *Arch Surg* 1996;131(6):604–610; discussion 611.
6. Clarke TA, Coen RW, Feldman B, et al. Esophageal perforations in premature infants and comments on the diagnosis. *Am J Dis Child* 1980;134(4):367–368.
7. Seefelder C, Elango S, Rosbe KW, et al. Oesophageal perforation presenting as oesophageal atresia in a premature neonate following difficult intubation. *Paediatr Anaesth* 2001;11(1):112–118.
8. Sapin E, Gumpert L, Bonnard A, et al. Iatrogenic pharyngoesophageal perforation in premature infants. *Eur J Pediatr Surg* 2000;10(2):83–87.
9. Nagaraj HS, Mullen P, Groff DB, et al. Iatrogenic perforation of the esophagus in premature infants. *Surgery* 1979;86(4):583–589.

10. Panieri E, Millar AJ, Rode H, et al. Iatrogenic esophageal perforation in children: patterns of injury, presentation, management, and outcome. *J Pediatr Surg* 1996;31(7):890–895.

11. Allewelt M, Schuler P, Bolcskei PL, et al. Study Group on Aspiration Pneumonia. Ampicillin + sulbactam vs clindamycin +/- cephalosporin for the treatment of aspiration pneumonia and primary lung abscess. *Clin Microbiol Infect* 2004 10(2): 163–170.

12. Asher MI, Spier S, Beland M, et al. Primary lung abscess in childhood: the long-term outcome of conservative management. *Am J Dis Child* 1982;136:491–494.

13. Pena Grinan N, Munoz Lucena F, Vargas Romero J, et al. Yield of percutaneous needle lung aspiration in lung abscess. *Chest* 1990;97:69–74.

14. Al-Salem AH, Ali EA. Computed tomography-guided percutaneous needle aspiration of lung abscesses in neonates and children. *Ped Surg Int* 1997;12:417–419.

15. Cowles RA, Lelli JL Jr, Takayasu J, et al. Lung resection in infants and children with pulmonary infections refractory to medical therapy. *J Ped Surg* 2002;37:643–647.

16. Schrag SJ, McGee L, Whitney CG, et al. Emergence of streptococcus pneumoniae with very-high-level resistance to penicillin. *Antimicrob Agents Chemother* 2004;48(8):3016–3023.

17. Schultz KD, Fan LL, Pinsky J, et al. The changing face of pleural empyema in children: epidemiology and management. *Pediatrics* 2004;113(6):1735–1740.

18. Ray TL, Berkenbosch JW, Russo P, et al. Tissue plasminogen activator as an adjuvant therapy for pleural empyema in pediatric patients. *J Intensive Care Med* 2004;19(1):44–50.

19. Wells RG, Havens PL. Intrapleural fibrinolysis for parapneumonic effusion and empyema in children. *Radiology* 2003; 228(2):370–378.

20. Kern JA, Rodgers BM. Thoracoscopy in the management of empyema in children. *J Pediatr Surg* 1993;28(9):1128–1132.

21. Gates RL, Caniano DA, Hayes JR, et al. Does VATS provide optimal treatment of empyema in children? A systematic review. *J Pediatr Surg* 2004;39(3):381–386.

22. Roberts JR. Minimally invasive surgery in the treatment of empyema: intraoperative decision making. *Ann Thorac Surg* 2003;76(1):225–230; discussion 229–230.

23. Hilliard TN, Henderson AJ, Langton Hewer SC. Management of parapneumonic effusion and empyema [see comment]. *Arch Dis Child* 2003;88(10):915–917.

24. Chen LE, Langer JC, Dillon PA, et al. Management of late-stage parapneumonic empyema. *J Pediatr Surg* 2002;37(3):371–374.

25. Eastham KM, Fall AJ, Mitchell L, et al. The need to redefine non-cystic fibrosis bronchiectasis in childhood. *Thorax* 2004;59(4): 324–327.

26. Callahan CW, Redding GJ. Bronchiectasis in children: orphan disease or persistent problem? *Pediatr Pulmonol* 2002;33(6): 492–496.

27. Karakoc GB, Yilmaz M, Altintas DU, et al. Bronchiectasis: still a problem. *Pediatr Pulmonol* 2001;32(2):175–178.

28. Mazieres J, Murris M, Didier A, et al. Limited operation for severe multisegmental bilateral bronchiectasis. *Ann Thorac Surg* 2003; 75(2):382–387.

29. Balkanli K, Genc O, Dakak M, et al. Surgical management of bronchiectasis: analysis and short-term results in 238 patients. *Eur J Cardiothorac Surg* 2003;24(5):699–702.

30. Riordan JR, Rommens JM, Kerem B, et al. Identification of the cystic fibrosis gene: cloning and characterization of complementary DNA. *Science* 1989;245(4922):1066–1073.

31. Doull IJ. Recent advances in cystic fibrosis. *Arch Dis Child* 2001;85(1):62–66.

32. McKone EF, Emerson SS, Edwards KL, et al. Effect of genotype on phenotype and mortality in cystic fibrosis: a retrospective cohort study. *Lancet* 2003;361(9370):1671–1676.

33. Fitzgerald D. Non-compliance in adolescents with chronic lung disease: causative factors and practical approach. *Paediatr Respir Rev* 2001;2(3):260–267.

34. Long FR, Williams RS, Castile RG. Structural airway abnormalities in infants and young children with cystic fibrosis [see comment]. *J Pediatr* 2004;144(2):154–161.

35. McColley SA. Cystic fibrosis lung disease: when does it start, and how can it be prevented? [comment]. *J Pediatr* 2004;145(1):6–7.

36. Wagener JS, Headley AA. Cystic fibrosis: current trends in respiratory care. *Respir Care* 2003;48(3):234–245; discussion 246–247.

37. Flume PA. Pneumothorax in cystic fibrosis. *Chest* 2003;123(1): 217–221.

38. Stern RC, Wood RE, Boat TF, et al. Treatment and prognosis of massive hemoptysis in cystic fibrosis. *Am Rev Respir Dis* 1978; 117(5):825–828.

39. Godfrey S. Pulmonary hemorrhage/hemoptysis in children. *Pediatr Pulmonol* 2004;37(6):476–484.

40. Huddleston CB, Bloch JB, Sweet SC, et al. Lung transplantation in children. *Ann Surg* 2002;236(3):270–276.

41. Aigner C, Jaksch P, Seebacher G, et al. Cystic fibrosis and lung transplantation—determination of the survival benefit. *Wien Klin Wochenschr* 2004;116(9-10):318–321.

42. Rovin JD, Rodgers BM. Pediatric foreign body aspiration. *Pediatr Rev* 2000;21(3):86–90.

43. Vane DW, Pritchard J, Colville CW, et al. Bronchoscopy for aspirated foreign bodies in children. Experience in 131 cases. *Arch Surg* 1988;123(7):885–888.

44. Metrangelo S, Monetti C, Meneghini L, et al. Eight years' experience with foreign-body aspiration in children: what is really important for a timely diagnosis? *J Pediatr Surg* 1999;34(8): 1229–1231.

45. Zerella JT, Dimler M, McGill LC, et al. Foreign body aspiration in children: value of radiography and complications of bronchoscopy. *J Pediatr Surg* 1998;33(11):1651–1654.

46. DeRowe A, Massick D, Beste DJ. Clinical characteristics of aerodigestive foreign bodies in neurologically impaired children. *J Pediatr Otorhinolaryngol* 2002;62(3):243–248.

47. Black RE, Johnson DG, Matlak ME. Bronchoscopic removal of aspirated foreign bodies in children. *J Pediatr Surg* 1994;29(5): 682–684.

48. Tokar B, Ozkan R, Ilhan H. Tracheobronchial foreign bodies in children: importance of accurate history and plain chest radiography in delayed presentation. *Clin Radiol* 2004;59(7): 609–615.

49. Molik KA, Engum SA, Rescorla FJ, et al. Pectus excavatum repair: experience with standard and minimal invasive techniques. *J Pediatr Surg* 2001;36(2):324–328.

50. Daunt SW, Cohen JH, Miller SF. Age-related normal ranges for the Haller index in children. *Pediatr Radiol* 2004;34(4): 326–330.

51. Malek MH, Fonkalsrud EW, Cooper CB. Ventilatory and cardiovascular responses to exercise in patients with pectus excavatum. *Chest* 2003;124(3):870–882.

52. Shamberger RC. Cardiopulmonary effects of anterior chest wall deformities. *Chest Surg Clin N Am* 2000;10(2):245–252, v–vi.

53. Lawson ML, Cash TF, Akers R, et al. A pilot study of the impact of surgical repair on disease-specific quality of life among patients with pectus excavatum. *J Pediatr Surg* 2003;38(6):916–918.

54. Ravitch MM. Operation for correction of pectus excavatum. *Surg Gynecol Obstet* 1958;106(5):619–622.

55. Welch KJ. Satisfactory surgical correction of pectus excavatum deformity in childhood; a limited opportunity. *J Thorac Surg* 1958;36(5):697–713.

56. Haller AJ Jr, Katlic M, Shermeta DW, et al. Operative correction of pectus excavatum: an evolving perspective. *Ann Surg* 1976; 184(5):554–557.

57. Nuss D, Kelly RE Jr, Croitoru DP, et al. A 10-year review of a minimally invasive technique for the correction of pectus excavatum. *J Pediatr Surg* 1998;33(4):545–552.

58. Fonkalsrud EW, Dunn JC, Atkinson JB. Repair of pectus excavatum deformities: 30 years of experience with 375 patients. *Ann Surg* 2000;231(3):443–448.

59. Holcomb GW Jr, Surgical correction of pectus excavatum. *J Pediatr Surg* 1977;12(3):295–302.

60. Colombani PM. Recurrent chest wall anomalies. *Semin Pediatr Surg* 2003;12(2):94–99.

61. Prabhakaran K, Paidas CN, Haller JA, et al. Management of a floating sternum after repair of pectus excavatum. *J Pediatr Surg* 2001;36(1):159–164.

62. Dalrymple-Hay MJ, Calver A, Lea RE, et al. Migration of pectus excavatum correction bar into the left ventricle. *Eur J Cardiothorac Surg* 1997;12(3):507–509.

63. Hosie S, Sitkiewicz T, Petersen C, et al. Minimally invasive repair of pectus excavatum—the Nuss procedure. A European multicentre experience. *Eur J Pediatr Surg* 2002;12(4):235–238.

64. Fonkalsrud EW, Beanes S, Hebra A, et al. Comparison of minimally invasive and modified Ravitch pectus excavatum repair. *J Pediatr Surg* 2002;37(3):413–417.

65. Croitoru DP, Kelly RE Jr, Goretsky MJ, et al. Experience and modification update for the minimally invasive Nuss technique for pectus excavatum repair in 303 patients. *J Pediatr Surg* 2002;37(3):437–445.

66. Watanabe A, Watanabe T, Obama T, et al. The use of a lateral stabilizer increases the incidence of wound trouble following the Nuss procedure. *Ann Thorac Surg* 2004;77(1):296–300.

67. Hebra A, Gauderer MW, Tagge EP, et al. A simple technique for preventing bar displacement with the Nuss repair of pectus excavatum. *J Pediatr Surg* 2001;36(8):1266–1268.

68. Park HJ, Lee SY, Lee CS. Complications associated with the Nuss procedure: analysis of risk factors and suggested measures for prevention of complications. *J Pediatr Surg* 2004;39(3):391–395.

69. Saitoh C, Yamada A, Kosaka K, et al. Allergy to pectus bar for funnel chest. *Plast Reconstr Surg* 2002;110(2):719–721.

70. Niedbala A, Adams M, Boswell WC, et al. Acquired thoracic scoliosis following minimally invasive repair of pectus excavatum. *Am Surg* 2003;69(6):530–533.

71. Ostlie DJ, Marosky JK, Spilde TL, et al. Evaluation of pectus bar position and osseous bone formation. *J Pediatr Surg* 2003;38(6):953–956.

72. Khattak IU, Kimber C, Kiely EM, et al. Percutaneous endoscopic gastrostomy in paediatric practice: complications and outcome. *J Pediatr Surg* 1998;33(1):67–72.

73. Hament JM, Bax NM, van der Zee DC, et al. Complications of percutaneous endoscopic gastrostomy with or without concomitant antireflux surgery in 96 children. *J Pediatr Surg* 2001;36(9):1412–1415.

74. Patwardhan N, McHugh K, Drake D, et al. Gastroenteric fistula complicating percutaneous endoscopic gastrostomy. *J Pediatr Surg* 2004;39(4):561–564.

75. Segal D, Michaud L, Guimber D, et al. Late-onset complications of percutaneous endoscopic gastrostomy in children. *J Pediatr Gastroenterol Nutr* 2001;33(4):495–500.

76. Gauderer MW. A simple technique for correction of severe gastrostomy leakage. *Surg Gynecol Obstet* 1987;165(2):170–172.

77. Gordon JM, Langer JC. Gastrocutaneous fistula in children after removal of gastrostomy tube: incidence and predictive factors. *J Pediatr Surg* 1999;34(9):1345–1346.

78. Davies BW, Watson AR, Coleman JE, et al. Do gastrostomies close spontaneously? A review of the fate of gastrostomies following successful renal transplantation in children. *Pediatr Surg Int* 2001;17(4):326–328.

79. Kobak GE, McClenathan DT, Schurman SJ. Complications of removing percutaneous endoscopic gastrostomy tubes in children. *J Pediatr Gastroenterol Nutr* 2000;30(4):404–407.

80. Gonzalez-Ojeda A, Avalos-Gonzalez J, Mucino-Hernandez MI, et al. Fibrin glue as adjuvant treatment for gastrocutaneous fistula after gastrostomy tube removal. *Endoscopy* 2004;36(4):337–341.

81. Khoshoo V, Le T, Haydel RM Jr, et al. Role of gastroesophageal reflux in older children with persistent asthma. *Chest* 2003;123(4):1008–1013.

82. Jolley SG, Halpern LM, Tunell WP, et al. The risk of sudden infant death from gastroesophageal reflux. *J Pediatr Surg* 1991;26(6):691–696.

83. Orenstein SR. Management of supraesophageal complications of gastroesophageal reflux disease in infants and children. *Am J Med* 2000;108(Suppl 4a):139S–143S.

84. Spechler SJ, Lee E, Ahnen D, et al. Long-term outcome of medical and surgical therapies for gastroesophageal reflux disease: follow-up of a randomized controlled trial. *JAMA* 2001;285(18):2331–2338.

85. Fonkalsrud EW. Nissen fundoplication for gastroesophageal reflux disease in infants and children. *Semin Pediatr Surg* 1998;7(2):110–114.

86. Di Lorenzo C, Orenstein S. Fundoplication: friend or foe? [see comment]. *J Pediatr Gastroenterol Nutr* 2002;34(2):117–124.

87. Dalla Vecchia LK, Grosfeld JL, West KW, et al. Reoperation after Nissen fundoplication in children with gastroesophageal reflux:

88. Contini S, Zinicola R, Bertele A, et al. Dysphagia and clinical outcome after laparoscopic Nissen or Rossetti fundoplication: sequential prospective study. *World J Surg* 2002;26(9):1106–1111.

89. Papasavas PK, Keenan RJ, Yeaney WW, et al. Prediction of postoperative gas bloating after laparoscopic antireflux procedures based on 24-h pH acid reflux pattern [see comment]. *Surg Endosc* 2003;17(3):381–385.

90. Alexander F, Wyllie R, Jirousek K, et al. Delayed gastric emptying affects outcome of Nissen fundoplication in neurologically impaired children. *Surgery* 1997;122(4):690–697; discussion 697–698.

91. Okuyama H, Urao M, Starr GA, et al. A comparison of the efficacy of pyloromyotomy and pyloroplasty in patients with gastroesophageal reflux and delayed gastric emptying. *J Pediatr Surg* 1997;32(2):316–319; discussion 319–320.

92. Johnson DG, Reid BS, Meyers RL, et al. Are scintiscans accurate in the selection of reflux patients for pyloroplasty? *J Pediatr Surg* 1998;33(4):573–579.

93. Bianchi A. Total esophagogastric dissociation: an alternative approach. *J Pediatr Surg* 1997;32(9):1291–1294.

94. Islam S, Teitelbaum DH, Buntain WL, et al. Esophagogastric separation for failed fundoplication in neurologically impaired children. *J Pediatr Surg* 2004;39(3):287–291.

95. Bufler P, Ehringhaus C, Koletzko S. Dumping syndrome: a common problem following Nissen fundoplication in young children. *Pediatr Surg Int* 2001;17(5-6):351–355.

96. Graziano K, Teitelbaum DH, McLean K, et al. Recurrence after laparoscopic and open Nissen fundoplication: a comparison of the mechanisms of failure. *Surg Endosc* 2003;17(5):704–707.

97. Kimber C, Kiely EM, Spitz L. The failure rate of surgery for gastro-oesophageal reflux. *J Pediatr Surg* 1998;33(1):64–66.

98. Ludtke FE, Mende V, Kohler H, et al. Incidence and frequency or complications and management of Meckel's diverticulum. *Surg Gynecol Obstet* 1989;169(6):537–542.

99. St-Vil D, Brandt ML, Panic S, et al. Meckel's diverticulum in children: a 20-year review. *J Pediatr Surg* 1991;26(11):1289–1292.

100. Cullen JJ, Kelly KA, Moir CR, et al. Surgical management of Meckel's diverticulum. An epidemiologic, population-based study [see comment]. *Ann Surg* 1994;220(4):564–568; discussion 568–569.

101. Tashjian DB, Moriarty KP. Laparoscopy for treating a small bowel obstruction due to a Meckel's diverticulum. *JSLS* 2003;7(3):253–255.

102. Swaniker F, Soldes O, Hirschl RB. The utility of technetium 99m pertechnetate scintigraphy in the evaluation of patients with Meckel's diverticulum. *J Pediatr Surg* 1999;34(5):760–764; discussion 765.

103. Lee KH, Yeung CK, Tam YH, et al. Laparascopy for definitive diagnosis and treatment of gastrointestinal bleeding of obscure origin in children. *J Pediatr Surg* 2000;35(9):1291–1293.

104. Kellnar S, Till H, Boehm R. Laparoscopy combined with conventional operative techniques. *Eur J Pediatr Surg* 1999;9(5):294–296.

105. Onen A, Cigdem MK, Ozturk H, et al. When to resect and when not to resect an asymptomatic Meckel's diverticulum: an ongoing challenge. *Pediatr Surg Int* 2003;19(1-2):57–61.

106. Fa-Si-Oen PR, Roumen RM, Croiset van Uchelen FA. Complications and management of Meckel's diverticulum—a review. *Eur J Surg* 1999;165(7):674–678.

107. Matsagas MI, Fatouros M, Koulouras B, et al. Incidence, complications, and management of Meckel's diverticulum. *Arch Surg* 1995;130(2):143–146.

108. Ravitch M. Intussusception. In: Ravitch M, et al., ed. *Pediatric surgery*, Chicago, IL: Year Book Medical Publishers, 1979:992.

109. Murphy TV, Smith PJ, Gargiullo PM, et al. The first rotavirus vaccine and intussusception: epidemiological studies and policy decisions.[see comment]. *J Infect Dis* 2003;187(8):1309–1313.

110. Pumberger W, Dinhobl I, Dremsek P. Altered consciousness and lethargy from compromised intestinal blood flow in children. *Am J Emerg Med* 2004;22(4):307–309.

111. Stringer MD, Pablot SM, Brereton RJ. Paediatric intussusception. *Br J Surg* 1992;79(9):867–876.

112. Daneman A, Alton DJ. Intussusception. Issues and controversies related to diagnosis and reduction. *Radiol Clin North Am* 1996; 34(4):743–756.

113. Daneman A, Navarro O. Intussusception. Part 2: an update on the evolution of management. *Pediatr Radiol* 2004;34(2):97–108; quiz 187. Epub 2003 Nov 21.

114. Ein SH. Recurrent intussusception in children. *J Pediatr Surg* 1975;10(5):751–755.

115. Liu KW, MacCarthy J, Guiney EJ, et al. Intussusception—current trends in management. *Arch Dis Child* 1986;61(1):75–77.

116. Kia K, Mona V, Drongowski R, et al. Laparoscopic vs open surgical approach for intussusception requiring operative intervention. *J Pediatr Surg* 2004;40(1):281–284.

117. van der Laan M, Bax NM, van der Zee DC, et al. The role of laparoscopy in the management of childhood intussusception. *Surg Endosc* 2001;15(4):373–376; Epub 2001 Feb 06.

118. Schier F. Experience with laparoscopy in the treatment of intussusception. *J Pediatr Surg* 1997;32(12):1713–1714.

119. Abasiyanik A, Dasci Z, Yosunkaya A, et al. Laparoscopic-assisted pneumatic reduction of intussusception. *J Pediatr Surg* 1997; 32(8):1147–1148.

120. Hale DA, Molloy M, Pearl RH, et al. Appendectomy: a contemporary appraisal. *Ann Surg* 1997;225(3):252–261.

121. Semm K. Endoscopic appendectomy. *Endoscopy* 1983;15(2): 59–64.

122. Minne L, Varner D, Burnell A, et al. Laparoscopic vs open appendectomy. Prospective randomized study of outcomes. *Arch Surg* 1997;132(7):708–711; discussion 712.

123. Marzouk M, Khater M, Elsadek M, et al. Laparoscopic versus open appendectomy: a prospective comparative study of 227 patients. *Surg Endosc* 2003;17(5):721–724.

124. Sauerland S, Lefering R, Neugebauer E. Laparoscopic versus open surgery for suspected appendicitis. *Cochrane Database Syst Rev* 2004;(4):CD001546.

125. Vernon AH, Georgeson KE, Harmon CM. Pediatric laparoscopic appendectomy for acute appendicitis. *Surg Endosc* 2004;18(1): 75–79.

126. Vegunta RK, Ali A, Wallace LJ, et al. Laparoscopic appendectomy in children: technically feasible and safe in all stages of acute appendicitis. *Am Surg* 2004;70(3):198–201; discussion 201–202.

127. Blakely ML, Spurbeck W, Lakshman S, et al. Current status of laparoscopic appendectomy in children. *Curr Opin Pediatr* 1998; 10(3):315–317.

128. Paya K, Fakhari M, Rauhofer U, et al. Open versus laparoscopic appendectomy in children: a comparison of complications. *JSLS* 2000;4(2):121–124.

129. Erzurum VZ, Kasirajan K, Hashmi M. Stump appendicitis: a case report. *J Laparoendosc Adv Surg Tech A* 1997;7(6):389–391.

130. Bufo AJ, Shah RS, Li MH, et al. Interval appendectomy for perforated appendicitis in children. *J Laparoendosc Adv Surg Tech A* 1998;8(4):209–214.

131. Weiner D, Katz A, Hirschl RB, et al. Interval appendectomy in perforated appendicitis. *Pediatr Surg Int* 1995;10:82–85.

132. Yardeni D, Hirschl RB, Drongowski RA, et al. Delayed versus immediate surgery in acute appendicitis: do we need to operate during the night? *J Pediatr Surg* 2004;39(3):464–469.

133. Meier DE, Guzzetta PC, Barber RG, et al. Perforated appendicitis in children: is there a best treatment? *J Pediatr Surg* 2003;38(10): 1520–1524.

134. Emil S, Laberge JM, Mikhail P, et al. Appendicitis in children: a ten-year update of therapeutic recommendations. *J Pediatr Surg* 2003;38(2):236–242.

135. Curran TJ, Muenchow SK. The treatment of complicated appendicitis in children using peritoneal drainage: results from a public hospital. *J Pediatr Surg* 1993;28(2):204–208.

136. Lund DP, Murphy EU. Management of perforated appendicitis in children: a decade of aggressive treatment. *J Pediatr Surg* 1994;29(8):1130–1133; discussion 1133–1134.

137. Puri P, McGuinness EP, Guiney EJ. Fertility following perforated appendicitis in girls. *J Pediatr Surg* 1989;24(6):547–549.

138. Urbach DR, Cohen MM. Is perforation of the appendix a risk factor for tubal infertility and ectopic pregnancy? An appraisal of the evidence. *Can J Surg* 1999;42(2):101–108.

139. Heifetz CJ, Bilsel ZT, Gaus WW. Observations on the disappearance of umbilical hernias of infancy and childhood. *Surg Gynecol Obstet* 1963;116:469–473.

140. Lassaletta L, Fonkalsrud EW, Tovar JA, et al. The management of umbilicial hernias in infancy and childhood. *J Pediatr Surg* 1975;10(3):405–409.

141. Walker SH. The natural history of umbilical hernia. A six-year follow up of 314 Negro children with this defect. *Clin Pediatr (Phila)* 1967;6(1):29–32.

142. Haller JA Jr, Morgan WW Jr, White JJ, et al. Repair of umbilical hernias in childhood to prevent adult incarceration. *Am Surg* 1971;37(4):245–246.

143. Vohr BR, Rosenfield AG, Oh W. Umbilical hernia in the low-birth-weight infant (<1,500 gm). *J Pediatr* 1977;90(5):807–808.

144. Papagrigoriadis S, Browse DJ, Howard ER. Incarceration of umbilical hernias in children: a rare but important complication. *Pediatr Surg Int* 1998;14(3):231–232.

145. Chatterjee H, Bhat SM. Incarcerated umbilical hernia in children. *J Indian Med Assoc* 1986;84(8):238–239.

146. Keshtgar AS, Griffiths M. Incarceration of umbilical hernia in children: is the trend increasing? *Eur J Pediatr Surg* 2003;13(1): 40–43.

147. Vrsansky P, Bourdelat D. Incarcerated umbilical hernia in children. *Pediatr Surg Int* 1997;12(1):61–62.

148. Golby M. Acute abdominal wall hernias in infants and children. *Am J Surg* 1967;114(6):888–893.

149. Blanchard H, St-Vil D, Carceller A, et al. Repair of the huge umbilical hernia in black children. *J Pediatr Surg* 2000;35(5): 696–698.

150. Ikeda H, Yamamoto H, Fujino J, et al. Umbilicoplasty for large protruding umbilicus accompanying umbilical hernia: a simple and effective technique. *Pediatr Surg Int* 2004;20(2):105–107.

151. Harper RG, Garcia A, Sia C. Inguinal hernia: a common problem of premature infants weighing 1,000 grams or less at birth. *Pediatrics* 1975;56(1):112–115.

152. Rajput A, Gauderer MW, Hack M. Inguinal hernias in very low birth weight infants: incidence and timing of repair. *J Pediatr Surg* 1992;27(10):1322–1324.

153. DeCou JM, Gauderer MW. Inguinal hernia in infants with very low birth weight. *Semin Pediatr Surg* 2000;9(2):84–87.

154. Walsh SZ. The incidence of external hernias in premature infants. *Acta Paediatr* 1962;51:161–164.

155. Rescorla FJ, Grosfeld JL. Inguinal hernia repair in the perinatal period and early infancy: clinical considerations. *J Pediatr Surg* 1984;19(6):832–837.

156. Rowe MI, Clatworthy HW. Incarcerated and strangulated hernias in children. A statistical study of high-risk factors. *Arch Surg* 1970;101(2):136–139.

157. Choi DM, Davis L. Postoperative recovery after inguinal herniotomy in ex-premature infants and the use of caffeine. [comment]. *Br J Anaesth* 2002;88(2):301.

158. Miltenburg DM, Nuchtern JG, Jaksic T, et al. Meta-analysis of the risk of metachronous hernia in infants and children. *Am J Surg* 1997;174(6):741–744.

159. Burd RS, Heffington SH, Teague JL. The optimal approach for management of metachronous hernias in children: a decision analysis. *J Pediatr Surg* 2001;36(8):1190–1195.

160. Chertin B, De Caluwe D, Gajaharan M, et al. Is contralateral exploration necessary in girls with unilateral inguinal hernia? *J Pediatr Surg* 2003;38(5):756–757.

161. Holcomb GW III, Brock JW III, Morgan WM III. Laparoscopic evaluation for a contralateral patent processus vaginalis. *J Pediatr Surg* 1994;29(8):970–973; discussion 974.

162. Geiger JD. Selective laparoscopic probing for a contralateral patent processus vaginalis reduces the need for contralateral exploration in inconclusive cases. *J Pediatr Surg* 2000;35(8): 1151–1154.

163. Holcomb GW III. Diagnostic laparoscopy for congenital inguinal hernia. *Semin Laparosc Surg* 1998;5(1):55–59.

164. Steward DJ. Preterm infants are more prone to complications following minor surgery than are term infants. *Anesthesiology* 1982;56(4):304–306.

165. Liu LM, Cote CJ, Goudsouzian NG, et al. Life-threatening apnea in infants recovering from anesthesia. *Anesthesiology* 1983; 59(6):506–510.

166. Krieger NR, Shochat SJ, McGowan V, et al. Early hernia repair in the premature infant: long-term follow-up. *J Pediatr Surg* 1994;29(8):978–981; discussion 981–982.

167. Gollin G, Bell C, Dubose R, et al. Predictors of postoperative respiratory complications in premature infants after inguinal herniorrhaphy. *J Pediatr Surg* 1993;28(2):244–247.

168. Allen GS, Cox CS, White N Jr, et al. Postoperative respiratory complications in ex-premature infants after inguinal herniorrhaphy. *J Pediatr Surg* 1998;33(7):1095–1098.

169. Coren ME, Madden NP, Haddad M, et al. Incarcerated inguinal hernia in premature babies—a report of two cases. *Acta Paediatrica* 2001;90(4):453–454.

170. Holsclaw DS, Shwachman H. Increased incidence of inguinal hernia, hydrocele, and undescended testicle in males with cystic fibrosis. *Pediatrics* 1971;48(3):442–445.

171. Lukash F, Zwiren GT, Andrews HG. Significance of absent vas deferens at hernia repair in infants and children. *J Pediatr Surg* 1975;10(5):765–769.

172. Tiryaki T, Baskin D, Bulut M. Operative complications of hernia repair in childhood. *Pediatr Surg Int* 1998;13(2-3):160–161.

173. Bronsther B, Abrams MW, Elboim C. Inguinal hernias in children—a study of 1,000 cases and a review of the literature. *J Am Med Womens Assoc* 1972;27(10):522–525, passim.

174. Grosfeld JL, Minnick K, Shedd F, et al. Inguinal hernia in children: factors affecting recurrence in 62 cases. *J Pediatr Surg* 1991;26(3):283–287.

175. Sheynkin YR, Hendin BN, Schlegel PN, et al. Microsurgical repair of iatrogenic injury to the vas deferens. *J Urol* 1998;159(1):139–141.

176. Steigman CK, Sotelo-Avila C, Weber TR. The incidence of spermatic cord structures in inguinal hernia sacs from male children [see comment]. *Am J Surg Pathol* 1999;23(8):880–885.

177. Yavetz H, Harash B, Yogev L, et al. Fertility of men following inguinal hernia repair. *Andrologia* 1991;23(6):443–446.

178. Abasiyanik A, Guvenc H, Yavuzer D, et al. The effect of iatrogenic vas deferens injury on fertility in an experimental rat model. *J Pediatr Surg* 1997;32(8):1144–1146.

179. Davies BW, Fraser N, Najmaldin AS, et al. A prospective study of neonatal inguinal herniotomy: the problem of the postoperative hydrocele. *Pediatr Surg Int* 2003;19(1-2):68–70.

180. Phelps S, Agrawal M. Morbidity after neonatal inguinal herniotomy. *J Pediatr Surg* 1997;32(3):445–447.

181. Puri P, Guiney EJ, O'Donnell B. Inguinal hernia in infants: the fate of the testis following incarceration. *J Pediatr Surg* 1984;19(1):44–46.

182. Walc L, Bass J, Rubin S, et al. Testicular fate after incarcerated hernia repair and/or orchiopexy performed in patients under 6 months of age. *J Pediatr Surg* 1995;30(8):1195–1197.

183. Wantz GE. Complications of inguinal hernial repair. *Surg Clin North Am* 1984;64(2):287–298.

184. Balistreri WF, Grand R, Hoofnagle JH, et al. Biliary atresia: current concepts and research directions. Summary of a symposium. *Hepatology* 1996;23(6):1682–1692.

185. Sokol RJ, Mack C, Narkewicz MR, et al. Pathogenesis and outcome of biliary atresia: current concepts. *J Pediatr Gastroenterol Nutr* 2003;37(1):4–21.

186. Ohi R. Biliary atresia. A surgical perspective. *Clin Liver Dis* 2000;4(4):779–804.

187. Desmet VJ. Congenital diseases of intrahepatic bile ducts: variations on the theme "ductal plate malformation." *Hepatology* 1992;16(4):1069–1083.

188. Zerbini MC, Gallucci SD, Maezono R, et al. Liver biopsy in neonatal cholestasis: a review on statistical grounds. *Mod Pathol* 1997;10(8):793 799.

189. Kasai M, Kimura S, Asakura Y, et al. Surgical treatment of biliary atresia. *J Pediatr Surg* 1968;3:665.

190. Nio M, Ohi R, Miyano T, et al. Five- and 10-year survival rates after surgery for biliary atresia: a report from the Japanese Biliary Atresia Registry. *J Pediatr Surg* 2003;38(7):997–1000.

191. Wildhaber BE, Coran AG, Drongowski RA, et al. The Kasai portoenterostomy for biliary atresia: A review of a 27-year experience with 81 patients. *J Pediatr Surg* 2003;38(10): 1480–1485.

192. Lilly JR, Karrer FM, Hall RJ, et al. The surgery of biliary atresia. *Ann Surg* 1989;210(3):289–294; discussion 294-296.

193. Tagge DU, Tagge EP, Drongowski RA, et al. A long-term experience with biliary atresia. Reassessment of prognostic factors. *Ann Surg* 1991;214(5):590–598.

194. Meyers RL, Book LS, O'Gorman MA, et al. High-dose steroids, ursodeoxycholic acid, and chronic intravenous antibiotics improve bile flow after Kasai procedure in infants with biliary atresia. *J Pediatr Surg* 2003;38(3):406–411.

195. Dillon PW, Owings E, Cilley R, et al. Immunosuppression as adjuvant therapy for biliary atresia. *J Pediatr Surg* 2001;36(1):80–85.

196. Bu LN, Chen HL, Chang CJ, et al. Prophylactic oral antibiotics in prevention of recurrent cholangitis after the Kasai portoenterostomy. *J Pediatr Surg* 2003;38(4):590–593.

197. Rothenberg SS, Schroter GP, Karrer FM, et al. Cholangitis after the Kasai operation for biliary atresia [see comment]. *J Pediatr Surg* 1989;24(8):729–732.

198. Deguchi E, Iwai N, Yanagihara J, et al. Relationship between intraoperative cholangiographic patterns and outcomes in biliary atresia. *Eur J Pediatr Surg* 1998;8(3):146–149.

199. Chardot C, Carton M, Spire-Bendelac N, et al. Is the Kasai operation still indicated in children older than 3 months diagnosed with biliary atresia? *J Pediatr* 2001;138(2):224–228.

200. Karrer FM, Price MR, Bensard DD, et al. Long-term results with the Kasai operation for biliary atresia [see comment]. *Arch Surg* 1996;131(5):493–496.

201. Chardot C, Carton M, Spire-Bendelac N, et al. Prognosis of biliary atresia in the era of liver transplantation: French national study from 1986 to 1996 [see comment]. *Hepatology* 1999;30(3):606–611.

202. Goss JA, Shackleton CR, Swenson K, et al. Orthotopic liver transplantation for congenital biliary atresia. An 11-year, single-center experience. *Ann Surg* 1996;224(3):276–284; discussion 284-287.

203. Grosfeld JL, Fitzgerald JF, Predaina R, et al. The efficacy of hepatoportoenterostomy in biliary atresia. *Surgery* 1989;106(4):692–700; discussion 700–701.

204. Chiba T. Problems involved in re-laparotomy for congenital biliary atresia: with special reference to postoperative ascending cholangitis. *Z Kinderchir* 1988;43(2):95–98.

205. Chiba T, Ohi R, Nio M, et al. Late complications in long-term survivors of biliary atresia. *Eur J Pediatr Surg* 1992;2(1):22–25.

206. Houwen RH, Bijleveld CM, de Vries-Hospers HG. Ciprofloxacin for cholangitis after hepatic portoenterostomy. *Lancet* 1987;1(8546):1367.

207. Mones RL, DeFelice AR, Preud'Homme D. Use of neomycin as the prophylaxis against recurrent cholangitis after Kasai portoenterostomy. *J Pediatr Surg* 1994;29(3):422–424.

208. Ogasawara Y, Yamataka A, Tsukamoto K, et al. The intussusception antireflux valve is ineffective for preventing cholangitis in biliary atresia: a prospective study. *J Pediatr Surg* 2003;38(12):1 826–1829.

209. Altman RP. Portal decompression by interposition mesocaval shunt in patients with biliary atresia. *J Pediatr Surg* 1976;11(5):809–814.

210. Miyano T, Yamataka A. Choledochal cysts. *Curr Opin Pediatr* 1997;9(3):283–288.

211. de Vries JS, de Vries S, Aronson DC, et al. Choledochal cysts: age of presentation, symptoms, and late complications related to Todani's classification. *J Pediatr Surg* 2002;37(11):1568–1573.

212. Yu ZL, Zhang LJ, Fu JZ, et al. Anomalous pancreaticobiliary junction: image analysis and treatment principles. *Hepatobiliary Pancreat Dis Int* 2004;3(1):136–139.

213. Yamataka A, Segawa O, Kobayashi H, et al. Intraoperative pancreatoscopy for pancreatic duct stone debris distal to the common channel in choledochal cyst [see comment]. *J Pediatr Surg* 2000;35(1):1–4.

214. Stringer MD, Dhawan A, Davenport M, et al. Choledochal cysts: lessons from a 20 year experience. *Arch Dis Child* 1995;73(6):528–531.

215. Watanabe Y, Toki A, Todani T. Bile duct cancer developed after cyst excision for choledochal cyst. *J Hepatobiliary Pancreat Surg* 1999;6(3):207–212.

216. Jan YY, Chen HM, Chen MF. Malignancy in choledochal cysts. *Hepatogastroenterology* 2000;47(32):337–340.

217. Hamada Y, Tanano A, Takada K, et al. Magnetic resonance cholangiopancreatography on postoperative work-up in children with choledochal cysts. *Pediatr Surg Int* 2004;20(1):43–46.

218. Mackenzie TC, Howell LJ, Flake AW, et al. The management of prenatally diagnosed choledochal cysts. *J Pediatr Surg* 2001; 36(8):1241–1243.

219. Yamataka A, Ohshiro K, Okada Y, et al. Complications after cyst excision with hepaticoenterostomy for choledochal cysts and their surgical management in children versus adults. *J Pediatr Surg* 1997;32(7):1097–1102.

220. Miyano T, Yamataka A, Kato Y, et al. Hepaticoenterostomy after excision of choledochal cyst in children: a 30-year experience with 180 cases. *J Pediatr Surg* 1996;31(10):1417–1421.

221. Saing H, Han H, Chan KL, et al. Early and late results of excision of choledochal cysts. *J Pediatr Surg* 1997;32(11):1563–1566.

222. Tsuchida Y, Takahashi A, Suzuki N, et al. Development of intrahepatic biliary stones after excision of choledochal cysts. *J Pediatr Surg* 2002;37(2):165–167.

223. Bismuth H, Krissat J. Choledochal cystic malignancies. *Ann Oncol* 1999;10(Suppl 4):94–98.

224. Yamataka A, Kobayashi H, Shimotakahara A, et al. Recommendations for preventing complications related to Roux-en-Y hepatico-jejunostomy performed during excision of choledochal cyst in children. *J Pediatr Surg* 2003;38(12):1830–1832.

225. Weinberg AG, Finegold MJ. Primary hepatic tumors of childhood. *Hum Pathol* 1983;14(6):512–537.

226. Schnater JM, Aronson DC, Plaschkes J, et al. Surgical view of the treatment of patients with hepatoblastoma: results from the first prospective trial of the International Society of Pediatric Oncology Liver Tumor Study Group. *Cancer* 2002;94(4): 1111–1120.

227. Suita S, Tajiri T, Takamatsu H, et al. Improved survival outcome for hepatoblastoma based on an optimal chemotherapeutic regimen—a report from the study group for pediatric solid malignant tumors in the Kyushu area. *J Pediatr Surg* 2004;39(2): 195–198.

228. Katzenstein HM, Krailo MD, Malogolowkin MH, et al. Fibrolamellar hepatocellular carcinoma in children and adolescents. *Cancer* 2003;97(8):2006–2012.

229. Ortega JA, Douglass EC, Feusner JH, et al. Randomized comparison of cisplatin/vincristine/fluorouracil and cisplatin/continuous infusion doxorubicin for treatment of pediatric hepatoblastoma: a report from the Children's Cancer Group and the Pediatric Oncology Group. *J Clin Oncol* 2000;18(14):2665–2675.

230. Otte JB, Pritchard J, Aronson DC, et al. Liver transplantation for hepatoblastoma: results from the International Society of Pediatric Oncology (SIOP) study SIOPEL-1 and review of the world experience. *Pediatr Blood Cancer* 2004;42(1):74–83.

231. Molmenti EP, Nagata D, Roden J, et al. Liver transplantation for hepatoblastoma in the pediatric population. *Transplant Proc* 2001;33(1-2):1749.

232. Towu E, Kiely E, Pierro A, et al. Outcome and complications after resection of hepatoblastoma. *J Pediatr Surg* 2004;39(2):199–202.

233. Lodge JP. Hemostasis in liver resection surgery. *Semin Hematol* 2004;41(1 Suppl 1):70–75.

234. Copel L, Sosna J, Weeks D, et al. Use of three-dimensional CT in the abdomen: a useful preoperative planning tool. *Surg Technol Int* 2003;11:71–78.

235. Ding YT, Sun XT, Xu QX. Non-bleeding technique in resection of hepatoma: report of 49 cases. *Hepatobiliary Pancreatic Dis Int* 2002;1(1):52–56.

236. Liu DC, Vogel AM, Gulec S, et al. Hepatectomy in children under total hepatic occlusion. *Am Surg* 2003;69(6):539–541.

237. Smyrniotis VE, Kostopanagiotou GG, Contis JC, et al. Selective hepatic vascular exclusion versus pringle maneuver in major liver resections: prospective study. *World J Surg* 2003;27(7):765–769.

238. Barro C, Wrobleski I, Piolat C, et al. Successful use of recombinant factor VIIa for severe surgical liver bleeding in a 5 month-old baby. *Haemophilia* 2004;10(2):183–185.

239. Lowe ME. Pancreatitis in childhood. *Curr Gastroenterol Rep* 2004;6(3):240–246.

240. Jacombs AS, Wines M, Holland AJ, et al. Pancreatic trauma in children. *J Pediatr Surg* 2004;39(1):96–99.

241. Greenfeld JI, Harmon CM. Acute pancreatitis. *Curr Opin Pediatr* 1997;9(3):260–264.

242. Meier DE, Coln CD, Hicks BA, et al. Early operation in children with pancreas transection. *J Pediatr Surg* 2001;36(2):341–344.

243. Wales PW, Shuckett B, Kim PC. Long-term outcome after nonoperative management of complete traumatic pancreatic transection in children. *J Pediatr Surg* 2001;36(5):823–827.

244. Firstenberg MS, Volsko TA, Sivit C, et al. Selective management of pediatric pancreatic injuries. *J Pediatr Surg* 1999;34(7): 1142–1147.

245. Cooney DR, Crosfeld JL. Operative management of pancreatic pseudocysts in infants and children: a review of 75 cases. *Ann Surg* 1975;182(5):590–596.

246. Haluszka O, Campbell A, Horvath K. Endoscopic management of pancreatic pseudocyst in children. *Gastrointest Endosc* 2002;55(1):128–131.

247. Jackson WD. Pancreatitis: etiology, diagnosis, and management. *Curr Opin Pediatr* 2001;13(5):447–451.

248. Rollins MD, Meyers RL. Frey procedure for surgical management of chronic pancreatitis in children. *J Pediatr Surg* 2004;39(6): 817–820.

249. Dunne MJ, Cosgrove KE, Shepherd RM, et al. Hyperinsulinism in infancy: from basic science to clinical disease. *Physiol Rev* 2004;84(1):239–275.

250. Fekete CN, de Lonlay P, Jaubert F, et al. The surgical management of congenital hyperinsulinemic hypoglycemia in infancy. *J Pediatr Surg* 2004;39(3):267–269.

251. Dunne MJ, Kane C, Shepherd RM, et al. Familial persistent hyperinsulinemic hypoglycemia of infancy and mutations in the sulfonylurea receptor. *N Engl J Med* 1997;336(10):703–706.

252. Adzick NS, Thornton PS, Stanley CA, et al. A multidisciplinary approach to the focal form of congenital hyperinsulinism leads to successful treatment by partial pancreatectomy. *J Pediatr Surg* 2004;39(3):270–275.

253. Cretolle C, Fekete CN, Jan D, et al. Partial elective pancreatectomy is curative in focal form of permanent hyperinsulinemic hypoglycaemia in infancy: a report of 45 cases from 1983 to 2000. *J Pediatr Surg* 2002;37(2):155–158.

254. Shilyansky J, Fisher S, Cutz E, et al. Is 95% pancreatectomy the procedure of choice for treatment of persistent hyperinsulinemic hypoglycemia of the neonate? *J Pediatr Surg* 1997;32(2): 342–346.

255. McAndrew HF, Smith V, Spitz L. Surgical complications of pancreatectomy for persistent hyperinsulinaemic hypoglycaemia of infancy. *J Pediatr Surg* 2003;38(1):13–16.

256. Rangel SJ, Henry MC, Brindle M, et al. Small evidence for small incisions: pediatric laparoscopy and the need for more rigorous evaluation of novel surgical therapies. *J Pediatr Surg* 2003; 38(10):1429–1433.

257. Rescorla FJ, Engum SA, West KW, et al. Laparoscopic splenectomy has become the gold standard in children. *Am Surg* 2002;68(3):297–301; discussion 301–302.

258. Park A, Heniford BT, Hebra A, et al. Pediatric laparoscopic splenectomy. *Surg Endosc* 2000;14(6):527–531.

259. Reddy VS, Phan HH, O'Neill JA, et al. Laparoscopic versus open splenectomy in the pediatric population: a contemporary single-center experience. *Am Surg* 2001;67(9):859–863; discussion 863–864.

260. Berends FJ, Schep N, Cuesta MA, et al. Hematological long-term results of laparoscopic splenectomy for patients with idiopathic thrombocytopenic purpura: a case control study. *Surg Endosc* 2004;18(5):766–770.

261. Rescorla FJ, Breitfeld PP, West KW, et al. A case controlled comparison of open and laparoscopic splenectomy in children. *Surgery* 1998;124(4):670–675; discussion 675–676.

262. Bisharat N, Omari H, Lavi I, et al. Risk of infection and death among post-splenectomy patients. *J Infect* 2001;43(3):182–186.

263. Castagnola E, Fioredda F. Prevention of life-threatening infections due to encapsulated bacteria in children with hyposplenia or asplenia: a brief review of current recommendations for practical purposes. *Eur J Haematol* 2003;71(5):319–326.

264. Kumar RJ, Borzi PA. Splenosis in a port site after laparoscopic splenectomy. *Surg Endosc* 2001;15(4):413–414; Epub 2001 Mar 13.

Index

Page numbers followed by *f* refer to figures; those followed by *t* refer to tables.

A

Abdominal aortic aneurysm (AAA), 159, 364
  angiogram, patient undergoing endograft repair, 365*f*
  aortic endograft repair associated with low mortality rate, 370
  defective wound healing, 109
  elective, 31
  repair, 150, 322
  resections, colon ischemia, 323
Abdominal approaches, 503
  sutured rectopexy, Ripstein procedure, 503
Abdominal catastrophe, 221
Abdominal compartment syndrome, 151, 420
  ascites, immediate large-volume paracentesis, 421
  total renal failure, 151
Abdominal occlusive vascular disease, 154
Abdominal wall
  and hernia surgery, 523–544
  defects, 751–754
    surgery for, 774–776
  incisions, 528*f*
  wound infections, 525–526
  wounds, chronic, 543–544
Abruptio placenta, 190
Abscess drainage, 518
Absorption atelectasis, 268
  proximal airway occlusion, 268
Acalculous cholecystitis, 133
  acute, 442
ACC/AHA guidelines, 62
  management of vascular heart disease, 62
Access injury, 546–548
Accessory hepatic veins, 414
  evaluation for, 414
Accreditation Committee for Graduate Medical Education (ACGME), 5
  duty hour restrictions, effect of, 7
  educational outcomes, 13
  outcome project, 15
  patient care and medical knowledge, 6
  practice-based learning and improvement, 6
  residents' learning and patient outcomes, 6
  systems-based practice, 6
Accreditation Council for Continuing Medical Education (ACCME), 18
Accreditation Council for Graduate Medical Education (ACGME), 11, 26, 29
Acetylcysteine
  antioxidant, for reducing contrast nephropathy, 358

  glutathione precursor, and oxygen free-radical scavenger, 153
ACGME. *See* Accreditation Committee for Graduate Medical Education (ACGME)
Achalasia
  advanced, megaesophagus of, 246
  esophagomyotomy for, 261
  megaesophagus of, 261
  recurrent or persistent symptoms of, 262
Acid-base disturbances, 203
Acinetobacter baumannii, 165
Acquired immunodeficiency syndrome (AIDS), 212
Acryl cyanosis, 190
Activated partial thromboplastin time (APTT), 187*t*, 338
  global screening assay, for coagulation protein defect, 187
  high molecular weight kininogen (HK) deficiencies, 188
  lupus anticoagulant, 187
Activated protein C, 348
  antithrombotic activities, 127
Activated tissue macrophages, 105
Acute Physiology and Chronic Health Evaluation (APACHE), 167
Acute renal failure (ARF), 150–156
  definition of, 150–151
  due to radiocontrast dye for CT scans, or angiography, 150
  etiology of, 152, 371
  fractional excretion of sodium (FENa), 152
  nonoliguric, oliguric, and anuric renal failure, 152, 358
  perioperative risk factors, 151, 151*t*
  prerenal, intrarenal, postrenal causes, 152
  prevention of, 152–155, 153*t*
  septic surgical ICU patients, 151
  surgery and postoperative renal failure, 150
  urine osmolality, 152
Acute respiratory distress syndrome (ARDS), 132, 157, 166–167, 231
  acute and progressive respiratory disease, 166
  clinical phases, 166, 166*t*, 167
  increase in pulmonary capillary permeability, 167
  massive capillary leak, 166
  mechanical ventilation, 132
  pathophysiology of, 166
  prone positioning, improves oxygenation, 170
Acute tubular necrosis (ATN), 138, 152, 657
Addisonian crisis, 128

Adenosine antagonists, 154
  assessment of perfusion, 64
Administrative data sets, 46, 48
Adrenal incidentaloma, 566–567
Adrenal venous sampling, 561, 562*t*
Adrenalectomy, 559
  expected outcomes, 560–567
  for hypercortisolism, postoperative hypoadrenalism, 568
  therapeutic goals of, 559–560
Adrenergic blocking agents, 179–180
  clonidine, 179–180
Adrenocortical adenoma, 563
Adrenocortical carcinoma, 565–566, 568–569
  nonfunctioning low-grade, 570*f*
  open anterior adrenalectomy, 568
  resected by an open approach, 569
  resection of, 560
Adrenocorticotropic hormone (ACTH), 133, 562, 563
Adult education and learning, 19–22
Adult respiratory distress syndrome (ARDS), 208, 266, 311
  associated with reexploration, 292
Afferent loop obstruction, 394*f*
  surgical emergency, 393
  urgent reoperation, possibility of perforation, 393
Afferent loop syndrome, 393
Aganglionosis, 738
  due to ischemia, 738
Agency for Healthcare Research and Quality (AHRQ), 3, 36, 38*t*
Air embolism, 414–415
  atrial septal defect, 414
  division of the hepatic parenchyma, 414
Air embolus, massive, 283*t*
  management strategy for treating CPB, 283*t*
Air plethysmography, 340
  complex noninvasive venous assessment, calf muscle pump function, 340
Airway complications, 70–75
Airway compromise, acute, 319
  recurrent laryngeal nerve damage, 160
  superior laryngeal nerve injury, 160
  unilateral recurrent laryngeal injury, 161*t*
Airway edema, acute, 234
Airway erythema, upper, 163
Airway mucosa, upper, 161
Airway obstruction
  acute, 164
  upper, 234
Airway stenosis, critical, 231
Albumin
  infusion, 147
  preparations, 146

Alcohol intoxication, acute, 139
Allen test, 291
Allergic contact dermatitis, 513
Allergic reactions, 92
Allogeneic blood products, 140
    immunomodulatory effect of, residual
        leukocytes, 140
Allogeneic blood transfusion, 140
    immunosuppressive, 140
Allograft failure, acute, 700–702
Allograft fracture, 651
Allograft rejection, chronic, 694–695
Alloplastic
    implantations, 523
    materials, 526
    meshes, 533
    tissue implants, 533–534, 539
    under-lay technique, 540f
Alpha 2-adrenergic agonists, 66
Alveolar capillary permeability, 132
Alveolar collapse, 268
Alveolar-arterial gradient, 267
American Board of Colon and Rectal
    Surgery, 27
American Board of Medical Specialties
    (ABMS), 22, 25, 29
American Board of Surgery (ABS), 5, 11,
    22, 25–27
American Board of Thoracic Surgery
    (ABTS), 14, 27
American College of Physicians (ACP), 159
    preoperative pulmonary function testing
        (PFT), 159
American College of Surgeons Advanced
    Trauma Life Support cause, 21
American College of Surgeons Surgical
    Education and Self-Assessment
    Program (SESAP), 27
American College of Surgeons, 22, 23, 54
American health care system, 25
American Heart Association (AHA), 174
    task, force algorithm, 178t
American Medical Association (AMA), 19
    Physician Recognition Award
        (AMA-PRA), 18
American Society of Anesthesiologists (ASA),
    69, 71, 72f, 73t, 116, 117, 158,
    391, 604
American Society of Regional and
    Pain Medicine
    spinal or epidural anesthesia, 85
    systemic heparinization, 86t
American-European Consensus
    Conference, 166
Aminophylline administration, 154
Amiodarone, 300
Ampulla of Vater, 395, 726
Amputation, 372, 625
Anal fissure, 516–518
Anal sensation, 516
Analgesics, 80–81
Anaphylaxis, 92–93, 93t
Anaplastic cancer, 578
Anastomoses, distal, 506
    dilute epinephrine injections, or
        cautery, 506
Anastomosis, 413, 419, 451, 480, 596, 748
    anastomotic leak at, 471
    anastomotic strictures, 453
    hepatic resection, 436

principles for, 451t
reconstruction
Anastomotic
    aneurysms, 329
    bleeding, 601
    dehiscence, 398, 403–404
    disruption, 245
    healing, 505
    hemorrhage, 506–507
    infections, 689
    intimal fibrodysplasia, 328
    leakage, 256, 403, 511–512, 747
        aggressive management of, 505
        algorithm for, 506f
        prevention of, 257
        secondary mediastinitis, 246
    stenosis, 643, 689
    stricture, 256–257
Anatomy, aberrant, 425
Anesthesiology
    complications in, 69–97
    delivery systems, 76–77
Aneursymectomy, elective
    acute renal failure, 323
Aneurysms, false femoral, 329
Angina, unstable
    direct coronary angiography, 64
    left ventricular function
        carotid endarterectomy and
        CABG, 288
Angiodysplasia, 502
Angiogram, visceral, 465f
Angiography
    hemorrhage, localize lesion bleeding, 488
    intraoperative duplex examination, 331
    number of complications, during
        vascular interventions, 357
    therapeutic embolization and
        localization, 502
Angiography with embolization,
    emergent, 409
Angioplasty, 363
    deep vein, 354
    primary, 362
    venous and stenting, 376
Angiosarcoma, 608
    x-ray therapy (XRT), 608
Angiotensin II release, 284
Angiotensin-converting enzyme
    (ACE), 178
Ankle-brachial indices (ABIs), 331
Annular suturing technique, 302
Annuloplasty, 303, 305
Anomalies, venous
    duplication of the inferior vena cava, 323
Anoplasty, 516, 517f
Anorectal abscesses
    signs of inflammation, 518
Anorectal manometry, 735
Anorectal procedures
    complications of, 514–520
Anorectal surgery, 515
Anorectum, 519
Anterior adrenalectomy, open, 568, 569–571
Anterior mediastinal thyroid, 578
Anterior thoracic esophagostomy, 256, 257f
Antiarrhythmic agents, 289
Antibiotic(s)
    broad-spectrum, 155, 751
    irrigation, combating empyema, 269

prophylaxis, 122
therapy, empiric, 165
    patient data institution-specific, 166
use, empiric, 267
Antibodies, 216–217
Anticalcification fixation techniques, 299
Anticoagulation, 188–190
    alternative agents for, 346t
    anticoagulants, 188t, 189
    chronic, 368
    therapy, 207, 674
Antifibrin agents
    antiplatelet agents, increased use in
        clinical medicine, 188t
    interaction with thrombin active site, 189
    nonspecific and specific inhibitors, 189
Antifibrinolytics epsilon-aminocaproic
    acid, 281
Antigen presenting cells (APCs), 213
Antimicrobial agents, 122
Antimicrobial therapy, 123, 306
Antiphospholipid antibody syndrome, 338
Antiplatelet therapy, 182
Antiproliferative agents, 216
Antithrombin III
    repletion of, 281
Antithrombotic therapy, 181
Antithymocyte globulin
    persistent lymphopenia, 217
Antithyroid medications, chronic
    propylthiouracil or methimazole, 578
Antiviral therapy, 709
Antrectomy, 390
Anuria
    abdominal decompression, 151
Aorta, 321
    and aortotomy, 304
Aortic
    aneurysm, ruptured, 222
    cross clamping
        inadequate protection, 278
        vasodilators, decrease peripheral
        resistance and afterload, 323
    endograft systems, 364, 369
    neck, angulation of, 369
    reconstruction, 321, 325f, 329
    regurgitation lesions, 62
    stenosis
        aortic valve replacement, definitive
        therapy of choice, 62
        noncardiac surgery, 62
        percutaneous aortic balloon
        valvotomy, 62
        typical murmur, and diminished
        delayed upstroke of the
        carotid, 60
        valve-associated cardiovascular risk
        for patients, 60
    surgery, 323, 329
    surgery, elective, 323
    valve, 304
Aortobifemoral bypass grafting, 329f, 363
Aortoenteric graft intestinal erosion, 327
Aortogram, 367f, 368
Aortoiliac
    angioplasty and stenting, 362
    bifurcation reconstruction, 364
    interventions, 362
    occlusive disease, 329

Aortoiliofemoral arterial occlusive disease, 329
Aortoiliofemoral graft thromboses, 328
APACHE II score, 131
Appendectomy, 498–520, 774
  colon and rectal surgery, complications of, 498–520
  laparoscopic approach to, 499
Appendicitis, 498, 774
  clinical diagnosis, 499
  complications of, 499
  in elderly, 500
  miscarriage associated with, 500
  operative approach, 499
  pathophysiology of, 498–499
  postoperative complications, 499–500
  pregnancy, 500
  radiologic imaging, 499
  tumors of appendix, 500
Apprenticeship model
  sequential close working relationships, 14
Aprotinin, 281
  protease inhibitor, 292
ARDS patients. See Acute respiratory distress syndrome (ARDS)
Arrhythmias, 59, 182, 265–266, 702–703
  and cardiovascular collapse, 180
  etiology of, multifactorial, 278
  intraoperative, 309
  preoperative cardiac risk factors, 182
  ventricular sustained/symptomatic, 62
Arterial
  and portal venous injury, 413–414
  and venous blood supplies
    occlusion of, 413
  blood gas analysis, 162
  contrast phase, 407
  disruption, 371
  dissection, 360, 362, 371, 372
  following PTA, intra-arterial stent placement, 372
  interventions, 357–360
  ischemia, 338
  oxygen saturation, 136
  phase imaging
    hypervascular tumors, 410
  pseudoaneurysm, 419
  puncture site closure, 360
  repair, 413
  surgery, 317–334
  thrombosis, 192, 360, 640–641
    elevated plasma fibrinogen levels, major risk factor, 364
    elevation of lipoprotein(a) [Lp(a)], 192
  venous thrombosis, 192
Arterial occlusion, complete, 360
Arterial surgery, open, 317
Arterial-venous fistula, 222
Arteriolar hyalinosis, 221
Arteriotomy closure, 321
Arteriovenous fistula, 359
  development of, 359
  persistence of, 332
  with hemoptysis, or high output heart failure, 743
  with steal syndrome or rupture, 359
Arteroembolism, 323
Artery stenting, femoropopliteal, 372
Artery, subclavian, 361, 362
Arytenoid dislocation, 230

Arytenoidectomy, 231
Ascending venography, 340
Ascites, 420–421
  and encephalopathy, 440
  biliary, 417
  infected, 420
Aseptic meningitis, 217
Aspiration
  chronic, laryngeal dysfunction, 243
  mastectomy and axillary incisions are insensate, 606
Aspiration pneumonia, 163, 246
  amoxicillin-clavulanate, piperacillin-tazobactam, 164
  Gram-negative bacilli or *Staphylococcus aureus*, 164
  Haemophilus influenzae, and Gram-negative bacilli, 163
  impaired nutrition, 258
  pulmonary complication, 163
  pulmonary infection, altered clearance mechanisms of less virulent bacteria, 163
  Staphylococcus aureus and *Streptococcus pneumoniae*, 163
  suppuration and necrosis in lung, 164
Aspirin
  improving graft patency postoperatively, 292
Atelectasis, 267–268, 311
  desaturation and mechanical ventilation, 90
Atheroemboli or thromboemboli, distal carotid artery stent-related strokes, 361
Atheroembolism, peripheral, 259
Atherosclerosis, 364
  progressive downstream, 328
  statins, 66
Atherosclerotic aorta, 288
Atherosclerotic ascending aorta
  atheroemboli, severe ischemic strokes, 287
  mobile plaques, presence of, 287
Atonic megarectum
  after PSARP, resection by endorectal pull, 742
Atraumatic intubation technique, 242
Atrial arrhythmias, 265
  atrial fibrillation, occurrence after valve surgery, 300
Atrial cardioversion electrodes, 290
Atrial contraction, normal, loss of, 288
Atrial cuff, 684
Atrial dysrhythmias, 90, 696
Atrial fibrillation patients
  low-dose heparin drip, 290
Atrial fibrillation, 182, 266, 278, 299
  atrial and ventricular filling and pumping, disruption of, 128
  β-blocker or calcium channel blocker, 182
  CO suppression, 128
  pathophysiology of, 288
Atrial fibrillation, persistent or recurrent coumadin treatment, 290
Atrial natriuretic peptide
  potential renoprotective agents, 155
Atrioventricular (AV)
  node, 304
  block, 702

conduction disturbances, 304
  groove rupture, 300
Atypical hyperplasia
  high-risk lesions, 609
Atypical wounds, 109
Auto Suture Endo-GIA II Stapler, 250
Autogenous renal artery reconstruction
  following excision, 371
Autogenous tissue reconstruction, 614
Autogenous vascular reconstruction, 362
Autoimmune disease, 212
Autologous pericardium, 300
Autologous tissue repairs, 538–539
  Shouldice repair, 531–533
Autologous tissue transfers, 538
Autonomic neuropathy, 670
Avulsion of the sphincter of Oddi, 395, 395f
Awake endoscopy, 230
Awake fiberoptic intubation, 90
Awake intubation
  using fiberoptic technique, 71
Awake laryngoscopy
  bilateral postintubation laryngeal granulomas, 233f
  proliferative tissue, pale gray to red, 232
  unilateral small granuloma, 233f
Awake paralysis
  inadvertent, 81
Axillary
  metastases, 615
  nodal status
    staging patients, with invasive breast cancer, 609
  padding, 606
  staging
    complications of, 609–613
    via sentinel lymph node biopsy, 615
  surgery, 606, 610
  vein to popliteal vein valve transplant, 354
  webs, 611
Axillary artery cannulation, 282
Axillary fat pads, 607
Axillary lymph node dissection (ALND)
  complications associated with, 609–613
  level I/II, 609
  patients, 606
Axillary lymph node, 628–631
Axillary/subclavian vein thrombosis, 338–339
  prevention of, 344

B

Babcock or Alice clamps, 411
Backwash ileitis, 502
Bacteremia, 339
Bacterial pneumonia, 163, 164
Balanced Budget Act, 6, 12
  graduate medical education (GME), 12
Balloon angioplasty, 66
Balloon occluders, 361
Balloon tamponade, 506
Band gastroplasty, 549
Bariatric surgery, 28, 159
  dvt prophylaxis, 403
  improved patient outcome, 28
  specially designed operating tables, 402
Barium esophagogram, 251
Barium swallow examination, 254
Barrett esophagus patients
  surgical therapy for, 254

β-blockers
    prophylactic administration of, 289
β-blocking agents
    abrupt stoppage, 300
B-cell malignancy, 187
Beckwith-Wiedeman Syndrome, 753
Behçet disease
    and indwelling catheters, 339
Benzodiazepines, 77
β-blockade, 179
β-blocker therapy, long-term
    risk of increased adrenergic activity, 178
β-blockers, 65
    for improving patient safety, 177–179
    periprocedural complications, reduction
        of, 66
    use of, 181
Bile
    leak, 457
    peritonitis, 416–417
    reflux gastritis, 728
    stasis, 203
Bile drainage, persistent
    radiocontrast drain injection study, 417
Bile duct
    disruption, 409
    injury
        avoidance by intraoperative
            ultrasound, 414
        mechanism of, 424–425
    obstruction
        etiologies of, 417
    resection, 450
        complications of, 450–458
    stricture
        associated complications, 418
        avoidance of, 418
Bile duct stones, 448
    preoperative predictive factors for, 447t
    visualization of, 446
Bile duct, partial obstruction
    unrelieved choledo cholithiasis,
        hepatolithiasis, 416
Bile or biloma
    intra-abdominal collection of, 416
Bileaflet valve
    perivalvular leak, 300
Biliary
    obstruction, 418
        chronic extrahepatic, 440
Biliary drainage, permanent, 420
Biliary fistula, persistent
    no free-flowing drainage to the
        intestine, 417
Biliary stricture, recurrent
    risk factors for, 453t
Biliopancreatic diversion, 401, 404
Billroth II
    anastomosis, 391
    gastrojejunostomy, 392
    reconstruction, 393
Biloma, 416
Bioartificial liver methods, 415
Biologic prostheses, 299
Biologic sealants, 310
Biomaterial allografts, 527
Bioprosthetic valve
    dysfunction, 302
    structural valve degeneration, important
        complication of, 299

Biphasic stridor, 236
Bismuth I and II tumors, 456
Bismuth-Corlette classification, 455
Bismuth-Strasberg A-E injuries, 435–438
Bite block, 233
Björk flap, 235
Bladder
    catheter, 752
    continence, 742
    drainage, 678
        complications associated with,
            675–676
    dysfunction, 508
    injury
        delayed presentation of, 550
    leak, 649
Bleeding peptic ulceration, 388t
Bleeding, 185, 409–410, 465–466,
        515–516, 572
    active, 388
    control of, 409
    diathesis. *See* Coagulopathy
    disorders, differential diagnosis, 187t
    duodenal ulcer
        Kocher maneuver, to mobilize
            duodenum from
            retroperitoneum, 389
        operative maneuvers in
            management, 389f
    history
        factor VIII (VIII) deficiency, 187
    iatrogenic inferior vena cava stenosis, 572
    life-threatening, 192
    massive, management of, 191–192
    perihepatic, 410
    recurrent, prevention of, 390
Blind loop syndrome, 728
Blood coagulation system, 186f
Blood pressure cuff, 403
    noninvasive, 90
Blood pressure, systemic, 138
Blood transfusion, allogeneic, 140
Blood urea nitrogen (BUN), 138, 159, 189
    level, 155
Blue dye allergy
    characterized by blue-tinged
        hives, 612
Blue dye reactions, 623–624
Blue toe syndrome, 360
Board certification, 6, 25–26
Board-certified intensivists, 33
Bochdalek hernia, 749
Body fluid
    compartment distribution, 144
    depletion, 137
Body habitus, 255
Body mass index (BMI), 88, 398, 548
Boerhaave syndrome, 247
BOS. *See* Bronchiolitis obliterans syndrome
    (BOS)
Botulinum toxin (Botox), 737
Bovine pericardial strips, 310
Bovine pericardium, 270
Bowel
    fistulization, 526
    intraluminal bowel flora, 120
    preparation, 120
    preserving techniques, 485f
    rest, 204
    wall edema, 145

Brachial artery embolization, 362
Brachial artery thrombosis
    following upper extremity arterial
        access, 360
Brachial plexus (weakness or
        paresthesias), 362
Brachiocephalic angioplasty, and stenting,
    361–362
Brachytherapy, 608
Bradyarrhythmias, heart block, 128
Breast
    and axillary incisions
        rates of postoperative infection, 604
    cancer cases, 613t
    cancer patients, 607
    cancer surgery, 606
    conservation therapy, 608
    edema, delayed, 608
    fibrosis, 607
    lymphedema, 607
    preservation
        and monitoring of
            chemosensitivity, 614
    surgery
        chemical maneuvers, to decrease
            seroma formation, 606
        complication rates, 614
        electrocautery, reduced hematoma
            formation, 606
        selected studies evaluating wound
            infection rates, 605t
        seroma formation, 606
Breast cellulitis, recurrent, 607
Breast lesions, nonpalpable
    risk of sampling error greater, 609
Breast procedures, surgical
    brachial plexopathy related to stretch
        injury, 604
    chronic incisional pain, 604
Bronchial blocking balloon, 309
Bronchial carcinoid, 564
Bronchial cuff. *See* Bronchial blocking
    balloon
Bronchiectasis, 766
Bronchiolitis obliterans syndrome (BOS),
    694–695
Bronchoalveolar lavage culture, 163
Bronchopleural fistula, 268–270
    appropriate intervention, with
        thoracostomy tube
        placement, 309
    chronic, closure of, 270
    incidence of, 268
Bronchoscopy, 16, 268, 273, 765
Bronchospasm
    intravenous dipyridamole, avoidance
        of, 63
Bupivacaine
    blocks sodium channels, 83
    toxicity, 82
Burn ICU
    empiric antibiotic strategy for,
        nosocomial pneumonia, 166
Burn patient
    endotracheal tube, securing of, 161
Burns
    cutaneous, and associated
        complications, 161
Buttock claudication
    hypogastric artery occlusion, predominant
        complaint later, 365

Bypass Angioplasty Revascularization Investigation (BARI)
  evaluate incidence of, postoperative cardiac complications, 67
Bypass graft thrombosis, 331
Bypass surgery
  saphenous vein harvest site, 291
Bypassing or excluding native esophagus
  complications of, 260

C

CABG patients
  postoperative hypertension requiring therapy, 181
CABG. See Coronary artery bypass grafting (CABG)
Cachectic patients, 200
CAD. See Cardiovascular disease (CAD)
Cadaveric pancreas donor selection, 670–671
Calcific degeneration, 304
Calcineurin inhibitors (CNIs), 214–215, 715
  cyclosporine and tacrolimus, 214
  glucose intolerance, 215
  nephrotoxicity side effects, 215
  therapy, 222
Calcium blockers, 155
Calcium channel blockade, 568
Calcium channel blockers, 66, 139
  second-line agents to β-blockers, controlling angina or stress-induced ischemia, 66
  verapamil, 265
Calcium chloride, 580
Calcium gluconate, 580
Calf thrombi, 345
Calf vein excision, 352
Caliber tubes, use of, 208
Calorimetry, indirect, 199
Cancer
  gastric resection, postoperative complication and operative mortality, 385
  related to prolonged inflammation of, biliary epithelium, 450
Cancer cachexia
  delay in wound repair, 108
Cancer resection, 311–312
Cancer, primary hepatobiliary, 407
Candida species, 218
Canine model
  role of overhydration, 266
Cannula obstruction, 235
  suction or removal of inner cannula, 235
Capillary perfusion
  low tissue oxygen tension, 107
Capillary perfusion pressure, 524
Capnography monitoring, 97
Capsular tear, splenic, 507f
Carbon dioxide pneumoperitoneum
  effects of, 549t
Carbon monoxide poisoning, 162–163
  bloodstream, evaluation of HbCO level in, 162
  obtundation and loss of consciousness, 162
  signs and symptoms of, 162t
Carboxyhemoglobin (HbCO), 162
Carcinoid syndrome
  carcinoid crisis, 488

Carcinoid tumor, 500
  neuroendocrine tumors, 487–488
Carcinoma, basal-cell, 219
Cardiac allograft rejection, 703–706
Cardiac allograft vasculopathy, 711
Cardiac arrhythmias, 62
Cardiac catheterization, 177, 278
Cardiac complications, 174–182
  perioperative mortality, late postoperative death after aortic surgery, 322
Cardiac disease
  long-standing immunosuppression, patients on, 220
Cardiac herniation, 267
  left and right pneumonectomies, 267
Cardiac imaging, nuclear, 64
Cardiac index, 141
Cardiac ischemia, 309
  electrocardiography, cardiac monitoring, cardiac enzyme measurements, 180
  intraoperative Swan-Ganz catheter monitoring, 309
Cardiac output (CO), 127, 136
  optimization, improving splanchnic perfusion, 284
  preload, heart rate, manipulation of, 278
Cardiac preload, 139
  central venous pressure (CVP), 139
  direct measurement of, 137
  measures of, 139
  monitoring of, 139–140
  pulmonary capillary wedge pressure (PCWP), 139
Cardiac revascularization
  cardiac catheterization, 177
  occurrence of major cardiac predictors, 63
Cardiac risk
  definition of, high-risk surgical procedures, 61t
  intraoperative two-lead ECG monitoring, 181
  stepwise approach, preoperative assessment of, 60
  type of surgery, important implications for, 60
Cardiac risk indices
  quantify cardiac risk for patients with CAD, 175
Cardiac risk stratification
  surgery-specific and clinical factors, 174
Cardiac risk studies
  estimation of cardiac risk, using Goldman index, 175t
Cardiac surgery
  postoperative arrhythmias, 182
Cardiac testing, noninvasive and invasive, 176–177
Cardiac toxicity
  prolonged resuscitation measures, 83
Cardiac troponin
  I and T, 181
  levels, 181
Cardiac venous return
  resulting in hypotension, 412
Cardiogenic shock, 62, 128, 287
  arrhythmias, cardiomyopathies, mechanical abnormalities, 128
  pericardial tamponade, massive pulmonary embolism, 128
  tension pneumothorax, 128

Cardiology imaging, nuclear, 176
Cardiology test predictors, nuclear, 176, 176t
Cardiomyopathy, 62
  severe deficits in myocardial contractility, 128
  valvular insufficiency, 128
Cardiopulmonary bypass (CPB), 277–283
  activation of inflammatory mediators, 280t
  followed by stroke, risk factors of, 283t
  neurologic injury, use of technical strategies, 282, 283t
  treatment of bleeding, investigating causative factors, 281t
  vascular complications of, 278
Cardiopulmonary resuscitation (CPR), 87
  coronary perfusion pressure, 87
  early administration of vasopressors, 87
Cardiopulmonary Risk Index (CPRI), 307
Cardiopulmonary system, assessment of, 129
Cardiotomy and vent suctions
  turbulence and shear stress of blood elements, 281
Cardiovascular collapse, 77, 180, 377
  hypoxemia and acidosis, 83
Cardiovascular complications, 278–279
  perioperative blood pressure instability, 318
  prevention of, 278–279
  strategies preventing, 278
Cardiovascular conditions, management of, 60
Cardiovascular disease (CAD), 220
Cardiovascular hemodynamic alterations, 361
Cardiovascular resuscitation, 409
Cardiovascular risk
  and surgically induced weight loss, 401
Cardiovascular toxicity, 82
  peak blood levels, ranking of local anesthetics, 83f
Care model, 12
Careers, surgical, 11
Carnitine deficiency
  hepatic steatosis, cause of, 203
Carotid artery
  angioplasty, 361
  and stenting, 361
    dilation of carotid bulb, 361
  defect
    identification of, 319
  disease, 287
  dissection, 319
  false aneurysms
    management of, arterial closure with a saphenous vein patch, 321
  occlusion
    adequacy of cerebral flow, 318
  stenting, 361
Carotid artery stenosis, symptomatic
  endarterectomy, prior to bypass surgery, 287
Carotid bruit, 287
Carotid cross-clamping
  initiates neurologic dysfunction, 318
  intraoperative cerebral ischemia, 318
Carotid duplex
  intraoperative use, 319

Carotid endarterectomy (CEA), 317, 361
   acute thrombosis of the ICA, subintimal
      hemorrhage, 319
   alteration in heart rate, 361
   early and late complications, 318*t*
   false aneurysm formation, 321
   false aneurysm of right carotid artery, 322*f*
   following cardiopulmonary bypass,
      minimizing stroke, 287
   myocardial infarction, late deaths in
      patients, 318
   recurrent carotid stenosis, secondary to
      neointimal hyperplasia, 320*f*
   specific intraoperative processes,
      determinants of operative
      mortality, 35
Carotid sinus nerve activity
   interruption of, 320
Carotid stenosis
   symptomatic recurrence of, 320
Carotid stenting, 321
Carpal tunnel syndrome, 94
Case-finding methods, 7
Catecholamine dependence, 131
Catheter
   and guidewire related, 360
   chronic indwelling catheters
      development of thrombi, 207
   directed thrombolysis, 416
   directed venous thrombolysis, 350
   infections
      bacterial translocation, seeding
        from, 206
   related bloodstream infection, 155
   related sepsis
      potential complication, 753
   suction embolectomy, 349
Catheters, modern angioplasty, 363
Caustic injury
   esophageal sphincter mechanism
      failure, 260
   perforation in mid- and distal
      esophagus, following biopsy
      or dilatation, 249
Cautery devices
   mono or bipolar cautery, 553
Cautery injury
   tips for minimizing, 553
Caval tumor
   extent of, 568
Caval-atrial junction, 272
Cave Automatic Virtual Environment
      (CAVE), 17
   geowall stereoscopic projection system, 17*f*
Cavitron ultrasonic aspirator (CUSA)
      technique
   high-energy ultrasound, 412
Cavity dilation, or thallium lung uptake, 64
Cavography, 376
CEA. *See* Carotid endarterectomy (CEA)
CEA/CABG stroke
   diagnosis of, 318
CEAP system
   categorize venous insufficiency, 340
Celiotomy incision
   worsens surgical outcomes, 524
Cell-cell contact inhibition, 105
Cellular dissemination, 444
Cellular hypoxia, 127

Cellulitis, 608
   cause edema, localized pain, and
      erythema, 339
Centers for Disease Control (CDC), 38, 114
   superficial or deep incisional SSIs, 114
   surgical site infection depth
      classification, 115*f*
   surveillance criteria for SSIs, 114
Central line
   aspiration of air through, 415
Central neck dissection
   complications of, 633
   redo, 633
Central nervous system (CNS), 282–283
Central neuraxial blockade. *See* Neuraxial
      anesthesia
Central pontine myelinolysis, 201
Central venous access
   via a percutaneous route, 204
Central venous lines (CVLs)
   catheter insertion, 206
   multiple drugs use, and blood draws, 206
Central venous pressure (CVP), 146
   measure of right atrial pressure, 139
   right heart filling pressures, 153
Central venous pressure monitoring line
   diuretic or inotropic therapy, 267
Cerebral angiography, 319, 360–361
Cerebral blood flow autoregulation, 283
Cerebral protection devices
   efficacy of, 361
Cerebrovascular accident (CVA), 46
Certifying examination, 27
Cervical
   dysphagia, 246
   endocrine surgery
      risky area of clinical practice, 576
   esophagogastric
      anastomotic leaks, 257
   esophagogastric anastomosis,
      246, 255
   hematoma, 578
      risk of, 579
   spine injury, 234
   structures
      injury to, 584–585
CF. *See* Cystic fibrosis (CF)
Chemical debridement, 112
Chemical pneumonitis, 163–164
   diagnosis of, 163
   intense inflammatory response, 163
   lung parenchyma, grossly edematous and
      hemorrhagic, 163
Chemical stress thallium testing, 322
Chemokines, 127
Chemoreceptor trigger zone, 88
   antagonizing neurotransmitter receptors,
      for controlling vomiting, 88
Chemotherapy and radiation
   wound-healing problems, acute and
      chronic, 625
Chemotherapy, 268
   antibiotic, 111, 112
Chest
   decompression
      airway intubation and positive-
        pressure ventilation, 161
      collapsed lung, treatment with
        thoracostomy tube, 161

endoscopy, 306–307
   diagnostic and therapeutic
      procedures, 306
   minimally invasive surgery, 308
   physical therapy, 163
   physiotherapy
      postoperative prophylaxis, therapy for
        sputum retention, 311
   roentgenogram, 254
   surgery
      several complications, 309
   tube suction, 254
   tube thoracostomy, 311
   wall involvement, 307
   wall irradiation, 613
   wall reconstruction
      myocutaneous flaps, 274
      preventing flail chest, 274
   wall resection, 274
Chest x-ray (CXR), 310
Cheyne–Stokes respiration, 60
Chloride responsive alkalosis, 146
Cholangiocarcinoma, 779
   distant risk of, 419
   slow-growing tumor, 455
Cholangitis, 418, 419–420, 777
   acute, 448
   and biliary obstruction, 457
   early complication of liver resection, 419
   increased risk of, with intra-hepatic duct
      stone formation, 418
Cholecystectomy
   biliary dyskinesia, indication for, 423
   common biliary operation, 423
   complications of, 423–458
Cholecystectomy injury, open
   long-term results, 440
   restenosis, rate for repairs of laparoscopic
      injuries, 440
Cholecystitis, 292
   acute, 424, 442
Cholecystocholedochal fistulas, 443
Cholecystokinin (CCK)
   decreased secretion of, 203
Choledochal cyst, 778–779
Choledochoduodenostomy, 448–449
   long-term risk of cholangitis, 449
Choledochojejunostomy, 448–449
Choledocholithiasis
   elevated serum amylase, poor predictors
      for, 446
   preoperative predictors of, 446
Choledochoscopy
   direct visualization of duct system, 445
Cholelithiasis, 404
   gallbladder sludge, following bariatric
      surgery, 404
   risk of, 404
Cholelithiasis, symptomatic, 481
Cholestasis and hypoperfusion
   acalculous cholecystitis, 133
Cholestatic jaundice
   severely septic patients, 133
Cholesterol embolization, 364
Cholesterol syndrome
   dislodgement of cholesterol crystals, from
      atheromatous vessels, 360
Chordae tendineae rupture. *See* Valvular
      insufficiency
Chronic corticotrophin (ACTH), 563

Chronic obstructive pulmonary disease (COPD), 158, 288, 311
Chronotropic drugs
elimination of, 289
Chylothorax, 254, 259, 273
Chylous effusion, 254
C-indices, 54
Circulating mediators, endothelial cell damage, 132
Circulating monocytes
tissue macrophages, 104
Circulating-water mattresses, 91
Circumflex coronary artery injury
reinstitution of, cardiopulmonary bypass, 300
Circumflex coronary artery, 300
injury to, 300–301
Cirrhosis, 443
A and B cirrhotics, undergoing laparoscopic cholecystectomy, 443
gallstone disease, 443
infected ascites, treatment with spironolactone, loop diuretics, 420
warm ischemia, tolerated up to 30 minutes, 416
Cirrhosis, biliary, 441
Cirrhosis, secondary biliary, 419, 453
complicated by portal hypertension, bleeding due to varices, 450
development of, and hemodynamic derangements, 440
hepatitis B or C infection, 416
late complications of, 440
partially obstructing stones, 416
Cirrhotic livers
maintaining minimal inflow occlusion, 416
Claggett technique, 273
Clamp-crush technique, 412
Classic pancreaticoduodenectomy, 472
Clean base ulcers
low recurrent bleeding rate, 388
Clinical inflammatory response, 127
increased bacteremia, 127
Clinical markers, 64
Clinical outcomes, 52
coordination of care, 52
measures, 45
methodology, 46
reporting system, 46
surgical care coordination, 53
Clinical practice, evolution of, 11
Clinical risk factors, 175–176
Clinical trials, prospective
addressing melanoma surgical margins, 620t
Clopidogrel, 292
Closed Claims Project, 69, 97
limitations to, 70
Closed insurance claims, 87
Closed suction drains, 123
placement of, 420
Closed-claims analysis, 81
neuromuscular blocking agents, 81
recall during anesthesia, 81
Closure devices
increased complications with, 360
Closure, 524–525

Closure, secondary, 110
Clot and fluid
evacuation of, 415
CMV. See Cytomegalovirus (CMV)
CO₂ embolus, risk of
laparoscopic liver surgery, 415
Coagulation
abnormalities in, 185–194
cascade, 127
thrombin generated, 281
pathway, 347f
protein inhibitor, 189
protein system, 187
assessment of bleeding and clotting risk, 186t
Coagulopathy, 146
Cochrane Group
30 controlled trials, 147
albumin, increased mortality associated with, 141
Coding bias, 46
Cold fibrillatory arrest, 282
Colectomy, partial, 568
Collagen fiber bundles
basket-weave pattern, unwounded dermis, 105
Collagen synthesis, normal, 105
Collateral arterial flow, 413
Collis gastroplasty
esophagus-lengthening, 246
Collis gastroplasty-fundoplication operation, 255
Colloid administration
resuscitation, 146–148
Colloid infusions
acute volume expansion, 146
Colloid preparations, 148
resuscitation fluid, safety and efficacy of, 148
Colloid therapy
meta-analyses of clinical studies, 147f
resuscitation, 147
Colloids, 141, 146–148
albumin, Hetastarch, and Dextran-70, 141
volume expansion, with risk of hypersensitivity, 146
Coloanal anastomosis, 737
Colon
elective procedures of, 524
ischemia, 323–324
surgery, 774
Colonic
atresia, 752
lavage, 511
operations
left ureter injury, 507
Colorectal
carcinoma, 504
pathology, 529
resection, 501
surgery
complications of, 500–501
Colostogram, distal, 740
Colostomy closure, 742
Combination therapy, 166
Community-acquired pneumonia, 164
Comorbid diseases
importance of, on mortality, 321

Compartment syndrome, abdominal, 151, 420
ascites, immediate large-volume paracentesis, 421
total renal failure, 151
Competent valve leaflets, residual
cause of early graft thrombosis, 333
Complement-dependent cell lysis, 217
Complete blood count (CBC), 128
Complete heart block (CHB)
early risk, largely iatrogenic, 304
late, 305
Complication Conference, 7
faculty and residents attendance, 7
Complication rates, specific
early complications following intact abdominal aortic aneurysm repair, 321t
Complications of surgery for Fistula-in-Ano, 519–520
Compression therapy, 332
Computed tomography (CT) scan, 524
adrenocortical carcinomas, 567f
chronic pancreatitis, with intractable abdominal pain, 468f
confirms presence of pancreatic inflammation, 463
demonstrating active hemorrhage, 465f
intermittent hypertension, 565f
necrotizing pancreatitis, with evidence of extraluminal gas, 466f
sine qua non of small bowel intussusception, 486f
type II endoleak, 367f
Computed tomography (CT), 319
detection of infectious foci, 129
Computer-based educational programs, 11
Concomitant vascular injury, 438–440
Conduit harvest sites
complications of, 291
Confidence intervals (CIs), 51
Congenital cystic adenomatoid malformation (CCAM), 725, 742
Congenital diaphragmatic hernia (CDH), 725, 749–751, 749f
Congenital duodenal obstruction, 726
Congestive heart failure (CHF), 59, 174
secondary causes of venous thrombosis, 339
Conn syndrome, 560, 566
Connective tissue disorder, 187
Constipation or recurrent enterocolitis chronic, 738t
Consultative medicine
challenging aspects of, 188
Contact granuloma, 232
Contaminated bile
restricted drainage of, 419
Contemporary bariatric procedures
degree of gastric restriction, 399
Contemporary surgical training, 5–8
Continuing education, for practicing surgeons, 18–23
Continuing medical education (CME), 18, 19, 27
acquisition of new knowledge and skills, after residency or fellowship training, 18
content of, 18
for relicensure, 19

Continuing medical education
(CME) (*Continued*)
getting acquainted with, new or improved
surgical techniques, 18
improved surgical techniques, 18
industry and ethics, 22–23
keeping up with, changes in basic
pathophysiology of disease, 18
life-long learning, 18
offerings, 19
pharmacotherapeutic agents, learning
about new, 18
programs, 23
readily available sources of, 20*t*
Continuous venovenous hemofiltration
(CVVH), 189
Contraction, 106
Contralateral lung
overdistension of, 267
Contralateral ureteral patency, 551
Contrast agents, 358
Contrast enema
diagnostic and therapeutic, 734
examine for transition zone, 735
rule out obstruction in colon, 726
Contrast esophagogram, 247
Contrast nephropathy, 357–359
acute renal failure, 357
elevation in serum creatinine, 358
incidence of, 358
not a benign complication, 358
pathogenesis of, 358
risk factors for, 358*t*
Contrast phlebography, 339
Contrast radiography evaluation, 730
Contrast radiography, 387
intraperitoneal leakage of gastric
contents, 390
Contrast scans, 410
Contrast swallow or bronchoscopy, 747
Contrast venography, 568
Contrast-induced nephropathy, prevention
of, 153–154
Control-blockers, 65
Conventional ventilation
volume cycling, 169
Cooper ligament (McVay) repair, 533
treating femoral hernias, suturing of
inguinal ligament, 533
Coordination of care
programming and feedback, 53
Core needle biopsy, 609
Corneal abrasions, 94
lateral positioning, and operation on the
head or neck, 94
Coronary angiogram, 174
Coronary angiography, 360
for patients at high risk, 64
procedural risks of death and stroke, 177
Coronary arteriography, 322
abdominal aortic aneurysms, presence of
severe coronary disease, 322
Coronary artery bypass grafting (CABG), 31,
66, 177, 289, 318, 362
and carotid endarterectomy, 288
complications of stroke and in-hospital
mortality, 287
isolated coronary revascularization,
major complications, 287*t*
LV dysfunction, recommended for, 286

perioperative cardiac complications,
reduction of, 66
Coronary artery bypass surgery, 159, 286
pulmonary complications, lower risk
of, 158
Coronary artery disease (CAD), 64, 174
anti-ischemic therapy, on perioperative
prognosis, 65
cardiac troponin measurements, 24
hours postoperatively, 67
measurement of biomarkers, 67
perioperative cardiac complications, 64
perioperative myocardial ischemia,
MI, 65
preoperative risk markers, 64
Coronary artery disease, occult
presence of carotid or other vascular
bruits, 60
Coronary artery ischemia, 131
Coronary bypass surgery
postoperative arrhythmias, 288
Coronary endothelium
damage to, cardioplegic arrest and
reperfusion, 278
Coronary occlusion, acute, 67
Coronary revascularization, 278, 286–287
aorta, manipulation of, 287
development of stroke, 287
gastrointestinal complications, high
morbidity, 292
overall morbidity and mortality, 287
preoperative prophylaxis with
β-blockers, 289
therapy with aggressive β-blockade, 64
Coronary stent technology, 287
Coronary syndrome, acute, 190
Coronary thrombosis, 66
Cortical adenoma, 568
Corticosteroids, 131–132, 170, 213–214
delayed epidermal repair, 108
impair tissue repair, 109
Corticosteroids, stress-dose, 131
Cosyntropin challenge
detecting adrenal insufficiency, 128
CPB. *See* Cardiopulmonary bypass
Cranial nerve injury, 319
Creaticoduodenectomy
for pancreatic, or periampullary NETs, 595
Creatine kinase (CK), 181
Credentialing process, 27
delineation of clinical privileges, 28
Health Maintenance Organizations
(HMOs)
insuring reimbursement for services
provided, 28
Cricopharyngeal muscle dysfunction, 246
Cricothyroid membrane, 311
glottic scarring, 240
scarring of, 240
Cricothyroidotomy, 239–240
Cricothyrotomy, emergent, 70
Crohn
disease, 482, 502–503
anovaginal or rectovagina, 519
chronic, segmental, transmural,
T helper cell–mediated disease,
482–484
Crohn recurrence, 484
exacerbation and remission, 503
higher risk of SSI, 118

irradiated bowel, 484–486
malabsorption, 482–484
recurrence after fistulotomy, 519
risk factors for, postoperative
recurrence of, 484*t*
stricturing of, increase stomal
stenosis, 514
patients
intestinal obstruction, 483–484
postoperative fistula formation, 483
recurrence, 484
Crohn colitis, 503
Cronkite-Canada syndrome
hamartomas, 487
Cross-sectional imaging, 396
Cryoablation, 412–413
Cryoprecipitate infusion, 191
Cryoprecipitate or fresh frozen plasma, 350
Cryptococcus neoformans, 218
Cryptorchidism, 740
incidence of, 754
Crystalloid administration, excessive, 146
Crystalloid solutions, 145–148
advantages and disadvantages of, 146
mainstay in treating hypovolemia, 141
maintenance fluid, 145
replacement therapy in people, 145
types of, 145
Crystalloid use
first line treatment of shock, 146
resuscitation, 146
CT cystography
aid in diagnosis, 550
CT evaluation, 362
CT-guided drainage, 512
Cuff laceration, 233
Cuff leak, 233
Cure rates, 3
Current Advanced Trauma Life Support
guidelines, 73
Cushing disease, 563
Cushing syndrome, 563, 566
clinical presentation of, 563
Cushingoid features, 214
Cutaneous erythema
areas of, 333
Cutaneous melanoma
effectively and adequately excised, 620
margins for, 621*t*
Cutaneous thermal injury
potential complication, 352
CXR. *See* Chest x-ray (CXR)
Cyanosis, peripheral, 256
Cyclosporine, 214
cystadenoma, biliary, 416
hyperlipidemia, 215
microemulsion, 215
renal and peripheral
vasoconstriction, 215
Cystduodenostomy, 464
Cystgastrostomy, 464
Cystic duct
identification, 424
stump leaks, 426
Cystic fibrosis (CF), 218, 765, 766–767, 776
Cystjejunostomy, 464
used to internally drain
pseudocysts, 464
Cystoscopy, 551
Cystostomy tube placement, 742

Cystourethrogram
    to evaluate for vesicoureteral reflux, 740
Cytokine release syndrome, 217
Cytokine-dependant cell proliferation, 216
Cytokines interleukin-2, 214
Cytomegalovirus (CMV), 658, 690–692
    diagnosis of, 221
Cytoplasmic binding proteins, 214
Cytotoxic agents, 109
Cytotoxic chemotherapy, 624
Cytotoxicity
    evidence of cell injury, 358
Cytotoxin-associated gene (cagA), 387

D

Dacron grafts, 332
Data dictionary, 47
Data-collection system, 53
Data-reporting system, 46
    risk-adjustment methodology, 46
D-Dimer assay, 339
    confirmatory test, positive indicating
        thrombin and plasmin
        formation, 190
    measure of, plasmin-cleaved insoluble
        cross-linked fibrin, 190
De novo guanosine synthesis, 216
Debridement, 112
Decannulation, 235
    accidental, 235
Deceased donor organ procurement
    complications of, 655–656
Decompressive fasciotomy, 351
Decreased global perfusion, clinical signs
    of, 128
Deep and superficial perforator systems, 340
Deep vein thrombosis (DVT), 189,
        403, 594
    acute postoperative complications, 403
    acute, 350
    diagnosis of, edema of involved calf or
        ankle, 339
    fondaparinux, neutralization of factor Xa
        by antithrombin, 346
    hand-held Doppler examination, 339
    impedance plethysmography, 339
    incidence, risk factors and categories,
        337–339
    popliteal, femoral or iliac veins, effect
        on, 338
    pulmonary embolism, first
        manifestation, 338
    thrombolytic and surgical procedures,
        348–350
Deep venous thrombosis, recurrent
    incidence of, 377
Deflation lumen
    injection of carbon dioxide or
        saline, 363
Dehiscence, 111, 242
Dehydroepiandrosterone (DHEA), 566
Delay phenomenon, 362
Delayed capillary refill, 128
Delayed gastric emptying
    pancreaticoduodenectomy, for
        adenocarcinoma of
        pancreas, 601
    significant postoperative problem, 471
Delayed primary closure, 110

Delivery systems
    enteral feeding and preventive
        interventions, potential
        complications of, 205
    potential complications of central
        access, 204
Dental injury, acute, 229
Department of Veterans Affairs, 54
    and the NSQIP executive committee
        affairs, 54f
Departmental Complication Conference
    quality assessment in surgery,
        case-finding methods, 7
Dermal healing
    delay in, 108
Dermatitis, 513
Devascularization, avoidance of
    handling hilar blood vessels during
        operation, 416
Devitalized liver tissue
    removal of, 409
Dextran, 70, 146, 354
    volume expansion use, 146
Dextrose
    common additive to crystalloids, 145
Dextrose infusion
    increase in thiamine demands, 201
    lactate production, 145
    rate, 198
Dextrose overfeeding
    hypertriglyceridemia, 198t, 199
Dextrose oxidation, 198
Diabetes
    insipidus, 139
    mellitus
        endocrine abnormality,
            immunosuppression
            patients, 222
        impaired neutrophil chemotaxis and
            phagocytosis, 108
Diabetic retinopathy, 670
Diagnostic angiography, 357, 359
Diagnostic lobectomy, 578
Diagnostic open biopsy, 608
    complications of, 608–609
Diagnostic pitfalls, 139
    clinical assessment of, 139
Diagnostic related groups, 6
Diagnostic thyroid evaluation, 576–577
Dialysis, 292
    access
        management of, 222
    catheters
        complications of, 155
        pneumothorax, arterial cannulation,
            complications of, 155
    chronic, 150
    severe hyperkalemia, acidosis, and
        volume overload, 150
    therapy, 645
Diaphragmatic hiatus, 258
    obstruction, 258–259, 259f
Diaphragmatic injury, 415
Diaphragmatic repair, 552
    prosthetic replacement, rarely
        required, 415
Diarrhea, 137
DIC. *See* Disseminated intravascular
        coagulation (DIC)
Difficult airway, 71

Diffusing capacity of the lung for carbon
        dioxide (DLCO)
    diffusion defects and emphysematous
        changes, 265
    preoperative assessment, 265
    pulmonary capillary surface area, 265
Diffusion-weighted magnetic resonance
        imaging, 360
Digital ischemia, 190
Digoxin
    alternative agent, atrial fibrillation, 182
    and β-blockers, 265
    drug of choice, preventing postoperative
        arrhythmias, 265
Diltiazem
    calcium channel blocker, reducing atrial
        arrhythmias, 265
Diltiazem drip, 290
Dipyridamole thallium imaging
    preoperative screening, limitations of
        low specificity and positive predictive
        value, 64
Dipyridamole-thallium test predictors, 176
Direct thrombin inhibitor, 346
    lepirudin, bivalirudin, or
        argatroban, 280
D-isomer
    clinical toxicity, and adverse changes in
        leukocyte function, 141
Disseminated intravascular coagulation
        (DIC), 132, 188, 190
    sepsis, malignancy, obstetrical
        complications, 190
Distal intestinal obstruction syndrome
        (DIOS), 735
Distributive shock, 137
    low systemic vascular resistance
        (SVR), 128
    septic shock and neurogenic shock, 128
Diuretic therapy, 267
    decreases preload, 181
    furosemide use for acute CHF, 181
Diverticular disease, 501–502
Diverticuli
    lower gastrointestinal hemorrhage, 502
Diverticulosis, 502
Diverting ileostomy
    construction of, 512
DLCO. *See* Diffusing capacity of the lung for
        carbon dioxide (DLCO)
Dobutamine stress echocardiography, 63
    noninvasive imaging tool, resting
        and stress systolic heart
        function, 177
Dobutamine therapy
    myocardial contractility increase, 131
Doctor–Patient relationship, 12
Donabedian
    measuring institutional quality, 46
Donor hemodynamic stability, 671
Dopamine, 154
Doppler ultrasonography, 643
Doppler ultrasound
    with allograft rejection, 642f
Doppler waveform, 139
Dor (anterior) fundoplication, 261
Dosing, 213
Down syndrome, 73, 234
Drain fluid, 417
Drainage procedures, internal, 464

Drainage, incomplete, 518
Draining lymph node
evaluation and management of, 622
Drains/dead space management, 123
devitalized tissue or fluid, 123
Drotrecogin alfa treatment
multiple-organ dysfunction, lower
incidence of, 131
Drotrecogin-treated group, 131
Drug Enforcement Administration (DEA), 27
Drug-eluting devices, 287
Drug-induced wound complications,
possibility of, 108
Duct-to-duct repairs, 430
Duhamel procedure, 736
Martin modification of, 737
Dumping, 395–396, 395t
Dumping syndrome, 254, 401, 747
Duodenal
perforation
infectious complications of, 390
laparoscopic closure of, 391
laparoscopic repair of, and open
repair, 391
pyloromyotomy, opening in mucosa
adjacent to duodenum, 755f
stump, 394
ulcer disease
effective antibiotic therapy,
elimination of, 390
ulcer perforation
hospitalization rates for, 390
Duodenal atresia, 747
Duodenal dysmotility, 728
Duodenal fistula, 394–395
complication of gastric resection, 394
parenteral alimentation, maintaining
positive nitrogen balance, 394
Duodenoenteric anastomosis, 675
Duodenopancreatic NETs, 594, 599t
Duodenotomy, 389
Duplex imaging
accurate technique in symptomatic
patients, 339
Duplex ultrasound
hemorrhage, assessment with, 359
normal venous flow, demonstrated in
left external iliac vein, 340f
thrombosed left common femoral vein
dilated, 341f
unstable thrombus, right external
iliac vein, 348f
Duplex ultrasound imaging
B-mode image and Doppler flow
analysis, 339
Duplex ultrasound screening, 343
Duplex-detected reflux, 352
Duplex-directed varicose excision, 352
DVT prophylaxis, 403
Dye load, 154
Dysesthesia. See Back pain
Dysfibrinogenemias, 188, 338
Dyspeptic symptom, 770

E
Early Specialization Programs (ESP), 13–14
EBV. See Epstein-Barr virus
ECG. See Electrocardiogram (ECG)
Echocardiograms, 300

Echocardiographic image quality, poor
quality of
myocardial perfusion study, 63
Echocardiography, 278
demonstrate valve malfunction, 302
ECMO. See Extracorporeal membrane
oxygenation (ECMO)
Ectopic ACTH syndrome, 564
Ectopic parathyroid adenomas, 589
Edema, cerebral
limitation of, 283
Educational integration, 15
distance learning, 15
live telesurgery transmissions, 15
Ehlers-Danlos syndrome
abnormal wound healing phenotype, 109
genetic disorder, 109
EKG response, abnormal, 63
Electrical cardioversion, 309
for hemodynamic instability, 289
Electrocardiogram (ECG), 59, 176–177
ambulatory, 63
ischemic ST-segment depression, low risk
for perioperative cardiac
events, 176
12-Lead ECG, 63, 181
Electrocautery injury, 550
Electrocautery, 62, 629
tissue effects, risk factor for seroma
formation, 606
Electroencephalographic (EEG)
monitoring during carotid artery
occlusion, 319
Electrolyte abnormalities, 201
Eloesser flap, 270
Embolic phenomenon
cannulation of the aorta, 282
Embolism, 301, 371
Embolization, 323, 360, 372
and stroke, 361–362
consequence of, 360
distal, 371, 372
distal cerebral, 361
iliac artery PTA and stent
placement, 363
incidence and sequelae of, during
cerebral angiography, 360
vertebral artery, risk of, 362
Emergent operation. See Elective operation
Empyema cavity, obliteration
myoplasty and thoracoplasty, 270
Empyema, 310–311, 693–694, 765–766
bronchopleural fistula, after pulmonary
resection, 310
development of, serosanguinous sputum,
purulent chest tube, 310
En bloc nephrectomy, 568
Encephalopathy, 288
incidence of, 282
End organ function, 146
End results system
advocated by Codman, 45
Endarterectomized vessel
extensive platelet aggregation, 320
Endarterectomy
cerebral ischemia, 318
hypercellular responses, 321
End-bleeding vessel
figure-8 or horizontal mattress suture, 411

Endobronchial injury, 74
Endobronchial tumor, 307
Endocarditis
mycotic infections, cardiac conduction
defects, 300
Endocrine
abnormalities, 222
and oncologic surgery
complications of, 557–573
complications, 281
insufficiency, 472
pancreatic insufficiency, 600
pancreatic neoplasms
resection of, 600
surgical treatment of, 594
pancreatic surgery
complications of, 596–601
pancreatic tumors, 597
approach to resection, 596
delayed gastric emptying, with
reduced frequency, 601
general complications, 600–601
Endograft, 364–369
Endoleak
persistence of blood flow, outside of
endograft, 366
types of, 366, 366t
Endomyocardial biopsy, 705
End-organ perfusion, 127
Endoscopic retrograde
cholangiopancreatography
(ERCP), 428, 430f, 436, 468f
risk factors for unsuccessful stone
extraction, 448t
Endoscopy
biliary dilation
percutaneous stenting, 454
biopsy
cryptitis and crypt abscesses, 502
cervical esophageal perforation, 248f
dilation, 453
overall complication rate for, 454
drainage, 465
guidance, 239
hemostasis, 391
second attempt at, 388
injection therapy, 388
laryngeal surgery, 230
mucosal resection, 397
radial artery harvesting
new techniques of, 291
retrograde cholangiography, 418
sphincterotomy, 435
stone extraction, 446
surgery
jet ventilation, 234
techniques, 291
therapy, 387
failure of, surgery next alternative,
388
major complication of, delayed
rebleeding, 388
thermal coagulation, and injection of
vessel sclerosants, 388
treatment, 387–388
ulcer
appearance and risk of, recurrent
hemorrhage, 387t
ultrasound, 396
upper gastrointestinal, 387

urgent, 393
vein harvest techniques
  ability of, 291
Endothelial cell damage, 132
Endotracheal intubation
  dyspnea, stridor, and cyanosis, early
    control of airway, 161
Endotracheal tubation, 753
Endotracheal tube (ETT), 70
  oral airway, 72
Endotracheal tube migration
  complication of, 549
Endovascular aneurysm repair, 369
  AAA repair, 369
  aortic aneurysm repair, 321
  interventions, 357
  snares, 364
  therapy, 354
    arterial rupture, feared complications,
      362
    complications managed in
      noninvasive fashion, or
      conventional surgery, 377
    complications of, 357–377
    for pulmonary embolism, 376
    main complications, 357
  venoplasty and stenting
    definitive approach for, iliac vein
      compression syndrome, 354
Endovascular techniques, standard
  snares and catheters, 350
End-to-end repair
  advantage of, 430
Enteral intolerance, 196
Enteral nutrition, 195, 207
  aspiration leading to ARDS, 208
Enteral nutritional support, 207
Enteric-pancreatic drainage, 597
Enteric-pancreatic or enteric-biliary
    anastomosis
  failure of, 596
Enterococci
  complications in GI tract
    operations, 118
Enterocolitis, 737
Enterocutaneous fistula
  anastomotic leak, 753
  development of, 752
  management of, 483
  suture-induced intestinal injury, 753
Enterocutaneous fistulae
  complex abdominal wall defects, and
    large hernias, 542
  increased risk for, 527
  management of, 483t
Enteroenteric fistula, 490
Enzymatic collagen hydroxylation, 105
Enzyme-linked immunosorbent assay
  detects antiheparin antibody in
    plasma, 346
Epidural analgesia, 268
Epidural anesthesia, 180
Epidural hematomas
  epidural space, 85
Epidural venous plexus
  disruption of, 85
Epinephrine
  decrease in peak plasma
    concentration, 83
Epistaxis, 228

Epithelialization
  epithelial cells, proliferation and
    migration of, 106
  wound breaking strength, 106
Eplerenone therapy, 563
Epstein-Barr virus (EBV), 219, 695
Esophageal
  anastomotic disruption
    complication of, 246
  anatomy, 245
  anomaly
    predictors of survival from, 748t
  carcinoma
    oncologic treatment for, 259
  diverticulectomy, 260–261
  Doppler monitor
    small-caliber Doppler ultrasound, 139
  fistula
    high mortality and morbidity, 274
  injury, 235, 585
  intubation, 74
  obstruction
    aspiration pneumonia, 246
    chronic, 259
  perforation, 247–251, 765
    causes of, 247t
    chronic reflux stricture, development
      of postoperative
      dysphagia, 250
    diagnosis of, 247–248
    essentiality of oral hygiene, 249
    intravenous fluid resuscitation, 248
    mid- and distal esophagus,
      following biopsy or
      dilatation, 249f
    nonoperative conservative
      therapy, 249
    reapproximation of the muscle, over
      the staple suture line, 251f
    treatment algorithm for, 250f
    treatment, 248
  replacement
    complications of, 259
  resection, 255–259
    gastric outlet obstruction,
      development of, 258, 258f
  spasm, 254
  stricture
    precisely measured localization of
      stricture, 252f
  surgery, 245
  tears
    acute, 253
    primary repair of esophageal
      perforation, 250f
  varices, 191
Esophageal atresia (EA), 744–749
  repair of, 746f
Esophageal echocardiogram. See Swan-Ganz
    catheter
Esophageal edema, distal, 253
Esophageal fistula, 273
Esophageal motor dysfunction, distal
  manipulation of vagus nerves, 253
Esophageal replacement, substernal,
    259–260
Esophageal segment, distal, 747
Esophagectomy
  emergent, primary or delayed esophageal
    reconstruction, 250

followed by chylothorax, 259
  postoperative pancreatitis, 259
  spleen injury, 259
Esophagoduodenoscopy, 16
Esophagogastric junction, 255
Esophagogastric varices, 420
Esophagogastroscopy, 251
Esophagogram
  esophagopleural cutaneous
    fistula, 260f
Esophagojejunostomy
  proximal jejunum, 399f
Esophagomyotomy, 261–262
  testing inadvertent esophageal
    perforation, 261f
Esophagopleural cutaneous
  fistula, 250
Esophagopleural fistula, 273–274
Esophagoscopy, 251–252, 748
Esophagotomy, elective
  primary esophageal closure, 247
Esophagram, 765
Esophagus
  parasympathetic innervation of, 246
  pulsion diverticula of, 260
Esophagus, diseased native
  management of, 260
Etomidate, 77
Eurostar registry, 370
Euvolemia, 152
Excision
  current recommendations for, 621t
Exercise ECG testing, for detecting
    myocardial ischemia, 63
Exercise echocardiography, 63
Exercise myocardial perfusion imaging, 63
Exercise oximetry, 265
Exercise stress testing, 177
Exercise thallium scans, 63
Exocrine insufficiency, 472–473
Exocrine pancreatic insufficiency, 600
Exogenous tumors, 488
Expanded polytetrafluoroethylene
    (ePTFE), 321
  stentgraft, 372
Expectant management
  neuropraxia, traction injury, 240
Expiratory reserve volume (ERV), 89
Exploratory laparotomy, 480
Exploratory surgery
  therapeutic value, 488
Exposure keratitis, 94
Extended choledochotomy
  removal of, intrahepatic stones by
    lithotomy, 449
Extended Kocher maneuver, 596
Extended learning curve, 403
Extended lymphadenectomy
  therapeutic benefit of, treatment of
    gastric adenocarcinoma, 397
External biliary fistula
  bile peritonitis, related to anastomotic
    leak, 451
External branch of the superior laryngeal
    nerve (EBSLN), 581, 583
  protection of, 584f
External drainage, 466
External iliac artery or femoral artery, 369
External thrombosed hemorrhoids, 516
Extracellular fluid compartment, 144

Extracellular fluid space, 144
  intravascular and extravascular
    compartment, 144
Extracellular hyaluronic acid
  cell migration and proliferation, 105
Extracorporeal anastamosis, 553
Extracorporeal circulation, 277–278
  complications of, 277–284
  in-line oxygenator, 277
  nonphysiologic and nonpulsatile, 277
Extracorporeal life support (ECLS), 167,
    170–171, 743
  adult ECLS criteria
    greater risk of death from
      ARDS, 171t
  algorithm for treatment of severe
    ARDS, 171t
  severe ARDS, 170–171
  survival outcome in ARDS, 170t
Extracorporeal membrane oxygenation
    (ECMO), 267, 688, 743
Extracranlial carotid arteries, 317–321
  specific complications, 317
Extrahepatic bile duct injury, 414
Extrahepatic blood loss
  sources of, 410t
Extraperitoneal rectal cancer
  preoperative staging, transrectal
    ultrasound, or endorectal
    MRI, 504
Extremity lymphedema, upper, 609
Extruded polytetrafluoroethylene (PTFE), 527

F

Fabric tears
  managing leak site, 368
Factor V Leiden, 190, 338, 344
Factor VIIa inhibitors, 348
Factor XI (XI) deficiency, 187
Failed block, 87
False aneurysm, 321
False passage, 235–236
False-positive cultures, 165
Familial adenomatous polyposis (FAP), 503
  autosomal dominant disease,
    503, 504
Familial cancer syndrome, 595
Fascia lata, 274
Fascial dehiscence
  careful wound examination and
    immediate reclosure, 528f
  reported incidence of, 526
Fascial necrosis, 524
Fasting PN patients
  distended gallbladder, 203
Fatigue, stress, 369
Fecal fistula, 505
  necrotic appendiceal stump, 500
Fecal impaction, 515–516
Fellowship training program, 6
Femoral
  and peroneal neuropathies, 510–511
  artery cannulation, 282
  hernias, 532
    preperitoneal approach, 534
  nerve palsy, 742
  neuropathy, 510
    retroperitoneal hemorrhage, 360
  popliteal bypass stenosis, 332f
  pseudoaneurysm, 359

Femoropopliteal angioplasty, and stenting,
    371–372
Femoropopliteal venous reflux,
    diagnosing, 340
Fenoldopam mesylate
  dopamine-1 agonist, decreased risk of
    postoperative ARF, 154
  potent vasodilator, increases renal
    plasma flow, 358
Ferguson closed hemorrhoidectomy, 515
Fiberoptic
  bronchoscopic intubation, 234
  bronchoscopy, 73, 268
  cystoscopy, 648
  endoscopy, 391, 393
  laryngobronchoscope
    intubation, 583
  nasopharyngeal endoscopy
    upper airway erythema, 163
Fibrillar collagen, 105
Fibrillation, 265
Fibrin glue, 310
  sealant, 273
Fibrin sealant, 629
Fibrinolytic mechanisms
  plasminogen-activator inhibitor-1,
    release of, 127
Fibrinolytic system
  factor XII, 281
Fibrinolytics, 67
Fibrinous exudate, acute, 250
Fibronous empyema
  thoracoscopic view of, 766f
Fibroplasia, 105
Fibroproliferation, and remodeling,
    104–106
Fibroproliferative phase, 106
Fibroproliferative stage of ARDS
  corticosteroids, 170
Fibrotic and cirrhotic livers, 412
Fibrotic lung, 270
Field of error analysis, 12
Filter occlusion
  massive pulmonary embolism, trapping
    of, 349
Filter strut
  fracture, duplex ultrasonography, 350
  full thickness erosion of, 376
Filter tilt
  another potential complication, 349
Fine needle aspiration biopsy, 609
Finger-fracture technique
  liver parenchyma, crushed between
    fingers, 412
Fistula, 236, 467–468, 505–506, 519
  closure, factors preventing
    spontaneous, 483t
  formation, 483
  pancreatic parenchymal
    necrosis, 467
Fistula-in-Ano
  cryptoglandular infection, from anal duct
    obstruction, 519
Fistulography, 428
Fistulotomy, 519–520
Fistulous disease
  complexity of, 519
Flaccid paralysis. See Phase I block
Flail chest, 274
Flair, 424

Flank hernia repairs, 523
Flash sterilization
  implantable devices, not applicable
    for, 121
  rapid steam sterilization, 121
Flexible bronchoscopy
  routine use of, 268
Flexible fiberoptic bronchoscopy, 269
Flexible sigmoidoscopy
  identifying mucosal ischemia, 293
Fluid therapy, standard, 145
  slower resolution of ileus, and longer
    hospital stay, 145
Fluid third spacing. See Third space fluid
    losses
Fluid, 129
  administration
    isotonic crystalloids or colloids, 152
  and electrolyte abnormalities,
    144–148, 144
  balance
    and renal complications, 281–282
  compartments, 144–145
  loss, 128
    acid-base balance effect, 138
  management, 144
    electrolyte derangements, 144
  overload, 266
  restriction, 145, 267
  resuscitation, 129
    endpoints for, 141
    physiological parameters, laboratory
      values pH, 141
    treatment for hypovolemic
      shock, 140
  therapy, 144
Flutter, 265
Focal nodular hyperplasia, 409
Fogarty catheters, 747, 768
Foley catheter, 729
  for laparoscopic procedures, 550
  patency, 152
Food and Drug Administration (FDA)
    database, 552
Foot venous pressures
  invasive methods, to quantitate venous
    hypertension, 340
Forced air warming, 91
Forced vital capacity, 197
Foregut duplication cyst, 744
Foreign body aspiration
  Heimlich maneuver, treatment for
    children, 164
Frank diabetes
  development of, 215
Frank-Starling curve, 139
FRC. See Functional residual capacity (FRC)
Free water deficit, 201
French balloon catheter, 748
Fresh frozen plasma (FFP), 140, 191
  acid-citrate-dextrose anticoagulant, 191
  coagulation factor deficiencies, 140
Fresh gas flow, 77
Fulminant hepatic failure, 415
  coagulopathy, 415
  hepatic encephalopathy, development
    of, 415
  normal liver, total devascularization
    of, 416

Functional residual capacity (FRC), 89, 169, 268
Fundoplication, 748, 770
  sutures, site of, 254
Fungal infections, 300
  invasive, 218
Furosemide
  loop diuretics, converts oliguric renal failure into nonoliguric failure, 154
Future surgical training, 9–17
FVIIa therapy, 192

G

Ganther Tulip, 349
Gallbladder cancer
  complications following treatment of, 445
  highly lethal disease, 444
  peritoneal tumor seeding, 444
  recommended treatment for, 444–445
  unsuspected, 443–444
Gallbladder tumors
  pathologic TNM classification of, 444t
Gallstone pancreatitis, 424
Gamma amino butyric acid (GABA), 77
Gangrene, venous, 338
Gangrenous cholecystitis, 442–443
Gas delivery system, 77
Gas embolism, 552
  asymptomatic, 552
Gas-bloat syndrome, 770–771
Gastrectomy, 394
Gastric
  acid secretion, 208
  adenocarcinoma
    high rates of, 396
    operative treatment of, 396
  atony, 246
  cancer, 396
    decreased in incidence, 385
    diagnosis of, 396
    incidence of, gastric cancer resection in the United States, 386f
    intramural spread, extensive intramural capillary and lymphatic network, 397
    subsequent gastric resection, decline in, 385
    surgical resection, only curative treatment, 396
  cardia, 398
  contents, aspiration of, 230
  distension, acute, 207, 404
  emptying, 145, 258
    inadequate, and multifactorial, 601
  lavage
    prelude to endoscopy, 391
  mobilization, 259
  motility
    impaired, 254
  operations, 385
  outlet obstruction, 258, 391–393
  perforation, 744
  pH
    nosocomial pneumonia, significant role in, 165
  resection
    length of stay, from 1988 through 2000, 386f
    operative technique, and postoperative physiologic support, 397

surgery, 768–771
  anatomic failure, 771
  dysphagia, 770
  fundoplication, 770
  gas-bloat syndrome, 770–771
  gastrocutaneous fistula, 769
  gastrostomy, 768–769
tonometry
  multiorgan dysfunction syndrome, 128
ulceration, 253
Gastric bypass, open, 403
  range of postoperative complications, 403
Gastric resection, 385
Gastrinomas
  longitudinal duodenotomy, 596
Gastrocolic reflux, 747
Gastrocutaneous fistula, 769
Gastroduodenal diseases, non-neoplastic, 396
Gastroduodenal ulcer disease
  routine prophylaxis, 220
Gastroesophageal reflux disease (GERD), 230, 770
Gastroesophageal reflux, 246
  pathophysiology of, 246
Gastrohepatic ligament
  large variceal vessels, 411
Gastrointestinal (GI), 136
  bleeding, 137, 420
    noncirrhotic patient, 420
  complications, 283–284,292
    immunosuppression related, 221
    strategies controlling, using increased perfusion flow rate, 284
  diagnosis of complications, 221
  disease, 220–221
  glaucoma and cataracts, ocular complications of, 214
  hemorrhage, 506
  injury
    risk factors, 284
  ischemic colitis, 503
  surgery
    complications of, 385–404
  tract CMV disease, 221
Gastrointestinal stromal tumor (GIST), 488
Gastrojejunostomy
  construction of, 392f, 601
  retrocolic position, occlusion of anastomosis by transverse mesocolon, 392
Gastroparesis, 207, 670
Gastroschisis, 730
  omphalocele, 753
Gastrostomy, 768–769
Gelfoam, 413
General anesthesia (GA), 70, 75–81
  emergence from anesthesia, proper timing and criticality of endotracheal extubation, 70
  induction of, and emergence from, 70
  insensibility to surgical pain, 75
  positive pressure ventilation, maintenance of, 414
  potent inhaled anesthetics (PIAs), 75–76
General complications, 308

General health status
  determinant of overall fitness, for surgical intervention, 158
  pulmonary risk predictor, 158
General risks, 567–571
Genetic defects, 109
Geowall stereoscopic projection system
  increasing fidelity, enhancing evaluation of performance, 17
GERD. *See* Gastroesophageal reflux disease (GERD)
GIA stapler, 736
Giant ventral hernias, 541–542
  severe skin lymphedema, 541
Gianturco stent
  recanalize inferior vena caval, 349
Gingival hyperplasia, 215
Glisson capsule, 414
Glisson sheath
  injury of, 413
Global hypoperfusion, 282
Global ischemia, 278
Glomerular filtration rate (GFR), 138, 150
  decrease in, 358
Glottic stenosis, 231–232
Glucagonomas, 594
Glucocorticoid insufficiency, 572
Gluconeogenesis, 197
Glucose homeostasis
  preexisting impairment of, 600
Goal-directed supportive therapy, early, 131
  oxyhemoglobin saturation (CVo$_2$ sat), 131
  volume resuscitation, 131
Goiter, 578
  enlarged thyroid, benign processes affecting the gland, 578
  resection for, 578
Goiter, substernal
  enlargement of, 578
Goldman cardiac risk index, 175
  cardiac morbidity and mortality, study of, 175
  independent correlates of, perioperative cardiac events, 175t
  pulmonary and cardiac complications, 158
Goldman risk factors, 176
Gore-Tex, 270
GpIIb/IIIa antagonists (aciximab)
  decreasing dose of lytic therapy, 350
Graded elastic support stockings
  Dextran, lowering fatal pulmonary embolism, 343
Graduate medical education (GME) funding
  rigid limitations of, 15
Graduate medical training, 13
Graft
  dilation, 328
  erosion
    areas of, 369
  explantation suture disruption, 369
  infection, 332
    lower extremity revascularization, 332
  migration, 369
  rejection, 656
  thrombectomy
    patients treated, followed by endovascular repair, 369
  thromboses, 328–329
  versus host disease (GVHD), 658

Graft occlusion, late, 331–332
Graft thromboses, early
    poor arterial inflow and outflow,
        associated with, 331
Graft thromboses, late
    kinking or excessive angulation of graft
        limbs, 329
Gram-negative bacilli
    Acinetobacter baumannii, 165
    anaerobic bacteria, 118
    enterococci, 118
Gram-negative infections
    DIC with sepsis, 190
Gram-positive bacteria
    peptidoglycan and lipoteichoic
        acid, 127
Gram-positive Staphylococcus, 107
Granulation, 242
Granuloma, 237–238
Graves disease, 576, 578
    neoplastic nodule, 576
    operative therapy, indications for, 578*t*
    therapeutic options, 578
    total thyroidectomy, effective strategy
        for, 578
Greenfield filters, 376
Griffith point, 503
Gross domestic product (GDP), 3

H
H_2-blockers, 420
H_2-receptor antagonists, 598
Hancock or Carpentier-Edwards
    porcine valves, probability of structural
        failure, 299
Haptic feedback
    robust data capture, 16
Hashimoto thyroiditis, 576, 578
    operation for, 578
HAT. *See* Hepatic artery thrombosis (HAT)
HB. *See* Hepatoblastoma (HB)
HCC. *See* Hepatoblastoma carcinoma (HCC)
Health and Human Services (HHS), 667
Health care system, crisis in, 12
Health maintenance organizations
        (HMOs), 28
Health Resources and Services
        Administration (HRSA), 667
Heart failure
    ACE inhibitor or β-blocker, preoperative
        diagnosis of, 181
    acute
        pulmonary rales, pulmonary
            congestion, 60
    cardiac complication, after noncardiac
        surgery, 180–181
    chronic, 60
    myocardial ischemia assessment, 181
    new unstable cardiac ischemia,
        assessment of, 180
    preoperative and postoperative
        management of, 181
    preoperative identification of, 180
Heart transplantation
    abdominal complications, 717–719
    acute allograft failure, 700–702
    arrhythmias, 702–703
    cardiac allograft rejection, 703–706
    chronic renal insufficiency, 715–716
    complications after first year, 711–715
    complications in first year, 703–711

complications of, 700–719
    gastrointestinal complications,
        717–719
    hyperglycemia, 717
    hyperlipidemia, 716–717
    hypertension, 716
    infection in, 706–711
    major complications in, 715–719
    malignancies, 714–715
    osteoporosis, 717
    perioperative period complications in,
        700–703
    technical factors, 703
Heimlich valve, 310
Helicobacter pylori
    childhood acquisition of, 396
    direct cellular injury, changes in gastric
        secretory physiology, 387
    eradication
        effect of, 390
    infection
        gastric secretory responses to, 387*t*
    long-term infestation with, 396
    pathogenicity of, 387
    seropositivity for, 396
Hematologic complications, 280–281
    multiple strategies, 281
Hematologic diseases, 338
Hematoma, 606–607
    significant nerve compression, sensory
        and motor deficits, 360
Hematoma, retroperitoneal
    first sign of, major vascular injury, 551
Hematuria, 675
Hemobilia, 419, 420
    bleeding into the bile ducts, 419
    serious complication, massive
        hemorrhage and death, 449
Hemodilution, 281
    crystalloid prime solution and
        hyperglycemia, modest
        diuresis in patients, 282
Hemodynamic instability, 361, 527
Hemodynamic measurements
    pulmonary artery catheterization in
        septic shock, 128
Hemodynamic optimization
    normalizing lactate levels, 128
Hemoglobin concentration, 136
Hemolysis, 303–304, 303
    hemoglobin cast formation, 282
Hemolytic Uremic Syndrome (HUS),
        338, 697
Hemoptysis
    pulmonary infarction, 341
Hemorrhage, 235, 308, 319, 323, 331, 359,
        386, 467, 488–490, 641, 685
    acute postoperative
        after antireflux operation, 254
    fatal intracranial, 131
    fatal postembolectomy pulmonary, 351
    intraluminal, 391
    major, 242
    retroperitoneal, 350
Hemorrhagic shock
    lactic acid production, and metabolic
        acidosis, 138
Hemorrhoidectomy, 514–515
    early complications of, 515–516
    late complications of, 516

Hemorrhoids, primary internal, 514
Hemostasis, 103, 534
    complications related to, 292
Hemostatic agents
    oozing from raw liver surface, 411
Heparin
    exposure, 280
    induced thrombocytopenia, 279–280, 338
        bovine and porcine unfractioned
            heparin, associated with, 345
        diagnosis of, 280
        production of immunoglobulin G
            antibodies, 279
        prevention of, warfarin induced skin
            necrosis, 344
    rebound, 281
    resistance
        administration of fresh frozen
            plasma, 281
        antithrombin III depletion, 281
Hepatectomy, 779
Hepatic
    adenoma, 409, 410
    arterial blood supply
        ischemic bile duct injury after
            ligation, 418
    arteries
        thrombosis of, 416
    artery embolization
        treatment of persistent, or massive
            hemobilia, 419
    artery ligation, 419
    artery or portal vein thrombosis
        early detection of, 416
    artery pseudoaneurysm, 659
    bleeding, 411–412
    failure, chronic, 416
    hemangiomas
        rupture of, 409
    resection, 451
        complications of, 779–780
    steatosis
        fat accumulation, liver lipid
            exceeding its removal, 203
        role of choline deficiency, 203
    surgery
        complications of, 407–421
        intraoperative and postoperative
            complications, 409
        neoplastic disease, 407
        surgical complications, 407
    toxicity, 289
    vasculature
        doppler examination of, 658
    venous structures, 412
Hepatic artery thrombosis (HAT), 658–659
Hepatic failure, subacute
    onset of hepatic coma, 416
Hepaticojejunostomy
    partial hepatic resections, 435
Hepaticojejunostomy or gastrojejunostomy
    anastomotic failure, 600
Hepatitis serologies, 410
Hepatobiliary scintigraphy, 428
    role of, 428
Hepatobiliary, 718
Hepatoblastoma (HB), 779
Hepatoblastoma carcinoma (HCC), 779
Hepatocellular carcinoma, 407, 409
Hepatoduodenal ligament, 413

Hepatolithiasis, 449
    development of, secondary biliary
        cirrhosis, 450
Hepatomegaly, 777
Hepatorenal syndrome, 420
Hepatotoxicity, 632
Hepp-Couinaud approach, 450
    liver split technique, approach to biliary
        reconstruction, 439f
Hepp-Couinaud hepaticojejunostomy, 451
Hepp-Couinaud technique, 436
Hereditary cancer syndromes, 595
Hereditary endocrine neoplasia syndromes,
    594, 597
Hereditary nonpolyposis colon cancer
    (HNPCC), 504
Hernia, 572
    clinically disabling, 523
    operations
        preoperative risk factors, 529
    repair, 540
Hernia, indirect, 534
Hernia, recurrent, 540–541, 541f
    managed with transabdominal
        reoperation, 751
Herniation, 771
    recurrent, 529
Herniorrhaphy, 776
Hesselbach triangle, 531, 536
Heterozygous Factor V Leiden, 345
HHS. See Health and Human Services (HHS)
Hiatal hernia repair, 252–255
    chylothorax, 254
Hiatal herniorrhaphy, 252
    complications of, 253t
HIDA scanning, 436
High airway pressure, 309
High and low outliers, 51
    warning system, communicating to
        surgical chiefs, 51t
High dose focal liver irradiation
    induces hypertrophy, unirradiated
        liver, 409
High peak airway pressures, 161
High sympathectomy
    bradycardia, 86
High urine output (UOP), 266
Higher baseline serum creatinine
    renal replacement therapy, 154
Higher-volume hospitals
    radical prostatectomy, lower rates of late
        urinary stricture, 32
High-quality effective CME, sources and
    characteristics of, 19
Hilar cholangiocarcinoma, 414
    risk factors of, and resection of, 457t
Hilar dissection, 272
Hilar vasculature, 507
Hill posterior gastropexy, 246
Hilum, right, 272
Hirschsprung disease, 730, 735–742
    diagnosis of, 735
    perianal excoriation, 737
    posterior myotomy/myectomy
        (POMM), 735
    three common types of operations, 736f
Hirsutism, 215
Histamine receptor antagonists, 220
Histamine receptor blocking drugs, 208
HLA. See Human leukocyte antigens (HLA)

Hodgkin disease, 613
Holosystolic murmur, diagnosis by
    echocardiogram, 302
Holter monitoring, 66
Horizontal mattress technique, 415
Hormone replacement therapy, 338
Horner syndrome, 362, 583
Hospital
    and surgeon volume
        complications, different effects on
            different types of, 35
    credentialing, 25
    credentials committees
        appeals process, 29
    factors, 35
        relative importance of, 35
    mortality, 300
    procedural volume
        regionalization of high-risk
            procedures, 31
    volume
        adjusted operative mortality rates, 33f
        high-volume hospitals, 31, 32t
        in-hospital mortality, 386f
        inversely related to operative
            mortality, 35
        operative mortality rates, observed
            and adjusted, 32
Hospital-level variables, 31–33
    high nurse-staffing levels, associated with
        better surgical outcomes, 33
    intensive care unit staffing, 32–33
    other variables, 33
    procedure volume, 31–32
Hospitals, high-outlier
    per-diem nursing support, 52
    quality-of-care issues, 52
Hospitals, high-volume, 31
    attenuated strength of surgeon
        volume–outcome
            relationships, 36f
    better-staffed ICUs, 35
    complex perioperative care, for patients
        undergoing high-risk
            surgery, 35
    data currency, 31
    elective abdominal aortic aneurysm
        (AAA)
            mortality significantly lower, 31
    lower mortality rates, 31, 32
    quality of case mix adjustment, 31
    specialist and technology-based services,
        broader range of, 35
Host immune system, 116
HRSA. See Health Resources and Services
    Administration (HRSA)
H-type fistula, 747
Human anodal trypsinogen (HAT), 678
Human cells
    glucocorticoid receptors, 213
Human herpes virus 8 (HHV-8), 219
Human leukocyte antigens (HLA), 656
Human serum albumin, 146
Human-activated Protein C, 131
Humoral pathways, 127
    microbial pathogens, recognition of, 127
HUS. See Hemolytic uremic syndrome (HUS)
Hydrocortisone, 132
Hydrodissection
    bloodless field during liver
        transection, 412

Hydronephrosis, 651
Hydrothorax, 256
Hydroxyethyl starch, 146
Hygiene, poor airway
    hemodynamic embarrassment, 311
    life-threatening problem, after chest
        surgery, 311
Hyperaldosteronism, 567
    posterior view of a NP-59 adrenal
        scintigram, by Conn
            syndrome, 561f
Hyperaldosteronism, primary, 560–563
    CT scan of, 561f
    diagnosis of, 567
    polyuria and nocturia occur, 560
Hyperalimentation, 482
Hyperammonemia, 696
Hyperamylasemia, 390
Hyperbaric oxygen (HBO), 162
Hyperbilirubinemia, 777
    and preoperative biliary drainage,
        471–472
Hypercalcemia, 651
Hypercapnia, 200
Hyperchloremic acidosis
    normal saline use, 141
Hypercoagulability, 337
Hypercortisolism, 563–564, 567–568
Hypergastrinemia
    secondary to *Helicobacter pylori*
        infection, 387
Hyperglycemia, 139, 198–199, 665, 678, 717
    fluid and electrolyte imbalances, 198
    hyperglycemic hyperosmolar nonketotic
        coma, 198
    impairment of neutrophil
        chemotaxis, 198
    perioperative management of, 288
Hyperglycemia, stress-induced, 198
Hyperinflation, 693
Hyperinsulinism, 780–781
Hyperkalemia, 141
    mild postoperative, 572
Hyperlipidemia, 199–200, 716–717
Hypernatremia
    dehydration, 201
Hyperparathyroidism, 589
    asymptomatic, 585
    persistent appearance of hypercalcemia,
        and elevated PTH levels, 589
    persistent or recurrent, 589–591
    primary
        operation in patients, indications for,
            585–586
        parathyroidectomy, 585
    secondary
        indications for operation, in patients
            with, 586
        nature of, 586
    symptomatic, 585
    tertiary, 585
Hyperplasia, 563
Hyperplastic gastric polyps
    neoplastic potential, 396
Hypertension, 62, 572, 642, 716
    and hypotension, 319–320
    rebound β-blockers and clonidine,
        abrupt withdrawal of, 62
    venous, 351
Hyperthermia, 91–92
    malignant hyperthermia (MH), 91–94

Hypertonic saline, 148
  efficient volume expander, 148
  improves cerebral blood flow, 148
  infusion
    beneficial in head trauma, 148
    macrophage, neutrophil, and endothelial
      cell activation, 141
  microcirculatory perfusion, 148
  microvascular circulation, improves, 141
  prehospital resuscitation strategy, 148
  resuscitation, 141
    intravascular volume resuscitation, 141
  volume resuscitation decrease, with
    decreased tissue edema, 141
Hypertriglyceridemia
  carnitine deficiency, 200
Hypertriglyceridemia, severe
  precipitates acute pancreatitis, 199
Hypertrophic cardiomyopathy, 62
Hypertrophic pyloric stenosis, 754
Hypertrophic scars, 111
Hypertrophy
  induced by, percutaneous portal vein
    embolization, 409
Hypervascular tumors
  imaging, 407
Hypoalbuminemia, 145
  adverse outcomes, 147
  protein depletion, postoperative
    mortality, 196
Hypoaminoacidemia, 594
Hypocalcemia
  acute management of, 579
  Chvostek sign, 579
  controlled by, intravenous calcium
    administration, 580
  temporary, 580
  Trousseau sign, 579
Hypochloremia, 137
Hypochloremic metabolic alkalosis,
    138, 146
Hypoganglionosis, 735
Hypogastric artery
  embolization, 365
Hypogastric artery, 364
  coil embolization, 365
  embolization, higher risk of pelvic
    symptoms, 365
Hypoglossal nerve
  tongue deviation, 319
Hypoglycemia, 199, 594
Hypokalemia, 200
  continuous EKG monitoring, 201
  correction of, 203
  mild, 62
  onset of the arrhythmia, 300
  severe, 203
Hypomagnesemia, 200
  functional ileus, hyperreflexia, and
    seizures, 202
Hyponatremia
  hypotonic solutions, administration
    of, 201
Hypoparathyroidism, 576, 579, 587
  chronic complications of, 579
  symptoms of, severe hypocalcemia, 579
Hypoparathyroidism, permanent, 576, 580
Hypophosphatemia, 200
  PN initiation, 203
Hypophosphatemia, severe, 202

Hypotension, 126, 572
  acute, low cardiac output state, 288
Hypothermia, 90–91
  dilution of clotting factors, 140
  prevention of, 753
  triggering peripheral vasoconstriction,
    decrease of tissue
      oxygenation, 119
Hypothyroidism, 577
Hypoventilation (loss of airway), 235
Hypovolemia, 137
  β-adrenergic and calcium channel
    blockers, 139
  contributing to graft thrombosis, 331
  intrathoracic perforation, 249
  melena, hematemesis, and guaiac
    positive stool, 137
  subtle signs to cardiovascular
    collapse, 152
Hypovolemic shock, 127, 136–141
  adequate tissue perfusion, 139
  clinical diagnosis of, 137
  cool and clammy skin, 138
  decreased organ perfusion, 137
  diagnosis of, 137–139
  etiology of, 127, 136–137
  inadequate intravascular volume,
    decreased cardiac preload, 127
  low intravascular volume, hemodynamic
    derangement of, 137
  low urine output, 138
  oxygen delivery to tissue, 136
  physical signs of, 137
  rapid identification and treatment, or
    survival of patients, 141
  redistribution of intravascular fluid, 137
  response to drugs, increased intravascular
    capacity, 137
  resuscitation using Ringer solution, 141
  resuscitation, use of colloids, 140
  stages of hypovolemia, 138t
  treatment for, 139–141
  with or without total body fluid
    depletion, 137t
Hypoxemia, 685
Hysteroscopy, 16

I

Iatrogenic aortic dissection, 279
Iatrogenic biliary strictures, management
    of, 440
Iatrogenic hyperthyroidism or
    hypothyroidism, 585
Iatrogenic hyperthyroidism, 577
Iatrogenic intraoperative hyperthermia, 91
Iatrogenic lung injury, 167
Iatrogenic paraesophageal hiatal
    hernia, 254
  complication of, 253
Iatrogenic short bowel syndrome, 482
ICU setting
  monitoring shock patients, 128
Ideal intravenous (IV), 77
Idiopathic deep venous thrombosis, 345
Idiopathic hyperaldosteronism, 560, 562
Idiopathic venous thromboembolism, 338
Ileocolectomy
  indicated for tumors, 500
Ileocolic intussusception, 772
  barium enema, 773f

Ileostomy
  complications of, 491–494, 491t
Ileus, 480–481, 572
  postoperative complications, 504
Iliac artery
  aneurysms, 364
  angioplasty
    angiogram of patient, resulting in
      perforation, 363f
  PTA
    complications of, 363
  rupture, 364
    balloon dilation, and stent
      placement, 363
  stenosis
    predilated with balloon
      angioplasty, 364
  stent placement
    arterial dissection, 363
  thrombosis, 364
Iliac endarterectomy, 363
Iliac stent migration
  management options, emergent vascular
    surgery, observation, stent
      retrieval, 363
Iliac vein thrombolysis
  arterio-venous fistula, 351
Iliac vein thrombus, distal
  duplex assessment of, 348
Iliofemoral bypass, 363
Iliofemoral deep venous thrombosis,
    massive
  early thrombolysis, 350
  phlegmasia alba dolens and phlegmasia
    cerulean dolens, 338
Ilioinguinal nerve
  cremasteric layer, minimizing injury to
    neurolemmal sheath, 542
Image-guided percutaneous needle biopsy
  initial diagnostic strategy, 609
Imaging studies
  chest x-ray and lateral neck x-ray, 231
Imaging tests, noninvasive preoperative, 595
Immediate breast reconstruction
    (IBR), 613
  complications of, 613–614
  skin-sparing mastectomy, 613
Immune activation
  rapid treatment of, 213
Immune and allergic, 279
Immune cells
  receptor systems, 127
Immune system, 212
  compromised, 212
Immunodeficiency
  cause of, 212
Immunodeficiency states
  delayed wound healing, 108
Immunologic stenosis, 642
Immunosuppression
  agents, 212–218
    immunosuppressive medications,
      sites of inhibition, 214f
    treatment of an autoimmune
      flare, 212
  common problems, 218–222
  complications of, 212–222
  medication
    side effects, 212, 213t
  therapy, 214

Impaired leukocyte function
  increased risk of pneumonia, 197
Impaired wound healing, 216, 219–220
  corticosteroid therapy, consequence
    of, 220
  zinc, vitamin C (ascorbic acid), and
    vitamin A deficiencies, 197
Imperforate anus
  arrest of normal descent, 738
  in male, 739f
Impotence, 329
In situ saphenous vein bypass, 332–334
  retained vein graft fistula, 334f
Inadequate hemostasis
  platelet dysfunction, poor technique, 106
Inadequate pouch length, 511
Incarcerated inguinal hernia, 775f
Incision
  biopsy, 578
  care, 123
  cellulites
    treated with oral antibiotics, 604
  dog-ears, 607
  for axillary dissection, 610f
  hernia repair, 538
    risk factors for wound infection, 539t
    serious complications with, alloplastic
      mesh implantation, 540
    study of, 529
  hernia, 404, 524, 538, 572, 656
    abdominal operations, iatrogenic
      complications of, 523
  herniorrhaphy
    reoperative nature of, 538
  intrathoracic extension, improves
    proximal exposure, 524
  metastases, 554
  pain, 525
Incision placement, standard
  open approaches, to the adrenal gland,
    569f
Incontinence, 510, 516, 518
  incidence rates for, 519
Increased host age
  impairs wound healing, 108
Incurable lesions
  detection of, 397
Induction chemotherapy or prior
  irradiation, 308
Industry-sponsored CME opportunities, and
  inducements, 22
Infarction, 318
Infected pancreatic necrosis
  drainage of, 466
Infection, 218–219, 371, 419–420
Infectious complications, 206
Infectious foci, identification of, 129
Inferior mesenteric artery back pressure, 324
Inferior vena cava (IVC)
  anastamosis
    complications of, 659–660
  filters
    complications during placement of,
      375, 376
    occlusion rates, 349
    prophylactic placement of, for high-
      risk trauma patients, 348
  occlusion, 349
  placement, 349
  thrombosis, 350, 659
Inflammation, 103–104

Inflammatory mediator release, 132
Inflammatory mediators, removal of, 132
Inflatable balloon dissector, 572
Inflow occlusion, 411
Information technology, use of
  in clinical decision support, 55
Infrahepatic vena cava, 412
Infrapancreatic approach, 570f
Infrarenal abdominal aortic aneurysm repair
  early and late complications, 321t
Infundibular, method, 424
Inguinal
  hernia, 530–531, 775
    classification of, 531t
    herniorrhaphy, 531
      Shouldice clinic principles
        of, 532t
    lymph node dissection
      widespread lymphedema, 623
    lymphadenectomy, 631–633
      complications of, 631
    repairs
      nerve injuries, 542–543, 543f
      sentinel node biopsy, 632–633
Inhalation injury
  carbon monoxide poisoning, 163
Inhibitory hormone somatostatin
  local secretion of, 387
Initial endoscopy
  performance of, 388
Injection laryngoplasty
  endoscopic technique, 240
  injury, biliary, 414
    algorithm for diagnosis and
      treatment of, 432f
    Bismuth-Strasberg classification, 426f
    classification of, 426–427
    clinical presentation of, 427–428
    intraoperative identification
      of, 425
    risk factors for, 425
Injuries, bronchial, 684
Injury, visceral, 542
  risk of, during laparotomy, 525
Inotropic agents
  adjuvants to proper fluid
    administration, 153
Institute of Medicine, 3, 4 11
Institutional quality
  query administrative data sets, 46
Instrument sterilization, 121
Insufflation, 548–550
Insulin drip
  controlling severe hyperglycemia, 199
Insulin-like growth factor, 155
Insulinoma resections, benign, 595f
Insulinoma. See Hypoglycemia
Intensive and conventional insulin
  therapy, 198
Intensive care unit (ICU) patients
  hypovolemic shock, and increased
    interstitial fluid, 139
Intensive care unit (ICU), 151
  high intensity vs. low intensity, ICU
    physician staffing, 34f
  high-intensity staffing, associated with
    lower hospital mortality, 33
  intensivist or elective intensivist
    consultation, 33
  low-intensity ICU physician staffing, 33
  staffing, 32

Intensive insulin therapy
  cardiac surgery patients, reduced
    mortality of, 39
  critically ill patients, 38–39
Intercostal incisional bleeding, 272
Intercostal space
  narrowing of, 270
Intermediate-risk patients, 63
  guide to noninvasive testing in
    preoperative patients, 63t
  noninvasive testing, 63
Internal carotid artery (ICA)
  common carotid artery, 287
  focal dissection of, 361
  thrombosis, acute, 319
  vasospasm, 361
International Liaison Committee on
  Resuscitation
  algorithm and guidelines, for
    management of
    tachyarrhythmias, 182
International Pancreas Transplant Registry
  (IPTR), 666
Internet-enabled educational programs, 11
Intersphincteric abscess, 518
Interstitial
  bypass, 490
  failure
    due to postoperative ileus, 477
    medical therapy for, 478
    underlying etiologies of, 478t
  failure patients, 479f
  fibrosis, 221
  ischemia, 133, 489
  motility, 490–491
  pseudo-obstruction
    chronic, 490
  surgery
    therapeutic goals of, 479t
Intestinal disorders, specific, 481–495
Intestinal ischemia, early, 293
Intestinal neuronal dysplasia (IND), 738
Intestinal pseudo-obstruction, chronic, 490
Intra-abdominal abscess/peripancreatic fluid
  collection, 505, 599–600
Intra-aortic balloon pump (IABP), 279, 291
  use of, 291
Intra-aortic filters, 288
Intra-arterial stent
  placement of, 363
Intracaval tumor thrombus
  extension, 568
Intracellular fluid compartment, 144
Intracerebral hemorrhage
  presence of, 319
Intracranial hemorrhage, 361
  risk factors for, 350
Intractable Crohn colitis, 503
  proctocolectomy with ileostomy,
    treatment of, 503
Intrahepatic
  abscess, 420
  bile duct
    injury, 414
    operative injury, 414
    stenting of, 414
    stone formation, 418
  biliary injury, 414
  fluid collection, 418
  hematoma, 420

Intrahepatic (*Continued*)
 liver volume ratios
  CT for normal livers, 408*t*
 stone formation
  serum alkaline phosphatase, increase
   of, 418
 stones, 449
In-training/Surgical Basic Science
  Examination, 27
Intralesional steroid therapy, 111
Intralobar sequestrations, 743
Intraoperative
 angiography, 333
 arterial oxygen desaturation, 74
 arteriography, 333
 awareness, 81, 82*t*
 biopsy, 415
 bleeding, 410
 cardiogenic disturbances, 308–309
 cholangiography
  abnormal cholangiograms, 425
  postoperative ERCP, 447
  use of, 425
 complete liver devascularization, 413
 complications, 234, 240–242, 308–309,
   409, 550–553, 626
 Doppler confirmation of blood flow, 324
 Doppler examination, 333
 enteroscopy
  push enteroscopy, 488
 fiberoptic cholangioscopy, 449
 fluids, 515
 gallbladder perforation
  port site recurrence, 444
 hemorrhage, 272
 ischemia, 181
 management, 402–403
 PTH levels, 586
 renal artery perfusion, 323
 transesophageal echocardiogram
   (TEE), 301
 ultrasonography, 596
 ultrasound, 597
Intraoperative bleeding, massive, 410
Intraoperative hemorrhage, massive, 308
Intraparenchymal bleeding, 412
Intrapleural CO$_2$ insufflation
 hemodynamic consequences, 308
Intrapulmonary cysts, 744
Intrathoracic esophagogastric anastomotic
  leak, 246
Intrathoracic esophagus, 273
Intrathoracic fundoplication, 253
Intrathoracic gastric outlet obstruction, 258
Intratracheal pulmonary ventilation,
  167–169
Intravascular
 blood volume
  maintenance of, 152–153
 cannulae
  placement of, 278
  retroperitoneal hematoma, 278
 catheter-directed thrombolysis, 350
 coagulation, 132
 volume deficit
  discontinuation of pressors, 303
 volume, expansion of, 129
Intravenous
 calcium gluconate, 580
 cyclosporine, 215

fluid, 144, 145, 358
 hyperalimentation, 256
 lipid emulsions
  long-chain triglycerides (LCTs), 199
 support
  electrolyte abnormalities, 201
Intravenous amiodarone, administration
  of, 289
Intravenous immune globulins (IVIGs), 217
Intubation complications
 risk factors, 228*t*
Intubation, 228
 acute and chronic complications of, 227
 incorrect placement, 234
 upper aerodigestive tract injury, 228
Intubation, bronchial, 74
Intubation, long-term
 tracheal damage, 233
Intussusception, 486, 772–774
 and gall bladder disease, with cystic
  fibrosis, 735
Intussusceptum
 schemic necrosis of, 393
Inverse ratio ventilation, 169
Inversion pancreaticojejunostomy, 597
Ionized calcium measurements, 579
Ipsilateral greater saphenous vein
 harvesting of, 332
Ipsilateral hemidiaphragm
 elevation of, 309
Ipsilateral hemisphere, 318
Ipsilateral main pulmonary artery, 308
IPTR. See International Pancreas Transplant
   Registry (IPTR)
Irradiated tissue
 hypoperfused by microangiopathy, 107
Irretrievable liver
 devascularization
  emergency liver transplant, 413
Ischemia, 181–182, 489–490
 stress-induced, 177
 warm, 416
  inflow occlusion, better tolerated, 416
  liver cells injury, 416
  postoperative rise in transaminases, 416
  residual, 64
Ischemia-reperfusion injury, 686–688
Ischemic
 and thermal bile duct injury, 416
 chest pain, 181
 colitis, 503–504
  treatment for, degree of injury, 503
 extremities
  reperfusion of, 323
 heart disease, 311
 necrosis, 506
 optic neuropathy
  ischemic optic neuritis, 95
 preconditioning, 416
 testicle, 775*f*
Isolated abnormal PT, 188
Isosulfan blue, 623
Isotonic crystalloids, 147

J

Japanese Gastric Cancer Association
 early gastric cancer, tumor invasion
   restricted to mucosa or
   submucosa, 397

Japanese Research Society
 for gastric cancer, 397
Jejunal feedings
 septic complications, low rate
   of, 133
Jejunogastric intussusception, 393
Jejunoileal
 atresia, 731*f*
  anastomotic leak, 730
  end-to-back anastomosis, 732*f*
  primary anastomosis, 752
 obstruction, 730–735
  jejunoileal atresia, 730
Jejunostomy
 feeding tube, 253
 placement, 494
 tube
  complications of, 494–495
Jejunum
 Roux-en-Y limb of, 395
Jet ventilation, 234
Johns Hopkins Hospital surgery training
   program
 education of surgeons, 5
Joint Commission on Accreditation of
   Healthcare Organizations
   (JCAHO), 39
Joint Council on Accreditation of Healthcare
   Organizations (JCAHO), 28
Jugular vein abscess, 256
Jugular venous distension, 267
J-wire
 strut apex fixation, 350

K

Kaposi sarcoma, 219
Kasai portoenterostomy, 777
Keel procedure, 539
Keloids, 111
Keratinocyte growth factor (KGF), 105
Ketamine, 78
Ketorolac
 intravenous substitute for opiate
   analgesics, 607
Ketorolac tromethamine, 515
Kidney transplantation
 Doppler ultrasound, 642*f*
Klatskin tumors
 classification of, 455*t*
Kocher maneuver, 259, 389, 726
Krebs cycle, 76
Kwashiorkor protein deficiency, 197
 decreased polymorphonuclear leukocyte
   activity, 108

L

Laboratory tests
 etiology of patient's shock, 128
Lactated Ringer solution
 appropriate replacement fluid, 146
 diluent for blood, 145
 serum lactate measurements, 145
Lactic acidosis, 201
Ladd procedure, 726
Lag phase, 106–107
Laparoscopy, 396–397
 adrenalectomy, 568
 antireflux surgery, 255
 approaches, 443, 560

bariatric surgery, 403
camera, 553
cholecystectomy, 16, 424, 442, 549, 446t
bile duct injury, 424
endoscopic retrograde
cholangiopancreatography,
428f
gallbladder opened, detecting
possible malignancy, 444
gallbladder perforation, 443
less postoperative pain, treatment of
complicated gallstone disease,
424
management of injuries, 430–435
mechanisms of biliary injury, 424t
stone and bile spillage, 443, 443t
cystgastrostomy, 464
fundoplication
complications of, 255
paraesophageal hiatal hernias, 255
gastrectomy
for treatment of gastric malignancy,
397
long-term cancer control rates for,
397
gastric bypass, 403
inguinal hernia repairs, 538
inguinal herniorrhaphy, 536–538
liver resection, 412, 415
Nissen fundoplication
transdiaphragmatic herniation, 771f
omental patching or fibrin glue repair,
391
operation
trocar insertion and placement, 546
posterior adrenalectomy, 571–572
procedures, 550f
stapling devices, 552
surgery
complications of, 546–554
postoperative shoulder tip pain, 553
transperitoneal adrenalectomy, 571
transperitoneal approach, 572
Laparotomy incisions, 524
Large balloon-expandable stent, 368
Large introducer sheaths, 364
Large mattress sutures
occlude important blood inflow, 411
Large pseudoaneurysms
retroperitoneal incision, control of distal
external iliac artery, 359
Laryngeal
complications
acute, 229–230
chronic, 230
mask ventilation, 234
neoplasm, 234
nerve injury, 246
trauma, 234
Laryngeal electromyography (EMG), 230
vocal fold paralysis, 230
Laryngeal mask airway (LMA), 74
complications with, 74
pharyngolaryngeal and neurovascular
complications, 74
Laryngoscopy
direct, 72
indirect, 235
Laryngospasm, 230
following extubation, 230

Laryngotracheal stenosis, 230–231
prolonged intubation, for tracheal
resection, 227
Laser and radio frequency ablation
devices, 352
Laser probe ablation, 418
Latex allergy, 93
Latissimus dorsi muscle, 272, 628
Laudanosine
hypotension and bradycardia, 79
Laudanosine toxicity, 79
Leaflet entrapment
retained valvular tissue, 302
Leaflet looping
valve struts examined, 302
Leak, 505
Leapfrog Group
criteria for, evidence-based hospital
referral, 40t
direct outcomes assessment, 39
Leflunomide, 216
Left bundle branch block (LBBB), 176
dipyridamole or adenosine-thallium
imaging, 63
Left hilum, 272
Left mainstem bronchus
bronchoscopic view of, 767f
chest x-ray, 767f
Left ventricular (LV) dysfunction
geometric relationship, 302
hypertrophy, 62
outflow, 60
pulmonary artery catheters, 62
Left ventricular (LV) filling pressure, 139
Left ventricular (LV) function, 286
Left ventricular ejection fraction (LVEF)
transthoracic echo, 177
Left ventricular hypertrophy, 176
Left ventricular outflow tract
obstruction, 303
Leg deep venous thrombosis
warfarin, for prevention of, 343
Leg wound complications
incidence of, 291
Lesions
asymptotic benign, 487
Less invasive catheter-based technique
efficacy of catheter, 351
Leukocyte filters
use of, 279
Leukoembolization, 279
Leukoreduction products, 140
Libby Zion case, in New York State
work hour regulations, 11
Lidocaine, 83
Life-table analysis, 361
Ligament of Berry
vessels of, 579
Limb salvage, 364
Limb thrombosis, 369
Linton procedure, 353
Lipopolysaccharide (LPS), 127
Lipoprotein lipase (LPL), 200
Lithotripsy, 449
Liver
abscess, 418
arterial bleeding from within,
intrahepatic hematoma, 409
biopsy, 419
cell perfusion retrograde, 416

complications, 203–204
cryoablation
cracking of liver parenchyma, 412
devascularization, 415, 416
disease, 190–191
chronic, 108
failure, 415–416
function studies, 410
inflow occlusion, 416
parenchyma, 411
portal hypertension, 191
preoperative management of, 191
regeneration, 415
resection
ascites occurs, ascitic leak from
incisions, 420
associated liver anatomy, 415
bilateral subcostal incision, 410
decreasing blood loss, using inflow
occlusion, 416
incisions for optimal exposure for,
bilateral subcostal
incision, 410f
malignant liver disease, staging to
eliminate patients, 407
metastatic colorectal cancer, 407
steatosis, 416
surgery, 776–780
biliary atresia, 776–777
cholangitis, 419
complications in, 408t, 777
etiologies of Cholangitis, 419t
hepatoblastoma, 779
kasai portoenterostomy, 777
preexisting bleeding associated, 409
surgical diseases of, 408
transection
blood loss during, eliminated by total
vascular exclusion, 412
blood loss minimization methods, 412
factors in blood loss, 411t
pressure or cautery, control over
minor bleeding points, 411
transplantation
biliary complications, 660–662
complications of, 655–662
graft vs. host disease (GVHD), 658
graft rejection, 656
hepatic artery thrombosis (HAT),
658–659
incisional complications in, 656–657
infection in, 658
portal vein thrombosis, 659
primary nonfunction, 656
recurrent disease, 657
remaining option for bile duct
stricture, 419
renal failure, 657
vascular complications in, 658
Liver disease, serious
prolonged PT and APTTs, 190
Liver failure, subacute, 416
Liver function
compromised, 416
Liver mass, residual
biliary drainage of, 416
Liver remnant, residual
maintenance of venous drainage,
continued intraoperative
attention, 414

Liver toxicities, severe
    steatosis, steatohepatitis, cholestasis, and
        cholelithiasis, 203
Liver volume, residual functioning
    amount of, influenced by technical
        factors, 415
Liver, normal, 413
Living donor liver transplantation
    complications of, 662
Lobar
    bronchial fistula, 270
    bronchus
        small defects, 270
    collapse, 268, 311
    torsion, 267
Lobe resections, partial, 414
Lobectomy or trisegmentectomy
    bile ducts, in a Glissonian fashion, 414
Lobectomy, right hepatic, 416
    morbidity and mortality, preoperative
        APACHE II scores, 408
Local anesthetic toxicity, 81–83
    maximal dose, for each local
        anesthetic, 84t
Local anesthetic-induced seizures, 83
Local mural necrosis, 253
Local operative risk factors, 425
Local recurrence and associated
        mortality, 620t
Local tumor recurrence, 620
Logistic regression
    analysis, 176
        nuclear cardiology imaging, 176t
        procedure complexity and patient
            characteristics, 55
    models
        logistic regression, calculating
            probability of death, 49t
        observed-to-expected ratios, 50t
        order of entry of predictive
            preoperative risk variables, 47t
        univariate t-tests or chi-square tests, 49
Longitudinal pancreaticojejunostomy,
        468–469
Long-segment stenosis, 232
Long-standing immunosuppression
    patients on, 220
Loop diuretics, 154
Loop ileostomy, 493–494, 512
    incarcerated prolapse, 494
    formation, 493f
    prone to prolapse, 494
Loproteinase
    elevated expression of tissue metal, 540
Loss of airway, 160–161
Low cardiac output, 302
Low dose unfractionated heparin (LDUH), 37
Low molecular weight heparin (LMWH), 189
    reduced risk of venous
            thromboembolism, 37
Low outlier
    confidence intervals (CI) range
            less than 1, 51
    O/E ratio, 52
Low-density lipoproteins (LDLs), 200
Lower abdominal surgery, 159
Lower extremity
    bypass
        complication rates, 331t
        early and late complications, 330t

edema, 332
    interventions, 371–375
    lymphedema
        treatment of, 632
Lower extremity revascularization, 329–330
    serious hemorrhage, 331
    subject to, rigorous postoperative
        follow-up, 329
Lower operative mortality, and processes, 52
Low-molecular-weight heparin, 344
    primary therapy, for venous
        thromboembolism, 344
Low-osmolality contrast agents, 358
Low-outlier hospitals
    high level of integration with VAH
        faculty, and faculty of
        medical school, 52
Low-outlier O/E ratio
    better nurse-staffing ratios, 52
Luminal platelet aggregation, 333
Lumpectomy
    complications of, 607–608
Lung
    abscess, 765
    cancer patients, 268
        marginal pulmonary reserve, 265
    cancer, 274
        induction chemoradiation therapy, 270
    carcinoma
        lung resection, curative
            treatment, 264
    disease
        chronic, 159, 751
        ventricular dysfunction, 265
    injury
        limiting CPB duration, 279
    parenchyma
        compression of, 308
    resection, 264, 307
        clinical assessment, and pulmonary
            function tests, 264
        Gibbon and Gibbon, 266
    surgery patients
        pneumothorax, secondary to
            barotraumas, 309
Lung approach, open, 169–170
    recruiting collapsed alveoli, and
        increasing FRC using PEEP, 169
Lung resection, major
    pulmonary edema, development of, 266
Lung resection, open
    prolonged air leak, morbidity after lung
        resection, 309
LV end-diastolic pressure (LVEDP), 139
Lymph node
    anatomical location of, 397
    dissection
        complete and selective, 621
    metastases, 595
Lymph node dissection, elective, 621
Lymphadenectomy, 628
    abdominal, 634–635
    complications of, 593–635
    head, 633–634
    inguinal sentinel node biopsy, 632–633
    level of nodal dissection, 397
    neck, 633–634
    pelvic, 634–635
    saphenous vein-sparing inguinal, 632
    thoracic, 635

Lymphangiosarcoma, secondary, 630
Lymphatic mapping and sentinel lymph
    node biopsy, 609, 612t
    after neoadjuvant chemotherapy, 614t
    complication associated with, 611–613
Lymphatic mapping technology
    into neoadjuvant chemotherapy
        protocols, 614
Lymphatic metastasis
    presence of, 397
Lymphedema, 216, 630
    causes of, 630
    chronic
        upper extremity angiosarcoma, 610
    risk of, higher-level axillary
        dissection, 610
    sentinel node biopsy, for melanoma, 623
    treatment of, 630
Lymphedema-related extremity
        angiosarcoma, 608
Lymphocele, 646, 649–650
    and lymph drainage, 331
    ultrasound image of, 650f
Lymphocyte surface antigens, 217
    lymphocyte depletion and
        thrombocytopenia, 217
Lymphoma, 578
Lymphopenia, 217
Lynch syndrome type I, 504
Lytic bone lesions, 234

M

Morbidity and Mortality (M&M)
    surgical residency training programs,
        powerful educational tools, 8
MACIS thyroid cancer prognosis
    classification system, 577, 577t
Macrophage and fibroblast activity,
        modulation of, 170
Macrophage phagocytosis, 217
Macrophage synthesis
    tissue growth factors, release of, 104
Macrophage-produced cytokines
    adhesion markers, endothelial cell
        expression of, 127
Magnetic resonance angiography (MRA), 643
Magnetic resonance
        cholangiopancreatography
        (MRCP), 418, 469
    demonstrating cholangiocarcinoma,
        457f, 458f
    demonstrating common bile duct
        stones, 447f
Magnetic resonance imaging (MRI), 129,
    319, 407
    diagnose pelvic vein and caval
        thrombosis, 339
Magnetic resonance imaging-guided wire
        localization technology, 609
Maintenance of certification (MOC), 29
Maintenance ranitidine therapy, 390
Maintenance therapy, 212
Malignancy, 219
Malignant esophagorespiratory
        fistulas, 257
Malignant hyperthermia (MH), 76,
    91–94
    suggested treatment of, 92t
Malignant thyroid lesion
    lobectomy and isthmusectomy, 576

Malnutrition
    atelectasis and pneumonia, 197
    complications of, 196–198
    efficacy of correcting, 197–198
    forms of, 197
    impaired healing, wound dehiscence and
            infection, 108, 197
    marasmus and kwashiorkor, 195t
    septic complications, 197
    severe, 197
Malone antegrade continent enema
            procedure, 742
Maloney dilator, 257
Maloney tapered esophageal dilators, 252
Malrotation, 728–730
    duodenal atresia, 729
    heterotaxia or polysplenia
            syndrome, 729
    jejunal obstruction, due to Ladd bands
            or volvulus, 753
Malrotation, symptomatic, 728
Mammalian target of rapamycin (mTOR), 213
    inhibitors, 215, 216
    sirolimus and everolimus, 215
Mammary artery, internal
    skeletonization of, 290
Mannitol
    osmotic diuretic, flushes necrotic tubular
            debris, 155
Manual esophageal anastomosis, 245
    mucosal apposition, and anastomotic
            disruption, 246f
Marasmus, 197
Marfan syndrome, 109
Marginal mandibular nerve injury
    drooping of lower lip, 319
Mask ventilation
    maintenance of, 70
Mastectomy procedures
    complications of, 607
Mastery (Case-based) Model, 14
Maximal respiratory inhalation, 159
Maximum predicted heart rate (MPHR), 63
May–Thurner syndrome, 354, 376
Mayo clinic, 265
Mean airway pressure, 169
Mechanisms
    responsible for injury, 278
Meckel diverticulum, 771–774, 772f
Meconium
    ascites, 734
    ileus, 730
        cystic fibrosis, 733
        typical intestinal findings in setting
            of, 733f
    peritonitis, 730
    pseudocyst, 734
Medial venous perforator incompetence, 351
Medialization thyroplasty, 240
Median alveolar concentration (MAC), 75
Mediastinal
    blood loss, 281
    cysts, 744
    granulomatosis
        patients with prior silica exposure, 308
    lymphadenectomy, 269
    lymphatics
        interruption of, 266
    shift
        avoidance of, 267

Mediastinal tumors, 339
Mediastinitis, 764–765
    chronic, 250
Mediastinum and pleural cavity
    copious irrigation of, 250
Medical consumerism, 4
Medical information systems
    surgical complications, reduction of, 4
Medical IT users
    health commerce areas, sound
            information and convenience, 4
Medicare
    patients, 470f
    programs, 6
    SEER linked databases, 32
Medication(s), 77–81
    analgesics, remifentanil, 81
    barbiturates, 77
    benzodiazepines
        hypnotic and amnestic
            properties, 77
        midazolam, frequently used
            drug, 77
    in development, 217–218
        APC and the T lymphocyte, agents
            targeting immune synapse
            between, 214f
    interactions
        monitoring drug levels, 215t
    intravenous anesthetics, 77–78
    meperidine, histamine release like
            morphine, 81
    normeperidine, CNS excitation and
            convulsions, 81
    primary venodilation and pooling of
            blood, 77
Medicine and changes, social contract of, 12
MEDPAR database
    for Medicare patients, 46
    single hospital's inpatient mortality
            rate, 46
Medullary thyroid carcinoma, 564
Melanoma, 619–624
    primary, excision of, 620
    proper management of, primary
            lesion, 619
    risk of locoregional recurrence, 621
Membrane integrity, 92
Memorial Sloan-Kettering Cancer
            Center, 257
Mendelian recessive gene, 766
Meningococcus
    vaccination for, 507
Mesenteric artery angioplasty
    and stenting, 370
Mesenteric artery endovascular
            therapy, 370
Mesenteric defects, 480
Mesenteric revascularization, 151
Mesenteric vessels
    injury to, 551
Mesh plug, 534
    inguinal herniorrhaphy, 535f
Metabolic
    acidosis
        electrolyte disturbance, 146
    alkalosis, 203
    complications, 198–204
    disorders, 600
Metabolic equivalents (METs), 63

Metaiodobenzylguanidine (MIBG) scan
    pheochromocytoma, 566f
Metallic stent
    fracture, 369
    long-term effects of, 450
    nonoperative placement of, 453
    recommendations for use of, 450t
Metaplasia, 254
Metastasectomy
    management of, 311
Methicillin-resistant *Staphylococcus aureus*
            (MRSA), 165, 218
Methylene blue
    less allergic, 613
Meticulous hemostasis, closure of
            any sites, 420
Metoclopramide, 771
Microbial wound contamination
    minimizing of, 109
Microembolization, 282, 288
Micrometastases
    progressive tumor growth and
            recurrence, 398
Micronutrient deficiency
    impairs wound healing, 108
Microvascular thrombosis, 167
    hypotension, leading to tissue
            hypoperfusion, 127
Midgut volvulus, 728, 730
Midline celiotomy incisions
    emergency access and exposure, 524
Midline laparotomy incisions, 527
Midthoracic esophageal
            perforations, 249
Migratory superficial thrombophlebitis
    presence of cancer, 339
Mineralocorticoid insufficiency, 572–573
Minimally invasive parathyroidectomy
            (MIP), 586
Minitracheostomy tube
    immediate and repeated aspiration,
            tracheobronchial tree, 311
Minitracheostomy, 268
    prophylactic use of, 311
Mirizzi Syndrome, 443
Mitral
    repair, 303
    stenosis
        mild and asymptomatic, 62
        residual, 303
Mitral regurgitation (MR), 302
    lesions, 62
    persistent, 303
Mitral valve
    annulus, 301f
    anterolateral commissure, 301
    mechanical, thrombosis of, 302
    repair
        complications of, 303–304
    replacement of, 282, 302, 303
    surgery, 300–303
Mixed oxygen venous saturation, 141
Mobilization stage, 410
MOC. *See* Maintenance of certification
            (MOC)
Moderate tricuspid regurgitation, 305
Monitoring, invasive, 129
Monocyte expressed, class II major
            histocompatibility
            complex, 127

Monotherapy, empiric
  third-generation cephalosporins, with
        antipseudomonal activity, 166
Morphine sulfate
  decreases central sympathetic outflow, 181
Morquio syndrome, 234
Mortality, 364, 371, 372–373, 376–377,
        466–467, 469, 474
  rates, 31, 362, 370
Motor paralysis, 86
Mowry and Reynolds
  arrhythmias after pneumonectomy,
        report on, 265
MR, residual, 303
MR. *See* Mitral regurgitation (MR)
MRA. See Magnetic resonance
        angiography (MRA)
Mucosa to mucosa pancreatic-jejunal
        anastomosis, 597
Mucosal
  colonization, 387
  ischemia, 324
  prolapse
        and ectropion, 516
  tear
        defining limits of, 250
  ulceration, 220, 233
Mucosectomy
  for prolapsed hemorrhoidal tissue, 515
Mucous cystadenocarcinoma, 500
Multifactorial risk index model
  postoperative respiratory failure, 158t
  predicts postoperative respiratory
        failure, 158
Multiglandular disease, 589
Multimodality therapy
  complications of, 624–625
Multinodular goiter, 576
Multiorgan dysfunction syndrome, 128
Multiorgan trauma, major, 222
Multiple adenomatous polyps
  increase risk of cancer, 396
Multiple endocrine neoplasia type 1 (MEN),
        595, 597
Multiple hyperplastic nodules, 578
Multiple logistic and linear regression
        analyses, 529
Multiple organ failure (MOF), 127
  severe sepsis and septic shock, 133
Multiple pseudocysts, 466
Multiple strategies, 281
Multivessel disease, 287
Mural thrombus, 290
Muscle relaxants
  depolarizing and nondepolarizing, 78
Mycophenolate mofetil (MMF), 216
Mycophenolic acid (MPA), 216
  DNA replication, 216
Mycotic aneurysm, 641
Myeloproliferative disorders
  polycythemia vera and essential
        thrombocythemia, 338
Myocardial
  preservation, 304
  rupture
        mitral valve surgery complication, 301
  stunning
        fluid overload and edema, 278
        reversible postischemic contractile
        dysfunction, 278

Myocardial infarction (MI), 35, 174, 181,
        254, 317–318, 322, 330–331
  acute, 67
        transrectal aspirin, 182
  and death, 361
  low-dose heparin, deep venous
        thrombosis a risk, 344
  risk factors for, 192
Myocardial injury, acute, 67
Myocardial ischemia (MI), 59, 322, 330–331
  diagnosis of, 291
  postoperative, 291
Myoclonic movements, 77
Myocutaneous flaps
  closure by means of, 625
Myofascial dehiscence
  and evisceration, 526–529
        mechanical separation of coapted fascial
        wound edges, 526
  risk factors for, 527t
Myofascial hernia ring, 534
Myofascial wound failure, acute, 526
Myofibroblast
  programmed cell death, 105
Myofibroblast terminal differentiation
  reduction in wound fibroblast
        number, 106
Myopathy/neuropathy, visceral, 490–491
Myopectineal orifice, 531
Myxedema coma, 128
  occlusive vascular disease, abdominal, 154
  resection, biliary
        complications of, 450–453
  surgery, biliary
        anatomic variation, well-recognized
        risk of, 425
        complications of, 423–458
  tumors, biliary
        classification of, 455

N

Narrow-complex rhythms, 182
Narrow-complex tachycardias, 182
Nasal
  alar necrosis, 229
  complications, 228
  intubation, 73
  tube patients
        sinusitis and otitis media, 208
Nasogastric
  bolus feeding
        acute gastric distension, 207
  suction, 390, 740
Nasotracheal intubation, 228
  acute dental injury, 229
  chronic sinusitis, 228
  for transoral procedures, 234
  lip injury, 229
  longer-term intubation and sinusitis, 228
  mucosal injury, 229
  nasal alar necrosis, 229
  oral cavity, oropharyngeal
        complications, 229
  pressure necrosis, 229
  sinus effusion on ultrasound, 228
  temporomandibular joint injury, 229
Nasotracheal suctioning, 268
National Institute of Diabetes & Digestive &
        Kidney Diseases (NIDDK), 666
National Institutes of Health (NIH), 585, 666

National Institutes of Health Consensus
        Development Panel, 399
National Nosocomial Infection
        Surveillance (NNIS) system,
        115, 116–118, 164
  hospital risk of SSI, by procedure and
        risk index, 117t
  percentile distributions of hospitals,
        mean rate for, 117t
  US acute care hospitals, 115
National Practitioner Databank, 29
National risk-adjusted data-collection and
        reporting system
  improving patient care, 53
  pairings of NSQIP and PTF data, 46t
National Surgical Quality Improvement
        Program (NSQIP), 30, 46, 526
  30-day endpoint, 47
  application to the private sector, 54
  architecture
        nurse data collector, 47, 47t, 48
  blocking and tackling of outcomes
        measurement, 47
  business case for quality, 54
  decision support, 55
  Department of Veterans Affairs, 30
  evolution of, 55
  four complication groups, 51t
  functional outcome data, mortality and
        morbidity, 56
  Hawthorne effect, 53
  methodology, 54
  nonpsychiatric admissions, 55
  placing reliable numbers into the quality
        numerator, 55
  postoperative occurrences or
        complications, 47
  private sector, 54
  proprietary cost-accounting software, 55
  respiratory complications, costly
        postoperative problems, 55
  risk-adjusted outcomes, association with
        structures, processes of care, 52
  sensitivity and positive predictive value, 46
        postoperative adverse events, 46
  standardization of definitions and
        terms, 47
  support from participating surgeons, 49
  surgical morbidity and mortality rates, 30
  unadjusted mortality rate and risk-
        adjusted rates, 50f
  wound infection prevention protocol, 54
National surgical quality reporting system, 54
National VA Surgical Risk Study (NVASRS), 46
  data acquisition and analysis, 46
National Veterans Administration Surgical
        Quality Improvement
        Program, 158
Native esophagus, 260
Native renal function, 568
Natural coagulation inhibitors
  deficiencies of, 338
Nausea/vomiting, 553
Neck dissection, 633–634
Neck hematoma, 579
Neck operations, 160
Necrosectomy, after
  management of gastrointestinal
        fistulas, 467t
Necrosis, 514

Necrotic
  bowel
    thromboembolectomy, surgical
        intervention, 293
    tissue, 107, 300
      sharp debridement, increased wound
          healing, 109
    wounds
      aggressive surgical debridement, 112
Necrotizing
  enterocolitis (NEC), 756–758
    mortality associated with, 758
  perineal infections, 518–519
Needle core biopsy, 678
Needle paracentesis, 744
Negative pressure pulmonary edema, 180
Nelson syndrome, 573
Neoadjuvant chemotherapy, 608, 614–615
  surgical complications, 625
Neoadjuvant radiation therapy, 272
Neointimal hyperplasia
  distal anastomosis site, 332
Neonatal mechanical ventilation, 169
Neoplasia
  development of, 396
Neoplasms
  benign, 487
  nonhealing wound with biopsy, 111
  of small bowel, 486–495, 487t
Neovascularization
  role of VEGF and bFGF in, central
      regulatory roles, 105
Nephrectomy, 649
Nephrotic syndrome, 339
Nephrotoxic drugs or dyes
  avoidance of, 282
Nephrotoxicity, 132, 215, 657
Nerve injuries, 359, 581–582, 629
Nerve injury, peripheral
  and positioning of the patient, 93–94
Nerve transection, 542
Neuraxial anesthesia, 83–87
  anticoagulation and neuraxial
      blockade, 85
  bradycardia and hypotension, risk factors
      for, 86–87, 87t
  complications of, 83
  failed block, 87–91
  hypotension, 86
  nerve injury, 85–86
  postoperative urinary retention, 84
  spinal hematoma and abscess, 85
  transient minor backache, 84
  transient neurologic symptoms, 84–85
Neuraxial, regional nerve blocks, 81–87
Neuroendocrine liver metastases, 407
Neuroendocrine tumors (NETs)
  of the pancreas and duodenum, 594
Neurogenic dysphagia, 246
Neurogenic impotence, 329
Neurogenic shock, 137
Neurohypophyseal stores, exhaustion
    of, 131
Neurologic complications, 287–288
Neurologic deficits, 282
  leading to duplex scanning, 319
Neurologic injury
  global or regional hypoperfusion, 282
Neurologic morbidity, 300
Neuromotor dysfunction, 260

Neuromuscular blocking agents, 78–80
  complete apnea, and cessation of
      spontaneous breathing, 78
  endotracheal intubation, 78
  extrajunctional nicotinic receptors, 78
Neuropathy, 359–360
Neuropsychometric tests, 288
Neurosurgery deep venous thrombosis, 344
Neutropenia
  copper deficiency, 197
Neutrophils, sequestration of
  microvasculature, release of oxygen free
      radicals, 279
Newborn
  bowel obstruction, bilious vomiting, 725
  gastroschisis, 751
  intensive care unit (ICU), 752
  intestinal obstruction, 725–742
  severe perianal skin breakdown, 737
  strictures following necrotizing
      enterocolitis, 757f
  surgical complications in, 725,
      754–758
Newer coronary stents
  advantages of, 287
Nicotinic acetylcholine receptors, 78
NIDDK. See National Institute of Diabetes &
    Digestive & Kidney Diseases
    (NIDDK)
Night Float System
  night shift (on a rotating basis), 14
NIH ARDSNET research group
  mechanical ventilation in ARDS, 170
NIH. See National Institutes of Health (NIH)
Nissen fundoplication, 246, 255, 748
Nitrates channel blockers, 66
Nitrous oxide, 76
  anesthetic technique, cardiovascular
      depression, 76
  laparoscopic cholecystectomy, 76
  pulmonary vascular resistance, and
      pulmonary artery pressure, 76
Nocardia infections, 692
Nonanatomic liver resection
  isolated bile duct after, 417f
Nonbleeding visible vessel, 388
Noncardiac surgery
  detection of intraoperative
      ischemia, 181
  elective, additional testing required, 60
  high-risk, coronary artery bypass grafting
      (CABG), cardio-protective
      effect, 67
  thoracic, 158
Noncardiogenic pulmonary edema, 266
Nonchylous effusions, 254
Noncontiguous deep venous thrombosis
  superficial thrombophlebitis, association
      of, 339
Noncontrast scans, 410
Noncoronary cusp, aortic valve
  entrapment of, 301–302
Nondepolarizing muscle relaxants, 79, 80t
Noninfected venous stasis ulcer
  Unna boot, saline, colloid, or vacuum, 353
Nonoperative therapy, standard
  stocking compression, elevation, 351
Nonparenchymal structures, 412
Nonpyogenic pneumonia
  absence of rigors, 164

Nonrenal solid organ transplants
  chronic renal failure, cumulative
      incidence of, 221f
  development of renal failure, 221
Nonresponding cellulites
  intravenous therapy, 604
Nonspecific anticoagulants
  unfractionated heparin and
      warfarin, 189
Nonsteroidal anti-inflammatory drugs
    (NSAIDs), 387, 607
  cause of ulcerogenic actions, 387
Nonstroke-related mortality
  cardiac complications, 317
Normotensive patients, 320
Normothermia, maintenance of, 91
North American Symptomatic Carotid
    Endarterectomy Trial
    (NASCET), 361
NOS blockade, 104
NOS inhibitors
  delays healing of acute excisional
      wounds, 104
Nosocomial pneumonia, 163–166
Nothing by mouth (NPO), 229
Novel residency structures, and physician
    extenders, 14–15
Nurse data collector
  interrater reliability measurements, 47,
      47t, 48
Nuss procedure, 768
Nutrient supplementation, 110
Nutritional assessment and monitoring, 196
Nutritional assessment, 196
  evaluation of surgical patients, 196
Nutritional status, poor, 60
Nutritional support route
  parenteral or enteral, 204
Nutritional support, 195
  complications of, 195–208
  parenteral or enteral delivery of
      nutrients, 195
Nyhus
  classification system for inguinal
      hernias, 531

O

Obesity, 60
  accelerated atherosclerosis, 401t
  difficulty in intubating, increased risk of
      acid aspiration, 90
  eccentric hypertrophy, 90
  ejection fraction and diastolic function,
      decrease in, 401
  morbid, 88–90, 398–402
  pressure sores and neural injuries, 402
  severe, classified as morbid, 398
  systolic and diastolic blood pressure,
      increase of, 401
Oblique aortotomy, 304
Observed-to-expected (O/E Ratio)
  comparative evaluation of quality, 51f
  high and low outliers, 51
Obstruction, mechanical, 164
Obstructive endobronchial neoplasm
  distal pneumonitis, low-grade
      infection, 268
Occlusion of portal flow
  occluding by ligature, or stapling the
      portal triad, 412

Occult spinal dysraphism
  tethered cord, without associated lipoma
    of cord, 740
Occupational Safety and Health
    Administration (OSHA)
  regulations, 122
  surgical garb and gloves, laundering
    of, 122
Octreotide
  beneficial effects of, vasomotor
    symptoms of dumping, 395
Ocular injury, 94
  corneal abrasions, 94
  damage to retina or visual pathway, 94
Odds ratio (OR), 158, 159
Off-pump bypass surgery, 279
Off-pump coronary artery bypass surgery, 293
  postoperative atrial fibrillation,
    decreased incidence of, 293
Off-pump coronary artery bypass
    techniques, 282
  reduced microemboli, no
    touchaortatechnique, 283
Off-pump coronary revascularization
  beneficial in atherosclerotic aorta
    patients, 293
  blood transfusion requirements,
    limitation of, 293
  hypercoagulable state, associated with, 291
Ohm's law, 137
Oligoanuric renal failure, 644
Oliguria, 128
  septic, cardiogenic, and hepatic shock, 138
Oliguric patient
  Foley catheter patency, assessment of, 152
OLT. *See* Orthoptic liver transplantation (OLT)
Omentopexy, 635
Omentum, 274
Omphalocele, 753–754, 754*f*
  initial management of, 753
Oncologic laparoscopic cases
  minimizing desufflation episodes, 554
Oncologic surgery, 27
On-pump coronary artery bypass
    surgery, 293
Operating room
  environment, 120–121
  personnel, 121–122
    specific rituals, observation of, 121
    sterile gloves and gown, 122–123
    surgical garb and gloves, 122
Operation, elective, 157
Operative
  care, 122–123
    reduce risk of SSI, 123
  endoscopy, 231
  gastrostomy decompression, 404
  hypotension
    preventing by, accurate blood and
     fluid replacement, 323
  monitoring, 180
  portal vein ligation, 409
  procedures
    complications of, 463–474
  stenting, 453
  technique, 466
  therapy, 3
    bleeding is rapid, 388
  thrombectomy, 416
  treatment, 388–389

Opioid agonists
  preoperative sedatives, 81
Optimal perioperative management, 67
Optimal pulmonary function, 157
OPTN. *See* Organ Procurement and
    Transplant Network (OPTN)
Oral β-blockers, 179
  perioperative and dosing regimens, 179*t*
Oral cyclosporine and tacrolimus, 215
Oral intubation, 70
  direct laryngoscopy and intubation, 70
  laryngotracheal mask airway (LMA), 71
  tracheal intubation, 71
Oral tracheal intubation, 160
Organ dysfunction syndrome, 141
  chronic, 145
Organ Procurement and Transplant Network
    (OPTN), 666
Organ space infections
  management of, 123
  pedicled or free tissue transfer, for wound
    coverage and healing, 124
  percutaneous catheter drainage, 123
Organ transplants, 212
  leflunomide administration, 216
Oropharyngeal suctioning, 746
Orotracheal intubation, 73, 227–228
  development of, 227
Orthoptic liver transplantation (OLT), 658
Osmolarity-induced thrombosis, 204
Osmotic
  diuresis
    increased sodium and water
     excretion, 358
  diuretics
    hypovolemia, 139
  load, 145
Osteoplastic thoracoplasty, 271
Osteoporosis, 717
Outcome measures, primary, 166
Outcomes data, 8
  departmental practice improvement
    opportunities, 8
  local practice trends, examination of, 8
  to improve morbidity and mortality, 8
Outcomes research, 45
Outpatient chest tube management, 310
Outpatient thyroidectomy
  safety of, 579
Overly tight fundoplication
  early postoperative dysphagia, 255
Oxygen delivery index, 141
Oxygen delivery, 136
  arterial oxygen saturation, 136

P

PAC. *See* Pulmonary artery catheter
Packed red blood cell transfusion, 146
Paget-von Schrötter syndrome, 339
Pain control, adequate, 267
Pain, 515–516, 553
  chronic, 607
Palliation
  nonoperative palliation, 458
Palliation of symptoms. *See* Cure rates
Palliative bypass for obstruction, 490
Palliative pharmacologic treatment, 564
Palliative resection, 578
Palmaz airway stent, 749

Palpable breast masses
  risk of misdiagnosis, 608
Palpable lesions
  suspicious imaging, 608
Pancreas
  allograft rejection, 677
  graft loss
    causes of, 668–669
    incidence of, 668–669
  surgery, 780–781
    acute pancreatitis, 780
    hyperinsulinism, 780–781
Pancreatectomy
  complications of distal and subtotal, 472
  direct invasion of the distal pancreas, 398
Pancreatic
  and duodenal NETs
    complication rates in patients
     undergoing resection of, 597*t*
    operative approach to excision of, 596
  carcinoid, 564
  debridement
    hemorrhage, 467
  drainage, 598
  ductal disruption
    and anastomotic failure, 599
  endocrine neoplasm, 594
    resection of, incidence of DVT not
     addressed, 601
  endocrine surgery
    complications of, 595
  endocrine tumors, 601
  enteric anastomosis
    construction of, 599
  enteric anastomotic leak, 596
  fistula, 469–471
    formation of, 472
  NETs
    hereditary endocrine neoplasia
     syndromes, 595
    operative intervention for, 594
  or biliary fistula, 596
  pseudocysts, 466
    asymptomatic, management of, 463
    drainage of, 463
    internal drainage, pseudocyst
     excision, and external
     drainage, 464
    laparoscopic management of, 464
    pancreaticocutaneous fistula, 466
  resection, 32
    challenging sequela of, recurrent
     hypoglycemia, 600
    for endocrine tumors, 597
  secretions
    octreotide, reduction in volume
     of, 598
  surgery
    complications of, 463
  transplantation
    complications of, 665–681
    hemorrhage, 674–675
    immunologic complications in, 677
     diagnosis of, 678–679
     immunosuppression, 679–680
    immunological progress in, 680–681
    infection of, 676–677
    outcome measures of, 666–668
    postoperative setting, complications,
     673–680

rationale for patients with type 1
diabetes mellitus, 665–666
recipient selection, 669–670
surgery, 671–673
technical progress in, 680–681
thrombosis, 673–674
tumors
resection of, 600
Pancreaticoduodenal NETs, 601
enucleation of, biliary fistulas,
peripancreatic abscess, 599
Pancreaticoduodenal resections
for malignant disease, 598
Pancreaticoduodenectomy, 469, 598
for malignancy, 598
pancreatic fistula formation, 469
with enteric-pancreatic
anastomosis, 598
Pancreaticogastrostomy, 470, 600
Pancreaticojejunostomy, 469
Pancreatitis, 133, 259, 446
acute, 284, 780
and postsphincterotomy
bleeding, 448
nasogastric tube decompression
treatment, 259
risk of, 284
Papilla of Vater, 419
Papillary muscle-annular continuity
maintenance of normal cardiac
output, 302
Papillary thyroid carcinoma, 576, 577
Paracolostomy hernias, 514
Paraesophageal hiatal hernias
laparoscopic technique, 255
Parahepatic abscess, 420
infected biloma or infected
hematoma, 420
treatment of, 420
Parahepatic fluid collection, 418
Paraileostomy hernias, 514
Parallel peripheral angiography, 360
Paranasal sinus drainage
osteomeatal complex pathway, 228
Parastomal hernia, 514
nonprotruding stoma, associated with
obstruction, 514f
Parastomal herniation, 491
Parathyroid
autograft, 582f
glands
damage during thyroidectomy, 579
exposure and identification, in
normal anatomic positions,
588f, 589, 590f
relationship, and dissection of the
parathyroid gland, 581f
surgery, 585
Parathyroidectomy, 651
conventional approach to, 586
current procedure strategies, 586–587
hypocalcemia, 587
indications for, 586t
intraoperative localization, with a γ
radiation probe, 586
nerve injury, 587–589
potential complications of, 587
Parenchymal injuries, 684
Parenchymal resection
increase risk of residual air space, 309

Parenteral nutrition (PN), 133, 195, 733,
734, 737
complete and balanced nutrition, 195
infectious complications, higher rates
of, 196
life-saving therapy, intestinal failure
patients, 195
Parenteral nutrition support, 754
Parietal peritoneum
chemical irritation of, 390
Paroxysmal atrial fibrillation
preoperative history of, 288
Patch venoplasty
occurrence of, persistent venous
narrowing, 351
Patch-graft angioplasty, 321
Patency, 372
long term, 372
rates, 372
Patent gastrojejunostomy, 601
Pathogen-associated molecular
patterns, 127
Pathogenesis, 386–387, 396
Patient
history
exercise intolerance, dyspnea on
exertion, 159
life expectancy, 32
movement
sign of inadequate anesthesia, 81
outcomes, 13
positioning, 93
complications of various patient
positions, 95t
prone or steep lateral decubitus
positions, 170
safety in surgery study, 54
safety issues, 8
medical–legal concerns, 8
safety movement, 15
satisfaction, 3
selection
critical principles of, 568
training
use of incentive spirometry, 268
Patients, high-risk
β-blocker therapy, 67
integrated team approach, 67
management of, 67
Pattern-recognition receptors, 127
Peak inspiratory pressures, 267
Pectus excavatum, 768
Pediatric surgery, 723–758
Pediatric tracheotomy, 238–239
Pedicled muscle flaps, 269
Peer education, open, 7
Peer review, 8
quality of care, case-by-case basis, 8
Peer-review evaluation of care, and risk-
adjusted outcomes, 52
PEG. See Percutaneous endoscopic
gastrostomy (PEG)
Pelvic
abscess, 512
angiography, 136
devascularization
colonic ischemia, requiring bowel
resection, 365
embolization, 136

fractures
high risk of massive
hemorrhage, 136
loss of blood into retroperitoneum,
136
hemorrhage volume, 136
ischemia, 364
Pelvicalyceal leak, 649
Peptic ulceration, 386–396
benign, 396
bleeding, perforation, obstruction, major
complications of, 386
Gram-negative bacterium, *Helicobacter
pylori*, development of peptic
ulceration, 386
results of elective operation for, 390t
role of, *Helicobacter pylori* infection, 386
upper gastrointestinal hemorrhage, 387
Percutaneous
biopsy
image guidance, initial maneuver, 609
operation for bleeding, 409
vascular complications of, 641
catheter drainage, 465
complications of, 465
coronary intervention (PCI), 39, 66, 181
use of coronary stents, 66
coronary revascularization, 182
cricothyroidotomy
preventing atelectasis, 268
drainage, 464
of pancreatic pseudocysts, 464
endoscopic gastrostomy (PEG), 208, 769
needle biopsy
lumpectomy, 604
nephrostogram, 646f
or surgical thrombectomy, 360
removal of intrahepatic stones
adjunct to operative intervention, 449
revascularization, 66
techniques, 286
tracheostomy, 151, 239
bedside procedure, 239
transhepatic cholangiogram (PTC), 661
attempted balloon dilation of
stricture, 435f
bifurcation of the right and left
hepatic ducts (Klatskin
tumor), 456f
common hepatic duct stricture
following an open
cholecystectomy, 427f, 433f
following laparoscopic
cholecystectomy, 429f
following reconstruction of, 437f
strictured biliary-enteric
anastomosis, 442f
strictured hepaticojejunostomy, 441f
following resection of a
choledochal cyst, 452f
techniques, 436
transhepatic cholangiography (PTC),
418, 428
transhepatic cholangioscopic lithotomy
(PTCSL), 449
transhepatic dilation, 453
transluminal angioplasty (PTA), 362, 644
and stenting of iliac artery, 364
transluminal coronary angioplasty
(PTCA), 287

Perforated duodenal ulcer, 292
    comparison of laparoscopic, and open
        repair of, 391*t*
    nonoperative management of, 390
    omental patch closure of, 391
Perforated neoplasms, 391
Perforation, 390–391
Perforator sclerotherapy, deep, 352
Perfusion scans, nuclear, 267
Perfusionist manipulations
    injection of drugs into the CPB circuit, 282
Pericardial patch graft, 272
Pericardial resection
    lethal complication, 267
Pericardial tamponade, 128
Periesophageal fibrosis, 261
Perigastric lymph nodes, 396
    radical extirpation of, 397
Perigastric lymphadenectomy, 397
    extent of, 396
Perihilar resection
    positive biliary margins, neoadjuvant
        chemoradiation, 458
Perineal approaches
    Altemeier and Delorme, 503
Perineural invasion
    absence of, 445
Perioperative
    ACE inhibitor, 181
    antibiotic coverage
        minimizing infection rates, 604
    antibiotics, 38
        prevention of surgical site
            infections, 38
    ARF
        elevated intra-abdominal pressure, 151
        maintaining adequate intravascular
            volume, 152
    β-blockers, 178
        criteria for cardiac complications, 179*t*
        effectiveness of, 38
        postoperative therapy, 38
        quality indicators, 31
        use of, 31
    cardiac ischemia, 38
    cardiac risk
        β-blockers, effectiveness of, 65
    care
        optimal pulmonary function,
            maintenance of, 157
    cephalosporin, 604
    complications
        hypothermia, 90
    hyperthermia
        iatrogenic causes, 91
        list of etiologies, diagnosis of
            intraoperative hyperthermia, 91*t*
    hypotension
        thrombosis, risk of, 155
    ischemia
        estimation of biomarker elevation, 67
        incidence of, 65
    mortality
        linked to postoperative morbidity, 287
    myocardial infarction (MI), 59, 67
        diagnosis of, 181
        elevated serum troponin levels, 181
        identification of risk markers
            preoperatively, 59
        modifying cardiac risk, 59

    preoperative evaluation and
        management, 59
    nutrition support, 196
    octreotide, 471
        administration, to prevent fistula, 598
        effectiveness of, 470
    patients
        temporary dialysis, 155
    pharmacotherapy, 289
    risk, 151
        uncontrolled systemic hypertension,
            patients with, 60
    risk, assessment of, 59
    setting
        sepsis, risk of developing ARF, 151
    stroke, 288
        embolization of thrombus, 319
Peripancreatic
    abscess, 599
    fluid collections
        area of loculated fluid, 600
Peripheral vascular disease (PVD), 287
    dipyridamole myocardial perfusion
        imaging testing, 63
    dobutamine echocardiography,
        commonly used tests, 63
    nonexercise stress test, 63
Periprocedural anticoagulation, 359
Periprocedural myocardial infarction, 361
Periprocedural pulmonary embolism
    filter deployed through thrombus, 348
Peristomal fistulae, 492
Peritoneal cavity, 415
    unretrieved stones in, 443
Peritoneal cultures, 390
Peritoneal dialysis catheters, 222
Peritoneal drainage, 757
Peritoneal insufflation, 548
Peritonitis, 499
Peritonitis, fatal, 258
Peritransplant abscess, 650
Perivalvular leak, 300, 302
Permissive hypercapnia, 167
Peroneal nerve injury, 511
Peroneal occlusive disease, 330
Peutz-Jeghers syndrome, 487
PFT. *See* Pulmonary function testing (PFT)
pH stat method, 283
Pharmacologic agents
    decreasing gastric and pancreatic
        secretion, 598
    macrophages, fibroblasts, and epithelial
        cells, 108–109
Pharmacologic cardioversion
    amiodarone or electrical
        cardioversion, 290
Pharmacologic measures
    preventing PNAC, 204
Pharmacological stress imaging, 63
Pharyngoesophageal, 765
Phase I block, 78
Phelbectomy, open
    complications of, hematoma and
        lymphocele, 352
Pheochromocytoma, 564–565, 568
    adrenal, 565*f*
    clinical presentation of, 565
    Cushing syndrome, 564*f*
    patients, 560
    resection of, leading to hypotension, 572

Phlebectomy, 351, 352
    open, peripheral nerve injury, 352
Phlegmasia alba dolens, 338
Phlegmasia cerulea dolens, 349
Phosphate and magnesium, 201–203
Phosphate deficiency, 197
    neutrophil chemotaxis and phagocytosis,
        impairment of, 197
Phospholipid-to-triglyceride (PL/TG)
    ratio, 200
Phrenic nerve injuries, 684–685
Physical examination, 159
Physician behavior
    blame and fault finding, 8
Physician recognition award (PRA)
    50 hours of CME per year, 19
Physician replacements, 14
Physician–patient relationship, 10
    business of coding, billing and
        reimbursement, 11
    dehumanization of, 10
Physiologic hemostasis
    tissue factor-factor VIIa (TF-VIIa)
        activating factor IX, 186*f*
Physiological and Operative Severity Score
        for Enumeration of Mortality
        and Morbidity (POSSUM), 307
Pinch-off syndrome, 206
Placenta previa
    acute hemorrhagic, 190
Plasma brain natriuretic peptide (BNP), 181
Plasma kallikrein–kinin system, 127
    neutrophil-activating and chemotactic
        properties, 127
    vascular permeability, 127
Plasma prekallikrein (PK), 186
    activates factor XII to an active enzyme,
        186
    activation of more factor XII to factor
        XIIa (XIIa), 186*f*
Plasma protein fraction. *See* Albumin infusion
Plasminogen activator inhibitor-1, 338
Platelet derived growth factor (PDGF), 103
Platelet dysfunction
    hematoma formation, 106
Platelet infusion
    plasma replacement, and additional
        replacement with fresh frozen
        plasma, 190
Pledgeted sutures
    fragile or minimal annular tissue, 302
Pleural effusion, 693
Pleural opacity, 310
Pleural peritoneal shunt, 273
Pleural space, 271
Pleural tenting
    reduced air leaks duration, 310
Pleurectomy, 273
PN-associated cholelithiasis
    decreased gallbladder contractility, 203
PN-associated cholestasis (PNAC), 204
Pneumatic compression devices, 344
Pneumococcus, 507
Pneumocystis carinii, 218
Pneumocystis jiroveci, 218
Pneumomediastinum, 229, 236, 255, 552, 765
Pneumonectomy
    chest x-ray, volume overload, 265
    entire cardiac output, 266
    fistula, 270

mediastinal lymphatic interruption, canine model, 266
patients, 266
correlation between age and arrhythmia nil, 265
right, 310
risk of mediastinal shift, and compromise of ventilation, 743
Pneumonia, 573
Pneumonia, untreated aspiration, 164
Pneumoperitoneum, 640
treating air leaks and residual spaces, 310
used during laparoscopy, 403
Pneumothorax, 229, 235, 255, 256, 552, 573, 693, 766
development of, 310
estimates of, during laparoscopic surgery, 552
Polar artery occlusion, 641
Polyglycolic acid polymermesh, 526, 527
Polymorphic ventricular tachycardia, without QT prolongation secondary to ischemia, 182
Polypropylene mesh (PM), 274, 527
used in United States, 539
Polypropylene monofilament suture, 413
Polytetrafluoroethylene (PTFE), 274, 332, 413, 570
Popliteal artery stenosis
balloon angioplasty of, 375f
Popliteal thromboembolectomy
lower extremity angiogram, primary balloon angioplasty, 372f
Porcine valve, 300
Port placement, 571
Port site
hernia, 553
small bowel obstruction, due to a Richter-type defect, 553
incisional hernias, 404
metastasis
exfoliation of malignant cells, by instrument manipulation, 554
occurrence of, in laparoscopic cholecystectomy, 553
recurrence, 553–554
sterile water lavage, 312
tumor recurrences
development of, 312
Porta-caval shunt, 656
Portal gastropathy, 420
Portal hypertension, 440
hypersplenism with thrombocytopenia and granulocytopenia, 191
liver operations, 411
Portal vein
laceration of, 656
thrombosis, 659
hypertension, 411
Portal venous contrast phase, 407
Positive blood cultures, 127
Positive end-expiratory pressure (PEEP), 139, 161, 236
Positive exercise stress test, 176
Positive pressure ventilation, 164, 267, 311
Postamputation management
properly fitting prostheses, 625
Postanastomotic stenosis, 642
Postdeployment complications, 376

Postdural puncture headache (PDPH), 84
cerebrospinal fluid leak, 84
Postembolectomy rethrombosis
groin arterio-venous fistula, use of, 351
Postembolization angiogram, 465f
Postendarterectomy stroke
intracerebral hemorrhage, 319
Posterior adrenalectomy, open
hockey-stick type incision, 571
Posterior cordotomy, 231
Posterior glottic stenosis
challenging clinical problem, 231
mucosalized tract, posterior to scar band by passage of suction tip, 231f
severe stenosis, with dense posterior commissure scarring, 231f
simple interarytenoid scar band, 231f
Posterior mitral annulus
extensive calcification, 300
Posterior myocardial perforation, 301
Posterior myotomy/myectomy (POMM), 735
Posterior sagittal anorectoplasty (PSARP), 740
features of, 741f
procedure, 740
Posteroanterior chest radiograph, 267
Postherniorrhaphy neuralgia, 542
Post-hospital prophylaxis, 343
Postintubation laryngeal granulomas, 232
Postintubation tracheal stenosis
tracheal resection, 232
Postjunctional receptors
depolarization of, 78
Postlytic venous patency, 350
Postmastectomy lymphedema
and typically bluish-reddish macular lesions or nodules, 610
Postobstructive pulmonary edema, 236
Postoperative
acute renal failure
incidence of, 292
air leak
fibrin glue, 310
airway compromise
pulse oximetry, for patients with respiratory difficulties, 160
ARF
thoracoabdominal aneurysm repair, 150
arrhythmia
age as a risk factor, 265
arrhythmias, 265, 288–290
temporary pacing treatment, 279
atelectasis
treatment of, 268
atrial arrhythmias
amiodarone treatment, 266
atrial fibrillation
age a predictor, 288
decreasing rate of, amiodarone administration, 289
incidence of, 288
management of, 289t
prevention of
biatrial overdrive pacing, 289
perioperative pharmacotherapy, 289
bile fistula, 417
biliary injuries
diagnosis of, 428–429

bleeding, 272
cause of, 272
early complication of CABG, 292
reexploration for bleeding, 292
bowel obstruction, 753
CABG
intestinal ischemia postoperatively, 293
cardiac events, 176
cardiac tamponade, 292
cholangitis
anastomotic narrowing, 452
treatment of, 419
chylothorax, 273
coagulopathy, 420
avoidance of, primary means of preventing parahepatic abscess, 420
complications, 180–182, 308, 403, 415–416
identification and management of, 67, 572–573
empyema
diagnosis of, 311
ERCP stone extraction, 446
esmolol infusions
lower ischemic events, and total ischemic time, 65
fluid accumulation
factors predicting, obesity, female sex, diabetes mellitus, 282
fluid management
postsurgical ileus, effect on, 145
fulminant liver failure
no specific treatment, 415
heart failure
incidence of, 180
hematoma, 419
develop airway compromise, for emergent evacuation, 579
hemorrhage, 272–273, 391
hyperglycemia
clinical importance of, 39
in critically ill patients, 39
hypertension
in chronically hypertensive patients, 320
ileus
temporary bowel motor dysfunction, 504
incision, care of, 123
incisional hernias
open bariatric surgery, major problem in, 404
insulin sensitivity, 600
intestinal ischemia
common etiology of, 489
laparotomy within 6 hours, decreasing mortality rate, 293
intra-abdominal abscess, 420
development of, 600
ischemia
risk factors, 291
ischemic events, 177
liver dysfunction, 408
liver failure, hallmark of
persistently rising bilirubin, 415
mechanical ventilation, 752
morbidity
most important factor, cirrhosis and portal hypertension, 452

Postoperative (*Continued*)
  morbidity and mortality
    preoperative diffusing capacity
      (DLCO), 265
  mortality
    after intervention for irradiated
      intestine, 486*f*
    risk of, 397
  nausea and vomiting (PONV),
    87–88, 87
    algorithm for the management of, 89*f*
    antiemetic therapy for prophylaxis, 88
    multimodal approach, 88
    prophylactic antiemetics, 88
    strategies reducing baseline risk of
      postoperative nausea, 88*t*
  nausea, 553
    etiology and treatment of, in
      laparoscopic surgery, 553
  nutrition, 196
    aggressive postoperative
      feedings, 196
  pancreatic fistulas, 469
  pancreatic function, 600
  papillary strictures, 451
  percutaneous tranhepatic cholangiogram
    hepaticojejunostomy, to treat
      stricture, 438*f*
  period
    patients developing, prolonged air
      leak, 310
  peritonitis
    acute distension, 404
    diagnosis of, 403
  problems, 3
  pulmonary complications, 292
    age and obesity, common risk
      factors, 159
    body mass index, independent risk
      factor for, 159
    chronic lung disease, patient-related
      risk factor, 159
    incidence of, 255
    patients with severe COPD, 159
    risks of smoking, poor general health
      status, metabolic
      abnormalities, 158
    smoking risk, 158
  pulmonary edema, 180
  pulmonary infarct, 267
  setting, 151
  sputum retention, 311
  starvation
    prevention of, 197
  urinary retention
    preoperative dysfunction, 742
  visual loss registry, 96
  wound complications, identification
    of, 110–111
  wound infections, 196
Postoperative necrosis, 514
Postpartum back pain
  associated with antepartum back pain, 84
Postphlebitic disease, 353
Postpneumonectomy empyema, 273
  routine barium swallow, 273
Postprandial diarrhea, 254
Postprandial flushing
  incidence of dumping, and vasomotor
    effects, 390

Postprocedural anticoagulant therapy
  serious bleeding, 66
Postprocedural pseudoaneurysms
  using covered stents, 359
Postprocedure complications, 553
Postpulmonary resection patients, 266
Postpyloric feedings
  in early postoperative period, 208
Postrenal ARF
  hydronephrosis, 152
Postrepair MR, 303
  pathogenesis, 266–267
Postresection pulmonary edema (PPE),
  266–267
  acute hyperinflation of, 267
  development of, 267
  fluid overload, pathogenesis of, 266
  treatment of, 267
Postsplenectomy infection, 507
Postsplenectomy sepsis, 781
Poststenting therapy
  combination of aspirin and
    clopidogrel, 66
Postsurgical gastroparesis, 393–394
Post-transplant
  diabetes
    incidence of, 215
  hyperamylasemia, 678
  lymphoproliferative disease (PTLD), 219,
    695–696
  renal dysfunction, 644–645
Postural drainage, 163
Potassium, 201
Potent inhaled anesthetics (PIAs), 75
  fulminant hepatic failure, 76
  halogenated hydrocarbons, 75
  halothane-associated liver failure, 76
  respiratory depressants, 75
Potential distal pancreatectomy, 568
Potential residual pleural air space, 310
Pouch circular myotomy of Livaditis,
  distal, 746
Pouch failure
  pelvic sepsis, pouch fistulization, and
    Crohn disease, 513
Pouch function, poor, 513
Pouch reconstruction, 398
Pouchitis, 512–513
Pouch-vaginal fistula, 512
Power interruption, 278
Powered catheter phlebectomy, 352
PPE. *See* Postresection pulmonary edema
Practice-based learning, 29
Pre- and postoperative pulmonary
  function
  risk factors for pulmonary
    complications, 158*t*
Preclinical wound healing data, 529
Predicted postoperative product, 307
Predictive Respiratory Quotient (PRQ), 307
Preexisting bleeding, 409–410
Preexisting heart disease
  intraoperative cardiogenic disturbances,
    ischemia and arrhythmias, 309
Preformed, spring-loaded silo, 752*f*
Preganglionic sympathetic block
  hypotension, 86
Preoperative
  assessment, 159–160, 264–265
  β-blockade, 178

bronchoscopy, 269
carotid duplex, 287
contrast enema, 737
coronary angiography
  recommendations of American
    college of cardiology/American
    heart association, 65*t*
coronary artery angioplasty, 322
dipyridamole-thallium imaging, 177
evaluation, 174–176
  ECG, essential screening tool, 176
hair removal, 120
history
  bleeding diathesis, identification
    of, 292
imaging, 273
  for malignant tumor resection
    planning, 596*f*
interventions, 177–180
nutrition
  indications for, 196
nutritional repletion
  improves surgical wound
    outcomes, 110
planning imaging
  and function tests, 415
portal vein embolization, 409
  indications for, 409*t*
PTC catheter placement, 436
pulmonary function testing (PFT), 159
pulmonary function, 157–159
  high-risk patients, identification
    of, 157
pulmonary risk
  patient history and physical
    examination, 159
renal dysfunction, 282
revascularization
  infrainguinal surgeries, 67
risk factors
  contamination and infection, 107
  evaluation of, 265
  identification and modification of,
    567–571
  modification of, 109–110, 529–530
  wound complications, 107–109
risk modification, 479
risk stratification
  dipyridamole thallium scintigraphy, 64
spirometry testing, 160
testing, 177
ureteral stenting, 508
Preperitoneal
  approach
    hemostasis, 534
  inguinal hernia repair
    Nyhus types III and IV, 534–536
Preprocedural stenting
  of iliac arteries minimal, 364
Prerenal hypoperfusion, 152
Presacral fascia
  preservation of, 506
Presacral hemorrhage, 506
Pressure control ventilation, 169
Pressure injury
  cicatrical scarring, 233
Pressure waveforms, 278
Preventative maneuvers, 267
Primary axillary or subclavian vein thrombosis
  intermittent obstruction of the vein, 339

Primary breast angiosarcomas, 608
Primary care physicians, 6
Primary sclerosing cholangitis (PSC), 450, 453
Pringle maneuver
general inflow occlusion, 411
Procedural complications, 251–255
Procedure volume, 31
assessment easy and inexpensive, 39
evidence-based hospital referral, 39
operative mortality, 31
recognizable structural variable, 31
surgical mortality rates, 31
Process measures, 31
baseline risks of the procedure, 42
major limitation of, 41
particulars of patients' care, 31
Quadrant III, 42
strengths and weaknesses of, 41–42, 42f
Process of care measures, 41
Process of care variables
patient outcomes, 35
Proctectomy, 519
Proctocolectomy
Kock continent ileostomy, 502
Profession and educational process
external regulation of, 11–12
Prognostic scoring systems
MACIS system, 577
Progressive alveolar collapse
and atelectasis, 268
Progressive fibroplasias
mechanical failure (dehiscence), or abnormal tissue (neoplasia), 110f
prominent midwound healing ridge, 110
Progressive renal insufficiency
incapacity of kidney, 47
Proinflammatory cytokines, 127, 132
activate coagulation, 132
tissue factor release, 127
Prokinetic drug therapy
prolonged trial of, 394
Prolapse, 513
occurs in loop, 513
Prolonged air leaks
preoperative awareness of, 310
Prolonged balloon inflation
sufficient to provide hemostasis, 362
Prolonged balloon tamponade
placement of covered stent, for achieving hemostasis, 363
Prolonged intubation, 230
Prolonged suctioning
precipitates hypoxia, 268
Prolonged ventilation
increases barotrauma, bronchial stump dehiscence, 267
Prolylcarboxypeptidase (PRCP)
endothelial cell-associated enzyme, 186
Promotility agents, 490
Prone positioning, 170
Properative arterial blood gas analysis
identifying patients with hypercapnia, 160
Prophylactic amoxicillin/clavulinic acid, 604
Prophylactic antibiotics, 38
surgical site infections, prevention of, 38

Prophylactic antimicrobial therapy, 118
Prophylactic beta adrenergic blockade, 66
Prophylactic β-blockers, 38
Prophylactic cholecystectomy
postoperative cholelithiasis, high incidence of, 404
Prophylactic inferior vena caval filters, 349
Prophylactic IVC filter placement
long-term morbidity, 350
Prophylactic ursodiol, 404
Propofol
dose-dependent elevation, serum triglyceride concentrations, 199
microbial growth retardant, 78
respiratory depressant, 78
Propofol syndrome, 78
impairment of free fatty acid utilization, 78
Prostanoids, 127
Prosthetic aortic graft infection
aortoiliac or aortofemoral positions, amputation morbidity high, 324
Prosthetic heart valves, 299–300, 299
mechanical and tissue (biologic) valves, 299
perioperative antithrombotic therapy, 62, 62t
Prosthetic mesh reconstructions
management of infections, 274
Prosthetic mitral valve
obstruction of the left ventricular outflow tract, 303f
Prosthetic valve endocarditis (PVE), 299–300
manifestation, 300
Prosthetic valve thrombosis, 302–303
fluoroscopy diagnosis, 303
Prosthetic valves
interference from periannular structures, dysfunction of, 302f
single or double leaflets, opening and closing of either, 302
Protamine administration
severe catastrophic reaction, 279
Protamine reaction, 279
Protective lung strategy. See Open lung approach
Protein deficiency (kwashiorkor), 197
Protein-calorie malnutrition (marasmus), 197
Protein-rich chyle, 259
Prothrombin 20210A mutation, 344
Prothrombin time (PT), 187
Proton pump inhibitors, 208, 220, 232, 387, 420
Prototypical colloid solutions
albumin preparations, 146
Proximal aortic extension cuff, 366
Proximal colostomy
Hartmann pouch, 324
Proximal deep venous thrombosis
treatment of, inferior vena caval (IVC) filters, 343
Pseudoaneurysm, 359
development of, palpation of a pulsatile mass on physical exam, 359
formation, 363
nonsurgical treatment of, 359
Pseudocyst, 463
surgical options to treat, 464t

Pseudomembranous colitis, 292
Pseudomonas aeruginosa
patients at risk, 165
Pseudo-obstructed patients, 490
PTC. See Percutaneous transhepatic cholangiogram (PTC)
PTCA. See Percutaneous transluminal coronary angioplasty (PTCA)
PTLD. See Post-transplant lymphoproliferative disease (PTLD)
Puestow procedure, 468
Pulmonary and chest wall surgery
complications of, 264
Pulmonary angiography, 267
Pulmonary artery
blood flow, blockage of, 414
catheterization
fluid resuscitation, adequacy of, 128
injury, 684
risk of a difficult dissection, 308
occlusion pressure, 128
occlusion, 267
perforation of, 376
Pulmonary artery catheter (PAC), 139, 180
Pulmonary barotraumas
spring-loaded silo placement, 752
Pulmonary capillary pressure
resultant elevation in, 267
Pulmonary capillary wedge pressure (PCWP), 139, 146, 167
LV preload, poor predictors of, 139
Pulmonary complications, 157–171, 257–258, 279, 544
atelectasis, pneumonia, respiratory failure, 158
diagnosis of, 157
management of, 157
multiple levels at varying rates of clinical urgency, 157
poor exercise tolerance, 158
Pulmonary compromise, acute, 160
Pulmonary disease, advanced
arterial blood gas analysis, 63
chronic, 159
Pulmonary dysfunction, 279
prevention, 279, 280, 281
risk factors, 279
Pulmonary edema, 167, 266
acute, 181
Pulmonary embolectomy
for massive pulmonary embolism, 351
heparin anticoagulation, 377
Pulmonary embolism (PE), 339, 341, 344, 403
endovascular treatment of, 376
hypoventilation syndrome and *cor pulmonale*, increased in obesity, 403
national multicenter study (PIOPED II) role in the diagnosis of, 341f
risks of postoperative, 37
thrombolytic and surgical procedures, 350
use of thrombolytic therapy, 350
with high ligation, and sclerotherapy, 352
Pulmonary embolism, 337, 341, 349
Pulmonary embolus, fatal
risk of, 85
Pulmonary fibrosis, 289

Pulmonary function
    improvement in, surgical weight
        reduction, 401
Pulmonary function studies
    flow-volume loops, 231
Pulmonary function testing (PFT)
Pulmonary function, poor, 310
Pulmonary hypertension, 685
Pulmonary insufficiency, severe
    prevention and treatment of, 157
Pulmonary lobectomy, 310
Pulmonary nodules, Peripheral and densities
    biopsy of, 306
Pulmonary resection
    atrial and ventricular arrhythmias, 265
Pulmonary sequestration, 743–744
Pulmonary transplantation
    acute rejection, 694
    airway complications in, 688–689
    anastomotic infections, 689
    anastomotic stenosis, 689
    atrial dysrhythmias, 696
    bacterial infections in, 690
    complications during recipient
        operation, 684–686
    complications of, 683–697
    empyema, 693–694
    fungal infections in, 692–693
    gastrointestinal complications in, 695–696
    hyperammonemia, 696
    hyperinflation, 693
    infections in, 690
    nonpulmonary complications in, 695–697
    pleural effusion, 693
    pleural space complications in, 693–694
    pneumothorax, 693
    postoperative complications in, 686–693
    rejection in, 694
    renal failure in, 696
    sternal complications in, 685–686
    suboptimal donor procurements, 684
    technical complications in, 683–686
    viral infections in, 690–692
Pulmonary vein injuries, 684
Pulse oximetry, 97, 160
Pump coronary artery bypass techniques, 282
Puncture site complications, 359–360
Push enteroscopy, 488
PVE. See Prosthetic valve endocarditis (PVE)
Pyloromyotomy, 254
    to enhance gastric emptying, 747
Pyloroplasty, 254, 258, 390
Pylorospasm, 254
Pylorus preservation (PPPD), 472
Pylorus-preserving
        pancreaticoduodenectomy, 600
Pyrexia, leukocytosis, 339

Q

Q waves
    presence of, 291
QT prolongation, acute, 182
Qualifying examination
    readmissibility pathway, 27
Quality improvement consortiums, 42
Quality measurement
    improving quality of, 42–43
    patient-centered outcome measures,
        quality judged by, 42
    surgical, 43

Quality reporting system, 48
    validated mechanism for risk
        adjustment, 48
Quality-of-care issues, 52

R

Radial artery grafts, 291
Radial artery harvesting
    complications of, 291
    neurologic injury, 291
Radial artery spasm, 291
Radiation exposure
    therapeutic or accidental doses of, 576
Radiation, 268
Radiofrequency ablation, 414, 419
Radioiodine approach, 578
Radiolabeled fibrinogen scanning, 339
Radiologic dye
    complications of, 358
Radionuclide ventriculography, 63
Ramstedt pyloromyotomy, 755
Ramstedt-type extramucosal
        pyloromyotomy, 258
Random axillary sampling procedures, 609
Randomized controlled trial (RCT), 165
Rapamycin inhibitors
    mammalian target of, 215–216
Rate control
    calcium channel blockers, conversion to
        sinus rhythm, 289
Ravitch procedure
    complications of, 768
Recalcitrant sputum retention
    require transcricoid saline injection, 311
Recertification
    preparing for, 22
    recertification exam within 7 years,
        following certificate
        issuance, 26
Recombinant factor VIIa (rVIIa)
    activation of IX or X leading to thrombin
        formation, 191
    intravenous infusion of, patient
        becoming prothrombotic, 191
Recombinant factor VIIa infusion, 189
Reconstruction, venous, 568
Reconstructions, 332–334
Reconstructive techniques
    flaps and free grafts, 274
Recovery Nitinol filter, 349
Recredentialing
    annual or a biannual event, 28
    CME credits, in practice and expertise, 28
Recredentialing requirements, preparing
        for, 22
Rectal advancement flaps
    incontinence and perineal wound
        healing, 519
Rectal irrigation, 751
Rectal mucosal prolapse
    excision of redundant mucosa, managed
        by, 742
Rectal prolapse, 503
    oral enzyme therapy, or rectal cautery
        and sclerotherapy, 735
Rectobulbar urethral fistula, 739
Rectosigmoid junction, 502
Rectosigmoid muscularis, 737
Rectourethral fistulas, recurrent, 742

Recurrent carotid disease
    neointimal hyperplasia, proliferation of
        mesenchymal cells, 320
    prevention through antiplatelet
        drugs, 321
    recurrent atherosclerosis, 320
Recurrent hyperparathyroidism, 589
Recurrent intra-abdominal abscess, 467
Recurrent laryngeal nerve (RLN), 230, 240,
        577, 582–583, 633
    cuffed endotracheal tube, 230
    injury, avoidance of, 582
    ipsilateral vagus nerve, injury by
        retractor, 319
    paresis, 582
    vocal fold medialization, 240
Red-cell transfusion, 140
Redo central neck dissection, 633
Reexploration
    postoperative renal failure, higher rate
        of, 292
Reexploration, emergent
    patients with, postoperative cardiac
        tamponade, 292
Refeeding syndrome, 200–201
    anorexia nervosa and malabsorption
        syndromes, 200
Reflux pancreatitis, 676
Refractory atrial fibrillation, 266
Refractory septic shock, 131
Refractory short bowel disease, 482
Regenerative reepithelialization, 106
Regional pancreatic resection, 601
Regression techniques, 32
    hospital volume and mortality, 32
Reheparinization
    and reinstitution of CPB, for
        hemodynamic support, 279
Renal artery, 370–371
Renal atheroembolism
    causing renal failure, 323
Renal collecting system
    iatrogenic injury, prevention through
        preoperative planning, 151
Renal complications, 292, 371
Renal dysfunction, 132, 217, 640
    acute, 217
    oliguric acute renal failure, 132
Renal failure, 221, 420, 657
    as a complication of liver surgery, 420
    chronic, 657
        arteriovenous fistula, 155
    dialysis, 292
Renal infarction, 371
Renal injury
    management of, maintaining fluid and
        electrolyte balance, 282
Renal insufficiency, 221, 323
    and failure, 221–222
    chronic, 715–716
        important risk factor, 358
    hemodilution, low perfusion pressure,
        combination of, 282
Renal ischemia, 154
Renal replacement, 132
    intermittent hemodialysis, 155
Renal transplantation, 639–640
    allograft fracture, 651
    artery stenosis, 642
    bladder leak, 649
    complications of, 639–651

donor-related complications in, 640
    deceased donors, 640
    volunteer living donors, 640
hypercalcemia, 651
pelvicalyceal leak, 649
recipient-related complications in, 640–641
    arterial thrombosis, 640–641
    hemorrhage, 641
    polar artery occlusion, 641
    renal vein thrombosis, 641
spontaneous decapsulation, 651
subfascial abscess, 650–651
superficial wound infection, 650
ureteral leak, 648–649
ureteral obstruction, 645–647
urinary extravasation, 647–648
urologic complications in, 645–649
vascular complications in, 640–644
Renal vasoconstriction
    decreased blood flow, by rheologic changes, 358
Renal vein thrombosis, 641
Reoperation, 587
Reoperative liver surgery
    increased perihepatic blood loss, 411
Reoperative peritoneum, 525
Reoperative surgery, 411
Reperfusion injury
    hypertonic saline, 141
Reperfusion therapy, 181
Repetitive alveolar recruitment-
        derecruitment, 132
Repogle suction
    and gastrostomy tube, for delayed repair, 744
Repogle tube, 744
Resected iliac artery, 364
Resection planning
    postresection functioning liver remnant,
        estimation of, 408
Resection, 397–398
Resectional therapy, 253
    complications after, 264
Residency Review Committee (RRC), 5, 11, 26
Residency training program, 5
Residency training, formal, 28
Residency years
    rite of passage, 12
Resident education, 5
    attending staff, increasing pressures of, 6
    central goal, improvement in patient care, 5
    in-hospital services, 6
    operating room, 6
    outpatient clinic, 6
Resident work hours, 7
Residents, general surgery, 6
Residual air space
    bilobectomies and lobectomies, 309
    persistent air leak, absence of, 309
Residual air space and prolonged air
Leaks, 309–310
Respiratory
    complication
        acute, 161
            etiology of, 167
            pulmonary abnormality, 158
    decompensation, 200

failure
    intraoperative risk factors,
        cardiopulmonary bypass time, 292
    pulmonary complications, 292
foreign bodies, 767–768
insufficiency, 257
status
    preoperative assessment of, 157
workload
    acute respiratory acidosis and
        ventilator dependence, 200
Restenosis, 364, 370, 371
    and late stroke, 361
    and occlusion, 362
    development of, 362
    restenosis within stent, and stenosis at
        the end of stent, 361
Restorative proctocolectomy, 512
    pelvic abscess, 512
Resuscitation fluid
    autologous fresh blood, 140
    blood and blood products, colloids, and
        crystalloids, 140
    choice of, 140
Resuscitation, 109
    large-bore intravenous lines (16-gauge or
        larger), 140
Retained dead fetus
    inciting infectious focus, removal with
        antibiotics, 190
Retained instrument
    intraoperative radiograph, 525
    technical error, occurring during
        laparotomy, 525
Retention sutures
    mTOR inhibitor receivers, 220
Retractor injury, 525
Retractors
    unintended organ injury, 525
Retroperitoneum
    iliac vein obstruction, unilateral massive
        leg edema, 339
Retrosternal dysphagia, 253
Retrosternal neohiatus
    obstruction of, 259
Reverse-Trendelenburg position
    decrease central venous pressure, 414
Rhabdomyolysis, 155
Rhythm disturbances, 304–305
Right ventricular (RV) hemodynamic
        abnormalities, 304
Right ventricular end-diastolic volume
        (RVEDV)
    modified pulmonary artery catheter,
        measured by, 139
Right ventricular failure
    vasodilators and phosphodiesterase
        inhibitors, 304
Right ventricular failure, persistent, 304
Rigid atherosclerotic plaque
    removal of, 320
Ringer solution, 141
    racemic mixture of D and L
        stereoisomers, 141
    resuscitation, modulation of leukocyte
        function, 141
Ringplasties
    complex internal, 531

Risk assessment
    preoperative risk assessment, 307–308
Risk factors, 280, 281, 282
    etiology and prevention of, 164–165
    patient-related, 158
    preoperative identification, 287
    specific, 118–119
        diabetes, tighter perioperative glucose
            control, 118
        effect of laparoscopy on risk, 118
        tobacco use, delay in primary wound
            healing, 118
        use of steroid, 118–120
Risk index category, 117
Risk markers
    diagnostic testing, 55t, 60t, 62
    hemoglobin, platelet count, potassium
        level, 62
    identification of, 59
    laboratory tests, serum creatinine, 62
    major, intermediate, and minor, 59
    supplemental preoperative evaluation,
        when and which test, 61f
Risk stratification models
    development of, 287
    high risk patients, 56
Risk-adjusted outcomes, 52
    associated structure and processes of
        care, 52
Risk-stratify patients with suspected CAD
    dipyridamole thallium stress testing, 64
Rituximab
    CD20 marker on B cells, 217
    treatment against antibody-mediated
        immunity, 217
RLN. *See* Recurrent laryngeal nerve (RLN)
Routine cholangiography, 425
Roux-en-Y
    choledochojejunostomy, 448
    esophagojejunostomy, 398
    gastrectomy, 393
    gastric bypass, 399
        nutrient deficiencies, 404
        Roux limb, 402f
    hepaticojejunostomy, 443, 449
    jejunal loop, 597
    limb, 260
        of intestine, 414
    loop, 452
Royal College of Physicians and
        Surgeons, 27
Rumel tourniquet, 272
Rupture
    high-grade stenosis, with heavy
        calcification, 363
    perinephric hematoma, 370
    visualization of contrast extravasation,
        on completion angiogram, 362
RV systolic function
    recovery of, 304
RVEDV index. *See* Right ventricular end-
        diastolic volume (RVEDV)
        index

S
Safe airway management, 157
Safe health care delivery
    clinical information, collection and
        sharing of clinical
        information, 4

Safe health care delivery (*Continued*)
    computer-aided decision support
        systems, 4
    medical knowledge accessibility, 4
    patient and clinician communication, 4
Safe surgical care, 4
    foundations of, 4
    knowledge, technical skill and
        judgment, 4
Salivary fistula, 246
Salt poor albumin. *See* Albumin preparations
Sampling error, 608
Saphenopopliteal reflux
    persistent and recurrent venous
        varicosities, 340
Saphenous vein
    and leg wound complications, 291
    bypass graft, 301
    graft, 321
    harvesting
Sarcoma resections, 625–626
Savary-Gilliard guidewire, 252
Scapula entrapment, 274
Scar revision
    stricture-plasties, 113
    Z-plasties or W-plasties, 113
Scarless fetal healing, 103
Scientific Registry of Transplant Recipients
    (SRTR), 666
Sclerotherapy
    causes an intraluminal fibrotic
        response, 351
    primary complication of, 352
    transient pigmentation and
        neovascularity, 352
    with hypertonic saline, 351
Screening tests
    abnormal
        coagulation protein system,
            measuring of, 187*t*
    of APTT and PT
        coagulation protein system,
            measuring portions of, 187*f*
Scrotal hematoma, 543
Scrotal swelling, 776
Secondary axillary and subclavian vein
    thrombosis
    due to indwelling catheters, or
        pacemaker wires, 339
Segmental colonic
    colorectal resection, with a continent
        reconstruction, 501
Segmental endarterectomy, and
    decalcification
    to successfully close the aorta, 304
Seldinger technique, 465
Selective arteriography, 221
Selective operative cholangiography
    indications for, 425*t*
Sensitive epiaortic echocardiography, 288
Sentinel lymph node biopsy (SLNB), 620, 630
    radioactive colloid lymphoscintigraphy,
        for identifying lymph node
        basins, 622
Sentinel node biopsy
    in head and neck, 634
    vs. axillary dissection, 630–631
Sepsis
    infectious and inflammatory, 127
    systemic inflammatory response, 126

Sepsis, severe
    and endocrine, 132–133
    dysregulation in host responses, leading
        to shock, 127
    organ dysfunction, hypoperfusion, or
        hypotension, 126
Sepsis, systemic
    sepsis-associated encephalopathy, 133
Septic patients
    decreased mortality rate, 127
    pseudomembranous colitis, 133
    stress gastritis and ulceration, 133
Septic pulmonary emboli, 300
Septic shock, 126–133
    activated leukocytes, and coagulation
        cascade, 127
    arterial catheterization, 128
    blood lactate concentration, 128
    chest x-ray and electrocardiogram, 129
    clinical assessment of, 128
    complications of, 132–133
    corticosteroid therapy, 131
    decreased vasomotor tone, using
        vasopressors and inotropic
        agents, 129
    depressed level of consciousness, or
        encephalopathy, 129
    flow diagram for management of, 130*f*
    fluids, 129
    gastrointestinal and hepatic, 133
    hypotension, multifactorial in
        origin, 129
    inotropic or vasopressor support, 126
    intravascular hypovolemia
        loss of plasma volume, 129
        pulmonary capillary leak, 129
        restoration using boluses, 129
        vasopressors, 129
    intravascular volume
        fluid resuscitation, 129
    intubation for airway protection, 129
    laboratory tests and studies, 128–129
    management of, 129–132
    myocardial depression, decreased
        vasomotor tone, 129
    pathophysiology of, 127
    patient surgical history, 128
    pulmonary acute lung failure, 132
    recombinant human-activated
        protein C, 131
    renal dysfunction, 132
    resuscitative measures, 129
    sepsis with hypotension, 126
    tumor necrosis factor α, 131
Serial preoperative therapeutic
    pneumoperitoneum
    technique of, 541
SEROMA, 274, 606, 629
Serosanguinous drainage, 254
Serpin plasma protein inhibitors
    reduced procoagulants and
        anticoagulants, 191
Serratus anterior muscle, 272
Serum bilirubin
    rise in, 416
Serum creatinine, 292
Serum phosphate levels, 202
Seton, cutting, 519
Settings, high-risk, 441–442
Sexual dysfunction, 508
Shear stress, mechanical, 279

Shock, 127, 129
    evaluation of, 127–129
    hypovolemic, cardiogenic, and
        distributive, 127
    inadequate oxygen delivery and cellular
        hypoxia, 127
Short bowel syndrome, 481–482, 729, 753
    cholesterol gallstone formation, and
        calcium bilirubinate
        precipitation, 204
    combined liver and bowel
        transplantation, 204
Short focal lesions
    treated by endarterectomy, 360
Shoulder immobilization
    with slings or special wraps, decreases
        seroma formation, 606
Shouldice clinic
    and Shouldice technique, managing
        inguinal hernias, 531
    holistic concept of hernia surgery, 531
Sigmoid diverticulosis, 501
Sign-out sheet, 7
Simple prolapse
    mobilizing mucocutaneous junction, 513
Simulation training, 15–17
    assessment, 16
    endoscopic retrograde
        cholangiopancreatography,
        interaction with an image, 16
    simulation, interaction with an image, 16*f*
Sinusitis, chronic 228–229
Sirolimus
    anastomosis dehiscence in lung
        recipients, 220
    cause of, hyperlipidemia, 220
    macrocyclic antibiotic, 215
Site-review teams, 52
Skeletal deformities, tremor, and anxiety, 60
Skin cancer
    immunosuppressive therapy patients,
        serious morbidity and
        potential mortality, 219
Skin graft closure
    topical silver sulfadiazine, 753
Skin preparation, 120
    antiseptic agents, 120
    hair removal, 120
    operating room formalities, 120–121
    preoperative shower, 120
Skin-sparing mastectomy, 613
Sleep apnea, obstructive
    patients with, 89
    pharyngeal collapse, 89
Sleeve lobectomy, 270
SLNB. *See* Sentinel lymph node
    biopsy (SLNB)
SLWL. *See* Suture length to wound length ratio
SMA. *See* Superior mesenteric artery (SMA)
Small bowel
    complications of intestinal surgery,
        477–495
    obstruction, 391, 511
    resection, 221
Small-bowel surgery, 771–774
    intussusception, 772–774
    Meckel diverticulum, 771–774
Small functioning remnant liver, 415–416
Small intestinal bleeding
    etiologies of, 489*t*
Small intestinal bypass, 490

Smaller alveoli
  preferential collapse of, 268
Smoke inhalation, 161
  thermal injury, hypoxia, 161–162
Soave operation, 736
Society of American Gastrointestinal
      Endoscopic Surgeons (SAGES),
      22, 28
  surgical activity and outcomes
      reporting, 22
Society of Thoracic Surgeons (STS)
  database, 290
  development of, 287
Sodium bicarbonate
  free-radical scavenger, 154
Sodium, 201
  excess. *See* Hypoalbuminemia
  repletion, 737
Soft-tissue massage
  expedite resolution, 604
Soft-tissue sarcomas, 624–626
  treated with, surgery and radiation
      therapy, 624
Soft-tissue surgery
  complications associated with, 624
Soft-tissue tumor surgery
  complications of, 619–626
  management of cutaneous melanoma,
      619
Solid organ and visceral injury
  incidence of, 551
Solid organ cancers
  abdominal CT scan, cancer metastases in
      liver and spleen, 219f
Solid organ transplants, 212
Somatostatin receptor scintigraphy, 596
Somato-statinomas, 594
Spaces and air leaks, 270–272
Special to ablation procedures, 408–409
Specific factor Xa inhibitor, 346
Sphincterotomy
  endoscopic biliary drainage, 448
  internal complications of, 518
  passage of stone fragments, biliary
      sludge, or clots, 448
Spigelian, 523
Spinal and epidural catheters
  epidural and spinal hematoma
      formation, 344
Spinal anesthesia, 84
Spinal cord injury
  monitoring using
      somatosensory, 324
  pulmonary embolism, frequent cause of
      death, 344
Spinal cord ischemia, 86, 324
  injury to anterior spinal artery, with
      epidural catheter, 86
Spinal-epidural anesthesia
  painful lumbar puncture, and syrinx in
      the conus, 86
Spiral computed tomography (CT)
      scanning, 341
  primary diagnostic test, 339
Splanchnic arterial blood flow
  decreased, 413
Splanchnic ischemia, 131
Splanchnic oxygenation, 154
Splanchnic perfusion
  intraoperative monitoring of, 284

Spleen
  hemorrhage, 391
  hilum
    positive lymph nodes, 398
  injury, 254, 259, 507
  surgery, 781
    increases incidence of, pancreatic
        fistula, pancreatitis,
        subphrenic abscess, 391
    postoperative morbidity and
        mortality, adverse effect on,
        398
    postsplenectomy sepsis, 781
    splenectomy, 781
    splenosis, 781
  unrecognized injury to, postoperative
      hemorrhage, 391
Splenosis, 781
Spontaneous decapsulation, 651
Sporadic NETs, 594
Sporadic pancreatic endocrine
      neoplasms, 594
Sputum retention
  reduce the incidence of, 311
Sputum retention and pneumonia, 311
Squamous-cell skin cancers, 219
SRTR. *See* Scientific Registry of Transplant
      Recipients (SRTR)
Stable atrial fibrillation
  electrocardioversion for, 266
Standard Belsey Mark IV transthoracic hiatal
      hernia repair, 246
  sliding hiatus hernia with a peptic
      stricture, 247f
Standard pacing electrodes, 290
Standard saphenous stripping, 352
Standard therapy, volume resuscitation in, 131
Standard underwater-seal drainage
      system, 269
Staphylococcal organisms, 604
Staphylococcus aureus
  common etiologic agent, 85
  bacteremia, 362
Staphylococcus epidermidis, 299
Staple line disruption
  complication of gastric bypass
      techniques, 404
Stapled bronchial closure, 269
Statins
  reduction of ischemic events, stroke, and
      cardiac death, 66
Steatohepatitis
  advanced stage of severe hepatic
      inflammation, 203
Steatorrhea
  calcium supplementation intramuscular
      vitamin D, 404
Steep learning curve
  disadvantages of VATS, 306
ST-elevation acute coronary
      syndromes, 67
Stenoses, high-grade, 321
Stenosis, 514
  gastrojejunal, 404
  magnetic resonance angiogram, 643f
  recurrent, 361
  residual, diagnosed by TEE, 303
  treatment of, 646f
Stenotic segment
  anatomy of, 232

Stent, 450
  dislodgement, 371
  graft designs, 369
  infection, 362
    following iliac artery stent
        placement, 364
    proteus mirabilis, 371
    Klebsiella pneumoniae, 371
    treated with, intravenous antibiotic
        administration, and
        resuscitation, 371
    underlying etiology of, 362
  occlusion, 450
  placement
    complications related to, 450
  restenosis, 372
    rate, following carotid artery stenting,
        361
Stent-graft migration, distal
  complicates abdominal aortic
      endografting, 369
Stenting, 354
  nonsurgical, palliative for, local tumor
      recurrence after resection, 457
  of ampulla Vater, 435
Sternal osteotomy, 768
Sternal rewiring, 290
Sternal wound complications, 290–291
Sternotomy, upper partial, 237
Steroid resistant acute rejection, 217
Steroid-receptor complex, 213
Steroids
  immunosuppressive medication, 213
  monocyte migration, and suppression of
      chemokine production, 213
Steroids, stress, 222
Stewart-Treves syndrome, 610, 630
Stitches, deeper fascial, 525
Stoma complications, 513
Stomach, fasting human, 390
Stomal appliance, 256
Stomal complications, 404
Stomal retraction, 513–514
Stomal stenosis, 403, 514
  symptoms of gastroesophageal reflux, 404
  upper endoscopy, preferred means of
      investigation, 404
Stomal ulceration, 404
  proton pump inhibitors, failure to
      heal, 404
Strangulated hernias, 538
Strasberg Class E injuries,
      complex, 433
Strasberg classification, 426
Streptococcus pneumonia
      (pneumococcus), 507
Streptococcus, 107
Streptomyces hygroscopius, 215
Streptomyces tsukubaenis
  tolypocladium inflatum Gams, and
      tacrolimus, 214
Stress testing
  noninvasive, 220
  nuclear, 177
Stricture, 516
  at anastomosis, 512
  mucosa-to-mucosa anastomosis, 449
Stricture, high-grade
  obstructing bile egress, associated with
      jaundice, 418
Strictures, recurrent, 440

Stricturoplasty
for long-segment radiation-associated obstruction, 485
Stroke
feared complication of, cerebrovascular interventions, 361
risk factors, 282–283, 287
Stroke patients, and lower extremity paralysis
low-dose heparin and low-molecular-weight heparin, 344
Stroke volume, 137
Stroke, fatal, 361
Structural graft failure, 327
Structural measures
individual physicians, relative expertise of, 31
procedure volume, 31
Structural valve degeneration, 299
Structural variables, imperfect proxies for quality, 39
Structure and process measures
quality indicators, 39–42
strengths and weaknesses of the two measures, 41t
Structure measures, 39
related to, surgical outcomes, 39
strengths and weaknesses of, 39–41
Structure of care, 31–35
Structured protocol and scoring system, 52
Strut perforation, 376
STS. See Society of Thoracic Surgeons (STS)
ST-segment–elevation MI, acute
reperfusion therapy, 67
Stunned myocardium
intra-aortic balloon pump (IABP), and ventricular assist device, 278
Subcarinal lymphadenectomy, 273
Subcutaneous emphysema, 236, 552
Subfascial abscess, 650–651
Subfascial approach, open
ligation of perforating venous branches, 353
Subfascial perforator surgery
remote endoscopic access to visualize, and ligate subfascial perforators, 353
Subglottic stenosis, 230, 231–232
mild short-segment, 232f
Subjective global assessment (SGA)
history and physical examination, including evaluation of weight loss, 196
Subluxation, 230
voice therapy for dysphonia, 230
Submucosal noncholinergic nonadrenergic nerve hypertrophy, 735
Suboptimal donor procurements, 684
Subpleural lesions
effacement of, 308
Subspecialty training, 34
Subtotal gastrectomy, 397
Successful endovascular mesenteric intervention
recurrent symptoms, due to development of restenosis, 370
Succinylcholine
increase in serum potassium, 78
mean intraocular pressure (IOP), 79
open globe injury, contraindicated in, 79

Suction bronchoscopy, 311
Suction decompression, intraluminal, 398
Suction drainage
mean duration, 606
Sudek critical point, 503
Sulodexide
healing ulcers, relative to saline and compression, 353
Sunbelt Melanoma Trial, 622, 630
Superior laryngeal nerve (SLN)
injury, 242
Superior mesenteric artery (SMA), 671
Superior vena cava
stenting of, complications associated with, 376
Superselective arterial access
embolization of feeding vessels, 369
Supine positioning
microaspiration and nosocomial pneumonia, 165
Support brassiere
in postoperative period, 607
Supportive therapy, standard, 267
Suppurative superficial thrombophlebitis
intravenous catheter use, or multiple puncture sites, 339
Suppurative superficial thrombophlebitis, secondary
limit intravenous peripheral catheters, 352
Supra-aortic interventions, 360–362
Supradiaphragmatic ligation, 273
Suprarenal aorta
clamping of, results in Spinal cord ischemia, 324
Suprarenal filter placement
T12-L1, 349
Suprarenal Greenfield filter
failed infrarenal filter, 349
Supraventricular arrhythmias, 300
Supraventricular tachycardia, 265, 278
Surface echocardiogram
diagnosis by, 254
Surface-coating hemostatic agents
preventative measures, 413
Surgeon
factors, 35
level variables, 33–35
subspecialty training, 34–37
surgeon volume, 33–34
skill and experience, 425
Surgery
colorectal, 10
educators, creativity and investigation, passion of some surgeons, 7
elective, 30
endocrine, 10
hemodynamic stress, 60
plus radiation, 624
subspecialty practice
curriculum redesign, specialization and fellowship training, 10
emergence of, 10–11
type, important cardiac risk factor, 175
vascular, 10
versus Thrombolysis for Ischemia of the Lower Extremity (STILE), 374
Surgical accountability
minimal prospect, 4

Surgical attention
meticulous operative techniques, development of, 3
Surgical biopsies, open
nonpalpable, 609
Surgical care
balancing risk and benefit, focus on, 3
evidence-based referral, and quality improvement strategies, 30
financial constraints, 3
improving quality of, 30
information technology (IT)
effective and safer care, 4
surgical complications, reports on unnecessary deaths, 3
quality, risk adjustment influences, 49
Surgical coronary revascularization, 286–293
Surgical credentials, 25–29
Surgical culture
reexamination of, 4
Surgical debridement, 290
Surgical decision making, 15
Surgical diseases
of the pancreas, 463
resection of the pancreas, associated with morbidity and mortality, 463
Surgical drainage
complications of, 465
Surgical Education and Self-Assessment Program (SESAP), 22
educational program, to help surgeons maintain clinical knowledge, 22
recertifying examination, 100 hours of CME, 22
Surgical educators
resident hours, demand in reduction of hours, 7
Surgical faculty members, 7
reduced resident work hours, benefits on quality of life, 7
resident work hours and duty hour restrictions, 7
Surgical harm
learning environments, 4
minimization of, 4
Surgical Intensive Care Unit (SICU), 52
pulmonary artery catheter, use of, 139
Surgical intervention
general health status, 158
Surgical masks, 122
Surgical morbidity, 4
after elective or therapeutic regional lymphadenectomy, 622
and mortality, 196
low preoperative serum albumin level, 108
recognition and correction of malnutrition, prior to elective surgery, 196
Surgical mortality, 4
risk of, 159
Surgical outcomes, 31
Institute of Medicine report, societal interest in surgical outcomes, 3
process of care, 35–39
structure of care, evidence linking, 31
Surgical patient, 195–196
bleeding risk, assessment of, 185–188
diagnosis of bleeding in, 188–192

Surgical practice
  continuity of care, 13
  doctor–patient relationship, 13
Surgical quality, 30
  assessment of, 30, 45
  clinical outcomes, linking structure and
    process to, 52
  coordination, an important
    aspect, 52
  critical elements in, 46
  end results system, 45
  Leapfrog Group, 30
  measurement and quality improvement,
    53, 53f
  O/E Ratio, 51
  quality–cost relationship, 55
  risk-adjusted morbidity and mortality
    rates, 30
  risk-adjusted outcomes, as measures
    of, 55
  structure and process of care measures,
    30–43
  using outcomes approach, 46
  value relationship, 55
Surgical resection, 565
Surgical residency, 8, 13, 15
Surgical revascularization, 286
Surgical risk, 3
  intraoperative and postoperative events,
    assessment of, 3
  operative and nonoperative
    therapy, 3
Surgical scrub, 121–122
  hand bacterial colony counts, 121
Surgical simulation technology, 16
Surgical site infections (SSIs), 114–124
  anastomotic leakage, following bowel
    preparation, 120
  antibiotic prophylaxis, 122
  classification and risk of, 114–118
  classifications of, 114–116
  complications of operative
    interventions, 114
  contamination of wound, 115–118
  deep incisional SSIs, deeper invasive
    management, 115
  mechanical and antibiotic bowel
    preparation, 119t
  microbial contamination, occurrence
    of, 116
  microbiology of, 118
  minimizing wound contamination, 114
  prevention of, 118–123
  prophylactic antibiotics, 119t
  risking infection, 116
  skin preparation, for decrease of bacterial
    contaminant, 120
  surgical site infection pathogens, 119t
  tissue oxygenation, 119–120
    resuscitation with colloids, 120
    superadequate intravascular
      hydration, 120
  treat remote infections, 120
  treatment of, 123–124
  variety of host contaminating
    organism, 116f
Surgical studies
  patient selection, 3
  statistical analysis and molecular
    biology, 3

Surgical technique, 472
  advances in, 23
  cooperation with sales representatives,
    for using new tools and
    equipment safely, 23
  purchase agreements, and cost of
    training, 23
Surgical therapy, 396
  alternatives to, 464–465
Surgical training, 13–17
  programs, 5
    ABS and RRC in surgery, 6
    Accreditation Committee for
      Graduate Medical Education
      (ACGME), 5
    American Board of Surgery (ABS), 5
    board pass rates and patient
      outcomes, 7
    complication conference, for
      monitoring surgical
      practice, 7
    early and accurate trainees
      designation and ability for
      flexibility, 6
    educational tool for house staff, 7
    evolution of, 6
    faculty and resident, commitment to
      patient care, 7
    faculty members, efficiency in
      resident education, 7
    placing residents in responsible
      positions, 8
    primary care physicians, increase
      number of, 6
    priority of patient's welfare, 7
    quality and continuity of care,
      relationship to, 7
    reengineering systems of patient care,
      redesigning residents' roles, 8
    Residency Review Committee
      (RRC), 5
    residents, structured operative
      experience of, 6
    role in surgical education, 7
    societal influences, effects of, 6
    trained and competent physicians,
      production of, 5
Surgical wound classification scheme,
    115, 115t
Surgical wound complications
  risk factors for, 107, 107t
Surveillance esophagoscopy, 254
Suture
  disruption, 369
  ligature, 410
  line disruption
    incidence of, 253
  line leak, 403
  tension, 524
  vascular staple closure, 410
  venorrhaphy, 572
Suture length to wound length ratio
    (SLWL), 524
Suture, permanent
  two layers of, 415
Sutures, deep cavity
  disadvantage of, 607
Swan-Ganz catheter, 153, 167, 181
Swan-Ganz pulmonary artery catheters
  hemodynamic monitoring, with, 333

Swenson operation
  dissection of rectum, 736
Sympathetic chain, 583
Symptomatic coronary
  and aneurysmal disease, 323
Symptomatic internal carotid artery (ICA)
    disease, 318
  combined CEA/CABG, 318
Synthetic prostaglandin analog
    Misoprostol, 390
Systemic inflammatory response syndrome
    (SIRS), 126
Systemic perfusion
  during and after bypass, 292
Systemic vascular resistance (SVR), 128, 137
  increased SVR, restricts blood flow, 138
Systems-based practice, 29
Systolic anterior motion (SAM), 303

T
T cells
  activation of, 213
Tachycardia
  atrial fibrillation and flutter, narrow-
    complex tachycardias, 182
  symptom for hypovolemic shock, 137
  worsening abdominal or back pain, and
    hiccups, 404
Tacrolimus, 214
  neurologic side effects, 215
Tamponade
  and cardiopulmonary collapse, 254
  late, 303
Tapered Hurst-Maloney esophageal
    dilators, 252f
Target peak and plateau airway pressure, 169
T-cell activation, 213
Technetium sestamibi scanning, 586
Technical complications, 370
  conversion to open surgery, 369–370
Teflon bolster
  improve fixation of valve, 302
Teflon pledgets
  causing perivalvular leak, 300
Temperature control and blood component
    replacement therapy
  lessens incidence of coagulopathies, 323
Temporary and retrievable filters, 349
Tension-free anastomosis, 232
"Tension-free" hernioplasty, 533
Tension pneumothorax, 128, 161, 415
  mediastinal shift, 161
  timely clinical assessment, 161
  traumatic injury, spontaneous rupture of
    a pneumocele, 161
Tertiary care centers, better patients
    outcomes, 34
Tertiary wound closure
  transfer of viable autologous tissue, 110
Testicular infarct, 543
Testing, noninvasive, 174
  improved prediction of cardiac risk, 177
Tetracycline
  sclerosing agent, 606
Thal fundic patch esophagoplasty, 253
Thal-Woodward procedure, 253
Therapeutic intestinal bypass
  for weight loss, 490
Therapeutic lymph node dissections
  for thick melanomas, 621

Therapeutic rigid bronchoscopy. *See* Fiberoptic bronchoscopy
Therapeutic thyroidectomy, 577
  indications, 577*t*
Therapy, nonoperative, 3
Thermal injury, 161
  upper airway edema, 161
Thermoregulatory vasoconstriction, 90
Thiamine deficiency
  Wernicke encephalopathy lactic acidosis, 201
Third fluid space
  extracellular fluid, intravascular or interstitial, 144
  patient's response to acute injury, 145
Third space fluid accumulation, 145
Third space fluid losses, 144
Thompson
  prophylactic gallbladder excision, prior to hepatic changes, 481
Thoracentesis, 766
Thoracic anomalies, 742–751
Thoracic duct injury, 633
Thoracic duct ligation
  right posterolateral thoracotomy, 259
Thoracic epidural anesthesia, 267
Thoracic esophageal perforation, 765
Thoracic esophagus
  perforation of, 247
Thoracic nerve
  disruption of, loss of serratus anterior function, 610
Thoracic outlet decompression
  main complications of, bleeding, lymphatic leak, infection, 351
Thoracic outlet syndrome, 94
Thoracic Surgery Directors Association
  integrated 6-year programs, 14
Thoracic surgery, 764–768
  bronchiectasis, 766
  chest infections, 764
  complications of, 227
  cystic fibrosis, 766–767
  empyema, 765–766
  esophageal perforation, 765
  lung abscess, 765
  mediastinitis, 764–765
  pectus excavatum, 768
  respiratory foreign bodies, 767–768
Thoracoabdominal adrenalectomy, open, 571
Thoracoabdominal aneurysm
  repair, 150
  resection of, 323
Thoracoabdominal approach
  for large tumor, 568
  pneumothorax, potential complication of, 573
Thoracodorsal neurovascular bundle, 610, 622, 629
Thoracoepigastric vein
  thrombosis of, 604
Thoracoplasty, 274
  muscle flap obliteration, 271
Thoracoscopy, 767
  complications of, 306–312
  contraindications to, 307, 307*t*
  use of, 306
Thoracotomy
  open-window, 270
  with fistula ligation, 748

Thoracotomy, open, 308
  sponge-stick, utility incision or a port site, 308
Thrombin activable fibrinolysis inhibitor thrombin (IIa) clots fibrinogen to make fibrin, 186*f*
Thrombin activable fibrinolysis inhibitor (TAFIa), 186
Thrombin formation, 186*f*
Thrombin inhibitors
  prevention of thrombotic complications, 280
Thrombin-activatable fibrinolysis inhibitor, 127
Thromboangiitis obliterans, 339
Thromboembolectomy, open, 351
Thromboembolic disease, 489
Thromboembolic etiology, 288
Thromboembolism, recurrent, 377
Thrombolysis or Peripheral Artery Surgery (TOPAS), 374
Thrombolysis, 373–375
  distal, for arterial occlusion, 361
  intracranial hemorrhage, 350
Thrombolytic therapy, 303, 349
  active bleeding, systolic blood pressure, trauma, or drug allergy, 182
  contraindications to, 374*t*
  iliac artery stent placement, 364
  significant bleeding risk, 350
  streptokinase derivatives, urokinase compounds (UK), 373
  tissue plasminogen activator, urokinase plasminogen activator, 350
  treat acute arterial or venous occlusions, 373
Thrombolytic therapy, systemic, 350
Thrombomodulin expression
  progressive endothelial dysfunction, 127
Thrombophlebitis, primary superficial
  treatment for, venous duplex ultrasound scan, 352
Thrombophlebitis, superficial, 339
  hypercoagulability, 339
  immunocompromised and burn patients, 339
  risk of, 339
  treatment options for, 353*t*
  varicose veins, pregnancy, 339
Thrombosed mechanical prosthesis
  restricted leaflet motion, 302
Thrombosis prophylaxis, deep venous, 567
Thrombosis, 185, 360, 371
  acute, 362, 372
  anticoagulation therapy, low doses of Warfarin, 207
  assessing risk and prevention of, 192–194
  atherosclerotic disease, arterial bypass, 360
  episodes of, 360
  intracatheter lytic therapy, 207
  patients with hypercoagulable states, 339
  prevention, therapy for, 194
  risk, 186
  venous, 192–194
Thrombotic complications
  rates of, 299
  variety of symptoms, 360
Thrombotic thrombocytopenic purpura (TTP), 338, 697

Thrombus fragmentation device, mechanical, 349
Thrombus, acute, 349
THVE. *See* Total hepatic venous exclusion (THVE)
Thyroid and parathyroid, 575–591
Thyroid carcinoma, 577–578
  classification of, 577*t*
  follicular-cell derived, 577
Thyroid function tests
  thyroid stimulating hormone (TSH), 576
Thyroid gland
  follicular lesions of, 576
Thyroid hormone administration
  problems with, 585
Thyroid hormone replacement therapy, 577
Thyroid lobectomy, 576
Thyroid nodule
  diagnostic evaluation of, 576
  thyroid ultrasound, 576
Thyroid scintigraphy, 576
Thyroid stimulating hormone (TSH), 576
Thyroid surgery, 576–578
Thyroidectomy, 577
  cervical hematoma, potential complication, 578
  damage to, sympathetic chain and stellate ganglion, producing a Horner syndrome, 583
  hypocalcemia, 579
  potential complications of, 578–579
Tibial angioplasty
  and stenting, 373
Tibial PTA
  complications of, 373
Tissue damage
  full heparinization and vasodilation, 352
Tissue factor pathway inhibitor (TFPI), 185
Tissue failure, 110
Tissue handling, 123
  proper operative technique, 123
Tissue hypoperfusion, 107–108, 127
Tissue injury
  redistribution of fluid, 137
Tissue perfusion, 107
Tissue regeneration
  surface area epidermal wounds, and liver injuries, 104
Tissue repair, 102
  comorbid conditions and polypharmacy, 108
Tissue retention
  obstruction or regurgitation, 302
Tissue valves
  advantage of, 299
Tissue-factor pathway inhibitors, 348
Toll-like receptors (TLR), 127
Tortuosity
  iliac artery complications, 364
Total abdominal colectomy
  ileostomy and the Hartmann procedure, 502
Total body surface area (TBSA), 140
Total colonic Hirschsprung disease, 737
Total gastrectomy, 397
  complication of, 398
  gastric tumors at esophagogastric junction, 398
  substantial postoperative nutritional challenge, 398

Total hepatic venous exclusion (THVE), 412, 779

Total knee arthroplasty, elective, 65

Total pancreatectomy
   complications of, 473–474
   endocrine insufficiency, 474

Total parenteral nutrition (TPN), 197

Total proctocolectomy
   ileal pouch anal anastomosis, 511
   with ileostomy, 502

Total thyroidectomy, 576
   adjuvant therapy, 578
   improved disease-free survival, 577
   incidence of complications after, 580t

Total vascular exclusion
   complete inflow and outflow vascular
      occlusion, of the liver, 412

Totally extraperitoneal preperitoneal
      approach (TEPPA), 537
   advantages of, 537
   herniorrhaphy, 537
   inguinal herniorrhaphy, 538
   laparoscopic inguinal hernia
      repair, 537f
   repair, 538

Toupet (posterior) fundoplication, 261

Toxicity, systemic
   incidence of, 82
   symptoms associated with toxicity, due
      to local anesthetics, 83f

Trachea
   compression, loss of airway
      patency, 583

Tracheal collapse, 74

Tracheal complications, 233

Tracheal injuries, 585

Tracheal reanastomosis, 242

Tracheal rupture, 233

Tracheal stenosis, 232, 233, 236, 242–243
   diagnosis and management of, 236

Tracheal surgery, 240–243
   atraumatic intubation technique, 240
   complications of, 230
   postintubation tracheal stenosis, 240
   postoperative complications, 242
   primary tracheal tumors, 240
   tracheal resection, and primary
      anastomosis, 240
   tracheomalacia, exteriorization of the
      airway and stenting, 243

Tracheitis, 233

Tracheobronchial tree, 236, 744
   development of a fistula, 257
   injury to, 163

Tracheoesophageal fistula (TEF), 233,
      236–237, 740, 744–749
   epithelialized tract between tracheal
      mucosa and skin, 238f
   repair of, 746f

Tracheoesophageal groove
   lateral approach to, 591f

Tracheoesophagogastric anastomotic
      fistula, 256

Tracheoinnominate artery fistula (TIF),
      237, 243
   sentinel bleed, 237

Tracheomalacia, 74, 233, 243
   airway obstruction, 233
   results in stridor, and a barking cough, 749

Tracheotomy, 234–238
   cutting the trachea, 234
   late complications of, 233
   prolonged ventilation patients, 227

Traditional surgical teaching, 3
   cure rates, or palliation of symptoms
      representing benefit, 3
   operative complications represent risk, 3

Tranexamic acid, 292

Transabdominal esophagomyotomy, 261

Transabdominal preperitoneal (TAPP)
      approach, 538

Transcutaneous oxygen tension
   measuring nutritive skin perfusion, 109

Transduodenal sphincteroplasty, 448

Transesophageal echocardiography (TEE),
      181, 278
   application of, 288

Transfusion, massive, 191

Transhepatic catheters
   postoperative stents, 436
   preoperative placement of, 436

Transhiatal esophagectomy, 255
   thromboembolic sequelae, 259

Transient bacteremia, 299

Transient ischemic attacks (TIAs),
      287, 360

Trans-jugular intrahepatic portosystemic
      shunt (TIPS)
   for treating intractable ascites, 421

Transluminal balloon angioplasty, 643f

Transmural venous invasion
   partial caval resection required, 570

Transplant coronary artery disease,
      711–714

Transplant pancreatitis, 675

Transplant renal artery stenosis, 642
   diagnosis of, 642–644
   etiology of, 642
   incidence of, 642
   treatment of, 644

Transplant renal artery stenosis, 642f

Transthoracic approach, 253

Transthoracic esophagectomy, 253

Transthoracic hiatal hernia repair, 254

Transverse aortic arch, 272

Transverse rectus abdominus myocutaneous
      (TRAM), 613

Transversus abdominis aponeurotic
      arch, 537

Trap-Ease-type filter, 349

Trauma
   blunt, 128, 136, 409
   intraoperative or postoperative
      hemorrhage, common
      etiologies of, 151
   patients, operative intervention, and
      control of hemorrhage, 139
   risk factors, spinal cord injury, 343
   surgery maintenance of intravascular
      volume, 155

Traumatic liver injuries
   management of, 409

Trendelenburg position, 74, 548
   exposing upper abdominal organs, 549

Tricuspid regurgitation, recurrent/residual, 305

Tricuspid valve endocarditis
   septic pulmonary emboli, patchy
      infiltrates, 300

Tricuspid valve surgery, 304–305, 304

Trocar injury
   precautions for avoiding, and
      complications of, 547t

Trocar insertion
   veress needle technique, 548

Trocar site recurrence
   routine use of plastic retrieval bag, 444

True junctional tachycardias
   due to digitalis toxicity, 182
   exogenous cathecolamines and
      theophylline, 182

True platelet function defect, 188

Truncal vagotomy, 253, 393

TTP. See Thrombotic thrombocytopenic
      purpura (TTP)

Tube
   complications, 233
   displacement, 234
   drainage, 270
   obstruction, 233–234
   problems, 235
   thoracostomy, 273

Tubular atrophy, 221

Tucker dilators
   vigorous dilations with, 748

Tumor
   adrenal, 573
   benign, rupture of, 409
   intracapsular hematoma, 409
   two-stage hepatectomy, 409

Tumor cell dissemination
   oncologic surgical technique, and open
      thoracotomy, 311

Tumor downstaging
   benefits of, 608

Tumor histology, 457

Tumor location
   important determinant for survival, 457

Tumor necrosis factor α, 131

Tumor, primary hepatic
   incidence of, 779t

Tumor, retroperitoneal, 625

Tumors, submucosal
   ultrasound-directed biopsy of, 396

Turnage and Lunn
   Mayo Clinic, 266

TV replacement or annuloplasty, 305

Type B injuries
   asymptomatic or present late with
      abdominal pain, 426

Type E injuries, 427
   jaundice is a common presentation, with
      bile leakage, 428

Type I and type III endoleaks
   risk of aneurysm enlargement, and
      rupture, 366

Type I collagen
   in bone and tendon, 105

Type I endoleak, 366

Type II endoleaks, 366
   generally no intervention, but treated for
      aortic pulsatility, 368
   rarely associated with, aneurysm
      rupture, 368

Type II inguinal hernias, 531

Type II pneumocytes, 268

Type II strictures
   treated with hepaticojejunostomy, 451

Type III and type I collagens
   in elastic soft tissues, 105

Type III endoleaks, 366, 369
Type III tumors
    extensive extrahepatic biliary resection,
        456
Type IV endoleaks
    develop secondary to, diffuse leaking of
        blood, 366
Type V strictures, 451
Type VII strictures
    hepatic resection, 451
Type VIII strictures
    percutaneous dilation, provide
        temporary palliation, 451
Type-I thyroplasty. *See* Medialization
    thyroplasty

U

Ulcer prophylaxis, stress, 165
Ulcer resection
    gastric tissue, to evaluate presence of
        gastric cancer, 388
Ulceration, stress, 420
Ulceration, venous
    pathophysiology of, chronic deep vein
        obstruction, 353
Ulcerative colitis, 502
Ulcers
    clean base, flat spot, adherent clot, 388
Ulnar neuropathy
    cubital tunnel retinaculum, 94
Ultrasonographic imaging
    of biopsy specimen, 609
Ultrasonography
    diagnosis by, 416
    serve as an initial screen, 420
Umbilical hernia, 774–775
Uncontrolled hemorrhage, 391
Undernutrition
    depressed T-lymphocyte numbers and
        function, 197
Unfractioned heparin
    bleeding risks of, 344
Unifocal breast cancers
    receiving induction chemotherapy, 614
Unilateral embolization, 365
Unilateral thyroidectomy, 577
Unilateral, symptomatic lesions
    thyroid lobectomy, therapeutic procedure
        of choice, 577
Uninfected biloma
    right upper quadrant or epigastric
        discomfort and tenderness, 416
Unique provider identification numbers
    (UPINs), 28
United Network for Organ Sharing
    (UNOS), 666
Univariate t-tests or chi-square tests, 49
University Renal Research and Education
    Association (URREA), 667
University-based system, 5
Unna boot, 353
UNOS. *See* United Network for Organ
    Sharing (UNOS)
Unplanned visceral injury, 525
Unrecognized devascularization
    occurs intraoperatively, with hepatic
        artery thrombosis, 416
Upper abdominal surgery, 159
Upper-lobe bronchial fistula
    sleeve lobectomy, 270

Upright abdominal films
    demonstrate pneumoperitoneum, 390
Upstaging
    of tumors, 398
Uremia, 150, 155
Ureteral injury, 324, 507
    distal, primary end-to-end anastomosis,
        over a stent, 551
    incidence of, during laparoscopic pelvic
        surgery, 550
    intraoperative, 508f
    surgical options for repair of, 509f
Ureteral leak, 648–649
Ureteral obstruction, 645–647
Ureteral patency, 647
Ureteral stents, 151
Ureteral/bladder injury, 550–551
Ureteroneocystostomy, 645
    with a psoas hitch, 551
Ureteroureterostomy, 508
Ureterovaginal fistula
    leakage of urine, 551
Ureterovesical anastomosis, 646
Urethral stricture formation, 740
Urinary extravasation, 647–648
Urinary retention, 84, 515
    and delayed gastrointestinal function, 525
Urinary tract or catheter obstruction
    oliguria, postrenal cause, 138
Urinary-rectal fistula
    presence of, 740
Urine output
    circulating volume status, assessment
        of, 138
Urinoma inferior
    ultrasound image of, 648f
URREA. *See* University Renal Research and
    Education Association (URREA)
Ursodeoxycholic acid
    improves bile flow and reduces clinical
        symptoms of cholestasis, 204

V

VA cooperative study, 196
VA health-care delivery system
    national Surgical Quality Improvement
        Program (NSQIP), 54
VACTERL association, 744
Vacuolating cytotoxin (vacA), 387
Vagal nerve injury, 254
Vagotomy, 390
Valsalva maneuvers, 79, 160, 529
Valve debridement
    emboli, 301
Valve dysfunction, acute
    suture looping, 302
Valve replacement, 32
Valve surgery
    general and procedure-specific,
        complications of, 299t
Valves, mechanical, 299
Valvular cardiac, 298–305
Valvular diseases
    echocardiographic stress test, 63
    stress perfusion or stress
        echocardiography, 63
Valvular dysfunction, 353
Valvular heart disease, 60
    and prosthetic heart valves, 62
    increased risk of, 60

Valvular insufficiency, 128
Valvuloplasty, primary, 354
Valvulotome, 333
Vancomycin Resistant Enterococcus
    (VRE), 218
Variceal hemorrhage, 440
Varicose veins
    primary thrombotic complications of, 351
Varicosities, venous, 351–352
    complication of, 351
    primary etiology of, 351
Varicosity excision, venous
    using tumescent anesthesia, 352
Vascular Closure Device Complications, 360
Vascular endothelial growth factor
    (VEGF), 105
Vascular exclusion, partial, 412
Vascular injury, 413–414, 542, 630
    second-leading cause of mortality, from
        laparoscopic procedures, 551
Vascular surgery
    ACE inhibitors, 181
    peripheral, 64
    peripheral, myocardial infarction, 38
Vasculogenic impotence, 329
Vasoactive drugs
    stopgap measure, 140
Vasoactive intestinal peptide tumors
    (VIPomas), 594
Vasoconstriction, hypotension of, 256
Vasoconstrictors
    epinephrine, 83
Vasodilator nuclear stress testing, 63
Vasopressin
    therapy, 131
    treating hypotension in septic shock, 131
Vasopressors administration. *See* Packed red
        blood cell transfusion
Vasopressors, 129–131
    agents, 293
    therapy
        α- and β-adrenergic agonistic
            activity, 129
        maintaining perfusion, 129
VATS. *See* Video-assisted thoracic surgery
        (VATS)
    intraoperative complications, 308
Vein thrombophlebitis, superficial
    after varicosity excision, 352
Vena caval filters, 348–350, 375–376
    filter complications, periprocedural, early
            device-related, long-term
            device-related, 348
    filter designs, 348
    placement, indications and
            complications, 348t
    preventing pulmonary embolism, 348
Venous disease
    complications of, 337–354
    diagnosis, 339
    therapies
        levels of medical evidence, for
            specific therapies, 338t
Venous distension, superficial, 339
Venous incompetence, superficial
    ulcers related to varicose veins, 351
Venous insufficiency
    chronic, 352–354
        diagnosis of, 340
        venous hypertension, related to, 352

Venous interventions, 375–377
Venous perforators, incompetent
    diagnosis of, venous stasis ulceration
        treatment, 340
Venous pressure, ambulatory, 340
Venous reconstructive surgery
    primary valvular dysfunction, 353
Venous return
    obstruction of, and hemodynamic
        compromise, 309
Venous sampling, 561
Venous Severity Score, 340
Venous stasis
    effects of pneumoperitoneum, 403
    ulceration
        multimodality therapy, 353
        standard therapy, elevation,
            compression, and local wound
            care, 353
Venous thromboembolism (DVT),
    acquired risk factors for, 338
    deep venous thrombosis and pulmonary
        embolism, 337
    family history of, 338
    hypercoagulable testing, 338t
    hyperhomocystinemia, 338
    increased incidence of, 338
    in-hospital symptomatic, 343
    lifelong warfarin, second episode of, 344
    risks of postoperative, 37
    standard therapy for, 344–346, 345f
    systemic anticoagulation, treatment
        for, 344
Venous thromboembolism prophylaxis,
    37–38, 342–344
    pharmacologic, mechanical, and
        combinations, 342
    risk factor stratification for, 343
Venous thromboembolism, recurrent, 344
Ventilation, 121
    alveolar overdistension, 132
    management of, 157
    mechanical, 132, 274
Ventilation/perfusion (V/Q), 162
    and pulmonary arteriography, 341
    mismatch, 279
Ventilator-associated pneumonia
    quantitative bronchoalveolar lavage
        culture, antibiotic therapy
        for, 166
Ventilator-induced lung injury, 167
    permissive hypercapnia, 167
    Webb and Tierney, detrimental effects of
        ventilation, 167
Ventilatory complications, 309
Ventilatory support, mechanical
    for respiratory failure, 292
Ventral hernia repair, 544
    use of autologous local tissues, 541
Ventral incisional hernia
    development of, 527
Ventricular tachycardia, 278
    unstable, life-threatening rhythm, 182
Venuta
    pericardial strips, to complete interlobar
        fissures, 310
Verapamil
    right ventricular systolic and diastolic
        pressures, reduction of, 265
Very low-density lipoproteins (VLDL), 199

Vessel disruptions
    with uncontained hemorrhage, 363
Vessel injury
    balloon oversizing, 363
Vessel wall injury, 337
Vicryl suture, 730
Video-assisted thoracic surgery (VATS)
    anatomic resection, 310
    approach, 306
        adequate exposure, 308
        immediate postoperative pain,
            associated with, 311
    chest, minimally invasive procedures, 307t
    lobectomy with thoracotomy, 311
    resection, of a malignancy, 311
    therapeutic procedures of the lung,
        pleura, 306
Virchow triad of stasis, 337
Visual pathway or retina
    central retinal artery occlusion, 95
Vitamin E
    protein kinase C inhibitor, interferes
        with platelet function, 190
Vitamin K deficiency, 191
    anatomic bypass of the small intestine,
        malabsorption, biliary tract
        obstruction, 191
    parenteral nutrition and antibiotic
        treatment, 191
Vitamins and trace elements, 201
    vitamin deficiencies/toxicities with
        clinical characteristics, 202t
Vocal cord edema
    flexible fiberoptic
        nasopharyngoscope, 160
    hoarseness and stridor, 160
    humidification of inspired air, and close
        airway monitoring, 160
Vocal cord paralysis
    true hoarseness from nerve
        compression, 578
Vocal fold, 228
    mobility, 230
    paralysis, 230
        incomplete glottic closure,
            recurrent laryngeal nerve (RLN)
            injury, 241f
Vocal process granuloma, 232–233
Voice changes
    difficulty with, complete glottic closure
        during coughing, 160
Volume expansion
    crystalloid or colloid solutions, use
        of, 129
Volume overload, 265
Volume–outcome studies, 32
    annual volume cutpoints, 32
    cancer surgery, 31
    carotid endarterectomy, 31
    coronary artery bypass grafting (CABG),
        pediatric cardiac surgery, 31
    curve, varies widely by procedure, 32
    elective abdominal aortic aneurysm
        (AAA) repair, 31
Volumetric analysis
    normal liver, extended lobectomy, 409
Volvulus
    malrotation with, 728f
von Willebrand disease
    easy bruisability of soft tissues, 188

VTE prophylaxis
    for general surgery patients, 342f
    for trauma patients, 343f

W
Warfarin dosing
    international normalized ratio (INR), 344
Warfarin therapy, 189
Water-soluble contrast esophagogram
    followed by dilute barium, identification
        of perforation site, 248
Wheat and Burford, 265
Wide-complex tachycardias, 182
    atrioventricular dissociation, helpful
        markers, 182
Windsock deformity, 727
Witzel maneuver, 255
Witzelling, a jejunal feeding tube
    placement of sutures, in seromuscular
        layer, 494f
Work hour regulations, 11
World Health Organization (WHO)
    Melanoma Group study, 621
Wound
    adjuvants
        vacuum assisted wound closure, 112
    bursting strength, 524
    closure, 123
        deep incisional wound infections, 123
        hypertrophic scarring,
            prevention of, 110
        occlusive surgical glue dressings, use
            of, 123
        primary wound closure, 109–110
        superficial incisional wound
            infections, antimicrobial
            therapy, 123
    complications, 107, 603–607, 624f
        management of, 111
        nonoperative and operative principles,
            management of, 112f
    contamination, 107
        dependent clinical circumstances, 107t
    contraction, 106
    cultures, 290
    dehiscence, 623
    dressings, 111
        wound desiccation, protection
            from, 111
    failure, acute, 106
        clinical studies of, 524
        dehiscence or wound separation, 111
        suture pulling, 110
    fibroblasts, 105
    healing, 102–113
        acute, 105
        anastomotic leaks and fascial
            dehiscences, 102
        cellular and molecular events,
            sequence of, 102
        cellular and molecular repair
            pathways, 103f
        chronic disease, 108
        complications of, 102
        deposition of fibrinogen, 103
        failure, 106f
        fascial, 538
        macrophages, tissue leukocytes, 103
        normal, 102–107
        trajectory, 107
        vitamin C, critical in strength gain, 108

Wound (*Continued*)
  hematoma, 351, 544
  infection, 274, 457, 511, 573, 604–606
    deep, 540
    enucleations and pancreatic
        resections, 601
    fasciitis or myonecrosis, 110–111
    precise anatomical
        localization, 111*f*
    prevention of, 650
  rates, 107
  superficial, 650
malignancy
  factitious injury, recurrent trauma, 109
recurrence/nonhealing, 518
remodeling process, 106
repair cells
  fibroblasts and keratinocytes, 107
seroma, 274
surface coverage, 106

X
X-rays, abdominal, 404

Z
Zenker diverticulum, 260
    contrast esophagogram, 251
Zinc levels
    delayed epithelialization, and fibroblast
        proliferation, 108
    reduction in, 108